Essential Pathology

Essential Pathology

Third Edition

EDITED BY:

Emanuel Rubin, MD

The Gonzalo E. Aponte Professor of Pathology
and Chairman of the Department of Pathology, Anatomy, and Cell Biology

Jefferson Medical College

Thomas Jefferson University

Philadelphia, Pennsylvania

WITH 47 CONTRIBUTORS

LIPPINCOTT WILLIAMS & WILKINS
A **Wolters Kluwer** Company

Philadelphia · Baltimore · New York · London
Buenos Aires · Hong Kong · Sydney · Tokyo

Publisher: Susan Katz
Managing Editor: Ulita Lushnycky
Marketing Manager: Aimee Sirmon
Production Editor: Paula C. Williams

351 West Camden Street
Baltimore, Maryland 21201-2436 USA

530 Walnut Street
Philadelphia, Pennsylvania 19106 USA

Printed in the United States of American

FIRST EDITION   1989
SECOND EDITION   1995

Library of Congress Cataloging-in-Publication Data

Essential pathology/edited by Emanuel Rubin; with 36 contributors; illustrations by Dimitri Karetnikov.—3rd ed.
     p.; cm.
  Includes index.
  ISBN 0-7817-2395-7
   1. Pathology.   I. Rubin, Emanuel, 1928-
  [DNLM: 1. Pathology. QZ 4 E783 2000]
  RB111.E856 2000
  616.07—dc21

                                      00-042037

To purchase additional copies of this book, call our customer service department at **(800) 638-3030** or fax orders to **(301) 824-7390**. International customers should call **(301) 714-2324**.

4 5 6 7 8 9 10

Preface to Third Edition

The enthusiastic reception of the third edition of *Pathology* led us to the preparation of this third edition of *Essential Pathology*. The text is based on the larger one and represents a summary of contemporary general and systemic pathology. To accomplish this end, we have omitted most of the discussions of normal anatomy and physiology, as well as the descriptions of less frequently encountered diseases. In addition, many sections dealing with the clinical and experimental support for statements in the text have been shortened. Thus, *Essential Pathology* presents the reader with all the key concepts of the evolution and expression of disease and assigns priorities based on the clinical importance and heuristic relevance of individual disorders.

As in the earlier editions, *Essential Pathology* maintains the traditional custom of dividing the subject matter into general (Chapters 1–9) and systemic (Chapters 10–29) pathology. The text features distinctions between pathogenesis, pathology, and clinical features of the various diseases discussed. Throughout the text, key terms and the definitions of important disease entities have been highlighted by bullets, italics, bold, and color to add emphasis and aid review. Many of the original drawings have been revised, and new ones have been added. The importance of pattern recognition in the study of pathology has been stressed by the presentation of all photographs in full color.

This third edition recognizes the remarkable expansion of knowledge relevant to pathology in the last few years and contains a considerable amount of new information. We anticipate that this edition will continue to serve the needs of all students of pathology who wish to integrate the concepts of modern biology with the study of clinical medicine.

Sadly, attempting to edit a comprehensive textbook of pathology without missing any errors is like trying to live without sin—worth the effort, but probably impossible. However, the inevitability of human mistakes has not deterred us from including new and still controversial concepts. Some of these will stand the test of time; others will be corrected in the next edition.

Emanuel Rubin

To my parents:
    Jacob and Sophie Rubin

And my wife:
    Linda Anne

Acknowledgments

Specific acknowledgment is made for permission to use the following material:

Chapter 1, Figure 1-5. Okazaki H, Scheithauer BW. Atlas of neuropathology. New York: Gower Medical Publishing, 1988. By permission of Mayo Foundation.

Chapter 3, Figure 3-9. Okazaki H, Scheithauer BW. Atlas of neuropathology. New York: Gower Medical Publishing, 1988. By permission of Mayo Foundation.

Chapter 5, Figure 5-5. Bullough PG, Vigorita VJ. Atlas of orthopaedic pathology. New York: Gower Medical Publishing, 1984.

Chapter 5, Figure 5-12. Bullough PG, Boachie-Adjei O. Atlas of spinal diseases. New York: Gower Medical Publishing, 1988.

Chapter 6, Figure 6-18. Bullough PG, Vigorita VJ. Atlas of orthopaedic pathology. New York: Gower Medical Publishing, 1984.

Chapter 9, Figures 9-6, 9-13, 9-20A, and 9-20B. Farrar WE, Wood MJ, Innes JA, Tubbs H. Infectious diseases text and color atlas, 2nd ed. New York: Gower Medical Publishing, 1992.

Chapter 12, Figure 12-27. Courtesy of the Armed Forces Institute of Pathology.

Chapter 13, Figures 13-4, 13-6, 13-7, 13-10, 13-17, 13-19, 13-32, 13-34, 13-36, 13-41, 13-42, and 13-47. Mitros FA. Atlas of gastrointestinal pathology. New York: Gower Medical Publishing, 1988.

Chapter 13, Figure 13-8. Courtesy of Dr. Cecilia M. Fenoglio-Preiser.

Chapter 21, Figure 21-9. Courtesy of Sandoz Pharmaceutical Corporation.

Chapter 26, Figures 26-17C, 26-23A, 26-27B, 26-29B, 26-32B, and 26-38A. Bullough PG. Atlas of orthopaedic pathology, 2nd ed. New York: Gower Medical Publishing, 1992.

Chapter 26, Figures 26-5C and 26-27A. Bullough PG, Vigorita VJ. Atlas of orthopaedic pathology. New York: Gower Medical Publishing, 1984.

Chapter 28, Figure 28-44B. Okazaki H, Scheithauer BW. Atlas of neuropathology. New York: Gower Medical Publishing, 1988. By permission of the Mayo Foundation.

Contributors

Vernon W. Armbrustmacher, MD
Medical Examiner, Neuropathologist
Office of the Chief Medical Examiner
New York, New York

Adam Bagg
Associate Professor of Pathology and Medicine
Georgetown University Medical Center
Director of Hematopathology and Clinical Hematology
Georgetown University School of Medicine
Washington, DC

Károly Balogh, MD
Associate Professor of Pathology
Harvard Medical School;
Pathologist
New England Deaconess Hospital
Boston, Massachusetts

Sue A. Bartow, MD
Associate Professor of Laboratory Medicine and Pathology
University of Minnesota Medical School
Minneapolis, Minnesota

Earl P. Benditt, MD*
Professor of Pathology Emeritus
University of Washington School of Medicine;
Distinguished Physician
Veterans Administration Medical Center
Seattle, Washington

Hugh Bonner, MD
Adjunct Associate Professor of Pathology
University of Pennsylvania School of Medicine
Philadelphia, Pennsylvania;
Director of Anatomic Pathology
The Chester County Hospital
West Chester, Pennsylvania

Deceased

Thomas W. Bouldin, MD
Professor of Pathology and Ophthalmology
University of North Carolina School of Medicine;
Attending Pathologist
University of North Carolina Hospitals
Chapel Hill, North Carolina

Stephen W. Chensue, MD, PhD
Assistant Professor of Pathology
University of Michigan Medical School;
Staff Pathologist
Veterans Affairs Medical Center
Ann Arbor, Michigan

Wallace H. Clark, MD*
Visiting Professor of Pathology
Harvard Medical School;
Senior Pathologist
Beth Israel Hospital
Boston, Massachusetts

Daniel H. Connor, MD
Visiting Professor of Pathology
Georgetown University School of Medicine
Rockville, Maryland

Jeffrey Cossman, MD
Oscar Benwood Hunter Professor of Pathology
Georgetown University School of Medicine
Washington, DC

John E. Craighead, MD
Professor of Pathology Emeritus
University of Vermont College of Medicine;
Attending Pathologist
Fletcher Allen Health Care
Burlington, Vermont

Maire A. Duggan, MB, BCH, FRCP
Professor of Pathology
University of Calgary;
Consultant Pathologist
Calgary Laboratory Services
Calgary, Alberta, Canada

Hormoz Ehya, MD
Senior Member and Director of Cytopathology
Fox Chase Cancer Center
Clinical Professor of Pathology
MCP-Hahnemann School of Medicine;
Adjunct Clinical Professor of Pathology, Anatomy, and Cell
    Biology
Jefferson Medical College
Philadelphia, Pennsylvania

Joseph C. Fantone, MD
Professor of Pathology
University of Michigan Medical School;
Pathologist
University of Michigan Medical Center
Ann Arbor, Michigan

John L. Farber, MD
Professor of Pathology, Anatomy, and Cell Biology
Jefferson Medical College
Thomas Jefferson University
Philadelphia, Pennsylvania

Gregory N. Fuller, MD
Assistant Professor of Pathology
MD Anderson Cancer Center
Houston, Texas

Robert M. Genta, MD
Professor of Pathology, Medicine, Microbiology and
    Immunology
Bayler Medical College
Chief of Pathology and Laboratory Medicine
Veterans Administration Medical Center
Houston, Texas

Avrum I. Gotlieb, MD
Professor and Chairman
Department of Laboratory Medicine and Pathobiology
Faculty of Medicine
University of Toronto
Director of Vascular Research Laboratories
Toronto Hospital
Toronto, Ontario, Canada

Stanley R. Hamilton, MD
Head
Division of Pathology/Laboratory Medicine
University of Texas
MD Anderson Cancer Center
Houston, Texas

Terence J. Harrist, MD
Clinical Assistant Professor of Pathology
Harvard Medical School
Senior Pathologist
Beth Israel Hospital
Boston, Massachusetts

Arthur P. Hays, MD
Associate Professor of Pathology
College of Physicians and Surgeons
Columbia University
New York, New York

J. Charles Jennette, MD
Professor of Pathology and Laboratory Medicine
University of North Carolina School of Medicine
Chapel Hill, North Carolina

Robert B. Jennings, MD
James B. Duke Professor of Pathology
Duke University Medical Center
Durham, North Carolina

Kent J. Johnson
Professor of Pathology
University of Michigan Medical School;
Pathologist
University of Michigan Medical Center
Ann Arbor, Michigan

Robert Kisilevsky, MD, PhD, FRCP
Professor of Pathology and Biochemistry
Queen's University;
Attending Pathologist
Kingston General Hospital
Kingston, Ontario, Canada

Gordon K. Klintworth, MD, PhD
Professor of Pathology
Joseph A. C. Wadsworth Research Professor of
    Ophthalmology
Duke University Medical Center
Durham, North Carolina

Robert J. Kurman, MD
Professor of Pathology and Obstetrics and Gynecology
Johns Hopkins University School of Medicine
Director of Gynecologic Pathology
Johns Hopkins Hospital
Baltimore, Maryland

Ernest A. Lack, MD
Professor of Pathology
Georgetown University School of Medicine
Director of Anatomic Pathology
Georgetown University Medical Center
Washington, DC

Antonio Martinez-Hernandez, MD
Professor of Pathology
University of Tennessee College of Medicine;
Chief of Pathology and Laboratory Medicine
Veterans Administration Medical Center
Memphis, Tennessee

Wolfgang J. Mergner, MD, PhD
Professor of Pathology
University of Maryland School of Medicine;
Director of Anatomic Pathology
University of Maryland Medical Center
Baltimore, Maryland

Robert O. Petersen, MD, PhD
Professor of Pathology, Anatomy, and Cell Biology
Jefferson Medical College
Thomas Jefferson University;
Attending Pathologist
Thomas Jefferson University Hospital
Philadelphia, Pennsylvania

Timothy R. Quinn, MD
Instructor in Pathology
Harvard Medical School;
Pathologist
Beth Israel Hospital
Boston, Massachusetts

Stanley J. Robboy, MD
Professor of Pathology and Obstetrics and Gynecology
Duke University Medical School;
Vice-Chairman of Pathology
Duke University Medical Center
Durham, North Carolina

Emanuel Rubin, MD
Gonzalo E. Aponte Professor and Chairman
Department of Pathology, Anatomy, and Cell Biology
Jefferson Medical College
Thomas Jefferson University
Philadelphia, Pennsylvania

Dante G. Scarpelli, MD, PhD*
Earnest J. and Hattie H. Magerstadt Professor of Pathology
Northwestern University Medical School
Chicago, Illinois

Brian Schapiro, MD
Instructor in Pathology
Harvard Medical School;
Pathologist
Beth Israel Hospital
Boston, Massachusetts

Alan L. Schiller, MD
Irene Heinz Given and John LaPorte Given Professor and
    Chairman of Pathology
Mount Sinai School of Medicine;
Director of Pathology
The Mount Sinai Hospital
New York, New York

Stephen M. Schwartz, MD, PhD
Professor of Pathology
University of Washington School of Medicine
Seattle, Washington

Benjamin H. Spargo, MD
Professor of Pathology Emeritus
University of Chicago School of Medicine;
Emeritus Director of Renal Pathology
University of Chicago Medical Center
Chicago, Illinois

Charles Steenbergen, Jr., MD, PhD
Assistant Professor of Pathology
Duke University Medical Center
Durham, North Carolina

Steven L. Teitelbaum, MD
Messing Professor of Pathology
Washington University Medical Center
St. Louis, Missouri

William D. Travis, MD
Co-Chairman
Department of Pulmonary and Mediastinal Pathology
Armed Forces Institute of Pathology
Washington, DC

Benjamin F. Trump, MD
Professor and Chairman
Department of Pathology
University of Maryland School of Medicine
Baltimore, Maryland

F. Stephen Vogel, MD
Clinical Professor of Pathology
Medical College of Georgia;
Secretary-Treasurer and Executive Director
United States and Canadian Academy of Pathology
Augusta, Georgia

Peter A. Ward, MD
Godfrey D. Stobbe Professor and Chairman
Department of Pathology
University of Michigan Medical School
Ann Arbor, Michigan

*Deceased

Contents

Cell Injury

Emanuel Rubin
John L. Farber

Pathology, in its simplest sense, is the study of structural and functional abnormalities that are expressed as diseases of organs and systems. Rudolf Virchow, often referred to as the father of modern pathology, proposed that the basis of all disease is injury to the cell. In this perspective, pathology is the study of cell injury and the expression of a pre-existing capacity to adapt to such injury on the part of either injured or intact cells.

CELLULAR PATTERNS OF RESPONSE TO STRESS

When environmental changes exceed the capacity of the cell to maintain normal homeostasis, we recognize acute cell injury. If the stress is removed in time or if the cell is able to withstand the assault, cell injury is reversible, and complete structural and functional integrity can be restored. For example, this is the situation when circulation to the heart is interrupted for less than 30 minutes. The cell can also be exposed to persistent, sublethal stress, as in mechanical irritation of the skin or exposure of the bronchial mucosa to tobacco smoke. In such instances, the cell has time to adapt to reversible injury in a number of ways, each of which has its morphologic counterpart.

Sufficiently severe stress may lead to irreversible injury and death of the cell. The precise moment when reversible gives way to irreversible injury, or the "point of no return," cannot at present be identified. The morphologic pattern of cell death occasioned by disparate exogenous environmental stresses is coagulative necrosis. This type of necrosis is common to almost all forms of cell death and precedes the other forms described here.

REVERSIBLE CELL INJURY

■ *Hydropic swelling is a condition of reversible cell injury characterized by a large, pale cytoplasm and a normally located nucleus* (Fig. 1-1). The greater volume reflects an increased water content caused by various insults, such as chemical and biologic toxins, viral or bacterial infections, ischemia, excessive heat or cold, and so on.

Hydropic swelling results from impairment of cellular volume regulation, a process that controls ionic concentrations in the cytoplasm. This regulation, particularly for sodium, operates at three levels: (1) the plasma membrane itself, (2) the plasma membrane sodium pump, and (3) the supply of adenosine triphosphate (ATP). Injurious agents may interfere with these

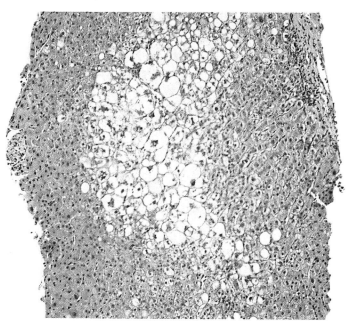

FIGURE   *1-1*
Hydropic swelling. A needle biopsy of the liver in a patient with toxic hepatic injury shows severe hydropic swelling in the centrilobular zone. The affected hepatocytes exhibit central nuclei and cytoplasm distended (ballooned) by excess fluid.

membrane-regulated processes by (1) increasing the permeability of the plasma membrane to sodium, thereby exceeding the capacity of the pump to extrude sodium; (2) damaging the pump directly; or (3) interfering with the synthesis of ATP, thereby depriving the pump of its fuel. In any event, accumulation of sodium in the cell leads to an increase in water to maintain isosmotic conditions, and the cell swells.

Ultrastructural Changes

- **Endoplasmic Reticulum.** The cisternae of the endoplasmic reticulum are distended by fluid in hydropic swelling (Fig. 1-2).
- **Mitochondria.** In some forms of acute injury, particularly ischemia, mitochondria swell (Fig. 1-3).
- **Plasma Membrane.** Blebs of the plasma membrane, that is, focal extrusions of the cytoplasm, are occasionally noted.
- **Nucleolus.** In the nucleus, reversible injury is reflected principally by changes in the nucleolus. The fibrillar and granular components of the nucleolus may segregate. Alternatively, the granular component may be diminished, leaving only a fibrillar core.

It is important to recognize that after withdrawal of an acute stress that has led to reversible cell injury, by definition, the cell returns to its normal state.

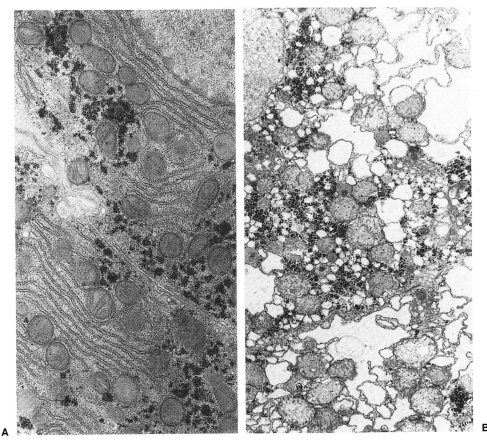

FIGURE   *1-2*
Ultrastructure of hydropic swelling of a liver cell. (A) Two apposed, normal hepatocytes with tightly organized, parallel arrays of rough endoplasmic reticulum. (B) Swollen hepatocyte in which the cisternae of the endoplasmic reticulum are dilated by excess fluid.

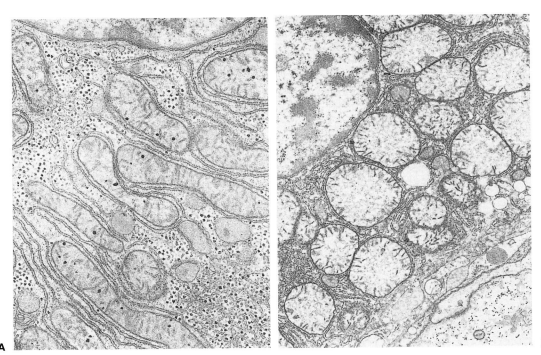

FIGURE   *1-3*
Mitochondrial swelling in acute ischemic cell injury. (A) Normal mitochondria are elongated and display prominent cristae, which traverse the mitochondrial matrix. (B) Mitochondria from an ischemic cell are swollen and round, and they exhibit a decreased matrix density. The cristae are less prominent than in the normal organelle.

MORPHOLOGIC REACTIONS TO PERSISTENT STRESS

In response to persistent stress, a cell dies or adapts. Cells experiencing persistent stress manifest few, if any, of the characteristic alterations described for acute cell injury. It is thus our view that at the cellular level, it is more appropriate to speak of chronic adaptation than of chronic injury (Fig. 1-4). The major adaptive responses are atrophy, hypertrophy, hyperplasia, metaplasia, dysplasia, and intracellular storage.

Atrophy

■ *Atrophy is a decrease in the size and function of a cell or organ.* Clinically, it is often recognized as a diminution in the size or function of an organ (Fig. 1-5). Atrophy is often seen in areas of vascular insufficiency or chronic inflammation, and it may result from disuse of skeletal muscle. Atrophy may be thought of as an adaptive response to stress in which the cell shrinks in volume and shuts down its differentiated functions,

thereby reducing its need for energy to a minimum. On restoration of normal conditions, atrophic cells are fully capable of resuming their differentiated functions. Their size increases to normal, and specialized functions, such as protein synthesis or contractile force, return to their original levels. Atrophy occurs under a variety of conditions outlined here.

Reduced Functional Demand

The most common form of atrophy follows reduced functional demand. For example, after immobilization of a limb in a cast as treatment for a bone fracture or prolonged bed rest, muscle cells atrophy, and muscular strength is reduced. With resumption of normal activity, normal size and function are restored.

Inadequate Supply of Oxygen

■ *Ischemia is interference with the blood supply to tissues.* Total ischemia, with cessation of oxygen perfusion of tissues, results in cell death. However, partial ischemia occurs after incomplete occlusion of a blood vessel. This results in a chronically reduced oxygen supply, a condition that is often incompatible with cell viability. Under such circumstances, cell atrophy is common. It is frequently seen around the inadequately perfused margins of ischemic necrosis (infarcts) in the heart, brain, and kidneys following vascular occlusion in these organs.

Insufficient Nutrients

Starvation or inadequate nutrition associated with chronic disease leads to cell atrophy, particularly in skeletal muscle.

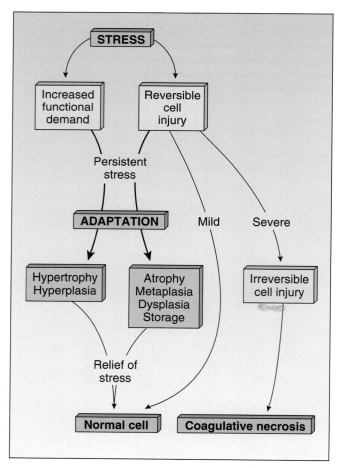

FIGURE *1-4*
Reactions of cells to stress.

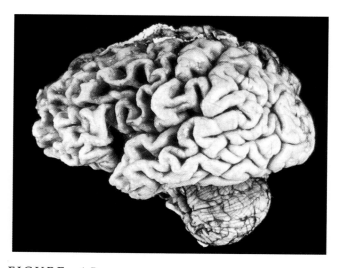

FIGURE *1-5*
Atrophy of the brain. Marked atrophy of the frontal lobes is noted in this photograph of the brain. The gyri are thinned and the sulci conspicuously widened.

Interruption of Trophic Signals

The functions of many cells depend on signals transmitted by chemical mediators. The endocrine system and neuromuscular transmission are the best examples. The demands placed on the cell by the actions of hormones or, in the case of skeletal muscle, by synaptic transmission can be eliminated by removing the source of the signal. This can be accomplished through, for example, ablation of an endocrine gland or denervation. If the anterior pituitary is surgically resected, the loss of thyroid-stimulating hormone (TSH), corticotropin, and follicle-stimulating hormone results in atrophy of the thyroid, adrenal cortex, and ovaries, respectively. Neurologic conditions resulting in denervation of muscle and, thus, in loss of the neuromuscular transmission necessary for muscle tone cause atrophy of the affected muscles. The wasting caused by poliomyelitis or traumatic paraplegia falls into this category.

Persistent Cell Injury

Persistent cell injury is most commonly caused by chronic inflammation associated with prolonged viral or bacterial infections. Cells in areas of chronic inflammation are often atrophic. Persistent toxic injury, as exemplified by the action of cigarette smoke on the bronchial mucosa, can also cause atrophy. Even physical injury, such as prolonged pressure in inappropriate locations, produces atrophy. Heart failure leads to increased pressure in the sinusoids of the liver, because the heart cannot efficiently pump the venous return from that organ. Accordingly, the cells exposed to the greatest pressure—those in the center of the liver lobule—become atrophic.

Aging

As discussed here, cell aging is a process independent of disease. One of the hallmarks of aging, particularly in nonreplicating cells such as those of the brain and heart, is cell atrophy. The size of all the parenchymal organs of the body decreases with age. The size of the brain is invariably decreased, whereas in very old patients, the size of the heart may be so diminished that the term **senile atrophy** has been used.

Hypertrophy

■ *Hypertrophy is an increase in the size of a cell accompanied by an augmented functional capacity.* It is a response to trophic signals or increased functional demands and is commonly a normal process.

Physiologic (Hormonal) Hypertrophy

Physiologic hypertrophy occurs during maturation under the influence of a variety of hormones. Sex hormones at puberty lead to hypertrophy of the juvenile sex organs and those organs associated with secondary sex characteristics. The lactating woman, under the influence of prolactin and estrogen, exhibits hypertrophy of the breast tissue.

Although hypertrophy results from certain normal hormonal signals, it is also a response to abnormal levels of hormones. Overproduction of TSH by the pituitary is responsible for the thyroid enlargement (goiter) that occurs with nutritional iodine deficiency. In the absence of sufficient iodine, thyroid hormone is not produced. Consequently, there is no feedback inhibition of TSH secretion, and the unopposed TSH, acting as a trophic hormone, induces hypertrophy of the thyroid follicular cells. Increased hormone levels can also result from abnormal hormone production by tumors. For example, oversecretion of corticotropin by pituitary tumors results in hypertrophy of the adrenal cortex.

Increased Functional Demand

Hypertrophy caused by an increased functional demand is exemplified by increased muscle size and strength following repeated exercise. Increased demand occurs under pathologic conditions as well. The heart may be called on to increase its contractile force because of mechanical interference with the aortic outflow or because of systemic hypertension, a condition requiring the heart to eject blood under higher pressure (Fig. 1-6). As in exercise-induced hypertrophy of

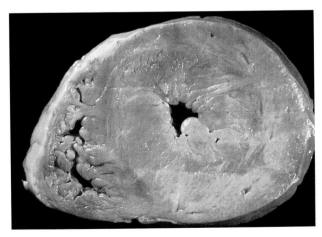

FIGURE *1-6*
Myocardial hypertrophy. Cross-section of the heart of a patient with longstanding hypertension shows pronounced, concentric left ventricular hypertrophy.

skeletal muscle, the myocardial cells enlarge, and the heart may double in weight. Increased demand also results from the loss of functional mass. If one kidney is surgically removed or rendered inoperative because of vascular occlusion, the contralateral kidney hypertrophies to accommodate the increased demand.

Hyperplasia

■ *Hyperplasia is an increase in the number of cells in an organ or tissue.* Hypertrophy and hyperplasia are not mutually exclusive and are often seen concurrently.

Hormonal Stimulation

Hormonal signals can induce a physiologic hyperplastic effect. For example, the normal increase in estrogen levels at puberty and during the early phase of the menstrual cycle leads to an increased number of both endometrial and uterine stromal cells. Hormones produced by tumors can also lead to hyperplasia. For example, secretion of erythropoietin by cancer of the kidney leads to an increase in the number of erythrocyte precursors in the bone marrow.

Increased Functional Demand

Hyperplasia, like hypertrophy, may follow increased physiologic demand. Residence at high altitude, where the oxygen content of the air is relatively low, leads to compensatory hyperplasia of erythrocyte precursors in the bone marrow and increased numbers of circulating erythrocytes (secondary polycythemia). The decrease in the amount of oxygen carried in each erythrocyte is balanced by an increase in the number of those cells.

Similarly, chronic blood loss, as in abnormal uterine bleeding, causes hyperplasia of erythrocytic elements. The immune system's response to many antigens—a vital mechanism for protection from foreign invaders—constitutes another example of demand-induced hyperplasia. Morphologically, lymphocyte hyperplasia is conspicuous in chronic inflammation caused by conditions such as bacterial infection or transplant rejection.

Persistent Cell Injury

Persistent cell injury may lead to hyperplasia. Chronic inflammation or chronic exposure to physical or chemical injury results in a hyperplastic response. For instance, pressure from ill-fitting shoes causes hyperplasia of the skin of the foot (so-called corns or calluses). Chronic inflammation of the bladder (chronic cystitis) commonly causes hyperplasia of the bladder epithelium, a condition that is easily viewed grossly by endoscopy as whitish plaques of the bladder lining. Abnormal hyperplasia can itself be harmful—witness the unpleasant consequences of psoriasis, a malady of unknown etiology characterized by conspicuous hyperplasia of the epidermis (Fig. 1-7).

Metaplasia

■ *Metaplasia is the conversion of one differentiated cell type to another.* The most common sequence is replacement of a glandular epithelium by a squamous one. It is almost invariably a response to persistent injury and can be thought of as an adaptive mechanism. Columnar or cuboidal lining cells committed to differentiated functions, such as mucus production, assume

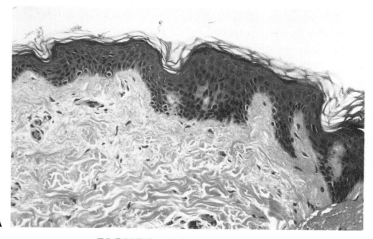
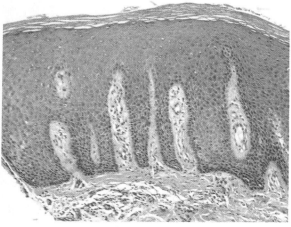

A   **B**

FIGURE   *1-7*
Epidermal hyperplasia. **(A)** Normal epidermis. **(B)** Epidermal hyperplasia in psoriasis, shown at the same magnification as in *panel A*. The epidermis is thickened, owing to an increase in the number of squamous cells.

a simpler form, thereby providing more protection against a pernicious chemical action or the effects of chronic inflammation. Prolonged exposure of the bronchi to tobacco smoke leads to squamous metaplasia of the bronchial epithelium. A comparable response associated with chronic infection occurs in the endocervix (Fig. 1-8).

Metaplasia is not restricted to squamous differentiation. In cases of chronic reflux of highly acidic gastric contents into the lower esophagus, the squamous epithelium is occasionally replaced by a gastric-like glandular mucosa (Barrett epithelium). This can be thought of as an adaptive response that protects the esophagus from the injurious effects of gastric acid and pepsin, to which the normal gastric mucosa is resistant.

It should be emphasized that metaplasia is not necessarily a harmless process. Neoplastic transformation may occur in metaplastic epithelium; indeed, cancers of the lung, cervix, stomach, and bladder have their origins in such areas. It is unlikely that the metaplastic epithelium itself is responsible for cancer formation. More probably, the noxious stimuli leading to metaplasia are also carcinogenic to metaplastic cells. Metaplasia is usually reversible if the stimulus is removed.

Dysplasia

■ *Cellular dysplasia is an alteration in the size, shape, and organization of the cellular components of a tissue.* The cells comprising an epithelium normally exhibit regularity of size, shape, and nucleus. Moreover, they are arranged in a regular fashion, as in the progression from plump basal cells to flat superficial cells in a squamous epithelium. When we speak of dysplasia, we

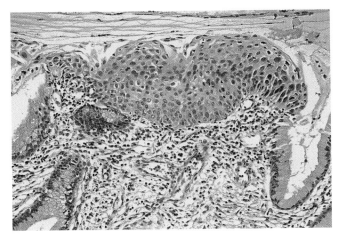

FIGURE 1-8
Squamous metaplasia. A section of endocervix shows the normal columnar epithelium at both margins and a focus of squamous metaplasia in the center.

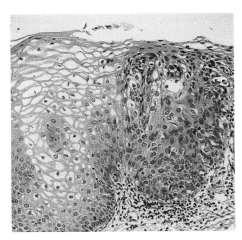

FIGURE 1-9
Dysplasia. A section of the cervix shows an area of epithelial dysplasia (*right*) adjacent to an area of normal squamous epithelium. The dysplastic epithelium lacks the normal polarity, and the individual cells show hyperchromatic nuclei, a larger nuclear:cytoplasmic ratio, and a disorderly arrangement.

mean that this monotonous appearance is disturbed by (1) variations in the size and shape of the cells; (2) enlargement, irregularity, and hyperchromatism of the nuclei; and (3) disorderly arrangement of the cells within the epithelium (Fig. 1-9). Dysplasia occurs most commonly in hyperplastic squamous epithelium, as seen in epidermal actinic keratosis (caused by sunlight), and in areas of squamous metaplasia, such as the bronchus or the cervix. It is not, however, exclusive to squamous epithelium. Ulcerative colitis, an inflammatory disease of the large intestine, is often complicated by dysplastic changes in the mucosal cells.

Dysplasia shares many cytologic features with cancer, and the line between the two may be very fine indeed. For example, a common diagnostic problem for the pathologist is the distinction between severe dysplasia and early cancer of the cervix. Dysplasia is a preneoplastic lesion, in the sense that it is a necessary stage in the multistep cellular evolution to cancer.

INTRACELLULAR STORAGE

Intracellular storage is a normal function of the tissues in multicellular organisms. Cells store nutritional constituents, including fat, glycogen, vitamins, and minerals, that are used at a later time. They also store the products of the turnover of endogenous membranes, principally in the form of degraded phospholipids. Furthermore, storage is the mechanism by which certain cells deal with substances that cannot be eliminated through intracellular digestion. For example, carbon particles inhaled in the form of soot cannot be metabolized or dissolved. They would accumulate indefinitely in the alveoli if they were not engulfed by macrophages. Finally, many inborn errors of metabolism lead to the accumulation of intermediate metabolites or abnormal material.

Fat

The abnormal accumulation of fat is most conspicuous in the liver (a subject treated in detail in Chapter 14). When the delivery of free fatty acids to the liver is increased, as in diabetes, or when the intrahepatic metabolism of lipids is disturbed, as in alcoholism, triglycerides accumulate in the liver cell. Fatty liver is identified morphologically by the presence of lipid globules in the cytoplasm. Other organs, including the heart and the kidney, also store fat.

Glycogen

Glycogen is a long-chain polymer of glucose formed in and largely stored in the liver and, to a lesser extent, in muscles. It is depolymerized to glucose and liberated as needed. The amount of glycogen stored in cells is regulated by the blood glucose concentration, and hyperglycemic states are associated with increased glycogen stores. Thus, in uncontrolled diabetes, hepatocytes and epithelial cells of the renal proximal tubules are enlarged by excess glycogen. Inherited defects of glycogen metabolism also lead to a variety of glycogen storage diseases.

Inherited Lysosomal Storage Diseases

Similar to the metabolism of glycogen, the breakdown of certain complex lipids and mucopolysaccharides (glycosaminoglycans) is accomplished by a sequence of enzymatic steps. Because these enzymes are located in the lysosomes, their absence results in the lysosomal storage of incompletely degraded lipids, such as cerebrosides (e.g., Gaucher disease) and gangliosides (e.g., Tay-Sachs disease), or products of the catabolism of mucopolysaccharides (e.g., Hurler and Hunter syndromes).

Iron

Approximately 25% of the body's total iron content is in an intracellular storage pool composed of the iron-storage proteins ferritin and hemosiderin. Hemosiderin is a partially denatured form of ferritin

that easily aggregates and is recognized microscopically as yellow-brown granules in the cytoplasm.

Total body iron may be increased by enhanced intestinal iron absorption, as in an anemia other than that produced by iron deficiency itself, or by parenteral administration of iron-containing erythrocytes in a transfusion. In either case, the excess iron is stored intracellularly as both ferritin and hemosiderin. Increasing the body's total iron content results in a progressive accumulation of hemosiderin, a condition termed **hemosiderosis**. In this condition, iron is present not only among the organs in which it is normally found but also throughout the body, in places such as the skin, pancreas, heart, kidneys, and endocrine organs. The intracellular accumulation of iron in hemosiderosis does not injure the cells. However, there are a number of situations during which the increase in total body iron is extreme, and we then speak of iron overload syndromes (see Chapter 14), or disorders in which iron deposition is so severe that it damages vital organs—the heart, liver, and pancreas. Severe iron overload can result from a genetic abnormality in iron absorption, a condition termed **hereditary hemochromatosis** (Fig. 1-10). Alternatively, severe iron overload may occur after multiple blood transfusions, such as those required in treating hemophilia or certain hereditary anemias.

Lipofuscin

■ *Lipofuscin , classically known as the "wear-and-tear" pigment, is composed of golden-brown granules found predominantly in cells that are either terminally differentiated (neurons and cardiac myocytes) or cycle only infrequently*

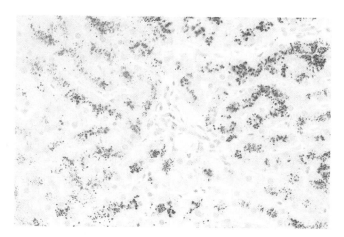

FIGURE *1-10*
Iron storage in hereditary hemochromatosis. A Prussian blue stain of the liver reveals large deposits of iron within hepatocellular lysosomes.

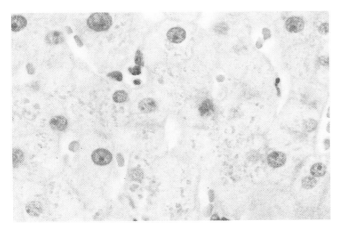

FIGURE *1-11*
Lipofuscin. A photomicrograph of the liver from an 80-year-old man shows golden cytoplasmic granules, which represent lysosomal storage of lipofuscin.

(hepatocytes) (Fig. 1-11). This material is a normal constituent of many cells and increases with age. Lipofuscin derives from the normal turnover of the membrane constituents of the cell. Peroxidation of unsaturated lipids and the formation of heterogeneous lipid-protein complexes, render these materials resistant to further digestion. The insoluble products are stored indefinitely as lysosome-derived residual bodies. Despite the occasional prominence of intracellular lipofuscin, there is no reason to believe that this pigment interferes, in any way, with the function of the cell.

Melanin

■ *Melanin is an insoluble, brown-black pigment found almost exclusively in the epidermal cells of the skin.* It is located in intracellular organelles known as melanosomes and is responsible for the differences in skin color among the various races.

Exogenous Pigments

■ *Anthracosis refers to the storage of carbon particles in the lung and regional lymph nodes.* Virtually all urban dwellers inhale particulates of organic carbon generated by the burning of fossil fuels. These particles accumulate in alveolar macrophages and are also transported to hilar and mediastinal lymph nodes, where the indigestible material is stored indefinitely within macrophages. Although the gross appearance of the lungs in persons with anthracosis may be alarming, the condition is entirely innocuous.

Tattooing involves the introduction of insoluble metallic and vegetable pigments into the skin, where they are engulfed by dermal macrophages and persist for a lifetime.

IRREVERSIBLE CELL INJURY

If the acute stress to which a cell must react is too great, the resulting changes in structure and function lead to the death of the cell. Among the more common causes of cell death are viruses, reduction in blood supply (ischemia), and physical agents such as ionizing radiation, extreme temperatures, or toxic chemicals. Cell death is classified into two types according to the presumed underlying mechanisms responsible for the loss of viability, namely necrosis and apoptosis. The latter is generally held to result from the expression of a genetically determined cell-death program, which can be activated by a variety of physiological signals or cellular injuries (discussed later). By contrast, necrosis is the consequence of a catastrophic injury to the mechanisms that maintain the integrity of the cell. At the level of light microscopy, both forms of cell death tend to be indistinguishable and have the appearance of coagulative necrosis.

Morphology of Necrosis
Coagulative Necrosis

Coagulative necrosis includes changes in both the cytoplasm and the nucleus (Figs. 1-12 and 1-13). When stained with the usual combination of hematoxylin and eosin, the cytoplasm is more eosinophilic than usual. The nucleus displays an initial clumping of the chromatin, followed by a redistribution along the nuclear membrane. The nucleus then becomes smaller and stains deeply basophilic as chromatin clumping continues. This process is termed **pyknosis**. The pyknotic nucleus may break up into many smaller fragments scattered about the cytoplasm, an appearance termed **karyorrhexis**. Alternatively, the pyknotic nucleus may be extruded from the cell, or it may manifest progressive loss of chromatin staining. We then use the term **karyolysis**.

Liquefactive Necrosis

There are circumstances in which the rate of dissolution of necrotic cells is considerably faster than the rate of repair. The polymorphonuclear leukocytes of the acute inflammatory reaction are endowed with potent hydrolases capable of completely digesting dead cells. A sharply localized collection of these acute inflammatory cells, generally in response to a bacterial infection, produces the rapid death and dissolution of tissue (so-called **liquefactive necrosis**). The result is often an **abscess**.

Coagulative necrosis of the brain as a result of cerebral artery occlusion is frequently followed by rapid

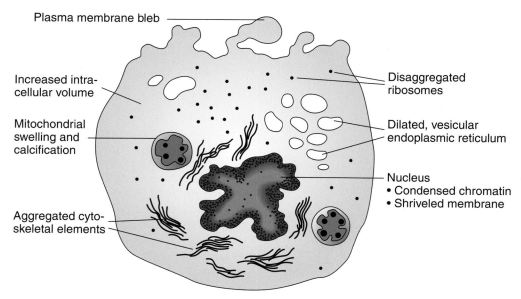

Plasma membrane bleb

Increased intra-
cellular volume

Mitochondrial
swelling and
calcification

Aggregated cyto-
skeletal elements

Disaggregated
ribosomes

Dilated, vesicular
endoplasmic reticulum

Nucleus
• Condensed chromatin
• Shriveled membrane

FIGURE   *1-12*
Ultrastructural features of coagulative necrosis.

dissolution—liquefactive necrosis—of the dead tissue by a mechanism that cannot be attributed to the action of an acute inflammatory response. The liquefactive necrosis of large areas of the central nervous system can result in formation of a cavity or cyst.

Fat Necrosis

Fat necrosis specifically affects adipose tissue and most commonly results from pancreatitis or trauma (Fig. 1-14). The unique feature determining this type of necrosis is the presence of triglycerides in adipose tissue.

The process begins when digestive enzymes, normally found only in the pancreatic duct and small intestine, are released from injured pancreatic acinar cells and ducts into the extracellular spaces. On extracellular activation, these enzymes digest the pancreas itself as well as the surrounding tissues, including adipose cells. Fatty acids are precipitated as calcium soaps, which accumulate microscopically as amorphous, basophilic deposits at the periphery of the irregular islands of necrotic adipocytes. On gross examination, fat necrosis appears as an irregular, chalky-white area embedded in otherwise normal adipose tissue.

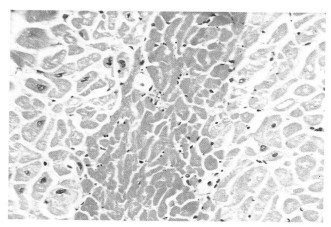

FIGURE   *1-13*
Coagulative necrosis. A photomicrograph of the heart in a patient with an acute myocardial infarction. In the center, the deeply eosinophilic necrotic cells have lost their nuclei. The necrotic focus is surrounded by paler-staining, viable cardiac myocytes.

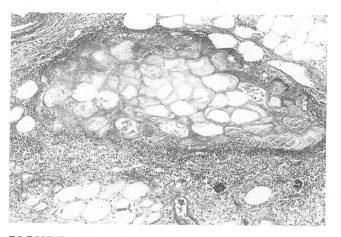

FIGURE   *1-14*
Fat necrosis. A photomicrograph of peripancreatic adipose tissue from a case of acute pancreatitis shows an island of necrotic adipocytes adjacent to an acutely inflamed area. Fatty acids are precipitated as calcium soaps, which accumulate as amorphous, basophilic deposits at the periphery of the irregular island of necrotic adipocytes.

Caseous Necrosis

■ *Caseous necrosis refers to the typical lesion of tuberculosis, in which the dead cells persist indefinitely as amorphous, coarsely granular, eosinophilic debris* (Fig. 1-15). The lesions of tuberculosis are the tuberculous granulomas, or tubercles. In the center of such a granuloma, the accumulated mononuclear cells mediating the chronic inflammatory reaction to the offending mycobacteria are killed. In caseous necrosis, unlike coagulative necrosis, the necrotic cells do not retain their cellular outlines. However, the cells fail to disappear by lysis, as in liquefactive necrosis. Grossly, caseous necrosis appears grayish-white and is soft and friable. It resembles clumpy cheese, hence the name caseous necrosis.

Fibrinoid Necrosis

■ *Fibrinoid necrosis refers to an alteration of injured blood vessels, in which the insudation and accumulation of plasma proteins causes the wall to stain intensely with eosin.* This term is something of a misnomer, however, because eosinophilia of the accumulated plasma proteins obscures the underlying alterations in the blood vessel, thereby making it difficult, if not impossible, to determine whether there truly is necrosis in the vascular wall.

PATHOGENESIS OF COAGULATIVE NECROSIS

The morphologic manifestation of cell death—coagulative necrosis—is the same regardless of whether the cells have been killed by a virus, ionizing radiation, or an interruption in blood supply. The concentration of calcium ions in extracellular fluids is in the millimolar range (10^{-3} M). By contrast, the concentration in the cytosol is some 10,000-fold lower (on the order of 10^{-7} M). This large concentration gradient is maintained both

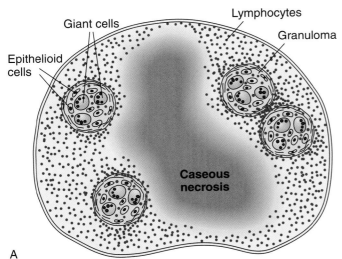

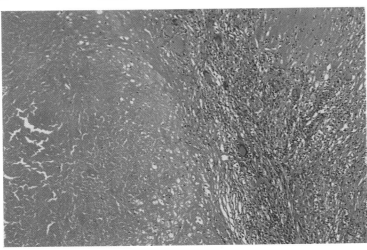

FIGURE *1-15*
Caseous necrosis in a tuberculous lymph node. (A) The typical amorphous, granular, eosinophilic, necrotic center is surrounded by granulomatous inflammation. (B) A photomicrograph shows a tuberculous granuloma with central caseous necrosis.

by the passive impermeability of the plasma membrane to calcium ions and by the active extrusion of calcium from the cell. It is not surprising, therefore, that coagulative necrosis is accompanied by the accumulation of calcium ions in the dead cells.

The influx and accumulation of calcium ions and the resultant morphologic changes of coagulative necrosis can account for the common morphology of cell death. The sequence of events leading to coagulative necrosis may then be described as (1) irreversible injury and cell death, (2) loss of the plasma membrane's ability to maintain a gradient of calcium ions, (3) an influx and accumulation of calcium ions in the cell, and (4) the morphologic appearance of coagulative necrosis. Under such a scheme, coagulative necrosis occurs after the point of no return, that is, after irreversible injury and "death" of the cell.

Alternatively, cell injury may lead to potentially reversible plasma membrane damage. In such a scheme the large gradient of calcium ions can no longer be maintained by the plasma membrane. Excess calcium ions then accumulate in the injured cells and cause coagulative necrosis. This scenario envisions the accumulation of calcium ions as the point at which potentially reversible cell injury becomes irreversible.

The previous discussion can be summarized as follows: **Whatever the role of calcium, the disruption of the permeability barrier of the plasma membrane seems to be a critical event in lethal cell injury.**

Ischemic Cell Injury

The interruption of blood flow—ischemia—is probably the most important cause of coagulative necrosis in human disease. The complications of atherosclerosis, for example, are generally the result of ischemic cell injury in the brain, heart, small intestine, kidneys, and lower extremities. Highly differentiated cells, such as the proximal tubular cells of the kidney, cardiac myocytes, and the neurons of the central nervous system, depend on aerobic respiration to produce ATP for the performance of their specialized functions. When ischemia limits the supply of oxygen and ATP is depleted, these cells rapidly manifest many changes in both structure and function.

The effects of ischemic injury are all reversible if the duration of ischemia is short. For example, changes in myocardial contractility, membrane potential, metabolism, and ultrastructure are short-lived if the circulation is rapidly restored. However, when ischemia persists, the affected cells become irreversibly injured; that is, the cells continue to deteriorate and become necrotic despite reperfusion with arterial blood.

Reperfusion Injury and Activated Oxygen

One popular theory postulates a role for partially reduced and, thus, activated oxygen species in the genesis of membrane damage in irreversible ischemia. It might seem paradoxical that oxygen species cause cell injury when that injury is attributed to an insufficient oxygen supply. This dilemma is more apparent, however, than real. Toxic oxygen species are generated not during the period of ischemia itself but rather on restoration of blood flow, or reperfusion, hence the term **reperfusion injury**.

Some event occurs during the period of ischemia that results in an overproduction of toxic oxygen species on later restoration of the oxygen supply. Two sources of activated oxygen species have been proposed, namely production by intracellular xanthine oxidase and extracellular release by activated neutrophils.

In some circumstances, xanthine dehydrogenase may be converted by proteolysis during the period of ischemia into xanthine oxidase. On return of the oxygen supply with reperfusion, the abundant purines derived from the catabolism of ATP during ischemia provide substrates for the activity of xanthine oxidase, which requires oxygen in catalyzing the formation of uric acid. Activated oxygen species are byproducts of this reaction.

A second source of activated oxygen species during reperfusion may be the neutrophil. It is thought that alterations in the cell surface occur during ischemia and, on reperfusion, induce the adhesion and activation of circulating neutrophils. These cells release large quantities of activated oxygen species, which then injure the previously ischemic cells.

The damage to the plasma membrane directly associated with irreversible ischemic injury and not dependent on reperfusion has been attributed to two mechanisms. One of these mechanisms relates to changes in the metabolism of the phospholipid bilayer, whereas the other emphasizes alterations in the cytoskeletal structures.

Altered Phospholipid Metabolism

Plasma membrane damage in irreversible ischemia has been attributed, at least in part, to accelerated degradation of membrane phospholipids. Experimental ischemia results in a loss of phospholipids from cell membranes, accompanied by a release of their fatty acids. Structural alterations in cellular membranes accompany this increased hydrolysis of phospholipids. Microsomal membranes prepared from ischemic livers

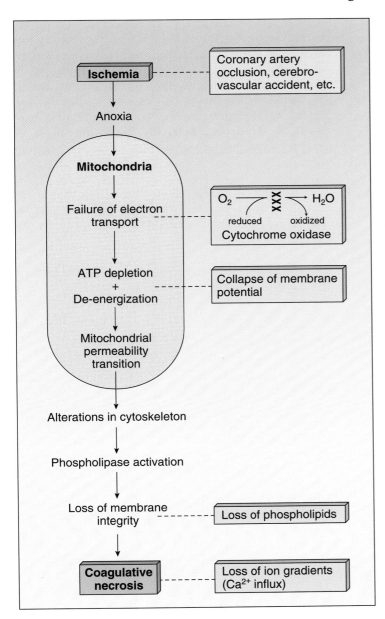

FIGURE **1-16**
Possible sequence of events in the pathogenesis of irreversible cell injury caused by anoxia-ischemia.

exhibit a 25- to 50-fold increase in their passive permeability to calcium.

Cytoskeletal Alterations

The intimate association of cytoskeletal elements with the plasma membrane of many cells suggests that the cytoskeleton plays a role in the regulation of the structure of the cell membrane. In a number of experimental systems, both ischemia and anoxia lead to the formation of prominent blebs of the plasma membrane, which have been attributed to cytoskeletal changes.

The events leading to irreversible ischemic cell injury are summarized in Figure 1-16.

Cell Injury Caused by Oxygen Free Radicals

Partially reduced oxygen species have been identified as the likely cause of cell injury in an increasing number of diseases (Fig. 1-17). We referred earlier to reperfusion injury when discussing the mechanism of cell injury in ischemia. The inflammatory process, whether acute or chronic, can cause considerable tissue destruction. Partially reduced oxygen species produced by phagocytic cells are important mediators of cell injury in such circumstances. Damage to cells resulting from oxygen radicals formed by inflammatory cells has been implicated in diseases of the joints and of many organs,

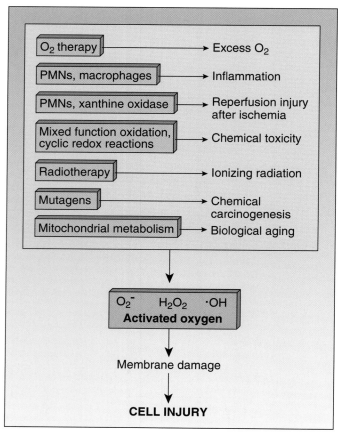

FIGURE   *1-17*
The role of activated oxygen species in human disease.

including the kidney, lungs, and heart. The toxicity of many chemicals may reflect the formation of toxic oxygen species. Killing of cells by ionizing radiation is most likely the result of the direct formation of hydroxyl radicals from the radiolysis of water. There is also evidence of a role for oxygen species in chemical carcinogenesis, during either initiation or promotion.

Cells also may be injured when oxygen is present at concentrations greater than normal. In the past, this occurred largely during those therapeutic circumstances in which oxygen was given to patients at concentrations greater than the normal 20% of inspired air. The lungs of adults and the eyes of premature newborns were the major targets of such oxygen toxicity.

Three partially reduced species are intermediate between O_2 and H_2O, representing transfers of varying numbers of electrons. They are O_2^-, superoxide (one electron); H_2O_2, hydrogen peroxide (two electrons); and OH^-, the hydroxyl radical (three electrons) (Fig. 1-18).

Superoxide. Components of the mitochondrial electron transport chain may be directly auto-oxidized by O_2 to yield superoxide anions (O_2^-). Superoxide an-

ions are also produced by enzymes such as xanthine oxidase and cytochrome P_{450}. Phagocytosis by polymorphonuclear leukocytes and macrophages is accompanied by increased oxygen consumption, which largely represents the formation of O_2^- by an oxidase in the plasma membrane. The O_2^- anions produced in the cytosol or mitochondria are catabolized by superoxide dismutase. Hydrogen peroxide is also produced directly by a number of oxidases in cytoplasmic peroxisomes.

Hydrogen Peroxide. Two different enzymes reduce H_2O_2 to water, namely catalase within the peroxisomes and glutathione peroxidase in both the cytosol and the mitochondria.

Hydroxyl Radical. Hydroxyl radicals are formed in biologic systems in two ways, namely by the radiolysis of water or by the reaction of hydrogen peroxide with ferrous iron (the Fenton reaction).

Role of Iron

A pool of free ferric iron seems to be required for partially reduced oxygen species to injure cells. Free ferric iron can be reduced by superoxide anions to ferrous iron. Hydrogen peroxide, formed either directly or (more commonly) by the dismutation of superoxide anions, then reacts with the ferrous iron by the Fenton reaction to produce hydroxyl radicals. This sequence, starting with superoxide anions and ferric iron and leading to the generation of hydroxyl radicals without consumption of ferric iron, is called an iron-catalyzed Haber-Weiss reaction:

$$H_2O_2 + O_2^- \xrightarrow{Fe^{2+}} \cdot OH + OH^- + O_2$$

Hydroxyl Radicals and Macromolecules

The hydroxyl radical ($\cdot OH$) is an extremely reactive species, and there are several mechanisms by which it might damage membranes.

- **Lipid Peroxidation.** The best-known effect of hydroxyl radicals relates to $\cdot OH$ as an initiator of lipid peroxidation (Fig. 1-19). The hydroxyl radical removes a hydrogen atom from the unsaturated fatty acids of the membrane phospholipids, a process that forms a free lipid radical. The lipid radical, in turn, reacts with molecular oxygen and forms a lipid peroxide radical. Like $\cdot OH$, this peroxide radical can function as an initiator, removing another hydrogen atom from a second unsaturated fatty acid. A lipid peroxide and a new lipid radical result, and a chain reaction is initiated.

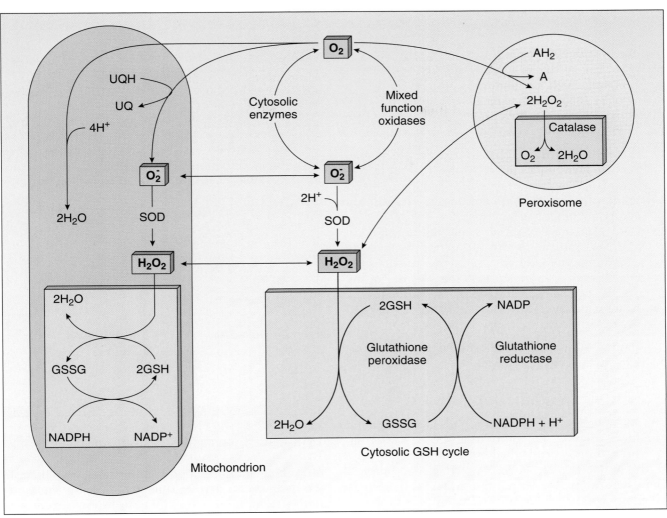

FIGURE 1-18
Cellular metabolism of oxygen and the accompanying antioxidant defense mechanisms.

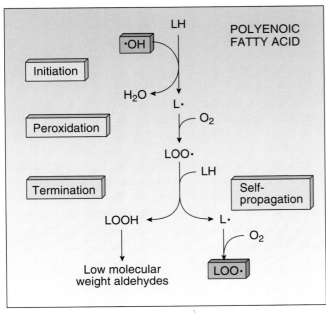

FIGURE 1-19
Lipid peroxidation initiated by the hydroxyl radical.

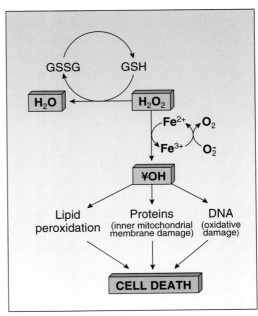

FIGURE 1-20
The mechanisms of cell injury by activated oxygen species.

The destruction of the unsaturated fatty acids of phospholipids results in a loss of membrane integrity. Antioxidants, such as vitamin E, prevent the injury that usually follows exposure of cells to partially reduced oxygen species. This protection is attributed to the inhibition of lipid peroxidation by antioxidants.

- **Protein Interactions.** Hydroxyl radicals also may damage membranes in ways other than lipid peroxidation. They may cause cross-linking of membrane proteins through formation of disulfide bonds and other mechanisms.
- **DNA Damage.** DNA is an important target of the hydroxyl radical. Structural alterations include strand breaks, modified bases, and cross-links between strands. In most cases, the integrity of the genome can be reconstituted by the various DNA repair pathways. However, if oxidative damage to DNA is sufficiently extensive, the cell dies.

Figure 1-20 summarizes the mechanisms of cell injury by activated oxygen species.

How Ionizing Radiation Kills Cells

The adjective *ionizing*, in reference to electromagnetic radiation, connotes an ability to effect the radiolysis of water, thus directly forming hydroxyl radicals. Hydroxyl radicals can interact with DNA and inhibit DNA replication. For a nonproliferating cell, such as a hepatocyte or a neuron, the inability to replicate DNA is of little consequence. For a proliferating cell, however, the inability to replicate DNA represents a catastrophic loss of function. Experimental data suggest that once a proliferating cell is prevented from replicating, a mechanism (apoptosis, discussed later) is set in motion that leads to its demise. Very large doses of ionizing radiation, however, can kill cells as a result of lipid peroxidation initiated by hydroxyl radicals.

Figure 1-21 summarizes the mechanisms of cell killing by ionizing radiation.

How Viruses Kill Cells

Viruses kill cells in two distinct ways. Infection of a cell by a **directly cytopathic virus** leads to lethal injury without the participation of the host immune system. **Indirectly cytopathic viruses,** on the other hand, require the participation of the immune system.

The poliovirus is typical of the group of viruses that is directly cytopathic. It consists of a single strand of RNA surrounded by a protein capsule. The viral genome in the cytosol is recognized by the protein synthetic apparatus as just another mRNA molecule. Virally coded proteins insert into the host-cell plasma

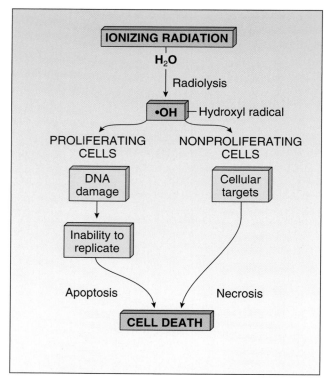

FIGURE   *1-21*
Mechanisms of cell injury by ionizing radiation.

membrane and form a pore, or channel, that disrupts the permeability barrier, thereby allowing equilibration of ionic gradients. Potassium ions leave, and sodium and calcium ions enter. The cell is then dead.

The hepatitis B virus is an example of an indirectly cytopathic virus. This agent consists of a double-stranded DNA genome enclosed in a protein capsule. Transcription of the viral DNA genome in the nucleus produces mRNAs, which are transported to the cytoplasm and translated into proteins. It is thought that the process of viral assembly or release exposes viral proteins on the external surface of the plasma membrane. These proteins are recognized by the immune system as nonself, or foreign, antigens. A cellular and humoral immune response develops in reaction to the viral proteins on the surface of the infected host cells. It is this immune response that seems to be responsible for the lethal injury of the virus-infected cell.

Figure 1-22 summarizes the mechanisms of cell killing by directly and indirectly cytopathic viruses.

How Chemicals Kill Cells

Toxic chemicals are divided into two general classes: those that interact directly with cellular constituents without requiring metabolic activation and those that are themselves not toxic but are metabolized to yield an ultimate toxin that interacts with the target cell.

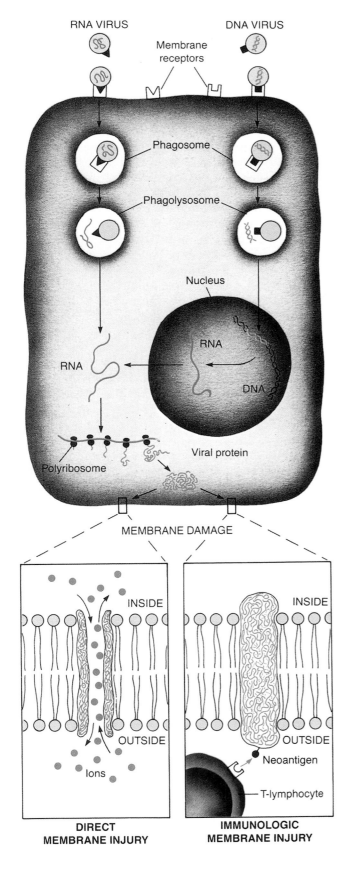

**DIRECT
MEMBRANE INJURY**

**IMMUNOLOGIC
MEMBRANE INJURY**

Liver Necrosis Caused by the Metabolism of Chemicals

Studies of a few compounds that produce liver cell necrosis in rodents have enhanced our understanding of how chemicals injure cells. These studies have focused principally on those compounds that are converted to toxic metabolites. Carbon tetrachloride, acetaminophen, and bromobenzene are well-studied hepatotoxins. Each is metabolized by the mixed-function oxidase system of the endoplasmic reticulum, and each causes liver cell necrosis.

Carbon Tetrachloride. The metabolism of carbon tetrachloride (CCl_4) is a model compound for toxicologic studies. After CCl_4 binds to cytochrome P_{450}, the mixed-function oxygenase involved in drug metabolism, the addition of an electron immediately results in the reductive cleavage of a carbon-chlorine bond. The products are a chlorine atom and a highly reactive, trichloromethyl free radical. The toxicity of CCl_4 relates to the formation of the trichloromethyl free radical and, thus, depends on metabolism of the parent compound. Like the hydroxyl radical, the trichloromethyl radical is a potent initiator of lipid peroxidation.

Acetaminophen and Bromobenzene. It has been suggested that the hepatotoxicity of the two model hepatotoxins, bromobenzene and the analgesic acetaminophen, might reflect covalent binding of electrophilic metabolites to critical cellular macromolecules. However, recent studies have shown that liver necrosis is actually related to the toxicity of activated oxygen species.

Like CCl_4, acetaminophen is metabolized by cytochrome P_{450}, and a number of electron transfer reactions result in the formation of superoxide and hydrogen peroxide. The liver cells may then be lethally injured by these activated oxygen species through mechanisms similar to those discussed earlier.

To summarize, the metabolism of hepatotoxic chemicals by mixed-function oxidation leads to irreversible cell injury. What is emerging is a common theme of membrane damage as a result of the peroxi-

FIGURE *1-22*
Mechanisms of cell killing by directly and indirectly cytopathic viruses. Membrane damage is the final common pathway by which both types of viruses produce cell death. The directly cytopathic viruses create a transmembrane channel by inserting their proteins into the plasma membrane, thereby disrupting its function as a permeability barrier. The indirectly cytopathic viruses also insert their proteins into the plasma membrane and create an antigenic target for cytotoxic T lymphocytes.

dation of the constituent phospholipids. Lipid peroxidation is initiated by a metabolite of the original compound (as with CCl_4) or by activated oxygen species formed during metabolism of the toxin (as with acetaminophen).

Chemicals That Are Not Metabolized

Directly cytotoxic chemicals do not have to be metabolized to injure the target cell. Such compounds combine directly with cellular constituents. The class of directly cytotoxic chemicals includes many of the cancer chemotherapeutic agents and toxic heavy metals, such as mercury, lead, and iron. Because of the inherent reactivity of directly cytotoxic chemicals, many constituents of the target cell are damaged.

Apoptosis (Programmed Cell Death)

■ *Apoptosis refers to a genetically determined, internal, self-destruct mechanism of cell death, which is activated under a variety of circumstances.* These include the following situations:

- Developmental morphogenesis
- Physiologic turnover of cells in renewable tissues
- Immune regulation, as exemplified by the deletion of self-reactive T cells in the thymus during development and of B cells in the germinal centers of peripheral lymph nodes
- Deprivation of hormones and other trophic factors
- Environmental hazards, including viral infections, ultraviolet exposure, ionizing radiation, and toxic cell injury
- Cancers, in which the vast majority of neoplastic cells undergo apoptosis, a feature that accounts for the slow growth of many malignant tumors

Multicellular organisms must control the elimination of damaged or surplus cells as strictly as they regulate the formation of new ones. Just as billions of hemopoietic elements, mucosal cells of the gastrointestinal tract, and epidermal cells of the skin are created daily, equal numbers of cells in the same tissues are simultaneously lost by apoptosis. In development, the formation of many structures (e.g., digits of the hands and toes) requires the elimination of tissues such as interdigital webs. Many newly formed neurons are actually surplus and, normally, die during development. Another example is the involution of the lactating breast, which is mediated by a reduction in prolactin secretion by the pituitary and consequent apoptosis of milk-producing cells. Finally, high doses of adrenal steroids (glucocorticoids) induce apoptosis

of T lymphocytes, thereby contributing to the anti-inflammatory and immunosuppressive actions of these hormones.

Morphology of Apoptosis

Apoptotic cells are shrunken and detached from their neighbors and are often engulfed by macrophages. The inflammatory response elicited by necrotic cells is absent or attenuated. By electron microscopy, apoptosis features (1) nuclear condensation and fragmentation, (2) segregation of cytoplasmic organelles into distinct regions, (3) surface membrane blebs, and (4) fragmentation of the dead or dying cell into membrane-bound bodies, which may or may not include nuclear components. The fragmentation of the nucleus characteristic of apoptosis (Fig. 1-23) has its counterpart in the electrophoretic pattern of DNA isolated from the dying cells. On electrophoresis, the cleaved DNA displays a characteristic "ladder" of bands.

Mechanisms of Apoptosis

Genes that control programmed cell death have been identified in the nematode worm *Caenorhabditis elegans*. They have been termed *ced* (*cell death*) genes. Homologues to these genes that involve cell death have been identified in mammalian tissues. At present, the two best-characterized models of programmed cell death are those that involve action of the Fas receptor and apoptosis induced by DNA damage (Fig. 1-24).

Cytotoxic T cells display a Fas ligand on the cell surface when the T cell interacts with a target cell. Binding of this ligand activates the Fas receptor on the surface membrane of the target cell, an effect that leads to a series of intracellular reactions. In turn, these intracellular reactions lead to the activation of endonucleases in the nucleus and subsequent fragmentation of DNA. In addition, the production of certain lipid messengers mediates mitochondrial injury.

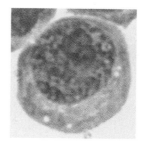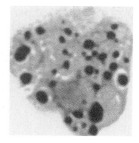

FIGURE   *1-23*
Apoptosis. A viable leukemic cell (*left*) contrasts with an apoptotic cell (*right*) in which the nucleus has undergone condensation and fragmentation.

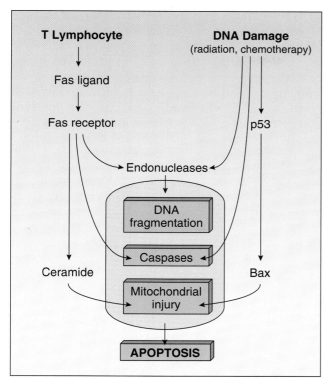

FIGURE   **1-24**
Mechanisms of apoptosis. Two major pathways that mediate cell death in apoptosis are illustrated. Cytotoxic T cells bear the Fas ligand, which binds and activates the Fas receptor on the surface of target cells. As a result, three biochemical consequences that collectively mediate apoptosis ensue: (1) activation of an endonuclease causes DNA fragmentation, (2) activation of caspases leads to proteolysis of a variety of substrates, and (3) generation of ceramide injures mitochondria. These same three events characterize the apoptosis induced by DNA damage. In this case, however, upregulation of p53 induces Bax synthesis, which leads to mitochondrial injury.

DNA damage upregulates the p53 nuclear protein, thereby leading to the expression of other genes involved in regulation of the cell cycle and, eventually, apoptosis. In particular, p53 induces the synthesis of Bax, a death-promoting protein that is thought to injure mitochondria. Cytoplasmic enzymes termed *caspases* also contribute to cell death initiated by DNA damage.

CALCIFICATION

The deposition of the mineral salts of calcium is, of course, a normal process in the formation of bone from cartilage. As we have learned, calcium entry into dead or dying cells is usual, owing to the inability of such cells to maintain a steep calcium gradient.

Dystrophic Calcification. This term refers to the macroscopic deposition of calcium salts in injured tissues. Dystrophic calcification does not simply reflect an accumulation of calcium derived from the bodies of dead cells; rather, it represents an extracellular deposition of calcium from the circulation or interstitial fluid. Dystrophic calcification is often visible to the naked eye and ranges from gritty, sand-like grains to firm, rock-hard material. In many locations, such as in cases of tuberculous caseous necrosis in the lung or lymph nodes, calcification has no functional consequences. However, dystrophic calcification may also occur in crucial locations, such as the mitral or aortic valves (Fig. 1-25). In such instances, calcification leads to impeded blood flow, because it produces inflexible valve leaflets and narrowed valve orifices (mitral and aortic stenosis). Dystrophic calcification in atherosclerotic coronary arteries contributes to narrowing of those vessels.

Metastatic Calcification. This process reflects deranged calcium metabolism, in contrast to dystrophic calcification, which has its origin in cell injury. Metastatic calcification is associated with an increased serum calcium concentration (hypercalcemia). In general, almost any disorder that increases the serum calcium level can lead to calcification in inappropriate locations, such as the alveolar septa of the lung, renal tubules, and blood vessels. Calcification is seen in various disorders, including chronic renal failure, vitamin D intoxication, and hyperparathyroidism.

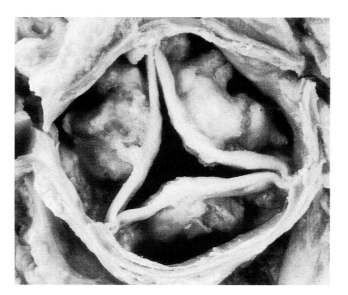

FIGURE   **1-25**
Calcific aortic stenosis. Large deposits of calcium salts are evident in the cusps and free margins of the thickened aortic valve as viewed from above.

Calcium Stones. Stones containing calcium carbonate in sites such as the gallbladder, renal pelvis, bladder, and pancreatic duct are another form of pathologic calcification. Under certain circumstances, the mineral salts precipitate from solution and crystallize about foci of organic material.

CELLULAR AGING

Although the biologic basis for aging is obscure, there is general agreement that its elucidation, as in all pathologic conditions, should be sought at the cellular level. Various theories of cellular aging have been proposed, but the evidence for each is, at best, indirect and often derived from data obtained in cultured cells.

Aging As a Genetic Program

Every species has an appointed life span that, within limits, is immutable. Given an adequate environment, life span may be genetically determined. In humans, the modest correlation in longevity between related persons and the excellent agreement among identical twins lend credence to this assumption. In addition, the entire process of aging, including features such as male pattern baldness, cataracts, and coronary artery disease, is compressed into a span of less than 10 years in the genetic syndrome of progeria.

Major support for the concept of a genetically programmed life span comes from studies of replicating cells in tissue culture. Unlike cancer cells, normal cells in tissue culture do not exhibit an unrestrained capacity to replicate. Cultured human fibroblasts undergo approximately 50 population doublings, after which they no longer divide, and the culture dies out (Fig. 1-26). If the cells are transformed into cancer cells, however, by exposure to simian virus 40 or a chemical carcinogen, they continue to replicate; in a sense, they become immortal. A rough correlation between the number of population doublings in fibroblasts and life span has been reported in several species. For example, rat fibroblasts exhibit considerably fewer doublings than human ones. Moreover, cells obtained from patients with precocious aging, such as those with progeria, also display a conspicuously reduced number of population doublings in vitro. Certain genes that influence cellular senescence have been identified, but the mechanisms by which they exert such effects are not understood.

An alternative explanation for in vitro cell senescence centers on the genetic elements at the tips of chromosomes, termed *telomeres*. These are short, repetitive nucleotide sequences, which are as long as 2000 bases in human chromosomes. Because DNA polymerase is unable to copy to the linear chromosomes all the way to the tip, the telomeres tend to shorten with each cell division, until a critical diminution in size may interfere with cell viability. To overcome this problem, cells utilize an enzyme termed *telomerase*, which is capable of extending the chromosome ends. However, many cells lack telomerase activity, and progressive telomere shortening occurs over the replicative life span of such cells in tissue culture. It has, therefore, been proposed that telomere shortening acts as a molecular clock that produces senescence after a defined number of cell divisions in vitro. However, in vivo, biologic aging also affects terminally differentiated cells, such as neurons and cardiac myocytes, and the telomerase theory of aging remains to be proved.

Aging As Accumulated Somatic Damage

Cell may sustain a variety of injuries during a lifetime, and the precise catalog of molecular lesions responsi-

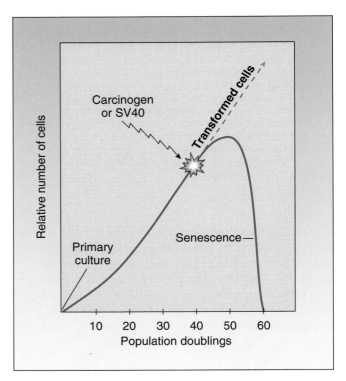

FIGURE   *1-26*
Cellular senescence in cultured human fibroblasts. The number of cultured cells is a function of the number of population doublings. After approximately 50 population doublings, the cells no longer divide, and the culture dies out. However, if the cells are transformed with a virus or a chemical, cellular senescence is not seen, and the cells are "immortalized" and continue to divide indefinitely.

ble for aging remains to be defined. Currently, most research is directed toward the molecular consequences of persistent oxidative stress, which may influence aging by causing irreversible accrual of molecular oxidative damage. Such lesions would include peroxidation of membrane lipids, DNA modifications, and protein oxidation. Interestingly, the generation rate of reactive oxygen species correlates crudely with the overall metabolic rate of an organism, which, in turn, relates inversely to body size (small animals tend to have higher metabolic rates than large ones). In this context, larger animals usually have longer life spans than smaller ones. Additional evidence for progressive oxidative damage with aging is the deposition of lipofuscin pigment, principally in postmitotic cells of organs such as the brain, heart, and liver. This brown pigment contains products of the peroxidation of unsaturated fatty acids, which is thought to reflect continuing lipid peroxidation of cellular membranes by activated oxygen species. Oxidative damage to mitochondria has also been proposed to play a role in aging, and more than a dozen large deletions in mitochondrial DNA have been identified in postmitotic tissues of older persons.

Current evidence supports the notion that the various hypotheses related to biologic aging are not mutually contradictory, and that all may contribute to this process (Fig. 1-27).

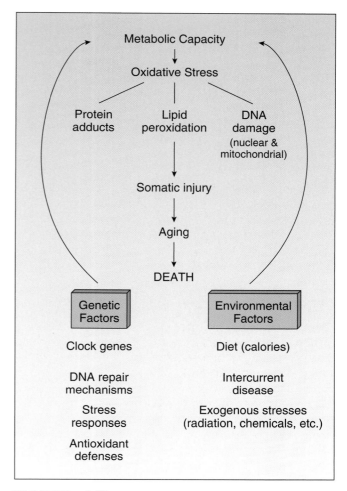

FIGURE *1-27*
Summary hypothesis of the mechanisms responsible for biologic aging. It is likely that aging represents the progressive accumulation of a variety of somatic injuries, including damage to proteins, membrane lipids, and nuclear and mitochondrial DNA. The extent of these injuries has been linked to the oxidative stress produced by cellular metabolism. In turn, both genetic and environmental factors have been invoked as determining the metabolic capacity and the antioxidant and other defenses of a cell.

Inflammation

Joseph C. Fantone
Peter A. Ward

■ *Inflammation is a reaction of the microcirculation characterized by movement of fluid and leukocytes from the blood into the extravascular tissues.* This is frequently an expression of the host's attempt to localize and eliminate metabolically altered cells, foreign particles, micro-organisms, or antigens. Inflammation can be thought to proceed as follows:

- **Initiation** of the mechanisms responsible for the localization and clearance of foreign substances and injured tissues is stimulated by the recognition that injury to tissues has occurred.
- **Amplification** of the inflammatory response, in which both soluble mediators and cellular inflammatory systems are activated, follows the recognition of injury.
- **Termination** of the inflammatory response, after generation of inflammatory agents and elimination of the foreign agent, is accomplished by specific inhibitors of the mediators.

Following injury to a tissue, changes in the structure of the vascular wall lead to:

- Loss of endothelial cell integrity
- Leakage of fluid and plasma components from the intravascular compartment
- Emigration of both erythrocytes and leukocytes from the intraluminal space into the extravascular tissue.

Specific inflammatory mediators produced at the sites of injury regulate this response of the vasculature to injury (Fig. 2-1). Among these mediators are vasoactive molecules that act directly on the vasculature to increase vascular permeability. In addition, chemotactic factors are generated that recruit leukocytes from the vascular compartment and into the injured tissue. Once present in the tissues, recruited leukocytes secrete additional inflammatory mediators that either enhance or inhibit the inflammatory response.

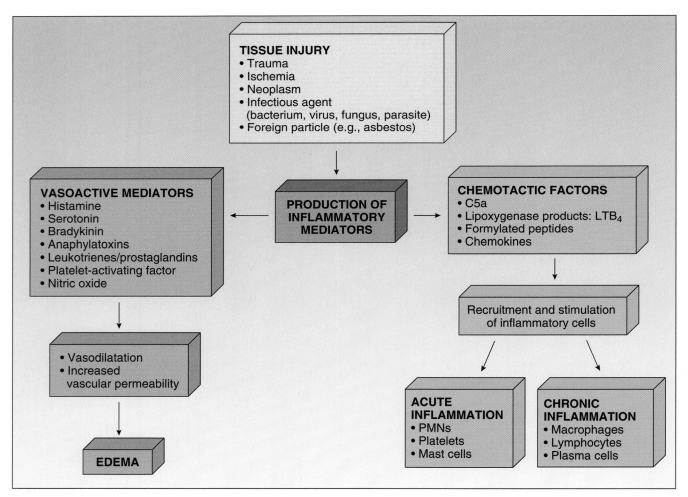

FIGURE *2-1*
Mediators of the inflammatory response.

ACUTE INFLAMMATION VERSUS CHRONIC INFLAMMATION

Historically, inflammation has been referred to as either **acute** or **chronic** inflammation, depending on the persistence of the injury, its clinical symptomatology, and the nature of the inflammatory response. The hallmarks of acute inflammation include (1) accumulation of fluid and plasma components in the affected tissue, (2) intravascular stimulation of platelets, and (3) presence of polymorphonuclear leukocytes (Fig. 2-2). By contrast, the characteristic cell components of chronic inflammation are lymphocytes, plasma cells, and macrophages (Fig. 2-3).

Activation of the inflammatory response results in a number of distinct outcomes:

- **Resolution.** Under ideal conditions, the source of the tissue injury is eliminated, the inflammatory response resolves, and the normal tissue architecture and physiologic function are restored.
- **Abscess.** If the area of acute inflammation is walled off by the collection of inflammatory cells, destruction of the tissue byproducts of the polymorphonuclear leukocytes (also known as neutrophils) takes place. This is the mechanism by which an abscess is formed.
- **Scar.** If the tissue is irreversibly injured, the normal architecture is often replaced by a scar, despite elimination of the initial pathologic insult.

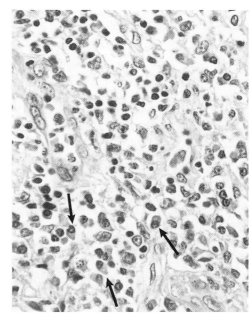

FIGURE 2-3
Chronic inflammation. Lymphocytes, plasma cells (*arrows*), and a few macrophages are present.

- **Persistent Inflammation.** Sometimes, the inflammatory cells fail to eliminate the pathologic insult, in which case the inflammatory reaction persists and may be associated with a cell-mediated immune reaction. This area of chronic inflammation often expands, leading to fibrosis and scar formation.

ACUTE INFLAMMATION

An understanding of the acute inflammatory process requires a discussion of vascular permeability and its mediators, recruitment of inflammatory cells, and mechanisms by which the inflammatory cells produce their effects.

Vascular Permeability and Edema
Normal Regulation of Fluid Transport

Under normal physiologic conditions, there is continuous movement of fluid from the intravascular compartment to the extravascular space. Fluid that accumulates in the extravascular space is normally cleared through the lymphatics and returned to the circulation.

Noninflammatory Edema

In certain conditions, the movement of fluid into the extravascular space exceeds the clearance ability of the lymphatics. The resulting increase in extravascular

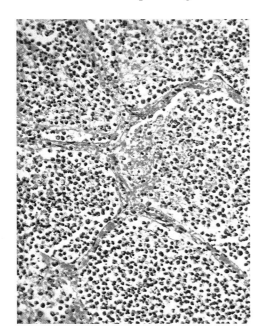

FIGURE 2-2
Acute inflammation. A photomicrograph of the lung from a patient with pneumonia shows densely packed polymorphonuclear leukocytes in the alveoli.

fluid is called **edema,** and its clinical manifestation is swelling. Examples of clinical conditions in which edema occurs include (1) pulmonary edema resulting from increased hydrostatic pressure in the pulmonary vasculature, secondary to left ventricular cardiac failure; (2) soft tissue edema in the leg as a consequence of increased hydrostatic pressure caused by thrombosis of the femoral vein; and (3) diffuse soft tissue edema secondary to decreased intravascular oncotic pressure in the hypoalbuminemia of the nephrotic syndrome.

Inflammatory Edema

Alterations in the anatomy and function of the microvasculature are among the earliest responses to tissue injury, and they may promote fluid accumulation in tissues (Figs. 2-4 and 2-5) as follows:

1. **Transient vasoconstriction of arterioles** at the site of injury is the earliest vascular response to mild injury of the skin. This process is mediated by the neurogenic and chemical mediator systems and usually resolves within seconds to minutes.
2. **Vasodilatation of precapillary arterioles** then increases blood flow to the tissue, a condition known as hyperemia. Vasodilatation is caused by the release of specific mediators and is responsible, in part, for the redness and warmth at sites of tissue injury.
3. **Increased permeability of the endothelial cell barrier** results in leakage of fluid from the intravascular compartment into the extravascular spaces, forming edema.

Vasoactive mediators, originating from both plasma and cellular sources, are generated at sites of tissue injury by a variety of mechanisms. These mediators bind to specific receptors on vascular endothelial and smooth muscle cells, causing vasoconstriction or vasodilatation. Vasodilatation of arterioles increases the blood flow and can exacerbate fluid leakage into the tissue. At the same time, vasoconstriction of postcapillary venules increases the hydrostatic pressure in the capillary bed, potentiating formation of edema.

The postcapillary venule is the primary site at which vasoactive mediators induce endothelial changes. Binding of vasoactive mediators to specific receptors on endothelial cells results in cell activation, causing endothelial cell contraction and gap formation. This break in the endothelial barrier leads to the extravasation (leakage) of intravascular fluids into the extravascular space.

In contrast to this action of vasoactive mediators, direct injury to the endothelium, such as that caused by burns or caustic chemicals, may result in irreversible damage. In such cases, the endothelium is separated from the basement membrane. This effect leads to cell blebbing (the appearance of blisters or bubbles between the endothelium and the basement membrane) and areas of denuded basement membrane. Mild direct injury to the endothelium results in a biphasic response: an early change in permeability occurs 15 to 30 minutes after the injury, followed by a second increase in vascular permeability after 3 to 5 hours. When damage is severe, the exudation of intravascular fluid into the extravascular compartment increases progressively, reaching a peak between 3 and 4 hours after the injury.

Several definitions are important for understanding the consequences of inflammation:

- An **effusion** is excess fluid in the cavities of the body, such as the peritoneum or pleura.
- A **transudate** describes edema fluid with a low protein content (specific gravity, <1.015).
- An **exudate** is edema fluid with a high protein concentration (specific gravity, >1.015), which frequently contains inflammatory cells. Exudates are observed early in acute inflammatory reactions and are produced by mild injuries, such as sunburn or traumatic blisters.
- A **serous** exudate or effusion is characterized by absence of a prominent cellular response and has a yellow, straw-like color.
- **Serosanguinous** refers to a serous exudate or effusion that contains erythrocytes and has a red tinge.
- A **fibrinous** exudate contains large amounts of fibrin as a result of activation of the coagulation system. When a fibrinous exudate occurs on a serosal surface, such as the pleura or pericardium, it is referred to as fibrinous pleuritis or pericarditis.
- A **purulent** exudate or effusion contains prominent cellular components. Purulent exudates and effusions are frequently identified with pathologic conditions such as pyogenic bacterial infections (Fig. 2-6), in which the predominant cell type is the polymorphonuclear leukocyte.
- **Suppurative inflammation** describes a condition in which a purulent exudate is accompanied by significant liquefactive necrosis. It is the equivalent of pus.

Mediators of Increased Permeability in Inflammatory Edema

The primary sources of vasoactive mediators are cells and plasma.

NORMAL VENULE

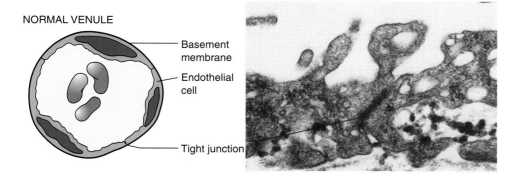

Basement
membrane

Endothelial
cell

Tight junction

VASOACTIVE MEDIATOR-INDUCED INJURY

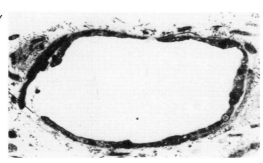

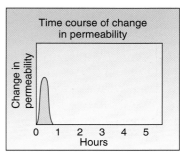

Endothelial
retraction
and gap
formation

Electrolytes,
fluid, protein

Time course of change
in permeability

Change in permeability

0 1 2 3 4 5
Hours

DIRECT INJURY TO ENDOTHELIUM

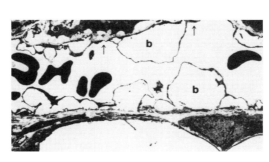

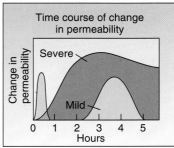

Denuded
basement
membrane

Gap formation

Blebbing

Time course of change
in permeability

Change in permeability

Severe

Mild

0 1 2 3 4 5
Hours

FIGURE   2-4

Responses of the microvasculature to injury. The wall of the normal venule is sealed by
tight junctions between adjacent endothelial cells. During mild vasoactive mediator–induced injury, the endothelial cells separate and permit passage of the fluid constituents
of the blood. With severe direct injury, the endothelial cells form blebs (*b*) and separate
from the underlying basement membrane. Areas of denuded basement membrane (*arrows*) allow prolonged escape of fluid elements from the microvasculature.

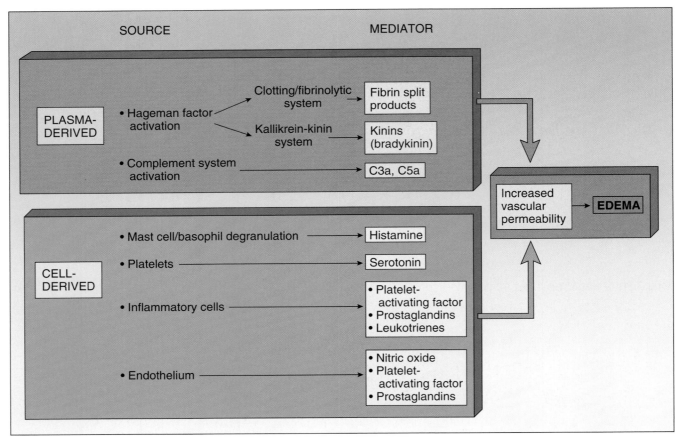

FIGURE   2-5
Vasoactive mediators of increased vascular permeability.

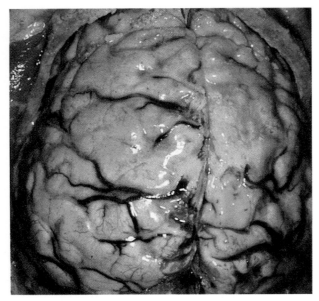

FIGURE   2-6
Purulent exudate. In this case of bacterial meningitis, a visicid, cream colored, acute inflammatory exudate is present within the subarachnoid space.

Cell-Derived Vasoactive Mediators

Circulating platelets, tissue mast cells, basophils, polymorphonuclear leukocytes, endothelial cells, monocytes/macrophages, and the injured tissue itself are all potent cellular sources of vasoactive mediators.

Phospholipid Metabolism and Arachidonic Acid Metabolites

Generation of Arachidonic Acid. Certain derivatives of phospholipids and fatty acids are among the mediators generated by inflammatory cells and injured tissues. Depending on the specific inflammatory cell and the nature of the stimulus, activated cells generate arachidonic acid (Fig. 2-7).

Cyclo-oxygenase. Inflammatory cells contain specific cyclo-oxygenase enzymes that generate derivatives of arachidonic acid, including prostaglandin (PG) I_2 (also known as prostacyclin), $PGF_{2\alpha}$, PGE_2, PGD_2,

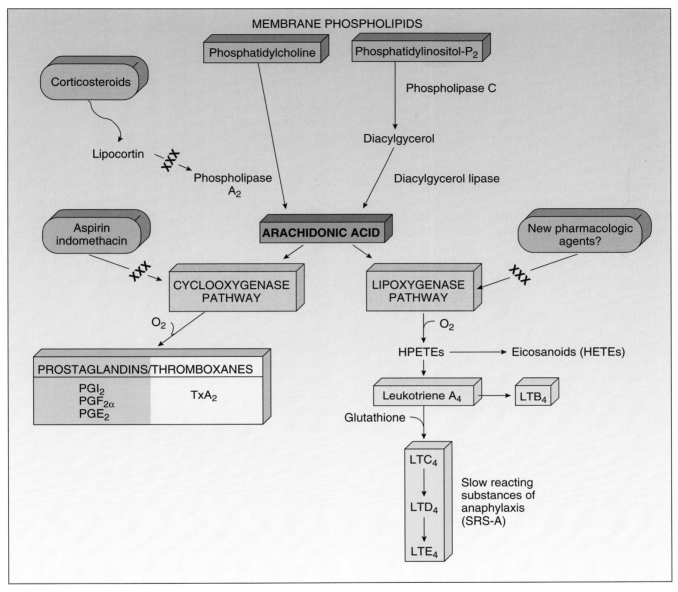

FIGURE 2-7
Arachidonic acid metabolism.

and thromboxane (Tx) A_2 (Table 2-1). The primary cyclo-oxygenase metabolite in platelets is TxA_2; endothelial cells secrete principally PGI_2. Monocytes/macrophages, depending on their state of activation, produce any or all of these derivative products.

Both PGI_2 and PGE_2, owing to their vasodilatory effects, enhance vascular permeability at sites of inflammation. A potent vasoconstrictor, TxA_2 plays an important role in mediation of the "second wave" of platelet aggregation. Both PGI_2 and PGE_2 bind to specific receptors on inflammatory cells and inhibit their functional responses to other inflammatory stimuli.

Lipoxygenase. A second pathway by which arachidonic acid is metabolized in inflammatory cells and tissues is lipoxygenation, with the formation of eicosanoids (HETEs) or leukotriene A_4. In the neutrophil and certain macrophage populations, leukotriene A_4 is metabolized to leukotriene B_4, a compound with potent chemotactic activity for neutrophils, monocytes, and macrophages. In other cell types, especially mast cells, basophils, and macrophages, leukotriene A_4 is converted to leukotriene C_4. Leukotrienes C_4, D_4, and E_4 are collectively known as slow-reacting substances of anaphy-

TABLE   2-1.   Biologic Activities of Arachidonic Acid Metabolites

Metabolite	Biologic Activity
PGE_2, PDG_2	Induce vasodilatation, bronchodilation; inhibit inflammatory cell function
PGE_2	Induces vasodilatation, bronchodilation; inhibits inflammatory cell function
$PGF_{2\alpha}$	Induces vasodilatation, bronchoconstriction
TxA_2	Induces vasoconstriction, bronchoconstriction; enhances inflammatory cell functions (especially platelets)
LTB_4	Chemotactic for phagocytic cells; stimulates phagocytic cell adherence; enhances microvascular permeability
LTC_4, LTD_4, LTE_4	Induce smooth muscle contraction; constrict pulmonary airways; increase microvascular permeability

laxis (SRS-As). They stimulate the contraction of smooth muscle and enhance vascular permeability. The generation of leukotriene B_4 at sites of tissue injury plays an important role in the recruitment of polymorphonuclear leukocytes, whereas the other leukotrienes are responsible for development of much of the clinical symptomatology associated with allergic-type reactions (see Table 2-1).

Platelets

Platelets play a primary role in normal homeostasis and in the initiation and regulation of clot formation. They are important sources of inflammatory mediators, including potent vasoactive substances and growth factors that modulate mesenchymal cell proliferation (Fig. 2-8). The platelet contains three distinct kinds of inclusions:

- **Dense granules,** which are rich in serotonin, histamine, calcium, and adenosine diphosphate
- **a-Granules,** containing fibrinogen, coagulation proteins, platelet-derived growth factor, and other peptides and proteins
- Lysosomes, which sequester acid hydrolases

Platelet adherence, aggregation, and degranulation occur when platelets come in contact with fibrillar collagen (following vascular injury that exposes the interstitial matrix proteins) or thrombin (following activation of the coagulation system). Degranulation is associated with the release of **serotonin** (5-hydroxytryptamine), which directly induces changes in vascular permeability. In addition, the arachidonic acid metabolite TxA_2 is produced by platelets. Not only does TxA_2 play a key role in the second wave of platelet aggregation, it also mediates smooth muscle constriction.

Mast Cells and Basophils

Mast cells are localized within the connective tissue of the body, whereas basophils are present in low numbers in the circulation. Mast cells are especially prevalent along mucosal surfaces of the lung and gastrointestinal tract and the dermis of the skin. This distribution places the mast cell at the interface between environmental antigens and the host for participation in a variety of allergic and inflammatory conditions.

Mast cells and basophils both contain receptors for immunoglobulin (Ig) E on their cell surface and are additional cellular sources of vasoactive mediators. When an IgE-sensitized mast cell or basophil is stimulated by an antigen, a variety of inflammatory mediators contained in dense cytoplasmic granules are secreted into extracellular tissues (Fig. 2-9). These

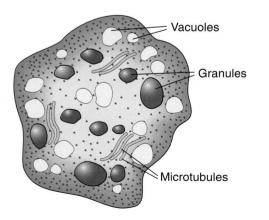

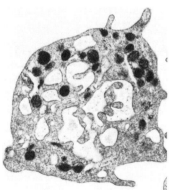

CHARACTERISTICS AND FUNCTIONS
- Thrombosis; promotes clot formation
- Regulates permeability
- Regulates proliferative response of mesenchymal cells

PRIMARY INFLAMMATORY MEDIATORS
- Dense granules
  - Serotonin
  - Ca^{2+}
  - ADP
- α-granules
  - Cationic proteins
  - Fibrinogen and coagulation proteins
  - Platelet-derived growth factor (PDGF)
- Lysosomes
  - Acid hydrolases
- Thromboxane A_2

FIGURE   2-8
Platelets: morphology and functions.

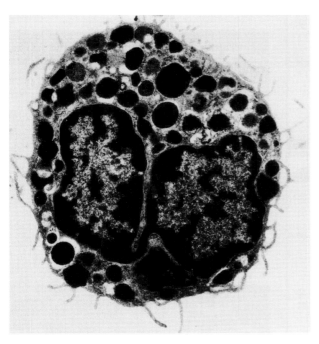

Mast Cell (Basophils)

CHARACTERISTICS AND FUNCTIONS
• Binds IgE molecules
• Contains electron-dense granules

PRIMARY INFLAMMATORY MEDIATORS
• Histamine
• Leukotrienes (LTC$_4$, LTD$_4$, LTE$_4$)
• Platelet activating factor
• Eosinophil chemotactic factors
• Cytokines (e.g., TNF-a IL-4)

FIGURE   2-9
Mast cells: morphology and functions.

granules contain histamine, acid mucopolysaccharides (including heparin), serine proteases, and chemotactic mediators for neutrophils and eosinophils. Because of their ability to secrete specific mediators following stimulation, both mast cells and basophils play an important role in the regulation of vascular permeability and bronchial smooth muscle tone, especially in many forms of allergic hypersensitivity reactions (see Chapter 4).

Histamine is also released from the dense granules when mast cells are stimulated with anaphylatoxins derived from complement. Both histamine and serotonin induce reversible endothelial cell contraction, gap formation, and edema. Stimulation of mast cells and basophils also leads to the release of SRS-As (leukotrienes C$_4$, D$_4$, and E$_4$).

Endothelial Cells
One of the important functions of endothelial cells is the regulation of tissue perfusion under physiologic

and pathologic conditions (Fig. 2-10). This regulation is mediated by the secretion of both vasoconstrictor and vasodilator substances as well as by the influence of platelet aggregation and the coagulation pathways.

• **PGI$_2$ has potent vasodilator and antiaggregatory effects.**
• EDRF is a vasodilator that inhibits platelet aggregation and regulates vascular tone by stimulating smooth muscle relaxation. It is either identical to the nitric oxide radical NO$^\bullet$ or a nitroso-compound that decomposes to NO$^\bullet$.
• **Endothelin** is a peptide produced by endothelial cells that induces prolonged vasoconstriction of vascular smooth muscle.

Coagulation. When exposed to bacterial lipopolysaccharide or specific cytokines (e.g., interleukin [IL]-1, tumor necrosis factor [TNF]-α), endothelial cells also play a central role in actively regulating blood coagulation. These cells secrete increased amounts of the procoagulant tissue factor that promotes thrombus formation through activation of the extrinsic coagulation pathway. When stimulated, mononuclear phagocytic cells also express increased tissue factor activity. By contrast, smooth muscle cells and fibroblasts constitutively express tissue factor. Thus, injury to a blood vessel wall that alters the endothelial barrier exposes a local procoagulant signal.

Monocytes/Macrophages
Both circulating and tissue mononuclear cells are included in the term **monocytes/macrophage system.** As previously noted, these cells are a direct source of potent vasoactive mediators. Moreover, monocytes/macrophages can act indirectly to modify vascular integrity by releasing cytokines (e.g., IL-1 and TNF-α) that activate endothelial cells.

Platelet-Activating Factor
Platelet activating factor (PAF) is a vasoactive mediator generated by the stimulation of virtually all activated inflammatory cells, endothelial cells, and injured tissue cells. PAF has a wide range of activities, among which are stimulatory effects on platelets, neutrophils, monocytes/macrophages, endothelial cells, and vascular smooth muscle cells. It induces platelet aggregation and degranulation at sites of tissue injury and enhances the release of serotonin, thereby causing changes in vascular permeability. In addition, PAF augments arachidonic acid metabolism in neutrophils and monocytes/macrophages, an effect associated with increased motility, superoxide production, and

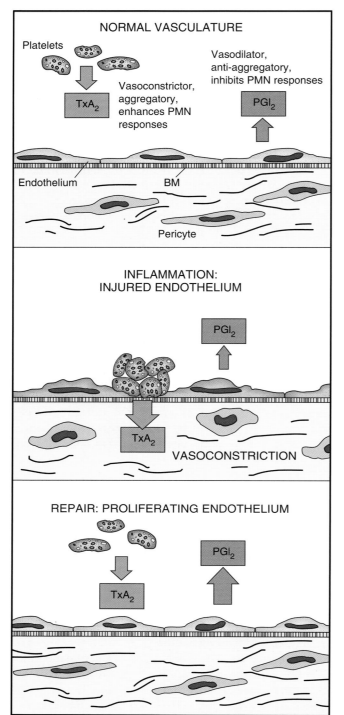

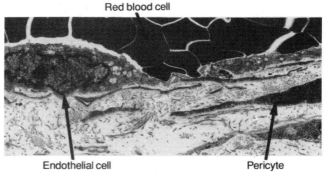

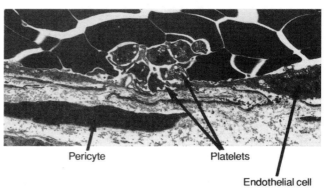

FIGURE   *2-10*
Regulation of platelet and endothelial cell interactions by thromboxane A_2 and prostaglandin I_2. During inflammation, the normal balance is shifted to vasoconstriction, platelet aggregation, and polymorphonuclear leukocyte responses. During repair, the prostaglandin effects predominate.

degranulation. Exposure of phagocytic cells to PAF "primes" them, resulting in enhanced responses (e.g., O_2^- production, degranulation) to a second stimulus. PAF is also an extremely potent vasodilator and enhances permeability of the microvasculature at sites of tissue injury.

Plasma-Derived Vasoactive Mediators

Plasma contains three major enzyme cascades in an inactive state, each of which is composed of a series of sequentially activated proteases. These interrelated systems include the coagulation cascade, kinin generation, and complement.

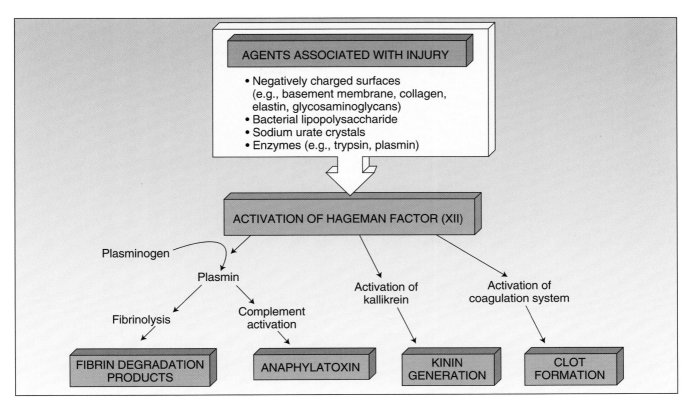

FIGURE *2-11*
Hageman factor activation and inflammatory mediator production.

Hageman Factor and the Kinins

Hageman factor (clotting factor XII), generated within the plasma, provides an additional source of vasoactive mediators (Fig. 2-11). Hageman factor is activated by exposure to negatively charged surfaces, such as basement membranes, proteolytic enzymes, bacterial lipopolysaccharide, and foreign materials (including urate crystals in gout). In turn, this process activates several additional plasma proteases, which lead to the following:

- Conversion of plasminogen to plasmin
- Conversion of prekallikrein to kallikrein
- Activation of the alternative complement pathway

Plasmin generated by activated Hageman factor induces fibrinolysis. In turn, the products of fibrin degradation (fibrin-split products) augment vascular permeability in both the skin and the lung. Plasmin also cleaves components of the complement system, thereby generating biologically active products that increase vascular permeability in the skin.

Plasma kallikrein cleaves kininogen, thereby producing **bradykinin,** which elicits reversible changes of the endothelium that lead to edema.

Complement System

The complement system consists of a group of 20 plasma proteins. In addition to being a source of vasoactive mediators, components of the complement system are an integral part of the immune system and play an important role in host defense against bacterial infection.

Classical Pathway. Activators of the classical pathway (Table 2-2) include antigen-antibody immune complexes and products of bacteria and viruses. The cascade leads from activation to formation of the mem-

TABLE 2-2. Activators of the Complement System

Classical	Alternative
Immune complexes (IgM, IgG)	Zymosan (yeast cell wall)
Aggregated antibody	Cobra venom factor
Proteases	Endotoxin
Urate crystals	Polysaccharides
Polyanions (polynucleotides)	Radiographic contrast media; dialysis membranes; parasites, fungi, viruses

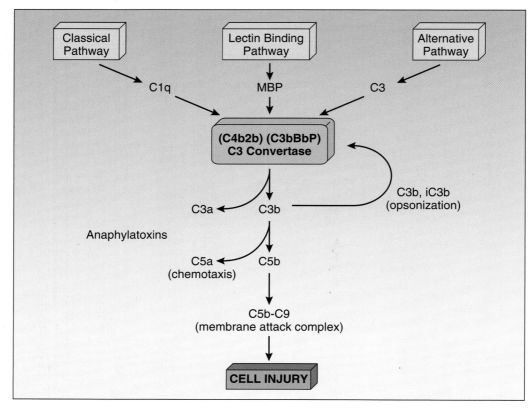

FIGURE   *2-12*
The complement system and its biologically active products.

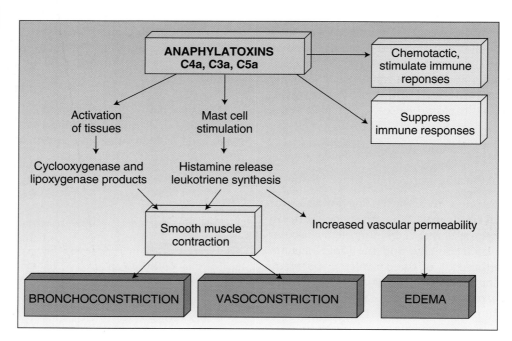

FIGURE   *2-13*
Biologic activity of the anaphylatoxins.

brane attack complex (Fig. 2-12). Insertion of the membrane attack complex into the plasma membrane creates a cylindrical hole in the limiting membrane. This effect destroys the barrier function of the plasma membrane and leads to cell lysis.

Alternative Pathway. Activation of the alternative pathway of the complement system is initiated by derivative products of infectious organisms and by foreign materials through a cascade-like interaction of specific plasma proteins (see Table 2-1).

Whether the alternative or the classical complement pathway is activated, the end result is the same: formation of a membrane attack complex capable of inducing cell lysis, and generation of the biologically active anaphylatoxins C3a and C5a.

Anaphylatoxins. The anaphylatoxins (C3a, C4a, C5a) are important products of complement activation through the classical pathway. Each of these molecules has potent effects on smooth muscle and the vasculature, including enhancement of smooth muscle contraction and an increase in vascular permeability (Fig. 2-13). Both C3a and C5a also induce degranulation of mast cells and basophils, and the consequent release of histamine further potentiates the increase in vascular permeability.

In addition, C5a is a potent chemotactic factor for neutrophils, monocytes, eosinophils, and basophils, and it induces low levels of neutrophil degranulation and superoxide anion production. Additional effects of C5a-induced stimulation of neutrophils include enhancement of the phagocytic response and, in response to a second stimulus, degranulation and superoxide anion production. This enhancement is referred to as "cell priming."

The complement system plays an important role in many forms of immunologic tissue injury (see Chapter 4) and is an important host defense mechanism against bacterial infection. Bacterial activation of the complement system may occur by direct activation of the alternative pathway or as an outcome of antibody binding to the surface of the organism and activation of the classical pathway. Once the complement system is activated, bacteriolysis may follow, either by means of the assembled membrane attack complex or by enhanced bacterial clearance following opsonization.

Bacterial opsonization is the process by which a specific molecule (e.g., IgG or C3b) binds to the surface of the bacterium. The process enhances phagocytosis by enabling receptors on the phagocytic cell membrane (e.g., the Fc receptor or the C3b receptor) to recognize and bind to the opsonized bacterium. Viruses, parasites, and transformed cells also activate the complement system by similar mechanisms, an effect that leads to their inactivation or death.

Cellular Recruitment

The second phase of the acute inflammatory response involves the accumulation of leukocytes, especially polymorphonuclear leukocytes, at the sites of tissue injury (Fig. 2-14). During the first 24 hours (and sometimes even during the first few hours) after the initiation of injury, many polymorphonuclear leukocytes accumulate. The sequence of events leading to this attraction of neutrophils to the inflammatory site is initiated by locally generated, soluble chemical mediators. These mediators, collectively referred to as **chemotactic factors,** are generated in high concentrations at sites of tissue injury, with a progressively decreasing gradient away from the injured tissue. The physiologic responses of circulating leukocytes exposed to chemotactic factors include margination, adherence, emigration, and chemotaxis.

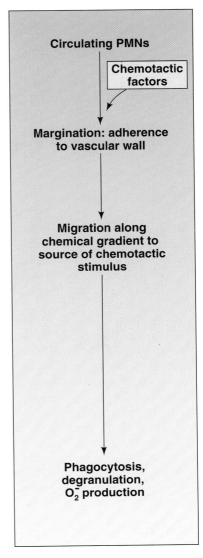

FIGURE   *2-14*
Leukocyte exudation and phagocytosis.

Margination

Under normal circumstances, blood flow in the venules is characterized by a central stream of formed elements and a clear, peripheral zone of plasma. On vasodilatation following injury, the blood flow slows, and leukocytes appear in the peripheral region that was previously acellular. This process, termed *margination*, concentrates the leukocytes adjacent to the endothelial cells.

Adherence

The adherence of inflammatory cells to the endothelium or vascular basement membrane is critical for recruitment of these circulating cells to the sites of tissue injury (Fig. 2-15). Importantly, the processes that mediate adherence within the vasculature are also crucial for the interaction of inflammatory cells with the extravascular targets they engulf (bacteria, necrotic cells, debris).

Cell Adhesion Molecules

Cell adhesion molecules are membrane glycoproteins that promote adherence and are among the factors that enhance phagocytic cell attachment to vascular walls and phagocytic particles (Fig. 2-16). Several distinct families of cell adhesion molecules participate in the regulation of leukocyte recruitment and platelet localization at sites of inflammation.

Lectin-Cell Adhesion Molecules. These molecules are expressed on the surface of endothelial cells, leukocytes, and platelets. They promote the adherence of circulating leukocytes to the endothelium at sites of inflammation. Three of the most important of these molecules are GMP-140, endothelial leukocyte adherence molecule (ELAM)-1, and leukocyte adhesion molecule (LAM)-1.

GMP-140 is expressed on the surface of activated endothelial cells and platelets. It binds to a glycoprotein on leukocyte surfaces, and it participates in the early interactions between neutrophils and endothelial cells and between platelets and neutrophils.

ELAM-1 is expressed by activated endothelial cells and enhances the later recruitment of leukocytes.

LAM-1 is constitutively expressed on the surfaces of lymphocytes and neutrophils and helps localize them to the sites of tissue injury. In addition, LAM-1 regulates lymphocyte binding to vascular endothelium in lymph nodes and, therefore, is considered to be a "homing" receptor.

Integrins. Integrins act in the regulation of cell-matrix and cell-cell adhesive interactions. Activation of phagocytic cells by chemotactic stimuli increases the expression of integrins on their cell surface. Expression of these integrins assists in the localization of circulating cells at the sites of tissue injury and in the host defense against bacterial infection.

Intercellular Adhesion Molecule-1. Intercellular adhesion molecule-1 is another molecule that helps localize leukocytes to areas of tissue injury. It is expressed on the surface of cytokine-stimulated endothelial cells and leukocytes, and it binds to integrins on the cell membranes of neutrophils and macrophages.

Chemotaxis

The most important chemotactic factors for polymorphonuclear leukocytes are:

- **C5a,** derived from complement
- **Bacterial and mitochondrial products,** particularly low-molecular-weight *N*-formylated peptides
- **Products of arachidonic acid metabolism,** especially leukotriene B_4
- **Cytokines,** notably IL-8.

Cytokine is a term that refers to a group of low-molecular-weight proteins that are secreted by cells, including (1) the interleukins, (2) certain growth factors and colony-stimulating factors, (3) TNF-α, and (4) lymphotoxin. Many of these cytokines are produced at the sites of inflammation and are chemotactic for a variety of cell types. Among their targets are neutrophils (IL-8), monocytes (macrophage chemotactic peptides), and lymphocytes.

Cytokine Networks in Inflammation

The recruitment of inflammatory cells to sites of tissue injury involves cell-cell communication networks (Fig. 2-17). This communication is effected both by direct cell contact and by the binding of cytokines to target cells. In addition, the expression by cells of certain classes of adherence proteins is regulated by cytokines that are produced at inflammatory sites.

The recruitment of neutrophils to sites of bacterial infection is an example of the interrelationship between adherence proteins, cytokines, and inflammatory cells at the sites of tissue injury. During the initial stages of bacterial infection, chemotactic peptides are produced and C5a is generated in response to activation of the complement system by the organisms. Each of these compounds is a potent chemotactic factor for neutrophils. In addition, other products of bacteria, such as endotoxin, activate tissue macrophages to produce (1) IL-8, (2) macrophage chemotactic peptides, and (3) other cytokines, such as TNF-α and IL-1.

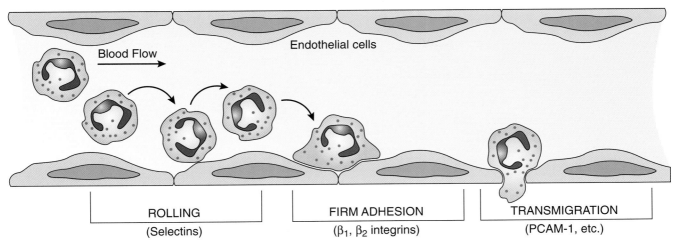

Blood Flow

Endothelial cells

ROLLING
(Selectins)

FIRM ADHESION
(β_1, β_2 integrins)

TRANSMIGRATION
(PCAM-1, etc.)

FIGURE 2-15
Mechanisms of leukocyte adherence.

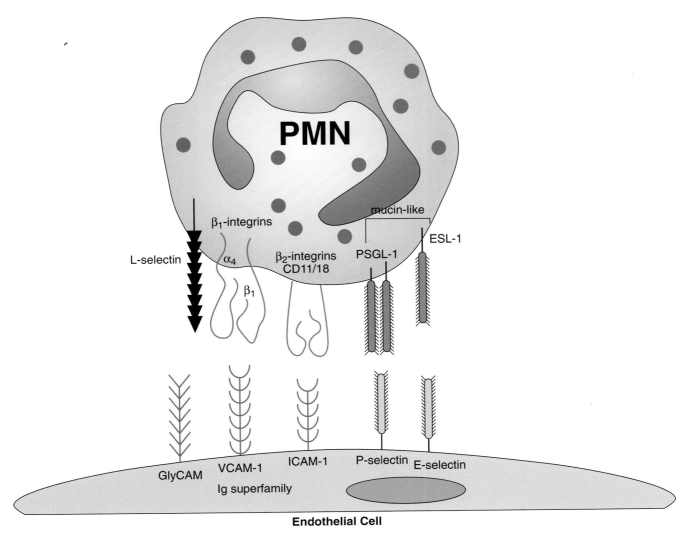

PMN

β_1-integrins

mucin-like

ESL-1

L-selectin

α_4

β_2-integrins
CD11/18

PSGL-1

β_1

GlyCAM   VCAM-1   ICAM-1   P-selectin   E-selectin

Ig superfamily

Endothelial Cell

FIGURE 2-16
Leukocyte and endothelial cell adhesion molecules.

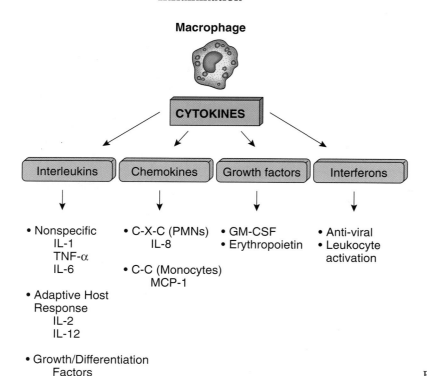

Macrophage

CYTOKINES

Interleukins   Chemokines   Growth factors   Interferons

• Nonspecific
  IL-1
  TNF-α
  IL-6

• Adaptive Host
  Response
  IL-2
  IL-12

• Growth/Differentiation
  Factors
  IL-5

• C-X-C (PMNs)
  IL-8

• C-C (Monocytes)
  MCP-1

• GM-CSF
• Erythropoietin

• Anti-viral
• Leukocyte
  activation

FIGURE   *2-17*
Cytokine activities.

Both IL-1 and TNF-α stimulate a variety of cell types, including endothelial cells, and induce the expression of adhesion molecules and the production of chemotactic cytokines. Maximum secretion of these chemotactic peptides requires several hours, in contrast to the rapid activation of complement and the generation of C5a.

On the basis of these observations, the initial recruitment of neutrophils to sites of tissue injury is thought to depend largely on C5a generation, whereas the prolonged recruitment from 6 to 48 hours following injury is mediated by the production of chemotactic cytokines.

Mechanisms of Inflammatory Cell Functions

Phagocytosis

Many inflammatory cells, including polymorphonuclear leukocytes, monocytes, and tissue macrophages, function by recognizing, internalizing, and digesting foreign material or the debris of injured cells. This process is termed **phagocytosis,** and the effector cells are known as **phagocytes.** In general terms, the critical events of phagocytosis proceed as follows (Fig. 2-18):

1. **Recognition.** The phagocytosis of most biologic agents is substantially enhanced by, if not dependent on, their coating (opsonization) with plasma components. Phagocytic cells possess specific receptors for C3b, C3bi, and the Fc fragment of immunoglobulin molecules, and the binding of opsonized particles to these receptors greatly facilitates the recognition process.
2. **Internalization.** The attachment of a particle to the surface of a phagocytic cell triggers its internalization.
3. **Digestion.** The phagosome containing the foreign material fuses with a cytoplasmic lysosomal granule to form a phagolysosome, into which lysosomal enzymes are released.

The cytoplasm of polymorphonuclear leukocytes contains primary, secondary, and tertiary granules, which can be differentiated both morphologically and biochemically (Fig. 2-19).

Bactericidal Activity of Inflammatory Cells

The bactericidal activity of polymorphonuclear leukocytes is mediated in part by the production of reactive oxygen species and in part by oxygen-independent mechanisms.

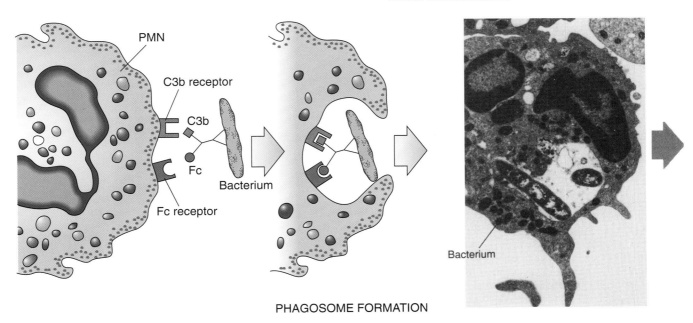

PHAGOSOME FORMATION

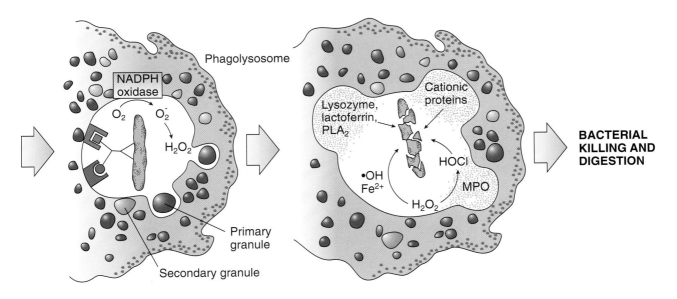

DEGRANULATION AND NADPH OXIDASE ACTIVATION

FIGURE *2-18*
Mechanisms of polymorphonuclear leukocyte bacterial phagocytosis and cell killing.

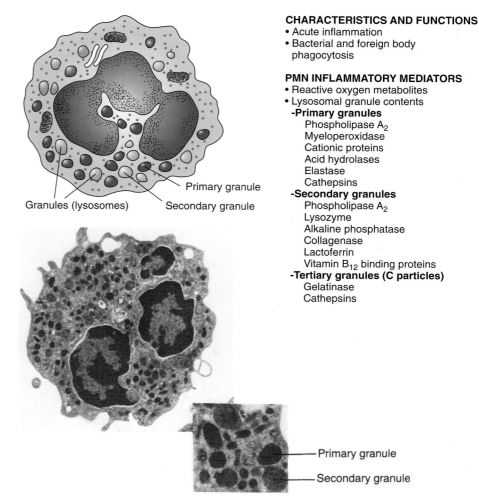

CHARACTERISTICS AND FUNCTIONS
- Acute inflammation
- Bacterial and foreign body phagocytosis

PMN INFLAMMATORY MEDIATORS
- Reactive oxygen metabolites
- Lysosomal granule contents
 -Primary granules
 Phospholipase A_2
 Myeloperoxidase
 Cationic proteins
 Acid hydrolases
 Elastase
 Cathepsins
 -Secondary granules
 Phospholipase A_2
 Lysozyme
 Alkaline phosphatase
 Collagenase
 Lactoferrin
 Vitamin B_{12} binding proteins
 -Tertiary granules (C particles)
 Gelatinase
 Cathepsins

Granules (lysosomes)

Primary granule

Secondary granule

Primary granule

Secondary granule

FIGURE 2-19
Polymorphonuclear leukocytes: morphology and function.

Bacterial Killing by Activated Oxygen Species

Phagocytosis is accompanied by metabolic reactions within inflammatory cells that lead to production of a number of oxygen metabolites. These products, which are more reactive than oxygen itself, are:

- **Superoxide (O_2^-).** Phagocytosis activates an NADPH oxidase in the cell membrane of polymorphonuclear leukocytes, which reduces molecular oxygen to the superoxide anion O_2^- as part of the "respiratory burst."
- **Hydrogen Peroxide (H_2O_2).** Superoxide is reduced to hydrogen peroxide by the superoxide dismutase reaction at the cell surface and within the phagolysosomes.
- **Hypochlorous Acid.** Hydrogen peroxide can react with myeloperoxidase in the presence of a halide to form hypochlorous acid (Table 2-3). This acid is a more potent oxidant than hydrogen peroxide itself and appears to be a major bactericidal agent produced by phagocytic cells.

TABLE 2-3. Reactions Involving Reactive Oxygen Metabolites Produced by Phagocytic Cells

Reduction of molecular oxygen	
$O_2 + e^- \rightarrow O_2^-$	Superoxide anion
Dismutation of O_2^-	
$O_2^- 1 O_2^- + 2H^- \rightarrow O_2 + H_2O_2$	Hydrogen peroxide
Haber-Weiss reaction	
$H_2O_2 + O_2^- \rightarrow OH^- + \cdot OH$	Hydroxyl radical
Fenton reaction (iron-catalyzed)	
$H_2O_2 + Fe^{2+} \rightarrow FE_3^- + OH^- + \cdot OH$	Hydroxyl radical
Myeloperoxidase reaction	
$H_2O_2 + Cl^- + H^- \rightleftarrows H_2O + HOCl$	Hypochlorous acid

- **Hydroxyl Radical ($\cdot OH$).** Hydrogen peroxide is further reduced to form the highly reactive hydroxyl radical ($\cdot OH$).

Monocytes, macrophages, and eosinophils also produce superoxide anion and hydrogen peroxide, depending on their state of activation and the stimulus to which they are exposed. The importance of oxygen-dependent mechanisms in the bactericidal function of

TABLE   2-4.   Congenital Diseases of Defective Phagocytic Cell Function Characterized by Recurrent Bacterial Infections

Disease	Defect
Leukocyte adhesion protein deficiencies (C3b receptor, MO-1, GP150, 95)	Poor adherence and chemotaxis
Hyper-IgE-recurrent infection (Job) syndrome	Poor chemotaxis
Chédiak-Higashi syndrome	Defective lysosomal granules (poor degranulation, deficient cathepsin G, elastase), poor chemotaxis
Neutrophil-specific granule deficiency	Absent neutrophil granules (poor chemotaxis, deficient O_2^- production, absent defensins)
Chronic granulomatous disease	Deficient NADPH oxidase, with absent H_2O_2 production
Myeloperoxidase deficiency	Deficient HOCl production

phagocytic cells is illustrated by a number of congenital diseases that render the victim subject to recurrent infections (Table 2-4).

Nonoxidative Bacterial Killing

Polymorphonuclear leukocytes and monocytes/ macrophages evidence substantial antimicrobial activity that is oxygen-independent:

- **Lysosomal Hydrolases.** The primary and secondary granules of neutrophils and the lysosomes of mononuclear phagocytes contain various hydrolases that possess antimicrobial activity.
- **Bactericidal/Permeability-Increasing Protein.** This cationic protein has been isolated from the primary granules of polymorphonuclear leukocytes and is potently bactericidal toward many gram-negative bacteria. It is not toxic to gram-positive bacteria, however, or to eukaryotic cells.
- **Defensins.** Primary granules of polymorphonuclear leukocytes and the lysosomes of some mononuclear phagocytes contain a family of cationic proteins, termed *defensins*, that kill a wide variety of bacteria, fungi, and some enveloped viruses.
- **Lactoferrin.** Lactoferrin is an iron-binding glycoprotein contained in the secondary granules of neutrophils and most secretory fluids in the body. Its antimicrobial properties are related to its iron-chelating capacity, by which it competes with bacteria for iron.
- **Lysozyme.** Lysozyme occurs in many tissues and fluids in the body and is contained in the primary and secondary granules of neutrophils and in the lysosomes of mononuclear phagocytes. The peptidoglycans of gram-positive bacterial cell walls are exquisitely sensitive to degradation by lysozyme, whereas gram-negative bacteria are resistant to its action.
- **Bactericidal Proteins of Eosinophils.** Eosinophils contain several granule-bound cationic proteins, the most important of which are major basic protein and eosinophilic cationic protein. Both proteins are relatively ineffective against bacteria but are cytotoxic for parasites.

Tissue Injury by Inflammatory Cells

Inflammatory cells, whose function evolved to combat micro-organisms and other foreign agents, are also capable of damaging the host tissue by the extracellular release of enzymes and activated oxygen.

Lysosomal Enzymes

Lysosomal enzymes involved in the intracellular degradation of phagocytosed material are also released into the extracellular environment. **The same enzymes that are beneficial when active intracellularly during phagocytosis are harmful to the tissues when released to the extracellular environment.**

Activated Oxygen

Similar to lysosomal enzymes, the activated oxygen species that mediate the bactericidal activity of phagocytes and phagocyte-derived NO can produce tissue injury in extracellular sites.

Phagocytic Cell Adherence

The ability of phagocytic cells to recognize a target and adhere to it serves to "focus" the functional responses of the cell along the adherent surface. For instance, when stimulated phagocytic cells adhere to basement membranes, production of reactive oxygen metabolites is greatest at the point of attachment. Moreover, this is also the site of greatest lysosomal degranulation.

Diseases Associated with Defects in Phagocytosis

The importance of the protection afforded by acute inflammatory cells is emphasized by the frequency and severity of infections in persons with defective phagocytic cells. **The most common defect is actually iatrogenic neutropenia as a result of cancer chemotherapy.**

Acquired diseases such as leukemia, diabetes mellitus, malnutrition, viral infections, and sepsis can also be accompanied by defects in inflammatory cell function.

CHRONIC INFLAMMATION

Chronic inflammation may occur as a sequela to acute inflammation or as an immune response to a foreign antigen. Under conditions in which the inflammatory response is unable to eliminate the injurious agent or restore injured tissue to its normal state, the process may become chronic. **Chronic inflammation primarily serves to contain and remove a pathologic agent or process within a tissue.**

The cellular components of the chronic inflammatory response are macrophages, plasma cells, lymphocytes, and in certain conditions, eosinophils. Chronic inflammation is mediated by both immunologic and nonimmunologic mechanisms and is frequently observed in conjunction with reparative responses, namely granulation tissue and fibrosis.

The **macrophage** is the pivotal cell in regulating the reactions that lead to chronic inflammation. It functions as a source of both inflammatory and immunologic mediators (Fig. 2-20). The accumulation of macrophages mainly reflects the recruitment of circulating monocytes by chemotactic stimuli and their differentiation in tissues (Fig. 2-21). In addition to generating inflammatory mediators, macrophages regulate lymphocyte responses to antigens and secrete other mediators that modulate the proliferation and function of fibroblasts and endothelial cells.

Plasma cells also participate in the chronic inflammatory response (Fig. 2-22). These lymphoid cells, which are rich in rough endoplasmic reticulum, are the primary source of antibodies. The production of antibody to specific antigens at the sites of chronic inflammation is important in antigen neutralization, clearance of foreign antigens and particles, and antibody-dependent cell cytotoxicity.

Lymphocytes are another prominent feature of chronic inflammatory reactions (Fig. 2-23) and perform vital functions in both humoral and cell-mediated immune responses. T lymphocytes function not only in the regulation of macrophage activation and recruitment through the secretion of specific mediators (lymphokines) but also modulate antibody production and cell cytotoxicity.

Eosinophils are occasionally a conspicuous component of the chronic inflammatory response. They are particularly evident during allergic-type reactions and parasitic infestations. Eosinophils share many functional features with the neutrophil. Their granules are rich in acid phosphatase and have a specific peroxidase activity (Fig. 2-24). As previously noted, the granules also contain unique basic proteins that are toxic to certain parasites and normal host cells.

Acute inflammation and chronic inflammation represent two ends of a dynamic continuum, in which the morphologic features of the inflammatory response frequently overlap.

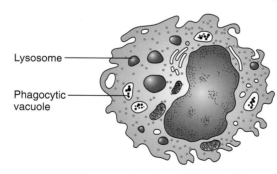

Lysosome

Phagocytic vacuole

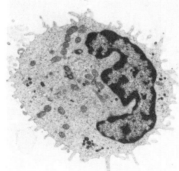

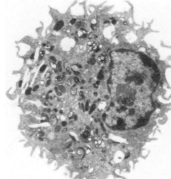

CHARACTERISTICS AND FUNCTIONS
• Regulates inflammatory response
• Regulates coagulation/fibrinolytic pathway
• Regulates immune response (see Chapter 4)

PRIMARY INFLAMMATORY MEDIATORS
• cytokines
  -IL-1
  -TNF-α
  -IL-6
  -Chemokines (e.g. IL-8, MCP-1)
• lysosomal enzymes
  -acid hydrolases
  -serine proteases
  -metalloproteases (e.g. collagenase)
• cationic proteins
• prostaglandins/leukotrienes
• plasminogen activator
• procoagulant activity
• oxygen metabolite formation

FIGURE   *2-20*
Monocytes/macrophages: morphology and function.

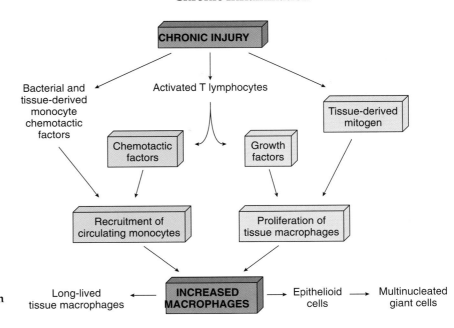

FIGURE *2-21*
Accumulation of macrophages in chronic inflammation.

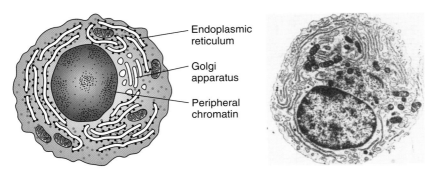

Endoplasmic reticulum

Golgi apparatus

Peripheral chromatin

CHARACTERISTICS AND FUNCTIONS
• Associated with:
  -antibody synthesis and secretion
  -chronic inflammation
• Derived from B lymphocytes

FIGURE *2-22*
Plasma cells: morphology and function.

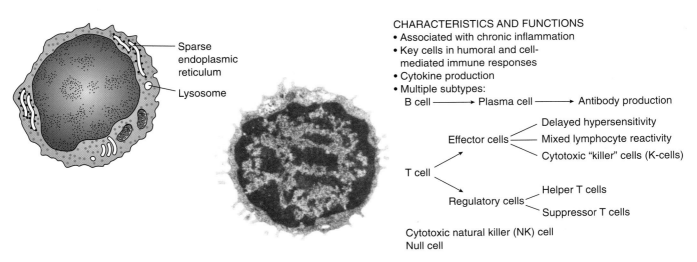

Sparse endoplasmic reticulum

Lysosome

CHARACTERISTICS AND FUNCTIONS
• Associated with chronic inflammation
• Key cells in humoral and cell-mediated immune responses
• Cytokine production
• Multiple subtypes:

B cell ⟶ Plasma cell ⟶ Antibody production

Effector cells ⟨ Delayed hypersensitivity
              Mixed lymphocyte reactivity
              Cytotoxic "killer" cells (K-cells)

T cell

Regulatory cells ⟨ Helper T cells
               Suppressor T cells

Cytotoxic natural killer (NK) cell
Null cell

FIGURE *2-23*
Lymphocytes: morphology and function.

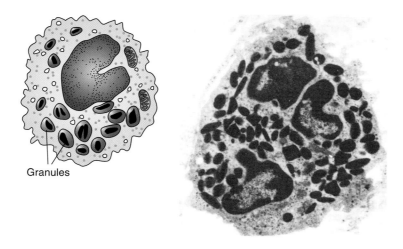

Granules

CHARACTERISTICS AND FUNCTIONS
• Associated with:
  -Allergic reactions
  -Parasite-associated inflammatory reactions
  -Chronic inflammation
• Modulates mast cell-mediated reactions

PRIMARY INFLAMMATORY MEDIATORS
• Reactive oxygen metabolites
• Lysosomal granule enzymes
  (primary crystalloid granules)
  -Major basic protein
  -Eosinophil cationic protein
  -Eosinophil peroxidase
  -Acid phosphatase
  -β-glucuronidase
  -Arylsulfatase B
  -Histaminase
• Phospholipase D
• Prostaglandins of E series
• Cytokines

F I G U R E   *2-24*
Eosinophils: morphology and function.

F I G U R E   *2-25*
Mechanism of granuloma formation.

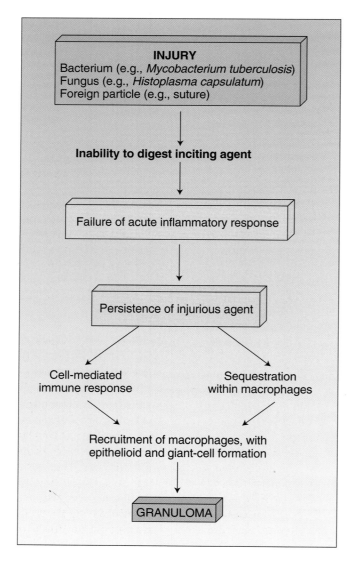

INJURY
Bacterium (e.g., *Mycobacterium tuberculosis*)
Fungus (e.g., *Histoplasma capsulatum*)
Foreign particle (e.g., suture)

Inability to digest inciting agent

Failure of acute inflammatory response

Persistence of injurious agent

Cell-mediated immune response

Sequestration within macrophages

Recruitment of macrophages, with epithelioid and giant-cell formation

GRANULOMA

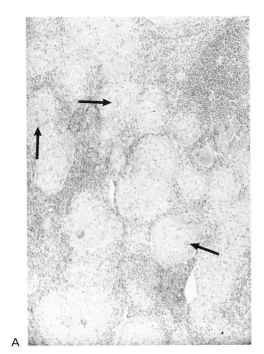

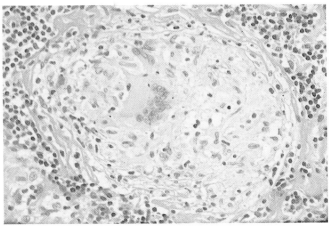

A   B

FIGURE   *2-26*
**Granulomatous inflammation. (A) A section of a lymph node from a patient with sar-
coidosis reveals numerous discrete granulomas in a lymphoid background. A granuloma
displays epithelioid cells in the center, surrounded by a rim of lymphoid cells. Several
multinucleated giant cells (*arrows*) are present. (B) A higher-power photomicrograph of
a single granuloma reveals a multinucleated giant cell amid numerous, pale epithelioid
cells. A thin rim of fibrosis separates the granuloma from the lymphoid cells of the node.**

Chronic Inflammation As a Primary Response

The presence of cells characteristic of chronic inflammation does not necessarily imply the existence of persistent inflammation. A chronic inflammatory infiltrate is usually observed as the primary response to viral infections, certain autoimmune diseases, parasitic infestations, and malignant tumors. Similarly, a chronic inflammatory response may be observed in association with certain cancers. In this circumstance, the presence of chronic inflammatory cells, especially macrophages and T lymphocytes, may be the morphologic expression of an immune response to the cancer. Many autoimmune diseases, including rheumatoid arthritis, chronic thyroiditis, and primary biliary cirrhosis, are also characterized by a chronic inflammatory response in the affected tissues.

GRANULOMATOUS INFLAMMATION

Neutrophils ordinarily remove agents that incite an acute inflammatory response by phagocytosis and digestion. However, there are circumstances in which the substances that provoke the acute inflammatory reaction cannot be digested by the reacting neutrophils. The mechanism for dealing with indigestible substances is termed *granulomatous inflammation* (Fig. 2-25).

The principal cells involved in granulomatous inflammation are macrophages and lymphocytes. Macrophages are much longer-lived than neutrophils. If they are not killed by the noxious agent that incites the inflammatory reaction, they can store the agent in their cytoplasm for indefinite periods, thereby preventing it from continuing to provoke an acute inflammatory reaction.

Recruitment of macrophages to the sites of injury, as well as their activation, is regulated by the local generation of chemotactic factors and lymphokines secreted by activated T lymphocytes. The latter include interferon-γ and, possibly, IL-4. On phagocytizing and storing substances that they cannot digest, the macrophages lose their motility and, thus, accumulate at the site of injury. Macrophages then undergo a characteristic change in their structure, which transforms them into **epithelioid cells**. The latter have considerably more pale cytoplasm than monocytes and tissue macrophages, and they are so named because of their resemblance to epithelial cells. **Nodular collections of epithelioid cells form the granulomas, which are the morphologic hallmark of granulomatous inflammation.**

Granulomas are small (<2 mm) collections of epithelioid cells, which are frequently surrounded by a rim of lymphocytes (Fig. 2-26). In addition, granulomas are populated by multinucleated giant cells, which are formed by the cytoplasmic fusion of macrophages. When the nuclei are arranged around the periphery of the cell in a horseshoe pattern, the cell is termed a **Langhans giant cell**. Frequently, a foreign pathogenic agent (e.g., silica or *Histoplasma* sp. spore) or other indigestible material is identified within the cytoplasm of a multinucleated giant cell, in which case the term **foreign body giant cell** is used. All the other cell types characteristic of chronic inflammation, including lymphocytes, eosinophils, and fibroblasts, may also be associated with granulomas.

Figure 2-25 summarizes the mechanisms in the generation of granulomatous inflammation. Granulomatous inflammation is typical of the tissue response elicited by fungal infections, tuberculosis, leprosy, schistosomiasis, and the presence of foreign material (e.g., suture or talc). It is characteristically associated with areas of caseous necrosis produced by infectious agents, particularly *Mycobacterium tuberculosis*. Some diseases of unknown cause, particularly sarcoidosis, are distinguished by florid granulomatous inflammation in which the inciting agent is not apparent.

SYSTEMIC MANIFESTATIONS OF INFLAMMATION

Fever

Fever is a clinical hallmark of inflammation. Bacteria, virus, or injured cells stimulate the production of endogenous pyrogens (IL-1 and TNF-α), and IL-1 promotes prostaglandin synthesis in the hypothalamic thermoregulatory center. Accordingly, inhibitors of cyclo-oxygenase, such as aspirin, block fever by preventing the synthesis of prostaglandins. TNF-α exerts a direct action on the hypothalamus and stimulates the release of IL-1 from macrophages.

Leukocytosis

Leukocytosis is defined as an increased number of circulating leukocytes and commonly accompanies acute inflammation. Leukocytosis presents as a two- to threefold increase in the number of leukocytes, which principally reflects an increase in polymorphonuclear leukocytes (neutrophilia).

Leukocytosis is caused by the release of specific mediators (IL-1 and TNF-α) by macrophages and, perhaps, other cells. These cytokines initially promote an accelerated release of polymorphonuclear leukocytes from the bone marrow. Subsequently, macrophages and T lymphocytes are stimulated to produce a group of proteins, referred to as **colony-stimulating factors,** that induce proliferation of bone marrow precursors.

Neutrophilia is most frequently seen in association with bacterial infections and tissue injury. On occasion, circulating leukocytes and their precursors may reach very high levels, even as much as 100,000 cells/μL. Such an event is referred to as a **leukemoid reaction** and is sometimes difficult to differentiate from leukemia.

In contrast to bacterial infections, viral infections (including infectious mononucleosis) are characterized by an absolute increase in the number of circulating lymphocytes (lymphocytosis). Parasitic infestations and certain allergic reactions cause an increase in the number of eosinophils in the peripheral blood (eosinophilia). Eosinophils, which normally constitute 1% to 3% of peripheral leukocytes, can reach levels as high as 90% in some parasitic infections, particularly trichinosis.

Acute Phase Response

The acute phase response is a regulated physiologic reaction that is associated with inflammatory conditions. It is characterized clinically by fever, leukocytosis, decreased appetite, altered sleep patterns, and changes in the plasma levels of **acute phase proteins.** These proteins (Table 2-5) are synthesized primarily by hepatocytes and are released in large amounts into the circulation in response to an acute inflammatory challenge. Changes in the level of acute phase proteins are mediated by IL-6. This cytokine is synthesized at sites of inflammation by a variety of cell types, including fibroblasts, macrophages, epithelial cells, and endothelial cells. IL-6 binds to specific receptors on hepatocytes, in which it induces synthesis of acute phase proteins. Increased plasma levels of some acute phase proteins are reflected in an accelerated erythrocyte sedimentation rate, which is a qualitative index used clinically to monitor the activity of many inflammatory diseases.

TABLE 2-5. Acute Phase Proteins

Protein	Function
C-reactive protein	Opsonization
α_1-Antitrypsin	Serine protease inhibitor
Haptoglobin	Binds hemoglobin
Ceruloplasmin	Antioxidant, binds copper
Fibrinogen	Coagulation
Serum amyloid A protein	Apolipoprotein
α_2-Macroglobulin	Antiprotease
Cysteine protease inhibitor	Antiprotease

CHAPTER 3

Repair, Regeneration, and Fibrosis

Antonio Martinez-Hernandez

Healing is a response to tissue injury, representing an attempt to maintain normal structure and function. It overlaps the inflammatory process, and it is only for didactic purposes that the two are separated. The major components of the repair reaction are the extracellular matrix and a variety of cells.

EXTRACELLULAR MATRIX

The extracellular matrix has five major components: (1) collagens, (2) basement membranes, (3) structural glycoproteins, (4) elastic fibers, and (5) proteoglycans.

Collagens

The collagens are a family of closely related proteins, which have common properties. At least 19 collagen types have been identified. The major types are:

- **Type I collagen** is the principal collagen of bone, skin, and tendon, and the predominant collagen in mature scars.
- **Type II collagen** is the major collagen in cartilage.
- **Type III collagen** is abundant in embryonic tissues. In the adult, it predominates in pliable organs, such as blood vessels, the uterus, and the gastrointestinal tract.
- **Type IV collagen** is found exclusively in basement membranes.

Basement Membranes

Basement membranes, which are delicate structures at the interface between cells and stroma, contain type IV collagen, laminin, and other matrix components. By light microscopy, basement membranes appear as pale, amorphous bands.

All epithelia (epidermal, endocrine, genitourinary, respiratory, gastrointestinal) are separated from the stroma by continuous basement membranes. The liver is an exception, however, because hepatocytes lack a basement membrane. In the peripheral nervous system, Schwann cells are surrounded by a basement membrane. **All vascular endothelial cells are separated from the underlying stroma by a basement membrane, except for the sinusoidal endothelium of the bone marrow, lymphoid organs, and liver.** Adipocytes and cardiac, skeletal, and smooth muscle cells are individually surrounded by basement membranes. All other cells of mesodermal origin (fibroblasts, macrophages, synovial cells, lymphoid cells, and other blood cells) lack basement membranes.

Elastic Fibers

Tissues such as the uterus, blood vessels, skin, and lung require elasticity in addition to tensile strength. Whereas tensile strength is provided by members of the collagen family, the ability to recoil after transient stretching is provided by the elastic fibers. Elastic fibers vary in size from large sheets visible by light microscopy (elastic lamellae of large arteries) to delicate fibers demonstrable only by electron microscopy.

Fibronectin

The fibronectins are a family of glycoproteins in which specialized binding sites allow avid binding to a variety of structures, including collagen, proteoglycans, glycosaminoglycans, fibrinogen, fibrin, cell surfaces, bacteria, and DNA. The varied binding properties of fibronectin permit it to connect cells with other components of the extracellular matrix, thereby integrating the tissue into a functional unit. Fibronectin is ubiquitous in the extracellular matrix, where it is found (1) as delicate filaments or small aggregates, (2) attached to collagen fibers, and (3) on cell surfaces.

Proteoglycans

Proteoglycans are molecules of the extracellular matrix formed by long, unbranched polysaccharide chains, which are covalently bound to a protein core. They are widely distributed in all extracellular matrices, and they are also found in cell surfaces and in most biologic fluids. The carbohydrate polymers were formerly termed **mucopolysaccharides** but are more properly referred to as **glycosaminoglycans,** because one of the sugar residues in the repeating disaccharide unit is always an amino sugar. Glycosaminoglycans are negatively charged, extended molecules that occupy large volumes. They are also highly hydrophilic and form hydrated gels, even at low concentrations.

Proteoglycans participate in organization of the extracellular matrix by binding to collagen fibers, elastic fibers, and fibronectin. As organizers of the extracellular matrix, these molecules are deposited during the early phases of wound healing, before collagen deposition becomes prominent.

CELL PROLIFERATION

Tissues periodically renew their cell populations, except for organs composed of nondividing (permanent) cells. This orderly renewal is under rigorous control, as expressed in the cell cycle.

Cell Cycle

Maintenance of the structure of tissues composed of short-lived cells (e.g., gastrointestinal epithelium, epidermis, neutrophils) and regeneration of injured tissues require rigorously controlled cell proliferation to maintain an appropriate cell number. The factors that regulate cell division are only partially understood. The cell cycle, that is, the period of time between two successive cell divisions, is divided into four unequal phases (Fig. 3-1):

- **M Phase** (M = mitosis). This term describes the interval between the onset of the mitotic prophase and the conclusion of the telophase, at which time the cell has divided.
- **G_1 Phase** (G = gap). Following mitosis, the cell enters the G_1 phase, during which time it is devoted to its own specialized activities. The main difference between rapidly dividing and slowly dividing cells is in the length of the G_1 phase.
- **S Phase** (S = synthesis). After the G_1 phase, a doubling of DNA takes place during the S phase.
- **G_2 Phase.** After the completion of nuclear DNA duplication, the cells enter the G_2 phase, which is followed by the next mitosis (or M) phase.

- **G_0 Phase.** Some cells remain quiescent after an M phase and do not divide unless stimulated. After an appropriate stimulus, they may re-enter the cell cycle at the G_1 phase and continue through the cycle to mitosis.

Classification of Cells by Their Proliferative Potential

The cells of the body divide at different rates. Some mature cells do not divide at all, whereas other cells complete a cycle every 16 to 24 hours.

- **Labile cells** comprise tissues that are in a constant state of renewal, such as the epithelial lining of the gastrointestinal tract or the hemopoietic system.
- **Stable cells** form tissues that normally are renewed very slowly but are capable of more rapid renewal after tissue loss. The liver and the proximal renal tubules are examples of stable cell populations.
- **Permanent cells** are terminally differentiated and have lost all capacity for regeneration. Neurons and cardiac myocytes are representative of permanent cells.

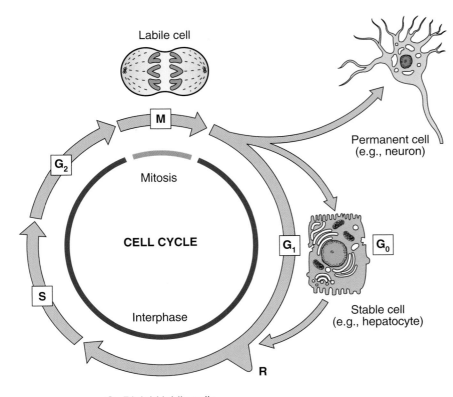

Labile cell

M

G_2

Mitosis

CELL CYCLE

G_1 G_0

S

Interphase

R

G_1-Diploid labile cells
(e.g., stem cells of intestinal crypts)

Permanent cell
(e.g., neuron)

Stable cell
(e.g., hepatocyte)

FIGURE *3-1*
The cell cycle. Labile cells (e.g., intestinal crypt cells) undergo continuous replication, and the interval between two consecutive mitoses is designated as the cell cycle. After division, the cells enter a gap phase (G_1), in which they pursue their own specialized activities. If they continue in the cycle, after passing the restriction point (R), they are committed to a new round of division. The G_1 phase is followed by a period of nuclear DNA synthesis (S) in which all chromosomes are replicated. The S phase is followed by a short gap phase (G_2) and then by mitosis. After each cycle, one daughter cell will become committed to differentiation, and the other will continue cycling. Other cell types, such as hepatocytes, are stable; that is, after mitosis, the cells take up their specialized functions (G_0). They do not re-enter the cycle unless stimulated by the loss of other cells. Permanent cells (e.g., neurons) become terminally differentiated after mitosis and cannot re-enter the cell cycle.

Labile Cells

Tissues in which more than 1.5% of the cells are in mitosis are composed of labile cells. Such tissues include the epidermis; the mucosa of the gastrointestinal, respiratory, urinary, and genital tracts; the bone marrow; and the lymphoid organs.

Stem cells are constituents of labile tissues that are programmed to divide continuously. One daughter cell of each division becomes another stem cell, whereas the other follows an irreversible path to terminal differentiation. The basal cells of the epidermis and the gastrointestinal crypts are examples of stem cells.

Tissues composed of labile cells regenerate after injury, provided that enough stem cells remain.

Stable Cells

Stable cells populate tissues in which fewer than 1.5% of the cells are in mitosis. Stable tissues, such as endocrine glands and endothelium, do not have stem cells. (The liver may or may not have stem cells.) The cells of these stable tissues require an appropriate stimulus to divide. **It is the potential to replicate, not the actual number of steady-state mitoses, that determines an organ's ability to regenerate.** For example, the liver, a stable tissue with less than one mitosis for every 15,000 cells, regenerates rapidly after a loss of as much as 70% of its mass.

Permanent Cells

Permanent cells are terminally differentiated and do not enter the cell cycle. Neurons, cardiac myocytes, and cells of the lens are permanent cells. **If lost, permanent cells cannot be replaced.**

CELL-MATRIX INTERACTIONS

The structure of normal mature tissues is dependent on a close relationship between cells and their surrounding connective tissue matrix, as exemplified by the relationship between epithelial, endothelial, and muscle cells and their basement membranes. In addition, close interactions between cells and matrix components are crucial for cell migration and differentiation during embryogenesis and wound healing.

Cell Migration

Embryonic development and wound healing require the orderly movement of both cells and extracellular matrix. For example, during repair of a wound, inter-actions between the extracellular matrix and the cells are critical for the "directed" migration of the respective cell types into the area of injury. Whereas soluble factors attract inflammatory and fibrogenic cells to the wound site (chemotaxis), the distribution, organization, and orientation of these cells are determined by information contained in the insoluble matrix.

Integrins

Integrins comprise a family of cell surface receptors that bind components of the extracellular matrix, including collagen, laminin, and fibronectin. By interacting with integrins, the extracellular matrix can modify cell behavior. In turn, the matrix is reciprocally modified by the cells with which it is in contact. The association of integrins with cytoskeletal filaments has been suggested as a possible route of communication between the matrix and the intracellular compartments.

CELL-CELL INTERACTIONS

In addition to the influence exerted by physical contact between cells and between cells and the extracellular matrix, many cells secrete soluble proteins termed **cytokines.** These factors (1) bind to specific cell surface receptors, (2) are mitogenic (growth factors), and (3) modulate cell behavior. The programmed elaboration of many cytokines is important in embryogenesis, normal tissue maintenance, inflammation (see Chapter 2), immune responses, and wound healing.

Macrophage-Derived Growth Factor

Macrophages produce macrophage-derived growth factor (MDGF), a molecule that stimulates the proliferation of quiescent fibroblasts, endothelial cells, and smooth muscle cells. Secretion of MDGF is stimulated by fibronectin and products of Gram-negative bacteria (endotoxin).

Platelet-Derived Growth Factor

Platelet-derived growth factor (PDGF) is a polypeptide that is a potent mitogen for mesodermal-derived cells, including smooth muscle cells, fibroblasts, and microglia. This cytokine is stored in the α-granules of platelets and is released after platelet aggregation during hemostasis. Several other cells, including macrophages, endothelial cells, smooth muscle cells, and transformed fibroblasts, produce PDGF-like molecules. PDGF is also a potent chemotactic signal for inflammatory cells, including monocytes/macrophages and neutrophils.

The chemotactic and mitogenic properties of PDGF may be important for processes such as (1) recruitment of inflammatory cells, fibroblasts, endothelial cells, and smooth muscle cells to a wound site; (2) activation of neutrophils and monocytes; and (3) proliferation of connective tissue cells.

Epidermal Growth Factor

Epidermal growth factor (EGF) is a small polypeptide that exhibits a wide range of physiologic effects. It binds to a transmembrane receptor present in most mammalian cell types but that is most abundant on epithelial cells. After binding EGF, the cell assumes a less differentiated appearance and begins to proliferate. EGF accelerates the healing of corneal and skin wounds as well as gastrointestinal ulcers. It also enhances collagen deposition during wound healing by stimulating the proliferation of fibroblasts and other cells.

Fibroblast Growth Factor

Fibroblast growth factor (FGF) promotes the growth of capillaries and is mitogenic for fibroblasts, endothelial cells, smooth muscle cells, and several other mesenchymal cells. This cytokine leads to an increase in collagen, protein, and DNA content, thereby accelerating wound healing. FGF exists in two forms, namely basic and acidic, with the basic form being 10-fold more active than the acidic one.

Transforming Growth Factor-β

Transforming growth factor-β (TGF-β) is a cytokine whose name is derived from its secretion by transformed cells in culture. Platelets also have high concentrations of TGF-β in their α-granules, and activation of lymphocytes induces transcription of the *TGF-β* gene. Whereas TGF-β is involved in terminating cellular proliferation within the regenerating liver and inhibits the growth of many cell types in culture, it is mitogenic for fibroblasts and increases the amount of collagen and other proteins during wound healing. It also induces the formation of granulation tissue (discussed later) when injected subcutaneously.

WOUND HEALING

■ *Healing is the restoration of integrity to an injured tissue.* Following creation of a wound, an initial inflam-

matory phase leads to formation of an exudate that is rich in fibrin and fibronectin. Before necrotic tissue is replaced, the dead cells and all other debris resulting from the injury are removed by phagocytic cells of the inflammatory response.

After the inflammatory phase, wound healing is accomplished by three mechanisms: (1) **contraction**, (2) **repair**, and (3) **regeneration.** In most instances, all three mechanisms are operative simultaneously. Thus, in a skin wound, part of the defect is closed by wound contraction, part by repair, and part by regeneration of epithelial cells. Figure 3-2 summarizes events in the healing of a skin wound.

Wound Contraction

■ *Contraction is a reduction in the size of a wound mediated principally by myofibroblasts.* This process is most prominent in the skin, but it also contributes to wound healing in the gastrointestinal and genitourinary tracts. The decrease in wound size is achieved by the inward migration of the surrounding mesenchymal cells. Under some circumstances, contraction reduces the size of an open defect by as much as 70%. **Wound contraction results in faster healing, because only one-third to one-half of the original defect has to be repaired.** If contraction is prevented, large and unsightly scars result.

Myofibroblasts

Myofibroblasts migrate into the wound 2 or 3 days after injury, and their active contraction decreases the size of the defect. They have features intermediate between those of fibroblasts and smooth muscle cells. The origin of myofibroblasts is not entirely clear, but they probably derive either from perivascular cells (pericytes) or from mesenchymal stem cells.

Repair

■ *Repair is the orderly process by which a wound is eventually replaced by a scar.* Wounds in which only the lining epithelium is affected are termed **erosions** and heal exclusively by regeneration. In such cases, proliferation of the epithelial cells surrounding the erosion covers the defect, without formation of a scar. By contrast, wounds that extend through the basement membrane to the connective tissue, such as the dermis in the skin or the submucosa in the gastrointestinal tract, lead to formation of granulation tissue and eventual scarring.

Granulation Tissue

■ *Granulation tissue is the initial response to a wound. It consists of a richly vascular connective tissue that contains*

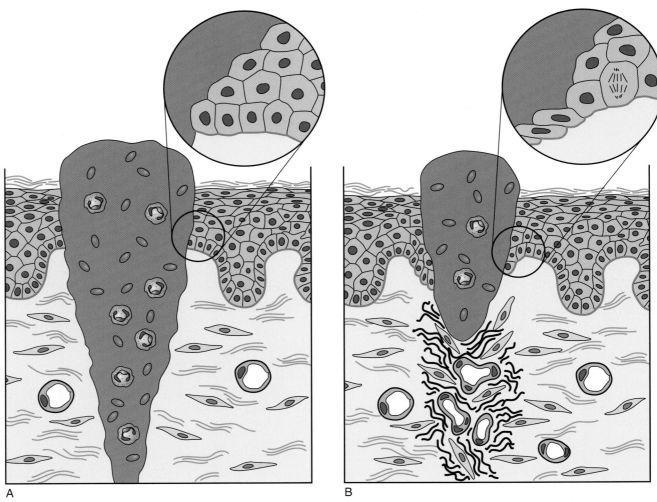

FIGURE   3-2

Skin healing. **(A)** In any wound, the initial gap is filled by blood that, on clotting (formation of fibrin polymers), provides the initial stability to the wound. Plasma fibronectin, present in the clot, can be cross-linked with extracellular matrix components and fibrin to bridge the clot and tissues. **(B)** The epidermal cells at the edges of the wound lose contact with other epithelial cells and with their basement membranes. At the same time, this loss of contact probably acts as a signal to trigger migration of the cells. Concurrently, basal epidermal cells adjacent to the migrating cells undergo division. The result of this co-ordinated migration and cell division is gradual covering of the epidermal defect. The breakdown products from the injured cells, fibronectin, and lysosomal enzymes from leukocytes act as chemoattractants, resulting in an influx of macrophages, myofibroblasts, and fibroblasts. Simultaneously, endothelial cells proliferate, and neovascularization begins. The phagocytic cells attracted to the wound remove part of the clot, whereas fibroblasts and myofibroblasts begin to deposit a new extracellular matrix. **(C)** The concentric migration of epidermal cells, sustained by the mitotic activity of the trailing cells, fills the wound gap and displaces the remnants of the original clot (scab) toward the surface. Contact with other epidermal cells is the signal that stops migration. The trailing cells not only divide but also secrete basement membrane components. In this manner, the continuity of the epidermal basement membrane is restored. In a similar fashion, the concerted activity of fibroblasts, myofibroblasts, macrophages, and endothelial cells fills the dermal gap. At this point, the number of macrophages and myofibroblasts declines. Those capillaries that failed to establish a definitive flow pattern begin to be obliterated, and accumulation of the definitive extracellular matrix is initiated. **(D)** The gap created by the wound has been repaired. Mitotic activity of the epidermal cells will restore the epidermal thickness. Most capillaries of the initial granulation tissue have been reabsorbed, and the dermal gap has been filled with a dense, almost avascular extracellular matrix composed predominantly of type I collagen.

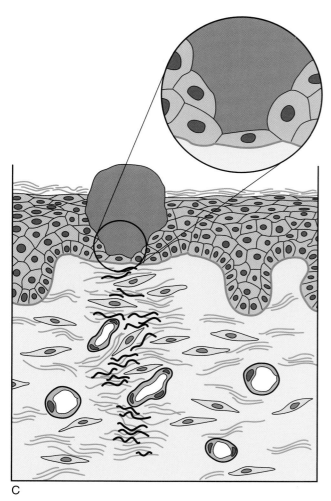

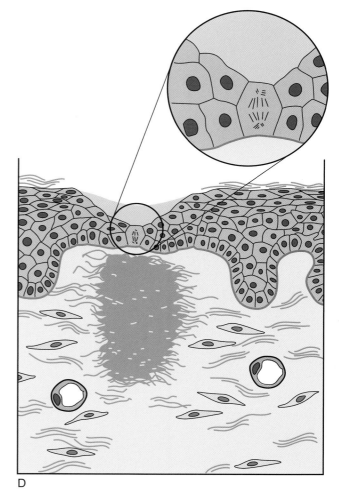

FIGURE   **3-2**   *(Continued)*

new capillaries, abundant fibroblasts, and variable numbers of inflammatory cells (Fig. 3-3). Formation of granulation tissue is a regulated process that involves a number of events, including the growth of new capillaries, fibrogenesis, and involution during maturation of the scar.

Angiogenesis

A striking vascular proliferation starts 48 to 72 hours after injury and lasts for several days. Endothelial cells near the injury divide and form solid sprouts extending from pre-existing vessels. The vascular sprouts arborize and anastomose to form a new capillary bed. These sprouting capillaries tend to protrude from the surface of the wound as minute red granules, imparting the name "granulation" tissue. Eventually, portions of the new capillary bed differentiate into arterioles and venules.

The cellular sources of angiogenesis factors in wound healing have not been conclusively identified. Macrophages produce angiogenesis factors in vitro,

but they probably are not the only cells responsible for endothelial proliferation. Basic FGF is a potent angiogenesis factor, but its precise cell of origin is still being debated. Interestingly, malignant tumors depend on neovascularization for their continuous growth, and many cancers secrete factors that induce the growth of endothelial cells. Angiogenesis probably is also modulated by inhibitory factors. Thus, it is likely that angiogenesis is controlled by combinations of signals rather than by a single factor.

Cell Proliferation

Early wound healing exhibits not only debris, inflammatory cells, and capillaries but also abundant fibroblasts. Following the initial influx of inflammatory cells from the blood into a wound site, a second wave of fibroblasts moves into the injured area within 2 to 3 days. Resting fibroblasts are oval cells, with an indistinct cytoplasm and an elongated, homogeneous nucleus. Activated fibroblasts have a distinct cytoplasm and an intensely basophilic nucleus, and they show

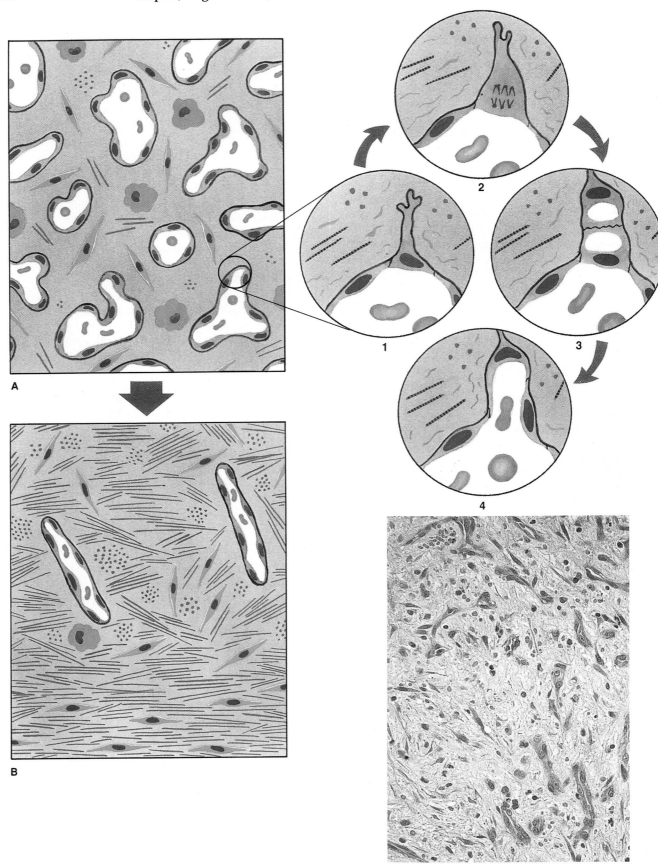

frequent mitoses. Activated fibroblasts secrete extracellular matrix components, including fibronectin, proteoglycans, and collagen (types I and III).

The factors responsible for fibroblast proliferation are not all known, but FGF, TGF-β, and PDGF likely are important. In addition, plasma fibronectin, extravasated as a consequence of an injury, is chemotactic for mesenchymal cells. Fibroblast proliferation is, in large part, also dependent on the presence of macrophages, which presumably secrete specific growth factors.

Deposition of Noncollagenous Extracellular Matrix

Fibroblasts secrete components of the extracellular matrix. Fibronectin and hyaluronic acid are the first fibroblast glycoproteins to be deposited in the healing wound, and proteoglycans appear later. Because proteoglycans are very hydrophilic, their accumulation contributes to the edematous appearance of the wound. Concentrations of proteoglycans and fibronectin in the wound peak 4 to 6 days after the injury and then decline to normal levels by day 12.

Collagen Synthesis

Significant collagen deposition in the wound is apparent by 4 days after injury. Initially, type III collagen predominates, but after a week, type I is abundant and, eventually, becomes the major collagen of mature scar tissue.

Scar Formation

As healing of the wound progresses, the rate of collagen synthesis exceeds its rate of degradation. As a result, collagen accumulates steadily during scar formation, usually reaching a maximum in 2 to 3 months. However, the tensile strength of the wound continues to increase for many months after the collagen content has peaked. This physical change is related to an increase in collagen cross-linking. As the scar matures, vascular involution continues, thereby transforming richly vascularized granulation tissue into a pale, avascular scar.

Figures 3-4, 3-5, and 3-6 summarize the repair mechanisms during wound healing.

Regeneration

■ *Regeneration is the renewal of a lost tissue or part in which the missing cells are replaced by identical ones.* This process has been well studied in the skin. As long as the basement membrane beneath the epidermis is not breached, damage to the epidermis is easily repaired by proliferation of epithelial cells at the wound margin. Epidermal reserve cells detach from the underlying basement membrane and increase their surface area by flattening. Mitosis occurs in cells that are slightly behind the advancing edge, and the epithelium advances across the wound. When the wound surface is completely covered, and the migrating cells are in contact with each other, the cells recover their usual shape, and they attach themselves to the basement membrane. Squamous differentiation proceeds, and the normal thickness of the epithelium is restored. Although there are variations depending on the cell type and organ, most tissues that are capable of regeneration show a similar pattern.

A number of growth factors, including EGF, FGF, PDGF, TGF-β, and nerve growth factor, have been implicated in the regeneration of various tissues. Insulin, glucagon, thyroid hormones, and even the extracellular matrix components fibronectin and laminin also play a role.

FIGURE *3-3*
Granulation tissue. (A) Granulation tissue has two major components, namely cells and proliferating capillaries. The cells are mostly fibroblasts, myofibroblasts, and macrophages. The macrophages derive from monocytes and fixed macrophages. The fibroblasts and myofibroblasts derive from mesenchymal stem cells, and the capillaries arise from adjacent vessels by division of the lining endothelial cells (*detail*) in a process termed *angiogenesis*. Endothelial cells put out cell extensions (pseudopodia) that grow toward the wound site. Cytoplasmic growth enlarges the pseudopodia, and eventually the cells divide. Vacuoles formed in the daughter cells eventually fuse to create a new lumen. The entire process continues until the sprout encounters another capillary, with which it will connect. At its peak, granulation tissue is the most richly vascularized tissue in the body. (B) Once repair has been achieved, most of the newly formed capillaries are obliterated and then reabsorbed, leaving a pale, avascular scar. (C) A photomicrograph of granulation tissue shows thin-walled vessels embedded in a loose, connective tissue matrix containing mesenchymal cells and occasional inflammatory cells.

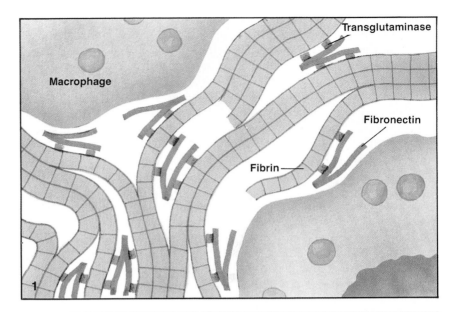

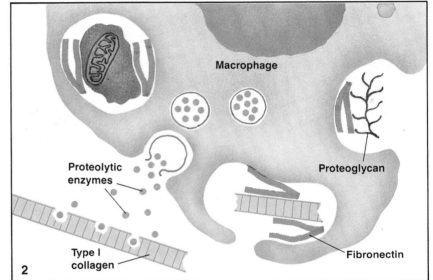

FIGURE   *3-4*

Summary of the healing process: The initial phase of the repair reaction, which typically begins with hemorrhage into the tissues. 1. A fibrin clot forms and fills the gap created by the wound. Fibronectin in the extravasated plasma is cross-linked to fibrin, collagen, and other extracellular matrix components by the action of transglutaminases. This cross-linking provides a provisional mechanical stabilization of the wound. 2. Macrophages recruited to the wound area process cell remnants and damaged extracellular matrix. The binding of fibronectin to cell membranes, collagens, proteoglycans, DNA, and bacteria (opsonization) facilitates phagocytosis of these elements; collagenases and other proteases secreted by leukocytes and macrophages contribute to the removal of debris. 3. Fibronectin, cell debris, and bacterial products are chemoattractants for a variety of cells, which are recruited to the wound site

The intermediate phase of the repair reaction. (1) As a new extracellular matrix is deposited at the wound site, the initial fibrin clot is lysed by a combination of extracellular proteolytic enzymes and phagocytosis. (2) Concurrent with fibrin removal, there is deposition of a temporary matrix formed by proteoglycans, glycoproteins, and type III collagen. (3) Final phase of the repair reaction. Eventually, the temporary matrix is removed by a combination of extracellular and intracellular digestion, and the definitive matrix, which is rich in type I collagen, is deposited.

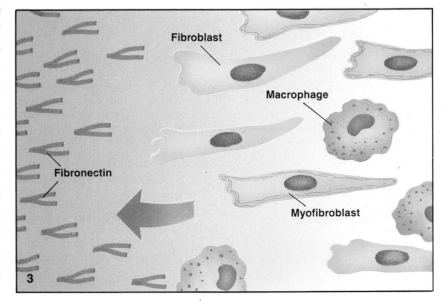

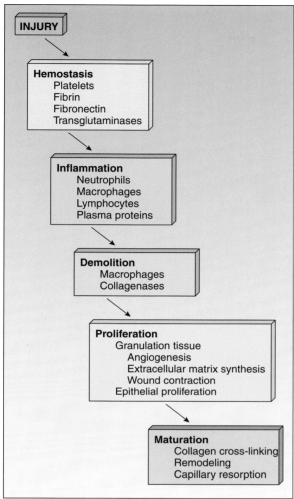

FIGURE 3-5
The repair cascade. Repair can be viewed as a chain of events, each stage completing the previous one and initiating the subsequent one.

The complexity of the problem is illustrated by liver regeneration. Liver regeneration is influenced by insulin, glucagon, calcitonin, thyroid hormone, parathormone, glucocorticoids, EGF, hepatotropin, several amino acids, and probably laminin. The mammalian liver regenerates after a loss of 70% of the original mass. In the rat, more than 40% of the removed mass has been replaced by 48 hours after partial hepatectomy, and in 6 days, regeneration has been completed.

Healing of Wounds with Apposed Edges (Primary Intention)

Immediately after an incision, a hematoma rich in fibrin and fibronectin forms. The hematoma is rapidly followed by acute inflammation and dissolution of the clot. Within 48 hours for a well-approximated wound, a continuous layer of epithelial cells covers the site of injury. By the third or fourth day, granulation tissue invades the wound, and collagen deposition begins. For the first month, tensile strength closely parallels the collagen content of the wound. Granulation tissue prevents epithelial migration deep into the wound, but the epithelial cells on the surface divide and differentiate, thereby restoring a multilayered epithelium. After 1 to 3 months, as the granulation tissue is devascularized, the linear scar decreases in size and changes from red to white, and the permanent scar is formed. **Healing by primary intention is the desired result in all surgical incisions.**

Healing of Wounds with Separated Edges (Secondary Intention)

Extensive tissue loss, or simple failure to approximate the wound edges, results in a defect that is filled by granulation tissue. The degree of inflammation and the amount of granulation tissue are considerably greater in gouged wounds than in surgical incisions. Whereas healing of a wound with apposed edges is fast and leaves a small, often inapparent scar, healing of wounds with separated edges is slow and can result in large, deforming scars.

Factors That Influence Wound Healing

Factors that influence wound healing are divided into local and systemic factors.

Local Factors

- **Type, Size, and Location of the Wound.** A clean, aseptic wound produced by the surgeon's scalpel heals faster than a wound produced by blunt trauma. Injuries in richly vascularized areas (e.g., the face) heal faster than those in poorly vascularized ones (e.g., the foot). In areas where the skin adheres to bony surfaces, such as with injuries over the tibia, wound contraction and adequate apposition of the edges are difficult.
- **Vascular Supply.** Wounds with impaired blood supply heal slowly. For example, healing of leg wounds in patients with varicose veins is prolonged. Ischemia caused by pressure produces bedsores and then prevents their healing. Ischemia caused by arterial obstruction, often in the lower extremities of patients with diabetes, also prevents healing.

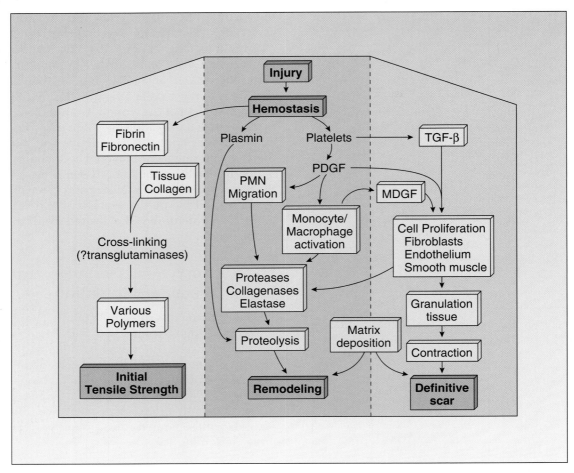

FIGURE 3-6
The major steps and interactions in three phases of wound healing.

- **Infection.** Wounds provide a portal of entry for micro-organisms. Infection delays or prevents healing, promotes the formation of excessive granulation tissue, and may result in large, deforming scars.
- **Movement.** Early motion, particularly before tensile strength has been established, subjects a wound to persistent trauma, thereby preventing or retarding its healing.

Systemic Factors

- **Circulatory Status.** Because it determines the blood supply to the injured area, cardiovascular function is important for wound healing. Poor healing attributed to old age is often due largely to impaired circulation.
- **Infection.** Systemic infections delay wound healing.
- **Metabolic Status.** Poorly controlled diabetes mellitus is associated with delayed wound healing. Wounds in patients with diabetes often become in-

fected, and in turn, an infection makes the control of diabetes difficult.
- **Malnutrition.** Nutritional deficiencies (e.g., scurvy) impair wound healing.

Complications of Wound Healing

Abnormalities in any of the three basic healing processes—contraction, repair, and regeneration—result in complications of wound healing.

Deficient Scar Formation

Inadequate formation of granulation tissue or inability to form a suitable extracellular matrix leads to deficient scar formation and its complications.

Wound Dehiscence and Incisional Hernias. Dehiscence (bursting of a wound) is of most concern after abdominal surgery. Dehiscence of an abdominal wound can be a life-threatening complication, carrying a mortality rate as high as 30% in some studies.

Increased mechanical stress on the wound from vomiting, coughing, or ileus is a factor in most cases of abdominal dehiscence. Systemic factors that predispose to dehiscence include poor metabolic status, such as vitamin C deficiency, hypoproteinemia, and the general inanition that often accompanies metastatic cancer. An incisional hernia, usually of the abdominal wall, refers to a defect caused by previous surgery into which the intestines protrude. Such hernias from weak scars are often the consequence of insufficient deposition of extracellular matrix or inadequate cross-linking of the matrix.

Ulceration. Wounds ulcerate because of an inadequate intrinsic blood supply or insufficient vascularization during healing. For example, leg wounds in persons with varicose veins or severe atherosclerosis typically ulcerate.

Excessive Scar Formation

An excessive deposition of extracellular matrix at the wound site results in a **hypertrophic scar** or a **keloid** (an exuberant scar that tends to progress and recur after excision). Histologically (Fig. 3-7), both types of scars exhibit abundant, broad, and irregular collagen bundles, with more capillaries and fibroblasts than expected for a scar of the same age.

Excessive Contraction

Exaggerated healing results in **contracture**, a severe deformity of the wound and surrounding tissues. Contractures are particularly conspicuous in the healing of serious burns. Contractures of the skin and the underlying connective tissue can be severe enough to compromise the movement of joints. In the alimentary tract, a contracture (stricture) can obstruct the passage of food in the esophagus or block the flow of intestinal contents.

HEALING IN SPECIFIC TISSUES

The general principles of wound healing apply to all tissues. Each organ, however, contains specialized cells and distinctive extracellular matrices, and these differences impart some organ specificity to the healing response (Fig. 3-8).

Liver

Liver injury is followed by complete parenchymal regeneration, formation of scars, or a combination of both. The outcome depends on the extent and chronicity of the insult. The hepatocytes lost after acute focal or zonal necrosis of the liver are restored by regeneration. The normal architecture is also re-established, and no fibrosis occurs. By contrast, chronic hepatic injury (e.g., chronic viral hepatitis, alcoholic liver injury) elicits a combination of regeneration and fibrosis, an appearance that is termed **cirrhosis** (Fig. 3-9).

Kidney

The kidney has a limited regenerative capacity. If the injury is not extensive and the extracellular matrix frame-

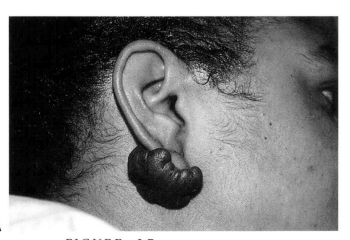

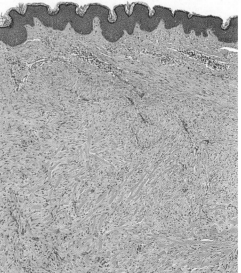

A   **B**

FIGURE *3-7*
Keloid. (A) A light-skinned black woman developed a keloid as a reaction to having her earlobe pierced. (B) Microscopically, the dermis is markedly thickened by the presence of collagen bundles with random orientation and few cells.

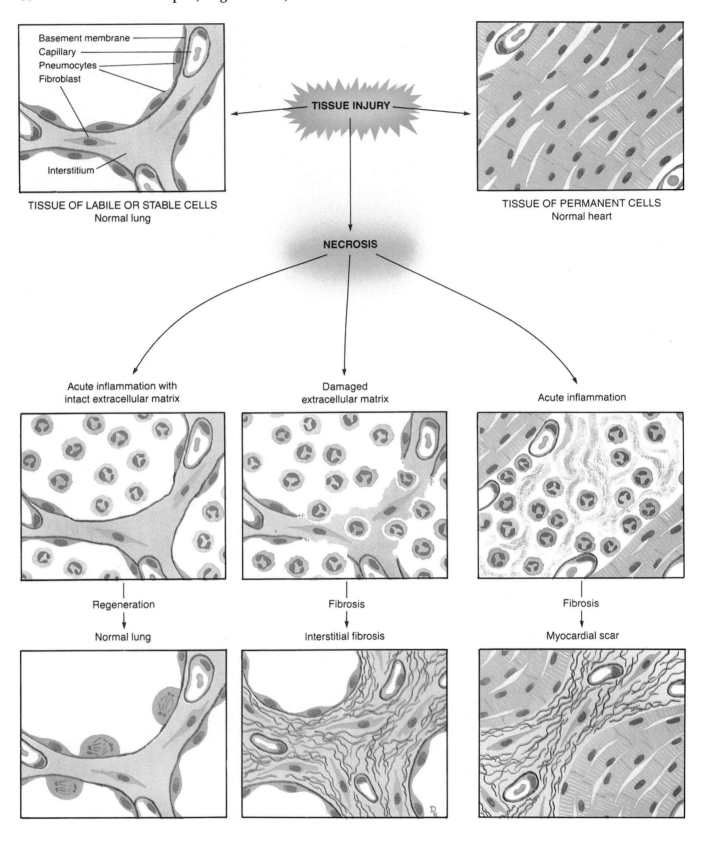

TISSUE INJURY

TISSUE OF LABILE OR STABLE CELLS
Normal lung

Basement membrane
Capillary
Pneumocytes
Fibroblast
Interstitium

TISSUE OF PERMANENT CELLS
Normal heart

NECROSIS

Acute inflammation with
intact extracellular matrix

Damaged
extracellular matrix

Acute inflammation

Regeneration

Fibrosis

Fibrosis

Normal lung

Interstitial fibrosis

Myocardial scar

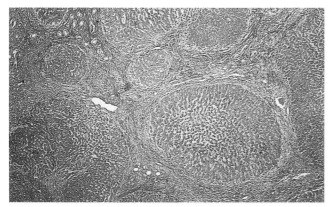

FIGURE *3-9*
Cirrhosis of the liver. The consequence of chronic hepatic injury is the formation of regenerating nodules separated by bands of fibrous connective tissue (*blue*).

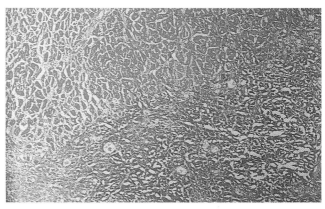

FIGURE *3-10*
Healed myocardial infarct. Tissues with permanent cells can only replace dead cells with scar tissue. After a myocardial infarct, the lost cardiac myocytes are replaced with dense connective tissue (*blue*)

work is not destroyed, the tubular epithelium regenerates. In most clinically relevant lesions, however, there is some destruction of the extracellular matrix framework. Regeneration is incomplete, and repair with scar formation is the usual outcome. The regenerative capacity of renal tissue is maximal in the cortical tubules, less in the medullary tubules, and nonexistent in the glomeruli.

Lung

The epithelium lining the respiratory tract has an excellent regenerative capacity, provided that the underlying extracellular matrix framework is not destroyed. Superficial injuries to tracheal and bronchial epithelia heal by regeneration from the adjacent epithelium. The outcome of alveolar injury ranges from complete regeneration of structure and function to incapacitating fibrosis. The determining factors are, again, the degree of cell necrosis and the extent of damage to the extracellular matrix framework.

Heart

Myocardial cells have no significant regenerative capacity. Myocardial necrosis, from whatever cause, heals by formation of granulation tissue and eventual scarring (Fig. 3-10). Myocardial scarring (e.g., after coronary occlusion) results in the loss of contractile elements, and the fibrous tissue also decreases the effectiveness of contraction in the surviving myocardium.

Nervous System

Because mature neurons are permanent postmitotic cells and cannot divide, neuronal connections damaged by trauma can be re-established only by regrowth and reorganization of the cell processes of the surviving neurons. Whereas the peripheral nervous system has the capacity for axonal regeneration, the central nervous system lacks this property.

FIGURE *3-8*
Possible outcomes of the healing response. A crucial factor in determining the outcome of any injury is the constituent cells of the injured tissue. In this figure, the lung represents tissues composed of labile or stable cells, and the heart represents tissues composed of permanent cells. If the injury to the lung produces cell necrosis but the framework of the organ remains intact, the surviving cells will proliferate. They migrate along the intact basement membrane, and they reconstruct the normal organ structure. On the other hand, if the injury destroys not only cells but also the basement membrane, the surviving cells, when they proliferate, will lack the master plan provided by the extracellular matrix. As a consequence, the repair reaction fails to duplicate the normal structure, and scarring of the lung ensues, with varying degrees of functional impairment. In tissues composed of permanent cells, as exemplified by the heart, lost parenchymal cells cannot be restored. Therefore, cell necrosis invariably results in permanent loss of parenchymal cells, fibrosis, and if extensive enough, functional impairment.

CHAPTER 4

Immunopathology

Kent J. Johnson
Steven W. Chensue
Peter A. Ward

During evolution, plants and animals have acquired a variety of mechanisms to defend themselves from invasion by a vast spectrum of micro-organisms, ranging from viruses to multicellular parasites. These defenses extend from simple phagocytosis and digestion in protozoa to the exquisitely complex network of cellular and humoral elements in the mammalian immune system.

The body's defense against micro-organisms consists of two interrelated but conceptually distinct systems, namely **natural immunity** and the more specific **acquired immunity.** Natural immunity is mediated principally by cells involved with the inflammatory responses discussed in Chapter 2. Natural immunity does not require previous exposure to the offending agent, nor is it enhanced by such exposure. Moreover, natural immunity is relatively nonspecific; that is, it does not discriminate among various foreign materials. By contrast, acquired immunity is specific. The functions of the cells that participate in acquired immune responses require a sensitizing exposure to the offending agent, and their response is magnified by subsequent exposures to that same macromolecule (antigen).

CELLULAR COMPONENTS OF THE IMMUNE RESPONSE

Lymphocytes

■ *Lymphocytes are the primary directors of antigen-specific immune responses, because they have the capacity to recognize and react with specific foreign molecules.* All lymphocytes originate from primitive yolk sac stem cell precursors that become either T cells (thymus-derived) or B cells (bone marrow–derived) (Fig. 4-1). A third class of lymphocytes (null cells) lacks the defining characteristics of T and B cells. Natural killer cells (described later) belong in this category.

T Lymphocytes

The stem cell precursors of lymphocytes interact with the thymic epithelium. In turn, the latter provides the molecular signals that cause the sequential expression of genes that confer the functional and phenotypic characteristics of T cells.

T cells at different stages of maturation are characterized by their expression of specific surface markers, and **cluster designation** (CD) or differentiation numbers have been assigned to distinguish between lymphocyte subsets. T-cell development begins with the proliferation of antigen-specific clones in the cortical regions of the thymic lobes. The differentiation of T lymphocytes proceeds as follows:

- **Early Cortical T Cells.** The early, or least mature, cortical thymocytes make up 10% of the lymphocytes.
- **Late Cortical T Cells.** Late cortical thymocytes account for 80% of the thymic population.
- **Medullary T Cells.** In the thymic medulla, the CD4 and CD8 antigens are distributed among two separate cell populations, which display helper (CD4) and cytotoxic/suppressor (CD8) functions, respectively. The medullary T cells also acquire the CD3 membrane marker, which is associated with the antigen receptor and persists for the life of the cell.
- **Peripheral T Cells.** The final stages of T-cell development occur with the migration of T cells to the blood and the lymphatic system, where the CD38 antigen is lost. **In the blood and peripheral lymphoid organs, CD4+ (helper) cells make up 65% of all T cells and CD8+ (cytotoxic/suppressor) cells 35%.**

T lymphocytes recognize specific antigens—usually proteins or haptens bound to proteins—and respond as directed by intrinsic factors that dictate maturational events and by exogenous signals delivered via extracellular molecules. The CD4+ and CD8+ cells are subsets of T cells that have varied effector or regulatory functions. Effector functions include secretion of proinflammatory mediators and cytotoxic responses to cells containing foreign or altered membrane antigens. Examples of regulatory functions are augmentation and suppression of immune responses, usually by secretion of specific helper or suppressor molecules.

An interesting aspect of T-cell antigen recognition is the requirement for antigens to be presented on the surface of another cell in association with a histocompatibility membrane protein. In other words, T cells have a membrane receptor complex (the T-cell receptor) on their surface that, for maximal immune response, must interact not only with the foreign antigen but also with histocompatibility molecular structures. As a consequence, antigens are presented to T cells by accessory cells (antigen-presenting cells) that bear appropriate histocompatibility antigens. These include macrophages, B lymphocytes, dendritic cells, Langerhans cells, and endothelial cells. Antigens may also be presented to certain T cells by a variety of cells, which are not normally antigen-presenting cells, when they express on their surface a foreign or altered self-protein in association with a histocompatibility molecule.

The relevant histocompatibility antigens are derived from genes in the major histocompatibility complex. This region codes for human leukocyte antigen (HLA) class I and class II membrane proteins. In general, CD8+ cells (cytotoxic T cells) recognize antigens

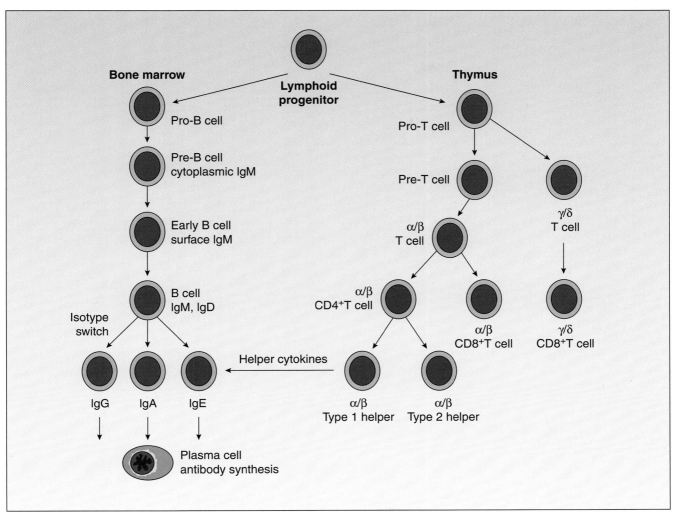

FIGURE *4-1*
Major maturational stages of lymphocytes.

in conjunction with class I molecules, whereas CD4+ cells (helper T cells) recognize antigen together with class II molecules. It should be noted that foreign class I and class II molecules, which are not histocompatible with the host (e.g., transplanted histocompatibility antigens), are themselves potent immunogens and are recognized by host T cells. Figure 4-2 illustrates some of the interactions between CD4+ T-helper cells and antigen-presenting cells.

B Lymphocytes

B lymphocytes are cells that bear membrane immunoglobulins and, under appropriate conditions, differentiate into antibody-secreting cells as follows:

- **Pre-B Cells.** Following development in the embryonic yolk sac, precursor B cells (pre-B cells) migrate to the fetal liver and, later, to the bone marrow,

where they multiply and diversify into a vast number of clones. Pre-B cells contain cytoplasmic heavy-chain immunoglobulins but no light-chain or surface immunoglobulins. However, receptors for complement fragment C3b and HLA class II proteins are present on the plasma membrane.

- **Early B Cells.** Immature B cells are recognized by the appearance of surface monomeric immunoglobulin (Ig) M. With subsequent maturation involving gene rearrangements, B cells acquire surface IgD.

- **Mature B Cells.** Mature B lymphocytes are primarily in a resting state, awaiting activation by foreign antigen. Activation involves cross-linking of membrane immunoglobulin receptors by antigens that are presented on accessory cells. This initial stimulus leads to the proliferation and clonal expansion of B cells, which are amplified by factors

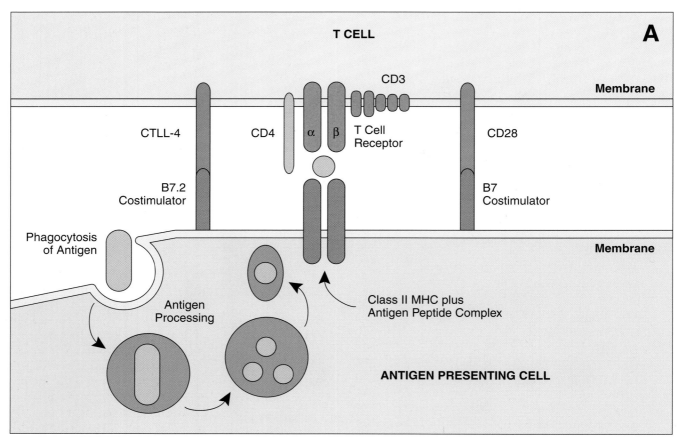

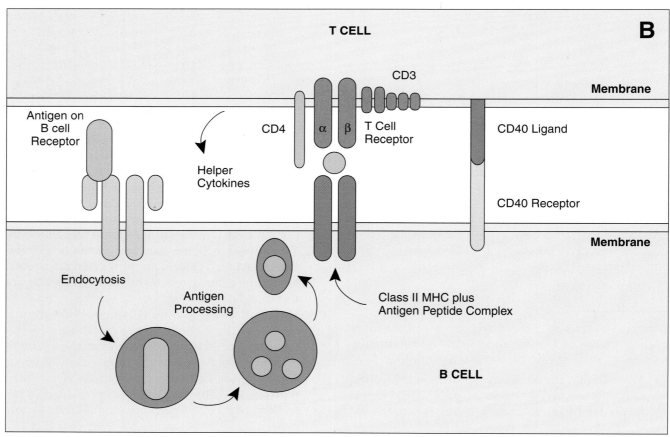

derived from macrophages and T cells, such as interleukin (IL)-1 and IL-4. If no further signal is provided, the proliferating B cells return to the resting state and enter the memory cell pool.

- **Isotype Switching.** The next stage of B-cell development involves further gene rearrangements, a process that results in isotype switching. The term **isotype** refers to the class of the defining heavy chain of an immunoglobulin molecule. In the absence of antigenic stimulation, a proportion of the B-cell clones proceed to express other heavy-chain isotypes, such as IgG (c1, c2, g3), IgA (1 or 2), or IgE (e). T cells are also involved in the differentiation of B cells. In the presence of antigen, T cells produce differentiation factors that either stimulate B-cell isotype switching or induce proliferation of particular committed isotype populations.

- **Plasma Cells.** The final stage of B-cell differentiation into antibody-synthesizing plasma cells generally requires exposure to additional T-cell products (e.g., B-cell differentiation factors). This is the case for responses to most protein antigens. However, some polyvalent agents directly induce B-cell proliferation and their differentiation to plasma cells, bypassing the requirements for B-cell growth and differentiation factors. Such agents are called **polyclonal B-cell activators**, because they do not interact with antigen-binding sites and, hence, are not specific antigens. Examples of polyclonal B-cell activators are bacterial products (lipopolysaccharide, protein A) and certain viruses (Epstein-Barr virus, cytomegalovirus).

The spectrum of immunoglobulins produced during immune responses changes with age. Newborns tend to produce predominantly IgM; by contrast, older children and adults show rapid shifts toward IgG synthesis following antigenic challenge.

Natural Killer Cells

■ *Natural killer (NK) cells comprise a population of lymphocytes with the capacity to recognize and kill various tumor and virus-infected cells in vitro.* These large lymphocytes cannot be precisely classified as T, B, or myelomonocytic cells. **Thus, NK cells represent a subset of so-called null cells.**

The NK cells are affected by several molecular mediators. For example, IL-2 supports their growth, and interferons promote their killing activity. By contrast, prostaglandin E_2 is highly suppressive of NK cell activity. NK cells also have Fc receptors and, thus, can kill target cells by antibody-dependent, cell-mediated cytotoxicity.

Mononuclear Phagocytes

■ *Mononuclear phagocyte is a general term applied to populations of phagocytic cells found in virtually all organs and connective tissues.* Among these cells are macrophages, monocytes, Kupffer cells of the liver, and so-called histiocytes (fixed tissue macrophages). Mononuclear phagocytes are identified by their nonsegmented nuclei, abundant cytoplasm, and phagocytic function.

In the lung, liver, and spleen, large numbers of macrophages populate the sinuses and capillaries to form an effective filtering system that removes effete cells and foreign particulate material from the blood. This system was formerly known as the **reticuloendothelial system,** but it is now termed the **mononuclear phagocytic system.** In addition to their housekeeping functions, macrophages play a critical role in the induction of immune responses and in the maintenance and resolution of inflammatory reactions.

Macrophages are important accessory cells by virtue of their expression of class II histocompatibility antigens. They actively ingest and process antigens for presentation to T cells in conjunction with class II antigens. The subsequent T-cell responses are further amplified by macrophage-derived monokines. One of the best characterized of these monokines is IL-1, which promotes expression of the IL-2 receptor by T cells. As a result, T-cell proliferation that is driven by IL-2 is augmented. IL-1 also has a broad spectrum of effects on other tissues and, in general, prepares the body to combat infection. For example, it induces fever and promotes catabolic metabolism.

Macrophages are dominant participants in subacute and chronic inflammatory reactions. During persistent inflammation, increased numbers of monocytes are recruited from the bone marrow. Under chemotactic influences, they migrate to sites of inflammation, where they mature into macrophages. Both recruited and local-tissue macrophages proliferate at these foci. Box 4-1 summarizes some of the many secretory products of macrophages that can function at sites of inflammation.

FIGURE 4-2
Interactions of T cells with antigen-presenting cells (APCs) and B cells. (A) CD4 T cells are activated by APCs via the T-cell receptor and CD28 or CTLL-4. (B) Antigen-specific B cells are activated via interaction with the T-cell receptor and CD40.

The functional activity of macrophages and the spectrum of molecules they produce are regulated by external factors, such as T cell–derived lymphokines. Macrophages exposed to such factors become "activated"; that is, they acquire a greater capacity to release oxygen metabolites and kill tumor cells and intracellular micro-organisms.

If the agent that incites an inflammatory process is poorly digestible, a **granulomatous reaction** may ensue. Under such conditions, macrophages show additional maturation and become epithelioid cells and multinucleated giant cells. Epithelioid cells are macrophages with abundant eosinophilic cytoplasm, which appear to be predominantly secretory. Giant cells are produced by macrophage fusion, resulting in syncytia containing multiple nuclei. Depending on the inciting agent, different types of giant cells may form. For example, granulomas elicited by mycobacteria often contain Langhans-type giant cells, which have a circular arrangement of nuclei. Giant cells of foreign body granulomas have a random distribution of nuclei. Both epithelioid cells and giant cells are poorly phagocytic; they mainly sequester and digest foreign material.

Human Major Histocompatibility Complex

The major histocompatibility complex (MHC) *is an intricate system of membrane proteins that is highly polymorphous within the human population and is the main target for the rejection of transplanted organs.* Individual MHC antigens are referred to as **human leukocyte antigens (HLA)**. Such antigens allow for self-recognition during cell-cell interactions, especially during immune responses.

The MHC genes are located on the short arm of chromosome 6 (Fig. 4-3), where they code for three major classes of molecules, which are designated as I, II, and III. The class III antigens represent certain complement components and are not histocompatibility antigens.

Cell surface histocompatibility molecules bind fragments of foreign proteins and then present these molecules to antigen-specific T cells. Class I molecules are present on all nucleated cells and are recognized by cytotoxic T cells during graft rejection or during killing of virus-infected cells. Class II molecules are limited principally to (1) cells involved in antigen presentation (e.g., macrophages and dendritic cells), (2) B cells, and (3) subsets of activated T cells. Thus, class II MHC molecules are important for interactions between immune cells, particularly in antigen presentation to T cells. Importantly, some cells (e.g., bile duct epithelial cells, renal tubular epithelium, and endothelial cells) may express class II molecules after stimulation by certain cytokines or other factors. In this situation, they then may become targets for an autoimmune attack.

IMMUNOLOGICALLY MEDIATED TISSUE INJURY

Although immune responses combat invasion by foreign organisms, they also often lead to tissue damage. An immune response that results in tissue injury is broadly referred to as a **hypersensitivity reaction** and

BOX *4-1* **Major Macrophage Products**

Proteins	Angiogenesis factor
Enzymes	**Reactive Oxygen Species**
Neutral proteinases (e.g., plasminogen activator	Superoxide anion
elastase collagenases)	Hydrogen peroxide
Lysozyme	Oxygen radicals
Arginase	Nitric oxide
Lipoprotein lipase	**Bioactive Lipids**
Angiotensin-converting enzyme	Prostaglandin E_2
Acid hydrolases	Prostacyclin I_2
Plasma proteins	Thromboxane B_2
Coagulation proteins	Leukotriene B_4, C_4, D_4, and E_4
Complement components	Hydroxyeicosatetraenoic acids (HETEs)
α_2-Macroglobulin	**Nucleotides**
Fibronectin	Thymidine
Cytokines	Uracil
IL-1, -10, and -12	cAMP
Tumor necrosis factor	Uric acid
Interferon-α	

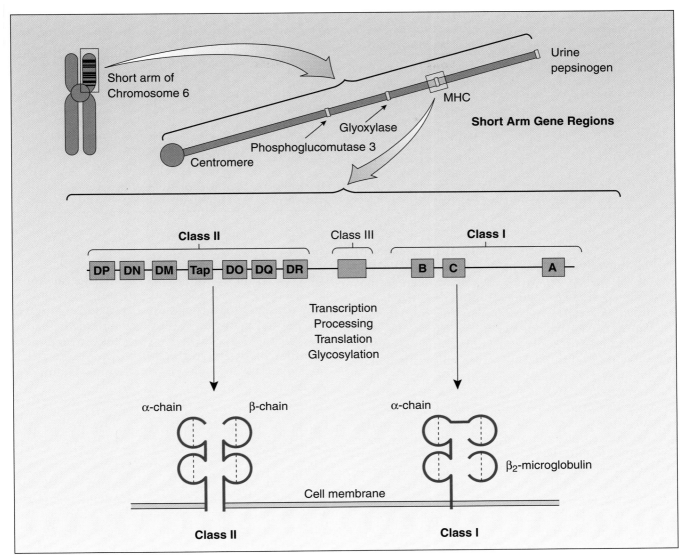

FIGURE   4-3
Genes of the human major histocompatibility complex (MHC) and their protein products.

is associated with diseases that are categorized as immune disorders or immunologically mediated conditions. Such diseases are common and include asthma, hay fever, hepatitis, glomerulonephritis, and arthritis. The most useful classification lists reactions according to which type of immune mechanism is involved (Table 4-1).

Type I Hypersensitivity (Immediate Type or Anaphylaxis)

■ *Immediate-type hypersensitivity or anaphylaxis* is manifested by a localized or a generalized reaction that occurs immediately (within minutes) after exposure to an antigen to which the person has previously become sensitized. These reactions depend on the site of antigen exposure. For example, when such reactions involve the skin, the characteristic local reaction is swelling and edema (**hives**). When the localized manifestations of immediate hypersensitivity involve the upper respiratory tract and conjunctiva, causing sneezing and conjunctivitis, we speak of **hay fever.** In its generalized, most severe form, namely the **anaphylactic syndrome**, an immediate hypersensitivity reaction is associated with bronchial constriction, airway obstruction, and circulatory collapse.

□ Pathogenesis: **The mechanism involved in all type I hypersensitivity reactions is related to the formation of IgE antibody.** These antibodies are

TABLE 4-1. Classification of Hypersensitivity Reactions

Type	Immunologic Mechanism	Examples
Type I (anaphylactic type): immediate hypersensitivity	IgE antibody-mediated mast cell activation and degranulation	"Hay fever" asthma, anaphylaxis
Type II (cytotoxic type): cytotoxic antibodies	Cytotoxic (IgG, IgM) antibodies formed against cell surface antigens. Complement is usually involved.	Autoimmune hemolytic anemias, ADCG, Goodpasture disease
Type III (immune complex type): immune complex disease	Antibodies (IgG, IgM, IgA) formed against exogenous or endogenous antigens. Complement and leukocytes (neutrophils, macrophages) are often involved	Autoimmune diseases (SLE, rheumatoid arthritis), most types of glomerulonephritis
Type IV (cell-mediated type): delayed-type hypersensitivity	Mononuclear cells (T lymphocytes, macrophages) with interleukin and lymphokine production	Granulomatous disease (tuberculosis, sarcoidosis)

formed by a CD4+, Th2 T cell-dependent mechanism and bind avidly to Fc receptors on mast cells and basophils. A person exposed to a specific allergen that has resulted in the formation of IgE is **sensitized;** that is, subsequent responses to the allergen induce the immediate hypersensitivity reaction. Once IgE antibodies are formed, re-exposure to the antigen often results in production of additional IgE antibodies rather than formation of other antibody classes, such as IgG or IgM ("isotype switching"). It should also be stressed that IgE bound to receptors on mast cells and basophils persists for weeks, a feature unique to IgE. Binding of the antigen-IgE complex to the IgE receptor activates mast cells and basophils, an event that, in turn, releases the potent inflammatory mediators responsible for development of the hypersensitivity reactions.

Cells can also be activated by agents other than antibodies. As shown in Figure 4-4, the complement anaphylatoxin peptides, C3a and C5a, directly stimulate mast cells by a different receptor-mediated process to cause release of granule constituents or rapid synthesis and release of other mediators. Of the granule constituents, histamine is perhaps the most important. In the lung, histamine is responsible for the classic early manifestations of immediate hypersensitivity, namely bronchospasm, vascular congestion, and edema.

Other preformed products released from mast cell granules are heparin, proteolytic enzymes, and at least two chemotactic factors, namely a neutrophil chemotactic factor and an eosinophil chemotactic factor. The latter is responsible for the accumulation of eosinophils, a characteristic effect of immediate hypersensitivity.

When the mast cell is activated, the synthesis of potent inflammatory mediators is also initiated. Foremost among these are the various products of the arachidonic acid pathway, which include prostaglandins, thromboxane, and leukotrienes. Stimulated mast cells also synthesize platelet-activating factor.

Summary

The type I (immediate) hypersensitivity reaction is characterized by a specific antibody (IgE) that binds to receptors on basophils and mast cells and that reacts with a specific antigen. This results in the activation of mast cells and basophils, which then release preformed (granule) products and synthesize mediators that cause the classic manifestations of immediate hypersensitivity.

Type II Hypersensitivity (Cytotoxic Type)

■ *Type II hypersensitivity* is caused by IgG and IgM cytotoxic antibodies directed against antigens on cell surfaces or in connective tissues. IgG and IgM are the classes of antibody usually involved in these reactions. The most important characteristic of these antibodies is their ability to activate the complement system through Fc receptors.

Complement-Mediated Cytotoxicity

The classic model of antibody-mediated cytotoxicity directed against erythrocytes is illustrated in Figure 4-5. IgM or IgG antibody binds to an antigen on the surface of the erythrocyte membrane. As discussed in Chapter 2, this antibody binding induces activation of the complement system through the classical pathway. Once activated, complement leads to destruction of the target cell by two distinct mechanisms.

Direct Lysis. Complement products directly lyse the target cells by formation of a complex of C5b-9 complement components, referred to as the **membrane attack complex**. This molecule inserts into the plasma membrane and forms "holes" or ionic channels, thereby destroying the permeability barrier and inducing lysis of the cell. Direct complement-mediated cell

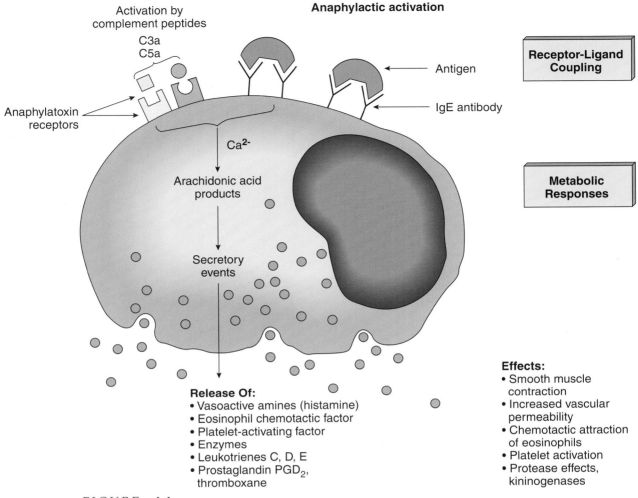

Receptor-Ligand Coupling

Metabolic Responses

Release Of:
- Vasoactive amines (histamine)
- Eosinophil chemotactic factor
- Platelet-activating factor
- Enzymes
- Leukotrienes C, D, E
- Prostaglandin PGD$_2$, thromboxane

Effects:
- Smooth muscle contraction
- Increased vascular permeability
- Chemotactic attraction of eosinophils
- Platelet activation
- Protease effects, kininogenases

FIGURE 4-4
Type I hypersensitivity. Activation of the mast cells and the potent inflammatory mediators released or synthesized by the cell.

lysis is exemplified by certain types of autoimmune hemolytic anemias that involve the formation of cold-reactive antibodies against erythrocyte blood group antigens. In transfusion reactions that result from major blood group incompatibilities, hemolysis occurs, because the activation of complement leads to erythrocyte destruction.

Opsonization. Complement also indirectly enhances destruction of a target cell by opsonization, a process in which complement interaction on the target cell surface leads to the formation of C3b (Fig. 4-6). Many phagocytic cells, including neutrophils and macrophages, express receptors for C3b on their cell membranes. By binding to its receptor, C3b connects the effector (phagocytic) cell to the target cell, thereby enhancing destruction of the complement-coated cell and phagocytosis of the debris. Certain types of autoimmune hemolytic anemias and some drug reactions

are mediated by this type of complement-associated opsonization.

Antibody-Dependent, Cell-Mediated Cytotoxicity (ADCC). There is another type of antibody-mediated cytotoxicity that does not require participation of the complement system. ADCC involves cell-destroying leukocytes that attack antibody-coated target cells through Fc receptors. Phagocytic cells and null or killer lymphocytes are the effector cells in this process. ADCC may be involved in the pathogenesis of some autoimmune diseases (e.g., autoimmune thyroiditis).

Antibody-Mediated Functional Changes

In some type II reactions, antibody binding to a specific target cell receptor does not lead to death of the cell but rather to physiologic changes. As shown in Figure 4-7, the autoimmune diseases myasthenia gravis and

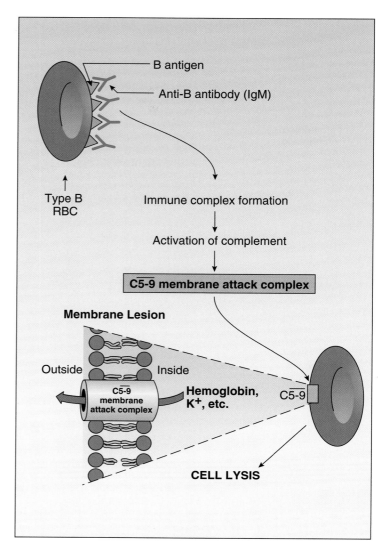

FIGURE *4-5*
Type II hypersensitivity. Antibody- and comple-ment-mediated red blood cell lysis due to comple-ment activation and the formation of the C5b-9 mem-brane attack complex (MAC).

Graves disease (hyperthyroidism) feature autoanti-bodies against hormone receptors. In Graves disease, the autoantibody against the thyroid-stimulating hor-mone (TSH) receptor mimics the effect of TSH, thereby stimulating thyroid acinar cells. By contrast, in myas-thenia gravis, the autoantibody competes with acetyl-choline for the acetylcholine receptor in the neuromus-cular end plate, thereby inhibiting synaptic transmission.

Antibody-Mediated Connective Tissue Injury

Some type II hypersensitivity reactions result from the formation of antibody against a connective tissue com-ponent. Classic examples are Goodpasture syndrome and the bullous skin diseases pemphigus and pem-phigoid. In these diseases, circulating antibody binds to a fixed connective tissue antigen, thereby evoking a local inflammatory response. In Goodpasture disease (Fig. 4-

8), an autoantibody binds to an antigen(s) in pulmonary and glomerular basement membranes. Local comple-ment activation recruits neutrophils into the site, result-ing in both lung hemorrhage and glomerulonephritis.

Summary

Type II hypersensitivity reactions are directly or indi-rectly cytotoxic and involve the formation of antibod-ies against antigens on cell surfaces or in connective tis-sues. Complement is required for many of these cytotoxic events. Lysis is mediated directly by comple-ment or indirectly by opsonization or the chemotactic attraction of phagocytic cells. Complement-indepen-dent reactions, such as ADCC, also fall into this cate-gory. Many human diseases, including autoimmune hemolytic anemias, Goodpasture syndrome, pemphi-gus and pemphigoid, Graves disease, and myasthenia gravis, are mediated by type II hypersensitivity reac-tions.

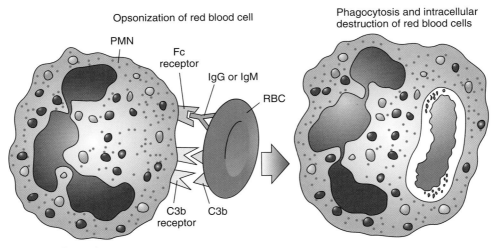

FIGURE 4-6
Type II hypersensitivity. Antibody-dependent and complement-dependent opsonization. Immunoglobulins and complement coating the surface of red blood cells (opsonization) bind to receptors on the surface of polymorphonuclear leukocytes, thereby facilitating phagocytosis.

Type III Hypersensitivity (Immune Complex Diseases)

■ *Type III hypersensitivity reactions* involve tissue injury mediated by immune complexes.

☐ **Pathogenesis:** IgM, IgG, or IgA is formed against a circulating antigen or one that is present in tissues. Antigen-antibody complexes formed in the circulation are then deposited in tissues, including the renal glomerulus, skin venules, choroid plexus, lung, and synovium. Once deposited, immune complexes call forth an inflammatory response by activating complement, thereby leading to chemotactic recruitment of neutrophils and macrophages to the site. These inflammatory cells are then activated and release their tissue-damaging mediators, such as proteases and oxygen radicals.

A convincing example of type III hypersensitivity is periarteritis nodosa associated with hepatitis B, in

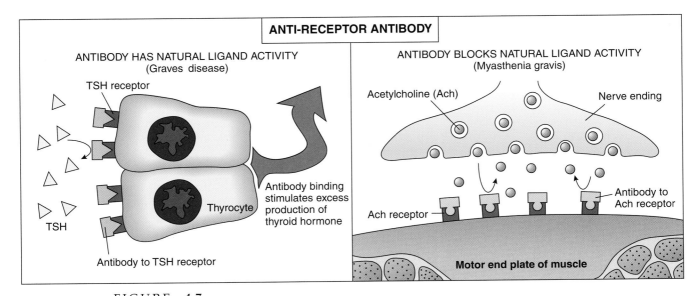

FIGURE 4-7
Type II hypersensitivity. Noncytotoxic antireceptor antibodies in Graves disease and myasthenia gravis. Binding of the antibody to the TSH receptor in Graves disease results in hyperthyroidism, whereas inhibition of synaptic transmission in myasthenia gravis leads to profound muscle weakness.

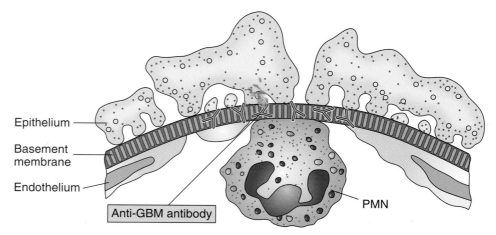

FIGURE *4-8*
Type II hypersensitivity. Antibody against glomerular basement membrane antigens in Goodpasture disease. The binding of antibody to antigens of basement membrane activates complement, thereby recruiting polymorphonuclear leukocytes and provoking tissue injury.

Epithelium

Basement membrane

Endothelium

Anti-GBM antibody

PMN

which medium-size arteries contain immune complexes of IgG and the hepatitis B virus antigen (HbsAg) in the vessel wall. **Diseases that seem to be most clearly attributable to the deposition of immune complexes are autoimmune diseases of connective tissue, such as systemic lupus erythematosus and rheumatoid arthritis, some types of vasculitis, and most varieties of glomerulonephritis.**

Serum Sickness

■ *Serum sickness is an acute, self-limited disease that occurs 6 to 8 days after the injection of a foreign protein (bovine albumin) and is characterized by fever, arthralgias, vasculitis, and an acute glomerulonephritis.* As shown in Figure 4-9, the levels of exogenously injected antigen in the circulation remain constant until approximately day 6, at which time they fall rapidly. At the same time, immune complexes (containing IgM or IgG and the antigen) appear in the circulation. Simultaneously, some of these circulating immune complexes begin to deposit in tissues such as the renal glomeruli and blood vessels.

Once immune complexes are deposited in tissues, they induce an inflammatory response. Experimental injury associated with serum sickness, such as that seen in the renal glomerulus, mimics the histologic appearance of many types of human glomerulonephritis.

Arthus Reaction

■ *The Arthus reaction is an experimental vasculitis model in which a localized injury is induced by immune complexes* (Fig. 4-10). This reaction is classically seen in the dermal blood vessels after local injection of an antigen to which the animal has been previously sensitized (against which it has circulating antibody). The circulating antibody and locally injected antigen form immune complex deposits in the walls of small blood vessels. The ensuing vascular injury is mediated by

complement activation, followed by recruitment and stimulation of neutrophils. Histologically, the affected vessels show numerous neutrophils and evidence of damage to the vessel, with edema and hemorrhage into the surrounding tissue.

Several experimental models of immune complex damage allow a precise definition of the mediator involved in this type of injury. Foremost among these models is acute serum sickness in the rabbit. In addition, the presence of fibrin in the vessel wall creates the classic appearance of an immune complex–induced vasculitis, which is referred to as **fibrinoid necrosis.** This experimental model of localized vasculitis is the prototype for many forms of vasculitis seen in humans (e.g., the cutaneous vasculitides present in drug reactions).

Summary

The type III hypersensitivity reaction is a type of immune complex–mediated injury in which antigen-antibody complexes, which are not organ specific, are formed in the circulation and deposited mainly in the tissues. These complexes then induce a localized inflammatory response by activating the complement system, thereby attracting neutrophils and macrophages. Activation of these cells by the immune complexes is directly responsible for the injury. **Many human disorders, including autoimmune diseases such as systemic lupus erythematosus and most types of glomerulonephritis, appear to be mediated by type III hypersensitivity reactions.**

Type IV Hypersensitivity (Cell-Mediated Immunity)

■ *Cell-mediated hypersensitivity is an antigen-elicited cellular immune reaction that results in tissue damage but does not require the participation of antibodies.*

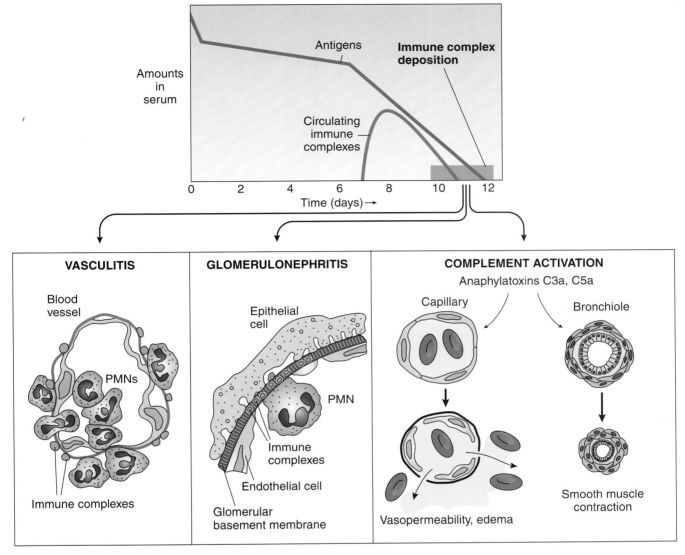

FIGURE *4-9*
Type III hypersensitivity. In the serum sickness model of immune complex tissue injury, antibody is produced against a circulating antigen, and immune complexes form in the blood. These complexes deposit in tissues such as blood vessels and glomeruli and, augmented by complement activation, induce tissue injury or dysfunctional responses.

Delayed-Type Hypersensitivity

■ *Delayed-type hypersensitivity is classically defined as a tissue reaction, primarily involving lymphocytes and mononuclear phagocytes, that occurs in response to subcutaneous injection of a soluble antigen and that reaches greatest intensity 24 to 48 hours after injection.* A naturally occurring example of this reaction is the contact sensitivity response to poison ivy.

Figure 4-11 summarizes the main stages of the delayed-type hypersensitivity reaction. In the initial phase, foreign protein antigens or chemical ligands in-teract with macrophages bearing class II HLA-D molecules. Protein antigens are processed by macrophages and then presented in conjunction with HLA-D molecules. By contrast, chemical ligands interact directly with membrane proteins. In either case, the foreign antigens are then recognized by antigen-specific T lymphocytes. The latter are called T-effector or delayed hypersensitivity cells, and they usually have the CD4 phenotype. These cells become activated and synthesize a spectrum of lymphokines, which, in turn, recruit and activate lymphocytes, monocytes, fibroblasts, and other inflammatory cells.

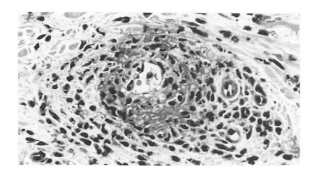

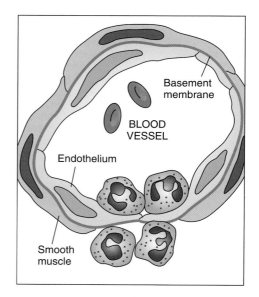

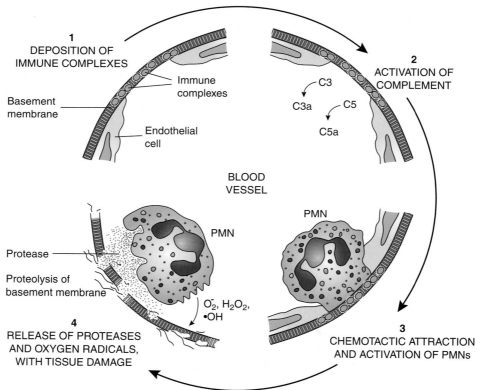

FIGURE   *4-10*
Type III hypersensitivity. Localized immune complex-induced vasculitis in the Arthus reaction is depicted. The deposition of immune complexes in the vessel wall leads to localized complement activation and recruitment of polymorphonuclear leukocytes, as shown in the photomicrograph. The leukocytes produce injury to the vessel wall, with edema and fibrin deposition.

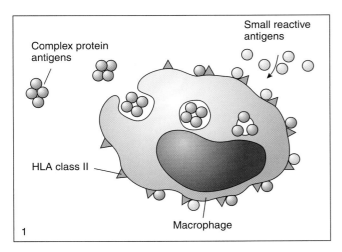

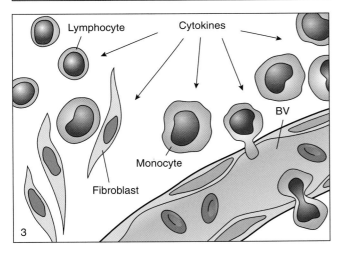

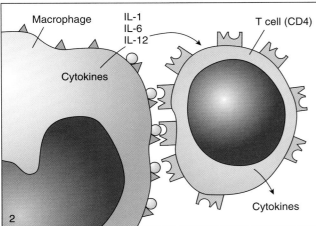

FIGURE *4-11*
Delayed-type hypersensitivity reaction. (Panel 1) Complex antigens are phagocytosed and "processed" by macrophages, then presented on the membrane complexed with class II (Ia) antigens. By contrast, chemically reactive ligands bind directly to macrophage membrane proteins. (Panel 2) Antigen-specific T cells recognize the membrane protein-antigen complexes and receive growth-promoting signals (monokines), such as IL-1, from macrophages. T cells then become activated and begin the synthesis and secretion of molecular mediators (lymphokines). (Panel 3) The lymphokines and monokines recruit additional inflammatory cells and initiate local cellular proliferation and activation.

Figure 4-12 summarizes the events in T cell-mediated cytotoxicity. In contrast to delayed hypersensitivity reactions, cytotoxic or killer T cells simultaneously interact with both the target antigen and class I MHC antigens. Self-MHC antigens of virus-infected cells or tumor cells are recognized in addition to the viral antigens or tumor neoantigens. In graft rejection, foreign MHC antigens are potent activators of T-killer cells, which bear the CD8 phenotype marker. Once activated by the antigenic stimulus, the proliferation of these T-killer cells is promoted by helper or amplifier cells and is mediated by soluble growth factors such as IL-2. An expanded population of antigen-specific killer cells is thus generated for attacking target cells. The killer cell binds to the target cell and delivers a molecular signal that disrupts the permeability barrier of the target membrane.

NK Cell-Mediated Cytotoxicity

The defining characteristics of NK cells have been described, but the extent to which such cells participate in tissue-damaging immune reactions is unclear. Mounting evidence, however, indicates that they exert both effector and immunoregulatory functions.

Figure 4-13 summarizes the events of target-cell killing by NK cells. Unlike killer T cells, NK cells bear receptors that recognize antigens on a variety of target cells. The target antigens are membrane glycoproteins that are expressed by certain virus-infected cells or tumor cells. In a series of events similar to that described for killer T cells, NK cells bind to the target cell and deliver a molecular signal that results in its lysis. NK cells also have membrane Fc receptors. Thus, they acquire antibodies that allow for the binding and killing of target cells by an antibody-directed mechanism (ADCC).

Summary

The type IV hypersensitivity reaction, unlike the other types of hypersensitivity reactions, is not an antibody-

T Cell-Mediated Cytotoxicity

Another mechanism by which T cells effect tissue damage is the direct cytolysis of target cells. This immune mechanism is important for the elimination of virus-infected cells and tumor cells that express neoantigens. Cytotoxic T cells also play an important role in graft or transplant rejection.

Immunopathology

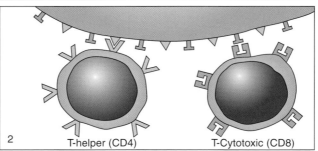

TARGET CELLS

Viral	HLA	Tumor

1

TARGET ANTIGENS
- Virally-coded membrane antigen
- Foreign or modified histocompatibility antigen
- Tumor-specific membrane antigens

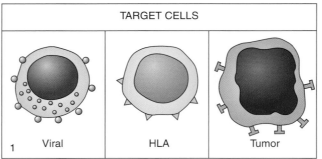

T-helper (CD4)   T-Cytotoxic (CD8)

2

RECOGNITION OF ANTIGEN BY T CELLS
- T-helper cells recognize antigen plus class II molecules
- T-cytotoxic/killer cells recognize antigen plus class I molecules

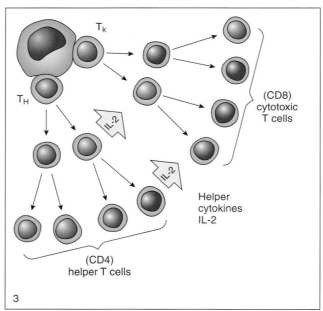

T_k

T_H

IL-2

IL-2

(CD8) cytotoxic T cells

Helper cytokines IL-2

(CD4) helper T cells

3

ACTIVATION AND AMPLIFICATION
- T-helper cells activate and proliferate, releasing helper molecules (e.g., IL-2)
- T-cytotoxic/killer cells proliferate in response to helper molecules

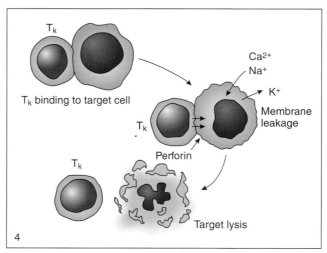

T_k

T_k binding to target cell

T_k

Ca^{2+}
Na^+
K^+
Membrane leakage

Perforin

T_k

Target lysis

4

TARGET CELL KILLING
- T-cytotoxic/killer cells bind to target cell
- Killing signals perforin release and target cell loses membrane integrity
- Target cell undergoes lysis

FIGURE *4-13*
Natural killer (NK) cell-mediated cytotoxicity. (Panel 1) Potential targets of NK cells include virally infected cells and tumor cells. (Panel 2) Recognition of antigen. NK cells bear receptors for a variety of membrane glycoproteins, allowing for cell-cell binding. (Panel 3) Following binding, the NK cell delivers the killer signal. The target cell sodium-potassium pump is disrupted, and the target cell is lysed.

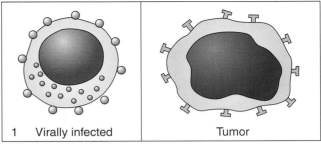

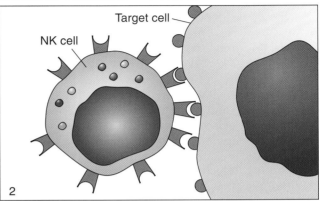

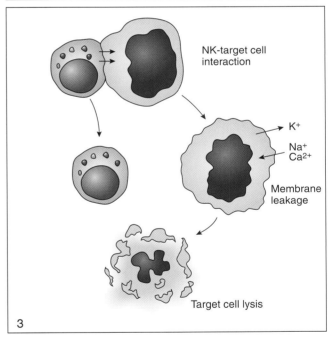

mediated response. Rather, antigens are processed by macrophages and presented to antigen-specific T lymphocytes. These lymphocytes become activated and then release a variety of mediators, or lymphokines, that recruit and activate lymphocytes, macrophages, and fibroblasts. The resulting injury is caused by the T lymphocytes themselves, the macrophages, or both. The chronic inflammation of a wide variety of presumably autoimmune diseases, such as chronic thyroiditis, Sjögren syndrome, and primary biliary cirrhosis, are examples of type IV hypersensitivity reactions.

IMMUNE REACTIONS TO TRANSPLANTED ORGANS AND TISSUES

Histocompatibility antigens are the critical immunogenic molecules that stimulate rejection of transplanted organs.

Host-Versus-Graft Reactions

The histopathologic features of graft rejection are well demonstrated in renal allografts. Three major types of rejection, categorized according to the time of onset of the rejection episode and the corresponding histologic features, have been described (Fig. 4-14).

Hyperacute Rejection. This reaction occurs within minutes to hours after transplantation. It is manifested clinically as a sudden cessation of urine output accompanied by fever and pain in the area of the graft site. It necessitates prompt resection of the kidney. The histologic features of hyperacute rejection within the trans-

FIGURE *4-12*
T cell-mediated cytotoxicity. (Panel 1) Potential target cells of T cells include virally infected cells, histoincompatible cells (e.g., transplanted organ), and tumor cells expressing neoantigens. (Panel 2) T cells recognize foreign antigens and class I histocompatibility antigens. (Panel 3) T cells become activated and begin to proliferate. T-helper cells release lymphokines that amplify proliferation. (Panel 4) T-killer cell binds to target cell and delivers a signal, resulting in disruption of the sodium-potassium pump. The target cell is then lysed.

planted kidney are (1) vascular congestion, (2) fibrin-platelet thrombi within capillaries, (3) neutrophilic vasculitis with fibrinoid necrosis, (4) prominent interstitial edema, and (5) neutrophilic infiltrates. This rapid form of rejection is mediated by **preformed** antibodies and products of complement activation.

Acute Rejection. Acute rejection occurs in the first few weeks or months after transplantation. Clinically, there is a sudden onset of azotemia and oliguria, which may be associated with fever and graft tenderness. The microscopic findings of acute graft rejection include (1) interstitial infiltrates of lymphocytes and macrophages, (2) edema, (3) lymphocytic tubulitis, and (4) tubular necrosis. The most severe form also shows vascular damage manifested as arteritis, fibrinoid necrosis, and thrombosis. Acute rejection likely involves both cell-mediated and humoral mechanisms of tissue damage.

Chronic Rejection. The transplanted kidney may undergo rejection several months to years after transplantation. Clinically, the patient develops progressive azotemia, oliguria, hypertension, and weight gain. The dominant features of chronic rejection are (1) arterial and arteriolar intimal thickening, causing stenosis or obstruction; (2) thick glomerular capillary walls; (3) tubular atrophy; and (4) interstitial fibrosis. The interstitium also often has scattered mononuclear infiltrates and tubules containing proteinaceous casts.

Graft-Versus-Host Reactions

Bone marrow transplantation to bone marrow-depleted or immunodeficient patients may result in graft versus host disease (GVD). In this condition, immunocompetent lymphocytes in the grafted marrow reject the host tissues. GVD also occurs when immunodeficient patients are transfused with blood products containing HLA-incompatible lymphocytes.

In GVD, the skin and intestine reveal mononuclear cell infiltrates and epithelial cell necrosis. The liver shows periportal inflammation, damaged bile ducts, and liver cell injury. Clinically, GVD manifests as rash, diarrhea, abdominal cramps, anemia, and liver dysfunction. A chronic form of GVD is characterized by dermal sclerosis, sicca syndrome (dry eyes and dry mouth secondary to chronic inflammation of the lacrimal and salivary glands), and immunodeficiency. Treatment of GVD requires immunosuppressive therapy.

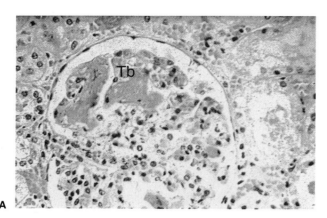

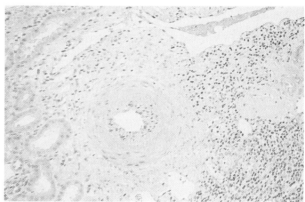

FIGURE *4-14*
Histologic features of major forms of renal transplant rejection. (A) Hyperacute rejection occurs in minutes to hours after transplant. This glomerulus shows intravascular fibrin-platelet thrombi and infiltrates of polymorphonuclear leukocytes. There is interstitial edema of surrounding tissue. *Tb*, thrombi. (B) Acute cellular rejection occurs within weeks to months after transplant. There is infiltration by mononuclear leukocytes with associated tubular damage. The small artery in the middle of the photo is also infiltrated, indicating vasculitis. (C) Chronic rejection is observed months to years after transplant. There is extensive deposition of fibrous tissue (blue) between tubules and around glomeruli. Tubules show atrophy and there are patchy interstitial infiltrates of mononuclear cells. Glomerular capillary walls are focally thickened.

IMMMUNODEFICIENCY DISEASES

Deficiencies of Antibody-Producing Cells (B Cells)

Congenital X-Linked Infantile Hypogammaglobulinemia. Also termed **Bruton disease,** this disorder is observed in male infants at 5 to 6 months of age, the time when maternal antibody levels begin to decline. The infant presents with recurrent pyogenic infections, severe hypogammaglobulinemia, and an absence of mature B cells in the peripheral blood. Pre-B cells, however, can be detected. **Thus, congenital X-linked hypogammaglobulinemia is caused by a defect early in the maturation of B cells** (see Fig. 4-1, step 2). An inactivating mutation of the gene for a B-cell tyrosine kinase is responsible for the disease.

Common Variable Immunodeficiency. Common variable immunodeficiency is characterized by a severe hypogammaglobulinemia (IgG) in which patients present with recurrent severe pyogenic infections, especially pneumonia and diarrhea, with the latter often resulting from *Giardia lamblia*. The mean age at onset is 30 years. A remarkable incidence of malignant disease is seen in common variable immunodeficiency, including a 50-fold increase in stomach cancer and a high incidence of lymphoma, especially in women. These patients are also susceptible to a variety of autoimmune disorders. Common variable immunodeficiency actually reflects a variety of maturational and regulatory defects of the immune system. Thus, this disorder probably represents several diseases rather than one.

Selective IgA Deficiency. An inadequate amount of IgA is the most common immunodeficiency syndrome, occurring in one of every 700 persons. Those with IgA deficiency are asymptomatic or present with respiratory or gastrointestinal infections of varying severity. There is also a strong predilection for allergies and collagen vascular diseases. Patients with IgA deficiency have normal numbers of IgA-bearing B cells, and their defect seems to be an inability to synthesize and secrete IgA (see Fig. 4-1, step 4).

Deficiencies of Cell-Mediated (T-Cell) Immunity

DiGeorge Syndrome. DiGeorge syndrome is one of the most severe forms of deficient T-cell immunity. The disease usually presents in infants with congenital heart defects and severe hypocalcemia (due to hypoparathyroidism) and is recognized shortly after birth. Infants who survive the neonatal period are subject to recurrent or chronic viral, bacterial, fungal, and protozoal infections. **DiGeorge syndrome is caused by defective embryologic development of the third and fourth pharyngeal pouches, which become the thymus and the parathyroid glands.** In the absence of a thymus, T-cell maturation is interrupted at the pre-T cell stage (see Fig. 4-1, stage A). Most patients have a point deletion in the long arm of chromosome 22.

Chronic Mucocutaneous Candidiasis. This congenital defect in T-cell function is characterized by susceptibility to candidal infections and is associated with an endocrinopathy (hypoparathyroidism, Addison disease, diabetes mellitus). Although most T-cell functions are intact, there is a defective response to *Candida* antigens.

Combined T-Cell and B-Cell Deficiencies

Severe Combined Immunodeficiency. This disease of both T and B lymphocytes is characterized by recurrent viral, bacterial, fungal, and protozoal infections. A virtually complete absence of T cells is associated with severe hypogammaglobulinemia. The disease occurs in X-linked and autosomal recessive (Swiss-type) forms, typically appearing at approximately 6 months of age.

Adenosine Deaminase Deficiency. This enzyme defect caused by mutations of the adenosine deaminase gene on chomosome 20q13, is present in approximately half of patients with the autosomal recessive form of combined immunodeficiency.

Wiskott-Aldrich Syndrome. This rare X-linked disorder is characterized by (1) recurrent infections, (2) hemorrhages secondary to thrombocytopenia, and (3) eczema. It typically presents within the first few months of life. Both cellular and humoral immunity are impaired. The Wiskott-Aldrich syndrome is caused by numerous mutations in a gene on the X chromosome, which encodes an effector for a GTPase that is important in maintaining a number of cell functions, including that of the actin cytoskeleton. A characteristic feature of this disorder is impaired CD43 glycoprotein expression on lymphocytes. Interestingly, Wiskott-Aldrich syndrome is the only immunologic disease characterized by complete failure to produce antibodies to an entire class of antigens, namely polysaccharides.

Acquired Immunodeficiency Syndrome

■ *Acquired immunodeficiency syndrome (AIDS) is a fatal, chronic disease caused by the human immunodeficiency virus (HIV)-1 and -2 and is characterized by a variety of immunologic defects, the most devastating of which is the complete loss of cellular immunity.* The vast majority of AIDS cases represent infection with HIV-1. As a result of HIV infection, catastrophic opportunistic infections are virtually inevitable. **The fundamental lesion in AIDS is infection of CD4+ (helper) T lymphocytes by HIV, leading to depletion of this cell population and consequent impaired immune function.** As a result, patients with AIDS usually die of opportunistic infections. There is also a high incidence of malignant tumors associated with AIDS, principally **B-cell lymphomas** and **Kaposi sarcoma.** Finally, infection of the central nervous system with HIV often leads to a form of encephalopathy termed **AIDS dementia complex.**

Transmission of HIV

AIDS is transmitted principally as a venereal disease, both homosexually and heterosexually. The infection is also transmitted directly through blood or blood products, as in intravenous drug abusers and transfusion recipients. HIV has also been isolated from semen, vaginal secretions, breast milk, and cerebrospinal fluid. Except for cerebrospinal fluid, occurrence of HIV in these fluids reflects the presence of lymphocytes.

Among homosexual men, the receptive partner in anal intercourse is at particularly high risk of becoming infected with HIV. The virus is transmitted from semen through tears in the rectal mucosa. It is also possible that HIV can infect the epithelial cells of the rectum directly. In heterosexual contact, transmission from male to female is more likely than the reverse, perhaps reflecting the greater concentration of HIV in semen than in vaginal fluids.

☐ **Pathogenesis:** The etiologic agent of AIDS (HIV-1) is an enveloped RNA retrovirus that contains a reverse transcriptase (RNA-dependent DNA polymerase). The RNA core is enveloped by a phospholipid bilayer that contains virally encoded glycoproteins (gp120 and gp41). The specific target cell for HIV-1 is the CD4+ T lymphocyte, although infection of other cells, such as B lymphocytes, macrophages, glial cells, and intestinal epithelial cells, has been described. The replicative life cycle of HIV-1 is shown in Figure 4-15.

The mechanism by which HIV kills infected T lymphocytes is still poorly understood. Whatever the mechanism, however, there is a clear association between increasing amounts of viral burden and decline in the CD4+ lymphocyte counts.

Immunology of AIDS

The destruction of CD4+ T cells by HIV-1 constitutes an attack on the Achilles heel of the entire immune system, because this subset of lymphocytes exerts critical regulatory and effector functions that involve both cellular and humoral immunity. **Thus, in the typical patient with AIDS, all the elements of the immune system are eventually perturbed, including T cells, B cells, NK cells, and monocytes/macrophages.**

T Cells. CD4+ lymphocytes include two functional types, namely helper and amplifier (or inducer) cells. Eventually, total CD4 counts fall to less than 500 cells/μL, and the helper:suppressor T-cell ratio declines from a normal of 2.0 to as little as 0.50. **The patient with AIDS cannot generate the antigen-specific, cytotoxic T cells that are required for the clearance of viruses and other infectious agents.**

B Cells. In persons infected with HIV, humoral immunity is also abnormal. Production of antibodies in response to specific antigenic stimulation is markedly decreased, often to less than 10% of normal. B cells also demonstrate a decreased proliferative response in vitro to mitogens and antigens. The lack of CD4+ lymphocytes impairs the proliferation of cytotoxic T cells that normally would eliminate B cells infected with Epstein-Barr virus. This defect contributes to the development of lymphoma in patients with AIDS.

NK Cells. NK cell activity is severely decreased in patients with AIDS. Because these cells kill both virus-infected and tumor cells, this defect may also contribute to the appearance of malignant tumors and the viral infections that plague these patients.

Monocytes/Macrophages. Macrophages are infected with HIV-1 and may serve as a reservoir for dissemination of the virus. Unlike T lymphocytes, which are killed by HIV, infected macrophages display little, if any, cytotoxicity. However, they do show impaired phagocytosis of immune complexes and opsonized particles, decreased chemotaxis, and impaired responses to antigenic challenges.

☐ **Pathology and Clinical Features:** Persons infected with HIV begin with an acute, self-limited illness and, months to years later, culminate in fulminant immunodeficiency and its fatal complications (Fig. 4-16).

Acute HIV Infection. Two to 3 weeks after exposure to HIV, and before the appearance of antibodies against HIV, infected persons often present with an acute illness that resembles infectious mononucleosis. Most of these symptoms resolve within 2 to 3 weeks.

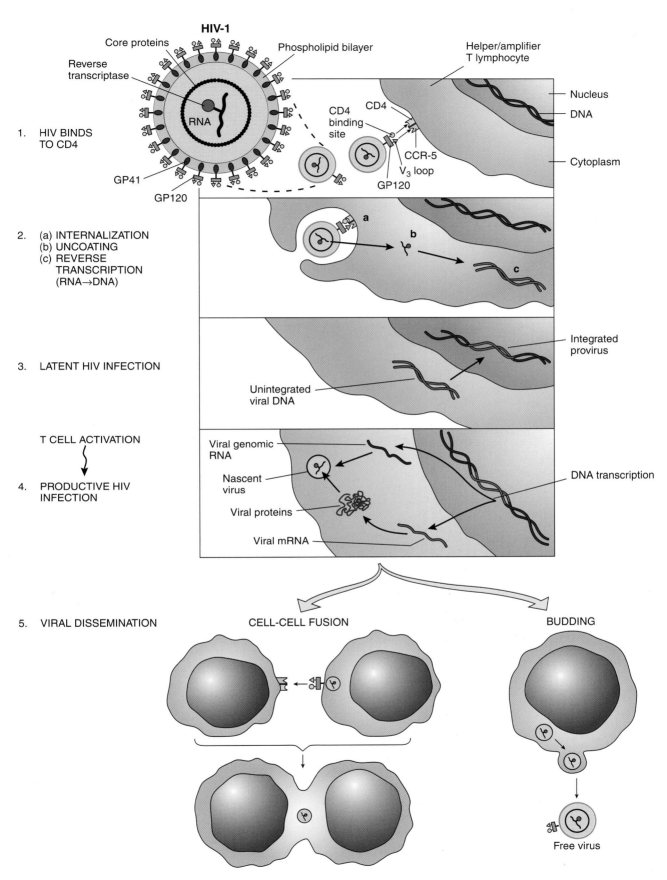

FIGURE 4-15
Life cycle of HIV-1.

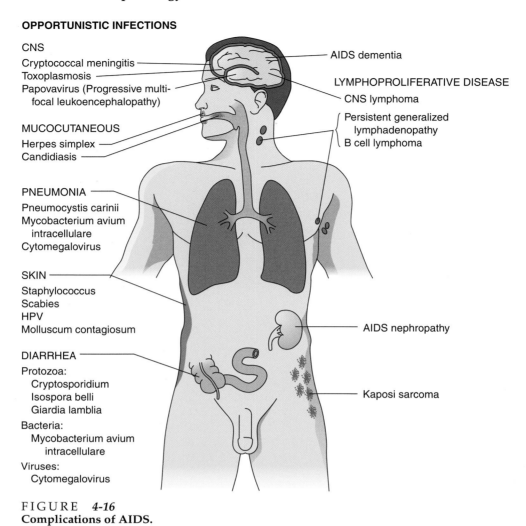

OPPORTUNISTIC INFECTIONS

CNS
Cryptococcal meningitis
Toxoplasmosis
Papovavirus (Progressive multi-
    focal leukoencephalopathy)

MUCOCUTANEOUS
Herpes simplex
Candidiasis

PNEUMONIA
Pneumocystis carinii
Mycobacterium avium
    intracellulare
Cytomegalovirus

SKIN
Staphylococcus
Scabies
HPV
Molluscum contagiosum

DIARRHEA
Protozoa:
    Cryptosporidium
    Isospora belli
    Giardia lamblia
Bacteria:
    Mycobacterium avium
        intracellulare
Viruses:
    Cytomegalovirus

AIDS dementia

LYMPHOPROLIFERATIVE DISEASE
CNS lymphoma

Persistent generalized
    lymphadenopathy
B cell lymphoma

AIDS nephropathy

Kaposi sarcoma

FIGURE   4-16
Complications of AIDS.

Seroconversion occurs 1 to 10 weeks after the onset of this acute illness.

Persistent Generalized Lymphadenopathy. Palpable lymphadenopathy occurs at two or more extrainguinal sites, persisting for longer than 3 months in persons infected with HIV. The most common sites of involvement are the axillary, inguinal, and posterior cervical nodes.

Progression to AIDS. Most persons infected with HIV exhibit viral antigens and antibodies within 6 months. **Viral replication remains at minimal levels for variable times (as long as 10 or more years), during which time the infected person is asymptomatic.** However, viral replication virtually always resumes at some time, and the number of helper T cells begins to decrease. Patients generally remain asymptomatic until the total number of CD4+ lymphocytes falls below 500 cells/μL, at which time symptoms begin to appear.

With CD4+ numbers of less than 150 cells/μL and CD4:CD8 ratios of less than 0.8, the disease progresses rapidly. A wide variety of bacteria, viruses, fungi, and protozoa attack the immunocompromised patient, Kaposi sarcoma and lymphoproliferative disorders may appear, and neurologic disease is common. AIDS has been uniformly fatal.

Opportunistic Infections. The diversity of infectious agents that ravage patients with AIDS reads like a textbook of microbiology:

- **Lungs.** The large majority of patients with AIDS suffers from opportunistic pulmonary infections. *Pneumocystis carinii* **pneumonia** occurs at some time in more than two-thirds of patients, and pulmonary infection with cytomegalovirus and *Mycobacterium avium-intracellulare* is common. Patients with AIDS are also susceptible to tuberculosis and *Legionella* infections.

- **Central Nervous System.** Cryptococcal meningitis is a devastating and usually fatal complication, representing 5% to 8% of all opportunistic infections in patients with AIDS. Toxoplasmosis of the brain is the most common cause of intracerebral mass lesions. Herpes encephalitis also occasionally complicates AIDS.
- **Gastrointestinal Tract.** Diarrhea is the single most common gastrointestinal symptom of AIDS, occurring in more than 75% of patients. The most frequent pathogens are protozoans, including *Cryptosporidium, Isospora belli,* and *Giardia. Mycobacterium avium-intracellulare* and *Salmonella* sp. are the most common bacterial causes of diarrhea in patients with AIDS.
- **Skin.** Virtually all patients with AIDS develop some form of skin disease, with infections being prominent causes. *Staphylococcus aureus* is the most common cutaneous bacterial offender, causing bullous impetigo, deeper purulent lesions (ecthyma), and folliculitis. Chronic mucocutaneous herpes simplex infection is so characteristic of AIDS that it is considered to be an index infection for establishing the diagnosis.

Neurologic Manifestations of AIDS. Postmortem studies of patients who died of AIDS have disclosed pathologic findings in more than three-fourths of the cases. Clinically, neurologic symptoms occur in 30% to 40% of patients. Direct infection of the brain with HIV leads to a subacute encephalopathy, also termed the **AIDS dementia complex.** Progressive multifocal leukoencephalopathy, reflecting infection with a papovavirus, is also a lethal complication.

AIDS-Associated Cancers. Kaposi sarcoma is an otherwise rare, multicentric, malignant neoplasm. It is characterized by cutaneous and, less commonly, visceral nodules in which endothelium-lined channels and vascular spaces are admixed with spindle-shaped cells. Patients with AIDS (particularly homosexual men rather than intravenous drug abusers) are at very high risk of developing Kaposi sarcoma. **In fact, the occurrence of Kaposi sarcoma in an otherwise healthy person younger than 60 years is considered to be strong evidence for the diagnosis of AIDS.** The cutaneous tumor in AIDS is commonly aggressive, often involving the gastrointestinal tract or lungs. Lung involvement frequently leads to death. Recent studies have incriminated a new strain of herpesvirus (HHV8) in all forms of Kaposi sarcoma. It seems that this virus is sexually transmitted, because almost all homosexual HIV carriers are infected.

Patients with AIDS are at substantial risk for the development of B-cell proliferative diseases. B-cell hyperplasia and generalized lymphadenopathy are common in patients infected with HIV and precede the appearance of malignant lymphoproliferative disease. HIV-associated lymphomas usually present as the large-cell variety, typically noted in other immunodeficient conditions, although a few small-cell lymphomas are encountered. A conspicuous feature of lymphomas associated with AIDS is the predilection for extranodal disease, particularly primary lymphomas of the brain. In addition, lymphomas of the gastrointestinal tract, liver, and bone marrow are frequent. The Epstein-Barr virus genome has been demonstrated in many of the lymphomas occurring with AIDS.

Other Acquired Immunodeficiencies

Acquired immunodeficiency states can be secondary to many conditions, including infections (viral, bacterial, and fungal), malnutrition, autoimmune diseases (systemic lupus erythematosus, rheumatoid arthritis), nephrotic syndrome, uremia, sarcoidosis, cancer, lymphomas, and treatment with immunosuppressive agents (e.g., radiation, corticosteroids, chemotherapy, cyclosporin A). **The widespread use of immunosuppressive agents is the main cause of immunodeficiency and the resulting increased risk for opportunistic infections.**

AUTOIMMUNITY

■ *Autoimmunity implies that an immune response has been generated against self-antigens (autoantigens) as a result of a breakdown in the ability of the immune system to differentiate between self- and nonself-antigens (loss of tolerance).* The normal development of anti-idiotype antibodies (antibodies against immunoglobulins), which serve as important regulatory proteins for the immune response, is, by definition, an autoimmune response. **Thus, the regulated production of autoantibodies is actually a normal event.** When these regulatory mechanisms are in some way deflected, the uncontrolled production of autoantibodies or the appearance of abnormal cell-cell recognition produces disease.

Theories of Autoimmunity

The most popular theories explaining the loss of tolerance in autoimmune disease are listed in Table 4-2.

Sequestered Antigens. Tissue antigens are usually contained within cells and are not exposed or released

TABLE 4-2. Postulated Mechanisms by Which Autoimmunity Develops

Mechanism	Examples
Release of sequestered antigens	Antibodies to spermatozoa, lens tissue, myelin
Abnormal T-cell function: diminished suppressor-cell function	Systemic lupus erythematosus and other autoimmune diseases
Enhanced helper-cell function	
Polyclonal B-cell activation	Drug-induced hemolytic anemias
	Systemic lupus erythematosus, other autoimmune diseases; Epstein-Barr virus-induced anti-DNA antibody

TABLE 4-3. Primary Organ System Involvement in Systemic Lupus Erythematosus

Organ System	Percentage of Cases	Characteristic Pathology
Joints	90	Nonerosive synovitis with neutrophils and mononuclear cells
Kidney	75	Immune complex glomerulonephritis, interstitial nephritis
Serosal membranes	35	Pleuritis, pericarditis, peritonitis secondary to immune complex deposition
Heart	45–50	Pericarditis, myocarditis, endocarditis

until some type of tissue injury occurs. When these antigens are released into the circulation, an immune response may develop. Examples of this type of response include antibodies against spermatozoa, lens tissue, and myelin. **Although autoantibodies may form against normally "sequestered antigens," there is little evidence that they are pathogenic.**

Abnormal T-Cell Function. Autoimmune reactions have been claimed to develop as a result of abnormalities in the T-lymphocyte system. Most immune responses require T-cell participation to activate antigen-specific B cells. Thus, alterations in the number or functional activities of helper or suppressor T cells would be expected to influence the ability of the host to mount an immune response. In fact, defects in T cells, particularly suppressor T cells, have been described in many autoimmune diseases. However, it is not clear whether these alterations in suppressor cell function are the primary cause of these diseases or merely a secondary response.

A possible mechanism by which helper T-cell tolerance of self-antigens may be overcome involves antibodies against foreign antigens that cross-react with self-antigens. An example is rheumatic heart disease, in which antibodies formed against streptococcal antigens cross-react with antigens from cardiac muscle in a process known as **biologic mimicry.**

Polyclonal B-Cell Activation. Another postulated mechanism to explain the loss of tolerance involves polyclonal B-cell activation, in which B lymphocytes are directly activated by complex substances that contain many antigenic sites (e.g., bacterial cell walls and viruses). **There is some evidence that polyclonal B-cell activation may be involved in the formation of autoantibodies.** The development of rheumatoid factor in rheumatoid arthritis, anti-DNA antibodies in lupus erythematosus, and other autoantibodies has been described after bacterial, viral, and parasitic infections.

Systemic Lupus Erythematosus

■ *Systemic lupus erythematosus (SLE) is a chronic, autoimmune, multisystemic inflammatory disease that may involve almost any organ but characteristically affects the kidneys, joints, serous membranes, and skin* (Table 4-3). It is the prototype of a systemic autoimmune disease in which autoantibodies are formed against a variety of self-antigens, including (1) plasma proteins (complement components and clotting factors), (2) cell surface antigens (lymphocytes, neutrophils, platelets, erythrocytes), (3) intracellular cytoplasmic components (microfilaments, microtubules, lysosomes, ribosomes, RNA), and (4) nuclear DNA, ribonucleoproteins, and histones. The most important diagnostic autoantibodies are those against nuclear antigens—in particular, antibody to double-stranded DNA and to the Sm antigen, a soluble nuclear antigen. These antinuclear antibodies are usually not directly cytotoxic. Tissue injury is caused by antigen-antibody complexes that form in the circulation and deposit in the tissues, creating the characteristic injury of **vasculitis, synovitis, and glomerulonephritis.** For this reason, SLE is considered to be the prototype of type III hypersensitivity reactions.

□ **Pathogenesis:** The cause of SLE is unknown. The characteristic feature of the disease—the presence of numerous autoantibodies, particularly antinuclear antibodies—suggests that there is a breakdown in the normal immune surveillance mechanisms. Presumably, this defect leads to a loss of normal self-tolerance.

Hormonal Factors. There is a clear female predisposition for SLE, with 90% of cases occurring in women between 12 and 40 years of age. For unknown reasons, this female predominance is true for all autoimmune diseases.

Genetic Factors. There appears to be some genetic predisposition to lupus, and a higher incidence is described in families and monozygotic twins. The incidence of lupus (and of the other autoimmune diseases) is higher among persons who express certain antigens of the MHC—in the case of lupus, DR2 and DR3.

Immunologic Abnormalities. Production of autoantibodies against nuclear antigens is characteristic of SLE. This immune response is linked to B-cell hyperreactivity, the major effector mechanism of this disease.

Type III Hypersensitivity. There is good reason to believe that the bulk of the injury in lupus is due to immune complexes formed against self, particularly against DNA. Although most of this multisystemic involvement in SLE can be traced to the deposition in tissues of the circulating, preformed immune complexes, under certain conditions the formation of immune complexes occurs in situ—that is, in the tissues rather than in the circulation. Examples include antibody formed against connective tissue components and, perhaps, the membranous form of lupus glomerulonephritis. Type II hypersensitivity reactions may also participate in lupus, because cytotoxic antibodies against leukocytes, erythrocytes, and platelets have been described. Current theories regarding the pathogenesis of SLE are outlined in Figure 4-17.

☐ **Pathology and Clinical Features:** Because circulating immune complexes deposit in almost all tissues, virtually every organ in the body can be involved. The organs with the most serious involvement by SLE are shown in Figure 4-18 and Table 4-3.

Skin. Skin involvement is common and is manifested by an erythematous rash in sun-exposed sites, with a "butterfly" malar rash being the most characteristic. Microscopically, the skin exhibits a perivascular lymphoid infiltrate and liquefactive degeneration of the basal cells.

Joints. Joint involvement is the most common manifestation of SLE, and more than 90% of patients have polyarthralgias. An inflammatory synovitis occurs, but unlike rheumatoid arthritis, there is usually no injury to the joint itself.

Kidneys. Renal involvement, in particular glomerulonephritis, is very common. Three-fourths of patients with SLE have evidence of renal disease at autopsy.

Serous Membranes. Involvement of the serous membranes is common in SLE. More than a third of patients have a pleuritis and a pleural effusion. Pericarditis and peritonitis occur less frequently.

Heart. Cardiac involvement is also frequent in SLE, although congestive heart failure is rare and, when present, is usually associated with a myocarditis. All layers of the heart may be involved, with pericarditis being the most common finding. Endocarditis, which is usually not clinically significant, is characterized by small, nonbacterial vegetations on the valve leaflets, termed **Libman-Sacks endocarditis.**

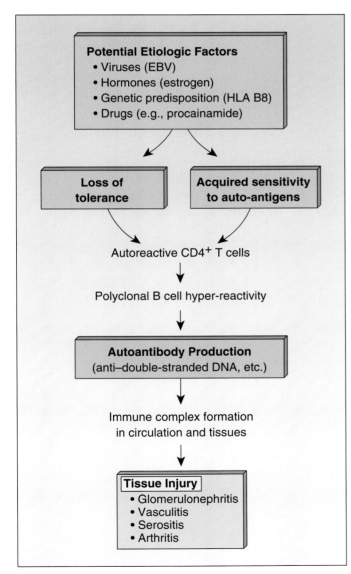

FIGURE *4-17*
Pathogenesis of systemic lupus erythematosus.

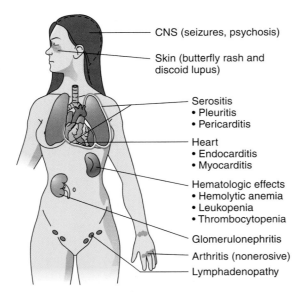

CNS (seizures, psychosis)

Skin (butterfly rash and discoid lupus)

Serositis
• Pleuritis
• Pericarditis

Heart
• Endocarditis
• Myocarditis

Hematologic effects
• Hemolytic anemia
• Leukopenia
• Thrombocytopenia

Glomerulonephritis

Arthritis (nonerosive)

Lymphadenopathy

FIGURE 4-18
Complications of systemic lupus erythematosus.

Brain. Involvement of the central nervous system is a life-threatening complication of lupus. Vasculitis, hemorrhage, and infarction of the brain are often lethal.

Course and Prognosis

The clinical course of SLE is highly variable and typically exhibits exacerbations and remissions. Before the advent of corticosteroids and other immunosuppressive therapies, SLE was considered to be a rapidly fatal disease. However, with the recognition of mild forms of the disease, improved antihypertensive medications, and use of immunosuppressive agents, the overall 10-year survival rate is now 70%. The worst prognosis is found in patients with severe disease of the kidneys and brain.

Summary

The primary abnormality in SLE is polyclonal B-cell hyperactivity, which is associated with a loss of normal self-tolerance and autoantibody formation to a variety of self-antigens, the most important of which is DNA (Fig. 4-17). The systemic injury seen in patients with SLE is mainly caused by the deposition of immune complexes in tissues, a process that triggers acute inflammation.

Sjögren Syndrome

■ *Sjögren syndrome is an autoimmune disorder characterized by keratoconjunctivitis sicca (dry eyes) and xerosto-*

mia *(dry mouth) in the absence of other connective tissue diseases.* Primary Sjögren syndrome is the second most common connective tissue disorder, after SLE. Like most autoimmune diseases, it occurs primarily in women 30 to 65 years of age. There are strong associations between primary Sjögren syndrome and certain MHC types, notably HLA-Dw3, HLA-DR3, HLA-Dw2, and MT2. Familial clustering occurs, and in these families, there is also a high incidence of other autoimmune diseases.

☐ **Pathogenesis:** The cause of Sjögren syndrome is unknown. Production of autoantibodies, particularly antinuclear antibodies, typically occurs in patients with Sjögren syndrome. These autoantibodies may be directed against DNA, histones, or nonhistone proteins in the nucleus. Rheumatoid factor is also commonly found in the saliva, tears, and circulation.

Production of autoantibodies appears to reflect a polyclonal B-cell activation, possibly triggered by the Epstein-Barr virus, which is commonly present in the salivary glands. However, direct proof to incriminate the Epstein-Barr virus in the pathogenesis of Sjögren syndrome is lacking.

☐ **Pathology and Clinical Features:** Sjögren syndrome is characterized by an intense lymphocytic infiltrate in the salivary and lacrimal glands (Fig. 4-19). The majority of lobules, and especially the centers of the lobules, are affected. Well-defined germinal centers are rare. The lymphoid infiltrates destroy acini and ducts, and the latter often become dilated and filled with cellular debris. The lymphocytic infiltrates in the

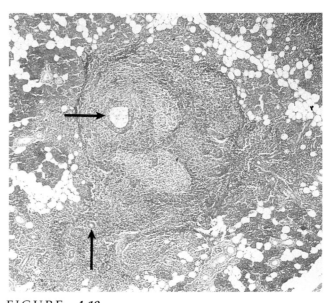

FIGURE 4-19
Sjögren syndrome involving a major salivary gland. An intense lymphoid infiltrate destroys the gland acini but spares the ducts (*arrows*).

glands are predominantly T cells. In the late stage of the disease, the glands atrophy and may be replaced by hyalinized tissue and fibrosis. Owing to the absence of tears, the cornea becomes dry and fissured, and it may ulcerate. The lack of saliva causes atrophy, inflammation, and cracking of the oral mucosa. The pathology of the salivary and lacrimal glands is described in greater detail in Chapter 25.

Involvement of extraglandular sites, including the lungs, gastrointestinal tract, liver, kidneys, and thyroid, is also common in Sjögren syndrome. **Sjögren syndrome is associated with a 40-fold increased risk of malignant lymphoma.** There is reason to believe that B-cell clonal expansion plays an integral role in the pathophysiology of the lymphoid infiltrates and may explain the increased incidence of malignant lymphoma associated with this disorder.

Scleroderma (Progressive Systemic Sclerosis)

■ *Scleroderma (progressive systemic sclerosis) is an autoimmune disease of connective tissue characterized by excessive collagen deposition in the skin and internal organs.* The disease occurs four times as often in women as in men, and mostly in persons between 25 and 50 years of age.

☐ **Pathogenesis:**

Immunologic Abnormalities. Patients with scleroderma exhibit abnormalities of the humoral and cellular immune systems. The number of circulating B lymphocytes is normal, but there is evidence of hyperactivity, as manifested by hypergammaglobulinemia and cryoglobulinemia. Antinuclear antibodies are common but are usually in a lower titer than that found in patients with SLE. Antibodies virtually specific for scleroderma include (1) nucleolar autoantibodies; (2) antibodies to ScL-70, a nonhistone nuclear protein; and (3) anticentromere antibodies. Rheumatoid factor is commonly present in scleroderma, and autoantibodies are occasionally directed against other tissues, such as smooth muscle, thyroid gland, and salivary glands. Antibodies against collagen (types I and IV) have also been described and may be relevant to the pathogenesis of this disease.

Cellular immune derangements in progressive systemic sclerosis include (1) a decrease in the number of circulating T cells, (2) a decrease in the number of helper T cells, and (3) an increase in the number of suppressor T cells. Although functional lymphocyte studies have been inconclusive, lymphocytes from patients with this disease are sensitized to skin extracts or collagen. They respond to these substances by proliferat-ing and by producing lymphokines, which may cause chemotaxis and enhanced collagen synthesis by fibroblasts.

Circulating male fetal cells have been demonstrated in the blood of many women with scleroderma who bore male children many years before the onset of disease. It has been suggested that scleroderma in these patients is similar to graft-versus-host reaction.

Other disorders associated with autoimmune phenomena, such as thyroiditis and primary biliary cirrhosis, have an increased incidence in patients with scleroderma.

Fibrosis. Progressive systemic sclerosis is characterized by excessive collagen deposition in many tissues. It is thought that this fibrosis may result from an abnormality in fibroblast function.

☐ **Pathology:** The skin in scleroderma displays early edema and then induration, with the latter being characterized by the following:

- A striking increase in collagen fibers in the reticular dermis
- Thinning of the epidermis, with loss of rete pegs
- Atrophy of dermal appendages
- Hyalinization and obliteration of arterioles
- Variable mononuclear infiltrates, consisting primarily of T cells

The stage of induration may progress to atrophy or revert to normal. Similar histologic alterations occur in the synovium, lungs, gastrointestinal tract, heart, and kidneys.

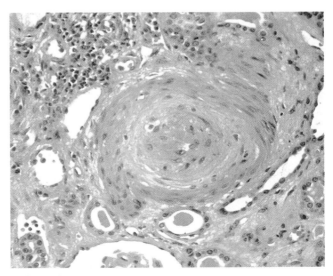

FIGURE *4-20*
Scleroderma with characteristic renal vascular involvement. The interlobular artery shows a marked intimal thickening, with virtual obliteration of the lumen

Blood Vessels. Lesions in the arteries, arterioles, and capillaries are typical and, in some cases, may be the first effect of the disease. Initial subintimal edema with fibrin deposition is followed by thickening and fibrosis of the vessel and reduplication or fraying of the internal elastic lamina (Fig. 4-20). The involved vessels usually are severely restricted in terms of blood flow and may actually be thrombosed.

Kidneys. The kidneys are involved in more than half of patients with scleroderma. They show marked vascular changes, often with focal hemorrhage and cortical infarcts. Among the most severely affected vessels are the interlobular arteries and afferent arterioles. Early fibromuscular thickening of the subintima causes luminal narrowing, which is followed by fibrosis. "Fibrinoid" necrosis is commonly seen in afferent arterioles.

Lungs. Diffuse interstitial fibrosis is the primary abnormality in the lungs. The disease progresses to end-stage pulmonary fibrosis, eventuating in a "honeycomb" lung.

Heart. The large majority of patients with scleroderma have patchy myocardial fibrosis, and in approximately one-fourth of cases, more than 10% of the myocardium is involved. These lesions result from focal myocardial necrosis, which may reflect focal ischemia complicating a Raynaud-like reactivity of the coronary microvasculature.

Gastrointestinal Tract. Progressive systemic sclerosis can involve any portion of the gastrointestinal tract. Esophageal dysfunction is the most common and troublesome gastrointestinal complication. Atrophy of the smooth muscle and fibrous replacement are seen in the lower esophagus. The small bowel is often involved with patchy fibrosis, principally of the muscular layers.

☐ **Clinical Features:** Generalized scleroderma is characterized by severe and progressive disease of the skin and by the early onset of all, or most, of the associated abnormalities of the visceral organs. Symptoms usually begin with Raynaud phenomenon (intermittent episodes of ischemia of the fingers, marked by pallor, paresthesias, and pain). This condition is accompanied or followed by edema of the fingers and hands, tightening and thickening of the skin, polyarthralgia, and complaints referable to involvement of specific internal organs.

The typical patient with generalized scleroderma has a "stone facies," owing to tightening of the facial skin and restricted motion of the mouth. Progression of vascular lesions in the fingers is reflected in the appearance of ischemic ulcerations of the fingertips in 10% to 20% of patients annually, with subsequent shortening and atrophy of the digits. Many patients suffer from painful tendonitis, and joint pain is common. Involvement of the esophagus leads to hypomotility and dysphagia, and fibrosis in the small bowel interferes with intestinal motility, with consequent overgrowth of bacteria and secondary malabsorption.

Dyspnea on exertion is the initial symptom of pulmonary fibrosis in scleroderma, occurring in more than half of the patients. The pulmonary disease progresses to dyspnea at rest and, eventually, to respiratory failure. Patients with longstanding disease are at risk for development of pulmonary hypertension and cor pulmonale. Although most patients with scleroderma have some degree of myocardial fibrosis, congestive heart failure is uncommon. However, ventricular arrhythmias are a cause of sudden death.

Vascular involvement of the kidneys in generalized scleroderma is responsible for the so-called scleroderma renal crisis, which is characterized by sudden onset of malignant hypertension and progressive renal insufficiency and is frequently associated with microangiopathic hemolytic anemia.

Polymyositis/Dermatomyositis

■ *Polymyositis/dermatomyositis is a multisystemic autoimmune disease primarily involving the skin and muscle.* It occurs in both children and adults, and there is an increased frequency of the MHC antigens HLA-B8 and HLA-DR3 in the childhood form of the disease. Women are affected twice as frequently as men. **In many patients, particularly adult men, polymyositis/dermatomyositis is associated with an underlying visceral cancer.** This disease is discussed in detail in Chapter 27.

CHAPTER 5

Neoplasia

Emanuel Rubin
John L. Farber

Cancer is an uncontrolled proliferation of cells that express varying degrees of fidelity to their precursors. In a sense, it may be viewed as a "burlesque" of normal development. The incidence of neoplastic disease increases with age, and the greater longevity in modern times necessarily enlarges the population at risk. Hence, for this reason alone, the overall incidence of cancer is increasing. Despite assertions that contemporary society is or will be subject to an "epidemic" of cancer, the epidemiologic data do not support such a concept. If all deaths from cancers caused by tobacco smoke are removed from the statistics, there has been no increase in the overall, age-adjusted cancer death rate among men during the past five decades and, in fact, a continually decreasing rate among women.

BENIGN VERSUS MALIGNANT TUMORS

By definition, benign tumors do not penetrate (invade) adjacent tissue borders, nor do they spread (metastasize) to distant sites. They remain as localized overgrowths at the area in which they arise. As a rule, benign tumors are more differentiated than malignant ones—that is, they more closely resemble their tissue of origin. **By contrast, malignant tumors, or cancers, have the added property of invading contiguous tissues and metastasizing to distant sites, where subpopulations of malignant cells take up residence, grow anew, and again invade.**

BENIGN TUMORS

The primary descriptor of any tumor, benign or malignant, is its cell or tissue of origin. Benign tumors are often identified by the suffix *-oma*, which is preceded by reference to the cell or the tissue of origin. For instance, a benign tumor that resembles chondrocytes is called a **chondroma** (Fig. 5-1). Tumors of epithelial origin are given a variety of names based on what is believed to be their outstanding characteristic. Thus, a benign tumor of the squamous epithelium may simply be called an **epithelioma** or, when branched and exophytic, a **papilloma**. A benign tumor arising from the glandular epithelium, such as in the colon or the endocrine glands, is named an **adenoma**. Accordingly, we refer to a thyroid adenoma (Fig. 5-2) or an islet cell adenoma. In some instances, the predominating feature is the gross appearance, in which case we speak, for example, of an adenomatous polyp of the colon or the endometrium.

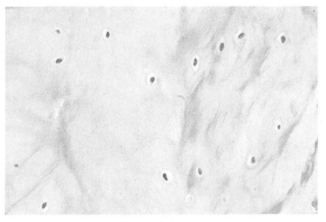
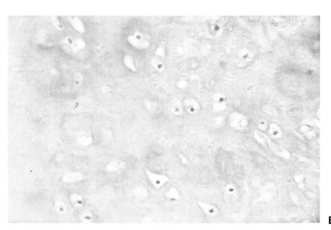

A   B

FIGURE *5-1*
Benign chondroma. (A) Normal cartilage. (B) A benign chondroma closely resembles normal cartilage.

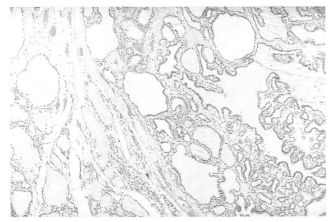

FIGURE 5-2
Benign thyroid adenoma. The follicles of a thyroid adenoma (*right*) contain colloid and resemble those of the normal thyroid tissue (*left*).

A benign tumor that arises from germ cells and contains derivatives of different germ layers is labeled a **teratoma**. These tumors occur principally in the gonads and, occasionally, in the mediastinum. They may contain a variety of structures, such as skin, neurons and glial cells, thyroid, intestinal epithelium, and cartilage. Localized, disordered differentiation during embryonic development results in a **hamartoma**, which is a disorganized caricature of normal tissue components (Fig. 5-3). Such tumors, which are not strictly neoplasms, contain varying combinations of cartilage,

ducts or bronchi, connective tissue, blood vessels, and lymphoid tissue.

MALIGNANT TUMORS

The malignant counterparts of benign tumors usually carry the same name, except that the suffix *carcinoma* is applied to epithelial cancers and *sarcoma* to those of mesenchymal origin. For instance, a malignant tumor of the stomach is a **gastric adenocarcinoma** or **adenocarcinoma of the stomach. Squamous cell carcinoma** is an invasive tumor of the skin (Fig. 5-4) or of the metaplastic squamous epithelium of the bronchus or endocervix. **Transitional cell carcinoma** is a malignant neoplasm of the bladder. By contrast, we speak of **chondrosarcoma** (Fig. 5-5) or **fibrosarcoma**. Sometimes, the name of the tumor suggests the tissue type of origin, such as in **osteogenic** or **bronchogenic carcinoma**.

The persistence of certain historical terms adds a note of confusion. **Hepatoma** of the liver, **melanoma** of the skin, **seminoma** of the testis, and the lymphoproliferative tumor **lymphoma** are all highly malignant. Tumors of the hemopoietic system are a special case, in

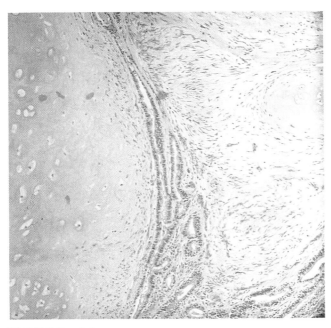

FIGURE 5-3
Hamartoma of the lung. The tumor contains islands of hyaline cartilage and clefts lined by a cuboidal epithelium embedded in a fibromuscular stroma.

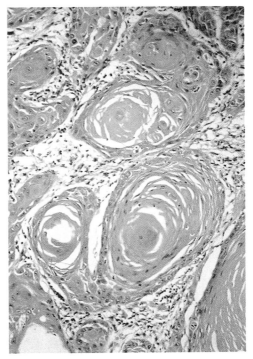

FIGURE 5-4
Squamous cell carcinoma of the skin. The tumor is composed of islands of neoplastic squamous cells. The well-differentiated tumor cells have formed concentric whorls of keratin and pyknotic nuclei, termed epithelial "pearls."

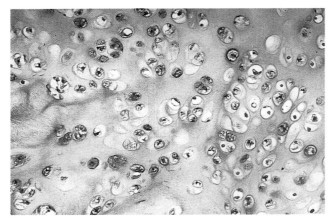

FIGURE   5-5
Chondrosarcoma of bone. The tumor is composed of malignant chondrocytes, which have bizarre shapes and irregular, hyperchromatic nuclei, embedded in a cartilaginous matrix. Compare with Figure 5-1.

which the relationship to the blood is indicated by the suffix *-emia*. Thus, **leukemia** refers to a malignant proliferation of leukocytes.

Secondary descriptors (again, with some inconsistencies) refer to a tumor's morphologic and functional characteristics. For example, the term **papillary** describes a frond-like structure (Fig. 5-6). **Medullary** signifies a soft, cellular tumor, with little connective tissue stroma, whereas **scirrhous** or **desmoplastic** implies a dense fibrous stroma (Fig. 5-7). **Colloid** carcinomas secrete abundant mucus, in which float islands of tumor cells. **Comedocarcinoma** is an intraductal neoplasm in which necrotic material can be expressed from the ducts. Certain visible secretions of the tumor cells (e.g., production of mucin or serous fluid) also lend their characteristics to the classification. A further designation describes the gross appearance of a cystic mass. From all these considerations, we derive such common

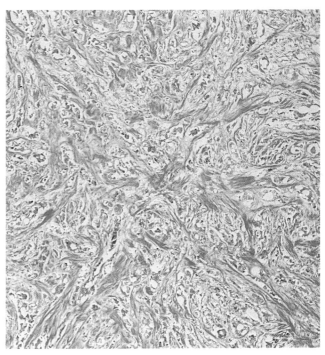

FIGURE   5-7
Scirrhous adenocarcinoma of the breast. A trichrome stain shows nests of cancer cells (*red*) embedded in a dense fibrous stroma (*blue*).

terms as **papillary serous cystadenocarcinoma** of the ovary, **comedocarcinoma** of the breast, **adenoid cystic carcinoma** of the salivary glands, **polypoid adenocarcinoma** of the stomach, and **medullary carcinoma** of the thyroid. Finally, tumors in which the histogenesis is poorly understood are often given an eponym, as in, for example, Hodgkin's disease, Ewing sarcoma of bone, or Brenner tumor of the ovary.

HISTOLOGIC DIAGNOSIS OF MALIGNANCY

Some of the histologic features that favor malignancy include:

- **Anaplasia or Cellular Atypia.** These terms refer to the lack of differentiated features in a cancer cell. In general, the degree of anaplasia correlates with the aggressiveness of the tumor. Cytologic evidence of anaplasia includes (1) variation in the size and shape of the cells and cell nuclei (**pleomorphism**); (2) enlarged and hyperchromatic nuclei, with coarsely clumped chromatin and prominent nucleoli; (3) atypical mitoses; and (4) bizarre cells, including tumor giant cells (Fig. 5-8).

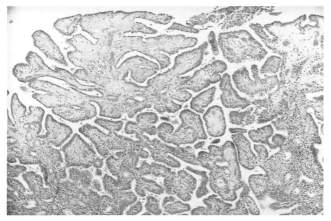

FIGURE   5-6
Papillary adenocarcinoma of the thyroid. The tumor exhibits numerous fronds lined by malignant epithelial cells.

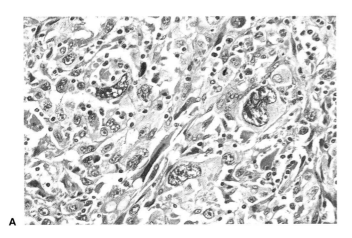

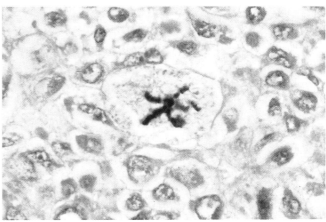

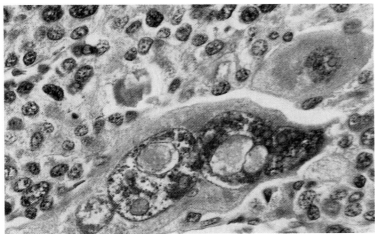

FIGURE 5-8
Anaplastic features of malignant tumors. (A) The cells of this anaplastic carcinoma are highly pleomorphic (vary in size and shape). The nuclei are hyperchromatic and are large relative to the cytoplasm. (B) A malignant cell in metaphase exhibits an abnormal mitotic figure. (C) Multinucleated tumor giant cell.

- **Mitotic Activity.** Abundant mitoses are characteristic of many malignant tumors but are not a necessary criterion. However, in some cases (e.g., leiomyosarcomas), the diagnosis of malignancy is based on the finding of even a few mitoses.
- **Invasion.** Malignancy is proved by the demonstration of invasion, particularly of the blood vessels and lymphatics. In some circumstances, such as squamous carcinoma of the cervix or carcinoma arising in an adenomatous polyp, the diagnosis of malignant transformation is made on the basis of local invasion.
- **Metastases.** It is intuitively obvious that the presence of metastases identifies a tumor as being malignant.
- **Tumor Markers.** Tumor markers are products of malignant neoplasms that can be detected in the cells themselves or in body fluids. Their presence indicates the preservation of characteristics of the progenitor cell or the synthesis of specialized proteins by the neoplastic cell. Tumor markers are often useful in identifying the origin of poorly differ-

entiated tumors, for which the appropriate therapies may be highly variable. For example, carcinomas, which are of epithelial origin, uniformly express cytokeratins. Lineage-associated markers include prostate-specific antigen (PSA) in prostatic cancers and carcinoembryonic antigen (CEA) in colon cancers. Neuroendocrine tumors often contain chromogranins, a family of proteins found in neurosecretory granules. An unpigmented malignant melanoma may not be distinguishable from a poorly differentiated carcinoma by routine staining, but the former usually contains S-100 protein and is not positive for cytokeratins. Malignant lymphomas generally display leukocyte common antigen. Tumor markers in the serum are not disease-specific but allow monitoring for tumor recurrence after surgery. For instance, an elevation of the serum CEA level suggests recurrence of colon cancer, whereas an increased serum level of PSA after prostatectomy indicates recurrence of prostatic carcinoma. Some examples of tumor markers are shown in Figure 5-9.

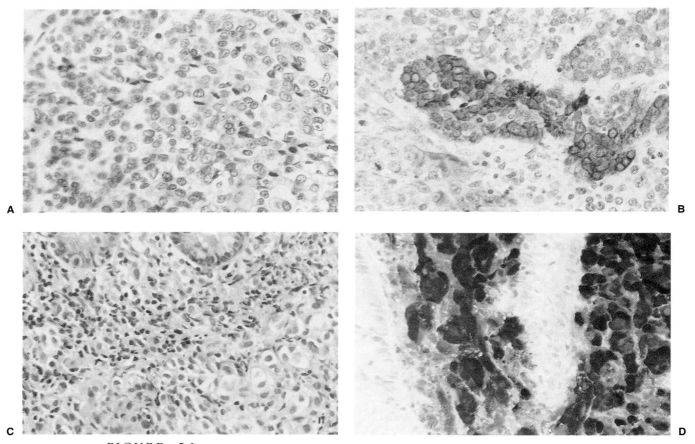

FIGURE 5-9

Tumor markers in the identification of undifferentiated neoplasms. (A) A poorly differentiated metastatic bladder cancer is difficult to identify as a carcinoma with the hematoxylin-and-eosin stain. (B) A section of the tumor depicted in *A* is positive for cytokeratin with an immunoperoxidase stain and is identified as carcinoma. (C) A metastasis to the colon of an undifferentiated malignant melanoma is not pigmented, and its origin is unclear. (D) An immunoperoxidase stain of the tumor shown in *C* reveals numerous cells positive for S-100 protein, a commonly used marker for cells of melanocytic origin.

INVASION AND METASTASIS

The two properties unique to cancer cells are the ability to invade locally and the capacity to metastasize to distant sites.

Patterns of Spread

Direct Extension

Most carcinomas begin as localized growths confined to the epithelium in which they arise. As long as these early cancers do not penetrate the basement membrane on which the epithelium rests, such tumors are termed **carcinoma in situ** (Fig. 5-10). When the in situ tumor acquires invasive potential, however, and extends directly through the underlying basement membrane, it is then in a position to compromise neighboring tissues and to metastasize.

Malignant tumors characteristically grow within the tissue of origin, where they enlarge and infiltrate normal structures. However, their invasive growth pattern often leads to their direct extension outside the tissue of origin, in which case the tumor may secondarily impair the function of an adjacent organ. For example, squamous carcinoma of the cervix often grows beyond the genital tract to produce vesicovaginal fistulas and obstruction of the ureters. Tumor cells that reach serous cavities (e.g., those of the peritoneum or pleura) spread easily by direct extension or can be carried by the fluid to new locations on the serous membranes. The most common example is seeding of the peritoneal cavity by certain types of ovarian cancer (Fig. 5-11).

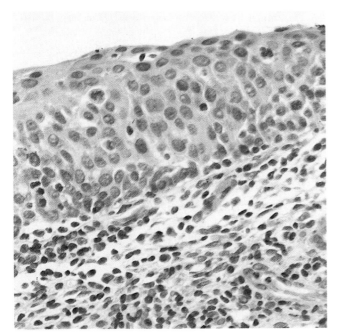

FIGURE 5-10
Carcinoma in situ. A section of the uterine cervix shows neoplastic squamous cells occupying the full thickness of the epithelium and confined to the mucosa by the underlying basement membrane.

Metastatic Spread

■ *Metastasis refers to the transfer of malignant cells from one site to another that is not directly connected with it.* The invasive properties of malignant tumors bring them into contact with blood and lymphatic vessels. In the same way that they can invade parenchymal tissue, neoplastic cells can also penetrate vascular and lym-

phatic channels, through which they are disseminated to distant sites.

Hematogenous Metastases

Cancer cells commonly invade the capillaries and venules, whereas the thicker-walled arterioles and arteries are relatively resistant. Before they can form viable metastases, circulating tumor cells must lodge in the vascular bed of the metastatic site (Fig. 5-12). This sequence of events explains why the liver and lung are so frequently the sites of metastases. Because abdominal tumors seed the portal system, they lead to hepatic metastases, whereas other tumors penetrate systemic veins that eventually drain into the vena cava and, hence, to the lungs. Neoplastic cells arrested in the microcirculation are believed to penetrate the vessel walls at the site of metastasis using the same mechanisms by which the primary tumor invades.

Lymphatic Metastases

Historical dogma of metastatic spread held that epithelial tumors (carcinomas) preferentially metastasized through lymphatic channels, whereas mesenchymal neoplasms (sarcomas) were distributed hematogenously. This distinction is no longer considered to be valid, however, because of clinical observations regarding metastatic patterns and the demonstration of numerous connections between the lymphatic and vascular systems.

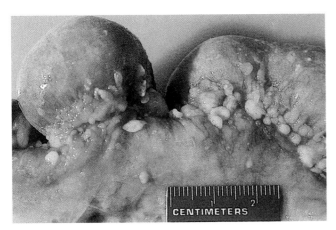

FIGURE 5-11
Peritoneal carcinomatosis. The mesentery attached to a loop of small bowel is studded with small nodules of metastatic ovarian carcinoma.

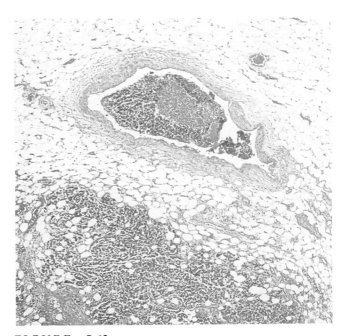

FIGURE 5-12
Hematogenous spread of cancer. A malignant tumor (*bottom*) has invaded the adipose tissue and penetrated into a small vein.

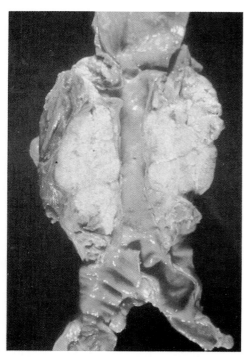

FIGURE *5-13*
Metastatic carcinoma in periaortic lymph nodes. The aorta has been opened and the nodes bisected.

Lymph nodes bearing metastatic deposits may be enlarged to many times their normal size, often exceeding even the diameter of the primary lesion. The cut surface of the lymph node usually resembles that of the primary tumor in color and consistency, and it may also exhibit the necrosis and hemorrhage commonly seen in primary cancers (Fig. 5-13).

The regional lymphatic pattern of metastatic spread is most prominently exemplified by cancer of the breast. Cancers arising in the lateral aspect of the breast characteristically spread to the lymph nodes of the axilla, whereas those arising in the medial portion drain to the internal mammary lymph nodes in the thorax.

Biology of Invasion and Metastasis

It is intuitively clear that for malignant cells to establish a metastasis, a number of steps are required:

1. Invasion of the basement membrane underlying the tumor.

2. Movement through the extracellular matrix.
3. Penetration of vascular or lymphatic channels.
4. Survival and arrest within the circulating blood or lymph.
5. Exit from the circulation into a new tissue site.
6. Survival and growth as a metastasis.

Invasion

Penetration of the basement membrane of the host tissue and invasion of the surrounding extracellular environment is believed to involve three steps (Fig. 5-14):

1. **Binding to the Extracellular Matrix.** The attachment of tumor cells to the underlying extracellular matrix is dependent on the expression of a number of different adhesion molecules. Among these are **integrins**, which comprise a family of transmembrane receptors that mediate the adhesive interactions between the cells themselves and between the cells and the extracellular matrix. A number of intercellular adhesion molecules belong to the immunoglobulin supergene family (e.g., intercellular adhesion molecule [ICAM]-1 and vascular cell adhesion molecule [VCAM]-1). **Cadherins** are adhesion molecules expressed on the surface of all epithelia. They interact with intracellular molecules known as **catenins**, thereby creating a mechanical linkage between extracellular molecules and the cytoskeleton. Expression of both cadherins and catenins is reduced or lost in most carcinomas, an effect that permits individual malignant cells to leave the main tumor mass and, thereby, metastasize.
2. **Degradation of Extracellular Matrix.** After binding to matrix components, the invading tumor cells secrete proteolytic enzymes that degrade the matrix components posing a barrier to their advance, namely type IV collagen, fibronectin, and proteoglycans. Such enzymes include the urokinase-type plasminogen activator and matrix metalloproteinases of the collagenase family.
3. **Movement through Interstitial Tissues.** Many of the steps in the metastatic cascade require locomotion by the malignant cell. An **autocrine motility factor** induces the protrusion of pseudopodia, which are enriched in receptors for laminin and fibronectin and appear to stimulate cell locomotion.

FIGURE *5-14*
Mechanisms of tumor invasion and metastasis. The mechanism by which a malignant tumor initially penetrates a confining basement membrane and then invades the surrounding extracellular environment involves several steps. The tumor first acquires the ability to bind components of the extracellular matrix. These interactions are mediated by the expression of a number of adhesion molecules. Proteolytic enzymes are then released from the tumor cells, and the extracellular matrix is degraded. After moving through the extracellular environment, the invading cancer penetrates blood vessels and lymphatics by the same mechanisms.

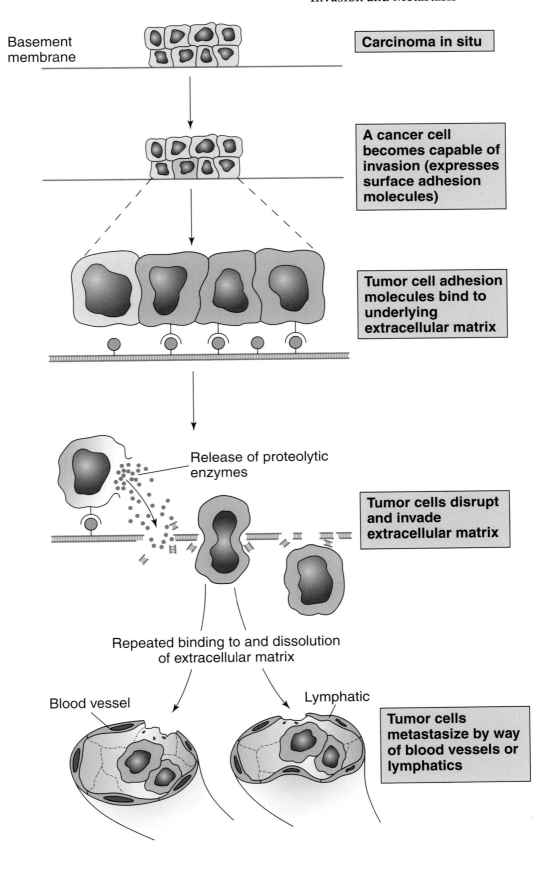

Basement membrane

Carcinoma in situ

A cancer cell becomes capable of invasion (expresses surface adhesion molecules)

Tumor cell adhesion molecules bind to underlying extracellular matrix

Release of proteolytic enzymes

Tumor cells disrupt and invade extracellular matrix

Repeated binding to and dissolution of extracellular matrix

Blood vessel

Lymphatic

Tumor cells metastasize by way of blood vessels or lymphatics

Metastasis

Following the invasion of surrounding tissue, malignant cells may spread to distant sites by a process that includes a number of steps:

1. **Invasion of the Circulation.** After invading the interstitial tissue, malignant cells penetrate the lymphatic or vascular channels.
2. **Escape from the Circulation.** Circulating tumor cells arrest mechanically in capillaries and venules and attach to endothelial cells. This adherence causes retraction of the endothelium, thereby exposing the underlying basement membrane, to which the tumor cells now bind. The tumor cells eventually extravasate by mechanisms similar to those responsible for local invasion.
3. **Angiogenesis and Local Growth.** A new vascular supply is necessary for the tumor to grow to a diameter greater than 0.5 mm. Thus, many tumors secrete polypeptides (e.g., platelet-derived growth factor [PDGF], fibroblast growth factor [FGF], transforming growth factor [TGF]-β) that stimulate the growth of new vessels in the host tissue, a process termed **angiogenesis** (see Chapter 3).

GRADING AND STAGING OF CANCERS

In an attempt to predict the clinical behavior of a malignant tumor and to establish criteria for therapy, many cancers are classified according to cytologic and histologic grading schemes or by staging protocols that describe the extent of spread.

Cancer Grading

Cytologic/histologic grading is based on the degree of anaplasia and the number of proliferating cells. The degree of anaplasia is determined from the shape and regularity of the cells and the presence of distinct, differentiated features, such as functioning gland-like structures in adenocarcinomas or epithelial pearls in squamous carcinomas. Evidence of rapid or abnormal growth is provided by large numbers of mitoses, atypical mitoses, nuclear pleomorphism, and tumor giant cells. Most grading schemes classify tumors into three or four grades that reflect increasing degrees of malignancy (Fig. 5-15).

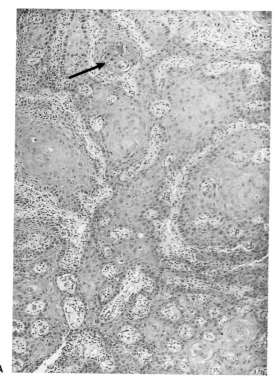
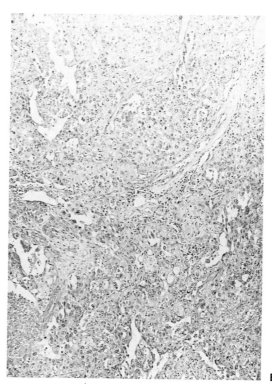

FIGURE 5-15
Cytologic grading of squamous cell carcinoma of the lung. (A) Well-differentiated (grade 1) squamous cell carcinoma. The tumor cells bear a strong resemblance to normal squamous cells and synthesize keratin, as evidenced by the epithelial pearl (arrow). (B) Poorly differentiated (grade 3) squamous cell carcinoma. The malignant cells are difficult to identify as being of squamous origin.

Cancer Staging

The choice of surgical approach or the selection of treatment modalities is influenced more by the stage of a cancer, which refers to the extent of spread, than by its cytologic grade. Moreover, most statistical data related to cancer survival are based on the stage rather than the cytologic grade of the tumor. Clinical staging is independent of cytologic grading and has been codified in the international TNM cancer staging system. **T** refers to the size of the primary tumor, **N** to the number and distribution of lymph node metastases, and **M** to the presence and extent of distant metastases.

GROWTH OF CANCERS

Cell Cycle Kinetics

Historically, cancer was considered to result from a totally unregulated growth of cells, and a logical corollary was that neoplastic cells proliferated grew more rapidly than normal ones. **However, it is now clear that tumor cells do not necessarily proliferate at a faster rate than their normal counterparts.** Tumor growth depends on other factors, such as the growth fraction (proportion of cycling cells) and the rate of cell death. In normal proliferating tissues, such as the intestine and bone marrow, an exquisite balance between cell renewal and cell death is strictly maintained. **By contrast, the major determinant of tumor growth is clearly that more cells are produced than die in a given time.**

Growth Factors and Neoplasia

Polypeptide growth factors (PGFs) have been implicated in the regulation of embryogenesis, growth and development, selective cell survival, hemopoiesis, tissue repair, immune responses, atherosclerosis, and neoplastic growth. Transformed cells are less dependent on exogenous growth factors than normal cells. Because some of the oncogenes (discussed later) of neoplastic cells code for products related to PGFs or their receptors, cancer cells are not subject to the normal control of growth and differentiation by exogenous growth factors.

Tumor Angiogenesis

□ **Angiogenesis:** refers to the sprouting of new capillaries from pre-existing blood vessels and is required for the continued growth of cancers, whether primary or metastatic. In the absence of new vessels to supply nutrients and remove waste products, malignant tumors do not grow larger then 1 to 2 mm in diameter. Among the molecules capable of stimulating an angiogenic response are FGF, TGF, tumor necrosis factor (TNF), vascular endothelial growth factor (VEGF), PDGF, and epidermal growth factor (EGF). Inhibitors of angiogenesis (e.g., angiostatin and endostatin) have been reported to eliminate malignant tumors in mice, but their effect in human tumors remains to be determined.

MOLECULAR GENETICS OF CANCERS

The unregulated growth of cancer cells results from the sequential acquisition of somatic mutations in genes that control cell growth and differentiation or that maintain the integrity of the genome. Similar mutations may also be present in the germline of persons with hereditary predispositions to a variety of cancers. Although mutations can be produced by environmental mutagens (e.g., chemical carcinogens or radiation) or as a consequence of normal cellular metabolism (possibly activated oxygen species), the most common mechanism relates to spontaneous errors in DNA replication and repair. Genes involved in the pathogenesis of cancer can be conveniently grouped into three categories:

- **Oncogenes** are altered versions of normal genes, termed *proto-oncogenes*, that regulate normal cell growth and differentiation.
- **Tumor suppressor genes** are normal genes whose products inhibit cellular proliferation.
- **Mutator genes** maintain the integrity of the genome and the fidelity of DNA replication. Inactivating mutations of these genes allow the successive accumulation of further mutations.

Retroviral Oncogenes

Although only one RNA retrovirus (human T-cell leukemia virus [HTLV]-I) has been linked to a human cancer, namely the rare T-cell leukemia/lymphoma noted in Japan and the Caribbean region, experimental studies of these viruses have added considerably to our understanding of the molecular biology of cancer. The oncogenic retroviruses can be divided into two general groups based on the interval between viral infection and the development of a tumor (Fig. 5-16). Acute transforming viruses produce tumors in a few weeks, whereas slow transforming viruses require months before cancers are evident.

Acute transforming viruses have acquired, by a process known as **transduction,** portions of cellular

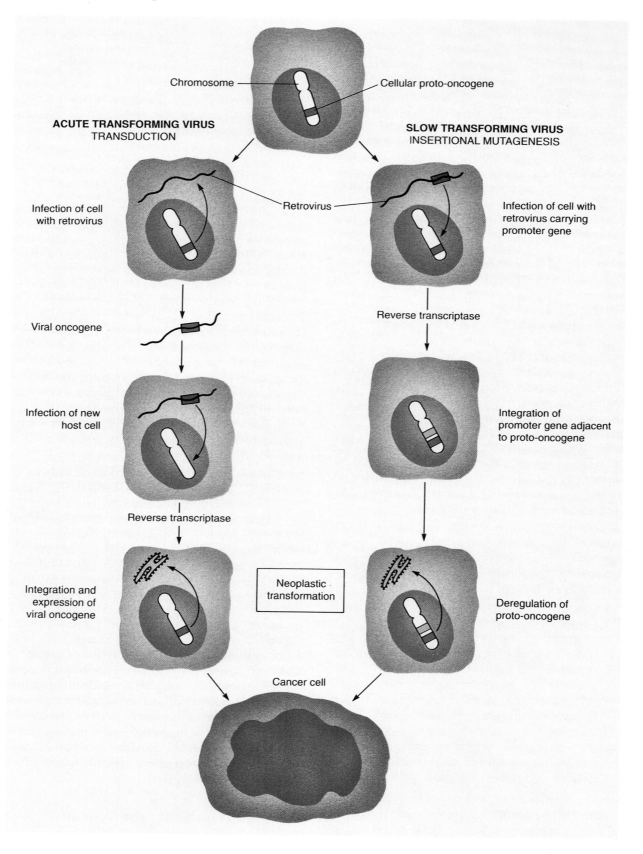

Chromosome — Cellular proto-oncogene

ACUTE TRANSFORMING VIRUS
TRANSDUCTION

SLOW TRANSFORMING VIRUS
INSERTIONAL MUTAGENESIS

Infection of cell
with retrovirus

Retrovirus

Infection of cell with
retrovirus carrying
promoter gene

Viral oncogene

Reverse transcriptase

Infection of new
host cell

Integration of
promoter gene adjacent
to proto-oncogene

Reverse transcriptase

Integration and
expression of
viral oncogene

Neoplastic
transformation

Deregulation of
proto-oncogene

Cancer cell

genes, whose expression in cells leads to the rapid development of tumors. Such transduced viral genes are termed **viral oncogenes** (v-onc), and the cellular genes from which they are derived are known as **cellular oncogenes** (c-onc) or **proto-oncogenes**. Infection with an acute transforming retrovirus leads to incorporation of a viral oncogene into the host DNA, where it is expressed as a transforming factor.

Slow transforming viruses do not possess viral oncogenes. Rather, they produce tumors by integrating the provirus (the DNA copy of the viral RNA genome) at critical sites in the cell genome, thereby deregulating a neighboring cellular oncogene. This integration of the provirus into host DNA and the resulting activation of a cellular oncogene are termed **insertional mutagenesis**.

Human Tumor Oncogenes

A search for cancer genes in human tumors not caused by viruses led to the discovery that such neoplasms also contain transforming and tumorigenic DNA sequences, again termed *oncogenes*. Importantly, the transforming oncogenes in human tumors are somatic mutants of normal proto-oncogenes. When proto-oncogenes, which control growth and differentiation, are converted to tumorigenic oncogenes, they are said to be "activated."

Mechanisms of Activation of Cellular Oncogenes

The similarity of oncogenes (both viral and tumor) to normal genes that code for proteins involved in growth and development poses the question of how these normal genes become oncogenes. There are two general mechanisms by which this activation is accomplished:

- A mutation in the structure of the proto-oncogene itself results in an abnormal gene product.
- An increase in the expression of the proto-oncogene causes overproduction of a normal gene product.

Activation by Mutation

It is now well documented that mutations of v-onc sequences increase the tumorigenic potential of acute transforming retroviruses. For example, the first oncogene identified in a human tumor was activated c-*ras* from a bladder cancer. This gene has a remarkably subtle alteration, namely a point mutation in codon 12, which results in the substitution of valine for glycine in the *ras* protein. Subsequent studies of other cancers revealed point mutations involving other codons of the *ras* gene, suggesting that these positions are critical for normal function of the *ras* protein. Point mutations in members of the *ras* proto-oncogene family have also been demonstrated in colorectal cancers and in adenocarcinomas of the lung.

Activation by Chromosomal Translocation

Chromosomal translocation—that is, the transfer of a portion of one chromosome to another—has been implicated in the pathogenesis of several human leukemias and lymphomas. The first (and still the best-known) example of an acquired chromosomal translocation in a human cancer is the **Philadelphia chromosome**, which is found in 95% of patients with chronic myelogenous leukemia (Fig. 5-17). The c-*abl* proto-oncogene on chromosome 9 is translocated to chromosome 22, where it is placed in juxtaposition to a site known as the breakpoint cluster region (bcr). The c-*abl* gene and bcr region unite to produce a hybrid oncogene that codes for an aberrant protein with very high tyrosine kinase activity. Tyrosine kinases are important in the normal regulation of cellular proliferation. The chromosomal translocation that produces the Philadelphia chromosome is an example of the activation of an oncogene by the formation of a mutant protein. Another example of activation by chromosomal translocation is removal of the c-*myc* proto-oncogene from its site on chromosome 8 to a position on chromosome 14, where it is placed adjacent to the genes that control transcription of the immunoglobulin heavy chains. As a result, the c-*myc* proto-oncogene is activated by the constitutively expressed promoter of the immunoglobulin genes. In this case, the translocation does not create a novel chimeric protein, but rather stimulates overproduction of a normal gene product.

FIGURE *5-16*
Mechanisms of tumorigenesis by RNA retroviruses. Acute transforming RNA viruses contain a viral oncogene formed by transduction of a cellular proto-oncogene. Infection of a cell by such a virus results in the integration and expression of the viral oncogene, presumably leading to neoplastic transformation. By contrast, slow transforming viruses do not contain a viral oncogene but, rather, a promoter gene. Integration of this promoter gene deregulates the expression of a cellular proto-oncogene (a process called insertional mutagenesis), again presumably leading to neoplastic transformation.

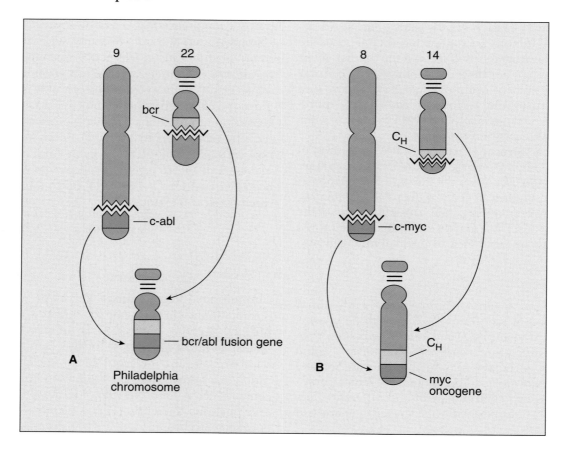

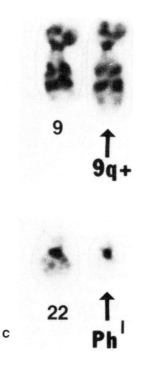

FIGURE 5-17

Oncogene activation by chromosomal translocation. (A) Chronic myelogenous leukemia. Breaks at the ends of the long arms of chromosomes 9 and 22 allow reciprocal translocations to occur. The c-*abl* proto-oncogene on chromosome 9 is translocated to the breakpoint region (bcr) of chromosome 22. The result is the Philadelphia chromosome, which contains a new fusion gene coding for a hybrid oncogenic protein (bcr/abl), which is presumably involved in the pathogenesis of chronic myelogenous leukemia. (B) Burkitt lymphoma. In this disorder, chromosomal breaks involve the long arms of chromosomes 8 and 14. The c-*myc* gene on chromosome 8 is translocated to a region on chromosome 14 adjacent to the gene coding for the constant region of an immunoglobulin heavy chain (C$_H$). The expression of c-*myc* is enhanced by its association with the promoter/enhancer regions of the actively transcribed immunoglobulin genes. (C) Karyotypes of a patient with chronic myelogenous leukemia showing the results of reciprocal translocations between chromosomes 9 and 22. The Philadelphia chromosome is recognized by a smaller-than-normal chromosome 22 (22q-). One chromosome 9 (9q+) is larger than its normal counterpart.

Activation by Gene Amplification

Chromosomal alterations that result in an increased number of copies of a gene (i.e., gene amplification) have been found primarily in human solid tumors. Such aberrations are recognized as (1) **homogeneous staining regions** (HSRs), (2) **abnormal banding regions** on chromosomes, or (3) **double minutes,** which are visualized as multiple, small, paired cytoplasmic bodies. In some cases, gene amplification has been shown to involve proto-oncogenes. For example, HSRs may be seen in neuroblastomas and are all derived from the N-*myc* proto-oncogene. The presence of N-*myc* HSRs is associated with as much as a 700-fold amplification of this gene and is a marker of advanced disease with a poor prognosis.

Mechanisms of Action of Oncogenes

Oncogenes can be classified according to the roles played by their normal counterparts (proto-oncogenes) in the biochemical pathways of signal transduction that regulate growth and differentiation. Representative examples of the various mechanisms of oncogene action are discussed here.

Oncogenes and Growth Factors

A retroviral oncogene, v-*sis*, encodes a growth factor with striking sequence similarity to the β-chain of PDGF. PDGF is the protein product of the c-*sis* proto-oncogene and is a potent mitogen for fibroblasts, smooth muscle cells, and glial cells. Cells derived from human sarcomas and glioblastomas (a malignant glial cell tumor) produce PDGF-like polypeptides, whereas their normal counterparts do not. Transfection of c-*sis* into cultured mouse fibroblasts results in their transformation. Thus, a normal human gene (c-*sis*) that encodes a growth factor (PDGF) acquires transforming capacity when it is constitutively expressed in a cell that responds to this signal. Synthesis of a PDGF-like growth factor by neoplastic cells that express a receptor for this activity is an example of autocrine growth stimulation, which is a mechanism implicated in oncogenesis.

Oncogenes and Growth Factor Receptors

Many growth factors stimulate cellular proliferation by interacting with a family of cell surface receptors that are integral membrane proteins. Binding of a ligand to such a receptor stimulates an intrinsic tyrosine kinase activity in the cytoplasmic domain of the molecule that phosphorylates tyrosine residues in other proteins. Because growth factor receptors can generate potent mitogenic signals, they harbor a latent oncogenic potential that, when activated, overrides the normal controls of signaling pathways. For example, the v-*erb* B oncogene codes for a truncated variant of the EGF receptor. In this mutation, one of the tyrosine residues is deleted, thereby permitting constitutive, rather than controlled, activation of the receptor.

Oncogenes and Membrane-Associated and Cytoplasmic Protein Kinases

A number of cytoplasmic protein kinases are loosely associated with the plasma membrane but are neither integral membrane proteins nor growth factor receptors. These include enzymes that phosphorylate either tyrosine or serine/threonine residues in proteins that regulate growth and differentiation (e.g., the v-*src* family). In human cancer, the best-studied example of an oncogene that codes for a cytoplasmic tyrosine kinase is activated c-*abl*. As previously discussed, in certain leukemias this proto-oncogene, which codes for a cytoplasmic tyrosine kinase, is translocated from chromosome 9 to the bcr of chromosome 22. The *bcr/abl* fused gene encodes a mutant protein with conspicuously elevated tyrosine kinase activity.

ras Oncogenes

The *ras* proto-oncogene codes for a product, p21, that belongs to a family of small cytoplasmic proteins that bind guanosine triphosphate (GTP) and guanosine diphosphate (GDP) (G proteins). These G proteins are distinct from the integral membrane G proteins that are involved in receptor-mediated signal transduction (Fig. 5-18). Point mutations in the *ras* proto-oncogene lead to maintenance of the active state in one of three ways: (1) loss of intrinsic GTPase activity, (2) loss of sensitivity to the G-activating protein (GAP), or (3) increased exchange of GTP for GDP. Whatever the cause, persistence of the GTP-bound state results in uncontrolled stimulation of *ras*-related functions, because p21 is "locked" in the "on" position.

Oncogenes and Nuclear Regulatory Proteins

There is a group of nuclear proteins encoded by proto-oncogenes intimately involved in the sequential expression of genes that regulate cellular proliferation and differentiation. Many of these proteins have the capacity to bind to DNA and are believed to regulate the expression of other genes. In models of stimulated cellular proliferation, the transitory expression of several proto-oncogenes is necessary for the cells to pass through specific points in the cell cycle.

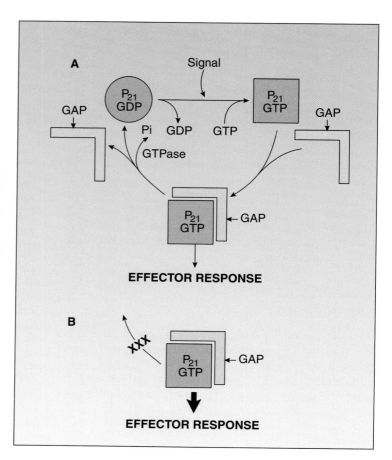

FIGURE *5-18*
Mechanism of action of *ras* oncogene. (A) Normal. The ras protein p21 exists in two conformational states, determined by the binding of either guanosine diphosphate (GDP) or guanosine triphosphate (GTP). Normally, most of the p21 is in the inactive GDP-bound state. An external stimulus, or signal, triggers the exchange of GTP for GDP, an event that converts p21 to the active state. Activated p21, which is associated with the plasma membrane, binds a GTPase-activating protein (GAP) from the cytosol. The binding of GAP has two consequences. First, in association with other plasma membrane constituents, it initiates the effector response. Second, and at the same time, the binding of GAP to p21-GTP stimulates by approximately 100-fold the intrinsic GTPase activity of p21, thereby promoting the hydrolysis of GTP to GDP and the return of p21 to its inactive state. (B) Mutated ras protein is locked into the active GTP-bound state because of an insensitivity of its intrinsic GTPase to GAP or because of a lack of GTPase activity itself. As a result, the effector response is exaggerated, and the cell is transformed.

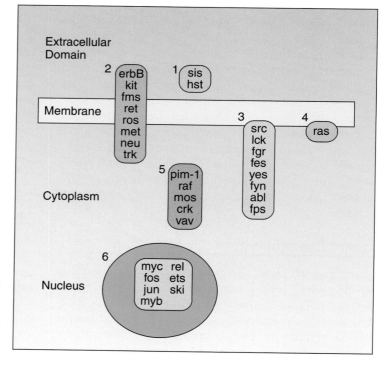

FIGURE *5-19*
Cellular compartments in which oncogene or proto-oncogene products reside. (1) Growth factors. (2) Transmembrane growth factor receptors (tyrosine kinase). (3) Integral membrane receptors. (4) *ras* GTPase family. (5) Cytoplasmic oncogenes. (6) Nuclear oncogenes.

As an example, binding of PDGF to cultured fibroblasts causes the cells to leave G_0 and enter the G_1 phase of the cell cycle. Shortly thereafter, several genes, including c-*myc* and c-*fos*, are expressed. However, the cells are not yet fully programmed to divide by the expression of these genes, and they will enter the S phase and mitosis only after further stimulation by other factors, such as EGF or insulin-like growth factor (IGF-I). Proto-oncogenes that are expressed early in the cell cycle, such as *myc* and *fos*, render the cells competent to receive the final signals for mitosis and are, therefore, termed **competence genes.** Overexpression of nuclear regulatory genes (e.g., c-*myc* in Burkitt lymphoma) can promote uncontrolled cell proliferation.

In summary, oncogenes augment the normal pathways controlling growth and differentiation. Virtually any step in the cascade of signal transduction, from the surface of the cell to the binding of regulatory proteins to DNA, may find its counterpart in the expression of an oncogene. The cellular compartments in which oncogenes reside are depicted in Figure 5-19.

Bcl-2 and Apoptosis

Follicular B-cell lymphomas display a characteristic chromosomal translocation, namely t(14;18). In this situation, the *bcl-2* gene on chromosome 18 is brought under the transcriptional control of the immunoglobulin light-chain gene promoter, thereby causing overexpression of bcl-2. *Bcl-2* is a unique oncogene that inhibits the programmed cell death (apoptosis) of the malignant B cells. As a result, the neoplastic clone accumulates in the affected lymph nodes. Other oncogenes with antiapoptotic properties have also been implicated in human tumorigenesis.

CAUSES OF CANCER

Chemical Carcinogenesis

The importance of chemicals as a cause of cancer has long been recognized in environmental medicine and is emphasized by the epidemic of tobacco-related lung cancer in the 20th century.

Chemical Carcinogens as Mutagens

■ *Mutagens are agents that can permanently alter the genetic constitution of a cell.* The most widely used screening test, the Ames test, uses the appearance of mutants in a culture of bacteria of the *Salmonella* species. Approximately 90% of known carcinogens are mutagenic in this system. Moreover, most (but not all) mutagens are carcinogenic. This close correlation between carcinogenicity and mutagenicity presumably occurs because both reflect damage to DNA. Although not infallible, the in vitro mutagenicity assay is a valuable tool in screening for the carcinogenic potential of chemicals. Cultured human cells are now being increasingly used for assays of mutagenicity.

Chemical Carcinogens and Their Metabolism

Chemicals cause cancer either directly or, more often, after metabolic activation. The direct-acting carcinogens are inherently sufficiently reactive to bind covalently to cellular macromolecules. In addition to a number of organic compounds, such as nitrogen mustard, bis(chloro-methyl)ether, and benzyl chloride, certain metals are included in this category. **The great majority of organic carcinogens, however, require conversion to an ultimate, more reactive compound.** This conversion is enzymatic and, for the most part, is effected by the cellular systems involved in drug metabolism and detoxification. Many cells in the body, particularly liver cells, possess enzyme systems capable of converting procarcinogens to their active forms.

Polycyclic Aromatic Hydrocarbons. The polycyclic aromatic hydrocarbons, originally derived from coal tar, are among the most extensively studied carcinogens. This class includes such model compounds as benzo(α)pyrene, 3-methylcholanthrene, and dibenzanthracene. These chemicals have a broad range of target organs and generally produce cancers at the site of application. Because polycyclic aromatic hydrocarbons have been identified in cigarette smoke, it has been suggested that they may be involved in the production of lung cancer.

Aflatoxin. Aflatoxin B_1, a natural product of the fungus *Aspergillus flavus,* is among the most potent liver carcinogens recognized, producing tumors in fish, birds, rodents, and primates. *Aspergillus* sp. are ubiquitous, and contamination of vegetable foods, particularly peanuts and grains exposed to the warm, moist conditions that favor growth of this mold, may result in formation of significant amounts of aflatoxin B_1. It has been suggested that aflatoxin-rich foods may also contribute to the high incidence of liver cancer in parts of Africa and Asia.

Aromatic Amines and Azo Dyes. Aromatic amines and azo dyes produce bladder and liver tumors, respectively, when fed to experimental animals. Both aromatic amines and azo dyes are primarily metabolized in the liver. Occupational exposure to aromatic amines in the form of aniline dyes has resulted in bladder cancer.

Nitrosamines. The simplest nitrosamine, dimethyl-nitrosamine, produces kidney and liver tumors in rodents. Nitrosamines are also potent carcinogens in primates, although unambiguous evidence of cancer induction in humans is lacking. The extremely high incidence of esophageal carcinoma in the Hunan province of China (100-fold higher than that in other areas), however, has been correlated with the high nitrosamine content of the diet. There is concern that nitrosamines may also be implicated in other gastrointestinal cancers, because nitrites, which are commonly added to preserve processed meats and other foods, may react with other dietary components to form nitrosamines.

Metals. A number of metals or metal compounds, such as Ni^{2+}, Pb^{2+}, Cd^{2+}, Co^{2+}, and Be^{2+}, can induce cancer. They are electrophilic and, therefore, can react with macromolecules. In addition, metal ions react with guanine and phosphate groups of DNA. Most metal-induced cancers occur in an occupational setting, and the subject is, therefore, discussed in more detail in Chapter 8, which deals with environmental pathology.

Factors Influencing Chemical Carcinogenesis

Metabolism of Carcinogens. Mixed function oxidases are enzymes whose activities are genetically determined. A correlation has been observed between levels of these enzymes in various strains of mice and sensitivity to chemical carcinogens. As already noted, most chemical carcinogens require metabolic activation. Thus, it follows that agents enhancing the activation of procarcinogens to ultimate carcinogens should lead to greater carcinogenicity, whereas those augmenting the detoxification pathways should reduce the incidence of cancer.

Sex and Hormonal Status. These factors are important determinants of susceptibility to chemical carcinogens but are highly variable. For example, pregnancy is associated with a decreased incidence of cancers of the breast, endometrium, and ovary, and women who have borne children at an early age are at a lesser risk than nulliparous woman for all of these tumors. Moreover, in the case of breast cancer, the earlier in life that the first pregnancy occurs, the less the risk of later disease. Conversely, early menarche, late menopause, and later age of first pregnancy all increase the risk of breast cancer.

Diet. Composition of the diet can affect the level of drug-metabolizing enzymes. A low-protein diet, which reduces the hepatic activity of mixed function oxidases, is associated with a decreased sensitivity to hepatocarcinogens. By contrast, obesity is associated with an increased number of tumors. Much attention has recently been focused on an alleged association between fat in the diet and the incidence of breast and colon cancers. There is a very large (greater than five-fold) variation internationally in the incidence of breast cancer and in the consumption of fat, and an excellent correlation has been demonstrated for these parameters. However, the results of case-control studies that have examined this association within individual populations, in which the amount of dietary fat varies far less than that between different populations, have been inconclusive. Thus, the relationship between breast cancer and fat consumption in humans remains controversial.

Dietary fiber has also been suggested to influence the occurrence of colorectal cancer. In this case, a plausible explanation lies in the effect of fiber on increasing the motility of the gut and, thereby, hastening the elimination of potentially harmful chemicals in the fecal stream. However, despite the recommendations of some health officials and the claims of manufacturers of certain foods, there is no clinical or epidemiologic evidence that the introduction of more fiber into the Western diet reduces the risk of colorectal cancer.

Chemical Carcinogenesis As a Multistep Process

Studies of chemical carcinogenesis among experimental animals have shed light on the individual stages in the progression of normal cells to cancer. From these studies, one can abstract four stages of chemical carcinogenesis:

1. Initiation is the first stage and likely represents mutations in a single cell (Fig. 5-20).
2. Promotion follows initiation and is characterized by clonal expansion of the initiated cell. The altered cells do not exhibit autonomous growth but remain dependent on continued presence of the promoting stimulus. This may be an exogenous chemical or physical agent or an endogenous mechanism, such as hormonal stimulation.
3. Progression is the third stage, in which growth becomes autonomous and is independent of the carcinogen or promoter. In this stage, genomic changes presumably endow cells with a relative growth advantage that, in turn, results in their further clonal expansion.
4. Cancer is the end result of the entire sequence and is established when the cells acquire the capacity to invade and metastasize.

Physical Carcinogenesis

The physical agents of carcinogenesis discussed here are ultraviolet (UV) light, asbestos, and foreign bodies. Radiation carcinogenesis is discussed in Chapter 8.

Ultraviolet Radiation

Cancers attributed to sun exposure (basal cell carcinoma, squamous carcinoma, and melanoma) occur predominantly in persons of the white race. The skin of persons of the darker races is protected by the increased concentration of melanin pigment, which absorbs UV radiation. The effects of UV radiation on cells include enzyme inactivation, inhibition of cell division, mutagenesis, cell death, and cancer.

Xeroderma pigmentosum, an autosomal recessive disease, exemplifies the importance of DNA repair in protecting against the harmful effects of UV radiation. In this rare disorder, a sensitivity to sunlight is accompanied by a high incidence of skin cancers, including basal cell carcinoma, squamous cell carcinoma, and melanoma. Both neoplastic and nonneoplastic disorders of the skin in xeroderma pigmentosum are attributed to an impairment in the excision of UV radiation–damaged DNA.

Asbestos

Pulmonary asbestosis and asbestosis-associated neoplasms are discussed in Chapter 12, which deals with diseases of the lungs. It is not conclusively established whether the cancers related to asbestos exposure should be considered as examples of chemical carcinogenesis or of physically induced tumors.

Sources of inhaled asbestos fibers include (1) mining and manufacturing of asbestos, (2) installation of asbestos insulation, (3) air in the vicinity of asbestos plants, (4) contaminated air in buildings undergoing repair or demolition, and (5) the clothing of asbestos workers.

The characteristic tumor associated with asbestos exposure is malignant mesothelioma of the pleural and peritoneal cavities. This cancer, which is exceedingly rare among the general population, has been reported to occur in 2% to 3% (and, in some studies, even more) of heavily exposed workers. The latent period—that is, the interval between exposure and the appearance of a tumor—usually is approximately 20 years but may be twice that figure. An association between cancer of the lung and asbestos exposure with pulmonary fibrosis has also been clearly established in smokers.

Foreign Body Carcinogenesis

A number of different sarcomas have been induced in rodents by the implantation of inert materials, such as plastic and metal films, various fibers (including fiberglass), plastic sponges, glass spheres, and dextran polymers. Foreign body carcinogenesis is highly species-specific. For example, rats and mice are highly susceptible to foreign body carcinogenesis, but guinea pigs are resistant. **Humans are certainly highly resistant to foreign body carcinogenesis, as evidenced by the lack of cancers following implantation of prostheses constructed of plastics and metals.**

Viruses and Human Cancer

The role of viruses in the spontaneous appearance and experimental induction of cancer among animals is thoroughly established, but it is estimated that viral infections are responsible for only 15% of all human cancers. The strongest associations between viruses and the development of cancer in humans are (1) the RNA retrovirus HTLV-I and human T-cell leukemia/lymphoma, (2) the human papillomavirus (DNA) and squamous carcinoma of the cervix, (3) the hepatitis B and C viruses and primary hepatocellular carcinoma, (4) the Epstein-Barr virus (EBV) and certain forms of lymphoma and nasopharyngeal carcinoma, and (5) human herpesvirus 8 and Kaposi sarcoma.

Human T-Cell Leukemia Viruses

The rare adult T-cell leukemia is endemic to parts of Japan, Africa, the Caribbean basin, and the southeastern United States. The causative agent, HTLV-I, has also been incriminated in the pathogenesis of a number of neurologic disorders. HTLV-I differs from other oncogenic retroviruses in two important respects. First, the genome of the virus contains no known oncogene. Second, it does not integrate at specific sites within the host genome. Thus, it is inappropriate to group HTLV-I with either the acute or the slow transforming retroviruses. On structural grounds, HTLV is analogous to a number of other retroviruses, including simian T-cell leukemia virus type I, bovine leukemia virus, and human immunodeficiency viruses (HIV)-1 and -2.

DNA Viruses

Four DNA viruses (human papillomavirus [HPV], Epstein-Barr virus [EBV], hepatitis B virus [HBV], and herpesvirus 8) are incriminated in the development of human cancers. **All oncogenic DNA viruses have genes that encode protein products that bind to specific host proteins (the products of tumor suppressor genes) involved in the regulation of cell proliferation.** Thus, they decouple cell proliferation from inhibitory control and play a role in creation of the transformed phenotype of a cancer cell.

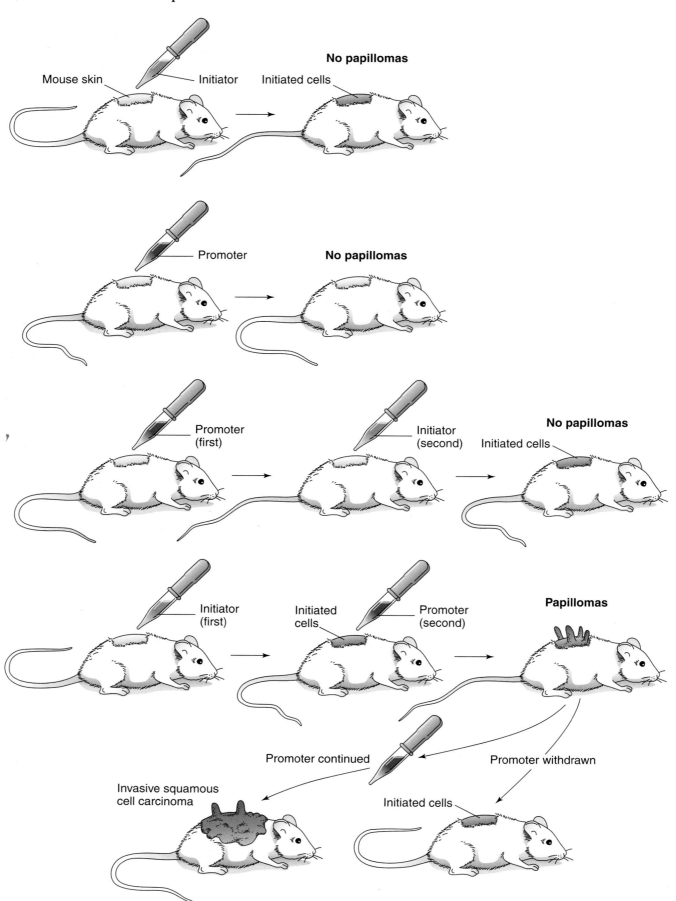

No papillomas

Mouse skin   Initiator   Initiated cells

Promoter   No papillomas

Promoter
(first)   Initiator
(second)   No papillomas
        Initiated cells

Initiator
(first)   Initiated
cells   Promoter
(second)   **Papillomas**

Promoter continued   Promoter withdrawn

Invasive squamous
cell carcinoma   Initiated cells

Infection of cultured cells with oncogenic DNA viruses almost always leads to the appearance of clones that express viral genes, and the expressed viral proteins are required for maintenance of the transformed state. **The transforming genes of oncogenic DNA viruses exhibit virtually no homology with cellular genes, whereas the transforming genes of retroviruses (oncogenes) are derived from, and are homologous with, their cellular counterparts (proto-oncogenes).**

Papillomaviruses

Human papillomaviruses (HPV) induce lesions in humans that progress to squamous cell carcinoma. HPV causes benign lesions of the squamous epithelium, including warts, laryngeal papillomas, and condylomata acuminata (genital warts) of the vulva, penis, and perianal region. Occasionally, condylomata acuminata and laryngeal papillomas undergo malignant transformation to squamous cell carcinoma.

Certain strains of HPV (particularly types 16 and 18) have now been associated with development of epithelial dysplasia of the uterine cervix, which can progress to carcinoma in situ and, eventually, to invasive squamous cell carcinoma. Importantly, HPV infection by itself is not sufficient for progression from dysplasia to carcinoma. This multistep sequence requires other factors, probably additional mutations. The role of HPV in the pathogenesis of squamous cancers of the female genital tract is discussed in detail in Chapter 18.

Epstein-Barr Virus

Epstein-Barr virus (EBV), a human herpesvirus, is so widely disseminated that 95% of adults in the world have antibodies to it. EBV infects B lymphocytes, transforming these cells into lymphoblasts with an indefinite life span. In a small proportion of primary infections with EBV, this lymphoblastoid transformation is manifested as infectious mononucleosis (see Chapter 9), a short-lived, lymphoproliferative disease. However, in three distinct situations, EBV is intimately associated with development of human cancers.

Burkitt Lymphoma

African Burkitt lymphoma is a B-cell tumor in which the neoplastic lymphocytes invariably contain EBV in their DNA and manifest EBV-related antigens. The tumor has also been recognized in non-African populations, but in those cases, only approximately 20% contain the EBV genome. The localization of Burkitt lymphoma to equatorial Africa is not understood, but it has been suggested that prolonged stimulation of the immune system by endemic malaria may be important.

In most instances, the EBV-stimulated proliferation of B lymphocytes is controlled by suppressor T cells. The lack of an adequate T-cell response that is often reported in chronic malarial infections might result in uncontrolled B-cell proliferation, thereby providing the background for further genetic events that lead to the development of lymphoma. One of these is a chromosomal translocation in which the c-*myc* proto-oncogene is deregulated by being brought into proximity of an immunoglobulin promoter region. In 75% of the cases, the c-*myc* proto-oncogene on chromosome 8 is translocated to chromosome 14, at the site of the immunoglobulin promoter. In 25% of the cases, the c-*myc* proto-oncogene remains in its normal location on chromosome 8, but an immunoglobulin promoter from either chromosome 2 or chromosome 22 is translocated to chromosome 8. A proposed sequence for the pathogenesis of Burkitt lymphoma is as follows:

1. Infection and polyclonal lymphoblastoid transformation of B lymphocytes by EBV.
2. Proliferation of B cells and inhibition of suppressor T cells induced by malaria.
3. Deregulation of the c-*myc* proto-oncogene by chromosomal translocation in a single transformed B lymphocyte.
4. Uncontrolled proliferation of a malignant clone of B lymphocytes.

Polyclonal Lymphoproliferation in Immunodeficient States. Congenital or acquired immunodeficiency states are often complicated by the development of EBV-induced, B-cell proliferative disorders. These lesions may be clinically and pathologically indistinguishable from true malignant lymphomas, but they differ in that most are polyclonal.

FIGURE *5-20*
The concept of initiation and promotion. (A) The single application of an initiator to the skin of a mouse produces initiated cells, but no papillomas form. (B) Likewise, the application of a promoter alone to the skin produces no papillomas. (C) If the promoter is applied to the skin before application of the initiator, no papillomas form, although initiated cells are present. (D) When the skin is first exposed to the initiator, subsequent application of the promoter results in papillomas. If the promoter is withdrawn, the papillomas regress, leaving initiated cells in their place. When the promoter is applied to mouse skin bearing papillomas, invasive squamous cell carcinomas are produced.

Nasopharyngeal Carcinoma. Nasopharyngeal carcinoma is a variant of squamous cell carcinoma that has a worldwide distribution and is particularly common in certain parts of Africa and Asia. EBV DNA and nuclear antigen (EBNA) are present in virtually all of these cancers.

Hepatitis B Virus

Chronic infection with HBV, a partially double-stranded DNA virus, is associated with the development of primary hepatocellular carcinoma. The risk for hepatocellular carcinoma in carriers of this virus is more than 200-fold greater than that in noncarriers (see Chapter. 14). The mechanism of carcinogenesis in HBV-related liver cancer is not apparent. Chronic liver cell injury may be sufficient to cause hepatocellular carcinoma, and HBV may be oncogenic in humans by virtue of its ability to induce chronic liver disease rather than by insertional mutagenesis. Alternatively, a protein product (HbX) of an *HBV* gene binds a tumor suppressor protein (p53) and, thus, may allow uncontrolled cell proliferation.

Tumor Suppressor Genes

The concept of oncogenes postulates a dominant genetic alteration that results in overproduction of a normal gene product or synthesis of an abnormally active mutant protein. A second general mechanism by which a genetic alteration contributes to carcinogenesis is a mutation that creates a deficiency of a normal gene product that suppresses tumor formation. In this circumstance, the heterozygous state is sufficient to protect against cancer. **Loss of heterozygosity by deletion or somatic mutation of the remaining normal allele predisposes to tumor development.**

Tumor suppressor genes are being increasingly incriminated in the pathogenesis of both hereditary and spontaneous cancers among humans. Two such genes have been particularly well studied. The retinoblastoma (*Rb*) and *p53* gene products serve to restrain cell division in many tissues, and their absence or inactivation is linked to the development of malignant tumors. Oncogenic DNA viruses also encode products that interact with these suppressor proteins, thereby inactivating their functions. **Thus, the mechanisms underlying development of some tumors associated with germline and somatic mutations or infections with DNA viruses involve the same cellular gene products.**

Retinoblastoma Gene

Retinoblastoma, a rare childhood cancer, is the prototype of a human tumor whose origin is attributed to the inactivation of a specific tumor suppressor gene. Approximately 40% of cases are associated with a germline mutation, whereas the remainder are not hereditary. In patients with hereditary retinoblastoma. all somatic cells carry one missing or defective allele of a gene (the *Rb* gene) located on the long arm of chromosome 13. By contrast, both alleles of the *Rb* gene are inactive in all the retinoblastoma cells. Thus, the *Rb* gene has a tumor suppressor function, and development of hereditary retinoblastoma has been attributed to two genetic events (the "two-hit" hypothesis) (Fig. 5-21). The *Rb* gene encodes a nuclear protein that exists in two phosphorylation states, thereby acting as a switch for entry of the cell into the S phase. It is thought that the function of the *Rb* gene is the most critical checkpoint in the cell cycle, and that inactivating mutations permit unregulated cell proliferation.

Children who inherit a mutant *Rb* gene also suffer a 200-fold increased risk of developing mesenchymal tumors during early adult life. More than 20 different cancers have been described, with osteosarcoma being by far the most common.

The *p53* Gene

The *p53* gene is located on the small arm of chromosome 17, and its protein product is present in virtually all normal tissues. This gene is deleted or mutated in 70% to 80% of colorectal cancers and frequently in cases of breast cancer, small cell carcinoma of the lung, hepatocellular carcinoma, astrocytoma, and numerous other tumors. **In fact, mutations of the *p53* gene seem to be the most common genetic change in human cancer.** In normal cells, p53 is a negative regulator of cell division. In response to DNA damage, p53 levels rise and prevent cells from entering the S phase of the cell cycle, thereby allowing time for DNA repair to take place. In this way, p53 acts as a guardian of the genome by restricting uncontrolled cellular proliferation under circumstances in which cells with abnormal DNA might propagate.

Other Tumor Suppressor Genes

A number of unrelated syndromes have been shown to harbor germline mutations in other tumor suppressor genes. Such tumors include colorectal cancers (*APC* gene) Wilms tumor (*WT-1* gene), neurofibromatosis type 1 (*NF-1* gene), breast cancer (*BRCA1* and *BRCA2* genes), and a number of other neoplastic conditions.

Tumor Suppressor Genes and Oncogenic DNA Viruses

The transforming genes of DNA viruses are not homologous with any cellular genes, but their gene products inactivate tumor suppressor proteins. The trans-

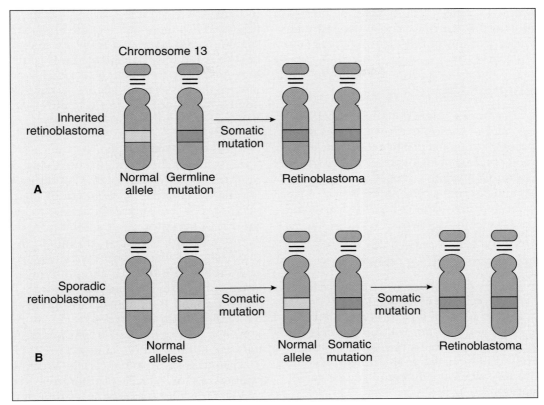

FIGURE 5-21
The "two-hit" origin of retinoblastoma. (A) A child with the inherited form of retinoblastoma is born with a germline mutation in one allele of the retinoblastoma gene located on the long arm of chromosome 13. A second somatic mutation in the retina leads to inactivation of the functioning *Rb* allele and the subsequent development of a retinoblastoma. (B) In sporadic cases of retinoblastoma, the child is born with two normal *Rb* alleles. It requires two independent somatic mutations to inactivate the *Rb* gene function and allow the appearance of a neoplastic clone.

forming proteins of DNA viruses inactivate both the Rb and p53 proteins by binding to these tumor suppressors. These observations indicate that oncogenic DNA viruses use a common mechanism for altering growth regulation and, thereby, transforming cells. Thus, oncogenic DNA viruses transform cells by coding for products that either inhibit tumor suppressor proteins or activate proto-oncogene functions.

Mutator Genes

Mutator genes exercise surveillance over the integrity of genetic information by participating in the cellular response to DNA damage. Loss of these gene functions renders the DNA susceptible to the progressive accumulation of mutations. Two hereditary syndromes associated with an increased risk of cancer have shed light on the roles of mutator genes. Patients with hereditary nonpolyposis colon cancer (HNPCC) display heterozygous germline mutations in at least one of four genes involved in the DNA mismatch repair systems. By contrast, the tumors themselves have lost

the function of both alleles in the affected gene. Ataxia telangiectasia (AT) is a rare hereditary syndrome that includes, among other abnormalities, a predisposition to a number of different cancers. The gene responsible for this condition, termed *ATM* (AT mutated), codes for a nuclear protein that participates in multiple responses to DNA damage, including control of checkpoints in the cell cycle, activation of DNA repair enzymes, and regulation of apoptosis. Considering the carrier rate of 1% in the general population, it has been suggested that *ATM* gene mutations may contribute to a significant number of sporadic cancers.

Telomerase and Cancer

As cells in tissue culture continue to divide, the tips of chromosomes, termed *telomeres*, progressively shorten (see Chapter 1). Because somatic cells do not normally express telomerase, an enzyme that maintains the length of the telomere, the telomere progressively shortens with each replication, thereby acting as a molecular clock that governs the life span of replicating cells. By contrast, cancer cells express telomerase, and reactivation of this enzyme may be necessary for the immortalization of cancer cells. However, the subject requires further study.

Clonal Origin of Cancer

Most cancers arise from a single transformed cell. The most common piece of clinical evidence for this statement is the production by neoplastic plasma cells of a single immunoglobulin that is unique to an individual patient with multiple myeloma. Indeed, such a "monoclonal spike" in the serum electrophoresis from a patient with suspected myeloma is regarded as being conclusive evidence of the disease.

Cancer As Altered Differentiation

In some cancers, the malignant cells are thought to result from a maturation arrest in the sequence of development from a stem cell to a fully differentiated cell. According to this theory, tumor cells accumulate because the mechanisms that control the total number of cells in the fully differentiated compartment of some tissues do not apply when less differentiated precursor cells fail to mature.

Squamous Cell Carcinoma. In many tumors, most of the neoplastic cells are outside the cell cycle and, thus, do not contribute to the malignancy of the tumor. For example, as previously noted, fewer than 3% of cells in a squamous carcinoma maintain the malignant potential of the tumor, and most differentiate and die spontaneously. When such terminally differentiated tumor cells are transplanted into appropriate hosts, they do not grow, whereas their undifferentiated counterparts from the same tumor form typical squamous carcinomas. Such observations support the theory that the initial step in the development of some cancers is failure of the stem cell to differentiate normally.

Teratocarcinoma. Further evidence to support the concept of cancer as a failure of differentiation has come from the study of experimental malignant germ cell tumors (teratocarcinomas). A single embryonal carcinoma cell, the stem cell of a teratocarcinoma, when transplanted into a mouse, gives rise to a tumor containing cells derived from all three germ layers. Clearly, the progeny of the original transplanted tumor cell differentiate into more mature cells, which express

recognizable phenotypes of more fully differentiated tissues. When these differentiated tissues of the teratocarcinoma are separated from the malignant embryonal cells and then transplanted into compatible hosts, they not only survive but also function with no detriment to the host. These cells are clearly benign, and the dogma that "once a cancer cell, always a cancer cell" does not hold in this case.

Leukemias and Lymphomas. In acute lymphoblastic leukemia of childhood, the neoplastic cells strongly resemble the lymphocytes that appear transiently during the developmental sequence of the normal lymphocyte. The leukemic cells appear to be "frozen" in the act of receptor gene assembly and expression. Acute myeloid leukemia is similar to acute lymphoblastic leukemia in that the malignant cells express phenotypes of transient, immature myeloid populations. Likewise, studies of chronic lymphocytic leukemias and lymphomas have revealed that these malignant disorders represent clonal expansions of lymphocyte populations corresponding to subsets found in normal lymphoid tissue.

The data suggest that certain leukemias and lymphomas are not truly proliferative disorders but, rather, reflect an uncoupling of differentiation from proliferation, with the resulting accumulation of cells that have not attained terminal differentiation.

TUMOR IMMUNOLOGY

Results of animal experiments suggest that immune defenses against malignant tumors exist, but there is a paucity of direct evidence in human cancers.

Immunologic Defenses Against Cancer in Experimental Animals

To invoke a role for an immune defense against cancer, it is necessary to postulate that tumor cells express antigens that differ from those of normal cells and are recognized as being foreign by the host (Fig. 5-22). When cells from a chemically or virally induced tumor are transplanted into a syngeneic mouse, the cells form a tumor. After cells from this tumor are passed into a second mouse, they again form a tumor. On the other hand, if the first transplanted tumor is removed before

FIGURE 5-22
Immunogenicity of tumors. Cancer cells injected into a syngeneic mouse form tumors, which then metastasize and kill the animal. Excision of the tumor before it has metastasized allows the rejection of a second tumor implant, presumably as a consequence of immunity acquired from exposure to the original tumor.

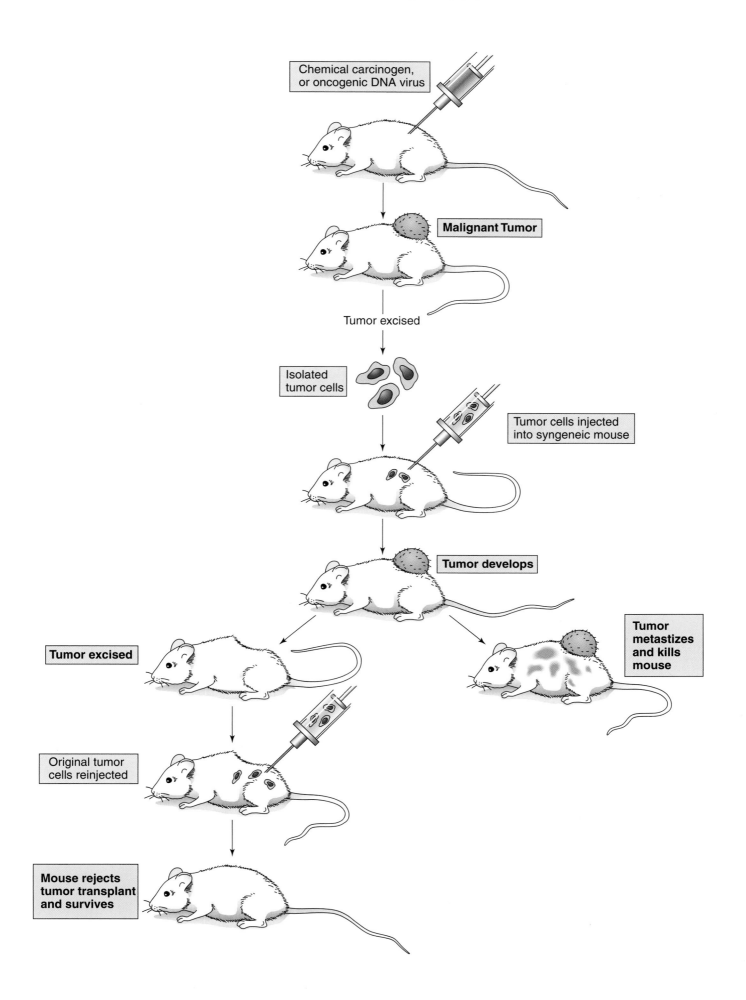

Chemical carcinogen, or oncogenic DNA virus

Malignant Tumor

Tumor excised

Isolated tumor cells

Tumor cells injected into syngeneic mouse

Tumor develops

Tumor excised

Tumor metastizes and kills mouse

Original tumor cells reinjected

Mouse rejects tumor transplant and survives

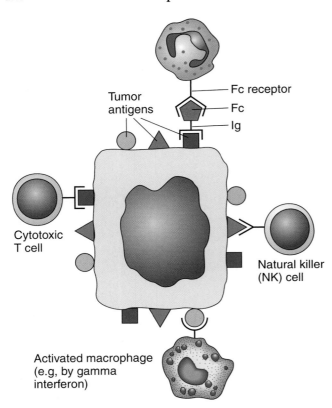

Tumor antigens

Fc receptor
Fc
Ig

Cytotoxic T cell

Natural killer (NK) cell

Activated macrophage (e.g, by gamma interferon)

FIGURE 5-23
Possible mechanisms of immunologic tumor cytotoxicity in animal studies

it metastasizes (i.e., the mouse is cured of its tumor), reinjection of the tumor cells back into the cured mouse will not produce a tumor. **The transplanted tumor is rejected because of an immunity acquired as a result of the first tumor transplant.**

Further evidence for the existence of immune mechanisms in the defense against cancer comes from studies in nude mice. These animals are devoid of T cell–mediated immunity and, thus, accept grafts from different species. Similarly, tumors from different species grow in an unrestrained fashion when transplanted into nude mice.

In experimental animals, tumors produced by chemicals and viruses display tumor-specific antigens. **The relevance of tumor-specific antigens to human cancer is suspect, because they have not been identified in human tumors.**

The contribution of any specific immunologic mechanism to tumor cell destruction in vivo has not been clearly defined. A number of possible mechanisms are recognized (Fig. 5-23):

- **T Cell-Mediated Cytotoxicity.** The capacity of cytotoxic T cells to mediate the specific rejection of transplanted tumors is evidenced by the demonstration that lymphocytes from tumor-bearing hosts can transfer tumor immunity when injected into normal animals.

- **Natural Killer Cell-Mediated Cytotoxicity.** Another set of lymphocytes, the natural killer cells, have tumoricidal activity that is not dependent on previous sensitization. These lymphocytes are generally more effective at killing tumor cells than untransformed cells.

- **Macrophage-Mediated Cytotoxicity.** Macrophages are capable of killing tumor cells in a nonspecific manner. However, their role in the control of malignant tumors is far from clear, because under some circumstances, in vitro factors derived from macrophages can actually stimulate the proliferation of tumor cells.

- **Antibody-Dependent Cell-Mediated Cytotoxicity.** Tumor-associated antigens are capable of eliciting a humoral antibody response, but these immunoglobulins by themselves do not kill tumor cells. However, as discussed in Chapter 4, such antibodies can participate in antibody-dependent cell-mediated cytotoxicity. The antibody binds to both the tumor antigen and the Fc receptor of the effector cell, thereby bringing the effector cell into direct contact with its target. Depending on the conditions, the effector cell may be a lymphocyte killer cell (null cell), macrophage, or neutrophil.

- **Complement-Mediated Cytotoxicity.** Tumor cells that have been coated with specific antibodies may be lysed by the activation of complement. This mechanism operates only on cells in suspension (e.g., leukemic cells) and has not been demonstrated to occur with solid tumors.

Immune Surveillance

The theory of immune surveillance holds that mutant clones with neoplastic potential frequently arise but are recognized and expunged by cell-mediated immune responses. The strongest evidence for such a scenario comes from the observation of increased susceptibility to tumor induction by oncogenic DNA viruses in T cell-deficient (nude) mice. However, these animals do not exhibit an increased incidence of spontaneous tumors, and they are not more susceptible to tumor induction by RNA viruses or chemicals. It is now thought that the susceptibility of nude mice to induction of tumors by oncogenic DNA viruses reflects an inability to control the viral infection rather than a defect of immune surveillance against the incipient neoplasms. **Thus, there is reason to believe that immune surveillance is either ineffective or nonexistent.**

Immunologic Defenses Against Cancer in Humans

Although some circumstantial evidence exists for the participation of immunologic defenses in the resistance to cancer among humans, it deserves emphasis

that conclusive proof for their clinical importance is lacking. Perhaps the strongest argument for immunologic tumor rejection in humans is the observation that immunodeficiency, whether acquired or congenital, is associated with an increased incidence of cancers, almost all of which are B-cell lymphomas. Three prominent examples are widely cited, namely X-linked lymphoproliferative syndrome (XLP), acquired immunodeficiency syndrome (AIDS), and patients who receive immunosuppressive therapy following organ transplantation. In patients with XLP or AIDS, the enormously increased risk can be attributed to a polyclonal lymphoid hyperplasia induced by infection with EBV, coupled with a lack of cytotoxic T cells that normally limit the proliferation of virus-infected B cells.

Evasion of Immunologic Cytotoxicity

That cancer is alive and well despite the presence of potential immunologic defenses implies that such mechanisms are ineffective or that tumor cells have the capacity to evade immunologic cytotoxicity. It is intuitively clear that an absence of tumor-specific antigens, or a lack of immunogenicity by such antigens, will permit unhampered growth of the neoplasm. **In this respect, tumor-specific antigens have not been found in the large majority of human tumors.**

Even in strongly antigenic tumors, it is thought that clones will arise that do not express tumor antigens or histocompatibility antigens and, thus, will be selected for survival. In this way, a tumor might develop resistance to immunologic defenses in a manner analogous to that of bacterial resistance to antibiotics.

SYSTEMIC EFFECTS OF CANCER ON THE HOST

In some patients, cancer produces remote effects that are not attributable to tumor invasion or metastasis. These are collectively termed **paraneoplastic syndromes.**

Fever

It is not uncommon for patients with cancer to present initially with fever of unknown origin that cannot be explained by an infectious disease. The cancers in which this most commonly occurs are Hodgkin's disease, renal cell carcinoma, and osteogenic sarcoma. Tumor cells may themselves release pyrogens, or the inflammatory cells in the tumor stroma can produce interleukin-1 or TNF.

Anorexia and Weight Loss

A paraneoplastic syndrome of anorexia, weight loss, and cachexia is very common in patients with cancer, often appearing before its malignant cause becomes apparent. Unlike starvation, which is associated with a lowered metabolic rate, cancer is often accompanied by an elevated metabolic rate. Much of this paraneoplastic syndrome is attributed to the effect of TNF-α.

Endocrine Syndromes

Malignant tumors may produce a number of peptide hormones whose secretion is not under normal regulatory control. Most of these hormones are normally present in the brain, gastrointestinal tract, or endocrine organs. Their inappropriate secretion can cause a variety of effects.

Cushing Syndrome. Ectopic secretion of corticotropin by a tumor leads to features of Cushing syndrome, including hypokalemia, hyperglycemia, hypertension, and muscle weakness. Corticotropin production is most commonly seen with cancers of the lung, particularly small cell (oat cell) carcinoma. It also complicates carcinoid tumors and other neuroendocrine tumors, such as pheochromocytoma, neuroblastoma, and medullary carcinoma of the thyroid.

Inappropriate Antidiuresis. Inappropriate production of arginine vasopressin (antidiuretic hormone) by a tumor may cause sodium and water retention to such an extent that it manifests as water intoxication, resulting in altered mental status, seizures, coma, and sometimes, even death. The tumor that most often produces this syndrome is small cell carcinoma of the lung. It is also reported with carcinomas of the prostate, gastrointestinal tract, and pancreas and with thymomas, lymphomas, and Hodgkin's disease.

Hypercalcemia. A paraneoplastic complication that afflicts 10% of all patients with cancer, namely hypercalcemia, is usually caused by metastatic disease of the bone. However, in approximately one-tenth of cases, it occurs in the absence of bony metastases. The most common cause of paraneoplastic hypercalcemia is secretion of a parathormone-like peptide by an epithelial tumor, usually squamous cell carcinoma of the lung or adenocarcinoma of the breast. In multiple myeloma and lymphomas, hypercalcemia is attributed to secretion of osteoclast-activating factor.

Gonadotropic Syndromes. Gonadotropins may be secreted by germ cell tumors, gestational trophoblastic tumors (choriocarcinoma, hydatidiform mole), and pituitary tumors. High gonadotropin levels lead to precocious puberty in children, gynecomastia in men, and oligomenorrhea in premenopausal women.

Hypoglycemia. The best-understood cause of hypoglycemia associated with tumors is excessive insulin production by islet cell tumors of the pancreas. Other tumors, especially large mesotheliomas and fibrosarcomas and primary hepatocellular carcinoma, are associated with hypoglycemia. The cause of hypoglycemia in nonendocrine tumors is not established, but the most likely candidate is production of somatomedins (insulin-like growth factors).

Neurologic Syndromes

A small group of patients with cancer suffer from a variety of neurologic complaints without any demonstrable cause. Such disorders are thought to reflect remote effects of cancer on the nervous system. Cerebral complications include dementia, subacute cerebellar degeneration, limbic encephalitis, and optic neuritis.

Spinal Cord

Subacute motor neuropathy, a disorder of the spinal cord, is characterized by slowly developing lower motor neuron weakness without sensory changes. It is so strongly associated with cancer that an intensive search for an occult neoplasm, often a lymphoma, should be made in patients who present with these symptoms.

Amyotrophic lateral sclerosis is well described among patients with cancer. Conversely, as many as 10% of patients with this disease are found to have cancer.

Peripheral Nerves

Sensorimotor peripheral neuropathy, which is characterized by distal weakness and wasting and sensory loss, is common in patients with cancer.

Purely sensory neuropathy, resulting from degenerative changes in the dorsal root ganglia, may also develop in persons with cancer.

Autonomic and gastrointestinal neuropathies, manifested as orthostatic hypotension, neurogenic bladder, and intestinal pseudo-obstruction, are associated with small cell carcinoma of the lung.

Skeletal Muscle

Patients with dermatomyositis or polymyositis have an incidence of cancer five- to sevenfold higher than that in the general population.

Hematologic Syndromes

Hematologic paraneoplastic syndromes are well described.

Erythrocytosis

Cancer-associated erythrocytosis is a complication of some tumors, particularly renal cell carcinoma, hepatocellular carcinoma, and cerebellar hemangioblastoma. Elevated erythropoietin levels are found in the tumor and in the serum of approximately half the patients with erythrocytosis.

Anemia

One of the most common findings in patients with cancer is normocytic and normochromic anemia, but the mechanism for this disorder is not clear. **Pure red cell aplasia,** often associated with thymomas, and megaloblastic anemia are sometimes encountered. **Autoimmune hemolytic anemia** may be associated with B-cell lymphomas and with solid tumors, particularly in elderly patients. In fact, autoimmune hemolytic anemia in an older person suggests the possibility of an underlying neoplasm.

Leukocytes and Platelets

Paraneoplastic granulocytosis, characterized by a peripheral granulocyte count of more than 20,000 cells/μL, is a finding that may lead to an erroneous diagnosis of leukemia. This condition usually results from secretion of a colony-stimulating factor by the tumor.

Eosinophilia is occasionally noted in association with cancer, particularly in Hodgkin's disease, in which it may occur in one-fifth of cases.

Thrombocytosis, with platelet counts of more than 400,000 cells/μL, occurs in one-third of patients with cancer.

Hypercoagulable State

The association between cancer and venous thrombosis was noted more than a century ago. Since then, other abnormalities resulting from a hypercoagulable state (e.g., disseminated intravascular coagulation and nonbacterial thrombotic endocarditis) have been recognized.

Venous Thrombosis. This condition is most distinctly associated with carcinoma of the pancreas, which carries a 50-fold increased incidence of this complication compared with that in cases of chronic pancreatitis. Venous thrombosis, commonly in the deep veins of the legs, is also particularly frequent in association with other mucin-secreting adenocarcinomas of the gastrointestinal tract and with lung cancer. Tumors of the breast, ovary, prostate, and other organs are occasionally complicated by venous thrombosis.

Disseminated Intravascular Coagulation. The widespread appearance of thrombi in small vessels in association with cancer may be noted because of the chronic occurrence of thrombotic phenomena or an acute hemorrhagic diathesis. This complication is most commonly found with acute promyelocytic leukemia and adenocarcinomas.

Nonbacterial Thrombotic Endocarditis. The presence of noninfected verrucous deposits of fibrin and platelets on the left-sided heart valves occurs in patients with cancer, particularly in those who were also debilitated. This form of endocarditis (also called marantic endocarditis) develops with or without disseminated intravascular coagulation. Although the effects on the heart are not of clinical importance, emboli to the brain present a great danger. This cardiac complication is most common with solid tumors but may occasionally be noted with leukemias and lymphomas.

Malabsorption

Malabsorption of a variety of dietary components is an occasional paraneoplastic symptom, and half of patients with cancer develop some histologic abnormalities of the small intestine. The classic tumor associated with malabsorption is lymphoma of the small intestine. However, such changes can occur even with tumors that do not directly involve the bowel.

Renal Syndromes

Nephrotic syndrome, as a consequence of renal vein thrombosis or amyloidosis, is a well-known complication of cancer. Nephrotic syndrome may also represent a paraneoplastic complication in the form of minimal change disease (lipoid nephrosis) or glomerulonephritis produced by the deposition of immune complexes. The antigens in this type of glomerulonephritis are not generally identified.

Cutaneous Syndromes

Pigmented lesions and keratoses are well-recognized paraneoplastic effects.

Acanthosis nigricans is a cutaneous disorder marked by hyperkeratosis and pigmentation of the axilla, neck, flexures, and anogenital region. **It is of particular interest, because more than half of patients with acanthosis nigricans have cancer.** More than 90% of the cases occur in association with gastrointestinal carcinomas.

EPIDEMIOLOGY OF CANCER

Incidence of Cancer in the United States

Cancer accounts for one-fifth of the total mortality in the United States and is the second-leading cause of death after cardiovascular diseases and stroke. For most cancers, death rates in the United States have largely remained flat during the past 50 years, but with some notable exceptions. The death rate from cancer of the lung among men has risen dramatically since 1930, when it was an uncommon tumor, to the present, when it is by far the most common cause of death from cancer in men. As discussed in Chapter 8, the entire epidemic of lung cancer deaths is attributable to smoking. Among women, smoking did not become fashionable until World War II. Considering the time lag needed between starting to smoke and development of cancer of the lung, it is not surprising that the increased death rate from lung cancer in women did not become significant until after 1965. In the United States, the death rate from lung cancer in women now exceeds that for breast cancer and is now, as in men, the most common fatal cancer.

By contrast, and for reasons difficult to fathom, cancer of the stomach, which in 1930 was by far the most common cancer among men and only slightly less common than breast cancer among women, has shown a remarkable and sustained decline in frequency. Similarly, there has been an unexplained decline in the death rate from cancer of the uterus, although better screening and diagnostic and therapeutic methods may account for some of this reduction.

Individual cancers have their own age-related profiles, but for most, increased age is associated with increased incidence. The most striking example of this dependency on age is carcinoma of the prostate, in which the incidence increases 30-fold between 50 and 85 years of age. Certain neoplastic diseases, such as acute lymphoblastic leukemia in children and testicular cancer in young adults, show different age-related peaks of incidence.

Geographic and Ethnic Differences in Cancer Incidence

Nasopharyngeal Cancer. Nasopharyngeal cancer is rare in most of the world, except for certain regions of China, Hong Kong, and Singapore. This tumor has been associated with infection by EBV.

Esophageal Carcinoma. The range in incidence of esophageal carcinoma varies from extremely low among Mormon women in Utah to a value some 300-fold greater among the female population of northern Iran. Particularly high rates of esophageal cancer are noted in a so-called Asian esophageal cancer belt, which includes the great land mass stretching from European Russia to eastern China. Esophageal cancer is also more common in certain regions of Africa inhabited predominantly by blacks and among blacks in the United States. The causes of esophageal cancer are obscure. It disproportionately affects the poor in many areas of the world, however, and the combination of alcohol abuse and smoking is associated with a particularly high risk.

Stomach Cancer. The highest incidence of stomach cancer occurs in Japan, where the disease is almost 10-fold as frequent as it is among U.S. whites. A high incidence has also been observed in Latin American countries, particularly Chile. Stomach cancer is also common in Iceland and Eastern Europe.

Colorectal Cancer. The highest incidence of colorectal cancer is found in the United States, where it is three- or fourfold more common than in Japan, India, Africa, and Latin America. It has been theorized that the high fiber content of the diet in low-risk areas and the high fat content in the United States are related to this difference, although this concept has been seriously questioned.

Liver Cancer. There is a strong correlation between the incidence of primary hepatocellular carcinoma and the prevalence of hepatitis B and hepatitis C infection. Endemic regions for both diseases include large parts of sub-Saharan Africa and most of the Orient, Indonesia, and the Philippines. It must be remembered, too, that levels of aflatoxin B_1 are high in the staple diets of many high-risk areas.

Skin Cancer. As previously noted, rates for skin cancers vary with skin color and exposure to the sun. Thus, particularly high rates have been reported in Northern Australia, where the population is principally of Celtic origin and sun exposure is intense. Increased rates of skin cancer have also been noted among the white population of the American Southwest. The lowest rates are found among persons with pigmented skin (e.g., Japanese, Chinese, and Indians). The rates for African blacks, despite their heavily pigmented skin, are occasionally higher than those for Asians because of the higher incidence of melanomas of the soles and palms in blacks.

Breast Cancer. Adenocarcinoma of the breast, which is the most common female cancer in many parts of Europe and North America, shows considerable geographic variation. The rates in Africa and Asia are only one-fifth to one-sixth of those prevailing in Europe and the United States. Epidemiologic studies have contributed little to our understanding of the cause of breast cancer. Although hormonal factors are clearly involved, except for a good correlation with age at first pregnancy, few confirmed hormonal correlations have surfaced. The role of dietary fat in the pathogenesis of breast cancer is still being debated.

Cancer of the Cervix. Striking differences in the incidence of squamous carcinoma of the cervix exist between ethnic groups and different socioeconomic levels. For instance, the very low rate in the Ashkenazi Jews of Israel contrasts with a 25-fold greater prevalence in the Hispanic population of Texas. In general, groups with low socioeconomic status have a higher incidence of cervical cancer than more prosperous and better educated groups. This cancer is also directly correlated with early sexual activity and multiparity, and it is rare among women who are not sexually active, such as nuns. It is also uncommon among women whose husbands are circumcised. A strong association with HPVs has been demonstrated, and cervical cancer may eventually be classed as a venereal disease.

Choriocarcinoma. Choriocarcinoma, an uncommon cancer of trophoblastic differentiation, is found principally in women following pregnancy, although it can present as a testicular tumor. The rates of this disease are particularly high in the Pacific Rim of Asia (Singapore, Hong Kong, Japan, and the Philippines).

Prostatic Cancer. Very low incidences of prostatic cancer are reported for Oriental populations, particularly Japanese, whereas the highest rates are described in U.S. blacks, in whom the disease occurs some 25-fold more often. The incidence in U.S. and European whites is intermediate.

Testicular Cancer. An unusual aspect of testicular cancer is its universal rarity among black populations. Interestingly, although the rate in U.S. blacks is only approximately one-fourth that in whites, it is still considerably higher than the rate among African blacks.

Cancer of the Penis. This squamous carcinoma is virtually nonexistent among circumcised men of any race, but it is common among uncircumcised men in Africa and Asia.

Cancer of the Urinary Bladder. The rates for transitional cell carcinoma of the bladder are fairly uniform. Squamous carcinoma of the bladder, however, is a special case. Ordinarily far less common than transitional cell carcinoma, it has a high incidence in areas where schistosomal infestation of the bladder (bilharziasis) is endemic.

Burkitt Lymphoma. Burkitt lymphoma, a disease of children, was first described in Uganda, where it accounts for half of all childhood tumors. Since then, a high frequency has been observed in other African countries, particularly in the hot and humid lowlands. These are areas where malaria is also endemic. High rates have been recorded in other tropical areas, such as Malaysia and New Guinea, but European and U.S. cases are encountered only sporadically.

Multiple Myeloma. This malignant tumor of plasma cells is uncommon among U.S. whites but displays a three- to fourfold higher incidence in U.S. and South African blacks.

Chronic Lymphocytic Leukemia. Chronic lymphocytic leukemia is common among elderly persons in Europe and North America but is considerably less common in Japan.

CHAPTER 6

Developmental and Genetic Diseases

Emanuel Rubin
John L. Farber

Multifactorial Inheritance	Erythroblastosis Fetalis and Neonatal Hemolytic Anemia
Cleft Lip and Cleft Palate	Birth Injury
Diseases of Infancy and Childhood	Sudden Infant Death Syndrome
Prematurity and Intrauterine Growth Retardation	**Neoplasms of Infancy and Childhood**
Organ Immaturity	Benign Tumors and Tumor-Like Conditions
Respiratory Distress Syndrome of the Newborn (Hyaline Membrane Disease)	Malignant Tumors

Developmental and genetic disorders are classified as follows:

- Errors of morphogenesis
- Chromosomal abnormalities
- Single-gene defects
- Polygenic inherited diseases.

The fetus may also be injured by adverse transplacental influences or by deformities and injuries caused by intrauterine trauma or during parturition. After birth, acquired diseases of infancy and childhood are also important causes of morbidity and mortality.

PRINCIPLES OF TERATOLOGY

■ *Teratogens are chemical, physical, and biologic agents that cause developmental anomalies.*

- **Susceptibility to teratogens is variable.** An example of human variability in vulnerability to teratogens is the fetal alcohol syndrome. This condition affects some children of alcoholic mothers whereas others are resistant.
- **Susceptibility to teratogens is specific for each developmental stage.** Most agents are teratogenic only during critical stages of development (Fig. 6-1). For example, maternal rubella infection causes abnormalities in the fetus only during the first 3 months of pregnancy.
- **The mechanism of teratogenesis is specific for each teratogen.** Teratogenic drugs inhibit the activity of crucial enzymes or receptors, interfere with formation of the mitotic spindle, or block energy production, thereby inhibiting metabolic steps critical for normal morphogenesis. Many drugs and viruses affect specific tissues (e.g., neurotropism, cardiotropism) and damage some developing organs more than others.
- **Teratogenesis is dose-dependent.**

- **Teratogens produce death, growth retardation, malformation, or functional impairment.** The specific outcome depends on the interaction between the teratogenic influences, the maternal organism, and the fetal-placental unit.

ERRORS OF MORPHOGENESIS

Normal intrauterine and postnatal development depends on sequential activation and repression of genes inherited from the parents. Although the fertilized ovum (zygote) has all the genes found in the adult organism, most of them are inactive. As the zygote enters the cleavage stages of development, individual genes (or sets of genes) are activated in a stage-specific manner. Initially, activation involves only those genes essential for cellular replication and growth, cell-to-cell interaction, and regulation of important morphogenetic movements. **Abnormally activated or structurally abnormal genes in the zygote and early embryonic cells result in early death.**

Cells that form the two- and four-cell embryos (blastomeres) are developmentally equipotent, and each can give rise to an adult organism. Thus, adverse environmental influences on preimplantation-stage embryos exert an all-or-nothing effect. Either the conceptus dies, or development proceeds uninterrupted (because the interchangeable blastomeres can replace the loss). The most common consequence of toxic exposure at the preimplantation stage is embryonic death, which often passes unnoticed or is perceived as heavy, albeit delayed, menstrual bleeding.

Most complex developmental abnormalities affecting several organ systems result from injuries inflicted from the time of implantation of the blastocyst through early organogenesis. **The formation of primordial organ systems is the stage of embryonic development most susceptible to teratogenesis.** Many major developmental abnormalities probably result from faulty gene activity or the deleterious effects of exogenous toxins on the embryo at this time (see Fig. 6-1).

■ *Agenesis is the complete absence of an organ primordium.* It may present as (1) complete absence of an organ, as in unilateral or bilateral agenesis of kidneys; (2) absence of part of an organ, as in agenesis of the corpus callosum of the brain; or (3) absence of tissue or cells within an organ, as in the absence of testicular germ cells in congenital infertility ("Sertoli cell only" syndrome).

■ *Aplasia is absence of an organ coupled with persistence of the organ anlage or a rudiment that never developed completely.* Thus, aplasia of the lung refers to a condition in which the main bronchus ends blindly in nondescript tissue composed of rudimentary ducts and connective tissue.

■ *Hypoplasia refers to reduced size owing to the incomplete development of all or part of an organ.* Examples include microphthalmia (small eyes), micrognathia (small jaw), and microcephaly (small brain and head).

■ *Dysraphic anomalies are defects caused by the failure of apposed structures to fuse.* Spina bifida is an anomaly in which the spinal canal has not closed completely and the overlying bone and skin have not fused, thereby leaving a midline defect.

■ *Involution failures reflect the persistence of embryonic or fetal structures that should involute at certain stages of development.* A persistent thyroglossal duct is the result of incomplete involution of the tract that connects the base of the tongue with the developing thyroid.

■ *Division failures are caused by the incomplete cleavage of embryonic tissues when that process depends on the programmed death of cells.* Fingers and toes are formed at the distal end of the limb bud through the loss of cells located between the primordia that contain the cartilage. If these cells do not die in a programmed manner, the fingers will be conjoined or incompletely separated (syndactyly).

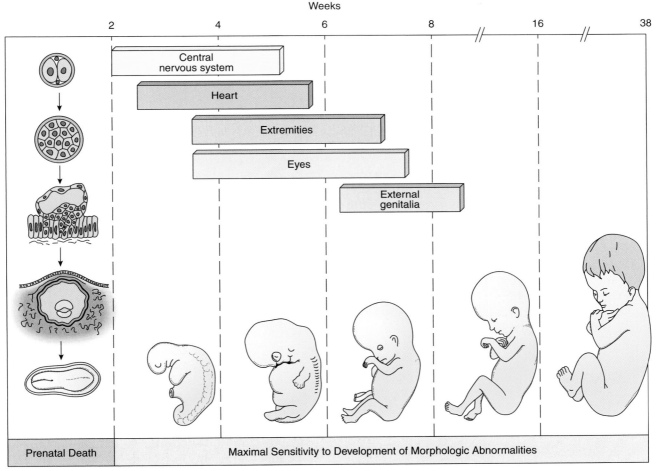

FIGURE *6-1*
Sensitivity of specific organs to teratogenic agents at critical stages of human embryogenesis. Exposure to adverse influences during the preimplantation and early postimplantation stages of development (*far left*) leads to prenatal death. Periods of maximal sensitivity to teratogens (*horizontal bars*) vary for different organ systems but, overall, are limited to the first 8 weeks of pregnancy.

■ *Atresia refers to defects caused by the incomplete formation of a lumen.* Many hollow organs originate as strands and cords of cells, the centers of which are programmed to die, thus forming a central cavity or lumen. Atresia of the esophagus is characterized by partial occlusion of the lumen, which was not fully established during embryogenesis.

■ *Dysplasia is caused by abnormal organization of cells into tissues, a situation that results in abnormal histogenesis.* (Dysplasia has a different meaning here from that used in characterizing the precancerous lesion epithelial dysplasia [see Chapter 1].) Tuberous sclerosis is a striking example of dysplasia and is characterized by abnormal development of the brain, which contains aggregates of normally developed cells arranged into grossly visible "tubers."

■ *Ectopia or* **heterotopia** *is an anomaly in which an organ is outside its normal anatomic site.* Thus, an ectopic heart is located outside the thorax.

■ *Dystopia refers to retention of an organ at the site where it is located during development.* For example, the kidneys are initially in the pelvis and then move into a more cranial lumbar position. Dystopic kidneys are those that remain in the pelvis.

After the third month of pregnancy, exposure of the human fetus to teratogenic influences rarely results in major errors of morphogenesis. However, morphologic and, especially, functional consequences are still found in children exposed to exogenous teratogens during the second and third trimesters. For example, the central nervous system does not attain functional maturity until several years after birth and, therefore, is susceptible to adverse exogenous influences not only during pregnancy but for some time after birth as well.

■ *Developmental sequence anomaly is a pattern of defects related to a single anomaly or pathogenetic mechanism.* In this anomaly, different factors lead to the same consequences through a common pathway. Such a situation is well illustrated by Potter complex (Fig. 6-2), in which pulmonary hypoplasia, external signs of intrauterine fetal compression, and morphologic changes of the amnion are all related to oligohydramnios (a severely reduced amount of amniotic fluid). A fetus enclosed in an amniotic sac develops the distinctive features of Potter complex regardless of the cause of the oligohydramnios.

Clinically Important Malformations

Anencephaly

■ *Anencephaly refers to congenital absence of the cranial vault, with cerebral hemispheres completely missing or reduced to small masses attached to the base of the skull.* This condition is a dysraphic defect of neural tube closure

(Fig. 6-3). Failure of the neural tube to close results in a lack of closure of the overlying bony structures of the cranium and an absence of the calvarium, skin, and subcutaneous tissues of this region. The exposed brain is incompletely formed or even entirely absent.

Genetic factors seem to play a role in the pathogenesis of anencephaly. The anomaly is twice as common in females as in males, and it occurs with higher frequency in certain families. The risk of a second anencephalic fetus is 2% to 5%, and after two anencephalic fetuses. the risk rises to 25% for each subsequent pregnancy.

Other Neural Tube Defects

The neural tube closes sequentially in a craniocaudad direction, and a defect in this process results in abnormalities of the vertebral column.

■ *Craniorachischisis occurs when defective closure extends from the cranium into the spinal cord and vertebral column.*

■ *Spina bifida refers to the incomplete closure of the spinal cord and vertebral column.* This anomaly is usually localized to the lumbar region and represents the mildest dysraphic abnormality of the central nervous system.

■ *Meningocele is a hernial protrusion of the meninges through a defect in the vertebral column.*

■ *Myelomeningocele refers to the same condition as meningocele, but in this case, it is complicated by hernial protrusion of the spinal cord itself.*

Neural tube defects are illustrated in Figure 6-3 and discussed in greater detail in Chapter 28.

Fetal Alcohol Syndrome

■ *Fetal alcohol syndrome describes a complex of abnormalities induced by maternal consumption of alcoholic beverages and includes (1) growth retardation, (2) central nervous system dysfunction, and (3) characteristic facial dysmorphology.* Because not all children adversely affected by maternal alcohol abuse exhibit the entire spectrum of abnormalities, the term **fetal alcohol effect** is also used.

Abnormalities related to fetal alcohol effect, particularly mild degrees of mental deficiency and emotional disorders, are far more common than the full-blown fetal alcohol syndrome. The minimum amount of alcohol that results in fetal injury is not well established, but children with the entire spectrum of fetal alcohol syndrome are usually born to mothers who are chronic alcoholics.

☐ **Pathology and Clinical Features:** Infants born to alcoholic mothers often exhibit prenatal growth retardation, which continues after birth. The facial dysmorphology of fetal alcohol syndrome includes microcephaly, epicanthal folds, short palpebral fissures, maxillary hypoplasia, a thin upper lip, a small jaw (micrognathia), and a poorly developed philtrum. Septal defects of the heart are described in as many as one-third of the patients, although many of these defects close spontaneously.

Fetal alcohol syndrome is perhaps the most common cause of acquired mental retardation. In a major study, one-fifth of children with fetal alcohol syndrome had IQs of lower than 70, and 40% of the children had IQs of between 70 and 85.

TORCH Complex

■ *TORCH refers to a complex of similar signs and symptoms produced by fetal or neonatal infection with a variety of micro-organisms. These include* Toxoplasma *(T)*, rubella *(R)*, cytomegalovirus *(C)*, and herpes simplex virus *(H)*. In the acronym TORCH, the letter "O" represents "others" (Fig. 6-4).

- **Toxoplasmosis.** Asymptomatic toxoplasmosis is common, and 25% of women in their reproductive years exhibit antibodies to this organism. By contrast, intrauterine *Toxoplasma* infection occurs in only 0.1% of all pregnancies.
- **Rubella.** Introduction of the rubella vaccine in the United States has virtually eliminated congenital rubella, and fewer than 10 cases are reported each year.
- **Cytomegalovirus.** Two-thirds of women at child-bearing age test positive for cytomegalovirus immunoglobulin G, and as many as 2% of newborns in the United States are congenitally infected with this virus.
- **Herpesvirus.** Intrauterine infection with herpes simplex virus type 2 is uncommon. Infection is most often acquired during passage through the birth canal of a mother with active genital herpes. Congenital herpes infection can be prevented by cesarean section of mothers who exhibit active genital lesions.

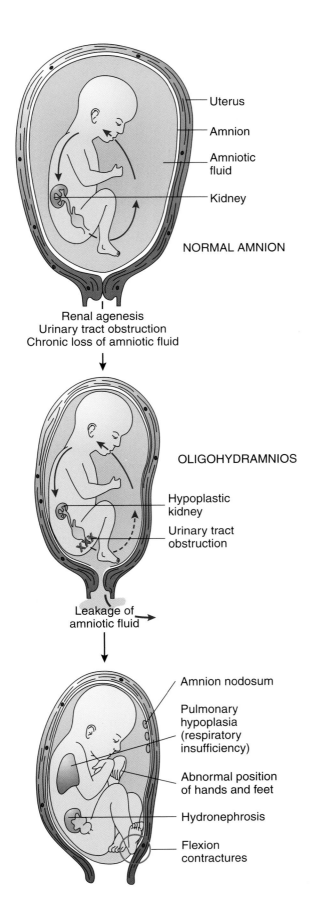

NORMAL AMNION

Renal agenesis
Urinary tract obstruction
Chronic loss of amniotic fluid

OLIGOHYDRAMNIOS

Hypoplastic kidney

Urinary tract obstruction

Leakage of amniotic fluid

Amnion nodosum

Pulmonary hypoplasia (respiratory insufficiency)

Abnormal position of hands and feet

Hydronephrosis

Flexion contractures

FIGURE   6-2
Potter complex. The fetus normally swallows amniotic fluid and, in turn, excretes urine, thereby maintaining a normal volume of amniotic fluid. In the face of urinary tract disease (e.g., renal agenesis or urinary tract obstruction) or leakage of amniotic fluid, the volume of amniotic fluid decreases, a situation termed *oligohydramnios*. Oligohydramnios results in a number of congenital abnormalities termed *Potter complex*, which includes pulmonary hypoplasia and contractures of the limbs. The amnion has a nodular appearance. In cases of urinary tract obstruction, congenital hydronephrosis is also seen, although this abnormality is not considered to be part of the Potter complex.

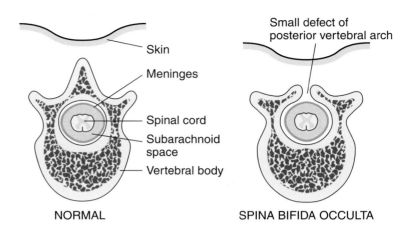

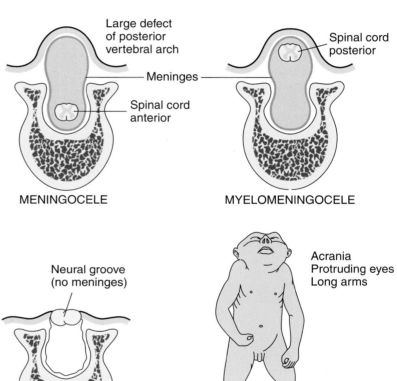

FIGURE   *6-3*
Dysraphic defects of the neural tube. Incomplete fusion of the neural tube and overlying bone, soft tissues, or skin leads to several defects, varying from mild anomalies (e.g., spina bifida occulta) to severe anomalies (e.g., anencephaly).

The specific organisms of the TORCH complex are discussed in greater detail in Chapter 9.

☐ **Pathology:** The clinical and pathologic findings in the symptomatic newborn vary, and only a minority present with multisystem disease and the entire spectrum of abnormalities.

Lesions of the brain represent the most serious pathologic changes in TORCH-infected children.

Acute encephalitis is associated with foci of necrosis, which are initially surrounded by inflammatory cells. Later, the lesions become calcified and are visualized radiologically, most prominently in congenital toxoplasmosis. Microcephaly, hydrocephalus, and abnormally shaped gyri and sulci (microgyria) are frequent. Severe brain damage is reflected in psychomotor retardation, neurologic defects, and seizures.

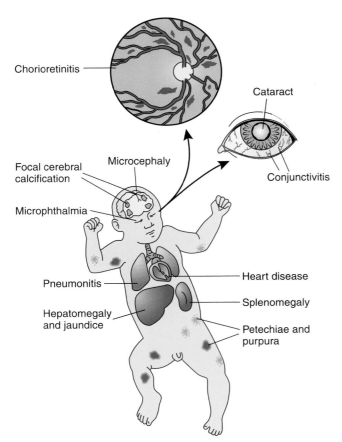

FIGURE 6-4
TORCH complex. Children infected in utero with *Toxoplasma*, **rubella, cytomegalovirus, or herpes simplex virus show remarkably similar symptoms.**

Ocular defects are also prominent in the TORCH complex, particularly in rubella embryopathy, in which more than two-thirds of patients present with cataracts and microphthalmus.

Cardiac anomalies occur in many children with the TORCH complex, most commonly in congenital rubella. Patent ductus arteriosus and various septal defects are the most frequent abnormalities.

STRUCTURAL CHROMOSOMAL ABNORMALITIES

The structural chromosomal abnormalities that originate during gametogenesis are important, because they are transmitted to all the somatic cells of the offspring and may result in heritable diseases. During normal meiosis, homologous chromosomes (e.g., two chromosome 1s) form pairs, termed **bivalents.** By a normal process known as crossing-over, parts of these chromosomes are exchanged, thereby rearranging the genetic constituents of each chromosome. Such an exchange of genetic material may also take place between nonhomologous chromosomes (e.g., between chromosomes 3 and 21) by an abnormal process termed **translocation** (Fig. 6-5).

Reciprocal Translocations

■ *Reciprocal translocations refer to the exchange of acentric chromosomal segments between two different (nonhomologous) chromosomes.* A reciprocal translocation is said to be **balanced** when there is no loss of genetic material—that is, when each chromosomal segment is translocated in its entirety. When such translocations are present in the gametes (sperm or ova), the progeny maintain the abnormal chromosomal structure in all somatic cells. Because balanced translocations are not associated with the loss of genes or the disruption of vital gene loci, most carriers of such balanced translocations are phenotypically normal. Carriers of balanced translocations, however, are at risk for producing offspring with unbalanced karyotypes and severe phenotypic abnormalities.

Robertsonian Translocations

■ *Robertsonian translocation (centric fusion) involves nonhomologous acrocentric chromosomes that are broken near the centromere. It is characterized by the exchange of two arms to form one large metacentric chromosome and a small chromosomal fragment.* The carrier is usually phenotypically normal but may suffer from infertility. When fertile, however, carriers of balanced robertsonian translocations are at risk of producing unbalanced translocations in their gametes, in which case the offspring may be born with congenital malformations.

Chromosomal Deletions

■ *Chromosomal deletions are the loss of a portion of a chromosome and involve either a terminal or an intercalary (middle) segment.* Deletion is related to several cancers in humans, including some hereditary forms of cancer. For example, some familial retinoblastomas are associated with deletions in the long arm of chromosome 13.

Chromosomal Inversions

■ *Chromosomal inversions refer to (1) the break of a chromosome at two points, (2) the inversion of the segment between the breaks, and (3) the rejoining of the two broken ends.* **Pericentric inversions** result from breaks on opposite sides of the centromere, whereas **paracentric inversions** involve breaks on the same arm of the chromosome.

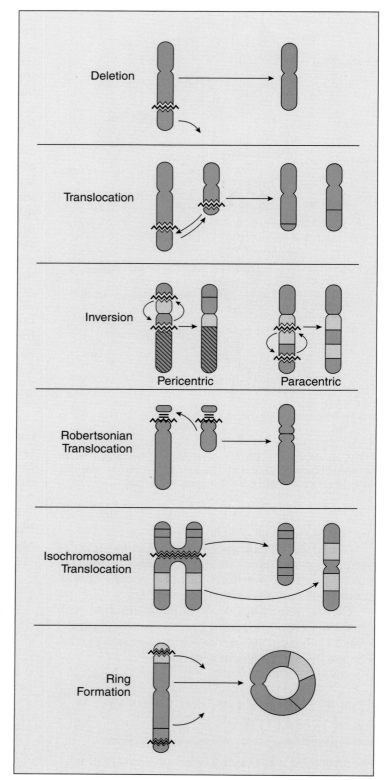

FIGURE 6-5

Structural abnormalities of human chromosomes.
Deletion of a portion of a chromosome leads to the
loss of genetic material and a shortened chromosome. A reciprocal translocation involves breaks on
two non-homologous chromosomes, with exchange
of the acentric segments. An inversion requires two
breaks in a single chromosome. If the breaks are on
opposite sides of the centromere, the inversion is
termed *pericentric*, whereas if the breaks are on the
same arm, the inversion is termed *paracentric*. A
robertsonian translocation occurs when two nonhomologous acrocentric chromosomes break near their
centromeres, after which the long arms fuse to form
one large metacentric chromosome. Isochromosomes
arise from faulty centromere division, which leads to
duplication of the long arm (iso q) and deletion of the
short arm, or the reverse (iso p). Ring chromosomes
involve breaks of both telomeric portions of a chromosome, deletion of the acentric fragments, and fusion of the remaining centric portion.

Ring Chromosomes

■ *Ring chromosomes are formed by a break involving both telomeric ends of a chromosome, followed by deletion of the acentric fragments and end-to-end fusion of the remaining centric portion of the chromosome.*

Isochromosomes

■ *Isochromosomes refer to faulty division of the centromere, in which it divides in a plane transverse to the long axis, thereby forming pairs of isochromosomes.* Normally, centromere division occurs in a plane parallel to the long axis of the chromosome, leading to the formation of two identical hemichromosomes. In the case of isochromosomes, one pair corresponds to the short arms attached to the upper portion of the centromere, and the other represents the long arms attached to the lower segment. The most important clinical condition involving isochromosomes is **Turner syndrome,** in which 15% of those affected have an isochromosome of the X chromosome.

NUMERIC CHROMOSOMAL ABNORMALITIES

A number of terms are important for understanding developmental defects associated with aberrations in the number of chromosomes:

- **Haploid.** *A single set of each of the chromosomes characteristic of a species (23 in humans).* Only germ cells have a haploid number (n) of chromosomes.
- **Diploid.** *A double set (2n) of each of the chromosomes (46 in humans).* Most somatic cells are diploid.
- **Euploid.** *Any multiple (from n to 8n) of the haploid number of chromosomes.* For example, many normal liver cells contain twice (4n) the DNA of diploid somatic cells and, therefore, are euploid or, more specifically, tetraploid.
- **Polyploid.** *A multiple of the haploid number greater than two (greater than diploid).*
- **Aneuploid.** *Karyotypes that are not exact multiples of the haploid number.* Many cancer cells are aneuploid, which is a characteristic often associated with an aggressive biologic behavior.
- **Monosomy.** *The absence in a somatic cell of one chromosome of a homologous pair.* For example, Turner syndrome is characterized by the presence of a single X chromosome.
- **Trisomy.** *The presence in a somatic cell of one extra copy of a normally paired chromosome.* For instance, Down syndrome is caused by the presence of three chromosomes.
- **Mosaicism.** *A condition caused by nondisjunction in which the body contains two or more karyotypically different cell lines.* Mosaicism involving sex chromosomes is common and is found in patients with gonadal dysgenesis who present with Turner or Klinefelter syndromes.

Nondisjunction

■ *Nondisjunction is a failure of paired chromosomes or chromatids to separate and move to opposite poles of the spindle at anaphase, during either mitosis or meiosis.* Numeric chromosomal abnormalities arise primarily from nondisjunction, which leads to aneuploidy if only one pair of chromosomes fails to separate. Nondisjunction results in polyploidy if the entire set does not divide and all the chromosomes are segregated into a single daughter cell.

NOMENCLATURE OF CHROMOSOMAL ABERRATIONS

Structural and numeric chromosomal abnormalities are classified according to (1) the total number of chromosomes, (2) the designation (number) of the affected chromosomes, and (3) the nature and location of the defect on the chromosome (Table 6-1). The karyotype is described sequentially in the following order: (1) the total number of chromosomes, (2) the sex chromosome complement, and (3) any abnormality. The short arm of a chromosome is designated **p** (petite), and the long arm is designated **q.** The addition of chromosomal material, whether an entire chromosome or only part of one, is indicated by a plus sign (+) before the number of the affected chromosome, and the loss of chromosomal material is indicated by a minus sign (—). Alternatively, the loss (deletion) of part of a chromosome may be designated by the symbol **del,** followed by the location of the deleted material on the affected chromosome. A translocation is written as **t,** followed by brackets containing the involved chromosomes.

SYNDROMES OF AUTOSOMAL CHROMOSOMES

Clinical syndromes that reflect disorders of the autosomal chromosomes may arise from numeric or structural abnormalities (Table 6-2).

Trisomy 21 (Down Syndrome)

■ *Trisomy 21 (Down syndrome) usually results from nondisjunction and is characterized by a constellation of distinctive morphologic abnormalities and mental retardation.*

TABLE 6-1.   Chromosomal Nomenclature

Numeric designation of autosomes	1–22
Sex chromosomes	X, Y
Addition of a whole or part of a chromosome	+
Loss of a whole or part of a chromosome	−
Numeric mosaicism (e.g., 46/47)	/
Short arm of chromosome (petite)	p
Long arm of chromosome	q
Isochromosome	i
Ring chromosome	r
Deletion	del
Insertion	ins
Translocation	t
Derivative chromosome (carrying translocation)	der
Terminal	ter

Examples

Male with trisomy 21 (Down syndrome)	47, XY, +21
Female carrier of fusion-type translocation between chromosomes 14 and 21	45, XX, −14, −21, +t (14q21q)
Cri-du-chat syndrome (male) with deletion of a portion of the short arm of chromosome 5	46, XY, del (5p)
Male with ring chromosome 19	46, XY, r (19)
Turner syndrome with monosomy X	45, X
Mosaic Klinefelter syndrome	46, XY/47, XXY

TABLE 6-2.   Clinical Features of the Autosomal Chromosomal Syndromes[a]

Syndromes	Features
Trisomic Syndromes	
Chromosomes 21 (Down syndrome 47,XX or XY,+21:1/800)	Epicanthic folds, speckled irides, flat nasal bridge, congenital heart disease, simian crease of paslm, Hirschsprung disease, increased risk of leukemia
Chromosome 18 (47,XX or XY,+18:1/8000)	Female preponderance, micrognathia, congenital heart disease, horseshoe kidney, deformed fingers
Chromosome 13 (47,XX or XY,+13:1/20,000)	Persistent fetal hemoglobin, microencephaly, congenital heart disease, polycystic kidneys, polydactyly, simian crease
Deletion Syndromes	
5p-syndrome (Cri-du-chat 46,XX or XY,5p-c)	Cat-like cry, low birth weight, microcephaly, epicanthic folds, congenital heart disease, short hands and feet, simian crease
11p-syndrome (46,XX or XY,11p-)	Aniridia, Wilms tumor, gonadoblastoma, male genital ambiguity
13q-syndrome (46,XX or XY,13q-)	Low birth weight, microcephaly, retinoblastoma, congenital heart disease

[a] All these syndromes are associated with mental retardation.

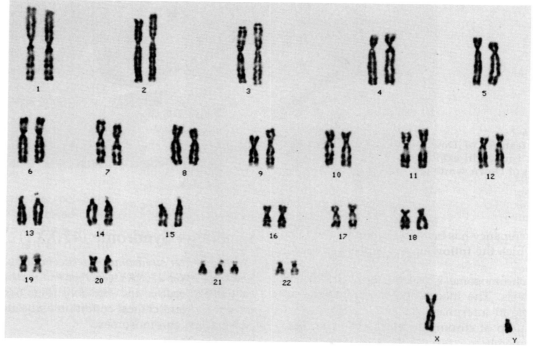

FIGURE 6-6
Trisomy 21 in the karyotype of a child with Down syndrome. All other chromosomes are normal.

In fact, trisomy 21 (Fig. 6-6) is the single most common overall cause of mental retardation.

The incidence of trisomy 21 correlates strongly with increasing maternal age—that is, older mothers are at substantially greater risk of giving birth to an infant with Down syndrome. Until their mid-thirties, women have a constant risk of giving birth to a trisomic child of approximately one per 1000 liveborn infants. The risk then increases dramatically and reaches an incidence of one in 30 at 45 years of age.

☐ **Pathology and Clinical Features:** As the child with Down syndrome develops, a typical constellation of abnormalities appears (Fig. 6-7).

Mental Status. Children with Down syndrome invariably suffer from severe mental retardation, with a relentless and progressive decline in their IQ with age. Beginning with a mean IQ of 70 before the age of 1 year, intelligence deteriorates during the first decade of life to a mean IQ of 30.

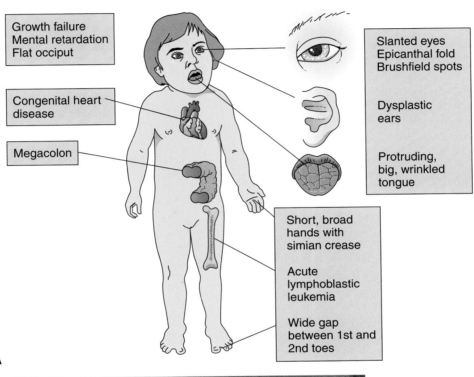

Growth failure
Mental retardation
Flat occiput

Congenital heart disease

Megacolon

Slanted eyes
Epicanthal fold
Brushfield spots

Dysplastic ears

Protruding, big, wrinkled tongue

Short, broad hands with simian crease

Acute lymphoblastic leukemia

Wide gap between 1st and 2nd toes

A

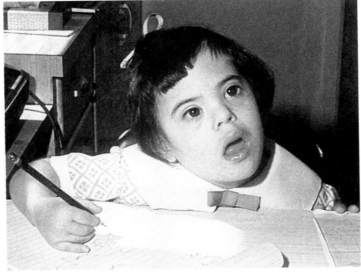

B

FIGURE 6-7. (A) Clinical features of Down syndrome. (B) A young girl exhibits the facial features of Down Syndrome.

Craniofacial Features. The face and occiput tend to be flat, with a low-bridged nose, reduced interpupillary distance, and oblique palpebral fissures. Epicanthal folds of the eyes impart an Oriental appearance, a feature that accounts for the obsolete term **mongolism.** A speckled appearance of the iris is referred to as **Brushfield spots.** The ears are enlarged and malformed, and a prominent tongue, which typically lacks a central fissure, protrudes through an open mouth.

Heart. A third of children born with Down syndrome suffer from congenital cardiac disease. The anomalies take the form of atrioventricular canal, ventricular and atrial septal defects, tetralogy of Fallot, and patent ductus arteriosus.

Skeleton. These children tend to be small owing to shorter than normal bones of the ribs, pelvis, and extremities. The hands are broad and short, and they exhibit a "simian crease" (a single transverse crease across the palm).

Gastrointestinal Tract. Duodenal stenosis or atresia, imperforate anus, and Hirschsprung disease (megacolon) occur in 2% to 3% of children with Down syndrome.

Immune System. Affected children are unusually susceptible to respiratory and other infections.

Hematologic Disorders. The risk of leukemia in children with Down syndrome younger than 15 years of age is approximately 15-fold greater than normal. In children younger than 3 years of age, acute nonlymphocytic leukemia predominates. After that age, when most of the leukemias in Down syndrome occur, the majority of cases are acute lymphoblastic leukemias.

Neurologic Disorders. One of the most intriguing neurologic features of Down syndrome is its association with Alzheimer disease. The morphologic lesions characteristic of Alzheimer disease progress in all patients with Down syndrome and are universally demonstrable by 35 years of age.

SYNDROMES OF SEX CHROMOSOMES

Y Chromosome

Historically, the sex of a person was believed to be determined by the number of X chromosomes. However, with the discoveries that the XXY phenotype (Klinefelter syndrome) is male and the XO phenotype (Turner syndrome) is female, the role of the Y chromosome in conferring the male phenotype was recognized. The testis-determining gene is located near the end of the short arm of the Y chromosome. It is thought to encode a transcription-activator protein that acts on autosomal genes whose expression controls development of the male phenotype.

X Chromosome

Although males carry only one X chromosome, both males and females produce the same amounts of gene products encoded by the X chromosome. This seeming discrepancy has been explained by the **Lyon effect,** on which the following principles are based:

- One X chromosome is inactivated early in embryogenesis. The inactivated X chromosome is detectable in interphase nuclei as a heterochromatic clump of chromatin attached to the inner nuclear membrane, termed the **Barr body.**
- Either the paternal or maternal X chromosome is inactivated randomly.

Klinefelter Syndrome (47,XXY)

■ *Klinefelter syndrome, or testicular dysgenesis, is the phenotype of the 47,XXY genotype and is characterized by male hypogonadism and infertility* (Fig. 6-8). It is the most important clinical condition associated with trisomy of sex chromosomes.

☐ **Pathology:** After puberty, the intrinsically abnormal testes do not respond to stimulation by gonadotropins and show sequentially regressive alterations. The seminiferous tubules display atrophy, hyalinization, and peritubular fibrosis. Germ cells and Sertoli cells are characteristically absent, and eventually, the tubules are represented by dense cords of collagen. Although Leydig cells usually appear to be increased in number, their function is impaired, as evidenced by low testosterone levels in the face of elevated luteinizing hormone and follicle-stimulating hormone levels.

☐ Clinical Features: Children with Klinefelter syndrome tend to be tall and thin, with long legs (eunuchoid body habitus). Normal testicular growth and masculinization at puberty do not occur, and the testes and penis remain small. Feminine characteristics are manifested as a high-pitched voice, gynecomastia, and a female pattern of pubic hair (female escutcheon). Azoospermia results in infertility. All of these changes are a consequence of hypogonadism and a resulting lack of androgens.

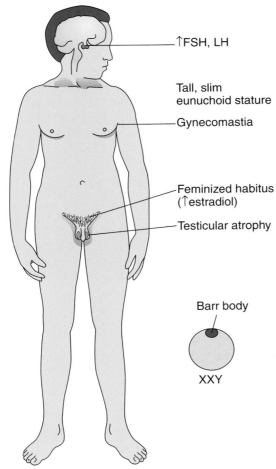

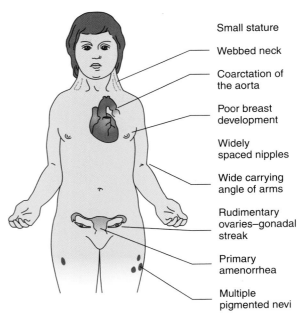

FIGURE   6-9
Clinical features of Turner syndrome.

normal urograms, with the most common anomalies being horseshoe kidney and malrotation. Many have facial abnormalities, including a small mandible, prominent ears, and epicanthal folds. Defective hearing and vision are common, and as many as one-fifth are reported to be mentally defective.

Cardiovascular anomalies are common in Turner syndrome, occurring in almost half of these patients. Coarctation of the aorta is seen in 15%, and a bicuspid aortic valve is detected by echocardiography in as many as one-third. Although the ovaries of fetuses with Turner syndrome initially contain oocytes, they are rapidly degraded, and none remain by 2 years of age. The ovaries are converted to fibrous streaks, whereas the uterus, fallopian tubes, and vagina develop normally. Children with Turner syndrome are treated with growth hormone and estrogens and enjoy an excellent prognosis for a normal life.

FIGURE   6-8
Clinical features of Klinefelter syndrome.

Turner Syndrome (45,X)

■ *Turner syndrome refers to the spectrum of abnormalities that results from complete or partial monosomy of the X chromosome in a phenotypic female.* Only approximately half of women with Turner syndrome lack an entire X chromosome (monosomy X). The remainder are mosaics or display structural aberrations of the X chromosome, such as isochromosome of the long arm, translocations, and deletions.

☐ **Pathology and Clinical Features:** The clinical hallmark of Turner syndrome is sexual infantilism, with primary amenorrhea and sterility (Fig. 6-9). In most cases, the disorder is not discovered until the absence of menarche brings the child to medical attention. Virtually all of these women are shorter than 5 feet (152 cm) in height. Other clinical features include a short and webbed neck (pterygium coli), a low posterior hairline, a wide carrying angle of the arms (cubitus valgus), a broad chest with widely spaced nipples, and hyperconvex fingernails. Half of the patients have ab-

SINGLE-GENE ABNORMALITIES

The classic laws of mendelian inheritance imply that single genes encode identifiable traits that segregate sharply within families.

- A **mendelian trait** is determined by two copies of the same gene, called alleles, which are located at the same locus on two homologous chromosomes.
- **Autosomal genes** refer to those located on one of the 22 autosomes.

- **Sex-linked genes** are important in the pathogenesis of heritable diseases and reside on the X chromosome.
- A **dominant phenotypic trait** requires the expression of only one allele of a homologous gene pair. In other words, the dominant phenotype is present whether the allelic genes are homozygous or heterozygous.
- A **recessive phenotypic trait** demands that both alleles be identical (homozygous).
- **Codominance** refers to a situation in which both alleles in a heterozygous gene pair are fully expressed (e.g., the AB blood group genes).

Mendelian traits are classified as (1) autosomal dominant, (2) autosomal recessive, (3) sex-linked dominant, or (4) sex-linked recessive.

Mutations

■ *Mutations are stable, heritable changes in DNA.* The major types of mutations encountered in the study of human genetic disorders (Fig. 6-10) are:

- **Point Mutation.** The replacement of one base by another.
- **Missense Mutation.** A situation in which the new codon codes for a different amino acid. In sickle cell anemia, an adenine-to-thymine substitution results in the replacement of glutamic acid (GAG) by valine (GUG) in the β-globin chain of hemoglobin.
- **Nonsense mutation** (4%). One in which the base substitution changes the normal codon to a termination codon, so that translation is halted at the site of the mutation. For example, UAU codes for tyrosine, but UAA is a stop codon.
- **Frameshift mutation.** Insertions or deletions of one or more bases into the coding region of DNA change the reading frame of the genetic code. In this situation, every codon in the same gene downstream from the mutation has a new sequence and codes for a different amino acid or a termination signal. Frameshift mutations can also alter the transcription, splicing, or processing of mRNA.

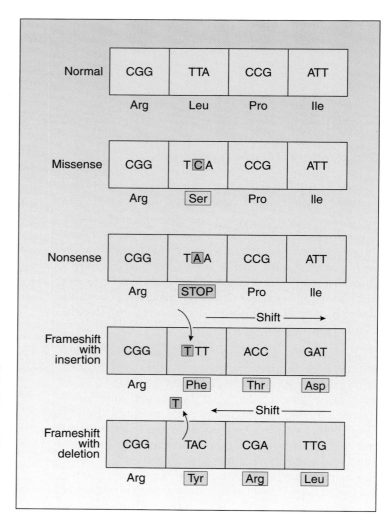

FIGURE *6-10*
Point mutations that alter the reading frame of DNA. A variety of mutations in the second codon of a normal sequence of four amino acids is depicted. With a missense mutation, a change from T to C substitutes serine for leucine. With a nonsense mutation, a change from T to A converts the leucine codon to a stop codon. A shift in the reading frame to the right results from an insertion of a T, thereby changing the sequence of all subsequent amino acids. Conversely, deletion of a T shifts the reading frame one base to the left and also changes the sequence of all subsequent amino acids.

- **Large Deletion.** When an extensive segment of DNA is deleted, the coding region of a gene may be entirely removed, in which case the protein product is absent. On the other hand, a large deletion may result in the approximation of neighboring genes, thereby producing a fused gene that codes for a hybrid protein—that is, one in which the initial sequence of one protein is followed by the terminal sequence of another.

AUTOSOMAL DOMINANT DISORDERS

■ *Autosomal dominant* disorders refer to single-gene abnormalities that are expressed in heterozygotes. In other words, a dominant disease occurs when only one defective gene (a mutant allele) is present; its paired allele on the homologous chromosome is normal. The salient features of autosomal dominant traits are (Fig. 6-11):

- Males and females are equally affected, because by definition, the mutant gene resides on one of the 22 autosomal chromosomes.
- The trait encoded by the mutant gene can be transmitted to successive generations.
- Unaffected members of the family do not transmit the trait to their offspring.
- The proportions of normal and diseased offspring of patients with the disorder are, on average, equal, because most affected persons are heterozygous and their normal mates do not harbor the defective gene.
- The human genome contains frequent tandem trinucleotide repeat sequences, the length varying among different persons. Above a certain threshold, the number of repeats can expand, and distinct trinucleotide expansions have been identified in human disease.

More than 1000 human diseases are inherited as autosomal dominant traits, although most of them are rare. Examples of human autosomal dominant diseases are given in Table 6-3.

Huntington Disease. An inherited neurodegenerative disorder, Huntington disease (HD) is caused by expansion of a CAG repeat within the coding sequence of the gene that codes for the protein Huntingtin. Whereas normal alleles contain 10 to 30 repeats, alleles in patients with HD exhibit 40 to 100 repeats. The abnormal expansion of the protein, in this case a polyglutamine segment, confers a toxic gain-of-function to Huntingtin.

Fragile X Syndrome. This genetic disorder, the most common cause of inherited mental retardation, results from expansion of a CGG repeat in a noncoding region of the X chromosome, where it silences an adjacent gene. The abnormal repeat is also associated with a fragile site on the X chromosome that is susceptible to a chromosomal break.

Myotonic Dystrophy. The most frequent autosomal muscular dystrophy, myotonic dystrophy (MD) is caused by expansion of a CTG repeat in the *MD* gene. Patients with MD display as many as 2000 repeats, compared with as few as 35 in normal persons.

Friedreich Ataxia. An autosomal recessive degenerative disease of the brain and heart, Friedreich ataxia is associated with expansion of a GAA repeat in the frataxin gene.

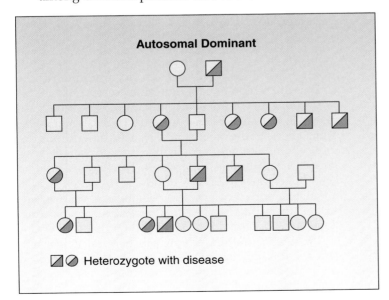

Autosomal Dominant

▨ ⊘ Heterozygote with disease

FIGURE *6-11*
Autosomal dominant inheritance. Only symptomatic persons transmit the trait to the next generation, and heterozygotes are symptomatic. Both males and females are affected.

TABLE 6-3.   Representative Autosomal Dominant Disorders

Disease	Frequency	Chromosome
Familial hypercholesterolemia	1/500	19p
von Willebrand disease	1/8000	12p
Hereditary spherocytosis (major forms)	1/5000	14,8
Hereditary elliptocytosis (all forms)	1/2500	1,1p,2q,14
Osteogenesis imperfecta (types I–IV)	1/10,000	17q,7q
Ehlers-Danlos syndrome, type III	1/5000	?
Marfan syndrome	1/10,000	?
Neurofibromatosis type 1	1/3500	17q
Hungtington disease	1/15,000	4p
Retinoblastoma	1/14,000	13q
Wilms tumor	1/10,000	11p
Familial adenomatous polyposis	1/10,000	5p
Acute intermittent porphyria	1/15,000	11q
Hereditary amyloidosis	1/100,000	18q
Adult polycystic kidney disease	1/1000	16p

Heritable Diseases of Connective Tissue

Marfan Syndrome

■ *Marfan syndrome is an autosomal dominant, inherited disorder of connective tissue characterized by a variety of abnormalities in many organs, including the heart, aorta, skeleton, eyes, and skin.*

☐ **Pathogenesis:** The cause of Marfan syndrome is a mutation in the gene coding for **fibrillin,** which has been mapped to the long arm of chromosome 15. Fibrillin is a family of connective tissue proteins that are widely distributed among many tissues in the form of a fiber system termed **microfibrils.** By electron microscopy, microfibrils are thread-like filaments that form larger fibers organized into rods, sheets, and interlaced networks. **Microfibrillar fibers** are believed to serve as a scaffold for the deposition of elastin during embryonic development, after which these fibers constitute part of the elastic tissues.

☐ **Pathology and Clinical Features:** Persons with Marfan syndrome are usually tall, and the lower body segment (pubis to sole) is longer than the upper body. A slender habitus, which reflects a paucity of subcutaneous fat, is complemented by long, thin extremities and fingers, which account for the term **arachnodactyly** (spider fingers).

Skeletal System. The skull in Marfan syndrome is characteristically long (dolichocephalic), with prominent frontal eminences. Disorders of the ribs are conspicuous and produce pectus excavatum (concave sternum) and pectus carinatum (pigeon breast). The tendons, ligaments, and joint capsules are weak, a condition that leads to hyperextensibility of the joints (double-jointedness), dislocations, hernias, and kyphoscoliosis. The last is often severe.

Cardiovascular System. Cardiovascular disorders are the most common causes of death in Marfan syndrome. The most important cardiovascular defect resides in the aorta, in which the principal lesion is a faulty media. Weakness of the media leads to variable dilatation of the ascending aorta and a high incidence of **dissecting aneurysms.** Dilatation of the aortic ring results in aortic regurgitation, which may be so severe as to produce angina pectoris and congestive heart failure. The mitral valve may exhibit redundant valve leaflets and chordae tendineae, which are changes that result in the mitral valve prolapse syndrome.

Eyes. Ocular changes are common in Marfan syndrome, reflecting the intrinsic lesion in the connective tissue. Ocular changes include dislocation of the lens (ectopia lentis), severe myopia owing to an elongation of the eye, and retinal detachment.

Untreated men with Marfan syndrome usually die in their thirties, and untreated women often succumb in their forties. However, with the use of drugs that reduce blood pressure and replacement of the aorta with prosthetic grafts, life expectancy approaches normal.

Ehlers-Danlos Syndrome

■ *Ehlers-Danlos syndrome (EDS) comprises a group of rare, autosomal dominantly inherited disorders of connective tissue that are characterized by remarkable hyperelasticity and fragility of the skin, joint hypermobility, and often, a bleeding diathesis.* More than 10 varieties of EDS have been distinguished, and the molecular lesions have been identified in several.

☐ **Pathogenesis: The common feature of all types of EDS is a generalized defect in collagen.** In some types (EDS I–IV, VI, X), electron microscopic studies of the skin have shown an increased size of collagen fibrils, with unusually small bundles, which are features that suggest the presence of abnormal collagen. Defects in the biochemical structure, synthesis, secretion, and degradation of collagen have been demonstrated in a number of cases. Such changes involve type III collagen in EDS IV and type I collagen in EDS VII. Deficiencies of specific collagen-processing enzymes, including lysyl hydroxylase and lysyl oxidase, have been identified in EDS VI and IX, respectively.

Whatever the underlying biochemical defect, the end result is deficient or defective collagen. Depending on the type of EDS, these molecular lesions are associated with conspicuous weakness of the supporting structures of the skin, joints, arteries, and visceral organs.

□ **Pathology and Clinical Features:** All types of EDS are characterized by a soft, fragile, and hyperextensible skin. Patients are typically able to stretch the skin many centimeters, and trivial injuries can lead to serious wounds. Hypermobility of the joints allows for unusual extension and flexion, a situation that accounted for the "human pretzel" and other contortionists in the freak shows of an earlier time. EDS IV is the most dangerous variety because of a tendency toward spontaneous rupture of large arteries, bowel, and gravid uterus. Death from such complications is common during the third and fourth decades of life.

Similarly, EDS VI also has major complications, including severe kyphoscoliosis, blindness from retinal hemorrhage or rupture of the globe, and death from aortic rupture. Severe periodontal disease, with loss of teeth by the third decade, characterizes EDS VIII. EDS IX features the development of bladder diverticula during childhood, with a danger of bladder rupture, and skeletal deformities.

Osteogenesis Imperfecta

■ *Osteogenesis imperfecta* (OI), *or brittle bone disease, comprises a group of inherited disorders in which a generalized abnormality of the connective tissue is expressed principally as fragility of bone.* Most cases of OI are inherited in an autosomal dominant pattern.

□ **Pathogenesis:** The genetic defects in all four types of OI are heterogeneous, but all affect the synthesis of type I collagen. OI type I, which may be the most common, is characterized by the synthesis of only half the normal amount of type I procollagen. A few patients with the type I phenotype of OI exhibit mutations in the *pro-α1(I)* gene that substitutes a residue other than glycine in the procollagen molecule. Mutations and deletions in type I procollagen genes are responsible for the defective collagens in OI types II, III, and IV.

□ **Pathology and Clinical Features:**

Type I OI is characterized by a normal appearance at birth, but fractures of many bones occur during infancy and at the time when the child learns to walk. Such patients have been described as being "as fragile as a china doll." Children with type I OI typically have blue sclerae as a result of the deficiency in collagen fibers, which imparts translucence to the sclera. A high incidence of hearing loss occurs, because fractures and fusion of the bones of the middle ear restrict their mobility.

Type II OI is usually fatal in utero or shortly after birth.

Type III OI is the progressively deforming variant, which ordinarily is detected at birth by the presence of short stature and deformities caused by fractures in utero.

OI is discussed in further detail in Chapter 26.

Neurofibromatoses

■ *Neurofibromatoses include two distinct autosomal dominant disorders characterized by the development of multiple neurofibromas, which are benign tumors of the peripheral nerves of Schwann cell origin.*

Neurofibromatosis Type I (von Recklinghausen Disease). Neurofibromatosis type I (NF1) is the most common autosomal dominant disorder, affecting one in 3500 persons of all races. The *NF1* gene has an unusually high rate of mutation, and half of the cases are sporadic rather than familial.

□ **Pathogenesis:** The *NF1* gene is located in the centromeric region of the long arm of chromosome 17. This very large gene encodes for a protein (neurofibromin) that is a member of the family of guanosine triphosphatase (GTPase)–activating proteins (GAP) involved in regulation of the *ras* protein (see Chapter 5). The normal *NF1* gene, a classic tumor-suppressor gene, probably suppresses activity of the *ras* protein following stimulation by nerve growth factor or other agents. Loss of this suppression owing to a mutation or translocation affecting the *NF1* gene presumably permits uncontrolled *ras* activation, an effect that may predispose to the formation of neurofibromas.

□ **Pathology and Clinical Features:** The typical features of NF1 include:

- **Neurofibromas.** More than 90% of patients with NF1 develop cutaneous and subcutaneous neurofibromas during late childhood or adolescence. These tumors, which may total more than 500, appear as soft, pedunculated masses, usually with a diameter of approximately 1 cm (Fig. 6-12). However, on occasion, they may reach alarming proportions and dominate the physical appearance of the patient, with lesions of 25 cm in the largest dimension. Subcutaneous neurofibromas present as soft nodules along the course of the peripheral nerves.

Plexiform neurofibromas occur only within the context of NF1 and are diagnostic of that condition. These tumors usually involve the larger peripheral nerves but, on occasion, may arise from the cranial or intraspinal nerves. Plexiform neurofibromas are often large, infiltrative tumors that cause severe disfigurement of the face or an extremity. The microscopic appearance of neurofibromas is discussed in Chapter 28.

One of the major complications of NF1, occurring in 3% to 5% of patients, is the appearance of a neurofibrosarcoma within a neurofibroma, usually a larger one of the plexiform type. NF1 is also associated with an increased incidence of other neurogenic tumors, including meningioma, optic glioma, and pheochromocytomas.

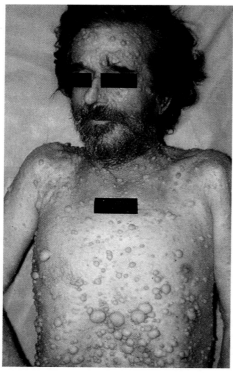

FIGURE   *6-12*
Neurofibromatosis type I. Multiple cutaneous neurofibromas are noted on the face and trunk.

- **Café-Au-Lait Spots.** Although normal persons may exhibit occasional light-brown patches on the skin, more than 95% of persons affected by NF1 display six or more such lesions. These are larger than 5 mm before puberty and greater than 1.5 cm thereafter.
- **Lisch Nodules.** More than 90% of persons with NF1 display pigmented nodules of the iris, which consist of masses of melanocytes.
- **Skeletal Lesions.** A number of bone lesions occur frequently in NF1. These include malformations of the sphenoid bone and thinning of the cortex of the long bones, with bowing and pseudarthrosis of the tibia, bone cysts, and scoliosis.
- **Mental Status.** Mild intellectual impairment is frequent in patients with NF1, but severe retardation is not part of the syndrome.

Neurofibromatosis Type II (Central Neurofibromatosis). Neurofibromatosis type II (NF2) is considerably less common than NF1, occurring in only one in 50,000 persons. Most patients suffer from bilateral acoustic neuromas, but the condition can be diagnosed in the presence of a unilateral eighth nerve tumor if two of the following are present: (1) neurofibroma, (2) meningioma, (3) glioma, (4) schwannoma, or (5) juvenile posterior lenticular opacity. Despite the superficial similarities between NF1 and NF2, they are not vari-

ants of the same disease and, indeed, have separate genetic origins. The *NF2* gene resides in the middle of the long arm of chromosome 22 and encodes a tumor suppressor termed *merlin* or *schwannomin*.

Achondroplastic Dwarfism

■ *Achondroplastic dwarfism is an autosomal dominant, hereditary disturbance of epiphyseal chondroblastic development that leads to inadequate enchondral bone formation.* This abnormality causes a distinctive form of dwarfism characterized by short limbs with a normal head and trunk. The affected person has a small face, a bulging forehead, and a deeply indented bridge of the nose. The pathology of achondroplasia is discussed in Chapter 26.

Familial Hypercholesterolemia

■ *Familial hypercholesterolemia is one of the most common autosomal dominant disorders and is characterized by a striking acceleration of atherosclerosis and its complications.* In its heterozygous form, the disease affects at least one in 500 adults in the United States. Only one in a million persons is homozygous for the disease. This subject is discussed in more detail in Chapter 10.

☐ **Pathogenesis:** Familial hypercholesterolemia results from abnormalities in a gene on chromosome 19 that codes for the cell surface receptor that removes low-density lipoprotein (LDL) from the blood. The defect reflects some 150 different mutations, including insertions, deletions, and nonsense as well as missense point mutations.

The LDL receptor resides on the surface of hepatocytes and, to some extent, on other cells. After binding to the receptor, LDL is internalized and degraded in lysosomes, thereby freeing cholesterol for further metabolism. A deficiency in LDL receptors leads to an increase in plasma LDL, because the rate of LDL clearance is inversely proportional to the number of LDL receptors. As a result, LDL cholesterol (some of which may be oxidized) is taken up via a scavenger pathway by tissue macrophages and accumulates to form occlusive arterial plaques (atheromas) and papules or nodules of lipid-laden macrophages (xanthomas).

☐ **Clinical Features:** Heterozygous and homozygous familial hypercholesterolemia constitute two distinct clinical syndromes. In heterozygotes, elevated blood cholesterol levels (mean, 350 mg/dL; normal, <200 mg/dL) are noted at birth. Symptoms of coronary heart disease often occur before the age of 40. In homozygotes, the blood cholesterol content reaches astronomic levels (600–1200 mg/dL), and virtually all patients exhibit generalized atherosclerosis in childhood. Homozygotes typically die of myocardial infarction before 30 years of age.

AUTOSOMAL RECESSIVE DISORDERS

Autosomal recessive diseases are associated with clinical symptoms only when both alleles at a given locus on homologous chromosomes are defective. In other words, the affected person is homozygous for the recessive trait (Fig. 6-13). **The large majority of genetic metabolic diseases exhibit an autosomal recessive mode of inheritance** (Table 6-4). Some of the salient features of autosomal recessive disorders are:

- The more infrequent the mutant gene in the general population, the less the probability that unrelated parents are heterozygous for the trait. **Thus, rare autosomal recessive disorders are often the product of consanguineous marriages.**
- Both parents are usually heterozygous for the trait and clinically normal.
- Symptoms appear, on average, in one-fourth of the offspring. Half of all offspring are heterozygous for the trait and, therefore, are asymptomatic.
- As in autosomal dominant disorders, autosomal recessive traits are transmitted equally to males and females, because by definition, the mutant gene resides on one of the 22 different autosomal chromosomes.

Biochemical Basis of Autosomal Recessive Disorders

Autosomal recessive diseases characteristically are caused by deficiencies in enzymes rather than by abnormalities in structural proteins. A mutation that results in the inactivation of an enzyme does not ordinarily produce an abnormal phenotype, because compensatory mechanisms readily correct the functional defect. For instance, because most cellular enzymes operate at substrate concentrations significantly below saturation, an enzyme deficiency is easily corrected simply by increasing the amount of substrate. By contrast, loss of both alleles in a homozygote results in complete loss of enzyme activity, a situation that is not amenable to correction by regulatory mechanisms. It follows, therefore, that diseases caused by the impairment of catabolic pathways and that involve the accumulation of dietary substances (e.g., phenylketonuria, galactosemia) or cellular constituents (e.g., Tay-Sachs, Hurler) are autosomal recessive, because the accumulation of substrate overcomes any partial enzymatic defect in the heterozygote.

Cystic Fibrosis

■ *Cystic fibrosis* (CF) *is an autosomal recessive disorder affecting children and is characterized by (1) chronic pulmonary disease, (2) deficient exocrine pancreatic function, and (3) other complications of inspissated mucus in a number of organs, including the small intestine, liver, and reproductive tract.* The disease results from abnormal electrolyte transport that, in turn, reflects impaired function of a chloride channel of the epithelial cells. **CF is the most common lethal autosomal recessive disorder in the white population, with an incidence of one in 2500 newborns.** More than 95% of cases have been reported in whites, and the disease is found only exceptionally in blacks—and almost never in Asians. It is estimated that one in 25 whites is a heterozygous carrier of the *CF* gene.

☐ **Pathogenesis:** The gene responsible for CF is located on the long arm of chromosome 7 and encodes a protein termed the **CF transmembrane conductance regulator (CFTR)** (Fig. 6-14). In normal mucus-secreting epithelia, chloride channels open in response to an increase in cyclic adenosine monophosphate (cAMP), which activates cAMP-dependent protein kinase. In

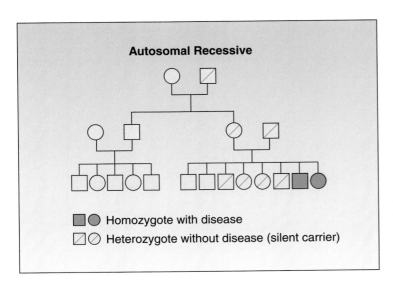

Autosomal Recessive

■ ● Homozygote with disease
◩ ⊘ Heterozygote without disease (silent carrier)

FIGURE *6-13*

Autosomal recessive inheritance. Symptoms of the disease appear only in homozygotes, male or female. Heterozygotes are asymptomatic carriers. Symptomatic homozygotes result from the mating of asymptomatic heterozygotes.

TABLE *6-4.* Representative Autosomal Recessive Disorders

Disease	Frequency	Chromosome
Cystic fibrosis	1/2500	7q
γ-Thalassemia	High	16p
β-Thalassemia	High	11p
Sickle cell anemia	High	11p
Myeloperoxidase deficiency	1/2000	17q
Phenylketonuria	1/10,000	12q
Gaucher disease	1/1000	1q
Tay-Sachs disease	1/4000	15q
Hurler syndrome	1/100,000	22p
Glycogen storage disease Ia (von Gierke disease	1/100,000	?
Wilson disease	1/50,000	13q
Hereditary hemochromatosis	1/1000	6p
γ₁-Antitrypsin deficiency	1/7000	14q
Oculocutaneous albinism	1/20,000	?
Alcaptonuria	<1/100,000	?
Metachromatic leukodystrophy	1/100,000	22q

turn, this enzyme phosphorylates the chloride channel (CFTR). As a consequence, secretion of chloride, together with that of associated fluid, is enhanced. In CF, mutations in the gene encoding CFTR that disturb the function of the chloride channel include failure of CFTR synthesis, failure of CFTR transport to the plasma membrane, defective adenosine triphosphate binding to CFTR, and defective chloride secretion by mutant CFTR. In any event, the cells do not secrete chloride and water efficiently and exhibit increased sodium absorption. These effects lead to a more viscid mucus. **All the pathologic consequences of CF can be attributed to the presence of this abnormally thick mucus, which obstructs the lumina of airways, pancreatic and biliary ducts, and fetal intestine. It also impairs mucociliary function in the airways.**

□ **Pathology:**

Respiratory Tract. Pulmonary disease is responsible for most of the morbidity and mortality associated with CF. The earliest lesion is obstruction of the bronchioles by mucus, with secondary infection and inflammation of the bronchiolar walls. Recurrent cycles of obstruction and infection result in **chronic bronchiolitis and bronchitis,** which increase in severity as the disease progresses. The mucous glands in the bronchi undergo hypertrophy and hyperplasia, and the airways are distended by thick and tenacious secretions. Widespread **bronchiectasis** becomes apparent by 10 years of age (and often earlier). In the late stages of the disease, large bronchiectatic cysts and lung abscesses are common.

Pancreas. The large majority (85%) of patients with CF have a form of **chronic pancreatitis,** and in long-standing cases, little or no functional exocrine pancreas remains. The inspissated secretions in the pancreatic ducts produce secondary dilatation and cystic change of the distal ducts (Fig. 6-15) as well as extensive fibrosis.

Liver. Inspissated mucous secretions in the intrahepatic biliary system obstruct the flow of bile and are responsible for the development of focal **secondary biliary cirrhosis,** which is seen in one-fourth of patients at autopsy.

Gastrointestinal Tract. Shortly after birth, the normal newborn passes the intestinal contents that have accumulated in utero (meconium). The most important lesion of the gastrointestinal tract in CF is small bowel obstruction in the newborn, which is termed **meconium ileus** and is caused by the failure to pass meconium in the immediate postpartum period. This complication, which occurs in 5% to 10% of newborns with CF, has been attributed to the failure of pancreatic secretions to digest meconium.

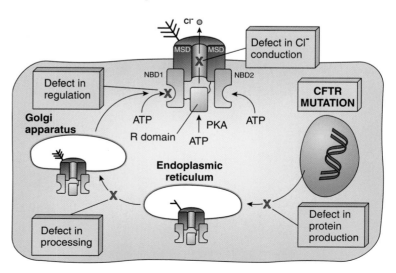

FIGURE *6-14*
Cellular sites of the disruptions in the synthesis and function of cystic fibrosis transmembrane conductance regulator (CFTR) in cystic fibrosis.

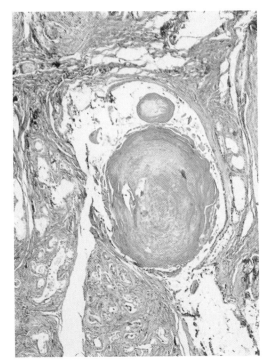

FIGURE   *6-15*
Intraductal concretion and atrophy of the acini in the pancreas of a patient with cystic fibrosis.

□ **Clinical Features:** The diagnosis of CF is most reliably made by the demonstration of increased concentrations of electrolytes in the sweat. The decreased chloride conductance that is characteristic of CF results in a failure of chloride reabsorption by cells of the sweat gland ducts and, hence, the accumulation of sodium chloride in the sweat (Fig. 6-16). Improved medical care and recognition of milder cases of CF have served to prolong the average life span, and half of these patients now survive to 25 years of age.

Lysosomal Storage Diseases

■ *Lysosomal storage diseases, inherited as autosomal recessive traits, are characterized by the accumulation ("storage") of unmetabolized normal substrates in the lysosomes owing to deficiencies of specific acid hydrolases.* Virtually all lysosomal storage diseases result from mutations in genes that encode lysosomal hydrolases. A deficiency in one of the more than 40 acid hydrolases can result in the inability to catabolize the normal macromolecular substrate of that enzyme. As a result, the undigested substrate accumulates in the lysosomes, thereby leading to engorgement of these organelles and expansion of the lysosomal compartment of the cell.

Gaucher Disease

■ *Gaucher disease is caused by a deficiency in glucocerebrosidase and is characterized by the accumulation of glucosylceramide, primarily in the lysosomes of macrophages.*

□ **Pathogenesis:** The deficiency of glucocerebrosidase activity can be traced to a variety of single-base mutations in the β-glucosidase gene, which resides on the long arm of chromosome 1. The glucosylceramide that accumulates in the Gaucher cells of the spleen, liver, bone marrow, and lymph nodes derives principally from the catabolism of senescent leukocytes. The membranes of these cells are rich in cerebrosides; when their degradation is blocked by the deficiency of glucocerebrosidase, the intermediate metabolite, glucosylceramide, accumulates. The glucosylceramide of Gaucher cells in the brain is believed to originate from the turnover of plasma membrane gangliosides of cells in the central nervous system.

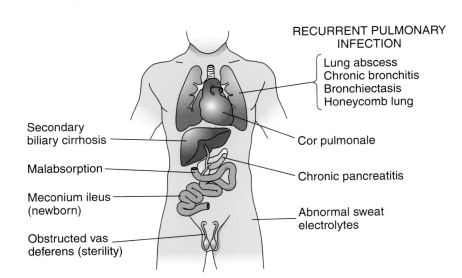

FIGURE   *6-16*
Clinical features of cystic fibrosis.

☐ **Pathology:** The hallmark of this disorder is the presence of **Gaucher cells,** which are lipid-laden macrophages that are characteristically present in the red pulp of the spleen, liver sinusoids, lymph nodes, lungs, and bone marrow. These cells are derived from the resident macrophages in the respective organs (e.g., Kupffer cells in the liver and alveolar macrophages in the lung).

The Gaucher cell is large (diameter, 20–100 μm) and has a clear cytoplasm and an eccentric nucleus (Fig. 6-17). By light microscopy, the cytoplasm has a characteristic fibrillar appearance that has been likened to wrinkled tissue paper and is intensely positive with the periodic acid-Schiff stain. By electron microscopy, the storage material is found within enlarged lysosomes and appears as parallel layers of tubular structures.

Enlargement of the spleen is virtually universal in Gaucher disease. In the adult form of the disorder, splenomegaly may be massive, with spleen weights of as much as 10 kg. The cut surface of the enlarged spleen is firm and pale, often containing sharply demarcated infarcts. Microscopically, the red pulp shows nodular and diffuse infiltrates of Gaucher cells together with moderate fibrosis. The liver is usually enlarged by the presence of Gaucher cells within the sinusoids, but the hepatocytes are unaffected. The extent of bone marrow involvement varies but leads to some radiologic abnormalities in 50% to 75% of cases (see Chapter 26).

☐ **Clinical Features:** Gaucher disease is the most common of all lysosomal storage diseases and is found principally in adult Ashkenazi Jews. The age at onset is highly variable, but the majority of cases are not diagnosed until adulthood and present initially as painless splenomegaly and complications of hypersplenism (anemia, leukopenia, and thrombocytopenia). Bone involvement in the form of pain and pathologic fractures is the leading cause of disability and may be severe

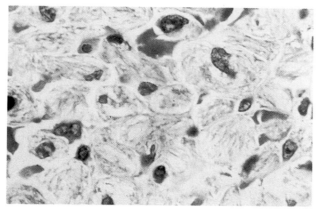

FIGURE   *6-17*
The spleen in Gaucher disease. Typical Gaucher cells have foamy cytoplasm and eccentrically located nuclei.

enough to confine the patient to a wheelchair. The life expectancy of most persons with Gaucher disease is normal. Rare types of infantile Gaucher disease involve the central nervous system.

Tay-Sachs Disease (GM₂ Gangliosidosis, Type 1)

■ *Tay-Sachs disease is an autosomal recessive disorder that reflects deposition of ganglioside GM₂ in the neurons of the central nervous system owing to a failure of lysosomal degradation.* It is predominantly a disorder of Ashkenazi Jews.

☐ **Pathogenesis:** Gangliosides are glycosphingolipids consisting of a ceramide and an oligosaccharide chain that contains *N*-acetylneuraminic acid. They are present in the outer leaflet of the plasma membrane of animal cells, particularly in brain neurons. Lysosomal catabolism of ganglioside GM₂ is accomplished through the activity of β-hexosaminidase. Tay-Sachs disease results from mutations in the gene on chromosome 15 that codes for the α-subunit of hexosaminidase A.

☐ **Pathology:** Ganglioside GM₂ accumulates in the lysosomes of all organs in Tay-Sachs disease, but it is most prominent in brain neurons and retinal cells. Microscopic examination reveals neurons that are markedly distended with storage material that stains positively for lipids. As the disease progresses, neurons are lost, and numerous lipid-laden macrophages are conspicuous in the gray matter of the cerebral cortex. Eventually, gliosis becomes prominent, and myelin and axons in the white matter are lost.

☐ **Clinical Features:** Symptoms of Tay-Sachs disease appear between 6 and 10 months of age and are characterized by progressive motor and mental deterioration. Vision is seriously impaired, and blindness (Gk. *amaurosis*) is the feature responsible for the original designation of the disease as familial amaurotic idiocy. Involvement of the retinal ganglion cells is detected by ophthalmoscopy as a **cherry-red spot** in the macula. Most children with Tay-Sachs disease die before 4 years of age.

Niemann-Pick Lipidoses

■ *Niemann-Pick lipidoses refer to a heterogeneous group of disorders characterized by lysosomal storage of sphingomyelin, cholesterol, and other glycolipids in macrophages of many organs, hepatocytes, and the brain.* Type I disease includes all affected persons who are deficient in sphingomyelinase activity. In type II disease, sphingomyelinase activity is normal, and the primary defect is, at present, uncertain. Three-fourths of all cases of Niemann-Pick disease are type I. A high frequency of type I disease is observed among Ashkenazi Jews, but the disorder is also present among other ethnic groups.

☐ **Pathogenesis:** Sphingomyelin is a membrane phospholipid composed of phosphorylcholine, sphingosine (a long-chain amino alcohol), and a fatty acid. It accounts for as much as 14% of the total phospholipids of the liver, spleen, and brain. The metabolic defect in all forms of type I Niemann-Pick disease reflects mutations in the gene (11p) that encodes **sphingomyelinase,** the lysosomal enzyme that hydrolyzes sphingomyelin to ceramide and phosphorylcholine.

☐ **Pathology:** The characteristic storage cell in Niemann-Pick disease is a foam cell, which is an enlarged (20–90 μm) macrophage in which the cytoplasm is distended by uniform vacuoles that contain sphingomyelin and cholesterol. Foam cells are particularly numerous in the spleen, lymph nodes, and bone marrow, but they are also found in other organs.

The brain is the most important organ involved in Niemann-Pick disease, and neurologic damage is the usual cause of death. At autopsy, the brain is atrophic and, in severe cases, may be reduced to as little as half the normal weight. Neurons are distended by vacuoles containing the same stored lipids found elsewhere in the body. Advanced cases are characterized by severe loss of neurons and, sometimes, by demyelination. Foam cells are noted in many locations. Half of the children demonstrate a cherry-red spot in the retina, similar to that seen in those with Tay-Sachs disease.

☐ **Clinical Features:** The acute form of Niemann-Pick disease presents in early infancy with conspicuous enlargement of the spleen and liver and with psychomotor retardation. There is progressive loss of motor and intellectual function, and the child invariably dies before the age of 5 years. ·

Mucopolysaccharidoses

■ *Mucopolysaccharidoses (MPS) comprise an assortment of lysosomal storage diseases characterized by the accumulation of glycosaminoglycans (GAGs; mucopolysaccharides) in many organs.* All types of MPS are inherited as autosomal recessive traits, with the exception of Hunter syndrome, which is X-linked recessive. These rare diseases are caused by deficiencies in any one of the 10 lysosomal enzymes involved in the sequential degradation of GAGs.

☐ **Pathogenesis:** GAGs are large polymers composed of repeating disaccharide units containing *N*-acetylhexosamine and a hexose or hexuronic acid. The accumulated GAGs (dermatan sulfate, heparan sulfate, keratan sulfate, and chondroitin sulfates) in MPS all derive from the cleavage of proteoglycans, which are important constituents of the extracellular matrix. A deficiency in any of the glycosidases or sulfatases results in the accumulation of undegraded GAGs.

☐ **Pathology:** The undegraded GAGs tend to accumulate in connective tissue cells, mononuclear phagocytes (including Kupffer cells), endothelial cells, neurons, and hepatocytes. The affected cells are swollen and clear, and stains for metachromasia confirm the presence of GAGs. The most important lesions of MPS involve the central nervous system, skeleton, and heart, although hepatosplenomegaly and corneal clouding are common.

The **central nervous system** initially demonstrates only the accumulation of GAGs. With advancing disease, there is extensive loss of neurons and increasing gliosis, changes that are reflected in cortical atrophy.

Skeletal deformities are a consequence of the accumulation of GAGs in chondrocytes, a process that eventually interferes with the normal endochondral sequence of ossification and deforms the skeleton.

Cardiac lesions are often severe and are characterized by thickening and distortion of the valves, chordae tendineae, and endocardium. The coronary arteries are frequently narrowed by intimal thickening caused by GAG deposits in smooth muscle cells.

Hepatosplenomegaly is secondary to the distention of Kupffer cells and hepatocytes in the liver and the accumulation of macrophages filled with GAGs in the spleen.

☐ **Clinical Features:** Hurler syndrome, the most severe clinical form of MPS, remains the prototype of these syndromes. The clinical features of the other varieties of MPS are summarized in Table 6-5. The symptoms of Hurler syndrome become apparent between 6 months and 2 years of age. These children typically exhibit skeletal deformities, an enlarged liver and spleen, a characteristic facies, and joint stiffness. The combination of coarse facial features and dwarfism is reminiscent of the gargoyle figures decorating Gothic cathedrals, accounting for the term **gargoylism** that was previously appended to this syndrome.

Children with Hurler syndrome suffer developmental delay, hearing loss, clouding of the cornea, and progressive mental deterioration. Increased intracranial pressure owing to communicating hydrocephalus can be troublesome. Most patients die before 10 years of age from recurrent pulmonary infections and cardiac complications.

Glycogenoses (Glycogen Storage Diseases)

■ *Glycogenoses are a group of at least 10 distinct, autosomal recessive disorders characterized by the accumulation of glycogen, principally in the liver, skeletal muscle, and heart.* Each entity reflects a deficiency of one specific

TABLE 6-5.   Mucopolysaccharidoses

Type	Eponym	Location of Gene	Clinical Features
I H	Hurler	4p16.3	Organomegaly, cardiac lesions, dysostosis multiplex, corneal clouding, death in childhood
I S	Scheie	4p16.3	Stiff joints, corneal clouding, normal intelligence, longevity
II	Hunter	x	Organomegaly, dysostosis multiplex, mental retardation, death earlier than 15 years of age
III	Sanfilippo	12q14	Mental retardation
IV	Morquio	16q24	Skeletal deformities, corneal clouding
V	Obsolete		
VI	Maroteaux-Lamy	5q13–14	Dysostosis multiplex, corneal clouding, death in second decade of life
VII	Sly	7q21.1–22	Hepatosplenomegaly, dysostosis multiplex

enzyme involved in the metabolism of glycogen. Although each of the glycogen storage diseases involves an accumulation of glycogen, the significant organ involvement varies with the specific enzyme defect. Some predominantly affect the liver, whereas others principally manifest by cardiac or skeletal muscle dysfunction. Importantly, the symptoms of a glycogenosis can reflect either the accumulation of glycogen itself (Pompe disease, Andersen disease) or lack of the glucose that is normally derived from glycogen degradation (von Gierke disease, McArdle disease).

Von Gierke Disease (Type IA Glycogenosis)

■ *Von Gierke disease is characterized by the accumulation of glycogen in the liver as a result of a deficiency in glucose-6-phosphatase.* Symptoms reflect the inability of the liver to convert glycogen to glucose, which results in hepatomegaly and hypoglycemia. The disorder is usually evident during infancy or early childhood. Although growth is commonly stunted, with modern treatment the prognosis for normal mental development and longevity is generally good.

Pompe Disease (Type II Glycogenosis)

■ *Pompe disease is a glycogen storage disease that involves virtually all organs and results in death from heart failure before 2 years of age.* The disorder is caused by a deficiency in the lysosomal enzyme acid α-glucosidase (17q23), which leads to the inexorable accumulation of undegraded glycogen in the lysosomes of many different cells.

McArdle Disease (Type V Glycogenosis)

■ *McArdle disease is characterized by the accumulation of glycogen in skeletal muscles owing to a deficiency of muscle phosphorylase (11q13), the enzyme responsible for release of glucose-1-phosphate from glycogen.* Symptoms usually appear during adolescence or early adulthood and consist of muscle cramps and spasms during exercise

and, sometimes, myocytolysis and resulting myoglobinuria.

Inborn Errors of Amino Acid Metabolism

Heritable disorders involving the metabolism of many amino acids have been described (Box 6-1). Some are lethal in early childhood, whereas others are asymptomatic biochemical defects with no clinical significance.

Phenylketonuria

■ *Phenylketonuria (PKU, hyperphenylalaninemia) is an autosomal recessive disorder caused by a deficiency of the hepatic enzyme phenylalanine hydroxylase (PAH) and is characterized by progressive mental deterioration during the first few years of life.* The severe brain damage in PKU results from high levels of circulating phenylalanine.

□ **Pathogenesis and Clinical Features:** Phenylalanine, an essential amino acid derived exclusively from the diet, is oxidized in the liver to tyrosine by PAH. A deficiency in PAH results in both hyperphenylalaninemia and the formation of phenylketones from the transamination of phenylalanine. Excretion in the urine of phenylpyruvic acid and its derivatives accounts for the original name of phenylketonuria. **However, it is now established that phenylalanine itself, rather than its metabolites, is responsible for the neurologic damage central to this disease.** Point mutations in the *PAH* gene, which is located on the long arm of chromosome 12, are responsible for the deficiency of PAH.

Hyperphenylalaninemia during infancy causes irreversible brain damage by impairing the development of neurons and the synthesis of myelin. The affected infant appears normal at birth, but mental retardation is evident within a few months. Treatment of PKU involves restriction of phenylalanine in the diet.

B O X   *6-1*   **Representative Inherited Disorders of Amino Acid Metabolism**

Phenylketonuria (hyperphenylalaninemia)
Tyrosinemia
Histidinemia
Ornithine transcarbamylase deficiency (ammonia
    intoxication)
Carbamyl phosphate synthetase deficiency (ammonia
    intoxication)

Maple syrup urine disease (branched-chain ketoacidemia)
Arginase deficiency
Arginosuccinic acid synthetase deficiency (citrulline
    accumulation)

Alkaptonuria (Ochronosis)

■ *Alkaptonuria is a rare autosomal recessive disease characterized by the excretion of homogentisic acid in the urine, generalized pigmentation, and arthritis.* A deficiency in hepatic and renal homogentisic acid oxidase prevents catabolism of homogentisic acid, an intermediate product in the metabolism of phenylalanine and tyrosine. Alkaptonuria has greater historical significance than clinical importance. Studies conducted almost a century ago by Garrod and others described the mode of inheritance of alkaptonuria and were among the first to define the concept of hereditary inborn errors of metabolism.

Patients with alkaptonuria excrete urine that darkens rapidly on standing, reflecting the formation of a pigment by the nonenzymatic oxidation of homogentisic acid (Fig. 6-18). In longstanding alkaptonuria, a similar pigment is deposited in numerous tissues, particularly the sclera, cartilage in many areas (ribs, larynx, trachea), tendons, and synovial membranes. Although the pigment appears bluish-black on gross examination, it is brown under the microscope, thereby accounting for the term **ochronosis** (color of ocher). A degenerative and frequently disabling arthropathy (ochronotic arthritis) often develops after years of alkaptonuria.

Albinism

■ *Albinism refers to a heterogeneous group of at least 10 inherited disorders of pigmentation characterized by absent or reduced biosynthesis of melanin.* The most common type is oculocutaneous albinism (OCA), a family of closely related diseases that (with a single, rare exception) represent autosomal recessive traits. OCA is characterized by a deficiency, or complete absence, of melanin pigment in the skin, hair follicles, and eyes. The two major forms of OCA are distinguished by the presence or absence of tyrosinase, which is the first enzyme in the biosynthetic pathway that converts tyrosine to melanin.

Tyrosinase-positive OCA is the most common type of albinism. These patients typically begin life with complete albinism, but with age, a small amount of clinically detectable pigment accumulates. The basic biochemical defect responsible for the impairment of melanin synthesis in tyrosinase-positive OCA is attributed to mutations in the *P* gene (15q), which is thought to encode a tyrosine transport protein.

Tyrosinase-negative OCA is the second most common type of albinism and is characterized by the complete absence of tyrosinase (11q) and melanin, although melanocytes are present and contain unpigmented melanosomes. The affected person has snow-white hair, pale pink skin, blue irides, and prominent red pupils owing to an absence of retinal pigment.

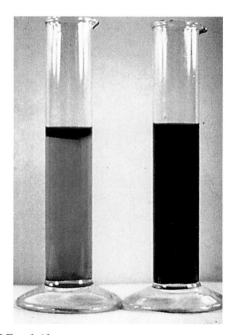

F I G U R E   *6-18*
Urine from a patient with alkaptonuria. A specimen that has been standing for 15 minutes (*left*) shows some darkening at the surface owing to the oxidation of homogentisic acid. After 2 hours (*right*), the urine is entirely black.

Persons with OCA typically have severe ophthalmic problems, including photophobia, strabismus, nystagmus, and decreased visual acuity. These patients are at greatly increased risk for development of squamous cell carcinoma of the skin in sun-exposed sites.

X-LINKED DISORDERS

Expression of X-linked disorders is different in males than in females. Females, having two X chromosomes, may be homozygous or heterozygous for a given trait. It follows, therefore, that the clinical expression of the trait in a female is variable, depending on whether it is dominant or recessive. By contrast, males have only one X chromosome and are said to be hemizygous for the same trait. **Thus, regardless of whether the trait is dominant or recessive, it is invariably expressed in the male.**

A cardinal attribute of X-linked inheritance, whether dominant or recessive, is the lack of transmission from father to son. The symptomatic father donates only his normal Y chromosome to his male offspring. By contrast, he always donates his X chromosome to his daughters, who, therefore, are obligate carriers of the trait. As a consequence, the disease classically skips a generation in the male, with the female carrier transmitting the trait to the grandsons of the original symptomatic male.

X-Linked Dominant Traits

X-linked dominance refers to the expression of a trait only in the female, because the hemizygous state in the male precludes a distinction between dominant and recessive inheritance (Fig. 6-19). The distinctive features of X-linked dominant disorders are:

- Females are affected twice as frequently as males.
- A heterozygous woman transmits the disorder to half her children, whether male or female.
- A man with a dominant X-linked disorder transmits the disease only to his daughters.
- Clinical expression of the disease tends to be less severe and more variable in heterozygous females than in hemizygous males.

Only a few X-linked dominant disorders have been described, among which are familial hypophosphatemic rickets and ornithine transcarbamylase deficiency. In such diseases, variations in the phenotypic expression of the trait in the female may be explained, at least in part, by the Lyon effect—that is, the inactivation of one X chromosome. This random inactivation results in mosaicism for the mutant allele, a condition that may be associated with inconstant expression of the trait.

X-Linked Recessive Traits

Most X-linked traits are recessive—that is, heterozygous females do not exhibit clinical disease (Fig. 6-20). The characteristics of this mode of inheritance are:

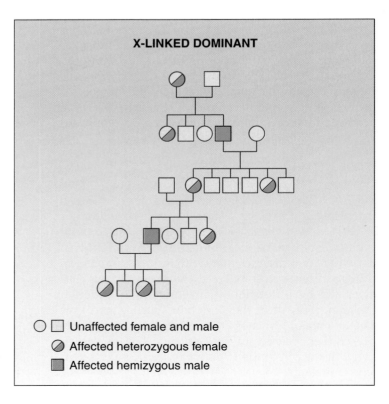

FIGURE *6-19*
X-linked dominant inheritance. A heterozygous woman transmits the trait equally to both sons and daughters, whereas men transmit the trait only to their daughters. Asymptomatic males and females do not carry the trait.

- Women who are carriers of the trait have a 50% chance of inheriting the disease, whereas the daughters are not symptomatic.
- All daughters of affected men are asymptomatic carriers, but the sons of these men are free of the trait and, thus, cannot transmit the disease to their children.
- Symptomatic homozygous females result only from the rare mating of an affected man and an asymptomatic, heterozygous woman.

Table 6-6 presents a list of representative X-linked recessive disorders.

Muscular Dystrophies (Duchenne and Becker Muscular Dystrophies)

■ *Muscular dystrophies comprise a number of devastating, wasting muscle diseases, most of which are X-linked.* The most common variant is Duchenne muscular dystrophy, a fatal, progressive degeneration of muscle that appears before the age of 4 years (Fig. 6-21). Duchenne muscular dystrophy is allelic with a less frequent and milder disorder known as Becker muscular dystrophy. Duchenne and Becker muscular dystrophies are among the most frequent human genetic diseases, occurring in one in 3500 boys, which is an incidence approaching that of cystic fibrosis.

☐ **Pathogenesis:** Duchenne and Becker muscular dystrophies are caused by a deficiency of dystrophin, a member of the family of membrane cytoskeletal proteins, which includes α-actinin and spectrin. The protein is located on the cytoplasmic face of the plasma membrane of muscle cells and is linked to it by an integral membrane glycoprotein. Dystrophin molecules form a network connecting actin fibers to the extracel-

TABLE 6-6. Representative X-Linked Recessive Diseases

Disease	Frequency in Males
Fragile X syndrome	1/2000
Hemophilia A (factor VIII deficiency)	1/10,000
Hemophilia B (factor IX deficiency)	1/70,000
Duchenne-Becker muscular dystrophy	1/3500
Glucose-6-phosphate dehydrogenase deficiency	≤30%
Lesch-Nyhan syndrome (HPRT deficiency)	1/10,000
Chronic granulomatous disease	Not rare
X-linked agammaglobulinemia	Not rare
X-linked severe combined immunodeficiency	Rare
Fabry disease	1/40,000
Hunter syndrome	1/70,000
Adrenoleukodystrophy	1/100,000
Menkes disease	1/100,000

lular matrix, which is important in maintaining both the mechanical properties of the cell and the flexibility that is needed during the contraction and relaxation of the muscle fibers.

☐ **Clinical Features:** The symptoms of muscular dystrophy progress with age. During the first year of life, the infant appears normal, but more than half fail to walk by 18 months of age. Proximal muscle weakness and pseudohypertrophy of the calf muscles become obvious, and more than 90% of afflicted boys are chair-bound by 11 years of age. In advanced disease, cardiac symptoms are almost universal. There is an overall decrease in intelligence, and one-fifth of patients are significantly retarded. The mean age at death in boys with Duchenne muscular dystrophy is 17 years.

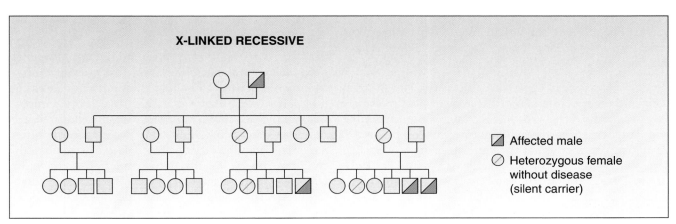

FIGURE 6-20
X-linked recessive inheritance. Only males are affected, whereas daughters of affected men are all asymptomatic carriers. Asymptomatic men do not transmit the trait. Clinical expression of the disease skips a generation.

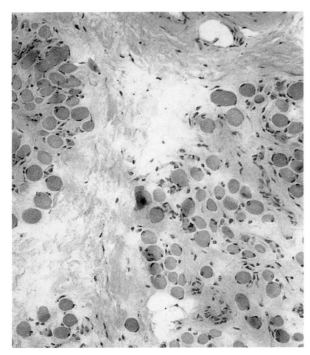

FIGURE   *6-21*
Dystrophic skeletal muscle in Duchenne muscular dystrophy. The muscle cells are atrophic and embedded in intrafascicular fibrosis. A few inflammatory cells are present.

Hemophilia A (Factor VIII Deficiency)

■ *Hemophilia A is an X-linked recessive disorder of blood clotting that results in spontaneous bleeding, particularly into the joints, muscles, and internal organs.* It is now clear that classic hemophilia is actually two distinct diseases, with one resulting from mutations in the gene encoding factor VIII (hemophilia A) and the other caused by defects in the gene encoding factor IX (hemophilia B). Because hemophilia A is the most frequently encountered sex-linked inherited bleeding disorder (one in 10,000 males), our discussion is limited to that variant.

☐ **Pathology and Clinical Features:** The mutations in the very large factor VIII gene at the tip of the long arm of the X chromosome include deletions, point mutations, and insertions. Patients with hemophilia A exhibit a mild, moderate, or severe bleeding tendency, depending on the amount of factor VIII activity in the blood. The most frequent complication of hemophilia A is a deforming arthritis caused by repeated bleeding into many joints. Although uncommon today, bleeding into the brain was formerly the most frequent cause of death in patients with hemophilia. Hematuria, intestinal obstruction, and respiratory obstruction all

may occur with bleeding into the respective organs. Treatment with human recombinant factor VIII maintains the levels of this clotting factor and generally controls the bleeding diathesis.

Fragile X Syndrome

■ *Fragile X syndrome is associated with expansion of a trinucleotide repeat on the X chromosome and is the most common form of inherited mental retardation.* In fact, it is second only to Down syndrome as an identifiable cause of retardation.

☐ **Pathogenesis:** A fragile site represents a specific locus, or band, on a chromosome that breaks easily, after which it is usually detected in cytogenetic preparations as a nonstaining gap or constriction. The fragile X locus represents a distinct kind of mutation characterized by amplification of a multiple triplet (CGG) repeat segment of the chromosome. Normal persons have approximately 30 CGG repeats at the X locus, whereas males with fragile X syndrome have more than 200 (and possibly as many as 4000) repeats. **In other words, expansion of the number of repeats is associated with the disease, and the severity of the syndrome seems to be related to the number of repeats.**

☐ **Clinical Features:** The male newborn afflicted with fragile X syndrome appears normal, but during childhood, characteristic features appear, including an increased head circumference, facial coarsening, joint hyperextensibility, enlarged testes, and abnormalities of the cardiac valves. Mental retardation is profound, with IQ scores varying from 20 to 60. **Interestingly, a significant proportion of autistic male children carry a fragile X chromosome.**

MULTIFACTORIAL INHERITANCE

■ *Multifactorial inheritance describes a disease process that reflects the additive effects of a number of abnormal genes and environmental factors.* Most normal human traits are inherited as neither dominant nor recessive mendelian attributes but, rather, in a more complex manner. For example, multifactorial inheritance determines intelligence, height, skin color, body habitus, and even emotional disposition. Similarly, most of the common chronic disorders of adults represent multifactorial genetic diseases and are well known to run in families. Such maladies include diabetes, atherosclerosis, many forms of cancer and arthritis, and hypertension. Inheritance of a number of birth defects is also multifactorial (e.g., cleft lip and palate, pyloric stenosis, and congenital heart disease) (Table 6-7).

TABLE 6-7. Representative Diseases

TABLE 6-7. Representative Diseases
Associated with Multifactorial Inheritance

Adults	Children
Hypertension	Pyloric stenosis
Atherosclerosis	Cleft lip and palate
Diabetes, type II	Congenital heart disease
Allergic diathesis	Meningomyelocele
Psoriasis	Anencephaly
Schizophrenia	Hypospadias
Ankylosing spondylitis	Congenital hip dislocation
Gout	Hirschsprung disease

The biologic basis of polygenic inheritance rests on the evidence that more than one-fourth of all genetic loci in normal humans contain multiple polymorphic alleles. Such genetic heterogeneity provides a background for the wide variability in the susceptibility to many diseases, which is compounded by a multiplicity of interactions with environmental factors. The following criteria are useful in characterizing multifactorial inheritance:

- Expression of symptoms is proportional to the number of mutant genes.
- Environmental factors influence expression of the trait. The risk in all first-degree relatives (parents, siblings, children) is the same (5–10%).
- The probability of expression in later offspring is influenced by whether the trait is expressed in earlier siblings. If one or more children are born with a multifactorial defect, the chances for recurrence are doubled. This contrasts with mendelian traits, in which the probability of expression is independent of the number of affected siblings.
- The more severe the defect, the greater the risk of transmitting it to offspring.
- Some abnormalities characterized by multifactorial inheritance show a sex predilection.

Cleft Lip and Cleft Palate

Cleft lip and cleft palate are excellent paradigms to illustrate the principles of multifactorial inheritance. Fusion of the frontal prominence with the maxillary process to form the upper lip is under the control of many genes. Hereditary or environmental disturbance in gene expression at the time of this closure results in cleft lip, with or without cleft palate (Fig. 6-22). This anomaly may also be part of a systemic malformation syndrome caused by teratogens (rubella, anticonvulsants) and is often encountered in children with chromosomal abnormalities.

If one child is born with a cleft lip, there is a 4% chance that the second child will exhibit the same defect. If the first two children are affected, the risk of cleft lip increases to 9% for the third child. Whereas 75% of cases of cleft lip occur in boys, the sons of women with cleft lip have a fourfold greater risk of acquiring the defect than the sons of affected fathers.

DISEASES OF INFANCY AND CHILDHOOD

Prematurity and Intrauterine Growth Retardation

The normal duration of human pregnancy is 40 ± 2 weeks, and most newborns weigh 3300 ± 600 g. Prematurity has been defined by the World Health Organization as being a gestational age of younger than 37 weeks (from the first day of the last menstrual period). The traditional definition of prematurity was a birth weight of less than 2500 g, regardless of the gestational age. However, it is now appreciated that full-term infants may weigh less than 2500 g because of intrauterine growth retardation rather than premature birth. Thus, low-birth-weight infants (<2500 g) are classed as being either appropriate for gestational age (AGA) or small for gestational age (SGA).

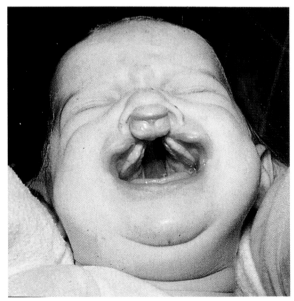

FIGURE 6-22
Cleft lip and cleft palate in an infant.

☐ **Etiology:** Factors that predispose to the premature birth of an infant (AGA) are (1) maternal illness, (2) uterine incompetence, (3) fetal disorders, and (4) placental abnormalities. When the life of a fetus is threatened by such conditions, it may be necessary to induce premature delivery to salvage the infant. Intrauterine growth retardation and the resulting birth of SGA infants are associated with disorders that (1) impair maternal health and nutrition, (2) interfere with placental circulation or function, or (3) disturb the growth or development of the fetus.

☐ **Clinical Features:** Prematurity is often associated with severe respiratory distress, metabolic disturbances (e.g., hyperbilirubinemia, hypoglycemia, hypocalcemia), circulatory problems (anemia, hypothermia, hypotension), and bacterial sepsis. By contrast, SGA infants comprise a much more heterogeneous group, including many infants with congenital anomalies and infections acquired in utero. In addition to many of the problems associated with prematurity, SGA infants also often suffer from perinatal asphyxia, meconium aspiration, necrotizing enterocolitis, pulmonary hemorrhage, and disorders related to birth defects or inherited metabolic diseases.

Organ Immaturity

Maturity of the newborn can be defined in both anatomic and physiologic terms.

Lungs. Immaturity of the lungs poses one of the most common and immediate threats to the viability of a low-birth-weight infant. The lining cells of the fetal alveoli do not differentiate into type I and type II pneumocytes until late pregnancy. The amniotic fluid, which fills the fetal alveoli, drains from the lungs at birth, after which air expands the respiratory spaces. Often, the sluggish respiratory movements of the immature infant do not suffice to evacuate the amniotic fluid from the lungs. As a result, such newborns die of respiratory failure, with incompletely expanded lungs. On gross examination, the lungs are not crepitant, and microscopically, the alveoli are variably expanded. The air passages contain desquamated squamous cells (squames) and lanugo hair from the fetal skin and protein-rich amniotic fluid (Fig. 6-23). Although this appearance is often termed **amniotic fluid aspiration,** it actually represents retained amniotic fluid.

Liver. The fetal liver is deficient in glucuronyl transferase, and the resulting inability of the organ to conjugate bilirubin often leads to **neonatal jaundice.** This enzyme deficiency is aggravated by rapid destruction of fetal erythrocytes, a process that results in an increased supply of bilirubin.

Brain. Incomplete development of the central nervous system is often reflected in poor vasomotor control, hypothermia, feeding difficulties, and recurrent apnea.

Respiratory Distress Syndrome of the Newborn (Hyaline Membrane Disease)

■ *Respiratory distress syndrome (RDS) of the newborn is a life-threatening disorder of the lungs principally associated with prematurity.* More than half of newborns younger than 28 weeks of gestational age are afflicted with RDS, whereas only one-fifth of infants between 32 and 36 weeks of gestational age are affected. In addition to prematurity, other risk factors for RDS include (1) neonatal asphyxia, (2) maternal diabetes, (3) delivery by cesarean section, (4) precipitous delivery, and (5) twin pregnancies.

☐ **Pathogenesis:** The pathogenesis of RDS of the newborn is intimately linked to a deficiency of surfactant (Fig. 6-24). In the normal newborn, the onset of breathing is associated with a massive release of stored surfactant. This material lowers the surface tension of the alveoli at low lung volumes and, thereby, prevents

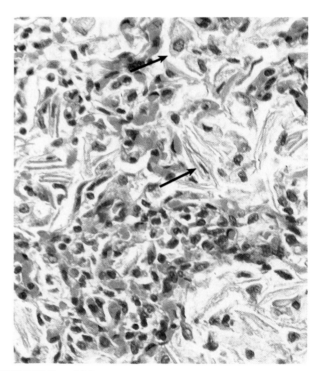

FIGURE   *6-23*
Retention of amniotic fluid in the lung of a premature newborn. The incompletely expanded lung contains squames (*arrows*) consisting of squamous epithelial cells shed into the amniotic fluid from the fetal skin.

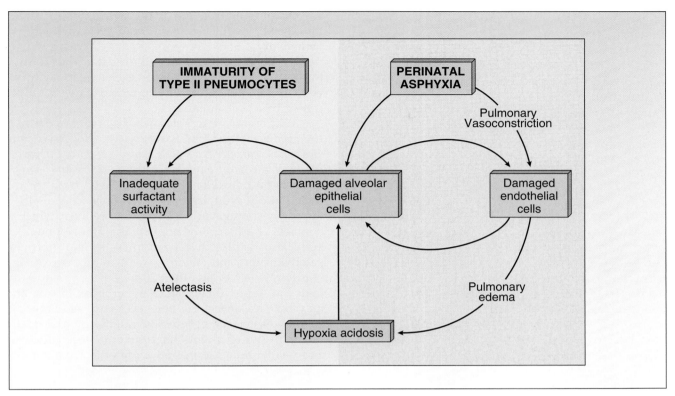

FIGURE *6-24*
Pathogenesis of the respiratory distress syndrome of the neonate. Immaturity of the lungs and perinatal asphyxia are the major pathogenetic factors.

collapse (atelectasis) of the alveoli during expiration. The immature lung, however, is deficient in both the amount and the composition of surfactant. Moreover, any damage to type II pneumocytes (e.g., from asphyxia) will interfere with the synthesis and secretion of surfactant. Atelectasis secondary to surfactant deficiency results in perfused, but not ventilated, alveoli. This leads to hypoxia and acidosis, with further compromise in the ability of type II pneumocytes to produce surfactant. Moreover, hypoxia produces pulmonary arterial vasoconstriction, thereby increasing right-to-left shunting through the ductus arteriosus and foramen ovale and within the lung itself. The resulting pulmonary ischemia further aggravates alveolar epithelial damage and injures the endothelium of the pulmonary capillaries. The leak of protein-rich fluid into the alveoli from the injured vascular bed contributes to the typical clinical and pathologic features of RDS.

☐ **Pathology:** On gross examination, the lungs are dark red and airless. Microscopically, the alveoli are collapsed, and the alveolar ducts and respiratory bronchioles are dilated. Within these expanded spaces, cellular debris, proteinaceous edema fluid, and erythrocytes are evident. The alveolar ducts are lined by conspicuous, eosinophilic, fibrin-rich amorphous

structures termed **hyaline membranes,** thereby accounting for the original designation of RDS as **hyaline membrane disease** (Fig. 6-25).

☐ **Clinical Features:** The first symptom, usually appearing within an hour after birth, is increased respiratory effort, with forceful intercostal retraction and use of accessory neck muscles. The respiratory rate increases to more than 100 breaths per minute, and cyanosis becomes apparent. Long periods of apnea ensue, and the infant eventually dies of asphyxia. Despite advances in neonatal intensive care, the overall mortality rate of RDS remains approximately 30%, and half of infants born before 30 weeks of gestational age die of this disorder.

The major complications of RDS relate to anoxia and acidosis. They include intraventricular cerebral hemorrhage, persistence of the patent ductus arteriosus, necrotizing enterocolitis, and bronchopulmonary dysplasia.

Erythroblastosis Fetalis and Neonatal Hemolytic Anemia

■ *Erythroblastosis fetalis is a hemolytic disease of the fetus or newborn caused by the transplacental passage of maternal antibodies against fetal erythrocytes.* More than 60

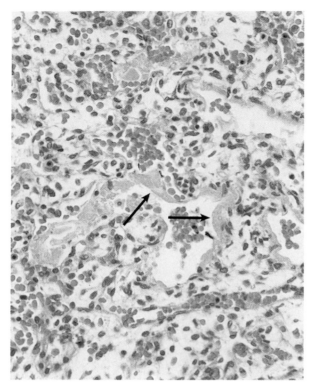

FIGURE   *6-25*
The lung in the respiratory distress syndrome of the neonate. The alveoli are atelectatic, and a dilated alveolar duct is lined by a fibrin-rich hyaline membrane (arrows).

antigens on the surface of erythrocytes can elicit an antibody response, but only the D antigen of the Rh group and the ABO system are associated with a significant incidence of hemolytic disease.

☐ **Pathogenesis:** Introduction of Rh-positive fetal erythrocytes (>1 mL) into the circulation of an Rh-negative mother at the time of delivery sensitizes her to an Rh antigen (Fig. 6-26). Erythroblastosis fetalis does not ordinarily occur during the first pregnancy, because the quantity of fetal blood necessary to sensitize the mother is introduced into her circulation only at the time of delivery, which is too late to affect the fetus. However, when the sensitized mother again bears an Rh-positive fetus, much smaller quantities of antigen elicit an increase in antibody titer. This cycle is exaggerated in multiparous women, and the severity of erythroblastosis tends to increase progressively with each succeeding pregnancy. Even after multiple pregnancies, only 5% of Rh-negative women ever deliver infants with erythroblastosis fetalis.

☐ **Pathology and Clinical Features:** The severity of erythroblastosis fetalis varies from a mild hemolysis to a fatal anemia, and the pathologic findings are determined by the extent of the hemolytic disease.

Death in utero occurs in the most extreme form of the disease, in which case severe maceration is evident on delivery.

Hydrops fetalis refers to the most serious form in liveborn infants. This condition is characterized by severe edema secondary to congestive heart failure caused by severe anemia.

■ *Kernicterus, also termed bilirubin encephalopathy, is a neurologic condition associated with severe jaundice and is characterized by bile staining of the brain, particularly of the basal ganglia, pontine nuclei, and dentate nuclei in the cerebellum.* Bilirubin derived from the destruction of erythrocytes in erythroblastosis fetalis is not easily conjugated by the immature liver, which is deficient in glucuronyl transferase. Development of kernicterus is directly related to the level of unconjugated bilirubin and, in term infants, is rare with serum bilirubin levels of less than 20 mg/dL. Premature infants are more vulnerable to hyperbilirubinemia and may develop kernicterus at levels as low as 12 mg/dL. Severe kernicterus progresses to lethargy and death. Most surviving infants have severe choreoathetosis and mental retardation, and a minority have varying degrees of intellectual and motor retardation.

Birth Injury

Birth injury is a broad term that spans the spectrum of mechanical trauma to anoxic damage. Some of these injuries relate to poor obstetric manipulation, whereas many are unavoidable sequelae of routine delivery. Birth injuries occur in approximately five in 1000 live births. Factors that predispose to birth injury include cephalopelvic disproportion, dystocia (difficult labor), prematurity, and breech presentation.

Cranial Injury

Cephalohematoma is a subperiosteal hemorrhage confined to a single cranial bone and becomes apparent within the first few hours after birth. It may or may not be associated with a linear fracture of the underlying bone. Most cephalohematomas resolve without complications and require no treatment.

Skull fractures during birth result from the impact of the head on the pelvic bones or pressure from obstetric forceps.

Intracranial hemorrhage is one of the most dangerous birth injuries. It may be traumatic or secondary to asphyxia. Traumatic intracranial hemorrhage occurs in the setting of (1) significant cephalopelvic disproportion, (2) precipitous delivery, (3) breech presentation, (4) prolonged labor, or (5) inappropriate use of forceps. These traumas can result in **subdural or subarachnoid hemorrhage,** which commonly are sec-

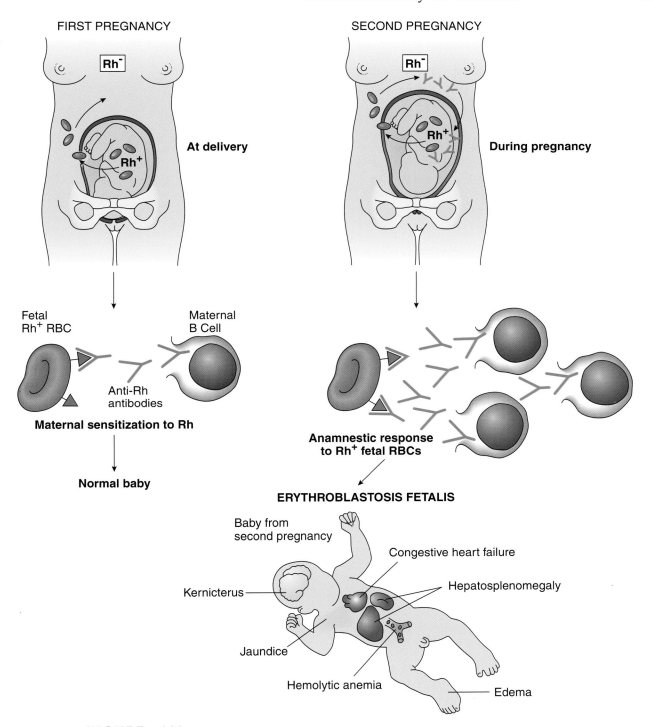

FIRST PREGNANCY

SECOND PREGNANCY

Rh⁻

At delivery

Rh⁺

Rh⁻

During pregnancy

Rh⁺

Fetal
Rh⁺ RBC

Maternal
B Cell

Anti-Rh
antibodies

Maternal sensitization to Rh

Normal baby

**Anamnestic response
to Rh⁺ fetal RBCs**

ERYTHROBLASTOSIS FETALIS

Baby from
second pregnancy

Congestive heart failure

Hepatosplenomegaly

Kernicterus

Jaundice

Hemolytic anemia

Edema

FIGURE   *6-26*
**Pathogenesis of erythroblastosis fetalis due to maternal-fetal Rh incompatibility.
Immunization of the Rh-negative mother with Rh-positive erythrocytes during the first
pregnancy leads to the formation of anti-Rh antibodies of the immunoglobulin G type.
These antibodies cross the placenta and damage the Rh-positive fetus in subsequent
pregnancies**

ondary to lacerations of the falx cerebri or tentorium cerebelli that involve the vein of Galen or the venous sinuses. Anoxic injury from asphyxia, particularly in the premature infant, is often associated with intraventricular hemorrhage.

The prognosis for a newborn with intracranial hemorrhage varies with the extent. Massive hemorrhage is often rapidly fatal. If the infant survives, recovery may be complete, or the child may be afflicted with chronic neurologic residuals, usually in the form of cerebral palsy or hydrocephalus. It deserves emphasis, however, that many cases of cerebral palsy have been shown by ultrasound studies to relate to brain damage acquired at least 2 weeks before birth rather than to birth trauma.

Peripheral Nerve Injury

Brachial palsy refers to varying degrees of paralysis of the upper extremity and is caused by excessive traction on the head and neck or shoulders during delivery.

Phrenic nerve paralysis, and associated paralysis of a hemidiaphragm, may be associated with brachial palsy. It results in breathing difficulties and generally resolves spontaneously within a few months.

Facial nerve palsy usually presents as a unilateral, flaccid paralysis of the face caused by injury to cranial nerve VII during labor or delivery, especially with forceps.

Sudden Infant Death Syndrome

■ *Sudden infant death syndrome (SIDS) is defined as the sudden death of an infant or young child that is unexpected by the history and in which a thorough postmortem examination fails to demonstrate an adequate cause of death.* Typically, the victim is an apparently healthy young infant who has been asleep without any hint of impending calamity. The infant does not awake spontaneously at the usual time, and when the baby cannot be aroused, the parent realizes that it has died. Postmortem examination does not disclose a cause of death, such as pneumonia, food aspiration, sepsis, or cerebral hemorrhage.

Beyond the neonatal period, SIDS is the leading cause of death during the first year of life, accounting for more than a one-third of all deaths in this time. The large majority of deaths occur at night or during periods associated with sleep. It has recently been proposed that infants who sleep in the prone position are at greater risk of SIDS. A number of cases also have recently been shown to be examples of homicide rather than unexplained death.

The strongest **maternal risk factors** appear to be the following:

- Low socioeconomic status (limited education, unmarried mother, poor prenatal care)
- Maternal age younger than 20 years at first pregnancy
- Cigarette smoking during pregnancy
- Use of illicit drugs during pregnancy.

The risk factors for the **infant** are controversial. The consensus includes the following:

- Low birth weight
- Prematurity
- An illness, often gastrointestinal, within the last 2 weeks before death
- Subsequent siblings of SIDS victims
- Survivors of an apparent life-threatening event, defined as an episode characterized by some combination of apnea, color change, marked alteration in muscle tone, and choking or gagging.

☐ **Pathogenesis:** It is unclear whether SIDS is a single entity or represents the common end point of several different conditions. The most popular hypothesis relates SIDS to a prolonged spell of apnea, followed by a cardiac arrhythmia or shock, in susceptible, sleeping infants who cannot arouse themselves and prevent the process from progressing to a fatal outcome. However, it deserves emphasis that fewer than 10% of parents of SIDS victims report an episode of apnea or an apparent life-threatening event at any time before the fatal event. **Thus, although sleep apnea may contribute to the sequence of events leading to SIDS, available data do not support a strong and predictable relationship between the two conditions.**

☐ **Pathology:** At autopsy, a number of morphologic alterations have been described in victims of SIDS, but their relevance to the cause and pathogenesis of this disorder remains unclear. Chronic hypoxia is said to be evidenced by gliosis of the brainstem, medial hypertrophy of the small pulmonary arteries, persistence of extramedullary hemopoiesis in the liver, retention of periadrenal brown fat, and right ventricular hypertrophy. However, with the exception of brainstem gliosis, none of these changes occurs with any regularity. Petechiae on the surfaces of the lungs, heart, pleura, and thymus, which have been reported in most infants dying of SIDS, are probably terminal events.

NEOPLASMS OF INFANCY AND CHILDHOOD

Malignant tumors between the ages of 1 and 15 years are distinctly uncommon, but cancer remains the leading cause of death from disease in this age group. In children, 10% of all deaths are due to malignancies, and only accidental trauma kills a larger number. **Unlike adults, in whom the large majority of cancers are of epithelial origin (e.g., carcinomas of the lung, breast, and gastrointestinal tract), most malignant tumors in children arise from the hemopoietic, nervous, and soft tissues.** Another feature that distinguishes childhood tumors from adult ones is that many of the former are part of developmental complexes. Examples include Wilms tumor associated with aniridia, genitourinary malformations, and mental retardation (WAGR complex); hemihypertrophy of the body associated with Wilms tumor, hepatoblastoma, and adrenal carcinoma; and tuberous sclerosis in association with renal tumors and rhabdomyomas of the heart. Some tumors are apparent at birth and, obviously, are developmental tumors that have evolved in utero. In addition, abnormally developed organs, persistent organ primordia, and displaced organ rests are all vulnerable to neoplastic transformation.

Benign Tumors and Tumor-Like Conditions

Hamartomas. These lesions represent focal, benign overgrowths of one or more of the mature cellular elements of a normal tissue, often with one element predominating.

Hemangiomas. These lesions, which are of varying size and in diverse locations, are the most frequently encountered tumors in childhood. Whether hemangiomas are true neoplasms or hamartomas is unclear, although half are present at birth and most regress with age. Occasionally, large, rapidly growing hemangiomas can be serious lesions, especially when they occur on the head or neck. A **port wine stain** is a congenital capillary hemangioma that involves the skin of the face and scalp and often is large enough to be disfiguring, imparting a dark-purple color to the affected area. Unlike many small hemangiomas, they persist for life and are not easily treated.

Lymphangiomas. Also termed **cystic hygromas,** lymphangiomas are poorly demarcated swellings that usually are present at birth and, thereafter, rapidly increase in size. Most lymphangiomas occur on the head and neck, but the floor of the mouth, mediastinum, and buttocks are not uncommon sites. Lymphangiomas appear as unilocular or multilocular cysts, with thin, transparent walls and straw-colored fluid. Microscopically, myriads of dilated lymphatic channels are separated by fibrous septa. Unlike hemangiomas, these lesions do not regress spontaneously and should be resected.

Sacrococcygeal Teratomas. Although rare, these germ cell neoplasms are the most common solid tumors in the newborn. At least 75% of sacrococcygeal teratomas occur in girls, and a substantial number have been encountered in twins. The tumors are usually noticed at birth as a mass in the region of the sacrum and buttocks. They commonly are large, lobulated masses, often as large as the infant's head. Microscopically, sacrococcygeal teratomas are composed of numerous tissues, particularly of neural origin. The large majority (90%) of sacrococcygeal teratomas detected before the age of 2 months are benign, but as many as half of those diagnosed later in life are malignant. Associated congenital anomalies of the vertebrae, genitourinary system, and anorectum are common. The lesion should be resected promptly.

Malignant Tumors

Cancers in the pediatric age group are uncommon, with an incidence of 1.3 in 10,000 per year in children younger than 15 years of age. The mortality rate clearly varies with the intrinsic behavior of the tumor and the response to therapy, but as an overall figure, the death rate for childhood cancer is only approximately one-third of the incidence. **Almost half of all malignant diseases in patients younger than 15 years of age are acute leukemias and lymphomas.** Leukemias alone, particularly acute lymphoblastic leukemia, account for one-third of all cases of childhood cancer. Most of the other malignant neoplasms are neuroblastomas, brain tumors, Wilms tumors, retinoblastomas, bone cancers, and various soft-tissue sarcomas.

Hemodynamic Disorders

Wolfgang J. Mergner
Benjamin F. Trump

The metabolism of organs and cells depends on an intact circulation, both for the continuous delivery of oxygen, nutrients, hormones, electrolytes, and water and for the removal of metabolic waste and carbon dioxide. Delivery and elimination at the cellular level are controlled by exchanges between the intravascular, interstitial, cellular, and lymphatic spaces.

HEMORRHAGE

■ *Hemorrhage (bleeding) is a discharge of blood from the vascular compartment to the exterior of the body or to nonvascular body spaces.* The most common and obvious cause is trauma; however, an artery may be ruptured in ways other than laceration. For instance, severe atherosclerosis may weaken the wall of the abdominal aorta so that it balloons to form an aneurysm, which then ruptures and bleeds into the retroperitoneal space. By the same token, an aneurysm may complicate a congenitally weak cerebral artery (berry aneurysm) and lead to subarachnoid hemorrhage. Certain infections (e.g., pulmonary tuberculosis) erode blood vessels; a similar vascular injury is caused by invasive tumors.

Hemorrhage also results from damage at the level of the capillaries. For instance, rupture of capillaries by blunt trauma is evidenced by the appearance of a bruise. Increased venous pressure also causes extravasation of blood from capillaries in the lung. Vitamin C deficiency is associated with capillary fragility and bleeding owing to a defect in the supporting structures. A severe decrease in the number of platelets (thrombocytopenia) or deficiency of a coagulation factor (e.g., factor VIII in hemophilia) is associated with spontaneous hemorrhages unrelated to any apparent trauma.

A person may also exsanguinate into an internal cavity, as in the case of gastrointestinal hemorrhage from a peptic ulcer (arterial hemorrhage) or esophageal varices (venous hemorrhage). In such cases, large amounts of fresh blood fill the entire gastrointestinal tract. Bleeding into a serous cavity can result in the accumulation of a large amount of blood, even to the point of exsanguination. A few definitions are now in order:

■ *Hemothorax: Hemorrhage into the pleural cavity.*
■ *Hemopericardium: Hemorrhage into the pericardial space.*
■ *Hemoperitoneum: Bleeding into the peritoneal cavity.*
■ *Hemarthrosis: Bleeding into a joint space.*
■ *Hematoma: Hemorrhage into the soft tissues.* Such collections of blood can be merely painful, as in a muscle bruise, or fatal, if located in the brain.

■ *Purpura: Diffuse superficial hemorrhages in the skin, as large as 1 cm in diameter.*
■ *Ecchymosis: A larger superficial hemorrhage.* Following a bruise or in association with a coagulation defect, an initially purple discoloration of the skin turns green, and then yellow, before resolving. This sequence reflects the progressive oxidation of bilirubin released from the hemoglobin of degraded erythrocytes. A good example of an ecchymosis is a black eye.
■ *Petechia: A pinpoint hemorrhage, usually in the skin or conjunctiva.* This lesion represents the rupture of a capillary or arteriole. It occurs in conjunction with coagulopathies or vasculitis, with the latter being classically associated with infections of the heart valves (bacterial endocarditis).

HYPEREMIA

■ *Hyperemia is an excess amount of blood in an organ.*

Active Hyperemia

■ *Active hyperemia is an augmented supply of blood to an organ, usually as a physiologic response to increased functional demand, as in the case of the heart and skeletal muscles during exercise.* Neurogenic and hormonal influences play a role in active hyperemia, as exemplified at both extremes of the female reproductive span—namely, in the form of the "blushing bride" and the menopausal flush. The increased blood supply is brought about by arteriolar dilatation and recruitment of inactive or latent capillaries.

The most striking active hyperemia occurs in association with inflammation. Vasoactive materials released by inflammatory cells cause dilatation of the blood vessels; in the skin, this results in the classic "tumor, rubor, and calor" of inflammation. In pneumonia, alveolar capillaries are engorged with erythrocytes as a hyperemic response to inflammation.

Passive Hyperemia (Congestion)

■ *Passive hyperemia, or congestion, refers to the engorgement of an organ with venous blood.* Clinically, acute passive congestion is a consequence of acute failure of the left ventricle. The resulting venous engorgement of the lung leads to accumulation of a transudate in the alveoli, a condition termed **pulmonary edema.** A generalized increase in venous pressure, typically from chronic heart failure, results in slower blood flow and consequent increase in the volume of blood in many organs, including the liver, spleen, and kidneys.

Passive congestion may also be confined to a limb or an organ as a result of more localized obstruction to the venous drainage. Examples include deep venous thrombosis of the leg, with resulting edema of the lower extremity, and thrombosis of the hepatic veins (Budd-Chiari syndrome), with secondary chronic passive congestion of the liver.

Lung. Chronic failure of the left ventricle impedes the exit of blood from the lungs and leads to chronic passive congestion of that organ. As a result, pressure in the alveolar capillaries is increased, and these vessels become engorged with blood. This increased pressure in the alveolar capillaries has four major consequences:

1. Microhemorrhages release erythrocytes into the alveolar spaces, where they are phagocytosed and degraded by alveolar macrophages. The released iron, in the form of hemosiderin, remains in the macrophages, which are then called "heart failure cells."
2. The increased hydrostatic pressure forces fluid from the blood into the alveolar spaces, thereby resulting in pulmonary edema, a dangerous condition that interferes with gas exchange in the lung.
3. The increased pressure, together with other poorly understood factors, stimulates fibrosis in the interstitial spaces of the lung. The presence of fibrosis and of iron is viewed grossly as a firm, brown lung ("brown induration").
4. The increased capillary pressure is transmitted to the pulmonary arterial system, a condition labeled

pulmonary hypertension. This disorder leads to right-sided heart failure and consequent generalized venous congestion.

Chapter 12 discusses the morphologic changes associated with chronic passive congestion of the lungs.

Liver. The liver, with the hepatic veins emptying into the vena cava immediately inferior to the heart, is particularly vulnerable to chronic passive congestion. The central veins of the hepatic lobule become dilated, and the increased venous pressure is transferred to the sinusoids, where it leads to dilatation of the sinusoids, with blood and pressure atrophy of the centrilobular hepatocytes (Fig. 7-1).

Grossly, the cut surface of a chronically congested liver exhibits dark foci of centrilobular congestion, which are surrounded by paler zones composed of unaffected peripheral portions of the lobules. The result is a curious reticulated appearance, resembling the cross-section of a nutmeg and appropriately called "nutmeg liver" (see Fig. 7-1).

Spleen. Increased pressure in the liver, either from cardiac failure or an intrahepatic obstruction to the flow of blood (e.g., cirrhosis), results in higher pressure in the portal vein, which is transmitted to the splenic vein and leads to congestion of the spleen. The organ becomes enlarged and tense, and the cut section oozes dark blood. In longstanding congestion, diffuse fibro-

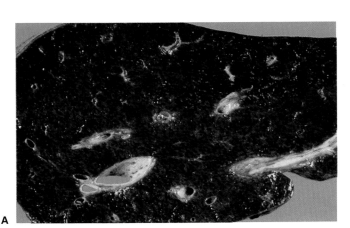
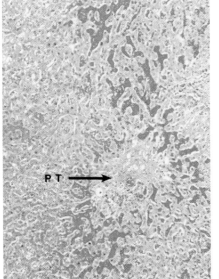

FIGURE **7-1**
Passive congestion of the liver. (A) A gross photograph shows the pattern of chronic passive congestion, in which lighter-appearing tissue segments form an interlacing pattern with dark-staining. centrilobular blood spaces. (B) A photomicrograph of the liver shows centrilobular sinusoids dilated with blood. The intervening plates of hepatocytes show pressure atrophy. *PT,* **portal tract.**

sis of the spleen is observed, together with iron-containing, fibrotic, and calcified foci of old hemorrhage (Gamna-Gandy bodies). Fibrocongestive splenomegaly may result in an organ that weighs from 250 to 750 g (compared with a normal weight of 150 g).

Edema and Ascites. Venous congestion impedes the flow of blood in the capillaries, thereby increasing hydrostatic pressure and promoting formation of edema. Accumulation of edematous fluid in heart failure is particularly noticeable in the dependent tissues, namely the legs and feet in ambulatory patients and the back in bedridden persons. Ascites, which is the accumulation of fluid in the peritoneal space, reflects (among other factors) the lack of tissue rigor, a condition in which there is no countervailing external pressure to oppose the hydrostatic pressure.

THROMBOSIS

■ *Thrombosis refers to the formation within a vascular lumen of a thrombus, which is an aggregate of coagulated blood containing platelets, fibrin, and entrapped cellular elements.* A **thrombus** is, by definition, adherent to the vascular endothelium and should be distinguished from a simple blood clot. The latter only reflects activation of the coagulation cascade and can form in vitro or in situ in the postmortem state.

Thrombosis in the Arterial System

☐ **Pathogenesis:** The most common cause of arterial thrombosis is atherosclerosis, and the most important vessels involved are the coronary, cerebral, mesenteric, and renal arteries, as well as the arteries of the lower extremities. Uncommonly, arterial thrombosis occurs in other disorders, including inflammation of the arteries (arteritis), trauma, and diseases of the blood. Thrombi are common in aneurysms (localized dilatations of the lumen) of the aorta and its major branches, in which the distortion of blood flow, combined with intrinsic vascular disease, promotes thrombosis.

The pathogenesis of arterial thrombosis involves three principal factors:

- **Damage to the endothelium,** usually by atherosclerosis, disturbs the anticoagulant properties of the vessel wall and serves as the nidus for platelet aggregation and fibrin formation.
- **Alterations in the flood of blood,** whether from turbulence in an aneurysm or at the sites of arterial bifurcation or from slowing in narrowed arteries, tend to favor thrombosis.
- **Increased coagulability of the blood,** as seen in polycythemia vera or after the use of oral contra-

ceptives, is associated with increased risk of thrombosis.

☐ **Pathology:** Initially, an arterial thrombus, which is attached to the vessel wall, is soft, friable, and dark red. It exhibits fine, alternating bands of yellowish platelets and fibrin, the so-called **lines of Zahn.** Once formed, arterial thrombi have several outcomes:

- **Lysis of an arterial thrombus** may occur owing to the potent thrombolytic activity of the blood.
- **Propagation of a thrombus** (an increase in size) may ensue, because the thrombus serves as the focus for further thrombosis.
- **Organization** refers to the eventual invasion of connective tissue elements, which causes the thrombus to become firm and grayish-white.
- **Canalization** is the process by which new lumina, lined by endothelial cells, form in an organized thrombus.

The organized structure of a thrombus reflects a tight interaction between platelets and fibrin. It differs in appearance from that of a postmortem clot or one formed in a test tube. The lines of Zahn stabilize a thrombus formed during life, whereas a postmortem clot has a more gelatinous structure.

☐ **Clinical Features:** Arterial thrombosis is the most common cause of death in Western industrialized countries. Because most arterial thrombi occlude the vessel, they often lead to ischemic necrosis of the tissue supplied by the artery—that is, an **infarct.** Thus, thrombosis of a coronary or a cerebral artery results in a **myocardial infarct** (heart attack) or **cerebral infarct** (stroke). Other end arteries that are affected by atherosclerosis and often suffer thrombosis include the mesenteric arteries (intestinal infarction), renal arteries (kidney infarcts), and arteries of the leg (gangrene).

Thrombosis in the Heart

As in the arterial system, endocardial injury and changes in the blood flow of the heart are associated with mural thrombosis (thrombi attached to the endocardium of a cardiac chamber). The disorders in which mural thrombosis occurs include:

- **Myocardial Infarction.** Adherent mural thrombi form in the cavity of the left ventricle over areas of myocardial infarction, owing to damaged endocardium and alterations in blood flow associated with an adynamic myocardial segment.
- **Atrial Fibrillation.** A disorder of atrial rhythm (atrial fibrillation) leads to slower blood flow in the left atrium, which predisposes to the formation of mural thrombi in that location.

- **Cardiomyopathy.** Primary diseases of the myocardium are associated with mural thrombi in the left ventricle. The reasons are poorly understood but, presumably, relate to endocardial injury and altered hemodynamics associated with poor myocardial contractility.
- **Endocarditis.** Small thrombi, termed **vegetations,** may also develop on cardiac valves, usually mitral or aortic, that are damaged by a bacterial infection (bacterial endocarditis).

The major complication of thrombi at any location in the heart is the detachment of fragments and their transport to distant sites (embolization), where they lodge and occlude arterial vessels.

Thrombosis in the Venous System

☐ **Pathogenesis:** At one time, venous thrombosis was widely referred to as **thrombophlebitis,** implying that an inflammatory or infectious process had injured the vein, thereby causing thrombosis. However, because most cases have no evidence of inflammation, the term **phlebothrombosis** is more accurate. Nevertheless, both terms have been replaced, for the most part, by the expression **deep venous thrombosis.** This phrase is particularly appropriate for the most common manifestation of the disorder, namely thrombosis of the deep venous system of the legs.

Deep venous thrombosis is generally caused by the same factors that dispose toward arterial and cardiac thrombosis, namely endothelial injury, stasis, and a hypercoagulable state. Conditions that favor development of deep venous thrombosis include:

- **Stasis** (heart failure, chronic venous insufficiency, postoperative immobilization, prolonged bed rest)
- **Injury** (trauma, surgery, childbirth)
- **Hypercoagulability** (oral contraceptives, late pregnancy, cancer)
- **Advanced age**
- **Sickle cell disease**

☐ **Pathology:** The large majority (>90%) of venous thromboses occur in the deep veins of the legs, with the remainder usually involving the veins of the pelvis. Most venous thrombi begin in the calf veins, usually in the sinuses above the venous valves. In this location, venous thrombi have several potential fates:

- **Lysis.** Venous thrombi generally remain small and, eventually, are lysed, thereby posing no further threat to health.
- **Organization.** Many thrombi undergo organization similar to thrombi of arterial origin. Small organized venous thrombi may be incorporated into the wall of the vessel, whereas larger ones may undergo canalization, with partial restoration of venous drainage.
- **Propagation.** It is not uncommon for venous thrombi to serve as a nidus for further thrombosis and, thereby, to propagate proximally and involve the larger iliofemoral veins.
- **Embolization.** Large venous thrombi or those that have propagated proximally represent a significant hazard to life, because they may dislodge and be carried to the lungs as pulmonary emboli.

☐ **Clinical Features:** Small thrombi in the calf veins are ordinarily asymptomatic, and even larger thrombi in the iliofemoral system may cause no symptoms. Occlusive thrombosis of the femoral or iliac veins leads to severe congestion, edema, and cyanosis of the lower extremity.

Function of the venous valves is always impaired in a vein subjected to thrombosis, organization, and canalization. As a result, chronic deep venous insufficiency (failure of venous drainage) is virtually inevitable. If the lesion is restricted to a small segment of the deep venous system, the condition may remain asymptomatic. More extensive involvement, however, results in pigmentation, edema, induration, and even ulceration of the skin of the leg.

EMBOLISM

■ *Embolism is the passage through the venous or arterial circulations of any material capable of lodging in a blood vessel and, thereby, obstructing the lumen.* The usual embolus is a thromboembolus—that is, a blood clot formed in one location that detaches from the vessel wall and then travels to a distant site.

Pulmonary Emboli

The large majority of pulmonary emboli (90%) arise from the deep veins of the lower extremities; most of the fatal ones originate in the iliofemoral veins (Fig. 7-2).

The clinical features of acute pulmonary emboli can be divided into the following syndromes:

- Asymptomatic small pulmonary emboli
- Transient dyspnea and tachypnea without other symptoms
- Pulmonary infarction, with pleuritic chest pain, hemoptysis, and pleural effusion
- Cardiovascular collapse with sudden death

Massive Pulmonary Embolism

One of the most dramatic—and tragic—calamities typically complicating hospitalization is the sudden collapse and death of a patient who appeared to be well

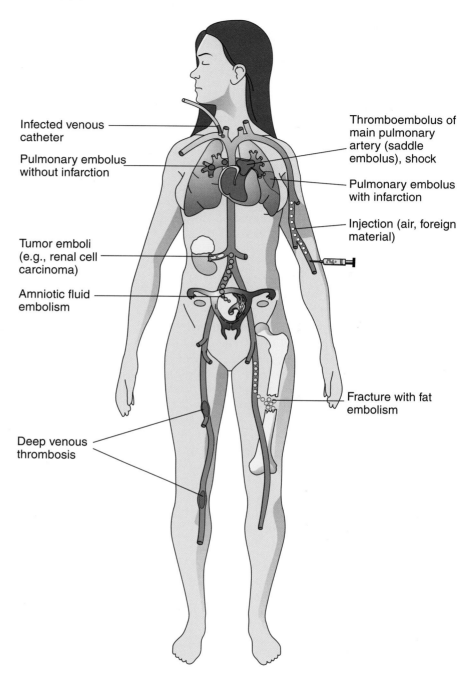

FIGURE   7-2
Sources and effects of venous emboli.

on the way to an uneventful recovery. The cause of this catastrophe is often a massive pulmonary embolism because of the release of a large deep venous thrombus from a lower extremity. Massive pulmonary embolism is the most frequent nonobstetric cause of postpartum death. It is also an especially common cause of death in patients with chronic heart and lung diseases and in those who are subjected to prolonged immobilization for any reason.

A large pulmonary embolus often lodges at the bifurcation of the main pulmonary artery (saddle embo-

lus), thereby obstructing the flow of blood to both lungs (Fig. 7-3). Somewhat smaller lethal emboli may be found in the right or left pulmonary arteries or in multiple primary and secondary branches. With acute obstruction of more than half the pulmonary arterial tree, the patient often goes into shock immediately and may die within minutes.

The hemodynamic consequences of such massive pulmonary embolism result from acute right ventricular failure because of sudden obstruction to outflow and a pronounced reduction in left ventricular cardiac

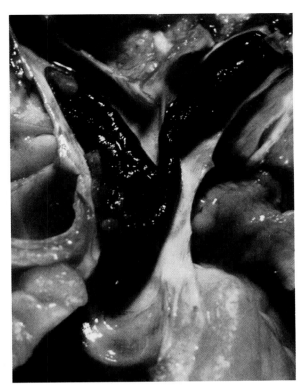

FIGURE   7-3
Pulmonary embolism. The main pulmonary artery and its bifurcation have been opened to reveal a large saddle embolus.

output secondary to the loss of right ventricular function. The low cardiac output is responsible for the sudden appearance of cardiogenic shock.

Pulmonary Infarction

Small pulmonary emboli tend to lodge in the peripheral pulmonary arteries, and in some patients produce infarcts of the lung. Because the lung has a dual circulation, being supplied by the bronchial arteries and the pulmonary artery, the large majority (75%) of small pulmonary emboli do not produce infarcts. Clinically, pulmonary infarction is usually seen in congestive heart failure or chronic lung disease. Pulmonary infarcts are typically hemorrhagic, because the bronchial artery pumps blood into the necrotic area. The infarcts are pyramidal, with the base of the pyramid on the pleural surface. Patients experience cough, stabbing pleuritic pain, shortness of breath, and occasional hemoptysis. Pleural effusion is common and often bloody. With time, the blood in the infarct is resorbed, and the center of the infarct becomes pale. Granulation tissue also forms on the edge of the infarct, after which it is organized to form a fibrous scar.

Paradoxical Embolism

■ *Paradoxical embolism refers to an embolism that arises in the venous circulation and bypasses the lungs by traveling through an incompletely closed foramen ovale, subsequently entering the left side of the heart and blocking the flow in systemic arteries.*

Arterial Emboli

The heart is the most common source of arterial emboli (Fig. 7-4), which usually arise from mural thrombi (Fig. 7-5) or diseased valves. Emboli tend to lodge at points where the vessel lumen narrows abruptly (e.g., at bifurcations or in the area of an atherosclerotic plaque). The organs that suffer the most from arterial embolism include:

- **Brain.** Arterial emboli to the brain cause strokes.
- **Intestine.** In the mesenteric circulation, emboli cause infarction of the bowel, a complication that presents as an acute abdomen and that requires immediate surgery.

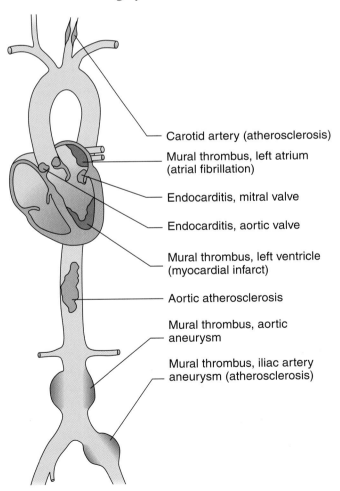

- Carotid artery (atherosclerosis)
- Mural thrombus, left atrium (atrial fibrillation)
- Endocarditis, mitral valve
- Endocarditis, aortic valve
- Mural thrombus, left ventricle (myocardial infarct)
- Aortic atherosclerosis
- Mural thrombus, aortic aneurysm
- Mural thrombus, iliac artery aneurysm (atherosclerosis)

FIGURE   7-4
Sources of arterial emboli.

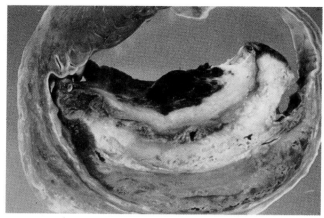

FIGURE *7-5*
Mural thrombus of the left ventricle. A laminated thrombus adheres to the endocardium overlying a healed aneurysmal myocardial infarct.

- **Lower Extremity.** Embolism in an artery of the leg leads to sudden pain, absence of pulses, and a cold limb. In some cases, the limb must be amputated.
- **Kidney.** Renal artery embolism may infarct the entire kidney but, more commonly, results in small peripheral infarcts.
- **Heart.** Coronary artery embolism and its resulting myocardial infarcts are rare.

The more common sites of infarction from arterial emboli are summarized in Figure 7-6.

Air Embolism

Air may be introduced into the venous circulation through neck wounds, thoracocentesis, punctures of the great veins during invasive procedures, and hemodialysis. Small amounts of circulating air in the form of bubbles are of little consequence, but quantities of 100 mL or more can lead to sudden death. Air bubbles tend to coalesce and physically obstruct the flow of blood in the right side of the heart, the pulmonary circulation, and the brain.

Persons exposed to increased atmospheric pressure, such as scuba divers and workers in underwater occupations (e.g., tunnels, drilling-platform construction), are subject to **decompression sickness,** a unique form of gas embolism. When a diver descends, large amounts of inert gas (nitrogen or helium) are dissolved in the body fluids. When the diver then ascends, the gas is released from solution and exhaled. However, if the ascent is too rapid, gas bubbles form in the circulation and within the tissues, thereby obstructing the flow of blood and directly injuring cells.

Acute decompression sickness, commonly known as **the bends,** is characterized by temporary muscular and joint pain owing to small vessel obstruction in these

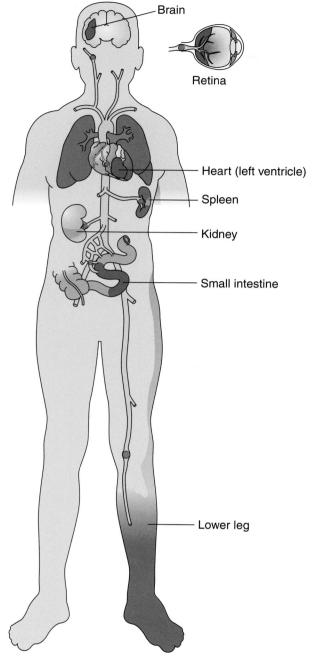

FIGURE *7-6*
Common sites of infarction from arterial emboli.

tissues. Involvement of the cerebral blood vessels may be severe enough to cause coma or even death.

Amniotic Fluid Embolism

■ *Amniotic fluid* embolism refers to the entry of amniotic fluid containing fetal cells and debris into the maternal circulation through the open uterine and cervical veins. It is a rare maternal complication of childbirth, but when it occurs, it is often catastrophic. This disorder usually begins at the end of labor, when amniotic fluid containing fetal cells and debris enters the maternal circulation, as mentioned, through the open uterine and cervical veins. The pulmonary emboli are composed of the solid epithelial constituents (squames) contained in the amniotic fluid. Of greater importance is the initiation of a potentially fatal consumptive coagulopathy caused by the high thromboplastin activity of the amniotic fluid.

Fat Embolism

■ *Fat embolism describes the release of emboli of fatty marrow into damaged blood vessels following severe trauma to fat-containing tissue, particularly accompanying bone fractures.* In most instances, fat embolism is clinically inapparent. However, cases of severe fat embolism are marked by a **fat embolism syndrome,** which appears 1 to 3 days after the injury. In its most severe form, which may be fatal, this syndrome is characterized by respiratory failure, mental changes, thrombocytopenia, and widespread petechiae. At autopsy, innumerable fat globules are seen in the microvasculature of the lungs, brain, and sometimes, other organs. The lungs typically exhibit the changes of adult respiratory distress syndrome (see Chapter 12). Lesions in the brain include cerebral edema, small hemorrhages, and occasionally, microinfarcts.

Bone Marrow Embolism

Bone marrow emboli, complete with hemopoietic cells and fat, are often seen in the lung at autopsy. They are usually encountered after cardiac resuscitation, a procedure in which fractures of the bones of the thorax, sternum, and ribs are common. No symptoms are attributed to bone marrow embolism.

INFARCTION

■ *Infarction is the process by which coagulative necrosis develops after distal occlusion of an end artery.*

☐ **Pathology:** The gross and microscopic appearance of an infarct depends on its location and its age. On vascular occlusion, the area supplied by the vessel rapidly becomes swollen and deep red. Microscopically, vascular dilatation and congestion and, occasionally, interstitial hemorrhage are noted. Subsequently, two types of infarcts are distinguishable on gross examination, namely pale and red infarcts.

Pale infarcts are typical in the heart, kidneys, brain, and spleen (Fig. 7-7). On gross examination, the

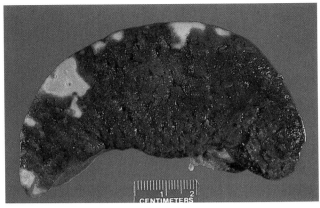

FIGURE 7-7
Spleen infarcts. A cut section of spleen shows multiple pale, wedge-shaped infarcts beneath the capsule.

infarct becomes soft, sharply delineated, and light yellow 1 or 2 days after the initial hyperemia (Fig. 7-8). The border tends to be dark red, reflecting hemorrhage into the surrounding viable tissue. Microscopically, a pale infarct exhibits uniform coagulative necrosis.

Red infarcts, which may result from either arterial or venous occlusion, are also characterized by coagulative necrosis but are distinguished by bleeding into the necrotic area from adjacent arteries and veins. This occurs principally in organs with a dual blood supply, such as the lung, or those with an extensive collateral circulation, such as the small intestine and brain. Grossly, red infarcts are sharply circumscribed, firm, and dark red to purple (Fig. 7-9). During a period of several days, acute inflammatory cells infiltrate the necrotic area from the viable border. The cellular debris is phagocytized and digested by polymorphonuclear leukocytes and, later, by macrophages.

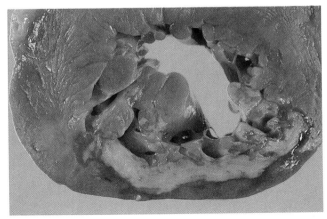

FIGURE 7-8
Acute myocardial infarction. A cross-section of the left ventricle reveals a sharply circumscribed, soft, yellow, acute myocardial infarct in the posterior wall.

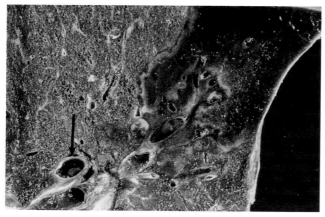

FIGURE   *7-9*
Pulmonary infarct. A section of lung shows a well-demarcated, subpleural, red infarct. An embolus (*arrow*) occludes the lumen of a small pulmonary artery at the base of the infarct.

Granulation tissue eventually forms, which is ultimately replaced by a scar. In a large infarct of organs such as the heart or kidney, the necrotic center remains inaccessible to the inflammatory exudate and may persist for months. In the brain, an infarct typically undergoes liquefactive necrosis and may become a fluid-filled cyst (Fig. 7-10).

A **septic infarct** results when the necrotic tissue of an infarct is seeded by pyogenic bacteria and becomes infected. Pulmonary infarcts are not uncommonly infected, presumably because the necrotic tissue offers little resistance to inhaled bacteria. In the case of bacterial endocarditis, the emboli themselves are infected, and the resulting infarcts are often septic. A septic infarct may become a frank abscess.

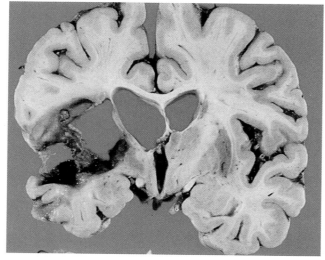

FIGURE   *7-10*
Cystic infarct of the brain. A section of the brain shows cystic transformation of an old infarct.

EDEMA

■ *Edema* refers to the presence of excess fluid in the interstitial spaces of the body and may be local or generalized.

Local edema, in most instances, occurs with inflammation, or the "tumor" of "tumor, rubor, and calor." Local edema of a limb, usually the leg, results from venous or lymphatic obstruction. Burns cause prominent local edema by disrupting the permeability of the local vasculature.

Generalized edema, affecting the visceral organs and the skin of the trunk and lower extremities, reflects a global disorder of fluid and electrolyte metabolism, most often occasioned by heart failure. Generalized edema is also seen in certain renal diseases associated with a loss of serum proteins to the urine (nephrotic syndrome) and in cirrhosis of the liver. **Anasarca** refers to extreme generalized edema, as evidenced by conspicuous fluid accumulation in the subcutaneous tissues, visceral organs, and body cavities. Edematous fluid may accumulate in the body spaces, such as the pleural cavity (hydrothorax), peritoneal cavity (ascites), or pericardial cavity (hydropericardium).

Mechanisms of Edema Formation

Normal Capillary Filtration

Normal formation and retention of interstitial fluid depend on filtration and reabsorption at the level of the capillaries (Starling forces). In the arteriolar segment of the capillary, the internal (or hydrostatic) pressure is 32 mm Hg, and at the middle of the capillary, it is 20 mm. Because the interstitial hydrostatic pressure is only 3 mm Hg, there is an outward fluid filtration of 14 mL/min. The hydrostatic pressure is opposed by the oncotic pressure of the plasma (26 mm Hg), which results in an osmotic reabsorption of 12 mL/min at the venous end of the capillary. Thus, interstitial fluid is formed at a rate of 2 mL/min and is reabsorbed by the lymphatics, so that in equilibrium, there is no net fluid gain or loss in the interstitium.

Sodium and Water Metabolism

Total body sodium is the principal determinant of the extracellular fluid volume, because sodium is the major cation that determines the osmolality of the extracellular fluid. In other words, an increase in total body sodium must be balanced by more extracellular water to maintain a constant osmolality. Control of the extracellular fluid volume depends, to a large extent, on the regulation of renal sodium excretion, which is influenced by (1) atrial natriuretic factor, (2) the renin-angiotensin system of the juxtaglomerular apparatus, and (3) activity of the sympathetic nervous system.

Edema Caused by Increased Hydrostatic Pressure

It is intuitively clear that an unopposed increase in hydrostatic pressure will result in a greater filtration of fluid into the interstitial space and its retention as edema. Such a situation is particularly prominent in the case of decompensated heart disease, in which backpressure in the lungs secondary to failure of the left ventricle leads to acute pulmonary edema and failure of the right side of the heart contributes to systemic edema. Similarly, backpressure caused by venous obstruction in the lower extremity causes edema of the leg. Obstruction to the portal blood flow in cirrhosis of the liver contributes to the formation of abdominal fluid (ascites).

Edema Caused by Decreased Oncotic Pressure

The difference in pressure between the intravascular and the interstitial compartments is largely determined by the concentration of plasma proteins, especially albumin. Any condition that lowers the plasma albumin levels (e.g., albuminuria in the nephrotic syndrome or reduced albumin synthesis in chronic liver disease) tends to promote generalized edema.

Edema Caused by Lymphatic Obstruction

Under normal circumstances, more fluid is filtered into the interstitial spaces than is reabsorbed into the vascular bed. This excess interstitial fluid is removed by the lymphatics. Thus, obstruction of the lymphatic flow leads to localized edema. Lymphatic channels can be obstructed by (1) malignant tumors, (2) fibrosis resulting from inflammation or radiation, and (3) surgical ablation. For instance, the inflammatory response to filarial worms (Bancroftian and Malayan filariasis) can result in lymphatic obstruction that produces massive lymphedema of the scrotum and lower extremities (elephantiasis) (Fig. 7-11). In the past, lymphedema of the upper extremity complicated radical mastectomies for cancer of the breast, owing to removal of the axillary lymph nodes and lymphatics.

Sodium Retention in Edema

Generalized edema and ascites invariably reflect an increased total body sodium content as a conse-

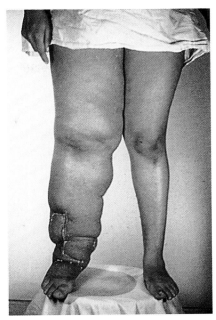

FIGURE **7-11**
Edema secondary to lymphatic obstruction. Massive edema of the right lower extremity (elephantiasis) in a patient with obstruction of the lymphatic drainage.

quence of sodium retention by the kidneys. When peripheral edema is first clinically detectable, the extracellular fluid volume has already expanded by at least 5 L. The most common conditions in which generalized edema is found include congestive heart failure, cirrhosis of the liver, nephrotic syndrome, and some cases of chronic renal insufficiency. The mechanisms of edema formation and representative disorders associated with them are summarized in Figure 7-12 and in Table 7-1.

Congestive Heart Failure

■ *Congestive heart failure is a syndrome that occurs when the heart does not pump a volume of blood adequate to meet the needs of the body.* In the United States, this disorder is most commonly associated with ischemic heart disease and carries a grave prognosis. Half of all patients with congestive heart failure who require admission to the hospital die within 1 year.

□ **Pathogenesis:** Both systolic and diastolic dysfunction may contribute to the low cardiac output and high ventricular filling pressure characteristic of congestive heart failure (see Chapter 11), although systolic dysfunction is more important in the majority of patients.

The inadequacy of cardiac output in patients with congestive heart failure stimulates arterial barorecep-

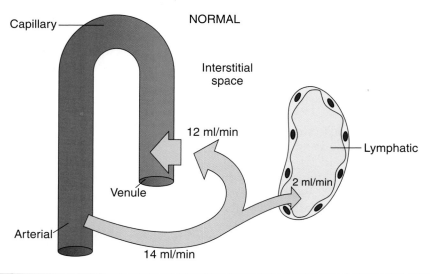

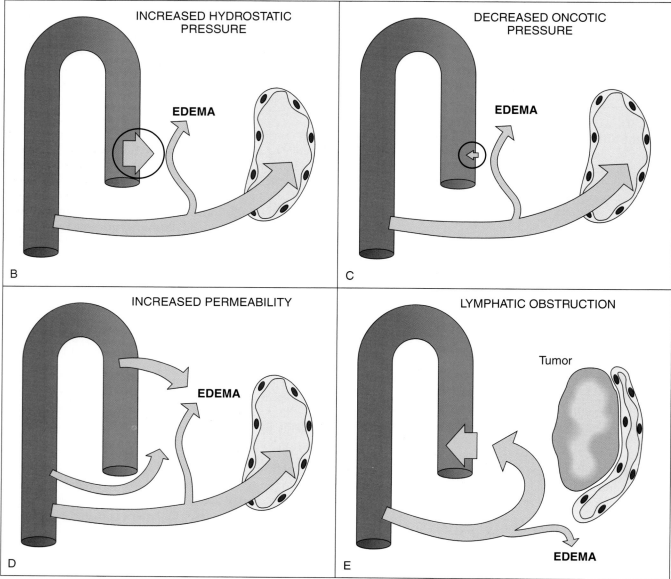

TABLE 7-1. Disorders Associated with Edema

Increased hydrostatic pressure	
Arteriolar dilatation	Inflammation
	Heat
Increased venous pressure	Venous thrombosis
	Congestive heart failure
	Cirrhosis (ascites)
	Postural inactivity (e.g., prolonged standing)
Hypervolemia	Sodium retention (e.g., decreased renal function)
Decreased oncotic pressure	
Hypoproteinemia	Nephrotic syndrome
	Cirrhosis
	Protein-losing gastroenteropathy
	Malnutrition
Increased capillary permeability	Inflammation
	Burns
	Adult respiratory distress syndrome
Lymphatic obstruction	Cancer
	Postsurgical lymphedema
	Inflammation

tors, thereby increasing renal sympathetic discharge. The latter effect promotes constriction of the renal arterioles and consequent tubular fluid reabsorption. Sympathetic activity and decreased renal perfusion stimulate the juxtaglomerular apparatus to activate the renin-angiotensin system, thereby leading to secretion of aldosterone and subsequent sodium retention.

For a time, these compensatory mechanisms expand the plasma volume and preserve an adequate intracardiac filling pressure. As long as cardiac output and blood pressure are maintained, the stimulus for renin release is decreased, and normal baroreceptor function restores the usual sympathetic tone. Distention of the atria by the increased blood volume promotes release of atrial natriuretic factor, which stimulates sodium excretion. However, with deteriorating cardiac function, these compensatory mechanisms eventually fail, and renal sodium retention again becomes important. Moreover, free water clearance is decreased (antidiuresis), an effect that results in hyponatremia and reduced plasma osmolarity. Finally, further expansion of the plasma volume leads to an increase in the pulmonary and the systemic venous pressure, which produces increased hydrostatic pressure in the respective capillary beds.

☐ **Pathology:** Failure of the left ventricle is principally associated with passive congestion of the lungs and pulmonary edema (Fig. 7-13). In turn, chronic passive congestion leads to pulmonary hypertension and, eventually, failure of the right ventricle. Right ventricular failure is characterized by generalized subcutaneous edema, which is most prominent in the dependent portions of the body, ascites, and pleural effusions. The liver, spleen, and other splanchnic organs are typically congested. At autopsy, the heart is enlarged, and its chambers are dilated.

☐ **Clinical Features:** Patients in congestive heart failure complain of shortness of breath (dyspnea) on exertion and when recumbent (orthopnea). They also may be awakened from sleep by sudden episodes of shortness of breath (paroxysmal nocturnal dyspnea). Physical examination usually reveals distended jugular veins and pitting edema of the lower extremities. The liver is enlarged and tender; when ascites is present, the abdomen is distended. Patients in congestive heart failure with pulmonary edema have crackling breath sounds (rales) caused by the expansion of fluid-filled alveoli.

Edema in Cirrhosis of the Liver

Cirrhosis of the liver is often accompanied by ascites and peripheral edema. Scarring of the liver obstructs

---

FIGURE 7-12

The capillary system and mechanisms of edema formation. (A) Normal. The differential between the hydrostatic and oncotic pressures at the arterial end of the capillary system is responsible for the filtration into the interstitial space of approximately 14 mL of fluid per minute. This fluid is reabsorbed at the venous end at the rate of 12 mL/min. It is also drained through the lymphatic capillaries at a rate of 2 mL/min. Proteins are removed by the lymphatics from the interstitial space. (B) Hydrostatic edema. If the hydrostatic pressure at the venous end of the capillary system is elevated, reabsorption is decreased. As long as the lymphatics can drain the surplus fluid, no edema results. If their capacity is exceeded, however, edematous fluid accumulates. (C) Oncotic edema. Edematous fluid also accumulates if reabsorption is diminished by a decrease in oncotic pressure of the vascular bed owing to a loss of albumin. (D) Inflammatory and traumatic edema. Edema, either local or systemic, results if the vascular bed becomes leaky following injury to the endothelium. (E) Lymphedema. Lymphatic obstruction causes the accumulation of interstitial fluid because of insufficient reabsorption and deficient removal of proteins, with the latter increasing the oncotic pressure of the fluid in the interstitial space.

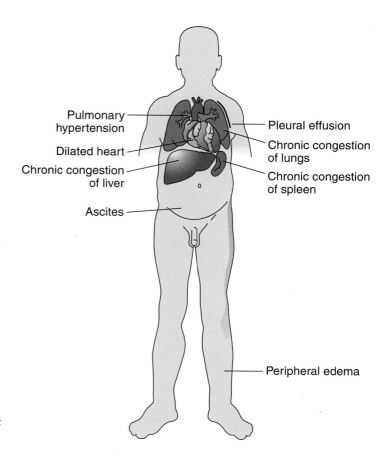

Pulmonary hypertension

Dilated heart

Chronic congestion of liver

Ascites

Pleural effusion

Chronic congestion of lungs

Chronic congestion of spleen

Peripheral edema

FIGURE   *7-13*
Pathologic consequences of chronic congestive heart failure.

the portal blood flow and leads to portal hypertension, a condition that increases the hydrostatic pressure in the splanchnic circulation. This situation is compounded by decreased hepatic synthesis of albumin as a result of liver dysfunction. The consequent accumulation of peritoneal fluid leads to a decreased effective blood volume, which, in turn, results in renal retention of sodium by mechanisms similar to those in congestive heart failure. Alternatively, chronic liver disease itself causes renal retention of sodium. Subsequent expansion of the extracellular fluid volume further promotes ascites and edema, thereby establishing a "vicious circle." In addition, increased transudation of lymph from the liver capsule adds to the accumulation of fluid in the abdomen.

Nephrotic Syndrome

Nephrotic syndrome is caused by a massive loss of protein to the urine, the magnitude of which exceeds the rate of replacement by the liver. The resulting decline in the concentration of plasma proteins, particularly albumin, reduces the oncotic pressure of the plasma and promotes edema. The ensuing decrease in

blood volume stimulates the renin-angiotensin-aldosterone mechanism, thereby leading to sodium retention. The edema is generalized but appears preferentially in the soft connective tissues, eyes, eyelids, and subcutaneous tissue. Ascites and pleural effusions also occur.

Cerebral Edema

Edema of the brain is dangerous, because the confined space of the cranium allows little room for expansion. Increased intracranial pressure from edema compromises the blood supply, distorts the gross structure of the brain, and interferes with the function of the central nervous system.

Pulmonary Edema

■ *Pulmonary edema refers to increased fluid in the alveolar spaces and interstitium of the lung.* This condition leads to decreased gas exchange in the lung, causing hypoxia and retention of carbon dioxide (hypercapnia).

□ **Pathogenesis and Pathology:** The most common causes of pulmonary edema relate to hemodynamic alterations in the heart that increase the perfusion pressure in the pulmonary capillaries and block effective lymphatic drainage. These include left ventricular failure (the most common cause), mitral stenosis, and mitral insufficiency. Disruption of capillary permeability is the cause of pulmonary edema in acute lung injury associated with adult respiratory distress syndrome, inhalation of toxic gases, aspiration of gastric contents, viral infections, and uremia. Acute lung injury is reflected in destruction of endothelial cells or disruption of their tight junctions.

When fluid can no longer be contained in the interstitial space, it spills into the alveoli.. The patient becomes acutely short of breath, and bubbly rales are heard. Sections of the edematous lung reveal severely congested alveolar capillaries and alveoli filled with a homogeneous, pink-staining fluid permeated by air bubbles (Fig. 7-14). In cases of pulmonary edema caused by alveolar damage, cell debris, fibrin, and proteins form films of proteinaceous material, called **hyaline membranes,** in the alveoli.

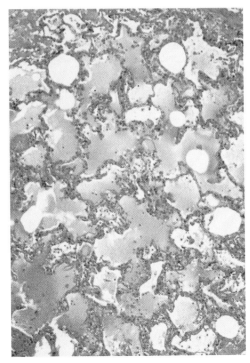

FIGURE *7-14*
Pulmonary edema. A photomicrograph of the lung from a patient in acute, left-sided heart failure shows pink-staining fluid filling the alveoli.

Fluid Accumulation in Body Cavities

Body cavities, such as the pericardium and the pleural and peritoneal spaces, are extensions of the interstitial space.

Pleural Space

Pleural effusion (fluid in the pleural space) is a straw-colored transudate of low specific gravity that contains few cells (mainly exfoliated mesothelial cells). Fluid commonly accumulates as an expression of a generalized tendency to form edema in diseases such as nephrotic syndrome, cirrhosis of the liver, and congestive heart failure. Pleural effusion is also a frequent response to an inflammatory process or tumor either in the lung or on the pleural surface.

Pericardium

Fluid in the pericardial cavity may result from either hemorrhage (hemopericardium) or injury to the pericardium (pericardial effusion). Pericardial effusions occur with pericardial infections, metastatic tumors to the pericardium, uremia, and systemic lupus erythematosus. They also are occasionally encountered after cardiac operations (postpericardiotomy syndrome) or after radiation therapy for cancer.

Pericardial fluid may accumulate rapidly, particularly with hemorrhage caused by a ruptured myocardial infarct, dissecting aortic aneurysm, or trauma. In this circumstance, pressure in the pericardial cavity rises to exceed the filling pressure of the heart, a condition termed **cardiac tamponade** (Fig. 7-15). The resulting precipitous decline in cardiac output is often fatal. When fluid in the pericardium accumulates rapidly, the tolerable limit may be only 90 to 120 mL, but 1 L or more of fluid can be accommodated when the process is gradual.

Peritoneum

Peritoneal effusion, also called ascites, is caused mainly by cirrhosis of the liver, abdominal tumors, pancreatitis, cardiac failure, nephrotic syndrome, and hepatic venous obstruction (Budd-Chiari syndrome). Obstruction of the thoracic duct by cancer may lead to chylous ascites, in which the fluid has a milky appearance and a high fat content.

Patients with severe ascites accumulate many liters of fluid and have a conspicuously distended abdomen. Complications of ascites derive from increased abdominal pressure and include anorexia and vomiting, reflux esophagitis, dyspnea, ventral hernia, and leakage of fluid into the pleural space.

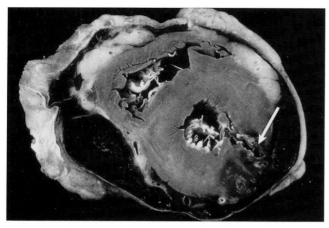

FIGURE *7-15*
Cardiac tamponade. A cross-section of the heart shows rupture of a myocardial infarct (*arrow*) with accumulation of a large quantity of blood in the pericardial cavity.

SHOCK

■ *Shock is a condition of profound hemodynamic and metabolic disturbance characterized by failure of the circulatory system to maintain adequate perfusion of vital organs.*

☐ **Pathogenesis:** Decreased perfusion in shock is generally the result of decreased cardiac output, resulting from either inability of the heart to pump the normal venous return or decreased volume of blood secondary to a decreased venous return.

Cardiogenic shock is usually caused by myocardial infarction, myocarditis, or pericardial tamponade. In these conditions, depressed systolic cardiac function (ejection fraction, <20%) is responsible for the decreased cardiac output.

Hypovolemic shock is secondary to a pronounced decrease in blood volume, which is caused by loss of fluid from the vascular compartment. Hemorrhage, diarrhea, excessive urine formation, and perspiration are the major mechanisms of external fluid loss. Internal fluid loss usually results from an increase in permeability of the microvasculature caused by endotoxemia, burns, trauma, or anaphylaxis. In the case of burns or trauma, direct damage to the microcirculation increases vascular permeability.

Anoxic injury is the common cellular consequence of the initial decrease in tissue perfusion (Fig. 7-16). A vicious circle of decreasing tissue perfusion and further cell injury is perpetuated by several mechanisms:

- Injury to endothelial cells, secondary to anoxia caused by decreased tissue perfusion, increases vascular permeability.
- Increased exudation of fluid from the circulation reduces (1) blood volume, (2) venous return, and

(3) cardiac output, thereby aggravating anoxic cell injury.
- Decreased perfusion of the kidneys and skeletal muscles results in metabolic acidosis, which further decreases cardiac output and tissue perfusion.
- Decreased perfusion of the heart injures the myocardial cells and decreases their ability to pump blood, thereby further reducing cardiac output and tissue perfusion.
- Hypovolemic shock is caused by a pronounced decrease in blood volume, which reduces venous return to the heart and, consequently, decreases cardiac output.

■ *Septic shock (endotoxic shock) refers to the vascular collapse that results from bacterial septicemia.* Infection with gram-negative organisms is the most common cause of septic shock. Invading bacteria are responsible for the release of **endotoxin,** a term used historically to describe the cell-associated toxin found in gram-negative bacteria. On entry into the circulation, endotoxin binds to a specific protein, after which the complex binds to a receptor on the surface of monocytes/ macrophages. This latter binding causes these cells to secrete large quantities of tumor necrosis factor (TNF), a cytokine that mediates the overwhelming cardiovascular collapse that is characteristic of septic shock. The pathogenesis of septic shock is summarized in Figure 7-17.

Systemic Inflammatory Response Syndrome/ Multiple Organ Dysfunction Syndrome. In patents who survive the acute manifestations of shock, multiple organ failure may result from a systemic inflammatory response. The latter is defined as being two or more signs of systemic inflammation, such as fever, tachycardia, tachypnea, leukocytosis, or leukopenia. The most important cause of systemic inflammatory response syndrome (SIRS) is the systemic release of cytokines, particularly TNF, interleukin (IL)-1, IL-6, and PAF. SIRS/multiple organ dysfunction syndrome now accounts for most deaths in noncoronary intensive care units in the United States.

☐ **Pathology:** Shock is associated with specific changes in a number of organs (Fig. 7-18).

Heart. The heart shows petechial hemorrhages of the epicardium and endocardium. Microscopically, necrotic foci in the myocardium range from the loss of single fibers to large areas of necrosis. Prominent contraction bands are visible by light microscopy.

Kidney. Acute tubular necrosis (acute renal failure) is a major complication of shock. During acute renal failure, the kidney is large, swollen, and congested, although the cortex may be pale. A cross-section re-

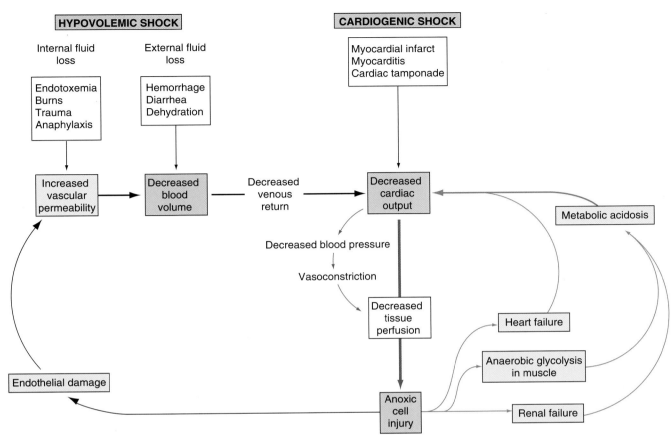

FIGURE *7-16*
Pathogenesis of shock. This drawing shows the integration of many factors in the progression of shock. Shock is initiated by one of two principal events: pump failure, or "cardiogenic shock"; and loss of circulatory volume, or "hypovolemic shock." Hypovolemic shock follows internal fluid loss, such as that in endotoxemia, burns, trauma, or anaphylaxis, or external fluid loss, such as that caused by hemorrhage, diarrhea, and dehydration. The effect of both events is decreased cardiac output and decreased tissue perfusion. The resulting anoxic cell injury sets into motion several "vicious circles." Metabolic acidosis (renal failure, increased anaerobic glycolysis) and heart failure lead to a further decline in cardiac output. Endothelial damage increases vascular permeability and decreases effective blood volume, thereby reducing venous return and, again, decreasing cardiac output.

veals blood pooling in the outer stripe of the medulla. Microscopically, fully developed acute tubular necrosis is evidenced by dilatation of the proximal tubules and focal necrosis of cells. Frequently, pigmented casts in the tubular lumina indicate the leakage of hemoglobin or myoglobin. Coarse, ropy casts are seen in the distal nephron and distal convoluted tubules. Interstitial edema is prominent in the cortex, and mononuclear cells accumulate within the tubules and the surrounding interstitium. Acute tubular necrosis is discussed in greater detail in Chapter 16.

Lung. Following the onset of severe and prolonged shock, injury to the alveolar wall results in focal or generalized interstitial pneumonitis. This condition is referred to as **shock lung** and is considered to be a variety of adult respiratory distress syndrome (see Chapter 12). Chronic changes may lead to persistent respiratory distress and even death. The sequence of changes is mediated by polymorphonuclear leukocytes and includes interstitial edema, necrosis of endothelial cells, microthrombi, and necrosis of the alveolar epithelium.

Gastrointestinal Tract. Shock often results in diffuse gastrointestinal hemorrhage. Erosions of the gastric mucosa and superficial ischemic necrosis in the intestines are the usual sources of this bleeding.

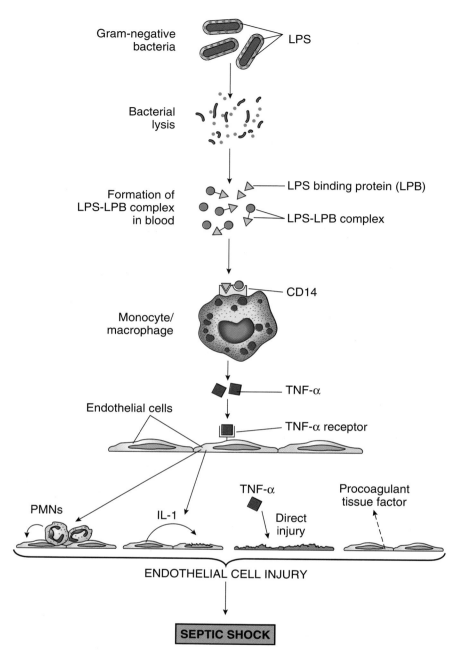

FIGURE 7-17

Pathogenesis of endothelial cell injury in endotoxic shock. In sepsis caused by gram-negative bacteria, the lysis of the organisms releases endotoxin (lipopolysaccharide [LPS]) into the circulation, where it binds to the LPS-binding protein (LBP). The LPS-LBP complex binds to CD14 on the surface of monocytes/macrophages, which are stimulated to secrete substantial quantities of tumor necrosis factor-α (TNF-α). TNF-α mediates septic shock by causing endothelial cell injury by a number of mechanisms: (1) direct cytotoxicity; (2) enhancing the adherence of polymorphonuclear leukocytes; (3) stimulating the release of interleukin-1 (IL-1), a cytokine that injures endothelial cells; and (4) promoting the expression of procoagulant tissue factor, thereby leading to thrombosis and local ischemia.

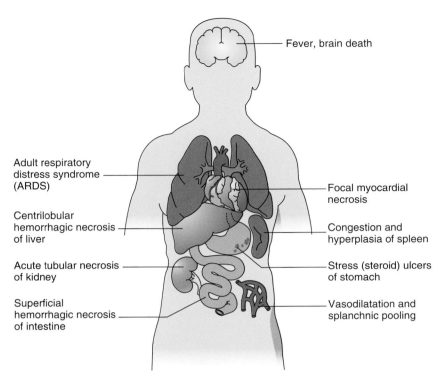

Fever, brain death

Adult respiratory distress syndrome (ARDS)

Focal myocardial necrosis

Centrilobular hemorrhagic necrosis of liver

Congestion and hyperplasia of spleen

Acute tubular necrosis of kidney

Stress (steroid) ulcers of stomach

Superficial hemorrhagic necrosis of intestine

Vasodilatation and splanchnic pooling

FIGURE *7-18*
Complications of shock.

Liver. In patients who die during shock, the liver is enlarged and has a mottled, cut surface that reflects a marked centrilobular pooling of blood. The most prominent histologic lesion is centrilobular congestion and necrosis.

Pancreas. The splanchnic vascular bed, which supplies the pancreas, is particularly affected by impaired circulation during shock. The resulting ischemic damage to the exocrine pancreas unleashes activated catalytic enzymes from the exocrine pancreas and causes acute pancreatitis, a complication that further promotes shock.

Adrenals. During severe shock, the adrenal glands exhibit conspicuous hemorrhage in the inner cortex. Frequently, this hemorrhage is only focal. However, it can be massive and accompanied by hemorrhagic necrosis of the entire gland, as seen in the Waterhouse-Friderichsen syndrome (Fig. 7-19), which is typically associated with overwhelming meningococcal septicemia.

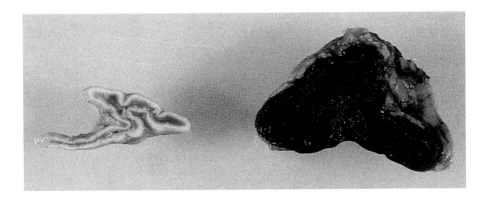

FIGURE *7-19*
Waterhouse-Friderichsen syndrome. A normal adrenal gland (*left*) is contrasted with an adrenal gland enlarged by extensive hemorrhage obtained from a patient who died of meningococcemic shock.

CHAPTER 8

Environmental and Nutritional Pathology

Emanuel Rubin
John L. Farber

Environmental pathology is the field that deals with diseases caused by exposure to harmful external agents and deficiencies of vital substances. In a sense, it encompasses all nutritional, infectious, chemical, and physical causes of illness.

SMOKING

Smoking is the single largest preventable cause of death in the United States, with direct health costs to the economy of at least $25 billion a year. **Approximately 350,000 deaths a year—one-sixth of the total yearly mortality in the United States—occur prematurely because of smoking.** Life expectancy is shortened, and overall mortality is proportional to the duration of cigarette smoking. Excess mortality associated with cigarette smoking declines after cessation of the habit, and after 15 years of abstinence from cigarettes, the mortality rate of ex-smokers compared to those who have never smoked at all is comparable.

Cardiovascular Disease

Cigarette smoking is a major independent risk factor for myocardial infarction and acts synergistically with other risk factors, such as high blood pressure and elevated blood cholesterol levels. Atherosclerosis of the coronary arteries and aorta is more severe and extensive among cigarette smokers than among nonsmokers, and the effect is dose-related. As a consequence, cigarette smoking is a strong risk factor for atherosclerotic aortic aneurysms, with the mortality ratio (death rate of smokers versus nonsmokers) for this disorder being approximately 8 : 1. Both the incidence and severity of atherosclerotic peripheral vascular disease are also remarkably increased by smoking.

During the earlier part of this century, a peculiar inflammatory and occlusive disease of the lower leg vasculature was described in a patient population consisting principally of Eastern European Jews, almost all of whom were heavy smokers. This disorder, termed **Buerger disease,** was characterized by inflammation, fibrosis, and thrombosis of both the artery and its accompanying vein, thereby leading to gangrene and amputation of the lower extremities. Although Buerger disease is unquestionably related to smoking, it is infrequently reported today.

Cancer

Death from cancer of the lung is the single most common death from cancer in both men and women in the United States today. Although the precise offenders in cigarette smoke have not been identified, cigarette smoke is clearly toxic to the bronchial mucosa. When cigarette smoke is passed through a filter, it is separated into gas and particulate phases. Cigarette tar, the material that is deposited on the filter, contains more than 2000 compounds, many of which have been identified as being carcinogens and ciliotoxic agents. The risk of developing lung cancer is directly related to the number of cigarettes that are smoked (Fig. 8-1).

Cancers of the lip, tongue, and buccal mucosa occur principally in tobacco users. All forms of tobacco use—cigarette, cigar, and pipe smoking as well as tobacco chewing—expose the oral cavity to the compounds found in raw tobacco or tobacco smoke.

Cancer of the larynx, which accounts for approximately 1% of all deaths from cancer in the United States, involves a similar situation. Among white male smokers, the mortality ratio (compared with that in nonsmokers) varies from 6 to 13, and in some large studies, all deaths from cancer of the larynx have occurred in smokers.

Cancer of the esophagus among smokers in the United States and Great Britain carries a risk ratio between 2 and 9.

Cancer of the bladder is twice as great a cause of death among cigarette smokers as it is among nonsmokers. In fact, 30% to 40% of all bladder cancers are attributable to smoking.

Adenocarcinoma of the kidney is increased by 50% to 100% (incidence rate) among smokers.

Cancer of the pancreas has shown a steady increase in incidence, which, at least in part, is related to cigarette smoking. The risk ratio in male smokers for pancreatic adenocarcinoma is 2 to 3, and a dose-response relationship exists. In fact, men who smoke more than two packs a day have a fivefold greater risk than nonsmokers of developing pancreatic cancer.

Cancer of the uterine cervix is significantly increased in women smokers, and it has been estimated that approximately one-fourth of cervical cancer mortality is attributable to this habit.

Nonneoplastic Diseases in Smokers

Smoking is the principal cause of **chronic bronchitis and chronic obstructive lung disease** (see Chapter 12). There is a 70% greater prevalence of **peptic ulcer disease** in male cigarette smokers than in nonsmokers. The converse has also been shown: the proportion of smokers is higher among patients with peptic ulcer disease than among controls.

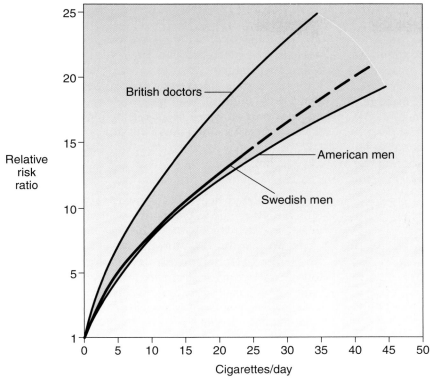

Relative risk ratio

British doctors

American men

Swedish men

Cigarettes/day

FIGURE 8-1
Dose-dependent relationship between cigarette smoking and risk of lung cancer. Prospective studies of three different populations of smokers found that the risk of lung cancer depended on the number of cigarettes smoked per day. For example, there is an approximately threefold greater risk of developing lung cancer in those who smoke 15 cigarettes a day as opposed to those who smoke five. The dashed line is an extrapolation of the data for Swedish men who smoke from 25 to 50 cigarettes a day.

Smoking and Women

Osteoporosis in women is exacerbated by smoking, which is, therefore, a risk factor for a variety of bone fractures. **Thyroid diseases**, particularly Graves disease (hyperthyroidism) with exophthalmos, has also been linked to smoking. Women who smoke experience **earlier menopause** than nonsmokers, possibly because of the effects of tobacco on estrogen metabolism.

Fetal Tobacco Syndrome

The most dangerous effect of smoking that affects women in particular occurs during pregnancy. The dangers to the fetus are so varied that, in an analogy to fetal alcohol syndrome, the term **fetal tobacco syndrome** has been suggested. Infants born to women who smoke during pregnancy are, on average, 200 g lighter than those who are born to comparable women who do not smoke. **These offspring are not born preterm; rather, they are small for gestational age at every stage of pregnancy.** The prevalence of newborns weighing less than 2500 g is much greater among mothers who smoke. In fact, 20% to 40% of the incidence of low-birth-weight newborns can be attributed to maternal cigarette smoking.

Perinatal mortality is increased among the offspring of smokers, with the increase amounting to almost 40% among the babies of those who smoke more than one pack per day. This excess mortality does not reflect specific abnormalities of the fetus but, rather, problems related to the uteroplacental system. **The incidences of abruptio placentae, placenta previa, uterine bleeding, and premature rupture of the membranes are all increased.** These complications of smoking tend to occur when the fetus is not yet viable or is at great risk, namely from 20 to 32 weeks of gestation.

There is substantial evidence that the injurious effects of maternal cigarette smoking are not limited to the fetus and the newborn but, rather, extend to the physical, cognitive, and emotional development of these children at older ages.

ALCOHOLISM

■ *Chronic alcoholism is the regular intake of a quantity of alcohol sufficient to injure a person socially, psychologically, or physically.* It is estimated that approximately 12 million persons in the United States, or approximately one-tenth of the population, are alcoholics and at risk.

The proportion may be even higher in other countries, particularly those in which wine is consumed in preference to water. Certain ethnic groups, such as Native Americans and Eskimos, have notoriously high rates of alcoholism. By contrast, other groups, for instance Chinese and Jews, experience little alcoholism. This addiction is more common in men, but the number of female alcoholics has been rapidly increasing.

Although there are no firm rules for most persons, daily consumption of more than 40 g of alcohol should probably be discouraged. Intakes of 100 g or more per day may be dangerous (10 g alcohol = 1 oz, or 30 mL, of 86 proof [43%] spirits).

Effects of Alcohol Ingestion on Organs and Tissues

Liver

Alcoholic liver disease, which is the most common medical complication of alcoholism (Fig. 8-2), accounts for a majority of the cases of liver cirrhosis in the industrialized countries. The nature of the alcoholic beverage is largely irrelevant; when consumed in excess, beer, wine, whiskey, hard cider, and so on all produce cirrhosis. Only the total daily dose of alcohol itself is relevant.

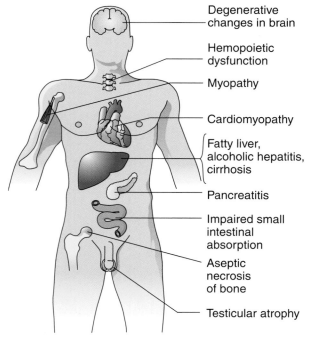

Degenerative changes in brain

Hemopoietic dysfunction

Myopathy

Cardiomyopathy

Fatty liver, alcoholic hepatitis, cirrhosis

Pancreatitis

Impaired small intestinal absorption

Aseptic necrosis of bone

Testicular atrophy

FIGURE   8-2
Complications of chronic alcohol abuse.

Pancreas

The relationship of acute pancreatitis to alcoholism is unclear, but such episodes occur with sufficient frequency to suggest it is also a complication of alcoholism. Chronic calcifying pancreatitis, on the other hand, is an unquestioned result of alcoholism as well as an important cause of incapacitating pain, pancreatic insufficiency, and pancreatic stones.

Heart

Alcohol-related heart disease was recognized more than a century ago in Germany, where it was referred to as "beer-drinker's heart." This degenerative disease of the myocardium is a form of dilated cardiomyopathy, termed **alcoholic cardiomyopathy,** and leads to low-output congestive heart failure. Although the pathogenesis is obscure, it is widely accepted as being a toxic effect of ethanol. Many cases of sudden death in persons with alcoholism are probably caused by sudden, fatal arrhythmias. It deserves mention, however, that moderate alcohol consumption is reported to exert a protective effect against coronary artery disease.

Skeletal Muscle

A wide range of changes in skeletal muscle occurs in persons with chronic alcoholism, varying from mild alterations in muscle fibers (evident only by electron microscopy) to severe, debilitating chronic myopathy, with degeneration of muscle fibers and diffuse fibrosis. On rare occasions, **acute alcoholic rhabdomyolysis**—that is, necrosis of muscle fibers and release of myoglobin to the circulation—also occurs. This sudden event can be fatal because of renal failure secondary to myoglobinuria.

Endocrine System

The principal endocrine effect of alcoholism in men is on the testes, which are reduced in size. Feminization of men with chronic alcoholism, together with loss of libido and potency, is common. The distribution of fat may also change, giving the alcoholic male a female habitus. The breasts become enlarged (gynecomastia), body hair is lost, and female distribution of pubic hair (female escutcheon) develops. Some of these changes can be attributed to impaired metabolism of estrogens due to chronic liver disease, but many—particularly atrophy of the testes—occur in the absence of any liver disease. Alcohol has a direct toxic effect on the testes; thus, sexual impairment in the male is one of the prices exacted by alcoholism.

Gastrointestinal Tract

Because the esophagus and stomach may be exposed to 10 mol/L ethanol, it is not surprising that a direct toxic effect on the mucosa of these organs is common. Injury to the mucosa of both organs is potentiated by hypersecretion of gastric hydrochloric acid stimulated by ethanol. **Reflux esophagitis** may be particularly painful, and peptic ulcers are also more common in persons with alcoholism. Violent retching leads to tears at the esophageal-gastric junction (**Mallory-Weiss syndrome**), which is sometimes so severe as to result in exsanguinating hemorrhage.

Blood

Megaloblastic anemia secondary to a deficiency of folic acid is not uncommon in malnourished patients with alcoholism. A nutritional deficiency of folic acid is the most important factor, but alcohol itself is considered to be a weak folic acid antagonist in humans. Moreover, absorption of folate in the small intestine may be decreased in alcoholics. Alcohol also interferes with the aggregation of platelets, thereby contributing to bleeding.

Nervous System

A general cortical atrophy of the brain is common in persons with alcoholism and may reflect a toxic effect of alcohol. By contrast, most of the characteristic brain diseases in alcoholics are probably a result of nutritional deficiency.

Wernicke encephalopathy is caused by thiamine deficiency and is characterized by mental confusion, ataxia, abnormal ocular motility, and polyneuropathy.

Korsakoff psychosis is characterized by retrograde amnesia and confabulatory symptoms.

Alcoholic cerebellar degeneration features progressive unsteadiness of gait, ataxia, and incoordination. The cerebellar vermis displays varying degrees of shrinkage of the folia and widening of the sulci. Microscopically, Purkinje cells in the cerebellum are the neuronal elements that are primarily destroyed, but in advanced cases, the molecular and granular cell layers are also affected.

Central pontine myelinolysis is another characteristic change in the brain of the patient with alcoholism and is, apparently, caused by an electrolyte imbalance, usually following electrolyte therapy after an alcoholic binge or during withdrawal. In this complication, progressive weakness of the bulbar muscles causes dysphagia and dysarthria and may be rapidly succeeded by an inability to swallow. Quadriparesis and coma eventually terminate in respiratory paraly-sis. Microscopic examination reveals foci of demyelination in the pons.

Polyneuropathy is common in chronic alcoholics. This condition is usually associated with deficiencies of thiamine and other B vitamins, but a direct neurotoxic effect of ethanol may play a role. The most common complaints include numbness, paresthesias, pain, weakness, and ataxia.

Fetal Alcohol Syndrome

Infants born to mothers who consume excess alcohol during pregnancy may show a cluster of abnormalities that, together, constitute the fetal alcohol syndrome. The disorder is discussed in detail in Chapter 6.

DRUG ABUSE

■ *Drug abuse has been defined as "the use of any substance in a manner that deviates from the accepted medical, social, or legal patterns within a given society."*

Heroin

Heroin, the potent diacetyl derivative of morphine, is the preferred illicit opiate in use today. It is ordinarily administered subcutaneously or intravenously and, in the usual dosage, is effective for approximately 5 hours. The drug produces euphoria and drowsiness, but overdoses are characterized by hypothermia, bradycardia, and respiratory depression.

Stimulants

Cocaine

Cocaine is an alkaloid derived from South American coca leaves. The processing of pure forms of cocaine has allowed both nasal and intravenous administration. The more potent freebase form of cocaine ("crack") is hard and "cracked" into smaller pieces, which are then smoked.

Cocaine users report extreme euphoria and a sense of heightened sensitivity to a variety of stimuli. The mechanism of action of cocaine is related to its interference with reuptake of the inhibitory neurotransmitter dopamine and the consequent, enhanced dopaminergic effects. Cocaine overdose leads to anxiety and delirium and, occasionally, to seizures. Cardiac arrhythmias and other effects on the heart may cause sudden death in otherwise apparently healthy persons.

Amphetamines

Amphetamines are sympathomimetic drugs and resemble cocaine in their effects, although they exhibit a longer duration of action. The most serious complications of amphetamine abuse are seizures, cardiac arrhythmias, and hyperthermia.

Hallucinogens

Hallucinogens comprise a group of chemically unrelated drugs that alter perception and sensory experience.

Phencyclidine (PCP) is an anesthetic agent with psychedelic or hallucinogenic effects. Other than the behavioral effects, PCP commonly produces tachycardia and hypertension, and high doses result in deep coma, seizures, and even decerebrate posturing.

Lysergic acid diethylamide (LSD) is a hallucinogenic drug whose popularity peaked during the late 1960s and is little used today. The drug causes a perceptual distortion of the senses, an interference with logical thought, an alteration of time perception, and a sense of depersonalization. Large overdoses cause coma, convulsions, and respiratory arrest.

Organic Solvents

Recreational inhalation of organic solvents is widespread, particularly among adolescents. Various commercial preparations, such as fingernail polish, glues, plastic cements, and lighter fluid, are all sniffed. Among the active ingredients are benzene, carbon tetrachloride, acetone, and toluene. Acute intoxication with organic solvents is similar to inebriation with alcohol.

Complications of Intravenous Drug Abuse

Apart from reactions related to the pharmacologic or physiologic effects of substance abuse, the most common complications (15% of directly drug-related deaths) result from the introduction of infectious organisms by a parenteral route. The most frequent of these complications are summarized in Figure 8-3.

IATROGENIC DRUG INJURY

Adverse drug reactions are surprisingly common, being found in as many as 5% of patients hospitalized on medical services, and of these reactions, 2% to 12% are fatal. The risk of an adverse reaction increases proportionately with the number of different drugs; for example, the risk of injury is at least 40% when more than 15 drugs are administered. Untoward effects of drugs result from (1) overdose, (2) exaggerated physiologic response, (3) genetic predisposition, (4) hypersensitiv-

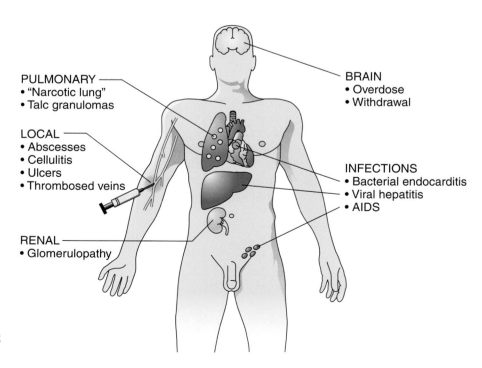

FIGURE 8-3
Complications of intravenous drug abuse.

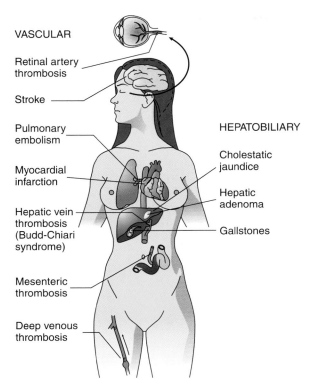

VASCULAR

Retinal artery
thrombosis

Stroke

Pulmonary
embolism

Myocardial
infarction

Hepatic vein
thrombosis
(Budd-Chiari
syndrome)

Mesenteric
thrombosis

Deep venous
thrombosis

HEPATOBILIARY

Cholestatic
jaundice

Hepatic
adenoma

Gallstones

FIGURE *8-4*
Complications of oral contraceptives.

ity mechanisms, (5) interactions with other drugs, and (6) other unknown factors.

Oral Contraceptives

Oral contraceptives act by either inhibiting the surge of gonadotropins at midcycle, thereby preventing ovulation, or preventing implantation by altering the phase of the endometrium. Most of the complications are produced by the estrogenic component, but some may be related to the progestin component or some combination of the two. The current preparations contain only one-fifth as much estrogen as earlier ones, and the incidence of side effects has progressively decreased as the amount of hormone in the proprietary oral contraceptives has been reduced. The major complications associated with use of these agents are shown in Figure 8-4.

ENVIRONMENTAL CHEMICALS

Humans inhale, bathe in, and eat a variety of chemical materials that are found as contaminants in foods and the food chain, the water supply, and the general ecosystem in which they live. Among the most important chemical hazards to which humans are exposed

TABLE *8-1*. Cancers Associated with Exposure to Occupational Carcinogens

Agent or Occupation	Site of Cancer
Arsenic	Lung cancer
Asbestos	Mesothelioma (pleura and peritoneum)
	Lung cancer (in smokers)
Aromatic amines	Bladder cancer
Benzene	Leukemia
bis-(Chloromethyl)ether	Lung cancer
Chromium	Lung cancer
Furniture and shoe manufacturing	Nasal carcinoma
Hematite mining	Lung cancer
Nickel	Lung cancer, paranasal sinus cancer
Tars and oils	Cancers of lung, gastrointestinal tract, bladder, and skin
Vinyl chloride	Angiosarcoma of liver

are environmental dusts and carcinogens. Inhalation of mineral and organic dusts primarily occurs in occupational settings (e.g., mining, industrial manufacturing, farming) and, occasionally, as a result of unusual situations (e.g., bird fanciers, pituitary snuff inhalation). Inhalation of mineral dusts leads to the pulmonary diseases known as pneumoconioses, whereas organic dusts produce hypersensitivity pneumonitis. Because of their importance, pneumoconioses and hypersensitivity pneumonitis are discussed in detail in Chapter 12.

Exposure to carcinogens in the workplace has been associated epidemiologically with a number of cancers (Table 8-1). Chemical carcinogenesis is reviewed in Chapter 5.

Toxic Versus Hypersensitivity Responses

Many substances elicit disease among a variety of animal species in a dose-dependent manner, with a regular time delay and a predictable target-organ response. Furthermore, morphologic changes in the injured tissues are both constant and reproducible. By contrast, other agents show great variability in the production of disease, with an irregular lag before any manifestation of injury, no dose dependency, and a lack of reproducibility. It has been assumed that the predictable dose-response reactions reflect a direct action of the compound or its metabolite on a tissue—that is, a "toxic" effect. The second, unpredictable type of reaction is believed to reflect "hypersensitivity" (presumably an immunologic response).

Responses to Chemical Substances

Volatile Organic Solvents and Vapors

Volatile organic solvents and vapors are widely used in industry, both to dissolve other compounds (degreasers) and as fuels. With few exceptions, these exposures are industrial or accidental, and they represent acute dangers rather than chronic toxicity. For the most part, exposure to solvents is by inhalation rather than ingestion.

- **Chloroform ($CHCl_3$) and Carbon Tetrachloride (CCl_4).** These solvents are hepatotoxins, and large doses lead to acute hepatic necrosis, fatty liver, and liver failure.
- **Trichloroethylene (C_2HCl_3).** A ubiquitous industrial solvent, trichloroethylene in high concentrations depresses the central nervous system, but hepatotoxicity is minimal.
- **Methanol (CH_3OH).** Methanol is used by some impoverished persons with chronic alcoholism as a substitute for ethanol—or by unscrupulous merchants as an adulterant of alcoholic beverages. In methanol poisoning, inebriation similar to that produced by ethanol is succeeded by gastrointestinal symptoms, visual dysfunction, coma, and death. The major toxicity of methanol is believed to arise from its metabolism to formaldehyde, followed by its oxidation to formic acid. The most characteristic effect of methanol toxicity in humans is blindness, which is characterized by necrosis of the retinal ganglion cells and subsequent degeneration of the optic nerve, a process that is presumably mediated by the metabolites of methanol oxidation.
- **Ethylene Glycol ($HOCH_2CH_2OH$).** Commonly used as an antifreeze, ethylene glycol has been ingested by persons with chronic alcoholism as a substitute for ethanol for many years. Poisoning with this compound came into prominence because it was used to adulterate wines in Austria and Italy owing to its sweet taste and solubility. The major toxicity relates to acute tubular necrosis in the kidney.
- **Benzene (C_6H_6).** Benzene is one of the most widely used chemicals in industrial processes, being employed both as the starting point for innumerable syntheses and as a solvent. It is also a constituent of fuels, accounting for as much as 3% of gasoline. Virtually all cases of acute and chronic benzene toxicity have occurred against the background of industrial exposure. Acute benzene poisoning primarily affects the central nervous system, and death results from respiratory failure. However, the chronic effects of benzene exposure on the bone marrow are what have attracted the most at-

tention. Those patients who develop hematologic abnormalities characteristically exhibit **hypoplasia or aplasia of the bone marrow and pancytopenia.** In a substantial proportion of the cases of benzene-induced anemias, **acute myeloblastic leukemia or erythroleukemia** develops. Overall the risk of leukemia is increased 60-fold in workers exposed to the highest atmospheric concentrations of benzene.

Agricultural Chemicals

Exposure to industrial concentrations of pesticides, fungicides, herbicides, and organic fertilizers or to inadvertently contaminated food can cause severe acute illness. A particularly common acute poisoning occurs in children who ingest home gardening preparations.

Symptoms of acute toxicity are often related to the mode of action of the toxin. For example, organophosphate insecticides exert their effect by inhibiting acetylcholinesterase; thus, acute toxicity among humans in this situation is principally reflected in symptoms referable to the nervous system. If the acute incident is not fatal, in most cases there are no chronic sequelae. However, delayed neurotoxicity has been reported with a few compounds, the most notorious of which is triorthocresyl phosphate (TOCP). Acute poisoning with this compound leads to a peripheral neuropathy that progresses to motor weakness of the limbs, which, in some cases, is only partially reversible. Contamination of illicit ginger liquor with TOCP in the United States during the 1930s led to an epidemic of "ginger jake paralysis." In Morocco, adulteration of cooking oil with lubricating oil containing TOCP produced an outbreak of a similar peripheral neuropathy.

Although a link between chronic toxicity of some agricultural chemicals and reproductive failure have been clearly established in predatory birds and fish, there are no reliable data to support a similar link in humans.

Aromatic Halogenated Hydrocarbons

The halogenated aromatic hydrocarbons that have received considerable attention include (1) polychlorinated biphenyls; (2) chlorophenols (pentachlorophenol, used as a wood preservative); (3) hexachlorophene, employed as an antibacterial agent in soaps; and (4) the dioxin tetrachlorodibenzodioxin (TCDD), a byproduct of the synthesis of herbicides and hexachlorophene and, therefore, a contaminant of these preparations. There is a lack of chronic effects after acute TCDD poisoning, but questions have been raised concerning the danger of chronic exposure to other halogenated hydrocarbons.

Air Pollutants

The most common atmospheric pollutants, in terms of human disease, are sulfur dioxide, ozone, and nitrogen dioxide. Sulfur dioxide results from the combustion of sulfur-containing petroleum and coal in power plants, oil refineries, and industries such as paper mills and smelters. Ozone and nitrogen oxides derive principally from the action of sunlight on the products of vehicular internal combustion engines. Automobiles and trucks emit unburnt hydrocarbons and nitrogen dioxide, after which ultraviolet irradiation leads to complex chemical reactions that produce ozone, various nitrates, and other organic and inorganic compounds. This mixture of pollutants comprises the smog that is characteristic of areas with numerous vehicles and abundant sunlight.

Episodes of unusually severe air pollution—such as occurred in the Meuse valley in Belgium (1930); Donora, Pennsylvania (1948); and London (1952)—were associated with striking increases in mortality. During each of these occurrences, concentrations of sulfur dioxide and particulates are believed to have increased remarkably. The adverse effects of this type of air pollution principally involve persons with existing respiratory ailments (asthma, chronic bronchitis, and emphysema) and cardiovascular disease. By contrast, evidence to incriminate sulfur oxides and particulates in the pathogenesis of chronic respiratory disease among previously normal people remains equivocal.

Carbon Monoxide

Carbon monoxide is an odorless, nonirritating gas that results from incomplete combustion of organic substances. It combines with hemoglobin with an affinity 240-fold greater than that of oxygen to form carboxyhemoglobin. In addition, binding of carbon monoxide to hemoglobin increases the affinity of the remaining heme moieties for oxygen. As a consequence, oxygen does not readily dissociate from carboxyhemoglobin in the tissues.

Environmental carbon monoxide is derived principally from automobile exhaust emissions, fires, and in some areas, home heating systems. A concentration of carboxyhemoglobin less than 10% is commonly found in smokers and, ordinarily, does not produce symptoms. Concentrations as great as 30% usually cause only headache and mild exertional dyspnea. Higher levels of carboxyhemoglobin, however, lead to confusion and lethargy. At concentrations greater than 50%, coma and convulsions ensue, and levels greater than 60% are usually fatal. In fatal cases of carbon monoxide poisoning, a characteristic cherry-red color is imparted to the skin by the carboxyhemoglobin in superficial capillaries. Treatment of acute carbon monoxide poisoning, as in persons who attempt suicide or are trapped in fires, consists principally of the administration of 100% oxygen.

Metals

Metals are an important group of environmental chemicals that have caused disease in humans, from ancient times to the present.

Lead

Lead is a ubiquitous heavy metal that is common in the environment of industrialized countries. Most dwellings built before 1940 were decorated on the interior and exterior with paint that contained lead (as much as 40% of dry weight). Children living in dilapidated older homes heavily coated with flaking paint were at significant risk for chronic lead poisoning. To these sources of lead was also added a heavy burden of atmospheric lead, in the form of dust derived from the combustion of lead-containing gasoline. Children and adults living near point sources of environmental lead contamination (e.g., smelters) were exposed to even higher levels.

In adults, occupational exposure to lead occurred primarily among those engaged in the smelting of lead, a process that releases metal fumes and deposits lead oxide dust in the industrial environment. Lead oxide is a constituent of battery grids, and occupational exposure to lead is a hazard in the manufacture and recycling of automobile batteries.

Toxicity. Classic lead toxicity, which is rarely encountered in the United States today, is manifested by the dysfunction of three important organ systems: (1) the nervous system, (2) the kidneys, and (3) the hemopoietic system (Fig. 8-5).

The brain is the target of lead toxicity in children; adults usually present with manifestations of peripheral neuropathy. Children with lead encephalopathy are typically irritable and ataxic. They may convulse or display altered states of consciousness, ranging from drowsiness to frank coma. Children with lead levels in the blood of greater than 80 μg/mL, but with concentrations lower than those in children with frank encephalopathy (120 μg/mL), exhibit mild symptoms involving the central nervous system, such as clumsiness, irritability, and hyperactivity.

Lead encephalopathy is a condition in which the brain is edematous and displays flattened gyri and compressed ventricles. Microscopically, congestion, petechial hemorrhages, and foci of neuronal necrosis are seen. A diffuse astrocytic proliferation in both the gray and white matter may accompany these changes.

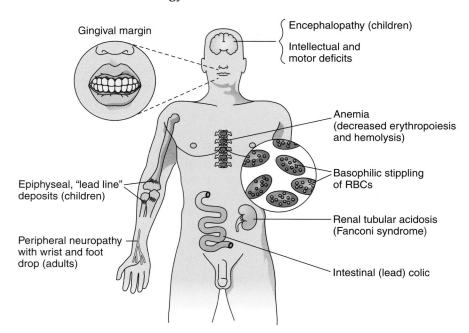

FIGURE   *8-5*
Complications of lead intoxication.

Vascular lesions in the brain are particularly prominent, with dilatation and proliferation of capillaries.

Peripheral motor neuropathy is the most common manifestation of lead neurotoxicity in the adult, typically affecting the radial and peroneal nerves and resulting in **wristdrop** and **footdrop**, respectively. Lead-induced neuropathy is probably also the basis for the paroxysms of gastrointestinal pain known as **lead colic.**

Anemia is a cardinal sign of lead intoxication, because lead disrupts heme synthesis in bone marrow erythroblasts. The defect is expressed as a microcytic and hypochromic anemia resembling that seen in patients with iron deficiency. Anemia of lead intoxication is also characterized by prominent basophilic stippling of the erythrocytes, which is related to the clustering of ribosomes. The life span of the erythrocytes is decreased; thus, the anemia of lead intoxication results from both ineffective hemopoiesis and accelerated erythrocyte turnover.

Lead nephropathy reflects the toxic effect of the metal on proximal tubular cells of the kidney. The resulting dysfunction features aminoaciduria, glycosuria, and hyperphosphaturia (Fanconi syndrome).

Effects of Chronic Exposure to Low Levels of Lead.
Low-level exposure to lead in children, though not producing recognizable symptoms, consistently decreases cognitive performance. Moreover, these deficits in intellectual and motor functions persist into adult life. The safe threshold for blood levels of lead in children is now thought to be less than 10 µg/dL.

Mercury
Although mercury poisoning still occurs in some occupations, there has been increasing concern regarding the potential health hazards posed by the contamination of many ecosystems following several well-known outbreaks of methylmercury poisoning. The most widely publicized episodes occurred in Japan, first in Minamata Bay during the 1950s and then in Niigata. In both cases, local inhabitants developed severe, chronic, organic mercury intoxication. This poisoning was traced to consumption of fish contaminated with mercury that had been discharged into the environment with the effluents from a fertilizer and a plastics factory. During the early 1970s, a more extensive outbreak of mercury poisoning occurred in Iraq, resulting from consumption of bread made with cereal grains that had been treated using organic mercury fungicides. Six-thousand persons were affected, 500 of whom died.

Mercury released into the environment may be bioconcentrated and enter the food chain. Bacteria at the bottoms of bays and oceans can convert mercury compounds released from industrial wastes into highly neurotoxic organomercurials. These compounds are then transferred up the food chain and, eventually, are concentrated in the large, predatory fish that comprise a substantial part of the diet in many countries.

Although inorganic mercury is not efficiently absorbed in the gastrointestinal tract, organic mercurial compounds are readily absorbed because of their lipid solubility. Both inorganic and organic mercury are preferentially concentrated in the kidney, and methylmercury also is distributed to the brain. **Although the kidney is the principal target of toxicity by inorganic mercury, the brain is damaged by organic mercurials.**

Nephrotoxicity. At one time, mercuric chloride was widely used as an antiseptic, and acute mercuric chloride poisoning was much more common. The compound was ingested by accident or for suicidal purposes. Under such circumstances, **proximal tubular necrosis** was accompanied by oliguric renal failure. Today, chronic mercurial nephrotoxicity is almost always a consequence of chronic industrial exposure. Proteinuria is common in chronic mercurial nephrotoxicity, and with more severe intoxication, there may be a nephrotic syndrome. Pathologically, there is a membranous glomerulonephritis with subepithelial, electron-dense deposits, suggesting immune complex deposition.

Neurotoxicity. The neurologic effects of mercury, now known as **Minamata disease,** are manifested as a constriction of visual fields, paresthesias, ataxia, dysarthria, and hearing loss. Pathologically, there is cerebral and cerebellar atrophy. Microscopically, the cerebellum exhibits atrophy of the granular layer, without loss of Purkinje cells, and spongy softenings in the visual cortex and other cortical regions.

Arsenic

Acute arsenic poisoning almost always results from accidental or homicidal ingestion, and death results from central nervous system toxicity. Chronic arsenic intoxication is characterized initially by such nonspecific symptoms as malaise and fatigue. Eventually, gastrointestinal disturbances develop, along with changes in the skin and a peripheral neuropathy. The latter is characterized by paresthesias, motor palsies, and painful neuritis. Cancers of the skin and respiratory tract have been attributed to both industrial and agricultural exposure to arsenic.

Nickel

Nickel is a widely used metal in electronics, coins, steel alloys, batteries, and food processing. Dermatitis ("nickel itch"), which is the most frequent effect of exposure to nickel, may occur from direct contact with metals containing nickel, such as coins and costume jewelry. The dermatitis is a sensitization reaction; the body reacts to nickel-conjugated proteins formed following penetration of the epidermis by nickel ions. Workers who are occupationally exposed to nickel compounds have an increased incidence of **lung cancer** and **cancer of the nasal cavities.**

THERMAL REGULATORY DYSFUNCTION

Hypothermia

Hypothermia—that is, a decrease in body temperature to below 35°C (95°F)—can result in systemic or focal injury. The latter is exemplified by **trenchfoot** or **immersion foot,** in which actual tissue freezing does not occur. **Frostbite,** by contrast, involves the crystallization of tissue water.

Generalized Hypothermia

Acute immersion in water at 4°C to 10°C leads to a reduction in central blood flow, coupled with decreased core body temperature and cooling of the blood perfusing the brain, which, in turn, results in mental confusion. Muscle tetany makes swimming impossible. Furthermore, an increased vagal discharge leads to premature ventricular contractions, ventricular arrhythmias, and even fibrillation.

Within 30 minutes, core temperature begins to fall. At less than 35°C, declines in respiratory rate, heart rate, and blood pressure ensue. The most important factor in causing death is cardiac arrhythmia or sudden cardiac arrest. A core temperature of less than 28°C (82.4°F) results in coma.

Focal Thermal Alterations

As discussed previously, local reduction in tissue temperature, particularly in the skin, is associated with local vasoconstriction. When freezing occurs slowly, tissue water crystallizes if the blood circulation is insufficient to counter persistent thermal loss.

The most biologically significant cell injury appears in the endothelial lining of the capillaries and venules, an effect that alters small vessel permeability. This injury initiates extravasation of plasma, formation of localized edema and blisters, and an inflammatory reaction. The target, again, seems to be the endothelial cell. Local thrombosis and changes caused by altered permeability are prominent, and vascular occlusion often leads to gangrene.

Hyperthermia

Tissue responses to hyperthermia are similar, in some respects, to those caused by freezing injuries. In both instances, injury to the vascular endothelium results in altered vascular permeability, edema, and blisters. Above a certain thermal limit, denaturation of enzymes and precipitation of other proteins occur.

The effect of mechanical trauma is related to the force transmitted to the tissue, the rate at which the transfer occurs, the surface area to which the force is transferred, and the area of the body that is injured.

Contusions

■ *Contusion refers to a localized area of mechanical injury with focal hemorrhage.* A force with sufficient energy may disrupt the capillaries and venules within an organ. If this occurs in the skin, loss of blood into the

■ *Radiation is the emission of energy by one body, its transmission through an intervening medium, and its absorption by another body.* Radiation encompasses the entire electromagnetic spectrum as well as certain charged particles emitted by radioactive elements. Alpha particles such as the radiation emitted by ^{32}P and beta particles of elements such as tritium (^{3}H) and ^{14}C are of immense use scientifically and diagnostically and pose few hazards for humans. High-energy radia-

Systemic Hyperthermia

In general, systemic temperature elevations to greater than 41° or 42°C (108°F) are not compatible with life. Systemic temperature elevations are commonly designated as "fever." During infectious processes and inflammatory responses, interleukin-1 and tumor necrosis factor, derived from macrophages, apparently reset the body's thermostat to permit a higher body core temperature level. Few, if any, defined pathologic

FIRST DEGREE

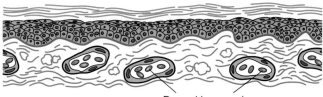

Dermal hyperemia

tion, in the form of gamma rays or x-rays, is the mediator of most of the biologic effects discussed here.

Radiation is quantitated in a number of ways:

- **Roentgen.** This unit is a measure of the emission of radiant energy from a source and refers to the amount of ionization produced in air.
- **Rad.** The absorption of radiant energy is biologically more important than its emission. A rad defines the energy, expressed as ergs, absorbed by a tissue.
- **Gray.** This measure corresponds to 100 rads.
- **Rem.** This term was introduced to describe the biologic effect produced by a rad of high-energy radiation, because for the same amount of radiation, low-energy particles produce more biologic damage than gamma rays or x-rays.
- **Sievert.** One sievert of radiation is equivalent in biologic effectiveness to one gray of gamma rays.

For this discussion of radiation-induced pathology, the roentgen, rad, and rem are considered to be comparable.

☐ **Pathogenesis:** At the cellular level, radiation essentially has two effects, namely a somatic effect (associated with acute cell killing) and the induction of genetic damage. Radiation-induced cell death is believed to result from the acute effects of the radiolysis of water (see Chapter 1). Production of activated oxygen species may result in lipid peroxidation, membrane injury, and possibly, interaction with macromolecules of the cell. Genetic damage to the cell, whether resulting directly from absorption of energy by DNA (the target theory) or indirectly from a reaction of DNA with oxygen radicals, is expressed either as a mutation or as reproductive failure. Both mutation and reproductive failure may lead to delayed cell death, and mutation has been incriminated in the development of radiation-induced neoplasia.

The differential sensitivity of tissues to radiation has been recognized since the beginning of the twentieth century. For example, both the intestine and the hemopoietic bone marrow are far more vulnerable to radiation than tissues such as bone and the brain. The vulnerability of a tissue to radiation-induced injury depends on its proliferative rate. Damage to the DNA of a long-lived, nonproliferating cell does not necessarily pose a threat to its function or viability. By contrast, short-lived, proliferating cells, such as intestinal crypt cells or hemopoietic precursors, must be rapidly replaced by the division of pre-existing cells. When radiation-induced DNA damage precludes mitosis of these cells, the mature elements are not replaced, and the tissue can no longer function.

Whole-Body Irradiation

Most of our information regarding whole-body irradiation has been derived from studies of Japanese survivors of the atomic bombs dropped on Hiroshima and Nagasaki.

- **300 Rads.** At this dose, a syndrome characterized by **hemopoietic failure** and pancytopenia develops within 2 weeks. A progressive decrease in formed elements of the blood eventually leads to bleeding, anemia, and infection. The last is often the cause of death.
- **1000 Rads.** With more intense radiation, the principal cause of death is related to the **gastrointestinal system.** Severe destruction of the entire epithelium of the gastrointestinal tract occurs within 3 days, which is the time that corresponds to the normal life span of the villous and crypt cells. As a result, fluid homeostasis of the bowel is disrupted, and severe diarrhea and dehydration ensue. Moreover, the epithelial barrier to intestinal bacteria is breached, and organisms invade and disseminate throughout the body. Septicemia and shock kill the victim.
- **2000 Rads.** Exposure to whole-body doses of 2000 rads or greater results in central nervous system damage and causes death within hours. In most cases, cerebral edema and loss of the integrity of the blood-brain barrier owing to endothelial injury predominate. With extreme doses, radiation necrosis of neurons can be expected. Convulsions, coma, and death follow.

Fetal Effects. Pregnant women exposed to doses of 25 rads or greater have given birth to infants with reduced head size, diminished overall growth, and mental retardation. Other effects of irradiation in utero include hydrocephaly, microphthalmia, chorioretinitis, blindness, spina bifida, cleft palate, clubfeet, and genital abnormalities.

Genetic Effects. The survivors of Hiroshima and Nagasaki have failed to manifest evidence of genetic damage in the form of either congenital abnormalities or hereditary diseases in subsequent offspring or their descendants. Even with the most pessimistic estimates, the risk of genetic damage to future generations from radiation appears to be vanishingly small.

Localized Radiation Injury Associated with Radiation Therapy

During the course of radiation therapy for malignant neoplasms, some normal tissue is inevitably included

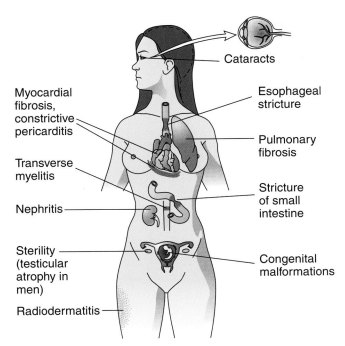

Cataracts

Myocardial fibrosis, constrictive pericarditis

Transverse myelitis

Nephritis

Sterility (testicular atrophy in men)

Radiodermatitis

Esophageal stricture

Pulmonary fibrosis

Stricture of small intestine

Congenital malformations

FIGURE 8-7
The nonneoplastic complications of radiation.

in the radiation field. Almost any organ can be damaged by radiation, but the clinically important tissues are the skin, lungs, heart, kidney, bladder, and intestine—that is, organs that are difficult to shield (Fig. 8-7).

□ **Pathology:** Persistent damage to radiation-exposed tissue can be attributed to two major factors, namely compromise of the vascular supply and a fibrotic repair reaction to acute necrosis and chronic ischemia. Radiation-induced tissue injury predominantly affects small arteries and arterioles. Endothelial cells are the most sensitive elements in the blood vessels and acutely exhibit both swelling and necrosis. Chronically, the walls become thickened by endothelial cell proliferation and subintimal deposition of collagen and other connective tissue elements. Striking vacuolization of intimal cells (the so-called foam cell) is typical. Fragmentation of the internal elastic lamina, loss of smooth muscle cells and scarring in the media, and fibrosis of the adventitia are seen in the small arteries. Bizarre fibroblasts with large, hyperchromatic nuclei are common.

□ **Clinical Features:** Acute necrosis from radiation is represented by disorders such as radiation pneumonitis, cystitis, dermatitis, and diarrhea from enteritis. Chronic disease is characterized by interstitial fibrosis in the heart and lungs, strictures in the esophagus and small intestine, and constrictive pericarditis. Chronic radiation nephritis, which simulates malignant nephrosclerosis, is primarily a vascular dis-

ease that leads to severe hypertension and progressive renal insufficiency.

Because radiation therapy inevitably traverses the skin, it often leads to radiation dermatitis. The initial damage is evidenced by the dilatation of blood vessels, which is recognized as erythema. Necrosis of the skin may follow and linger as indolent ulcers that do not heal, because the epithelium is unable to regenerate. Poorly healed or dehisced wounds and persistent ulcers often require full-thickness skin grafts. Chronic radiation dermatitis results from the repair and revascularization of the skin, and it is characterized by atrophy, hyperkeratosis, telangiectasia, and hyperpigmentation.

The gonads, both testes and ovaries, are similar to other tissues in their dependence on continuous cell cycling, and they are exquisitely radiosensitive. The combination of radiation-induced vascular injury and direct damage to the germ cells leads to progressive atrophy of the seminiferous tubules, peritubular fibrosis, and loss of reproductive function. Comparable injury is seen in the irradiated ovary. The follicles become atretic, and the organ eventually becomes fibrous and atrophic.

Cataracts (lenticular opacities) may be produced if the eye lies in the path of the radiation beam. Transverse myelitis and paraplegia occur when the spinal cord is unavoidably irradiated during treatment of certain thoracic or abdominal tumors. Vascular damage in the cord may produce localized ischemia.

Radiation and Cancer

High doses of radiation cause cancer in many organs (Fig. 8-8). However, few debates have engendered as much heat—and as little light—as that concerning the potential carcinogenic effect of low levels of radiation. The key question is whether there exists a threshold dose of radiation, below which no increase in the incidence of cancer occurs, or whether any exposure carries a significant risk.

Currently available data show that estimates of risk at low doses derived from a linear extrapolation of risk at high doses exaggerate the actual risk, perhaps by an order of magnitude. On the other hand, these data do not, by any means, show that the risk of radiogenic cancer from low-level radiation is zero. **When the data from atom bomb survivors are subjected to a linear-quadratic analysis, the lifetime risk from 1 rad of whole-body x-ray or gamma-ray radiation is one excess cancer death per 10,000 persons.**

Radon. The finding that some homes in the United States are contaminated with radon has elicited considerable public concern. Radon is a gas formed by the

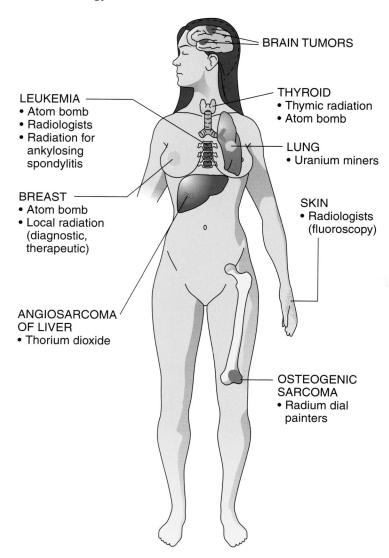

LEUKEMIA
• Atom bomb
• Radiologists
• Radiation for
  ankylosing
  spondylitis

BREAST
• Atom bomb
• Local radiation
  (diagnostic,
  therapeutic)

ANGIOSARCOMA
OF LIVER
• Thorium dioxide

BRAIN TUMORS

THYROID
• Thymic radiation
• Atom bomb

LUNG
• Uranium miners

SKIN
• Radiologists
  (fluoroscopy)

OSTEOGENIC
SARCOMA
• Radium dial
  painters

FIGURE   *8-8*
Radiation-induced cancers.

decay chain of the uranium-radium series of elements. The daughter products of radon emit alpha particles, which bind to dust in the home and may be inhaled and deposited in the lungs.

It has been estimated that 4% to 5% of homes in the United States have levels of radon at least fivefold greater than the average value and that, in as many as 2%, the concentrations are increased eightfold. However, a number of epidemiologic studies have found no increase in cancer incidence among persons exposed to residential levels of radon.

NUTRITIONAL DISORDERS

Obesity

■ *Obesity is an increase in adipose tissue beyond the requirements of the body.* It is the most common nutritional disorder in the industrialized countries. **If one defines obesity as beginning at 20% more than the mean adiposity, then 20% of middle-aged American men and 40% of middle-aged American women are obese.** Socioeconomic and cultural factors are important, because they influence not only the type and amount of food eaten but also the social acceptability of obesity. Genetic factors may also play a role in some ethnic and racial groups. For instance, blacks, particularly women, have a considerably higher prevalence of obesity than whites in the United States.

It is indisputable that obesity results from a chronic excess of caloric intake relative to the expenditure of energy. However, the reasons for this inappropriate intake of food are not at all clear. A gene (*LEP*) that encodes a protein termed *leptin* is produced by adipocytes and informs the brain of the amount of adipose tissue in the body. Although mutations of this gene have been detected in genetically obese mice, no such mutations have been found in obese humans, except for a heritable mutation in the *LEP* gene in a family of severely obese children. Other mechanisms that have been incriminated in the regulation of body adiposity include adrenergic receptors, central serotonergic systems, and a gene in a genetically obese mouse strain termed *TUB*. Although sharp distinctions cannot be made, there are two general types of obesity, namely that which occurs in children and is lifelong and that which begins in adults. Lifelong obesity is associated with a larger-than-normal number of adipocytes, which is presumably a genetically determined phenomenon. By contrast, obesity that begins in adult life develops against a background of larger—that is, hypertrophied—adipocytes, the number of which remains the same. In adult-onset obesity, fat is deposited principally on the trunk—that is, the hips and buttocks in women and the abdomen (pot belly) in men. In the type that begins in childhood, weight gain is distributed more peripherally and is readily measured as an increase in the skinfold thickness over the triceps muscle or in the subscapular area.

The most important consequence of obesity is type II (maturity-onset) diabetes, which is associated with normal or high levels of circulating insulin and peripheral resistance to the action of insulin (Fig. 8-9). In the United States, more than 80% of type II diabetes occurs in obese persons. Weight reduction usually ameliorates the glucose intolerance of type II diabetes, presumably owing to a decrease in the stimulus for insulin secretion by the pancreatic beta cells. This subject is more fully discussed in Chapter 22.

Obesity is also linked to atherosclerosis and my-ocardial infarction. It is noteworthy that obesity is associated with all major risk factors for myocardial infarction, including hypercholesterolemia, low levels of high-density lipoproteins, diabetes, and hypertension. **Obesity and hypercholesterolemia are associated with an increased incidence of gallstones, particularly in women.** For reasons that are not clear, blood levels of uric acid are increased in obese persons, as is the incidence of **gout**.

A number of complications can be traced simply to the physical effect of increased body weight and skinfold thickness. Osteoarthritis (degenerative joint disease) is common in weight-bearing joints, such as those of the hip, knee, and spine. Because the fat deposits place greater pressure on the veins, and possibly because tissue turgor is decreased, **varicose veins** of the lower extremities are more common in obese persons, and the incidence of **deep venous thrombosis** is correspondingly increased.

Obesity also has an important effect on the female reproductive system. **Oligomenorrhea and amenorrhea are common in premenopausal obese women.** Pregnant obese women have a higher incidence of toxemia of pregnancy, and postmenopausal obese women have higher rates of endometrial carcinoma and uterine fibroids. It has been postulated that the increased body fat provides a larger storage space for estrogens, and that the conversion of adrenal androgens to compounds with estrogenic activity is increased. Such mechanisms might lead to greater hormonal stimulation of the endometrium and myometrium.

Protein-Calorie Malnutrition

■ *Protein-calorie malnutrition is a direct result of inadequate dietary protein coupled with a deficient intake of the carbohydrates and lipids necessary to provide an adequate energy source.* A secondary form of this condition arises when digestive disease prevents the absorption of nutrients from the intestine or provokes an increased nutritional demand. A lack of carbohydrates and lipids results in the oxidation of endogenous protein, a complication that leads to wasting. Infants and children are particularly susceptible because of their requirements for growth.

There are two ends of the spectrum of protein-calorie malnutrition, reflecting the relative imbalance between components of the diet. **Marasmus** refers to a deficiency of calories from all sources. **Kwashiorkor** is a form of malnutrition in children caused by a deficiency in dietary protein alone.

Marasmus

■ *Marasmus is caused by global starvation—that is, by a deficiency in all elements of the diet.* The condition is com-

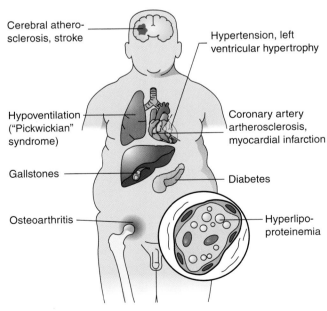

Cerebral athero-sclerosis, stroke

Hypertension, left ventricular hypertrophy

Hypoventilation ("Pickwickian" syndrome)

Coronary artery artherosclerosis, myocardial infarction

Gallstones

Diabetes

Osteoarthritis

Hyperlipo-proteinemia

FIGURE 8-9
Complications of obesity.

mon throughout the nonindustrialized world, particularly when breast feeding is stopped and a child must then subsist on a calorically inadequate diet. Pathologic changes are similar to those in starving adults, consisting of decreased body weight, diminished subcutaneous fat, protuberant abdomen, muscle wasting, and a wrinkled face. In general, the child is a "shrunken old person." The pulse, blood pressure, and temperature are low, and diarrhea is common. Because immune responses are impaired, the child suffers numerous infections. An important consequence of marasmus is growth failure. If these children are not provided with an adequate diet during childhood, they will not reach their full potential stature as adults. The effects on ultimate intelligence are controversial.

Kwashiorkor

■ *Kwashiorkor* (Fig. 8-10) *is a syndrome that results from a deficiency of protein in a diet that is relatively high in carbohydrates.* It is one of the most common diseases of

infancy and childhood in the nonindustrialized world. As in the case of marasmus, the disorder usually occurs after the infant is weaned, at which time a protein-poor diet, consisting principally of staple carbohydrates, replaces the mother's milk. Also as in marasmus, there is generalized growth failure and muscle wasting, but the subcutaneous fat is normal owing to an adequate caloric intake. Extreme apathy is a notable feature, in contrast to children with marasmus, who may be alert. Also in contrast to marasmus, severe edema, hepatomegaly, depigmentation of the skin, and dermatoses are usual. "Flaky paint" lesions of the skin, located on the face, extremities, and perineum, are dry and hyperkeratotic. The hair becomes a sandy or reddish color, and a characteristic, linear depigmentation of the hair ("flag sign") provides evidence for particularly severe periods of protein deficiency. The abdomen is distended because of flaccid abdominal muscles, hepatomegaly, and ascites. Along with generalized atrophy of the viscera, villous atrophy of the intestine may interfere with nutrient absorption, and diarrhea is common. Anemia is a usual feature, although it generally is not life-threatening. The nonspecific effects on growth, pulse, temperature, and the immune system are similar to those in patients with marasmus. Although it has been claimed that kwashiorkor not only impairs physical development but also stunts later intellectual growth, this subject requires further study.

Microscopically, the liver in kwashiorkor is conspicuously fatty, and the accumulation of lipid within the cytoplasm of the hepatocyte displaces the nucleus to the cell periphery. The adequacy of dietary carbohydrate provides lipid to the hepatocyte, but the inadequate protein stores do not permit synthesis of enough apoprotein carrier to transport lipid from the liver cell. The changes, with the possible exception of mental retardation, are fully reversible when sufficient protein is made available. In fact, the fatty liver reverts to normal after early childhood even when the diet remains deficient. In any event, the hepatic changes are not progressive, and they are not associated with development of chronic liver disease.

Vitamins

■ *Vitamin is a general term for a number of unrelated organic catalysts that are not endogenously synthesized but that are necessary in trace amounts for normal metabolic functions.* The body is, therefore, totally dependent on dietary sources for these crucial substances. Critical to the definition of a vitamin is the demonstration that a lack of the compound results in a clearly definable disease.

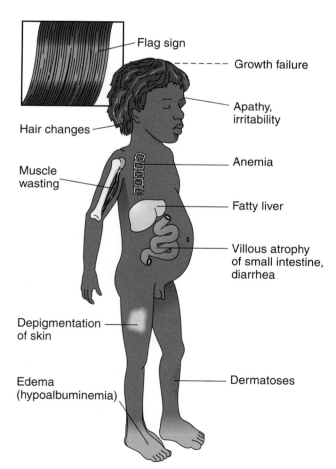

Flag sign

Growth failure

Apathy, irritability

Hair changes

Anemia

Muscle wasting

Fatty liver

Villous atrophy of small intestine, diarrhea

Depigmentation of skin

Dermatoses

Edema (hypoalbuminemia)

FIGURE   *8-10*
Complications of kwashiorkor.

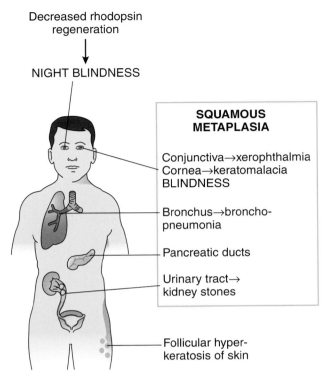

Decreased rhodopsin
regeneration

↓

NIGHT BLINDNESS

SQUAMOUS METAPLASIA

Conjunctiva→xerophthalmia
Cornea→keratomalacia
BLINDNESS

Bronchus→broncho-
pneumonia

Pancreatic ducts

Urinary tract→
kidney stones

Follicular hyper-
keratosis of skin

F I G U R E *8-11*
Complications of vitamin A deficiency.

Vitamin A

Vitamin A, a fat-soluble substance, is important for the maintenance of a number of specialized epithelial linings, skeletal maturation, and the structure of the cell membranes. In addition, it is an important constituent of the photosensitive pigments in the retina. Vitamin A occurs naturally as retinoids or a precursor (β-carotene). The source of the precursor, carotene, is in plants, principally leafy green vegetables. Fish livers are a particularly rich source of vitamin A itself.

Lack of vitamin A results principally in squamous metaplasia, especially glandular epithelium (Fig. 8-11). Stratified squamous epithelium keratinizes, and the keratin debris blocks the sweat and tear glands. Squamous metaplasia is common in the trachea and bronchi; as a result, bronchopneumonia is a frequent cause of death. The lining epithelia of the renal pelvis, pancreatic ducts, uterus, and salivary glands are also commonly affected. Epithelial changes in the renal pelvis are occasionally associated with kidney stones. With further diminution of vitamin A stores, squamous metaplasia of the epithelial cells in the conjunctiva and tear ducts occurs, which, in turn, leads to **xerophthalmia,** a dryness of the cornea and conjunctiva. The cornea becomes softened (**keratomalacia**) and vulnerable to ulceration and bacterial infection, which are

complications that may lead to blindness. **Follicular hyperkeratosis,** a skin disorder that results from occluded sebaceous glands, is also a feature of this disease.

Vitamin A is a necessary component in the pigment of the retinal rods, and it is active in light transduction. **Accordingly, the earliest sign of vitamin A deficiency is often diminished vision in dim light.**

Vitamin B Complex

The B group of water-soluble vitamins are numbered from 1 through 12, but most are not distinct vitamins. Members of the complex currently recognized as being "true" vitamins are vitamins B_1 (thiamine), niacin, B_2 (riboflavin), B_6 (pyridoxine), and B_{12} (cyanocobalamin). With the exception of vitamin B_{12}, which is derived only from animal sources, the vitamins of the B complex, although chemically distinct, are found principally in leafy green vegetables, milk, and liver.

Thiamine

Thiamine deficiency was classically seen in the Orient, where the staple food was polished rice that had been deprived of its thiamine content by processing. With increased awareness of the disease and improved nutrition in some areas, the disorder is less common now than in previous generations. In Western countries, thiamine deficiency occurs in persons with alcoholism, neglected persons with poor overall nutrition, and food faddists. **The cardinal symptoms of thiamine deficiency are polyneuropathy, edema, and cardiac failure** (Fig. 8-12). The deficiency syndrome is classically divided into **dry beri-beri,** in which symptoms are referable to the neuromuscular system, and **wet beri-beri,** in which edema and other manifestations of cardiac failure predominate.

☐ **Pathogenesis:** Patients with dry beri-beri present with paresthesias, depressed reflexes, and weakness as well as atrophy of the muscles of the extremities. Wet beri-beri is characterized by generalized edema, which is a reflection of severe congestive failure. The basic lesion is an uncontrolled, generalized vasodilatation and significant peripheral arteriovenous shunting. This combination leads to a compensatory increase in cardiac output and, eventually, to a large, dilated heart and congestive heart failure.

☐ **Pathology:** Thiamine deficiency in persons with chronic alcoholism may manifest by involvement of the brain in the form of **Wernicke syndrome,** in which progressive **dementia, ataxia,** and **ophthalmoplegia** (paralysis of the extraocular muscles) are prominent. **Korsakoff syndrome,** in which a thought disorder is conspicuous, at one time was attributed solely to thi-

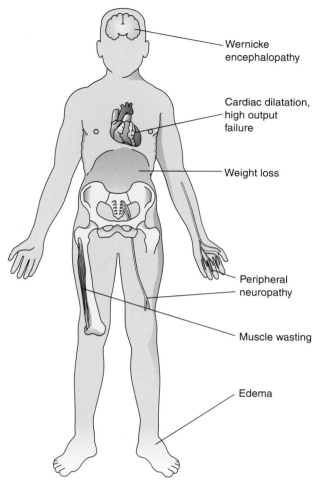

FIGURE *8-12*
Complications of thiamine deficiency (beri-beri).

ically active components are derived from dietary niacin or biosynthesized from available tryptophan. Niacin plays a major role in the formation of nicotinamide adenine dinucleotide (NAD) and its phosphate (NADP), which are compounds important in intermediary metabolism and a wide variety of oxidation-reduction reactions. Animal protein, as found in meat, eggs, and milk, is high in tryptophan and, therefore, a good source of endogenously synthesized niacin. Niacin itself is available in many types of grain.

Pellagra refers to clinical niacin deficiency and is uncommon today. It is seen principally in patients who have been weakened by other diseases and in malnourished patients with alcoholism. Pellagra is particularly prevalent in areas where corn (maize) is the staple food, because the niacin in corn is chemically bound and, thus, is poorly available. Corn is also a poor source of tryptophan.

☐ **Pathology:** Pellagra is characterized by the **three D's of niacin deficiency: (1) dermatitis, (2) diarrhea, and (3) dementia** (Fig. 8-13). Those areas exposed to light, such as the face and hands, and those subjected to pressure, such as the knees and elbows, exhibit a rough, scaly dermatitis. Involvement of the hands leads to so-called glove dermatitis. In the mouth, inflammation and edema cause a large, red tongue, which during the chronic stage is fissured and likened in appearance to raw meat. A chronic, watery diarrhea is a typical feature of the disease and, presumably, results from mucosal atrophy and ulceration in the entire gastrointestinal tract, particularly the colon. Dementia,

amine deficiency, but it now appears to be a finding both in persons with chronic alcoholism and in those with other organic mental syndromes.

A characteristic alteration is the degeneration of myelin sheaths, often beginning in the sciatic nerve and then involving other peripheral nerves and, sometimes, even the spinal cord itself. In Wernicke encephalopathy, the most striking lesions are found in the mamillary bodies and surrounding areas that abut the third ventricle. Microscopically, degeneration and loss of ganglion cells, rupture of small blood vessels, and ring hemorrhages are seen.

Grossly, the heart in beri-beri is flabby, dilated, and increased in weight. Microscopically, changes are nondescript and include edema, inconsistent fiber hypertrophy, and occasional foci of fiber degeneration.

Niacin

Niacin refers to two chemically distinct compounds, namely nicotinic acid and nicotinamide. These biolog-

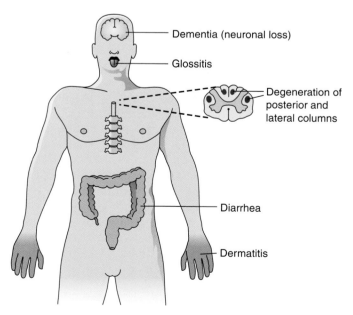

FIGURE *8-13*
Complications of niacin deficiency (pellagra).

which is characterized by aberrant ideation bordering on psychosis, is represented in the brain by degeneration of ganglion cells in the cortex. Myelin degeneration of tracts in the spinal cord resembles the subacute combined degeneration of vitamin B_{12} deficiency. Severe, longstanding pellagra adds another D, namely death.

Riboflavin

Riboflavin, a vitamin derived from many plant and animal sources, is important for the synthesis of flavin nucleotides, which play an important role in electron transport and other reactions in which the transfer of energy is crucial. Clinical symptoms of riboflavin deficiency are uncommon; they are usually seen only in debilitated patients with a variety of diseases and in poorly nourished patients with alcoholism.

☐ **Pathology:** Riboflavin deficiency is manifested principally by lesions of the facial skin and the corneal epithelium. **Cheilosis,** a term used for fissures in the skin at the angles of the mouth, is a characteristic feature (Fig. 8-14). These cracks in the skin may be painful, and they often become infected. **Seborrheic dermatitis,** which is an inflammation of the skin that exhibits a greasy, scaling appearance, typically involves the cheeks and areas behind the ears. The tongue is smooth and purplish in color owing to atrophy of the mucosa. The most troubling lesion may be an **interstitial keratitis of the cornea.** This process is followed by opacification of the cornea and, eventually, ulceration.

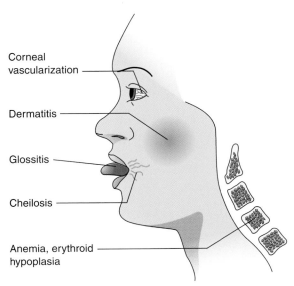

Corneal vascularization

Dermatitis

Glossitis

Cheilosis

Anemia, erythroid hypoplasia

F I G U R E   *8-14*
Complications of riboflavin deficiency.

Pyridoxine

Vitamin B_6 activity is found in three related, naturally occurring compounds: (1) pyridoxine, (2) pyridoxal, and (3) pyridoxamine. For convenience, they are all grouped under the heading of pyridoxine. These compounds are widely distributed in vegetable and animal foods.

Pyridoxine is converted to pyridoxal phosphate, which is a coenzyme for many enzymes, including transaminases and carboxylases. Pyridoxine deficiency is rarely caused by an inadequate diet, although infants who have been fed a poorly prepared, powdered formula in which the pyridoxine has been destroyed during preparation have suffered convulsions. A higher demand for the vitamin, such as may occur in pregnancy, may lead to a secondary deficiency state. Of particular concern is the deficiency of pyridoxine following prolonged medication with a number of drugs, particularly isoniazid, cycloserine, and penicillamine. A deficiency state also is occasionally reported in persons with alcoholism.

The primary expression of pyridoxine deficiency is in the central nervous system (hyperirritability and convulsions in infants), which is a feature consistent with the role of this vitamin in the formation of pyridoxal-dependent decarboxylase of the neurotransmitter γ-aminobutyric acid. Pyridoxine-responsive anemia is hypochromic and microcytic and, therefore, can be confused with iron-deficiency anemia.

Vitamin B_{12} and Folic Acid Deficiencies

Deficiencies of vitamin B_{12} are almost always seen in cases of pernicious anemia and result from the lack of secretion of intrinsic factor in the stomach, which prevents absorption of the vitamin in the ileum. Because vitamin B_{12} is found in almost all animal protein, including meat, milk, and eggs, dietary deficiency only is seen in rare cases of extreme vegetarianism—and even then only after many years of a restricted diet. Parasitization of the small intestine by the fish tapeworm *Diphyllobothrium latum* may lead to vitamin B_{12} deficiency, because the parasite absorbs the vitamin in the lumen of the gut.

Deficiency of folic acid, which is the trivial name for pteroylmonoglutamic acid, is commonly of dietary origin. Leafy vegetables, liver, kidney, and yeast are rich sources of folic acid. However, excessive cooking destroys much of the folic acid in foods. Folate deficiency is common in certain diseases of malabsorption, notably nontropical and tropical sprue. The latter condition is responsive to treatment with folic acid.

Deficiencies of both vitamin B_{12} and folic acid are associated with **megaloblastic anemia.** In addition, pernicious anemia is complicated by a neurologic condition called **subacute combined degeneration of the spinal cord.** Comprehensive discussions of vitamin B_{12} and folic acid deficiencies are found in Chapters 20 and 28.

Vitamin C (Ascorbic Acid)

Ascorbic acid is a powerful biologic reducing agent that is involved in numerous oxidation-reduction reactions and in the transfer of protons.

The clinical vitamin C deficiency state is termed **scurvy.** This disorder is uncommon in the Western world but is often noted in nonindustrialized countries in which other forms of malnutrition are prevalent. In the industrialized countries, scurvy is now a disease of persons afflicted with chronic diseases who do not eat well, the neglected aged, and malnourished persons with alcoholism. Elderly persons who consume a "tea-and-toast" diet are particularly vulnerable to ascorbic acid deficiency because of an inadequate intake of the vitamin.

☐ **Pathology:** Most of the events associated with vitamin C deficiency are caused by the formation of abnormal collagen that lacks tensile strength (Fig. 8-15).

Within 1 to 3 months, subperiosteal hemorrhages lead to pain in the bones and joints. Petechial hemorrhages, ecchymoses, and purpura are common, particularly after mild trauma or at pressure points. Perifollicular hemorrhages in the skin are especially typical of scurvy. In advanced cases, swollen and bleeding gums are a classic finding. Alveolar bone resorption results in the loss of teeth. Wound healing is poor, and dehiscence of previously healed wounds occurs. Anemia may result from prolonged bleeding, impaired iron absorption, or an associated folic acid deficiency. Effects on developing bone are conspicuous and relate principally to impaired function of osteoblasts (see Chapter 26).

Vitamin D

Vitamin D is a fat-soluble, steroid hormone found in two forms, namely vitamin D_3 (cholecalciferol) and

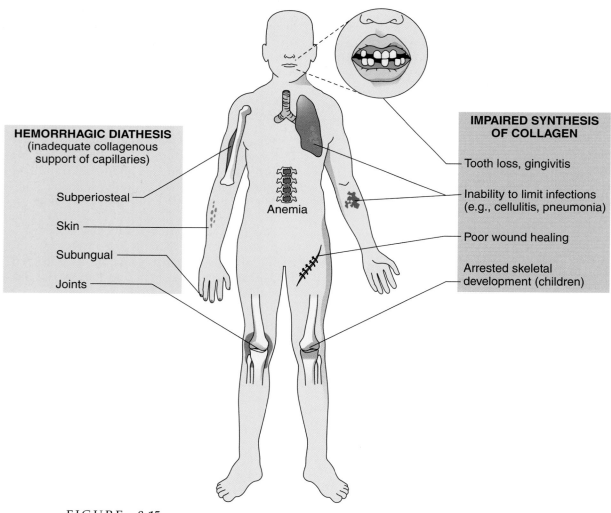

HEMORRHAGIC DIATHESIS
(inadequate collagenous
support of capillaries)

Subperiosteal

Skin

Subungual

Joints

Anemia

**IMPAIRED SYNTHESIS
OF COLLAGEN**

Tooth loss, gingivitis

Inability to limit infections
(e.g., cellulitis, pneumonia)

Poor wound healing

Arrested skeletal
development (children)

FIGURE   *8-15*
Complications of vitamin C deficiency (scurvy).

vitamin D_2 (ergocalciferol), both of which have equal biologic potency in humans. Vitamin D_3 is produced in the skin, and vitamin D_2 is derived from plant ergosterol. To achieve biologic potency, vitamin D must be hydroxylated to active metabolites in the liver and kidney. The active form of the vitamin promotes calcium and phosphate absorption from the small intestine.

Vitamin D deficiency results from (1) insufficient vitamin D in the diet; (2) insufficient production of vitamin D in the skin, because of limited sunlight exposure as a result of occupation or dress; (3) inadequate absorption of vitamin D from the diet (as in the fat malabsorption syndromes); or (4) abnormal conversion of vitamin D to its bioactive metabolites. The last occurs in patients with liver disease and chronic renal failure. **In children, vitamin D deficiency causes rickets; in adults, such deficiency causes osteomalacia.** A full discussion of the metabolism of vitamin D and its relationship to rickets and osteomalacia is found in Chapter 26.

Vitamin E

Vitamin E is an antioxidant that, at least experimentally, protects membrane phospholipids against lipid peroxidation by free radicals formed via cellular metabolism. The activity of this fat-soluble vitamin is found in a number of dietary constituents, principally in α-tocopherol. Corn and soybeans are particularly rich in vitamin E.

A dietary deficiency of vitamin E is rare, except among patients receiving total parenteral nutrition. Low levels of vitamin E have also been found in patients with disorders of fat absorption from the intestine. A clearly definable syndrome associated with vitamin E deficiency, however, has not been identified in adults. In premature infants, hemolytic anemia, thrombocytosis, and edema have been associated with a deficiency of this nutrient.

Vitamin K

Vitamin K, a fat-soluble material, occurs in two forms, namely vitamin K_1 (from plants) and vitamin K_2 (principally synthesized by the normal intestinal bacteria). Green leafy vegetables are rich in vitamin K, and liver and dairy products contain smaller amounts. Dietary deficiency is very uncommon in the United States; most cases are associated with other disorders.

Vitamin K deficiency is common in severe fat malabsorption, as seen in sprue and biliary tract obstruction. Destruction of intestinal flora by antibiotics may also result in vitamin K deficiency. Newborn infants frequently exhibit vitamin K deficiency, because the vitamin is not transported well across the placenta and because the sterile gut of the newborn does not have bacteria to produce it. Vitamin K, which confers calcium-binding properties to certain proteins, is important for the activity of four clotting factors: (1) prothrombin, (2) factor VII, (3) factor IX, and (4) factor X. Deficiency of vitamin K can be serious, because it can lead to catastrophic bleeding. Parenteral vitamin K therapy is rapidly effective.

Minerals

The essential trace minerals are, for the most part, components of enzymes and cofactors necessary for metabolic functions. These include iron, copper, iodine, zinc, cobalt, selenium, manganese, nickel, chromium, tin, molybdenum, vanadium, silicon, and fluorine. Dietary deficiencies of these minerals are clinically important in the case of iron and iodine and are discussed in Chapters 20 and 21, which deal with blood diseases and endocrinologic pathology, respectively.

CHAPTER 9

Infectious and Parasitic Diseases

Robert M. Genta
Daniel H. Connor

VIRAL INFECTIONS

Respiratory Viruses

Influenza

Respiratory Syncytial Virus

Viral Exanthems

Measles (Rubeola)

Rubella

Mumps

Intestinal Viruses

Rotavirus

Hemorrhagic Fevers

Yellow Fever

Herpesviruses

Varicella-Zoster Virus

Herpes Simplex Virus

Epstein-Barr Virus (Infectious Mononucleosis)

Cytomegalovirus

Human Papillomavirus

BACTERIAL INFECTIONS

Pyogenic Gram-Positive Cocci

Staphylococcus aureus

Streptococcus pyogenes

Streptococcus pneumoniae

Bacterial Infections of Childhood

Diphtheria

Pertussis

Haemophilus influenzae

Neisseria meningitidis

Sexually Transmitted Bacterial Diseases

Gonorrhea

Chancroid

Granuloma Inguinale

Enteropathogenic Bacteria

Cholera

Clostridia

(continued)

Clostridial Food Poisoning

Necrotizing Enteritis

Gas Gangrene (Clostridial Myonecrosis)

Tetanus

Botulism

Clostridium difficile Colitis

Bacterial Infections with Animal Reservoirs or Insect Vectors

Brucellosis

Plague

Tularemia

Anthrax

Listeriosis

Cat-Scratch Disease

Filamentous Bacteria

Actinomyocosis

Nocardiosis

SPIROCHETES

Syphilis

Lyme Disease

CHLAMYDIA

Chlamydia trachomatis

Genital and Neonatal Diseases

Lymphogranuloma Venereum

Trachoma

Psittacosis (Ornithosis)

RICKETTSIAE

Rocky Mountain Spotted Fever

Epidemic (Louse-Borne) Typhus

MYCOPLASMA

MYCOBACTERIA

Tuberculosis

Leprosy

Tuberculoid Leprosy

Lepromatous Leprosy

FUNGI

Candida

Aspergillosis

Cryptococcosis

Histoplasmosis

Coccidioidomycosis

Blastomycosis

PROTOZOAL INFECTIONS

Malaria

Toxoplasmosis

Pneumocystis carinii **Pneumonia**

Amebiasis

Giardiasis

Leishmaniasis

Chagas Disease (American Trypanosomiasis)

African Trypanosomiasis

HELMINTHIC INFECTIONS

Filarial Nematodes

Lymphatic Filariasis (Bancroftian and Malayan Filariasis)

Onchocerciasis

Intestinal Nematodes

Ascariasis

Hookworms

Strongyloidiasis

Tissue Nematodes

Trichinosis

Trematodes (Flukes)

Schistosomiasis

Clonorchiasis

Cestodes

Intestinal Tapeworms

Echinococcosis (Hydatid Disease)

Infectious diseases are disorders in which tissue damage or dysfunction is produced by a micro-organism. They are the most frequent afflictions of mankind worldwide, the most common reasons that people seek medical care, and the leading causes of death from disease. Bacterial and viral diarrheas, bacterial pneumonias, tuberculosis, measles, malaria, hepatitis B, pertussis, and tetanus kill more people each year than all cancers and cardiovascular diseases.

Virulence. Virulence refers to the capacity of an organism to achieve infection, which is a complex and, often, highly regulated process. The organism must (1) gain access to the body, (2) avoid multiple host defenses, (3) accommodate to growth in the human milieu, and (4) parasitize human resources.

Host-Defense Mechanisms. The means by which the body prevents or contains infections are known as **defense mechanisms.** Major anatomic barriers to infection—the skin and aerodynamic filtration system of the upper airway—prevent most organisms from ever penetrating the body. The mucociliary blanket of the airways is also an essential defense, providing a means of expelling organisms that gain access to the respiratory system. The microbial flora normally resident in the gastrointestinal tract and various body orifices compete with outside organisms, preventing them from gaining sufficient nutrients or binding sites in the host. The body's orifices are also protected by antimicrobial secretions, usually containing lysozyme and immunoglobulin A. Gastric acid and bile chemically destroy many ingested organisms.

Host Factors in Infection. A single infecting organism often causes a wide range of effects in exposed persons. An infectious agent, for instance the influenza virus, may (1) fail to infect some persons, (2) produce asymptomatic infections in others, (3) cause modest symptomatic disease in some, and (4) produce lethal infections in still others. This variability results from diverse host factors, heritable variability, age, integrity of host defenses, and behavior.

Heritable Differences in Response to Infecting Agents. The first step in infection is often a highly specific interaction of a binding molecule on the infecting organism with a receptor molecule on the host. If the host lacks the appropriate receptor molecule, attachment of the organism to the target cannot occur. An example is *Plasmodium vivax*, one of the organisms that causes human malaria. It infects human erythrocytes by using the Duffy blood group determinants on the cell surface as receptor molecules. These Duffy blood group determinants, however, are not conserved in all human populations. Many persons, particularly blacks, lack these determinants and, therefore, are not susceptible to infection with *P. vivax*. As a result, *P. vivax* malaria is absent from much of Africa.

Containment or elimination of an infecting organism also depends on specific molecular interactions between the host and the organism, as illustrated by the racial variations in the response to infection with *Coccidioides immitis*. This fungus is present in the environment in restricted geographic regions. In most persons infected with *C. immitis*, cell-mediated immunity rapidly controls the infection, and the disease is usually mild and self-limited. By contrast, some otherwise healthy persons do not contain the infection, because their immune system fails to respond to the organism. In these persons, infection spreads throughout the body and is potentially lethal. Whereas disseminated coccidioidomycosis is rare in healthy whites, it is 14-fold more common in blacks and 175-fold more frequent in persons of Filipino ancestry, a pattern that reflects heritable differences in the ability to contain the organism.

Effect of Age on Response to Infection. Age of the host affects the outcome of exposure to many infectious agents. This is well illustrated in the case of fetal infections. Some organisms produce more severe disease in utero than in children or adults. Infections of the fetus with cytomegalovirus, rubella virus, human parvovirus B19, and *Toxoplasma gondii* interfere with fetal development. Depending on the organism and the time of exposure, fetal infection can produce minimal damage, major congenital abnormalities, or even death. By contrast, when these organisms infect children or adults, they usually produce asymptomatic, or only minimally symptomatic, diseases.

Age also affects the course of common illnesses, such as the diverse viral and bacterial diarrheas. In older children and adults, these infections cause discomfort, inconvenience, and sometimes embarrassment, but rarely do they cause severe injury. The outcome can be different, however, in children younger than 3 years, who lack the capacity to compensate for the rapid volume loss that results from profuse diarrhea. Thus, if intense fluid replacement is not provided in small children, the fluid and electrolyte disturbances resulting from diarrheal disease can kill.

There are numerous other examples of how age influences the outcome of exposure to an infectious agent. For instance, infection with *Mycobacterium tuberculosis* often produces severe, disseminated tuberculosis in children younger than 3 years, probably because of the immaturity of the cell-mediated immune system. By contrast, older persons fare much better. Maturity, however, is not always an advantage during infection.

Epstein-Barr virus is more likely to cause symptomatic infections in adolescents and adults than in younger children, and varicella-zoster virus, the cause of chickenpox, produces more severe disease in adults, who are more likely to develop viral pneumonia.

Elderly persons fare more poorly than younger persons with almost all infections. Common respiratory illnesses, such as influenza and pneumococcal pneumonia, are more often fatal in those older than 65 years.

Effect of Behavior on Infection. Behavior is another host factor that influences infections. The link between behavior and infection is probably most obvious for sexually transmitted diseases. Syphilis, gonorrhea, urogenital chlamydial infections, acquired immunodeficiency syndrome (AIDS), and a number of other infectious diseases are transmitted primarily by sexual contact. Thus, the type and number of sexual encounters profoundly influence the risk of acquiring sexually transmitted diseases.

Other aspects of behavior also influence the risk of acquiring infections. Humans contract brucellosis and Q fever, which are primarily bacterial diseases of domesticated farm animals, by close contact with infected animals or their secretions. These infections occur in farmers, herders, meat processors, and in the case of brucellosis, persons who drink unpasteurized milk. Toxoplasmosis is a protozoan infection transmitted from animals to humans by ingestion of incompletely cooked, infected meat or by exposure to infected cat feces. Botulism, a food poisoning caused by a bacterial toxin, is usually acquired by ingestion of improperly canned food.

As humans change their behavior, they open up new possibilities for infectious diseases. Introduction of hyperabsorbent tampons during the late 1970s led to an epidemic of toxic shock syndrome, a previously unrecognized disease caused by *Staphylococcus aureus*. The novel tampons provided an excellent vehicle for the production and delivery of a staphylococcal toxin. Although the agent of legionnaires' disease is common in the environment, aerosols generated by cooling plants, faucets, and humidifiers have provided the means for causing human infections. Traditional behaviors are not necessarily health-promoting, either. Hundreds of thousands of cases of neonatal tetanus in less-developed countries are linked to coating umbilical stumps with dirt, dung, or even homemade cheese to stop the bleeding. These materials do stop the bleeding but often contain the spores of *Clostridium tetani*, which germinate and release the toxin that causes tetanus.

Effect of Compromised Host Defenses on Infection. The state of host defense mechanisms also affects susceptibility and response to infection. A disruption or absence of any of the complex host defenses results in both increased numbers and severity of infections. Disruptions of the skin surface by trauma or burns frequently lead to invasive bacterial or fungal infections. Injury to the mucociliary apparatus of the airways, as occurs in smoking or influenza, impairs the clearing of inhaled micro-organisms and produces an increased incidence of bacterial pneumonias. Congenital absence of complement components C5, C6, C7, and C8 prevents formation of a fully functional membrane attack complex and permits disseminated *Neisseria* infections. Diseases and drugs that interfere with neutrophil production or function increase the likelihood of bacterial infection.

The technologic capacity to prolong the lives of debilitated persons, the broad use of cytotoxic and immunosuppressive therapies, and the rapid expansion of the AIDS epidemic have led to an exponential increase in the number of patients with severe defects in their host defenses. Burn and trauma units, transplantation centers, and medical as well as surgical intensive care facilities are filled with patients who lack the normal capacity to ward off infections. Many of these patients are immunocompromised, meaning that their defects lie in the capacity to mount inflammatory or immunologic responses. Not only do compromised hosts more easily become infected, they are often attacked by organisms that are otherwise innocuous to a normal person. For instance, patients who are deficient in neutrophils frequently develop life-threatening bloodstream infections with commensal micro-organisms that normally populate the skin and gastrointestinal tract. Organisms that take advantage of impaired host immunity to cause disease are known as **opportunistic pathogens**. Most are part of the normal endogenous human or environmental microbial flora.

Viral Infections

Viruses, the smallest human pathogens, range in size from 20 to 300 nm and consist of RNA or DNA contained in a protein shell. **Viruses are incapable of independent metabolism or reproduction and, thus, are obligate intracellular parasites, requiring living cells in which to replicate.** After invading cells, these micro-organisms divert their biosynthetic and metabolic capacities to the synthesis of viral-encoded nucleic acids and proteins.

Viruses often cause disease by killing the infected cells. Many viruses, however, produce disease without killing the infected cells. For instance, rotavirus, a common cause of diarrhea, interferes with the function of infected enterocytes without immediately killing them.

The virus prevents enterocytes from synthesizing proteins that transport molecules from the intestinal lumen and, thereby, causes diarrhea.

Viruses also produce disease by promoting the release of chemical mediators that incite inflammatory or immunologic responses. The symptoms of common colds are due to the release of bradykinin from virally infected cells. Some viruses produce disease by causing cells to proliferate and form tumors. Human papillomaviruses, for instance, cause squamous cell proliferative lesions, which include common warts and anogenital warts.

Some viruses infect and persist in cells without interfering with normal cellular functions, which is a process known as **latency**. Viruses that establish latent infections can emerge to produce disease or transmit infection long after the primary infection. Opportunistic infections are frequently caused by viruses that have established latent infections. Cytomegalovirus and herpes simplex viruses are among the most frequent opportunistic pathogens, because they are commonly present as latent agents, which then emerge in persons with impaired cell-mediated immunity.

RESPIRATORY VIRUSES

Influenza

■ *Influenza* is an acute, self-limited infection of the upper airways caused by strains of influenza virus (RNA). Influenza is highly contagious, and epidemics often spread around the world from one original focus. The infection spreads from person to person by infected respiratory droplets and secretions that contain large amounts of virus. Sneezing, coughing, and even talking probably spread the virus.

☐ **Pathology:** Although infection is usually confined to the upper airway, the virus can spread to the lower respiratory tract, where it produces tracheitis, bronchitis, or pneumonitis. Destruction of the ciliated epithelium cripples the mucociliary blanket, predisposing to bacterial pneumonia.

In the upper airways, influenza virus causes necrosis and desquamation of the ciliated respiratory tract epithelium, associated with a predominantly lymphocytic inflammatory infiltrate. Extension of infection to the lungs leads to necrosis and sloughing of alveolar lining cells as well as the histologic appearance of viral pneumonitis.

☐ **Clinical Features:** Influenza presents as a rapid onset of fever, chills, myalgia, headaches, weakness, and nonproductive cough. The illness can be incapacitating for 3 to 5 days, followed by gradual improvement over 2 to 3 weeks. Influenza is especially injurious to elderly persons or those with underlying cardiopulmonary disease, who cannot tolerate further impaired respiratory function. Killed viral vaccines are 75% effective in preventing influenza.

Respiratory Syncytial Virus

■ *Respiratory syncytial virus (RSV)* is an RNA virus that is the major cause of bronchiolitis and pneumonia in children younger than 1 year. RSV spreads from child to child in respiratory aerosols and secretions.

☐ **Pathology:** RSV produces necrosis and sloughing of the bronchial, bronchiolar, and alveolar epithelium, associated with a predominantly lymphocytic inflammatory infiltrate. The virus can cause fusion of infected cells, and multinucleated syncytial cells are sometimes seen in infected tissues.

☐ **Clinical Features:** The respiratory illness is usually self-limited, resolving in 1 to 2 weeks. The mortality rate from RSV infection is very low, but it rises dramatically (to 20–40%) among hospitalized children who are compromised by congenital heart diseases or immunosuppression.

VIRAL EXANTHEMS

Measles (Rubeola)

■ *Measles results from* an RNA virus that causes an acute, highly contagious, self-limited illness characterized by upper respiratory tract symptoms, fever, and a rash. The infection is transmitted in respiratory aerosols and secretions. Measles virus produces necrosis of the infected respiratory epithelium, associated with a predominantly lymphocytic inflammatory infiltrate. In the skin, the virus produces a vasculitis of the small blood vessels.

☐ **Clinical Features:** After an incubation period of 10 to 21 days, skin lesions begin on the face as an erythematous, maculopapular rash, which usually spreads to involve the trunk and extremities. The rash fades in 3 to 5 days, and the symptoms gradually resolve. Measles often leads to secondary bacterial infections, especially otitis media and pneumonia.

Measles is a particularly severe disease when it affects very young, sick, or malnourished persons. In impoverished countries, the disease has a high mortality rate (10–25%). The currently available live, attenuated measles vaccines are highly effective in preventing measles and eliminating spread of the virus.

Rubella

■ *Rubella results from an RNA virus that causes a mild, self-limited systemic disease, usually associated with a rash.* In pregnant women, rubella virus is a destructive fetal pathogen. Infection early during gestation can produce fetal death, premature delivery, and congenital anomalies, including deafness, cataracts, glaucoma, heart defects, and mental retardation. The currently available live, attenuated viral vaccine prevents rubella, and vaccination programs have largely eliminated the disease from developed countries.

☐ **Pathology:** The pathology of congenital rubella is variable. The heart, eye, and brain are the organs most frequently affected. Cardiac lesions include pulmonary valvular stenosis, pulmonary artery hypoplasia, ventricular septal defects, and patent ductus arteriosus. Ocular abnormalities are characterized by cataracts, glaucoma, and retinal defects. Deafness is a common complication of fetal rubella. Severe brain involvement can produce microcephaly and mental retardation.

MUMPS

■ *Mumps results from an RNA virus that causes an acute, self-limited systemic illness characterized by parotid gland swelling and meningoencephalitis.* A live, attenuated vaccine prevents mumps, and the disease has been largely eliminated from most developed countries.

Mumps begins with viral infection of the respiratory tract epithelium. The mumps virus then disseminates through the blood and lymphatic systems to infect other sites, most commonly the salivary glands (especially the parotids), central nervous system, pancreas, and testes. The central nervous system is involved in more than half of cases, producing symptomatic disease in 10%. Epididymo-orchitis occurs in 30% of males infected after puberty.

☐ **Pathology:** Mumps virus causes necrosis of the infected cells, which is associated with a predominantly lymphocytic inflammatory infiltrate. The affected salivary glands are swollen, the ducts are lined by necrotic epithelium, and the interstitium is infiltrated with lymphocytes.

INTESTINAL VIRUSES

Many viruses cause gastrointestinal symptoms, but rotavirus is the most common cause of severe diarrhea worldwide.

Rotavirus

■ *Rotavirus is an RNA virus that usually infects young children, producing a profuse, watery diarrhea that can lead to dehydration and death if untreated.* Rotavirus infection spreads from person to person by the oral-fecal route. Pathologic changes in rotavirus infection are largely confined to the duodenum and jejunum, where there is shortening of the intestinal villi associated with a mild infiltrate of neutrophils and lymphocytes.

☐ **Clinical Features:** Rotavirus infection presents as vomiting, fever, abdominal pain, and profuse, watery diarrhea. Vomiting usually persists for 2 to 3 days, whereas the diarrhea continues for 5 to 8 days. Without adequate fluid replacement, the diarrhea can produce rapidly fatal dehydration in young children.

HEMORRHAGIC FEVERS

■ *Viral hemorrhagic fevers are a group of at least 13 distinct viral infections that cause varying degrees of hemorrhage, shock, and sometimes, death.* There are many similar viral hemorrhagic fevers in different parts of the world, which for the most part are named for the area where they were first described. Viral hemorrhagic fevers have been divided into four groups based on their mode of transmission (Table 9-1).

Yellow Fever

■ *Yellow fever is an acute hemorrhagic fever caused by an insect-borne RNA virus.* The disease is a febrile systemic illness sometimes associated with extensive hepatic necrosis, jaundice, and hemorrhages. Yellow fever is restricted to certain regions of Africa and South America, including both jungle and urban settings. The usual reservoir for the virus is tree-dwelling monkeys, with the agent being passed among them in the forest canopy by mosquitoes. Humans acquire yellow fever by entering the forest and being bitten by infected *Aedes* mosquitoes.

☐ **Pathology:** The virus has a tropism for liver cells, where it sometimes produces extensive acute hepatocellular destruction. Extensive damage to the endothelium of small blood vessels may lead to the loss of vascular integrity and, consequently, hemorrhages and shock. Yellow fever virus causes coagulative necrosis of hepatocytes, which begins among the cells in the middle of hepatic lobules and then spreads toward the central veins and portal tracts.

☐ **Clinical Features:** Yellow fever usually begins with the abrupt onset of fever, chills, headache, myal-

TABLE   9-1.   Viral Hemorrhagic Fevers

Vector	Viral Fever
Mosquitoes	Yellow fever
	Rift valley fever
	Dengue hemorrhagic fever
	Chikungunya hemorrhagic fever
Ticks	Omsk hemorrhagic fever
	Crimean hemorrhagic fever
	Kyasanur forest disease
Rodents	Lassa fever
	Bolivian hemorrhagic fever
	Argentine hemorrhagic fever
	Korean hemorrhagic fever
Undefined	Ebola virus disease
	Marburg virus disease

gias, nausea, and vomiting. After 3 to 5 days, some patients develop manifestations of hepatic failure, with jaundice (hence the term *yellow fever*), deficiencies of clotting factors, and diffuse hemorrhages. The overall mortality rate from yellow fever is 5%, but among those with jaundice, it rises to 30%.

HERPESVIRUSES

The virus family *Herpesviridae* includes a large number of DNA viruses, many of which infect humans.

Varicella-Zoster Virus

Varicella-zoster virus causes two distinct diseases, namely chickenpox and herpes zoster (Fig. 9-1). A person's first exposure to varicella-zoster virus produces chickenpox, an acute systemic illness whose dominant feature is a generalized vesicular skin eruption. The virus then becomes latent, and its reactivation causes herpes zoster ("shingles"), a localized vesicular skin eruption. Varicella-zoster virus spreads from person to person primarily by the respiratory route, but it can also be spread by contact with secretions from the skin lesions.

The virus initially infects cells of the respiratory tract or conjunctival epithelium. There, it reproduces and spreads throughout the body via the bloodstream and lymphatic system. The virus also spreads from the capillary endothelium to the epidermis, where viral replication destroys the basal cells. During primary infection with varicella-zoster virus, the agent establishes latent infection in perineuronal satellite cells of the dorsal nerve root ganglia.

Shingles occurs when replication of the virus is reactivated in the ganglion cells and the agent travels down the sensory nerve serving a dermatome. The agent then infects the epidermis of that dermatome, producing a localized, painful vesicular eruption.

□ **Pathology:** The skin lesions of chickenpox and shingles are indistinguishable from each other and from the lesions produced by herpes simplex virus. The vesicle fills with neutrophils and soon erodes to become a shallow ulcer.

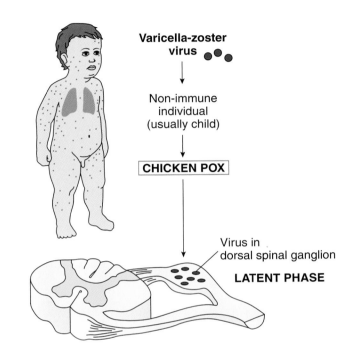

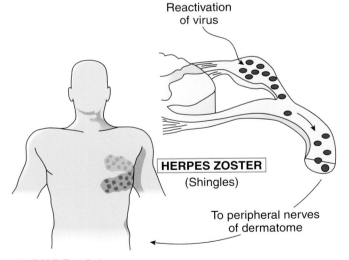

FIGURE   9-1
Varicella (chickenpox) and herpes zoster (shingles). Varicella-zoster virus (VZV) in droplets is inhaled by a nonimmune person (usually a child) and initially causes a "silent" infection of the nasopharynx. This progresses to viremia, seeding of fixed macrophages, and dissemination of VZV to skin (chickenpox) and viscera. VZV resides in a dorsal spinal ganglion, where it remains dormant for many years. Latent VZV is reactivated and spreads from ganglia along the sensory nerves to the peripheral nerves of sensory dermatomes, causing shingles.

☐ **Clinical Features:** After an incubation period of 11 to 21 days, chickenpox presents as fever, malaise, and a distinctive pruritic rash, which begins on the head and spreads to the trunk and extremities. Skin lesions begin as maculopapules that rapidly evolve into vesicles. The lesions heal in several weeks.

Herpes Simplex Virus

Herpes simplex viruses (HSVs) are common human viral pathogens, producing necrotizing infections at diverse body sites (Table 9-2). The virus spreads from person to person, primarily through direct contact with infected secretions or open lesions. HSV produces recurrent, painful vesicular eruptions of the skin and mucous membranes. Two antigenically and epidemiologically distinct HSVs, namely HSV-1 and HSV-2, cause human disease (Fig. 9-2).

- **HSV-1** is transmitted in oral secretions and causes disease "above the waist," including oral, facial, and ocular lesions.
- **HSV-2** is transmitted in genital secretions and produces disease "below the waist," including genital ulcers and neonatal herpes infection.

☐ **Pathology:** Primary HSV disease occurs at the site of initial viral inoculation, such as the oropharynx, genital mucosa, or skin. There, the virus infects the epithelial cells, producing progeny viruses and destroying the infected cells. Destruction of basal cells in the squamous epithelium disrupts the epithelium and leads to vesicle formation. The disease sometimes involves the brain, eye, liver, lungs, and other organs.

The virus invades sensory nerve endings in the oral or genital mucosa, ascends within axons, and establishes a latent infection in sensory neurons within the corresponding ganglia. From time to time, the latent infection is reactivated, and HSV travels back down the nerve to the epithelial site served by the ganglion, where it again infects the epithelial cells.

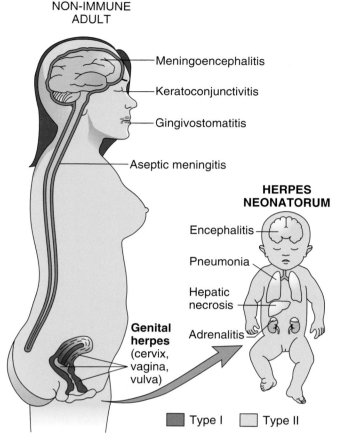

FIGURE 9-2
Herpesvirus infections. Herpes simplex virus type 1 (HSV-1) infects a nonimmune adult, causing gingivostomatitis ("fever blister" or "cold sore"), keratoconjunctivitis, meningoencephalitis, and aseptic spinal meningitis. Herpes simplex virus type 2 (HSV-2) infects the genitalia of a nonimmune adult, involving the cervix, vagina, and vulva. Herpes simplex virus type 2 infects the fetus as it passes through the birth canal of an infected mother. The infant's lack of a mature immune system results in disseminated infection with herpes simplex virus type 1. The infection is often fatal, involving lung, liver, adrenal glands, and central nervous system.

Herpes encephalitis is a rare (one in 100,000 HSV infections) but devastating manifestation of infection with HSV-1.

Neonatal herpes is a serious complication of maternal genital herpes. The virus is transmitted to the fetus from the infected birth canal, often the uterine cervix, and readily disseminates in the unprotected newborn.

☐ **Clinical Features:** In adults, clusters of painful, ulcerating vesicular lesions on the skin or mucous membranes are the most frequent manifestation of HSV infection. These lesions persist for 1 to 2 weeks and then resolve.

T A B L E   *9-2.*   Herpes Simplex Viral Diseases

Viral Type	Common Presentations	Infrequent Presentations
HSV-1	Oral-labial herpes	Conjunctivitis, keratitis Encephalitis Herpetic whitlow Esophagitis[a] Pneumonia[a] Disseminated infection[a]
HSV-2	Genital herpes	Perinatal infection Disseminated infection[a]

[a] These conditions usually occur in immunocompromised hosts.

Neonatal herpes typically begins 5 to 7 days after delivery, with irritability, lethargy, and a mucocutaneous vesicular eruption. The infection rapidly spreads to involve multiple organs, including the brain. The infected newborn develops jaundice, bleeding problems, respiratory distress, seizures, and coma. Treatment with acyclovir is often effective, but neonatal herpes still carries a high mortality rate.

Epstein-Barr Virus (Infectious Mononucleosis)

■ *Infectious mononucleosis results from infection with Epstein-Barr virus (EBV) and is characterized by fever, pharyngitis, lymphadenopathy, and increased circulating lymphocytes.* Infection with EBV has also been associated with several cancers, including African Burkitt lymphoma, B-cell lymphomas in immunosuppressed persons, and nasopharyngeal carcinoma. These neoplastic complications are discussed in Chapters 20 and 25.

☐ **Epidemiology:** In developed countries, many persons remain uninfected with EBV into adolescence or early adulthood. In such instances, two-thirds of those newly infected develop clinically evident infectious mononucleosis. EBV spreads from person to person primarily through contact with infected oral secretions. Once infected, persons remain asymptomatically infected for life, and a few (10–20%) intermittently shed EBV.

☐ **Pathogenesis:** The virus first binds to and infects nasopharyngeal cells and then B lymphocytes. Circulating B lymphocytes carry the virus throughout the body, producing a generalized infection of the lymphoid tissues. EBV induces a polyclonal activation of B cells. In turn, these activated B cells stimulate the proliferation of specific killer T lymphocytes and suppressor T cells. The former destroy virally infected B cells, whereas the suppressor cells inhibit production of immunoglobulins by the B cells.

☐ **Pathology:** The pathologic changes of infectious mononucleosis are prominent in the lymph nodes and spleen. Microscopically, the general architecture is preserved. The germinal centers are enlarged, and they have indistinct margins because of a proliferation of immunoblasts. They also contain frequent mitoses and scattered nuclear debris, presumably from degenerated B cells.

The spleen is large and soft owing to hyperplasia of the red pulp, and it is susceptible to rupture. Many immunoblasts are present throughout the pulp and infiltrate the walls of vessels, the trabeculae, and the capsule. The liver is almost always involved, and the sinusoids and portal tracts contain atypical lymphocytes.

One of the features of infectious mononucleosis is lymphocytosis with atypical lymphocytes, which display lobulated, eccentric nuclei, and vacuolated cytoplasm. These cells are activated T lymphocytes that suppress EBV-infected B lymphocytes.

☐ **Clinical Features:** Infectious mononucleosis presents as fever, malaise, lymphadenopathy, pharyngitis, and splenomegaly. In most patients, the lymphadenopathy is symmetric and most striking in the neck. Patients usually have an elevated leukocyte count, with a predominance of lymphocytes and monocytes. Treatment is supportive, and symptoms usually resolve in 3 to 4 weeks.

Cytomegalovirus

■ *Cytomegalovirus (CMV) is a congenital and opportunistic pathogen that infects many persons worldwide but only uncommonly produces disease.* The fetus and immunocompromised persons are particularly vulnerable to the destructive effects of the virus. CMV spreads from person to person by contact with infected secretions and fluids, including saliva, blood, urine, semen, breast milk, and cervical secretions. The normal immune response rapidly controls CMV infection. Infected persons usually show no ill effects, although they do shed virus periodically in body secretions. Similar to other herpesviruses, CMV can remain latent for years—and probably for life.

☐ **Pathology:** In the fetus with CMV disease, the most common sites of involvement are the brain, inner ears, eyes, liver, and bone marrow. The most severely affected fetuses may have microcephaly, hydrocephalus, cerebral calcifications, hepatosplenomegaly, and jaundice. Microscopically, lesions of fetal CMV disease show cellular necrosis and a characteristic cytopathic effect consisting of marked cellular and nuclear enlargement, with nuclear and cytoplasmic inclusions. The giant nucleus of the infected cell contains a large central inclusion surrounded by a clear zone. The cytoplasmic inclusions are less prominent.

In patients with AIDS and in immunosuppressed transplant recipients, CMV produces chorioretinitis, gastrointestinal ulcers, pneumonitis, hepatitis, encephalitis, and adrenal insufficiency.

HUMAN PAPILLOMAVIRUS

Human papillomaviruses (HPVs) are DNA viruses, which are members of the papovavirus group. They cause proliferative lesions of the squamous epithelium, including common warts, flat warts, plantar warts, anogenital warts (condyloma acuminatum), and laryngeal papillomatosis. Infection with HPV also contributes to the development of squamous cell dysplasias and squamous cell carcinomas of the genital tract (see Chapter 18).

Infection begins with viral inoculation into a stratified squamous epithelium, where the virus enters the nuclei of basal cells and then stimulates replication of the squamous epithelium, thereby producing the various HPV-associated proliferative lesions.

☐ **Clinical Features: Common warts** (verruca vulgaris) are firm, circumscribed, raised, rough-surfaced lesions that usually appear on surfaces subject to trauma, especially the hands. They are common in children but rare in elderly persons. **Plantar warts** are similar squamous proliferative lesions on the soles of the feet but are compressed inward by standing and walking.

Anogenital warts (condyloma acuminatum) are soft, raised, fleshy lesions found on the penis, vulva, vaginal wall, cervix, or perianal region.

Flat warts in the genital area are now recognized to be more common than typical raised anogenital warts. When caused by certain HPV types, these flat warts can develop into malignant squamous cell proliferations.

Bacterial Infections

Bacteria are the smallest living cells, ranging from 0.1 to 10 μm in greatest dimension. Most bacteria are classified according to the tinctorial properties of their cell walls into Gram-positive and Gram-negative types. Round or oval bacteria are termed **cocci,** whereas elongated ones are called **bacilli.** Curved bacteria are known as **vibrios,** and spiral-shaped ones are referred to as **spirochetes.**

PYOGENIC GRAM-POSITIVE COCCI

Staphylococcus aureus

■ *Staphylococcus aureus* is a Gram-positive coccus, which typically grows in clusters and is one of the most common bacterial pathogens. It normally resides on the skin and is readily inoculated into deeper tissues, where it causes suppurative infections. **In fact, S. aureus is the most common cause of suppurative infections involving the skin, joints, and bones, and it is a leading cause of infective endocarditis.**

Staphylococcus aureus elaborates at least five different membrane-damaging toxins that are capable of destroying erythrocytes, leukocytes, platelets, fibroblasts, and other human cells. The organism sometimes invades beyond the initial site, spreading by the bloodstream or lymphatic system to almost any location in the body.

☐ **Pathology:** When *S. aureus* is inoculated into a previously sterile site, the infection usually produces suppuration and abscess formation. Abscesses range from microscopic foci to lesions of several centimeters in diameter. They are filled with pus and bacteria, which can usually be identified on Gram stains.

☐ **Clinical Features:** The clinical manifestations of infection with *S. aureus* vary according to the sites and types of infection:

- **Furuncles (Boils) and Styes.** Boils are deep-seated infections with *S. aureus* in and around hair follicles, often in a nasal carrier. The boil begins as a nodule at the base of a hair follicle, followed by a pimple that remains painful and red for a few days. A yellow apex forms, and the central core becomes necrotic and fluctuant.
- **Carbuncles.** These lesions result from coalescing infections with *S. aureus* around hair follicles and produce draining sinuses. Most carbuncles are on the neck, but they also occur on the limbs, trunk, face, and scalp.
- **Scalded Skin Syndrome.** This disease affects infants and children younger than 3 years who develop a bullous eruption. Even gentle rubbing causes the skin to desquamate owing to the systemic effects of a specific exotoxin. The disease resolves in 1 to 2 weeks as the epithelium regenerates.
- **Osteomyelitis.** Acute staphylococcal osteomyelitis, usually in the bones of the legs, most commonly afflicts boys between 3 and 10 years of age, many of whom have a history of infection or trauma. Adults older than 50 years are more frequently afflicted with osteomyelitis of the vertebrae. It may follow staphylococcal infections of the skin or urinary tract, prostatic surgery, or pinning of a fracture.
- **Respiratory Tract Infections.** Staphylococcal infections of the respiratory tract are most common in infants younger than 2 years. The child often has an underlying skin infection and may be suffering from a viral respiratory disease.
- **Bacterial arthritis.** *S. aureus* is the causative organism in half of septic arthritis cases, most of which occur in patients older than 50 years. Rheumatoid arthritis and corticosteroid therapy are common predisposing conditions.
- **Septicemia.** Septicemia with *S. aureus* afflicts patients with lowered resistance who are in the hospital because of other diseases.

- **Bacterial Endocarditis.** Bacterial endocarditis is a common complication of *S. aureus* septicemia.
- **Toxic Shock Syndrome.** This disorder most commonly afflicts menstruating women, who present with high fever, nausea, vomiting, diarrhea, myalgias, and eventually, shock. The disease has been associated with use of hyperabsorbent tampons, which provide a site for *S. aureus* replication and toxin elaboration.
- **Staphylococcal Food Poisoning.** This intoxication typically presents less than 6 hours after a meal. Nausea and vomiting begin abruptly, usually resolving within 12 hours.

Streptococcus pyogenes

■ *Sreptococcus pyogenes, also known as group A Streptococcus, is one of the most frequent bacterial pathogens of humans and causes many diseases of diverse organ systems, which range from acute, self-limited pharyngitis to major illnesses such as rheumatic fever.* S. pyogenes is a Gram-positive coccus, which is frequently part of the endogenous flora that colonizes the skin and oropharynx.

Streptococcal Pharyngitis ("Strep Throat"). *S. pyogenes* is the common bacterial cause of pharyngitis. The invading organism incites an acute inflammatory response, often producing an exudate of neutrophils in the tonsillar fossae. Reactive hyperplasia of the tonsils and the cervical lymph nodes are common responses.

"Strep throat" presents as a sore throat, fever, malaise, headache, and an elevated leukocyte count. The disease is self-limited, usually lasting from 3 to 5 days. In a few cases, streptococcal pharyngitis leads to rheumatic fever or acute poststreptococcal glomerulonephritis.

Scarlet Fever. Scarlet fever (scarlatina) describes a punctate, red rash that appears on the skin and mucous membranes during some suppurative infections with *S. pyogenes*, most commonly pharyngitis. The skin manifestations are caused by an erythrogenic toxin elaborated by certain streptococcal strains.

Erysipelas. Erysipelas is an erythematous swelling of the skin caused chiefly by *S. pyogenes*. It is the classic cutaneous streptococcal infection, usually beginning on the face and then spreading rapidly. A diffuse, edematous, acute inflammatory reaction in the epidermis and dermis extends into the subcutaneous tissues.

Impetigo. Impetigo (pyoderma) is a localized, intraepidermal infection of the skin caused by *S. pyogenes* or *S. aureus*. The disease most commonly affects children from 2 to 5 years of age. Lesions begin on exposed body surfaces as localized erythematous papules, which then become pustules that erode within a few days to form a thick, honey-colored crust.

Streptococcal Cellulitis. *S. pyogenes* is one of the most common causes of cellulitis, which is an acute, spreading infection of the loose connective tissue in the deeper layers of the dermis. This suppurative infection results from traumatic inoculation of micro-organisms into the skin.

Puerperal Sepsis. Postpartum infection of the uterine cavity by *S. pyogenes*, termed *puerperal sepsis*, was formerly common but is now rare in developed countries. The infection originates from the contaminated hands of attendants at delivery, an association first established by the historic observations of Semmelweis.

Streptococcus pneumoniae

■ *Steptococcus pneumoniae, often simply called pneumococcus, causes pyogenic infections that primarily involve the lungs (pneumonia), middle ear (otitis media), sinuses (sinusitis), and meninges (meningitis).* **It is one of the most common bacterial pathogens of humans, and by 5 years of age, most children in the world have suffered at least one episode of pneumococcal disease (usually otitis media).** After infection with *Haemophilus influenzae*, infection with pneumococcus is the second leading cause of bacterial meningitis.

☐ **Pathogenesis and Pathology:** Pneumococcal disease begins when the organism gains access to sterile sites, usually those in proximity to its normal residence in the oropharynx. Pneumococcal sinusitis, otitis media, and pneumonia are usually preceded by a viral illness, such as the common cold. The lower respiratory tract is protected by the mucociliary blanket and the cough response, which normally expel organisms that are inhaled into the lower airway. Insults that interfere with the function of these defenses, including influenza, other viral respiratory illnesses, smoking, and alcoholism, allow access to *S. pneumoniae*. Once in the alveoli, the organisms proliferate and cause lobar pneumonia.

BACTERIAL INFECTIONS OF CHILDHOOD

Diphtheria

■ *Diphtheria is a necrotizing, upper respiratory tract infection sometimes associated with cardiac and neurologic disturbances. Corynebacterium diphtheriae, a Gram-positive rod, is the causative agent.* Although immunization programs have largely eliminated the disease in developed countries, it persists as a major health problem in less-developed ones.

☐ **Pathology:** Diphtheria begins with the entry of *C. diphtheriae* into the pharynx, where the organisms proliferate (commonly on the tonsils). The characteristic lesions are thick, gray, leathery membranes that line the affected respiratory passages. These membranes are composed of sloughed epithelium, necrotic debris, neutrophils, fibrin, and bacteria. The inflammatory process often produces swelling in the surrounding soft tissues, which can be sufficiently severe as to cause respiratory compromise. When the heart is affected by diphtheria toxin, the myocardium displays fat droplets in the myocytes and focal necrosis. In the case of neural involvement, the affected peripheral nerves exhibit demyelination.

☐ **Clinical Features:** Diphtheria begins with fever, sore throat, and malaise. The dirty gray membrane develops first on the tonsils but may spread throughout the posterior oropharynx. Cardiac and neurologic symptoms develop in a minority of infected persons, usually those with the most severe local disease. Diphtheria is treated by prompt administration of antitoxin and antibiotics.

Pertussis

■ *Pertussis, commonly called whooping cough, is a prolonged upper respiratory tract infection characterized by debilitating coughing paroxysms.* The paroxysm is followed by a long, high-pitched inspiration—the "whoop" that gives this disease its name. Whooping cough lasts from 4 to 5 weeks. The causative organism is *Bordetella pertussis*, a small, Gram-negative coccobacillus similar in appearance to *Haemophilus* sp. *B. pertussis* causes an extensive tracheobronchitis, with necrosis of the ciliated respiratory epithelium and an acute inflammatory response. In susceptible populations, pertussis is primarily a disease of children younger than 5 years, and many cases occur in children younger than 1 year. Vaccination protects against *B. pertussis*.

Haemophilus influenzae

■ *Haemophilus influenzae, a Gram-negative coccobacillus, causes pyogenic infections, primarily in young children, involving the middle ear, sinuses, facial skin, epiglottis, meninges, lungs, and joints.* The organism is a major bacterial pathogen in children and is the leading cause of bacterial meningitis worldwide.

☐ **Pathology:** *H. influenzae* incites a pronounced acute inflammatory response, and specific pathologic features vary according to the sites affected.

- *H. influenzae* **meningitis** resembles other acute bacterial meningitides, with a predominantly neutrophilic infiltrate in the leptomeninges.
- *H. influenzae* **pneumonia** usually complicates chronic lung disease and, in half of patients, fol-

lows a viral infection of the respiratory tract. The alveoli are filled with neutrophils, macrophages containing bacilli, and fibrin. The bronchiolar epithelium is necrotic and infiltrated by macrophages.

- **Epiglottitis** consists of swelling and acute inflammation of the epiglottis, aryepiglottic folds, and pyriform sinuses, which sometimes completely obstruct the upper airway.

Neisseria meningitidis

■ *Neisseria meningitidis, commonly termed meningococcus, causes pyogenic meningitis and disseminated blood-borne infections, often accompanied by shock and profound disturbances in coagulation.* The organisms appear as paired, bean-shaped, Gram-negative cocci. Meningococci spread from person to person, primarily by respiratory droplets; close contact facilitates dissemination. Meningococcal infections appear as sporadic cases, clusters of cases, and epidemics. Most infections in developed countries are sporadic and occur in children younger than 5 years. In industrialized countries, epidemic disease occurs most frequently in crowded quarters, such as among military recruits in barracks.

☐ **Pathology:** Meningococcal disease can be confined to the central nervous system or be disseminated throughout the body in the form of septicemia. In the case of meningococcal meningitis, the leptomeninges and subarachnoid space are infiltrated with neutrophils.

Meningococcal septicemia is characterized by diffuse damage to the endothelium of small blood vessels, thereby resulting in widespread petechiae and purpura in the skin and viscera. Affected blood vessels initially show dilatation, with hemorrhage into the adjacent perivascular tissue. This is soon followed by an intense neutrophilic infiltrate of the vessel walls. Small vessels throughout the body are also occluded by fibrin clots. Rarely (3–4% of cases), the vasculitis and thrombosis produce hemorrhagic necrosis of both adrenals, a phenomenon known as the **Waterhouse-Friderichsen syndrome.**

☐ **Clinical Features:** Meningococcal diseases, both meningitis and sepsis, most often present as fulminant illnesses. Meningitis begins with rapid onset of fever, stiff neck, and headache. In the case of meningococcal sepsis, fever, shock, and mucocutaneous hemorrhages appear abruptly. Patients can progress to shock within minutes, and treatment requires rapid support of blood pressure and administration of antibiotics. During the preantibiotic era, meningococcal disease was almost invariably fatal, but modern treatment has reduced the fatality rate to less than 15%.

SEXUALLY TRANSMITTED BACTERIAL DISEASES

Gonorrhea

■ *Neisseria gonorrhoeae, also termed gonococcus, causes gonorrhea, one of the oldest—and still one of the most common—sexually transmitted diseases.* N. gonorrhoeae is a Gram-negative diplococcus that is morphologically indistinguishable from N. meningitidis.

☐ **Pathology:** Gonorrhea is an acute suppurative infection of the genital tract, which is reflected in urethritis among men and endocervicitis among women. Infection among women often ascends the genital tract, producing endometritis, salpingitis, and pelvic inflammatory disease.

Neonatal infections derived from the birth canal of a mother with gonorrhea usually present as conjunctivitis. This complication has been largely eliminated in developed countries by routine instillation of antibiotics into the conjunctiva at birth, but it remains a major cause of blindness in much of Africa and Asia.

Gonorrhea is a suppurative infection characterized by a vigorous acute inflammatory response, which produces copious pus and, often, forms submucosal abscesses. If untreated, the inflammatory response becomes chronic, with macrophages and lymphocytes being predominant.

☐ **Clinical Features:** After an incubation period of 3 to 5 days, men exposed to N. gonorrhoeae present with a purulent urethral discharge and dysuria. With prompt antibiotic treatment, the infection is arrested, and the organism remains confined to the mucosa of the anterior urethra. However, if treatment is not instituted promptly, urethral stricture is a common complication.

Approximately half of infected women manifest endocervicitis, with vaginal discharge or bleeding. The infection often extends to the fallopian tubes, where it produces acute and chronic salpingitis and, eventually, pelvic inflammatory disease. The fallopian tubes swell with pus, causing acute abdominal pain, and infertility occurs when inflammatory adhesions block the tubes. Gonorrhea is readily eradicated with effective antibiotic regimens, especially penicillin, although resistant strains are encountered.

Chancroid

■ *Chancroid is an acute, sexually transmitted infection caused by* Haemophilus ducreyi. The organism is a small, Gram-negative bacillus that appears in tissue as clusters of parallel bacilli and as chains resembling schools of fish. Chancroid is characterized by painful genital ulcerations and associated lymphadenopathy.

The infection is most common in tropical and subtropical regions, especially in Africa and parts of Asia. It is more frequent in men than in women, and it is associated with promiscuity and poor personal hygiene.

☐ **Pathogenesis and Pathology:** The ulcers of chancroid are located on the skin and mucous membranes of the genitalia. A papule develops 1 to 14 days after sexual contact, becomes pustular, and then ulcerates. Seven to 10 days after appearance of the primary lesion, half of patients develop unilateral, painful, suppurative inguinal lymphadenitis (bubo). The overlying skin becomes inflamed, breaks down, and drains pus from the underlying node. Treatment of chancroid with erythromycin is usually effective.

Granuloma Inguinale

■ *Granuloma inguinale is a sexually transmitted, chronic, superficial ulceration of the genitalia and the inguinal and perianal regions.* It is caused by *Calymmatobacterium granulomatis,* a small, Gram-negative bacillus. Granuloma inguinale is rare in temperate climates but is common in tropical and subtropical areas.

☐ **Pathology:** The characteristic lesion of granuloma inguinale is a raised, soft, beefy-red, superficial ulcer. Microscopically, the dermis and subcutis are infiltrated by numerous macrophages and plasma cells and by fewer neutrophils and lymphocytes. The macrophages contain many bacteria, which are termed **Donovan bodies.**

☐ **Clinical Features:** The incubation period of granuloma inguinale varies from 1 week to 6 months. Early ulceration of the penile and scrotal skin commonly extends to the adjacent inguinal areas. In women, ulcerations spread to the perineal and perianal skin. Homosexual men display anal and perianal lesions. Untreated granuloma inguinale follows an indolent, relapsing course, often healing with an atrophic scar. Antibiotic therapy is effective in cases of early infection.

ENTEROPATHOGENIC BACTERIA

Escherichia coli is among the most frequent and important bacterial pathogens of humans. *E. coli* organisms are Gram-negative bacteria that are mostly intestinal commensals and are well adapted to growth within the human colon without causing harm to the host. However, E. coli can be aggressive when it gains access to usually sterile body sites, such as the urinary tract, meninges, or peritoneum. It is also the major cause of endotoxic shock. Strains of *E. coli* that produce diarrhea possess specialized virulence properties, usually plasmid-borne, that confer the capacity to cause intestinal disease. The diseases caused by *E. coli* are discussed in the various chapters dealing with specific organs.

■ *Typhoid fever is a severe, prolonged systemic illness caused by* Salmonella typhi. It is spread primarily through ingestion of contaminated water and food, especially dairy products and shellfish. Infected food handlers with poor personal hygiene are a notorious source of infection. The disease is also acquired from convalescing patients or chronic carriers.

■ *Shigellosis is an acute, bacterial dysentery characterized by a necrotizing infection of the distal small bowel and colon.* It is caused by any species of the Gram-negative rods *Shigella,* with *S. dysenteriae* being the most virulent. *Shigella* organisms spread from person to person by the fecal-oral route. Shigellosis is a self-limited disease that typically presents as abdominal pain and bloody, mucoid stools.

■ *Campylobacter jejuni is the leading bacterial agent of diarrhea in the United States.* It is a Gram-negative rod and causes an acute, self-limited illness. The infection is acquired by ingestion of organisms contained in contaminated food or water. Raw milk and inadequately cooked poultry and meat are also frequent sources of disease.

Typhoid fever, shigellosis, and *C. jejuni* diarrhea are discussed in greater detail in Chapter 13.

Cholera

■ *Cholera is a severe diarrheal illness caused by the enterotoxin of the Gram-negative rod* Vibrio cholerae. Infection causes profuse and watery diarrhea, rapid dehydration, and if fluids are not restored, shock and death within 24 hours of the onset of symptoms. Cholera is acquired by ingesting *V. cholerae* in contaminated food or water. Cholera epidemics spread readily in areas where human feces pollute the water supply. Cholera organisms do not invade the mucosa but cause diarrhea by elaboration of a potent exotoxin (cholera toxin).

☐ **Clinical Features:** Cholera begins with a few loose stools, usually evolving within hours to severe, watery diarrhea. With adequate volume replacement, infected adults can lose up to 20 L of fluid in a single day. Untreated cholera has a 50% mortality rate. With rehydration, the illness subsides spontaneously in 3 to 6 days. Antibiotic therapy shortens the duration of the illness.

CLOSTRIDIA

Clostridia are Gram-positive, spore-forming bacilli that are obligate anaerobes and cause a number of important diseases (Fig. 9-3).

FIGURE   *9-3*
Clostridial diseases. **Clostridia in the vegetative form (bacilli) inhabit the gastrointestinal tract of humans and animals. Spores pass in the feces, contaminate soil and plant materials, and are ingested or enter sites of penetrating wounds. Under anaerobic conditions, they revert to vegetative forms. Plasmids in the vegetative forms elaborate toxins that cause several clostridial diseases.**

Food poisoning and necrotizing enteritis. **Meat dishes left to cool at room temperature grow large numbers of clostridia ($>10^6$ organisms/g). When the contaminated meat is ingested, *C. perfringens* types A and C produce α-enterotoxin in the small intestine during sporulation, causing abdominal pain and diarrhea. Type C also produces β-enterotoxin.**

Gas gangrene. **Clostridia are widespread and may contaminate a traumatic wound or surgical operation. *C. perfringens* type A elaborates a myotoxin (α-toxin), which is a lecithinase that destroys cell membranes, alters capillary permeability, and causes severe hemolysis following intravenous injection. The toxin causes necrosis of previously healthy skeletal muscle.**

Tetanus. **Spores of *C. tetani* are in the soil and enter the site of an accidental wound. Necrotic tissue at the wound site causes spores to revert to the vegetative form (bacilli). Autolysis of vegetative forms releases tetanus toxin, which is transported in the peripheral nerves and (retrograde) through axons to the anterior horn cells of the spinal cord. The toxin blocks synaptic inhibition, and accumulation of acetylcholine in the damaged synapses leads to rigidity and spasms of the skeletal musculature (tetany).**

Botulism. **Improperly canned food is contaminated by the vegetative form of *C. botulinum*, which proliferates under aerobic conditions and elaborates a neurotoxin. After the food is ingested, the neurotoxin is absorbed from the small intestine and, eventually, reaches the myoneural junction, where it inhibits the release of acetylcholine. The result is a symmetric, descending paralysis of the cranial nerves, trunk, and limbs, with eventual respiratory paralysis and death.**

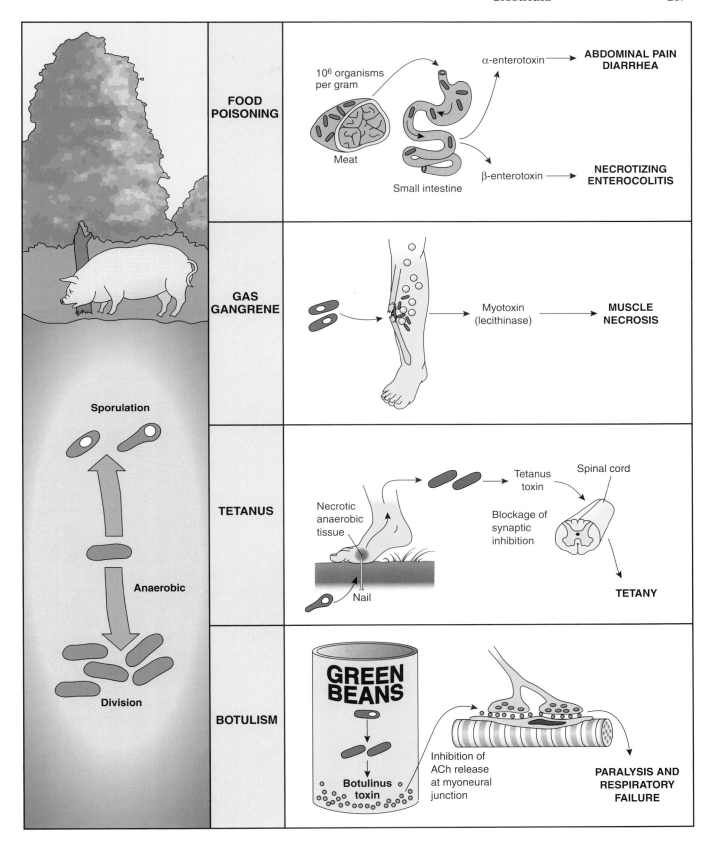

FOOD POISONING

10^6 organisms per gram

Meat

Small intestine

α-enterotoxin → **ABDOMINAL PAIN DIARRHEA**

β-enterotoxin → **NECROTIZING ENTEROCOLITIS**

GAS GANGRENE

Myotoxin (lecithinase) → **MUSCLE NECROSIS**

TETANUS

Necrotic anaerobic tissue

Nail

Tetanus toxin

Spinal cord

Blockage of synaptic inhibition

TETANY

BOTULISM

GREEN BEANS

Botulinus toxin

Inhibition of ACh release at myoneural junction

PARALYSIS AND RESPIRATORY FAILURE

Sporulation

Anaerobic

Division

Clostridial Food Poisoning

■ *Clostridium perfringens is one of the most common causes worldwide of bacterial food poisoning, an acute, generally benign diarrheal disease usually lasting less than 24 hours.* Spores of *C. perfringens* survive cooking temperatures and germinate to yield vegetative forms, which proliferate when food is allowed to stand without refrigeration. Clostridial food poisoning results from ingestion of food containing large numbers ($>10^5$/g) of these vegetative bacteria.

Necrotizing Enteritis

■ *C. perfringens type C produces an enterotoxin that causes a necrotizing enterocolitis.* This disorder is still endemic in the highlands of New Guinea, especially among children who have participated in pig feasts (hence the pidgin term **pigbel**).

□ **Pathology:** Necrotizing enteritis is a segmental disease that may be restricted to a few centimeters or involve the entire small intestine. Histologic sections reveal infarction of the intestinal mucosa, with edema, hemorrhage, and a suppurative, transmural infiltrate.

□ **Clinical Features:** Presenting symptoms include severe abdominal pain and distention, vomiting, and passage of bloody or black stools. Patients with fulminating pigbel usually die within 24 hours of the onset of symptoms.

Gas Gangrene (Clostridial Myonecrosis)

■ *Gas gangrene is a necrotizing, gas-forming infection that begins in contaminated wounds and spreads rapidly to the adjacent tissues.* The disease can be fatal within hours of onset. *C. perfringens* is the most common cause of gas gangrene, but other clostridial species occasionally produce the disease. The anaerobic conditions necessary to foster clostridial growth occur with severe trauma, wartime injuries, and septic abortions. The necrosis of previously healthy muscle is caused by the myotoxins elaborated by *C. perfringens*.

□ **Pathology:** Affected muscles become necrotic and may even liquefy. Edema and gas expand the soft tissues. Microscopic examination shows extensive tissue necrosis, with dissolution of the normal cellular architecture.

□ **Clinical Features:** The incubation period of gas gangrene is commonly from 2 to 4 days after injury. The skin darkens because of hemorrhage and cutaneous necrosis. The lesion develops a thick, serosan-guineous discharge, which has a fragrant odor and may contain gas bubbles, and hemolytic anemia, hypotension, and renal failure ensue. In the terminal stages, coma, jaundice, and shock supervene.

Tetanus

■ *Tetanus is a severe, acute neurologic syndrome of humans and other mammals caused by tetanus toxin and characterized by spastic contractions of the skeletal muscles.* *Clostridium tetani* is a common environmental organism and is present in the soil and the lower intestine of many animals. Tetanus occurs when the organism contaminates wounds and proliferates in tissue, releasing its exotoxin. A vaccine composed of inactivated tetanus toxin is highly effective in preventing tetanus, and immunization programs have largely eliminated the disease from developed countries.

Although the clostridial infection remains localized, the potent tetanus neurotoxin undergoes retrograde transport through the ventral roots of the peripheral nerves to the anterior horn cells of the spinal cord. Release of inhibitory neurotransmitters is blocked, thereby permitting unopposed neural stimulation and sustained contraction of skeletal muscles (tetany).

□ **Clinical Features:** The incubation period of tetanus is from 1 to 3 weeks. Spastic rigidity often begins in the muscles of the face, giving rise to "lockjaw" or spastic rigidity of several facial muscles and causing a fixed grin (risus sardonicus). Rigidity of the muscles of the back produces a backward arching (opisthotonos). Abrupt stimuli, including noise, light, or touch, can precipitate painful, generalized muscle spasms. Swallowing and breathing may be impaired by involvement of the associated muscles, and prolonged spasm of the respiratory and laryngeal musculature may lead to death. Administration of antibody to bind unabsorbed toxin, antibiotics to eliminate infection, and supportive care, including respiratory support, are the mainstays of therapy.

Botulism

■ *Botulism is a paralyzing illness that follows ingestion of food containing the preformed neurotoxins of* Clostridium botulinum. The disease is characterized by a symmetric, descending paralysis of the cranial nerves, limbs, and trunk. In the United States, the toxin is most commonly present in vegetables or other foods that have been improperly home-canned and stored without refrigeration. These circumstances provide suitable anaerobic conditions for growth of the vegetative cells that elaborate the neurotoxins.

Circulating toxin binds to nerve terminals and inhibits the release of acetylcholine, thereby producing a flaccid paralysis. Prompt administration of antitoxin prevents the action of botulinum toxin that has not been bound to the presynaptic membrane. Untreated botulism food poisoning is usually lethal, but treatment has reduced the mortality rate to 25%.

Clostridium difficile Colitis

■ *Clostridium difficile colitis is an acute, necrotizing infection of the terminal small bowel and colon.* The disease is responsible for a large fraction (25–50%) of antibiotic-associated diarrheas and is potentially lethal. The subject is treated in Chapter 13.

BACTERIAL INFECTIONS WITH ANIMAL RESERVOIRS OR INSECT VECTORS

Brucellosis

■ *Brucellosis is a zoonotic disease caused by one of four* Brucella *sp. that may present as an acute systemic disease or a chronic infection.* The latter is characterized by waxing and waning febrile episodes, weight loss, and fatigue. *Brucella* sp. are small, Gram-negative rods, which in humans primarily infect monocytes/macrophages.

☐ **Epidemiology:** Each species of *Brucella* has its own animal reservoir:

- *Brucella melitensis:* sheep and goats
- *Brucella abortus:* cattle
- *Brucella suis:* swine
- *Brucella canis:* dogs

Humans acquire the bacteria by several mechanisms, including (1) contact with infected blood or tissue, (2) ingestion of contaminated meat or milk, or (3) inhalation of contaminated aerosols. Brucellosis is an occupational hazard among ranchers, herders, veterinarians, and slaughterhouse workers. Elimination of infected animals and vaccination of herds have reduced the incidence of brucellosis in many countries, and only approximately 400 cases occur annually in the United States.

☐ **Pathology:** Bacteria enter the circulation through skin abrasions, the conjunctiva, oropharynx, or lungs. They then spread in the bloodstream to the liver, spleen, lymph nodes, and bone marrow, where they multiply in mononuclear macrophages. A generalized hyperplasia of these cells ensues, with conspicuous noncaseating granulomas, causing lymphadenopathy and hepatosplenomegaly. The most common complications of brucellosis involve the bones and joints, and they include spondylitis of the lumbar spine and suppuration in large joints. Peripheral neuritis, meningitis, orchitis, endocarditis, myocarditis, and pulmonary lesions are described. Prolonged treatment with tetracycline is usually effective.

Plague

■ *Plague is a bacteremic and often fatal infection usually accompanied by enlarged, painful regional lymph nodes (bubos).* It is caused by *Yersinia pestis*, a short, Gram-negative rod. Historically, devastating epidemics of plague made this disease the scourge of the civilized world.

☐ **Epidemiology:** *Y. pestis* infection is an endemic zoonosis in many parts of the world, including the Americas, Africa, and Asia. The organism is found in wild rodents, such as rats, squirrels, and prairie dogs. Fleas transmit the bacterium from animal to animal, and most human infections result from the bites of infected fleas.

☐ **Pathology:** After inoculation into the skin, *Y. pestis* organisms are carried to the regional lymph nodes, where they continue to multiply and produce extensive hemorrhagic necrosis. From the regional lymph nodes, they disseminate throughout the body via the bloodstream and lymphatics. Affected lymph nodes, known as **bubos**, are frequently enlarged and fluctuant owing to extensive hemorrhagic necrosis. Infected patients often develop necrotic, hemorrhagic skin lesions (hence the name "black death" for this disease).

☐ **Clinical Features:** There are three clinical presentations of infection with *Y. pestis*, although they often overlap:

- **Bubonic plague** begins within 2 to 8 days of the flea bite and progresses to septic shock within hours to days after appearance of the bubo.
- **Septicemic plague** (10% of cases) occurs when the bacteria are inoculated directly into the blood and do not produce bubos. Patients die from the overwhelming growth of the bacteria in the bloodstream.
- **Pneumonic plague** results from inhalation of airborne particles from the carcasses of animals or the cough of an infected person. Respiratory insufficiency and endotoxic shock kill the patient in 1 to 2 days.

All types of plague carry a high mortality rate (50% to 75%) if untreated. Tetracycline combined with streptomycin is the recommended therapy.

Tularemia

■ *Tularemia is an acute, febrile, granulomatous disease caused by* Francisella tularensis, *a small, Gram-negative coccobacillus.* The most important reservoirs for the organism are rabbits and rodents. Blood-sucking, infected ticks inoculate the organism into the skin on feeding. The bacteria may also be introduced into unnoticed breaks in the skin by direct contact with an infected animal.

Francisella tularensis multiplies at the site of inoculation, where it produces a focal ulceration. The bacteria then spread to the regional lymph nodes. Dissemination in the bloodstream leads to metastatic infections that involve the monocyte/macrophage system and, sometimes, the lungs, heart, and kidneys.

□ **Pathology:** Disseminated lesions undergo central necrosis and are surrounded by a perimeter of granulomatous reaction resembling the lesions of tuberculosis. The lymph nodes become large and firm owing to hyperemia and the presence of numerous macrophages in the sinuses. The nodes subsequently soften as necrosis and suppuration develop. The pulmonary lesions resemble those of primary tuberculosis.

Ulceroglandular tularemia is the most common form of the disease and begins as a tender, erythematous papule at the site of inoculation, usually on a limb. This develops into a pustule, which then ulcerates. The regional lymph nodes become large and tender. The duration of illness is from 1 week to 3 months, but this may be shortened by prompt treatment with streptomycin.

Anthrax

■ *Anthrax is a necrotizing disease that is rapidly fatal when it disseminates from localized sites of infection.* Bacillus anthracis, the cause of anthrax, is a large, spore-forming, Gram-positive rod.

□ **Epidemiology:** Anthrax is a zoonosis in which the major reservoirs are goats, sheep, cattle, horses, pigs, and dogs. Spores form in the soil and dead animals and can resist heat, desiccation, and chemical disinfection for years. Humans are infected when spores enter the body through breaks in the skin, by inhalation, or by ingestion.

□ **Pathology:** In 80% of cases of cutaneous anthrax, the infection remains localized, and the host immuno-

logic response eventually eliminates the organism. If the infection disseminates, as occurs when the organisms are inhaled or ingested, the resulting widespread tissue destruction is usually fatal.

Bacillus anthracis produces extensive tissue necrosis at the sites of infection, which is associated with only a mild infiltrate of neutrophils. Cutaneous lesions are ulcerated, contain numerous organisms, and are covered by a black scab. Pulmonary infection produces a necrotizing, hemorrhagic pneumonia associated with hemorrhagic necrosis of the mediastinal lymph nodes and widespread dissemination of the organism.

Listeriosis

■ *Listeriosis is a systemic infection caused by* Listeria monocytogenes, *a small, Gram-positive coccobacillus.* The organism grows at refrigerator temperatures, and outbreaks have been traced to contaminated cheese and other dairy products.

□ **Pathology and Clinical Features:** Most *Listeria* infections fall into one of two groups. Listeriosis of pregnancy includes prenatal and postnatal infections. Listeriosis of adults is characterized by meningoencephalitis and septicemia.

Maternal infection early in pregnancy leads to abortion or premature delivery. Infected liveborn, premature infants develop symptoms of infection within a few hours after birth, including respiratory distress, hepatosplenomegaly, cutaneous and mucosal papules, leukopenia, and thrombocytopenia. Widespread abscesses are found in many organs. Microscopically, foci of necrosis and suppuration contain many bacteria. Older lesions tend to be granulomatous. Neurologic sequelae are common, and even with prompt antibiotic therapy, the mortality rate is high.

Chronic alcoholics, patients with cancer, and those receiving immunosuppressive therapy are all susceptible to listeriosis. Meningitis is the most common form of the disease in adults and resembles other bacterial meningitides. Microscopically, the leptomeninges are infiltrated with lymphocytes, plasma cells, macrophages, and neutrophils. Prolonged treatment with antimicrobials is usually required, because patients tend to experience relapse if therapy is administered for less than 3 weeks.

Septicemic listeriosis is most common in immunodeficient patients. It is a severe, febrile illness that may lead to shock and disseminated intravascular coagulation, a situation that may be diagnosed erroneously as Gram-negative sepsis. A suppurative leptomeningitis can occur, and the brain may be seeded with miliary abscesses.

Cat-Scratch Disease

■ *Cat-scratch disease* *is a self-limited infection by* Bartonella henselae, *a small, Gram-negative rod.* Infection begins when the bacillus is inoculated into the skin by the claws of cats (and, rarely, other animals) or by thorns or splinters. At the site of inoculation, bacteria multiply in the walls of small vessels and about the collagen fibers. The organisms are then carried to the regional lymph nodes, where they produce a **suppurative and granulomatous lymphadenitis.**

□ **Clinical Features:** Most patients develop a papule at the site of inoculation from 3 to 14 days after the scratch, and this papule may persist for 2 months. Tenderness and enlargement of the regional lymph nodes ensue. The nodes remain enlarged for 3 to 4 months and may drain through the skin. Approximately half the patients have other symptoms, including fever and malaise, rash, brief encephalitis, and erythema nodosum. No antibiotic has been accepted as beneficial.

FILAMENTOUS BACTERIA

Actinomycosis

■ *Actinomycosis* *is a slowly progressive, suppurative, fibrosing infection involving the jaw, thorax, or abdomen.* The disease is caused by a number of anaerobic and microaerophilic bacteria, which are termed *Actinomyces.* These organisms are branching, filamentous, Gram-positive rods that normally reside in the human oropharynx, gastrointestinal tract, and vagina. Several *Actinomyces* sp. cause human disease, with the most common being *A. israelii.*

□ **Pathology:** *Actinomyces* are not ordinarily virulent, and the organisms reside as saprophytes in the body without producing disease. Two uncommon conditions must occur for *Actinomyces* to establish disease. First, the organism must be inoculated into the deeper tissues, because it cannot invade. Second, an anaerobic atmosphere is necessary for the bacteria to proliferate. Trauma can produce tissue necrosis, thereby providing an excellent anaerobic medium for the growth of *Actinomyces,* and can inoculate the organism into normally sterile tissue. Actinomycosis occurs at four distinct sites:

- **Cervicofacial actinomycosis** results from jaw injury, dental extraction, or dental manipulation.
- **Thoracic actinomycosis** is caused by aspiration of organisms contaminating dental debris.
- **Abdominal actinomycosis** follows traumatic or surgical disruption of the bowel, especially the appendix.
- **Pelvic actinomycosis** is associated with prolonged use of intrauterine devices.

Actinomycosis causes abscesses connected by sinus tracts, which burrow across normal tissue boundaries and into adjacent organs. Eventually, a tract may penetrate onto an external surface or mucosal membrane, producing a draining sinus. Within the abscesses and sinuses are pus and yellow colonies of organisms (sulfur granules) (Fig. 9-4). Actinomycosis responds to prolonged antibiotic therapy, and penicillin is a highly effective drug.

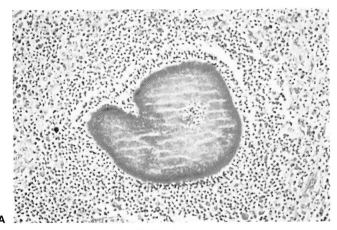
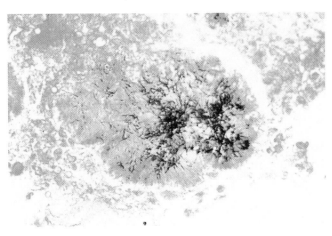

A   B

FIGURE   *9-4*
Actinomycosis. (A) A typical sulfur granule lies within an abscess. (B) The individual filaments of *A. israelii* are readily visible with the silver impregnation technique.

Nocardiosis

■ *Nocardiosis is a suppurative infection of the lung that may spread to the brain, skin, and less commonly, to the thyroid, liver, and other organs, frequently in immunocompromised persons.* Nocardia are Gram-positive, filamentous, branching bacteria. Human disease is caused by inhalation or inoculation of soil-borne organisms and is more common in persons with impaired immunity, particularly cell-mediated immunity. Organ transplantation, long-term corticosteroid therapy, lymphomas, leukemias, and various other debilitating diseases predispose to infection with *Nocardia*.

□ **Pathology:** The respiratory tract is the usual portal of entry for *Nocardia*. The organism incites a brisk infiltrate of neutrophils, and disease begins as a slowly progressive, pyogenic pneumonia. In immunocompromised persons, *Nocardia* produce pulmonary abscesses, which are frequently multiple and confluent. The brain is secondarily involved in one-third of infected persons. Untreated nocardiosis is usually fatal. Sulfonamides or related antibiotics, administered for several months, are often effective therapy.

Spirochetes

Spirochetes are long, slender, helical bacteria with specialized cell envelopes that permit them to move by flexion and rotation.

SYPHILIS

■ *Syphilis (lues) is a chronic, sexually transmitted, systemic infection caused* by Treponema pallidum. The infection is also spread from an infected mother to her fetus (congenital syphilis). The course of syphilis is classically divided into three stages (Fig. 9-5).

Primary Syphilis

The classic lesion of primary syphilis is the chancre (Fig. 9-6), a characteristic ulcer located at the site of *T. pallidum* inoculation, usually the penis, vulva, anus, or mouth. It appears 1 week to 3 months after exposure. Microscopically, chancres (and lesions of the other stages of syphilis) display a characteristic "luetic vasculitis," in which the endothelial cells proliferate and swell and the walls of the vessels become thickened by lymphocytes and fibrous tissue. The chancre lasts from 3 to 12 weeks and is frequently accompanied by inguinal lymphadenopathy. Penicillin remains effective therapy.

Secondary Syphilis

Secondary syphilis is characterized by lesions in a variety of organs, especially the skin, mucous membranes, lymph nodes, meninges, stomach, and liver. This stage results from the systemic dissemination and proliferation of *T. pallidum*. Histopathologically, the le-

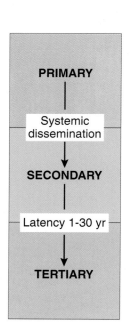
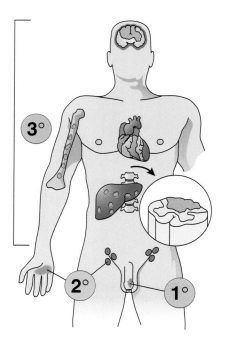
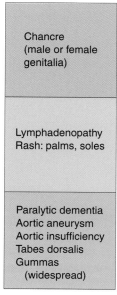

FIGURE   *9-5*
Clinical characteristics of the various stages of syphilis.

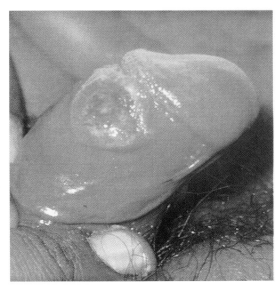

FIGURE 9-6
Syphilitic chancre. A patient with primary syphilis displays a rounded, raised penile chancre with central ulceration.

sions of secondary syphilis show a chronic, inflammatory infiltrate and endarteritis obliterans.

The most common presentation of secondary syphilis is a rash, accompanied by constitutional symptoms, that appears from 2 weeks to 6 months after the chancre heals. The rash is erythematous and maculopapular, involving the trunk and extremities and, often, the palms and soles as well. There are a variety of other skin lesions in secondary syphilis, including condylomata lata (exudative plaques in the perineum, vulva, or scrotum, which abound in spirochetes). Lesions on the mucosal surfaces of the mouth and genital organs, called "mucous patches," teem with organisms and are highly infectious. If untreated, secondary syphilis can relapse.

Tertiary Syphilis

After the lesions of secondary syphilis have subsided, an asymptomatic period lasts for years or decades. One-third of untreated patients with syphilis develop tertiary lesions. **Most of the pathologic processes associated with tertiary syphilis derive from focal ischemic necrosis secondary to obliterative endarteritis.** *T. pallidum* incites a mononuclear inflammatory infiltrate, predominantly composed of lymphocytes and plasma cells. These cells infiltrate the small arteries and arterioles, thereby producing a characteristic obstructive vascular lesion (endarteritis obliterans). The small arteries are inflamed, and their endothelial cells are swollen. They are also surrounded by concen-

tric layers of proliferating fibroblasts, which confer an "onion skin" appearance to the vascular lesions.

Syphilitic aortitis results from a slowly progressive endarteritis obliterans of the vasa vasorum that eventually leads to necrosis of the aortic media, gradual weakening and stretching of the aortic wall, and formation of an aortic aneurysm. The syphilitic aneurysm is saccular, and it involves the ascending aorta. The aorta gradually stretches, becoming progressively thinner to the point of rupture, massive hemorrhage, and sudden death. Damage to and scarring of the ascending aorta also commonly lead to dilatation of the aortic ring, separation of the valve cusps, and regurgitation of blood through the aortic valve (aortic insufficiency).

Neurosyphilis is a slowly progressive infection that damages the meninges, cerebral cortex, spinal cord, cranial nerves, or eyes. The lesions of neurosyphilis are discussed in detail in Chapter 28.

A **gumma** is a characteristic lesion of tertiary syphilis that may form in any organ or tissue. These granulomatous lesions are composed of a central area of coagulative necrosis, epithelioid macrophages, occasional giant cells, and peripheral fibrous tissue. Gummas are most commonly found in the skin, bone, and joints but, as mentioned, can occur at any body site.

LYME DISEASE

■ *Lyme disease is a chronic, systemic infection that begins with a characteristic skin lesion and later manifests as cardiac, neurologic, or joint disturbances.* The causative agent is *Borrelia burgdorferi*, a large spirochete. *B. burgdorferi* is transmitted from its animal reservoir to humans through the bite of the minute *Ixodes* tick. The insect is found in wooded areas, where it usually feeds on mice and deer. Disease is concentrated in three areas: (1) along the eastern seaboard, from Maryland to Massachusetts; (2) in the Midwest, in Minnesota and Wisconsin; and (3) in the West, in California and Oregon.

□ **Pathology and Clinical Features:** *B. burgdorferi* reproduces locally at the site of inoculation, spreads to the regional lymph nodes, and disseminates throughout the body in the bloodstream. *B. burgdorferi* incites a nonspecific, chronic inflammatory infiltrate composed of lymphocytes and plasma cells. Lyme disease is a prolonged illness with three distinct stages:

- **Stage 1.** A distinctive feature of the first stage of Lyme disease is the characteristic skin lesion, **erythema chronicum migrans,** which appears at the site of the tick bite. This begins as an erythematous macule or papule, which then grows to become an erythematous patch 5 to 50 cm in diameter. Erythema chronicum migrans is accompanied by fever, fatigue, headache, arthralgias, and regional lymphadenopathy. Treatment with tetracycline or erythromycin is effective in eliminating early Lyme disease.

- **Stage 2.** The second stage of Lyme disease begins within several weeks to months of the skin lesion and is characterized by migratory musculoskeletal pains as well as cardiac and neurologic abnormalities.
- **Stage 3.** The third stage of Lyme disease begins months to years after the tick bite and is manifested by joint, skin, and neurologic abnormalities. Joint abnormalities develop in more than half of infected persons and include severe arthritis of the large joints, especially the knee.

Chlamydia

Chlamydiae are obligate, intracellular parasites that are smaller than most other bacteria.

CHLAMYDIA TRACHOMATIS

Genital and Neonatal Diseases

■ *Chlamydia trachomatis causes a genital epithelial infection that is now among the most common sexually transmitted diseases in developed countries.* In men. the infection produces urethritis and, sometimes, epididymitis or proctitis. In women, the infection usually begins with cervicitis, which can progress to endometritis, salpingitis, and generalized infection of the pelvic adnexal organs (pelvic inflammatory disease). Repeated infections of the fallopian tubes are particularly associated with scarring, which may interfere with the passage of sperm or fertilized ova and result in infertility or ectopic pregnancy.

☐ **Pathology:** Chlamydial infection incites an inflammatory infiltrate of neutrophils and lymphocytes. In newborns, the conjunctival epithelium often contains characteristic vacuolar cytoplasmic inclusions, and the disease is frequently called **inclusion conjunctivitis.**

Lymphogranuloma Venereum

■ *Lymphogranuloma venereum is a sexually transmitted chlamydial disease that begins as a genital ulcer, progresses to a local necrotizing lymphadenitis, and may eventuate in local scarring.* The infection is uncommon in developed countries but is endemic in the tropics and subtropics. In North America and Europe, lymphogranuloma venereum is now primarily a disease of homosexual men.

☐ **Pathology:** The organism is introduced through a break in the skin. After an incubation period of 4 to 21 days, an ulcer appears, usually on the penis, vagina, or cervix, although the lips, tongue, and fingers may also be primary sites. The organisms are transported by the lymphatics to the regional lymph nodes, where a necrotizing lymphadenitis erupts from 1 to 3 weeks after the primary lesion. The necrotizing process produces enlarged and matted lymph nodes, containing multiple, coalescing abscesses that often develop a stellate shape. These abscesses have a granulomatous appearance, containing neutrophils and necrotic debris in the center that are surrounded by palisading epithelioid cells, macrophages, and occasional giant cells. The abscesses are rimmed by lymphocytes, plasma cells, and fibrous tissue. The nodal architecture is eventually effaced by fibrosis.

☐ **Clinical Features:** Most infections resolve completely, even without antimicrobial therapy. However, progressive ulceration of the penis, urethra, or scrotum, with fistulas and urethral stricture, develops in 5% of men. Women and homosexual men often present with hemorrhagic proctitis, and the large majority of late complications, such as rectal stricture, rectovaginal fistulas, and genital elephantiasis, occur in women. Tetracycline is recommended for treatment of acute lymphogranuloma venereum.

Trachoma

■ *Trachoma is a chronic chlamydial infection of the conjunctiva that progressively scars the conjunctiva and cornea and is a leading cause of blindness in many underdeveloped countries.* Trachoma occurs worldwide, is associated with poverty, and is most prevalent in dry or sandy regions. It remains a major problem in parts of Africa, India, and the Middle East. In endemic areas, infection is acquired during early childhood, becomes chronic, and eventually, progresses to blindness.

☐ **Pathology:** *Chlamydia trachomatis* is inoculated into the eye by contact, and the organism reproduces within the conjunctival epithelium, thereby inciting a mixed acute and chronic inflammatory infiltrate. Progressive scarring distorts the eyelids so that they abrade the cornea, and the distorted eye is subject to secondary bacterial infections. If not interrupted, this process of chronic inflammation, scarring, mechanical distortion, abrasion, and secondary bacterial infection eventuates in blindness.

PSITTACOSIS (ORNITHOSIS)

■ *Psittacosis is a self-limited, pneumonic illness transmitted to humans from birds.* The causative agent, *Chlamydia psittaci*, is spread by infected birds, and the resulting disease is known as both psittacosis (because of its association with parrots) or ornithosis (because of its association with birds in general). *C. psittaci* is present in the blood, tissues, excreta, and feathers of infected birds. Humans inhale the infectious excreta or dust from feathers.

□ Pathology: *C. psittaci* first infects the pulmonary macrophages, which carry the organism to the phagocytic cells of the liver and spleen, where it then reproduces. The organism is distributed from the liver and spleen by the bloodstream, thereby producing systemic infection, particularly diffuse involvement of the lungs. The pneumonia is predominantly interstitial, and the inflammatory infiltrate within the alveolar septa is composed largely of lymphocytes. Dissemination of the infection, which may be fatal, is characterized by foci of necrosis in the liver and spleen and by diffuse mononuclear cell infiltrates in the heart, kidneys, and brain. The mortality rate of psittacosis during the preantibiotic era exceeded 20%, but since the advent of tetracycline therapy, the disease is only rarely fatal.

Rickettsiae

Rickettsiae are small, Gram-negative coccobacillary bacteria that are obligate, intracellular pathogens. Humans are accidental hosts for most species of *Rickettsia*. The organisms reside in animals and insects and do not require humans for perpetuation. Human rickettsial infection results from insect bites.

Several species of *Rickettsia* cause different human diseases (Table 9-3), but rickettsial infections have many features in common. **The human target cell for all rickettsiae is the endothelial cell of the capillaries and other small blood vessels.** The organisms reproduce within these cells, killing them in the process and producing a necrotizing vasculitis.

ROCKY MOUNTAIN SPOTTED FEVER

■ *Rocky Mountain spotted fever is an acute, potentially fatal, systemic vasculitis usually manifested by headache, fever, and rash.* The causative organism, *Rickettsia rickettsii*, is transmitted to humans by tick bites. The infection occurs in various areas throughout North, Central, and South America. In the United States, most cases occur in a large cluster of states extending from the eastern seaboard (Georgia to New York) westward to Texas, Oklahoma, and Kansas. Cases in the Rocky Mountain region itself are uncommon.

The vascular lesions of Rocky Mountain spotted fever are found throughout the body and affect the capillaries, venules, arterioles, and sometimes, larger vessels. There is necrosis and reactive hyperplasia of the vascular endothelium, often associated with thrombosis of the smaller-caliber vessels, as well as microscopic infarctions and extravasation of blood into the surrounding tissues.

The rash of Rocky Mountain spotted fever begins as a maculopapular eruption, but it rapidly becomes petechial, spreading centripetally from the distal extremities to the trunk. If untreated, more than 20% to 50% of infected persons die. Prompt diagnosis and antibiotic treatment is lifesaving, and in the United States, the mortality rate has been reduced to less than 5%.

T A B L E 9-3. **Rickettsial Infections**

Disease	Organism	Distribution	Transmission
		Spotted-Fever Group	
Rocky Mountain spotted fever	*R. rickettsii*	Americas	Ticks
Queensland tick fever	*R. australis*	Australia	Ticks
Londonneuse fever, Kenya tick fever	*R. conorii*	Mediterranean, Africa, India	Ticks
Siberian tick fever	*R. sibirica*	Siberia, Mongolia	Ticks
Rickettsialpox	*R. akari*	United States, former Soviet Union, Korea, Africa	Mites
		Typhus Group	
Louse-borne typhus (epidemic typhus)	*R. prowazekii*	Latin America, Africa, Asia	Lice
Murine typhus (endemic typhus)	*R. typhi*	Worldwide	Fleas
Scrub typhus	*R. tsutsugamushi*	South Pacific, Asia	Mites
Q fever	*Coxiella burnetii*	Worldwide	Inhalation

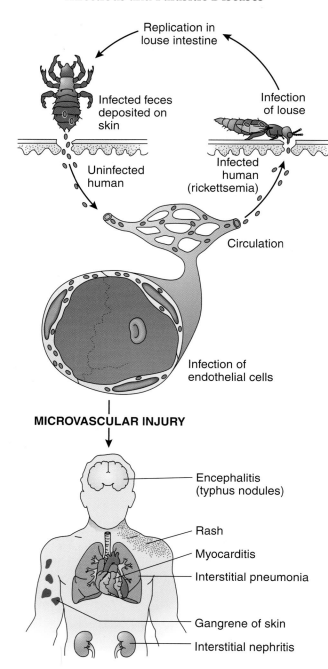

Replication in louse intestine

Infection of louse

Infected feces deposited on skin

Uninfected human

Infected human (rickettsemia)

Circulation

Infection of endothelial cells

MICROVASCULAR INJURY

Encephalitis (typhus nodules)

Rash

Myocarditis

Interstitial pneumonia

Gangrene of skin

Interstitial nephritis

FIGURE 9-7

Epidemic typhus (louse-borne typhus). *R. prowazekii* has a human-louse-human life cycle. The organism multiplies in endothelial cells, which detach, rupture, and release organisms into the circulation (rickettsemia). A louse taking a blood meal becomes infected with rickettsiae, which then enter the epithelial cells of its midgut, multiply, and rupture the cells, thereby releasing rickettsiae into the lumen of the louse intestine. Contaminated feces are deposited on the skin or clothing of a second host and either penetrate an abrasion or are inhaled. The rickettsiae then enter the endothelial cells, multiply, and rupture the cells, thus completing the cycle.

EPIDEMIC (LOUSE-BORNE) TYPHUS

■ *Epidemic typhus is a severe, systemic vasculitis transmitted by the bite of infected lice.* The disease is caused by *Rickettsia prowazekii*, an organism that has a human-louse-human life cycle (Fig. 9-7). The disease is widely distributed in some regions of Africa, Asia, Europe, and the Western Hemisphere. Devastating epidemics of typhus were associated with cold climates, poor sanitation, and crowding during natural disasters, famine, or war. Infrequent bathing and lack of changes of cloth-

ing lead to louse infestation of human populations and, consequently, epidemics of typhus. With the mass displacements of populations in Eastern Europe during World War I, epidemic typhus affected more than 30 million persons—and killed more than 3 million.

Epidemic typhus begins with localized infection of the capillary endothelium, and it progresses to a systemic vasculitis. The pathologic changes produced by *R. prowazekii* are similar to those of Rocky Mountain spotted fever and the other rickettsial diseases. Dying patients may exhibit the symptoms of encephalitis, myocarditis, interstitial pneumonia, interstitial nephritis, and shock.

Epidemic typhus can be controlled by large-scale delousing of the population using steam sterilization of clothing and insecticides. Typhus is treated with tetracycline or chloramphenicol.

Mycoplasma

Mycoplasmas, formerly known as pleuropneumonia-like organisms, are the smallest free-living prokaryotes, measuring less than 0.3 μm in the greatest dimension. *Mycoplasma pneumoniae* causes acute, self-limited, lower respiratory tract infections (tracheobronchitis and pneumonia), affecting mostly children and young adults. Most infections occur in small groups of persons who have frequent close contact, such as families, college fraternities, military units, and residents of closed institutions. The organism is spread by aerosol transmission from person to person over a period of several months, with an attack rate of greater than 50% within the group. Infection with *M. pneumoniae* occurs worldwide, and in developed countries, the organism causes 15% to 20% of all pneumonias.

☐ **Pathology:** Pneumonia caused by *M. pneumoniae* usually shows patchy consolidation of a single segment of a lower lung lobe, although the process can be more widespread. The alveoli display a largely interstitial process, with reactive alveolar lining cells and infiltration by mononuclear cells. The pneumonia tends to be milder than other bacterial pneumonias, which has earned the disease the appellation "walking pneumonia." Death from *M. pneumoniae* infection is rare, and the infection itself is treated with tetracycline or erythromycin.

Mycobacteria

Mycobacteria are distinctive organisms, from 2 to 10 μm in length, that share the cell wall architecture of Gram-positive bacteria. The waxy lipids of the cell wall make mycobacteria "acid fast"—that is, they retain carbolfuchsin after rinsing with acid alcohol.

Mycobacteria grow more slowly than other pathogenic bacteria, and mycobacterial diseases are all chronic, slowly progressive illnesses.

TUBERCULOSIS

Tuberculosis is a chronic, communicable disease caused principally by *Mycobacterium tuberculosis hominis* (Koch bacillus) but also occasionally by *M. tuberculosis bovis*. The lungs are the prime target, but any organ may be infected. Tuberculous diseases are discussed in detail in Chapters 12 and 13.

LEPROSY

■ *Leprosy (Hansen disease), an infection caused by* Mycobacterium leprae, *is a chronic, slowly progressive, destructive process involving the peripheral nerves, skin, and mucous membranes.* Leprosy is transmitted from person to person. However, years of close contact with an infected person are required for successful transmission of the disease. Leprosy is now rare in developed countries, but 15 million persons are infected worldwide, primarily in tropical areas.

Tuberculoid Leprosy

■ *Tuberculoid leprosy occurs in infected persons who manifest an effective immune granulomatous response that limits both proliferation of the bacillus and the extent of the disease.*

☐ **Pathology:** Tuberculoid leprosy is characterized by a single lesion (or by very few lesions) of the skin. Microscopically, they show well-formed, circumscribed dermal granulomas, which are composed of epithelioid macrophages, Langhans giant cells, and lymphocytes. Nerve fibers are almost invariably swollen and infiltrated with lymphocytes. The granulomas of leprosy lack caseous necrosis.

☐ **Clinical Features:** The skin lesions of tuberculoid leprosy on the face, extremities, or trunk appear as well-demarcated, hypopigmented or erythematous, dry, hairless patches, with raised outer edges. Nerve involvement causes diminished sensation or numbness within the patch. In contrast to lepromatous leprosy, the lesions of tuberculoid leprosy cause minimal disfigurement and are not infectious.

Lepromatous Leprosy

■ *Lepromatous leprosy occurs in persons who fail to develop an adequate immune response to the lepra bacillus.* This variant exhibits multiple, tumor-like lesions of the skin, eyes, testes, nerves, lymph nodes, and spleen. Nodular or diffuse infiltrates of foamy macrophages contain myriads of bacilli (Fig. 9-8). If unchecked, the dermal infiltrates expand slowly to distort and disfigure the face, ears, and upper airway and to destroy the eyes, eyebrows and eyelashes, nerves, and testes.

☐ **Clinical Features:** The nodular skin lesions of lepromatous leprosy sometimes ulcerate. Claw-shaped hands, hammertoes, saddle nose, and pendulous ear lobes are common deformities. Nodular lesions of the face may coalesce to produce a lion-like appearance

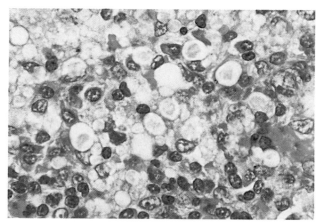

FIGURE   *9-8*
Lepromatous leprosy. A section of skin shows a tumor-like mass of foamy macrophages. The faint masses within the vacuolated macrophages are enormous numbers of lepra bacilli.

(leonine facies). The most commonly used drug, dapsone, effectively eliminates the lepra bacilli in 4 to 5 years, but administration must be continued indefinitely.

Fungi

Of more than 100,000 known fungi, only a few invade and destroy human tissue, and of these, most are opportunists—that is, they infect only persons with impaired immune mechanisms. **Thus, corticosteroid administration, antineoplastic therapy, and congenital or acquired T-cell deficiencies all predispose to mycotic infections.**

CANDIDA

The genus *Candida,* which comprises more than 20 species of yeasts, includes the most common opportunistic pathogens. Although the various forms of candidiasis vary in clinical severity, most are localized, superficial diseases limited to a particular mucocutaneous site. They include:

- **Intertrigo:** infection of opposed skin surfaces
- **Paronychia:** infection of the nail bed
- **Diaper Rash**
- **Vulvovaginitis**
- **Thrush:** oral infection
- **Esophagitis**

Candidal infections of the deep tissues are much less common than superficial infections, but they can be life-threatening. Antibiotic use is the most common

precipitating factor for candidiasis owing to suppression of the competing bacterial flora. The most common deep sites to be affected are the brain, eye, kidney, and heart. Candidal sepsis and disseminated candidiasis occur only in immunologically compromised persons and are often fatal. Candidal infections of specific organs are discussed in the appropriate chapters.

ASPERGILLOSIS

Aspergillus species are common environmental fungi that produce opportunistic infections, usually involving the lungs. One species, *A. fumigatus,* is by far the most frequent human pathogen. *Aspergillus* is present throughout the world, growing as saprophytes in soil, decaying plant matter, and dung. Pulmonary aspergillosis is acquired by inhalation of environmental organisms. The fungus reproduces by releasing numerous small (2–3 μm) spores, known as conidia, that are carried in the air and into almost every human environment. The pathology of pulmonary aspergillosis is described in Chapter 12.

CRYPTOCOCCOSIS

■ *Cryptococcosis is a systemic mycosis caused by* Cryptococcus neoformans *that principally affects the lungs and meninges.* The main reservoir for the fungus is pigeon droppings. The inhaled organisms penetrate to the terminal bronchioles. **Cryptococcosis almost exclusively affects persons with impaired cell-mediated immunity,** including patients with AIDS, lymphomas, Hodgkin's disease, leukemias, and sarcoidosis and patients receiving high doses of corticosteroids.

☐ **Pathology:** More than 95% of cryptococcal infections involve the meninges and brain. Lesions in the lungs can be demonstrated in half the patients. Cryptococcosis in the lung may present as diffuse disease or as isolated areas of consolidation. Affected alveoli are distended by clusters of organisms, usually with minimal associated inflammation. Because of its thick capsule, *C. neoformans* stains poorly with the routine hematoxylin-and-eosin stain and appears as bubbles or holes in tissue sections (Fig. 9-9).

In cryptococcal meningoencephalitis, the entire brain is swollen and soft, and the leptomeninges are thickened and gelatinous owing to infiltration by the thickly encapsulated organisms. Untreated cryptococcal meningitis is invariably fatal, and therapy requires

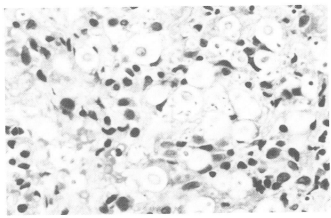
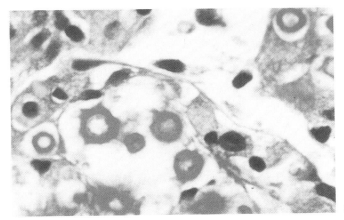

FIGURE   9-9
Cryptococcosis. (A) In a section of lung stained with hematoxylin and eosin, *C. neoformans* appears as holes or bubbles. (B) The same section stained with mucicarmine illustrates the capsule of the organism.

prolonged, systemic administration of antifungal medication.

HISTOPLASMOSIS

■ *Histoplasmosis is a worldwide, systemic mycosis caused by* Histoplasma *capsulatum that, in some respects, resembles tuberculosis.* Most cases (95%) of histoplasmosis are acute, self-limited lung infections and are completely asymptomatic. Progressive, disseminated infections do occur, however, in persons with impaired cell-mediated immunity.

Histoplasmosis is acquired by inhalation of infectious spores of *H. capsulatum*. The reservoir for the fungus is bird droppings and the soil. In the Americas, hyperendemic areas are the eastern and central United States, western Mexico, Central America, the northern countries of South America, and Argentina.

Histoplasmosis resembles tuberculosis in many ways. *Histoplasma* granulomas undergo caseation, develop progressively thicker fibrous capsules, and often, eventually calcify. The pathology of histoplasmosis is described in Chapter 12.

COCCIDIOIDOMYCOSIS

■ *Coccidioidomycosis is a chronic, necrotizing mycotic infection that both clinically and pathologically resembles tuberculosis.* The disease, caused by *Coccidioides immitis*, includes a spectrum of infections that begin as focal pneumonitis (Fig. 9-10). Most are mild, asymptomatic, and limited to the lungs and regional lymph nodes. Occasionally, *C. immitis* infections spread outside the lungs to produce life-threatening disease. The pathology of pulmonary coccidioidomycosis is discussed in Chapter 12.

Coccidioides immitis is present in the soil of restricted climatic regions, particularly the Lower Sonoran life zones of the Western Hemisphere. These are areas with sparse rainfall, hot summers, and mild winters. In the United States, large portions of California, Arizona, New Mexico, and Texas are a natural habitat for *C. immitis*.

A broad spectrum of illness ranges from acute, self-limited disease to disseminated infections. **The large majority of infections are produced by small inoculums of organisms in immunologically competent hosts and are both acute and self-limited.**

Disseminated coccidioidomycosis occurs in immunocompromised persons, either from a primary infection or from reactivation of old disease. Patients with lymphomas, leukemias, or AIDS and those receiving immunosuppressive therapy are at risk of dissemination. Certain racial groups, including Filipinos, other Asians, and blacks, are particularly susceptible to dissemination of coccidioidomycosis, probably because of a specific immunologic defect.

BLASTOMYCOSIS

■ *Blastomycosis is a chronic granulomatous and suppurative disease of the lungs and is often followed by dissemination to other body sites, principally the skin and bone.* The causative organism is *Blastomyces dermatitidis*, a dimorphic fungus that grows as a mold in warm, moist soil that is rich in decaying vegetable matter. In North America, the fungus is endemic along the distributions

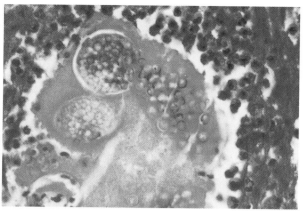

FIGURE   *9-10*
Coccidioidomycosis. A photomicrograph of the lung from a patient with acute coccidioidal pneumonia shows an acute inflammatory infiltrate surrounding spherules and endospores of *C. immitis*.

of the Mississippi and Ohio Rivers, the Great Lakes, and the St. Lawrence River.

☐ **Pathology:** Blastomycosis is usually confined to the lungs, where the infection most frequently produces small areas of pulmonary consolidation. *B. dermatitidis* incites a mixed suppurative and granulomatous inflammatory response, and even in the same patient, lesions may range from neutrophilic abscesses to epithelioid granulomas. The pulmonary disease usually resolves by scarring, but some patients develop progressive miliary lesions or cavities. When infection spreads outside the lungs, the skin (>50%), bones (>10%), and prostate are common sites of involvement.

Protozoal Infections

Protozoa cause human disease by diverse mechanisms. Some, such as *Entamoeba histolytica*, are extracellular parasites capable of digesting and invading human tissues. Others, such as the plasmodia, are obligate, intracellular parasites that replicate within human cells, thereby killing them. Still others, such as the trypanosomes, damage human tissue largely through the inflammatory and immunologic responses they incite. Some of the protozoa, such as *Toxoplasma gondii*, have the capacity to establish latent infections and produce reactivation disease among immunosuppressed hosts.

MALARIA

■ *Malaria is a mosquito-borne, hemolytic, febrile illness, which is one of the world's major health problems.* Malaria infects more than 200 million persons and yearly kills more than 1 million. Four species of *Plasmodium* cause malaria: (1) *P. falciparum*, (2) *P. vivax*, (3) *P. ovale*, and (4) *P. malariae*. These plasmodia all infect and destroy human erythrocytes, thereby producing chills, fever, anemia, and splenomegaly. *P. falciparum* causes more severe disease than the other plasmodial species, however, and accounts for most malarial deaths. Malaria has been eradicated in most developed countries but continues to be a scourge in tropical and subtropical areas, especially tropical Africa, parts of South and Central America, India, and Southeast Asia. Malaria is transmitted from person to person by the bite of the female *Anopheles* mosquito (Fig. 9-11).

The rupture of infected erythrocytes causes the chills and fever of malaria through release of as-yet-unidentified pyrogenic material. Anemia results both from the rupture of circulating infected erythrocytes and from the sequestration of cells in the enlarging spleen. Hepatosplenomegaly reflects the response of the fixed mononuclear phagocytes of the liver and spleen to the parasitism and destruction of the erythrocytes.

☐ **Pathology:** In all forms of malaria, the spleen and liver enlarge as erythrocytes are sequestered by the fixed mononuclear macrophage system. In falciparum malaria, capillaries of the deep organs become obstructed, thereby leading to ischemia of the brain, kidneys, and lungs. The brains of persons who die of cerebral malaria show congestion and thrombosis of small blood vessels in the white matter, which are rimmed with edema and hemorrhage ("ring hemorrhages") (Fig. 9-12). Obstruction of blood flow in the kidney produces acute renal failure, whereas intravascular hemolysis leads to hemoglobinuric nephrosis ("blackwater fever").

☐ **Clinical Features:** Recurrent bouts of chills and high fever, known as paroxysms, are characteristic of malaria. Paroxysms recur for weeks, eventually subsiding as the infected person mounts an immunologic response. Infection with *P. falciparum* frequently produces much graver disease than the other forms of malaria. Central nervous system disease is dangerous, with a mortality rate of 20% to 50%. Malarias other than falciparum malaria are treated with oral chloroquine, sometimes with the addition of primaquine. Therapy for falciparum malaria varies according to the likelihood of chloroquine resistance.

TOXOPLASMOSIS

■ *Toxoplasmosis is a worldwide disease caused by* Toxoplasma gondii. *Most infections are asymptomatic, but when they occur in the fetus or an immunocompromised host, devastating necrotizing disease may result.* In some areas (e.g., Paris), the prevalence of *T. gondii* infection exceeds 80% of adults, whereas in other (e.g., the southwestern part of the United States), only a small portion of the population is infected.

Toxoplasma gondii infects the cat's intestinal epithelium. In the tropics, where children are predominantly infected, oocysts in contaminated soil are the principal source of infection. By contrast, in developed countries the ingestion of incompletely cooked meat (lamb and pork) containing *Toxoplasma* tissue cysts is the major mechanism of infection. Another source of infection is cat feces. Oocysts contaminate the hands and food of persons who live in close association with cats. Congenital infection is acquired by transplacental transmission of infectious forms from an acutely infected (usually asymptomatic) mother to the fetus.

In most *T. gondii* **infections, little significant tissue destruction occurs before the immunologic response brings the active phase of the infection under control, and infected persons suffer few clinical effects.** *T. gondii* establishes latent infection, however, by forming dormant tissue cysts in some infected cells. If the infected person loses cell-mediated immunity, the organism can emerge from its encysted form and re-establish a destructive infection.

Congenital *Toxoplasma* Infections

Infection with *T. gondii* **in a fetus is much more destructive than in a child or adult.** The developing brain and eyes are readily infected, and the fetus lacks the immunologic capacity to contain the infection. Central nervous system infection produces a necrotizing meningoencephalitis, which, in the most severe cases, results in the loss of brain parenchyma, cerebral calcifications, and marked hydrocephalus (Fig. 9-13). Ocular infection causes chorioretinitis (necrosis and inflammation of the choroid and retina).

Toxoplasmosis in Immunocompromised Hosts

Devastating *T. gondii* infections occur in persons with decreased cell-mediated immunity (e.g., patients with AIDS or those immunosuppressed for transplantation). In most cases, the disease represents a reactivation of latent infection. In the brain, which is the most commonly affected organ, infection with *T. gondii* produces a multifocal necrotizing encephalitis.

PNEUMOCYSTIS CARINII Pneumonia

■ *Pneumocystis carinii causes progressive, often fatal pneumonias in persons with severely impaired cell-mediated immunity and is the most common serious opportunistic pathogen in persons with AIDS.* P. carinii is distributed worldwide, and because 75% of the population have acquired antibodies by 5 years of age, it is reasonable to assume the organisms are inhaled regularly by all. In persons with intact cell-mediated immunity, *P. carinii* infection is rapidly contained, without producing symptoms. **However, 80% of all patients with AIDS develop** *P. carinii* **pneumonia during the course of their illness.**

☐ **Pathogenesis:** *P. carinii* reproduces in intimate association with alveolar type 1 lining cells, and active disease is confined to the lungs. Infection begins with attachment of the *Pneumocystis* trophozoite to the alveolar lining cell. The trophozoite feeds on the host cell, enlarges, and transforms into the cyst form, which contains daughter organisms. The cyst then ruptures to release new trophozoites, which, in turn, attach to additional alveolar lining cells. If the process is not checked by the host immune system or antibiotic therapy, the infected alveoli eventually fill with organisms and proteinaceous fluid. The progressive filling of alveoli prevents adequate gas exchange, and the patient slowly suffocates. The pathology of *P. carinii* pneumonia is discussed in Chapter 12.

AMEBIASIS

■ *Amebiasis refers to an infection with* Entamoeba histolytica, *the most important intestinal ameba of humans.* Humans are the principal reservoir for *E. histolytica*, which reproduces in the human colon and passes in the feces. **Amebiasis is acquired by ingestion of materials contaminated with human feces** (Fig. 9-14).

Intestinal Amebiasis

☐ **Pathology:** Amebic lesions begin as small foci of necrosis, which progress to ulcers. Undermining of the

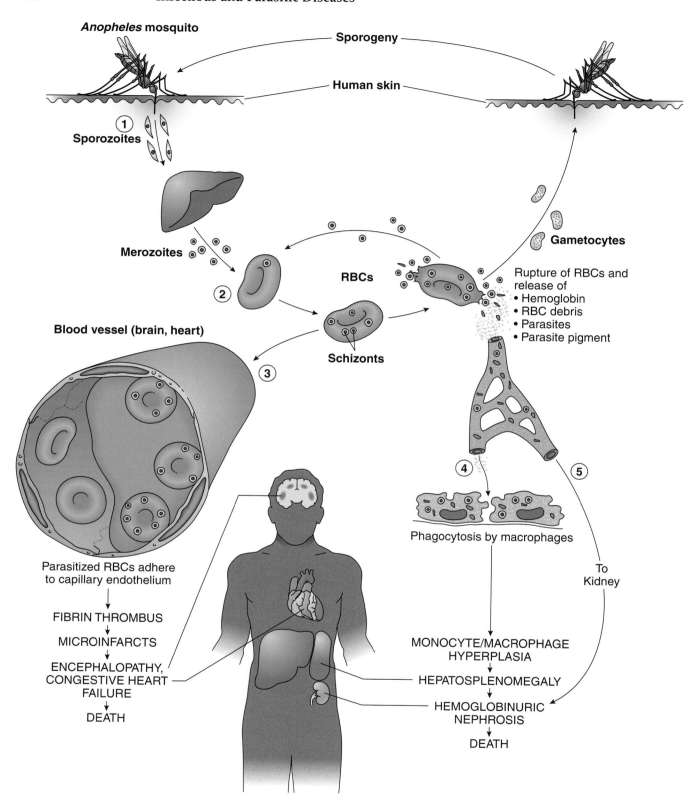

Anopheles mosquito

Sporogeny

Human skin

1 Sporozoites

Merozoites

RBCs

2

Gametocytes

Rupture of RBCs and release of
• Hemoglobin
• RBC debris
• Parasites
• Parasite pigment

Blood vessel (brain, heart)

Schizonts

3

Phagocytosis by macrophages

To Kidney

4

5

Parasitized RBCs adhere
to capillary endothelium

↓

FIBRIN THROMBUS

↓

MICROINFARCTS

↓

ENCEPHALOPATHY,
CONGESTIVE HEART
FAILURE

↓

DEATH

MONOCYTE/MACROPHAGE
HYPERPLASIA

↓

HEPATOSPLENOMEGALY

↓

HEMOGLOBINURIC
NEPHROSIS

↓

DEATH

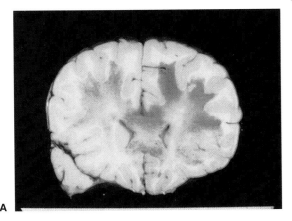

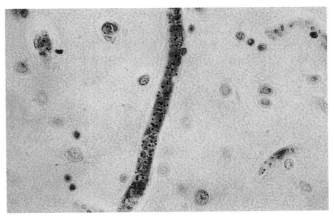

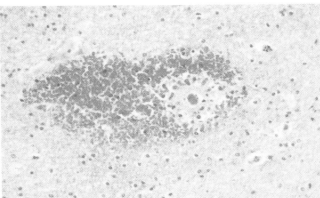

FIGURE 9-12

Acute falciparum malaria of the brain. (A) There is severe diffuse congestion of the white matter and focal hemorrhages. (B) A section of *panel A* shows a capillary packed with parasitized erythrocytes. (C) Another section of *panel A* displays a ring hemorrhage around a thrombosed capillary, which contains parasitized erythrocytes in a fibrin thrombus.

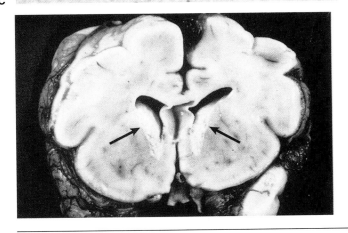

FIGURE 9-13

Congenital toxoplasmosis. The brain of a premature infant reveals subependymal necrosis, with calcification appearing as bilaterally symmetric areas of whitish discoloration (*arrows*).

FIGURE 9-11

Life cycle of malaria. An *Anopheles* mosquito bites an infected person, taking blood that contains micro- and macrogametocytes (sexual forms). In the mosquito, sexual multiplication ("sporogony") produces infective sporozoites in the salivary glands. (1) During the mosquito bite, sporozoites are inoculated into the bloodstream of the vertebrate host. Some sporozoites leave the blood and enter the hepatocytes, where they multiply asexually (exoerythrocytic schizogony) and form thousands of uninucleated merozoites. (2) Rupture of hepatocytes releases merozoites, which penetrate erythrocytes and become trophozoites, which then divide to form numerous schizonts (intraerythrocytic schizogony). In turn, schizonts divide to form more merozoites, which are released by the rupture of erythrocytes and re-enter other erythrocytes to begin a new cycle. After several cycles, subpopulations of merozoites develop into micro- and macrogametocytes, which are taken up by another mosquito to complete the cycle. (3) Parasitized erythrocytes obstruct capillaries of the brain, heart, kidney, and other deep organs. Adherence of parasitized erythrocytes to capillary endothelial cells causes fibrin thrombi, which produce microinfarcts. These result in encephalopathy, congestive heart failure, pulmonary edema, and frequently, death. Ruptured erythrocytes release hemoglobin, erythrocyte debris, and malarial pigment. (4) Phagocytosis leads to reticuloendothelial hyperplasia and hepatosplenomegaly. (5) Released hemoglobin produces hemoglobinuric nephrosis, which may be fatal.

ulcer margin and confluence of the expanding ulcers lead to sloughing of the mucosa in broad, irregular, geographic patterns. The ulcer bed is gray, necrotic, and composed of fibrin and cellular debris. The exudate raises the undermined mucosa, producing chronic amebic ulcers with a shape described as resembling a flask or a bottleneck.

Trophozoites are found on the surface of the ulcer, in the exudate, and in the crater. They are also frequent in the submucosa, muscularis, serosa, and small veins of the submucosa. There is little inflammatory response in early amebic ulcers. However, as the ulcer enlarges, there is an accumulation of neutrophils, lymphocytes, macrophages, plasma cells, and sometimes, eosinophils.

☐ **Clinical Features:** Intestinal amebiasis ranges from completely asymptomatic infection to severe dysenterial disease. Liquid stools (as many as 25 a day) contain bloody mucus, and prolonged diarrhea may result in dehydration. Amebic colitis often persists for months or years, and patients may become emaciated and anemic. In severe amebic colitis, massive destruction of the colonic mucosa may lead to fatal hemorrhage, perforation, or peritonitis. Therapy for intestinal amebiasis includes metronidazole, which acts against trophozoites, and diloxanide, which is effective against cysts.

Extraintestinal Amebiasis

☐ **Pathology: Liver abscess** is a major complication of intestinal amebiasis. *E. histolytica* trophozoites that have invaded into submucosal veins of the colon can enter the portal circulation and reach the liver. There, the organisms kill hepatocytes, producing a slowly expanding abscess filled with a dark-brown, odorless, semisolid material reported to resemble anchovy paste in consistency (Fig. 9-15). An amebic liver abscess may expand and rupture through the capsule, thereby extending into the peritoneum, diaphragm, pleural cavity, lungs, or pericardium. Extraintestinal amebiasis is treated with metronidazole and diloxanide.

GIARDIASIS

■ *Giardiasis is an infection of the small intestine caused by the flagellated protozoan* Giardia lamblia *and is characterized by abdominal cramping and diarrhea.* Giardiasis is acquired by ingestion of infectious cyst forms of the organism, which are shed in the feces of infected humans and animals. Infection spreads directly from person to person and in contaminated water or food. *Giardia* can be acquired from wilderness water sources, where infected animals, such as beavers and bears, serve as the reservoir of infection.

Giardia lamblia trophozoites are most numerous in the duodenum and upper small intestine. Microscopic examination shows *Giardia* trophozoites on the surface of villi and within crypts, with minimal associated mucosal changes. In some patients, symptoms resolve spontaneously in 1 to 4 weeks. Others complain for months of persistent abdominal cramping and poorly formed stools. The infection is effectively treated with various antibiotics, including metronidazole.

LEISHMANIASIS

■ *Leishmaniasis refers to a spectrum of clinical syndromes ranging from indolent, self-resolving, cutaneous ulcers to fatal disseminated disease.* Leishmania *are protozoans transmitted to humans by the bites of* Phlebotomus *sandflies, which acquire infection by feeding on infected animals.* In many subtropical and tropical areas, leishmanial infection is endemic in animal populations, which serve as a reservoir for infection.

Visceral Leishmaniasis (Kala-Azar)

■ *Visceral leishmaniasis, or kala-azar, is a disseminated infection produced by several subspecies of* Leishmania donovani.

☐ **Pathology:** Infection with *L. donovani* begins with a localized collection of infected macrophages at the

FIGURE　*9-14*

Amebic colitis and its complications. Amebiasis results from ingestion of food or water contaminated with amebic cysts. In the colon, amebae penetrate the mucosa and produce a flask-shaped ulcer of the mucosa and submucosa. The organisms may invade submucosal venules, thereby disseminating the infection to the liver and other organs. The liver abscess can also expand to involve adjacent structures.

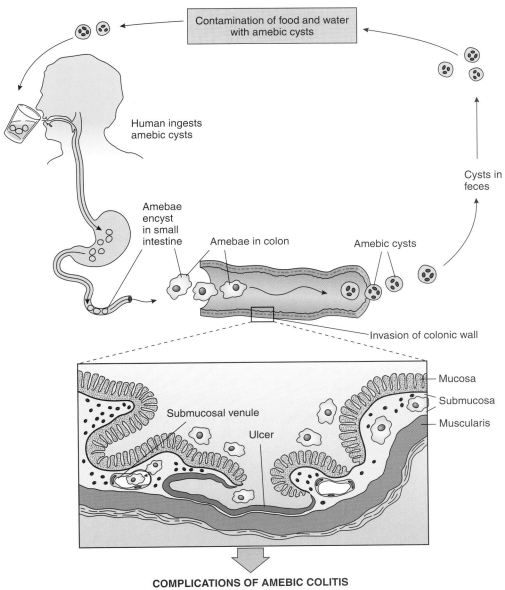

Contamination of food and water
with amebic cysts

Human ingests
amebic cysts

Amebae
encyst
in small
intestine

Amebae in colon

Amebic cysts

Cysts in
feces

Invasion of colonic wall

Mucosa

Submucosa

Muscularis

Submucosal venule

Ulcer

COMPLICATIONS OF AMEBIC COLITIS

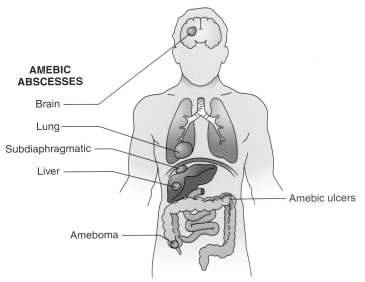

**AMEBIC
ABSCESSES**

Brain

Lung

Subdiaphragmatic

Liver

Ameboma

Amebic ulcers

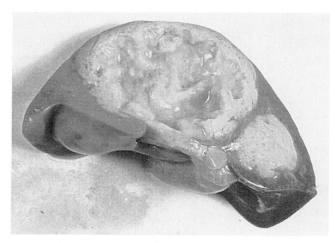

FIGURE   *9-15*
Amebic abscesses of the liver. The cut surface of the liver shows multiple abscesses containing "anchovy paste" material.

site of a sandfly bite. Unlike other leishmanial infections, in this case infected macrophages spread the organisms throughout the mononuclear macrophage system. Most infected persons destroy *L. donovani* by a cell-mediated immune response, but 5% of those infected cannot contain the organisms and develop disseminated disease.

In kala-azar, the liver, spleen, lymph nodes, and bone marrow become massively enlarged as the mononuclear phagocytes in these organs fill with proliferating leishmanial amastigotes. During the course of months, the patient with visceral leishmaniasis becomes profoundly cachectic, and the spleen enlarges massively. If untreated, the disease is invariably fatal. Treatment entails systemic antiprotozoal therapy.

CHAGAS DISEASE (AMERICAN TRYPANOSOMIASIS)

■ *Chagas disease is an insect-borne, zoonotic infection by the protozoan* Trypanosoma cruzi, *which causes a systemic infection of humans characterized by acute manifestations and delayed cardiac and gastrointestinal dysfunction.* T. cruzi infection is endemic among wild and domesticated animals in Central and South America, where the parasite is transmitted by the reduviid ("kissing") bug.

The most frequent and serious consequences of infection with *T. cruzi* develop years or decades after the acute infection. In this phase of the disease, *T. cruzi* is no longer present in the blood or tissue. Infected organs have been damaged, however, by a chronic, progressive inflammatory process.

Chronic myocarditis is characterized by a dilated heart. Microscopically, there is extensive interstitial fibrosis, hypertrophied myofibers, and focal lymphocytic inflammation, often involving the cardiac conduction system. Progressive cardiac fibrosis causes dysrhythmias or congestive heart failure.

Megaesophagus (dilatation of the esophagus caused by failure of the lower esophageal sphincter [achalasia]) is a common complication of chronic Chagas disease. It results from the destruction of parasympathetic ganglion cells in the wall of the lower esophagus, and leads to difficulty in swallowing, which may be so severe that the patient can consume only liquids.

Megacolon (massive dilatation of the large bowel) is similar to megaesophagus in that the myenteric plexus of the colon is destroyed. The progressive aganglionosis of the colon causes severe constipation.

Antiprotozoal chemotherapy is effective for acute Chagas disease but is of no value for the chronic sequelae.

AFRICAN TRYPANOSOMIASIS

■ *African trypanosomiasis, popularly termed sleeping sickness, is a chronic infection with* Trypanosoma brucei gambiense *or an acute infection with* T. brucei rhodesiense. These organisms are hemoflagellate protozoa transmitted by several species of blood-sucking tsetse flies of the genus *Glossina*.

☐ Pathology: Early in the course of the disease, there is prominent involvement of the lymph nodes and spleen, but infection eventually localizes to the small blood vessels of the central nervous system, where the replicating organisms incite a destructive vasculitis. In turn, the vasculitis of the brain and meninges produces the progressive decrease in mentation characteristic of sleeping sickness.

Helminthic Infections

Helminths, or worms, are among the most common human pathogens. Helminthic infections are acquired by ingestion, insect bites, or direct skin penetration. Eosinophils contain basic proteins toxic to some helminths and are a major component of inflammatory responses to these organisms. These cells are present in the acute infiltrates incited by helminths and in the chronic infiltrates and granulomas that form in response to helminth eggs, larvae, or adults.

Helminths are divided into three broad categories based on overall morphology and the structure of the digestive tissues:

- **Roundworms (nematodes)** are elongate, cylindrical organisms with tubular digestive tracts.
- **Flatworms (trematodes)** are dorsoventrally flattened organisms with digestive tracts that end in blind loops.
- **Tapeworms (cestodes)** are segmented organisms with separate head and body parts. They lack a digestive tract and absorb nutrients through their outer walls.

FILARIAL NEMATODES

Lymphatic Filariasis (Bancroftian and Malayan Filariasis)

■ *Lymphatic filariasis is an inflammatory, parasitic infestation of lymphatic vessels caused by the filarial roundworms* Wuchereria bancrofti *and* Brugia malayi. The adult worms inhabit the lymphatics, most frequently those in the inguinal, epitrochlear, and axillary lymph nodes, testis, and epididymis. There, they incite an inflammatory response that causes acute lymphangitis and eventual lymphatic obstruction, leading to massive lymphedema of the affected tissues (elephantiasis) (Fig. 9-16). Humans can acquire infection from the bites of at least 80 species of mosquitoes in southern Asia, the Pacific, Africa, and portions of South America. Diethylcarbamazine is the current chemotherapeutic agent of choice against lymphatic filariasis.

Onchocerciasis

■ *Onchocerciasis ("river blindness") is a chronic inflammatory disease of the skin, eyes, and lymphatics caused by the filarial nematode* Onchocerca volvulus. Blindness is the most severe consequence. *Simulium* blackflies transmit infectious larvae to humans on biting. These insects require rapidly running water for breeding, and onchocerciasis, therefore, is endemic along rivers and streams (hence the name river blindness) in parts of tropical Africa, South America, Guatemala, and Mexico. Gravid females produce millions of microfilariae, which migrate into the skin, eyes, lymph nodes, and deep organs, thereby producing the corresponding onchocercal lesions. Ocular onchocerciasis results from the migration of microfilariae into all regions of the eye, from the cornea to the optic nerve head. Systemic anthelminthic therapy, particularly with ivermectin, is effective in treating onchocerciasis.

INTESTINAL NEMATODES

Ascariasis

■ *Ascariasis refers to infection of the small intestine by the large roundworm* Ascaris lumbricoides. It is the most common helminthic infection of humans and affects one-fourth of the world's population, usually without causing symptoms. Humans acquire the infection by ingesting eggs in contaminated soil, food, or water. The worms mature in the small bowel and then live as adults within the lumen for 1 to 2 years. Adult worms (length, 15–35 cm) usually cause no pathologic changes, and patients are entirely asymptomatic. Heavy infestations may cause vomiting, malnutrition, and sometimes, intestinal obstruction. Ascaricidal drugs are effective.

Hookworms

Necator americanus and *Ancylostoma duodenale* ("hookworms") are intestinal nematodes that infect the human small bowel. These worms lacerate the bowel mucosa, thereby causing intestinal blood loss that can produce symptomatic disease in heavy infestations. Hookworm infection is commonly found among persons who walk barefoot in endemic areas.

On contact with human skin, filariform larvae in the soil directly penetrate the epidermis, enter the venous circulation, and travel to the lungs, where they lodge in alveolar capillaries. After rupturing into the alveoli, the larvae migrate up the trachea to the glottis and are then swallowed. They eventually reside in the duodenum, where they cause intestinal blood loss, resulting in anemia and hypoalbuminemia.

Strongyloidiasis

■ *Strongyloidiasis refers to a small intestinal infection with the nematode* Strongyloides stercoralis *("threadworm").* Although most cases of strongyloidiasis are asymptomatic, the infection can progress to lethal disseminated disease in immunocompromised hosts.

☐ **Pathogenesis and Pathology:** Eggs released by adult females in the intestine in turn release larvae, which are passed in the feces, become infective in the soil, and later, penetrate human skin. The rest of the cycle is similar to that of the hookworm.

Hyperinfection syndrome occurs in patients with suppressed immunity. Filariform larvae are found in the walls of the large and small intestine but may travel to any organ. The gut may exhibit ulceration, edema, and severe inflammation, and microabscesses may oc-

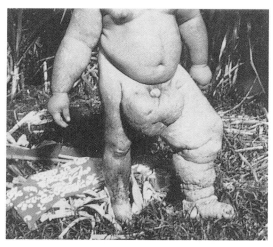

FIGURE   *9-16*
Bancroftian filariasis. Massive lymphedema (elephantitis) of the scrotum and left lower extremity are present.

cur in any organ. Obstruction from paralytic ileus and from thickening and immobility of the colon are characteristic of persistent *Strongyloides* hyperinfection. Malabsorption and hypoproteinemia with anasarca may be severe enough to kill the patient. Strongyloidiasis is treated with thiabendazole.

TISSUE NEMATODES

Trichinosis

■ *Trichinosis is a myositis produced by the roundworm* Trichinella spiralis, *which humans acquire from eating the muscles of domestic pigs or wild animals.*

☐ **Pathogenesis:** Within the small bowel, *T. spiralis* larvae emerge from the ingested tissue cysts and then burrow into the intestinal mucosa, where they develop into adult worms. The adults mate, and the female worm liberates larvae that invade the intestinal wall and enter the circulation. The larvae survive only in striated skeletal muscle, where they encyst and remain viable for years. The resulting myositis is especially prominent in the diaphragm, extraocular muscles, tongue, intercostal muscles, gastrocnemius, and deltoids. The larva grows to 10-fold its initial size, folds on itself, and develops a capsule. With encapsulation, the inflammatory infiltrate subsides. Eventually, the larva dies, and the cyst calcifies.

Symptomatic trichinosis is usually a self-limited disease from which patients recover in a few months. When large numbers of cysts are eaten, patients suffer severe pain and tenderness of the affected skeletal muscles, together with fever and weakness. Eosinophilia is the rule and may be extreme (>50% of all leukocytes). Severe cases of trichinosis are treated with corticosteroids to ameliorate the inflammatory response. Anthelminthic drugs are required to remove adult worms from the intestine.

TREMATODES (FLUKES)

Schistosomiasis

■ *Schistosomiasis (bilharziasis) is the most important helminthic disease of humans. Intense inflammatory and immunologic responses damage the liver, intestine, or bladder.* Three species of schistosomes, *Schistosoma mansoni, S. haematobium,* and *S. japonicum,* are responsible for the disease. **Schistosomiasis causes greater morbidity and mortality than all other worm infestations, and it ranks second only to malaria as a cause of disabling disease and death.** *S. mansoni* is found in much of trop-

FIGURE   *9-17*
Life cycle of *Schistosoma* and clinical features of schistosomiasis. The schistosome egg hatches in water and liberates a miracidium, which then penetrates a snail and develops through two stages to sporocyst to form the final larval stage, the cercaria. (1) The cercaria escapes from the snail into water, "swims," and penetrates the skin of a human host. (2) The cercaria loses its forked tail to become a schistosomule, which migrates through tissues and penetrates a blood vessel and (3) is carried to the lung and, later, to the liver. In hepatic portal venules, the schistosomule becomes sexually mature and forms pairs, each with a male and a female worm (the female worm lying in the gynecophoral canal of the male worm). The organism causes lesions in the liver, including granulomas, portal ("pipestem") fibrosis, and portal hypertension. (4) The female worm deposits immature eggs in small venules of the intestine and rectum (*S. mansoni* and *S. japonicum*) or (5) of the urinary bladder (*S. haematobium*). The bladder infestation leads to obstructive uropathy, ureteral obstruction, chronic cystitis, and bladder cancer. Embryos develop during passage of the eggs through the tissues, and larvae are mature when eggs pass through the wall of the intestine or urinary bladder. Eggs hatch in water and liberate miracidia to complete the cycle.

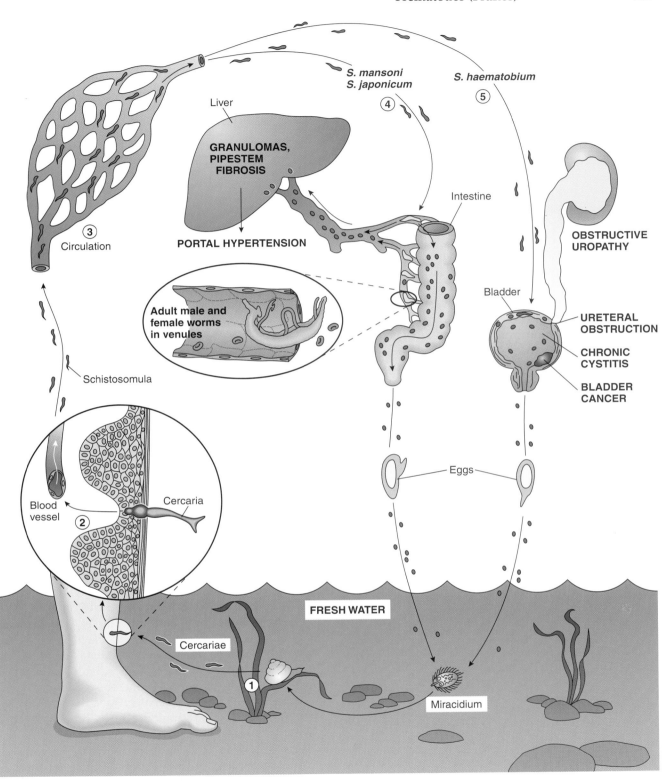

Liver

**GRANULOMAS,
PIPESTEM
FIBROSIS**

*S. mansoni
S. japonicum*   ④

S. haematobium   ⑤

Intestine

**OBSTRUCTIVE
UROPATHY**

③   Circulation

PORTAL HYPERTENSION

**Adult male and
female worms
in venules**

Bladder

**URETERAL
OBSTRUCTION**

**CHRONIC
CYSTITIS**

**BLADDER
CANCER**

Schistosomula

Blood
vessel   ②   Cercaria

Eggs

Cercariae

①

FRESH WATER

Miracidium

ical Africa, parts of southwest Asia, South America, and the Caribbean islands. *S. haematobium* is endemic in large regions of tropical Africa and parts of the Middle East. *S. japonicum* occurs in parts of Japan, China, the Philippines, southeast Asia, and India.

☐ **Pathogenesis and Pathology:** A schistosome egg hatches in fresh water, liberating a motile form (miracidium) that penetrates a snail, in which it develops to the final larval stage, the cercaria (Fig. 9-17). The cercaria escapes from the snail into the water and then penetrates the skin of the human host. In the intestinal venules of the portal drainage, the organisms mature. Female *S. mansoni* and *S. japonicum* deposit immature eggs in the intestinal venules, whereas female *S. haematobium* lay eggs in those of the urinary bladder.

The immunologic and inflammatory reactions to the schistosomal eggs in tissue cause the manifestations of schistosomiasis. **The basic lesion is a circumscribed granuloma or a cellular infiltrate of eosinophils and neutrophils around an egg.**

Liver disease caused by *S. mansoni* or *S. japonicum* begins as periportal granulomatous inflammation (Fig. 9-18) and progresses to dense periportal fibrosis (pipestem fibrosis) (Fig. 9-19). In severe cases of hepatic schistosomiasis, this eventuates in obstruction of the portal blood flow and portal hypertension. Hepatic involvement leads to portal hypertension, with splenomegaly, ascites, and bleeding esophageal varices.

Urogenital schistosomiasis, which is caused by *S. haematobium*, features eggs that are most numerous in the bladder. Schistosomiasis of the bladder causes

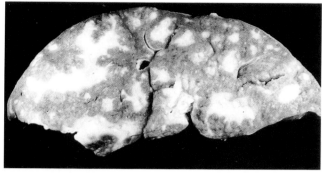

FIGURE   *9-19*
Hepatic schistosomiasis. Chronic involvement of the liver with *S. japonicum* has led to the characteristic "pipestem" fibrosis.

hematuria, recurrent urinary tract infections, and sometimes, progressive obstructive damage leading to renal failure. **The bladder disease produced by *S. haematobium* is related to the development of squamous cell carcinoma of the bladder.** Schistosomiasis is effectively treated with systemic anthelminthic agents.

Clonorchiasis

■ *Clonorchiasis is an infection of the hepatic biliary system by the Chinese liver fluke,* Clonorchis sinensis. Although presence of the fluke usually causes only mild symptoms, it is sometimes associated with bile duct stones, cholangitis, and bile duct cancer. Clonorchiasis is endemic in eastern Asia, from Vietnam to Korea. Human infection is acquired by ingestion of inadequately cooked freshwater fish containing *C. sinensis* larvae. When humans eat the fish, the cercariae emerge in the duodenum, enter the common bile duct through the ampulla of Vater, and mature in the distal bile ducts to an adult fluke.

The presence of *Clonorchis* in the bile ducts incites an inflammatory response, which fails to eliminate the worm but causes dilatation and fibrosis of the ducts. Sometimes, the worms cause calculus formation within the hepatic bile ducts, thereby leading to ductal obstruction. The adult *Clonorchis* persists in the ducts for decades, and longstanding infection is associated with an increased incidence of carcinoma of the bile duct epithelium (cholangiocarcinoma). Patients with clonorchiasis may die of a variety of complications, including biliary obstruction, bacterial cholangitis, pancreatitis, and cholangiocarcinoma. The infestation is effectively treated with systemic anthelminthic agents.

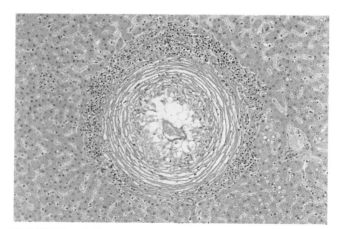

FIGURE   *9-18*
Hepatic schistosomiasis. A hepatic granuloma surrounds a degenerating egg of *S. mansoni*.

CESTODES

Intestinal Tapeworms

Taenia saginata, T. solium, and *Diphyllobothrium latum* are tapeworms that infect humans, growing to their adult forms within the intestine (Table 9-4).

Intestinal tapeworm infections are acquired by eating inadequately cooked beef (*T. saginata*), pork (*T. solium*), or fish (*D. latum*) containing the larval forms of the organisms. Intestinal tapeworm infection rarely harms the human host. The fish tapeworm (*D. latum*) competes for vitamin B_{12}, and a small number (<2%) of infected persons develop a deficiency of this nutrient. Adult tapeworm infections can be eliminated with niclosamide.

Echinococcosis (Hydatid Disease)

■ *Echinococcosis is a zoonotic infection caused by larval cestodes of the genus* Echinococcus. The most common offender is *E. granulosus,* which causes cystic hydatid disease. Infestation with the tapeworm *E. granulosus* is endemic in sheep, goats, cattle, and their attendant dogs. These animals, particularly dogs, contaminate their habitats (and their human keepers) with infectious eggs. Humans become infected when they inadvertently ingest the tapeworm eggs. Disease is especially common in Australia, New Zealand, Argentina, Greece, and the herding countries of Africa and the Middle East.

Larvae released from the eggs penetrate the wall of the gut, enter the bloodstream, and then disseminate to

TABLE 9-4. Tapeworm Infections

Species	Human Disease	Source of Human Infection
Taenia saginata	Adult tapeworm in intestine	Beef
Taenia solium	Adult tapeworm in intestine; cysticercosis	Pork, human feces
Diphyllobothrium latum	Adult tapeworm in intestine	Fish
Echinococcus granulosus	Hydatid cyst disease	Dog feces

the deep organs, where they grow to form hydatid cysts containing brood capsules and scolices. The most common sites of hydatid disease are the liver (75%), lungs (10%), and skeletal muscle (5%).

On gross examination, the unilocular hydatid cyst is a fluid-filled structure that varies from a few millimeters to as many as 20 cm in diameter (Fig. 9-20). The cyst is lined by daughter cysts, which bud from the internal cyst wall. Microscopically, the thin cyst wall is composed of an outer laminated layer and an internal germinal membrane, from which brood capsules and scolices develop. Fluid aspirated from the cyst often contains "hydatid sand," which consists of free daughter cysts and scolices.

Compression of intrahepatic bile ducts by the cyst may lead to obstructive jaundice. Pulmonary cysts are often asymptomatic and discovered incidentally on a chest radiograph. Treatment of echinococcal cysts frequently requires careful surgical removal.

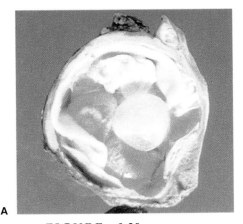 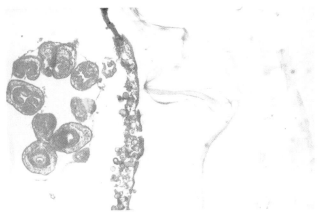

A   B

FIGURE 9-20
Echinococcal cyst. (A) An echinococcal cyst showing daughter cysts was resected from the liver of a patient infected with *E. granulosus*. (B) A photomicrograph of the cyst wall shows (from right to left) a laminated nonnuclear layer, a nucleated germinal layer with brood capsules attached, and numerous scolices in the cyst cavity.

CHAPTER 10

Blood Vessels

Avrum I. Gotlieb
Earl P. Benditt
Stephen M. Schwartz

At one time, blood vessels were considered to be mere passive conduits for the distribution of blood to organs of the body, and little attention was paid to the physiology and pathology of these structures. With the realization that vascular diseases are the most common causes of morbidity and mortality in Western countries, however, the study of the structure and function of the various components of blood vessels and their interactions with circulating elements has dramatically increased our understanding of this dynamic system.

HEMOSTASIS AND THROMBOSIS

■ *Hemostasis refers to the arrest of hemorrhage as a response to vascular injury.* It involves vasoconstriction, tissue swelling, coagulation, and thrombosis. The complex system that controls hemostasis is a network of activating and inactivating enzymes, as well as cofactors derived from different cells and tissues, some of which are circulating and some of which are locally produced (Table 10-1).

The hemostatic complex can be divided into several functional areas that combine coagulation of blood proteins and aggregation of platelets to form a hemostatic "plug":

- Contact activation of factors required for coagulation
- Blood coagulation
- Platelet aggregation
- Endothelial cell interactions
- Fibrinolysis

Coagulation refers to the formation of a clot as a result of activation of the clotting cascade, and it may occur in vitro. **Thrombosis**, by contrast, is the formation of a blood clot in situ. Thrombosis also involves (1) adherence and aggregation of platelets, (2) participation of cellular elements of the monocyte/macrophage system, and (3) endothelial cell functions.

Blood Coagulation

Generation of thrombin is probably the most important factor in progression and stabilization of the thrombus. Historically, the coagulation cascade was divided into two arms, termed the *intrinsic pathway* and the *extrinsic pathway*. However, it is today recognized that this partition into two distinct arms is arbitrary and does not accurately reflect the underlying mechanisms of clotting. The current view holds that after tissue injury, association of factor VIIa-TF complexes with tissue factor pathway inhibitor is crucial for generation of a thrombus. The entire scheme is shown in Figure 10-1.

TABLE   *10–1.*   Coagulation Factor Designations

Factor	Standard Name	Alternative Designations
I	Fibrinogen	
II	Prothrombin	
III	Tissue factor	Thromboplastin
IV	Calcium ions	
V	Proaccelerin	Labile factor, accelerator globulin (AcG), thrombogen
(VI)		No longer considered in the scheme of hemostasis
VII	Proconvertin	Stable factor, serum prothrombin conversion accelerator (SPCA)
VIII	Antihemophilic factor (AHF)	Antihemophilic globulin (AHG), antihemophilic factor A, platelet cofactor 1, thromboplastinogen
IX	Plasma thromboplastin (PTC)	Christmas factor, antihemophilic factor B, autoprothrombin II, platelet cofactor 2
X	Stuart factor	Prower factor, autoprothrombin III, thrombokinase
XI	Plasma thromboplastin antecedent (PTA)	Antihemophilic factor C
XII	Hageman factor	Glass factor, contact factor
XIII	Fibrin-stabilizing factor (FSF)	Laki-Lorand factor (LLF), fibrinase, plasma transglutaminase, fibrinoligase
—	Prekallikrein	Fletcher factor
—	High-molecular-weigh kininogen	High-molecular-weight kininogen, contact activation cofactor, Fitzgerald factor, Williams factor, Flaujeac factor, Reid factor, Washington factor

Platelet Adhesion and Aggregation

When vessels are injured, circulating platelets interact with one another to form a platelet thrombus—that is, an aggregate of activated platelets (Fig. 10-2). These platelet aggregates occlude injured small vessels and prevent the leakage of blood.

Once platelets are stimulated to adhere to the vessel wall, their granular contents are released. In turn, these contents promote aggregation with new platelets. Aggregation is enhanced by the release of von Willebrand factor from the endothelial cells. This substance is adhesive for the GpIb glycoprotein membrane receptor of platelets and for fibrinogen. Activated platelets also release adenosine diphosphate (ADP) and thromboxane A_2, which recruit additional platelets, thereby causing changes in platelet shape, re-

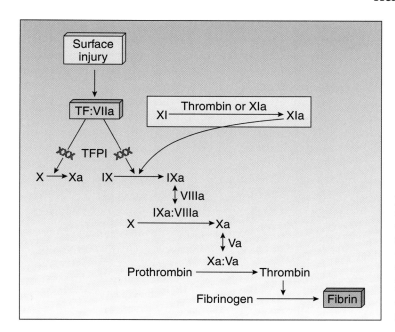

FIGURE *10-1*
Coagulation cascade. The coagulation cascade is initiated by endothelial injury, which releases tissue factor. The latter combines with activated factor VII (VIIa) to form a complex that activates small amounts of factor X to Xa and factor IX to IXa. The complex of IXa with VIIIa further activates factor X. The complex of Xa with Va then catalyzes the conversion of prothrombin to thrombin, after which fibrin is formed from fibrinogen.

lease of granule contents, and further aggregation. Activated platelets, in turn, release factors that initiate clotting, thereby resulting in formation of a complex thrombus on the vessel wall. Thrombin itself is sufficient to stimulate further release of platelet granules and subsequent recruitment of new platelets. Platelet membrane proteins GpIIb and GpIIIa adhere to fibrin and fibrinogen, a process that tends to stabilize the forming thrombus.

Endothelial Factors

The major initiating event for most thrombosis and coagulation is some form of injury to the endothelium (see Fig. 10-2). Thrombus formation is normally prevented by the flow of blood and the antithrombotic properties of the endothelium. Thrombi can form when (1) endothelial function is altered, (2) endothelial continuity is lost, or (3) blood flow is altered or becomes static. **Simple loss of endothelial cells or injury in a vessel with good flow produces platelet pavementing, but not thrombosis**.

For thrombosis to occur, endothelial continuity must be disrupted or the endothelial cell surface must change from an anticoagulant to a procoagulant one. Both processes are believed to occur. The most common denuding endothelial injury is progressive endothelial disruption of an advancing atherosclerotic lesion. Interactions of a thrombus with the underlying subendothelium may cause a further disturbance of endothelial integrity. Inflammatory agents released from monocytes can also activate procoagulant activities on the surface of an intact endothelium.

The endothelium plays an active rather than a passive role in the control of thrombosis (Box 10-1). The antithrombotic mechanisms of the endothelium include secretion of prostaglandin I_2 (prostacyclin), metabolites of ADP, and coating of the luminal surface by heparan sulfate. Endothelial cells may also lyse some clots as they form.

There are several other, more specific endothelial anticoagulant mechanisms. A cofactor on the endothelial cell surface inactivates thrombin by forming a complex with it and antithrombin 3, a plasma antiprotease. Thrombin itself activates protein C through an interaction with its receptor, called thrombomodulin, that is located on the surface of endothelial cells. Both protein C and thrombomodulin are synthesized by endothelial cells. Activated protein C destroys coagulation factors V and VII. The presence of these antithrombotic mechanisms on the endothelial surface raises the intriguing possibility that endothelial dysfunction might lead to thrombosis. One can envision that procoagulant injuries at the surface of blood vessels are produced by the loss of normal endothelial function or by the stimulation of an abnormal function.

Clot Lysis

The thrombus composed of aggregated platelets and clotted blood is made unstable by activation of the fibrinolytic enzyme plasmin (Fig. 10-3). During clot formation, plasminogen is bound to fibrin and, therefore, is an integral part of the forming platelet mass. Endothelial cells synthesize plasminogen activator, but in larger thrombi, circulating plasminogen may also be

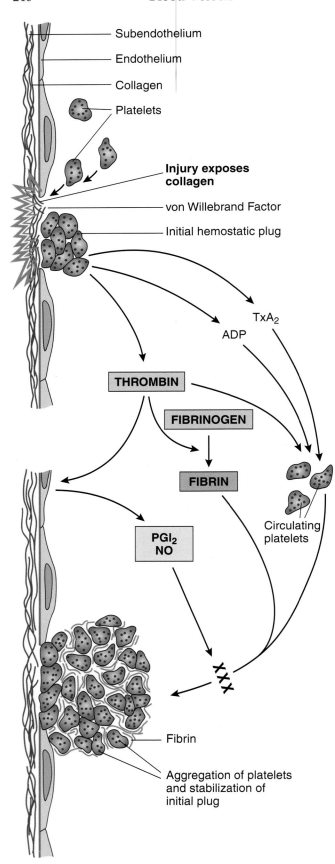

converted to plasmin by products of the coagulation cascade. Plasminogen activator bound to fibrin activates plasmin, and in turn, by digesting fibrin, plasmin lyses the clots and disrupts the thrombus. Synthesis of plasminogen activator represents still another antithrombotic mechanism of the endothelial cell, which also synthesizes an inhibitor of plasminogen activator. Thus, again, this cell possesses both procoagulant and anticoagulant properties.

ATHEROSCLEROSIS

■ *Atherosclerosis is a disease of large- and medium-size arteries that results in progressive accumulation within the intima of smooth muscle cells, lipids, and connective tissue.* Continued growth of the lesions encroaches on other layers of the arterial wall and narrows the lumen.

The major complications of atherosclerosis, including ischemic heart disease, myocardial infarction, stroke, and gangrene of the extremities, account for more than half the annual mortality rate in the United States. In fact, ischemic heart disease, by itself, is the leading cause of death. The incidence of ischemic heart disease in the United States and other Western countries rose progressively from the turn of the century to a peak during the late 1960s, but subsequently, it has fallen by more than 30%.

There are wide geographic and racial variations in the incidence of ischemic heart disease. For example, the mortality rate from ischemic heart disease is eightfold higher in Sweden than in Japan. The extent of coronary atherosclerosis found at autopsy and the mortality rate from ischemic heart disease in a given population are directly correlated.

☐ **Pathogenesis and Pathology:** Atherosclerotic lesions regularly develop in the tunica intima of elastic and muscular arteries as a result of the proliferation of intimal smooth muscle cells and the accumulation of lipid. As the lesion forms, the intima contains smooth muscle cells, macrophages, lymphocytes, and connective tissue. Later, as the lesion advances, the endothelium breaks down, and platelets are deposited. In more

FIGURE *10-2*
The role of platelets in thrombosis. Following vessel wall injury and alteration in flow, platelets adhere and then aggregate. Adenosine diphosphate and thromboxane A$_2$ are released and, along with locally generated thrombin, recruit additional platelets, causing the mass to enlarge. The growing platelet thrombus is stabilized by fibrin. Other elements, including leukocytes and red blood cells, are also incorporated into the thrombus. The release of prostacyclin (PGI$_2$) and nitric oxide (NO) by endothelial cells regulates the process by inhibiting platelet aggregation.

BOX *10-1*   **Regulation of Coagulation at the Endothelial Cell Surface**

Downregulation
1. Thrombin inactivators
   A. Antithrombin III
   B. Thrombomodulin
2. Activated protein C pathway
   A. Synthesis and expression of thrombomodulin
   B. Synthesis and expression of protein S
   C. Thrombomodulin-mediated activation of protein C
   D. Inactivation of factor Va and factor VIIIa by APC—protein S complex
3. Tissue factor pathway inhibition
4. Fibrinolysis
   A. Synthesis of tissue plasminogen activator, urokinase plasminogen activator, and plasminogen-activator inhibitor 1
   B. Conversion of GLU-plasminogen to LYS-plasminogen

C. APC-mediated potentiation
5. Synthesis of unsaturated fatty acid metabolites
   A. Lipoxygenase metabolites—13-HODE
   B. Cyclo-oxygenase metabolites—prostaglandins I_2 and E_2

Procoagulant Pathways
1. Synthesis of:
   A. Tissue factor (thromboplastin)
   B. Factor V
   C. Platelet-activating factor
2. Binding of clotting factors IX/IXa, X (prothrombinase complex)
3. Downregulation of APC pathway
4. Increased synthesis of plasminogen activator inhibitor
5. Synthesis of 15-HPETE

advanced lesions, small capillaries penetrate the vessel wall, thereby vascularizing the plaque with endothelialized channels called "vasa plaquorum." The expansion of this lesion, together with thrombosis, produces the final clinical result—that is, occlusion of a distributing artery.

It deserves emphasis that lipid deposition is a necessary, but not a sufficient, condition for the development of atherosclerosis. The presence of proliferated smooth muscle cells has called attention to peptides that stimulate proliferation of these cells. Other substances in the plaque may also act as signals that trigger a wide range of responses, both among the resident components of the arterial wall and between these and the blood. Such factors include cytokines that promote thrombosis or that cause the death of cells in the atherosclerotic plaque. In addition, some factors may promote immigration of leukocytes into the plaque. These cytokines and growth factors may be produced by all four cell types in the lesions. In addition, growth

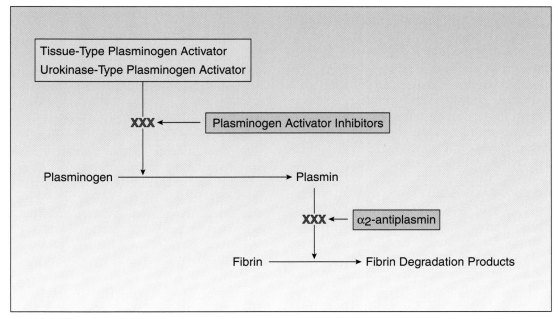

FIGURE *10-3*
Mechanisms of fibrinolysis. Plasmin formed from plasminogen lyses fibrin. The conversion of plasminogen to plasmin and the activity of plasmin itself are suppressed by specific inhibitors.

inhibitors of smooth muscle cells may be produced. Both genetic and hemodynamic factors could modify these responses. At this point, we must consider the main elements involved in production of an atherosclerotic plaque:

- **Vascular endothelium** interacts with macromolecules and formed elements of the blood, and it plays a role in the transport of plasma proteins.
- **Arterial smooth muscle cells** are important in (1) control of artery wall tone; (2) maintenance and repair; (3) metabolism of various blood-borne substances, including lipids; and (4) secretion of various cytokines.
- **Mononuclear phagocytes** have many functions, including uptake of low-density lipoproteins (LDLs) and secretion of various hydrolases and cytokines.
- **Lymphocytes and neutrophils** are involved in the response to tissue injury. They may participate in autoimmune reactions, such as may occur with viral infections in the vessels of transplanted organs.

Atherogenic Processes

At least six hypotheses have been proposed to explain the origins of atherosclerotic plaques.

Insudation Hypothesis. This theory states that the lipid in atherosclerotic lesions is derived from plasma lipoproteins. Although the insudation hypothesis explains the source of the plaque lipid, it does not provide a complete explanation for the pathogenesis of the atherosclerotic lesion itself.

Low-density lipoprotein (LDL) is the form of lipid in plasma that has been most closely associated with accelerated atherosclerosis. Endothelial cells have receptors for both LDL and modified forms of LDL. Recent studies of atherosclerosis in fat-fed animals have demonstrated that macrophages also play a major role during the early stages of lipid accumulation.

Encrustation Hypothesis. This theory holds that small mural thrombi represent the initial event in atherosclerosis and that the organization of these thrombi leads to the formation of plaques. We now know from experimental studies of hyperlipidemic animals, and from autopsy studies of children, that the mural thrombus is not the initial event in atherogenesis. **However, mural thrombosis is a critical part of the later progression of the atherosclerotic lesion and is probably the major event leading to vascular occlusion.**

Reaction to Injury Hypothesis. Another theory attempts to explain the accumulation of smooth muscle cells in atherosclerotic lesions, holding that smooth muscle proliferation depends on the release of polypeptide growth factors by platelets and monocytes that accumulate at sites of injury. The best known of these is **platelet-derived growth factor (PDGF),** which is not only mitogenic for smooth muscle cells but is also chemotactic for them. Thus, in addition to stimulating proliferation of cells already in the intima, PDGF may recruit smooth muscle cells from the media. Smooth muscle cells and endothelial cells also synthesize growth factors that stimulate proliferation of smooth muscle cells. Numerous growth factors that can potentially induce proliferation of cells are now known (Table 10-2). Although the reaction to injury hypothesis points to a mechanism for smooth muscle proliferation, it does not explain lipid accumulation.

Monoclonal Hypothesis. The monoclonal concept is also focused on smooth muscle proliferation and was originally derived from the observation that the fibrous caps of atherosclerotic plaques (discussed later) are composed of smooth muscle cells. Based on studies of women who are mosaic for X-linked markers, it has been established that many plaques are monoclonal—that is, they originate from one or very few smooth muscle cells. The monoclonality of the fibrous cap suggests that some unknown etiologic factor, perhaps circulating mutagens or viruses, might induce formation of atherosclerotic plaques by altering growth control in the smooth muscle cells of the arterial wall.

Intimal Cell Mass Hypothesis. The location of atherosclerotic lesions has been related to focal accumulation of smooth muscle cells in the normal intima at branch points and other sites in certain vessels, particularly the coronary arteries. The distribution of intimal cell masses in children resembles that of atherosclerotic lesions in adults, thereby suggesting that the intimal cell mass is either the early lesion of atherosclerosis or its precursor.

If the intimal cell mass is, indeed, the precursor of atherosclerosis, it is probable that all humans are susceptible to this disease. In that case, we would view other factors, such as hyperlipidemia or hypertension, as being critical for the progression of this disease to a clinically significant state.

Hemodynamic Hypothesis. The distribution of atherosclerotic lesions in large vessels and the differences in both the location and frequency of lesions in different vascular beds have encouraged a belief in the role of hemodynamic factors related to turbulence,

TABLE 10-2.   Growth Factors for Smooth Muscle Cells[a]

Molecule	Sources
Platelet-derived growth factor	Platelets, leukocytes
Fibroblast growth factor	Platelets, vessel wall cells, leukocytes
Epidermal growth factor	Epidermal growth factor
Transforming growth factor	Platelets, vessel wall cells
Insulin-like growth factor 1	Platelets, vessel wall cells
Catecholamines	Platelets
Angiotensin II	Platelets, vessel wall cells (stimulates mass change, not replication)
Low-density lipoprotein	Platelets
Neuraminidase	Leukocytes
Fibronectin	Platelets, vessel wall cells, leukocytes
Nicotine	Platelets
Leukotrienes	Leukocytes, platelets
Thrombospondin	Platelets
Thrombin	Platelets
Fibrin	Platelets
Interleukin-1	Leukocytes (interleukin-1 may work by eliciting platelet-derived growth factor expression)
Endothelin	Vessel wall cells, leukocytes
Serotonin	Platelets, leukocytes
Neurokinin A	Vessel wall cells
Substance K	Vessel wall cells
Substance P	Vessel wall cells

[a] Depending on the source of the cells and culture conditions, growth inhibition or stimulation may occur.

pressure, and shear forces. That hypertension enhances the severity of atherosclerotic lesions and low blood pressure is generally associated with increased longevity further encourage the idea that hemodynamic factors somehow play a role in development of sclerotic vascular disease.

A Unifying Hypothesis

We can construct a hypothetical sequence to tie the foregoing concepts together (Fig. 10-4):

1. The initial lesion is the intimal cell mass, which arises by the trapping of isolated smooth muscle cells in the intima. If the intimal mass arose as a mutation or from a few cells trapped in the intima, then monoclonality would be intrinsic to the early plaque.
2. Lipid accumulation in these foci might depend on the properties of the intimal smooth muscle cells. The types of connective tissue synthesized by the cells in the intima may render these sites prone to lipid accumulation.
3. Lipid insudation in these benign accumulations of intimal cells would produce cell injury, thereby leading to accumulation of macrophages and platelets.
4. In turn, these macrophages and platelets could release growth factors, as proposed in the reaction to injury hypothesis. Mononuclear macrophages could play a central role by participating in lipid accumulation and releasing growth factors, thereby stimulating further accumulation of smooth muscle cells.
5. As the lesion progresses, endothelial injury may lead to loss of the anticoagulant properties of the normal wall. The resulting mural thrombosis would promote the release of PDGFs, with further acceleration of smooth muscle proliferation. If the thrombus is large, it can lead directly to infarction of a vital organ.

Initial Lesion of Atherosclerosis

Fatty Streaks

■ *Fatty streaks are flat or slightly elevated lesions that contain accumulations of intracellular and extracellular lipid in the intima.* Fatty streaks are found in young children as well as in adults. In these simple, focal lesions, cells filled with lipid droplets ("foam cells") accumulate (Fig. 10-5). The cells with the greatest amount of lipid are macrophages, but smooth muscle cells also contain fat.

In children who die accidentally, significant numbers of fatty streaks are usually evident in many parts of the arterial tree. However, the distribution of these fatty streaks does not correspond to that of atherosclerotic lesions in adults. Nonetheless, fatty infiltration may represent the initial lesion of atherosclerosis, with other factors controlling distribution of the later, and more clinically significant, lesions.

Intimal Cell Masses

■ *Intimal cell masses are white, thickened areas at branch points in the arterial tree.* They are an alternative candidate for the initial lesion of atherosclerosis. Microscopically, they contain smooth muscle cells and connective tissue, but no lipid. The location of these lesions, which are also known as "cushions," at arterial branch sites correlates well with the location of later atherosclerotic lesions.

The concept of the intimal cell mass as the initial lesion is controversial. A gradual increase in thickness of the intima occurs diffusely throughout large arteries as a normal part of aging, and for this reason, many prefer to distinguish intimal thickening from atherosclero-

INTIMAL CELL MASS

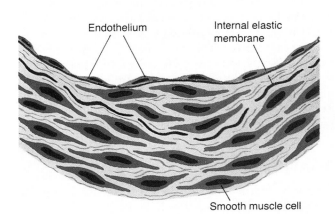

INSUDATION

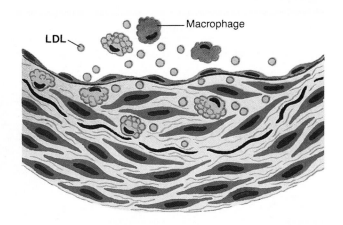

RESPONSE TO INJURY

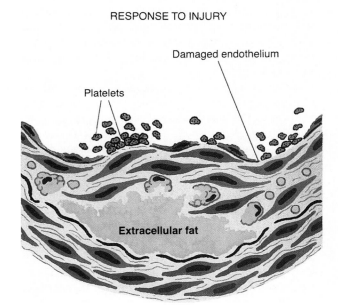

ENCRUSTATION AND THROMBOSIS

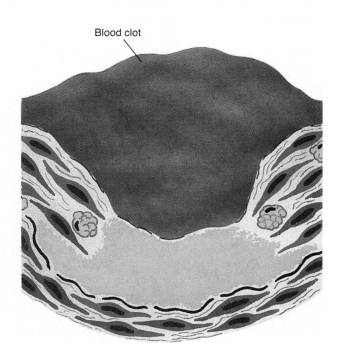

FIGURE   *10-4*

Unifying hypothesis for the pathogenesis of atherosclerosis. Monoclonality and the intimal cell mass occur very early in plaque development, and they are good candidates for the initial event. A single smooth muscle cell (*red*) proliferates in the intima, either because of a mutation or as part of an "intimal cushion," to form an intimal cell mass. Insudation of plasma lipids into the intimal cell mass occurs by direct passage of LDL across the endothelium and via macrophages that engulf LDL in the blood or intima. For reasons that are not clear, the expanding, early atherosclerotic lesion is complicated by damage to the endothelium. As a result, platelets adhere to the exposed subendothelial collagen. Platelets and macrophages release growth factors, thereby stimulating a polyclonal proliferation of smooth muscle cells (*blue*) to form the characteristic fibrous plaque. The continued insudation of lipid and its release by degenerating macrophages leads to further accumulation of extracellular lipid. Eventually, the surface of the plaque ulcerates, and a thrombus forms on the injured luminal surface.

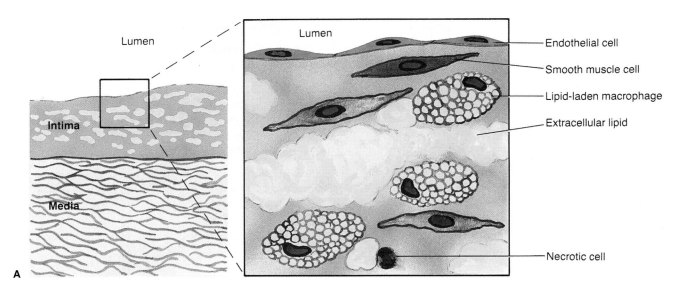

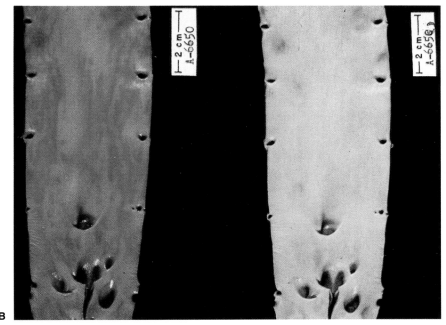

FIGURE   *10-5*

Fatty streak of atherosclerosis. (A) The fatty streak, composed largely of foamy macrophages, is presumed to be an early stage in the formation of atherosclerotic lesions. Note the intimal thickening (*left*) and infiltrating cells (*right*). (B) The aorta of the young man shows numerous fatty streaks on the luminal surface when stained with Sudan red. The unstained specimen is also shown (*right*).

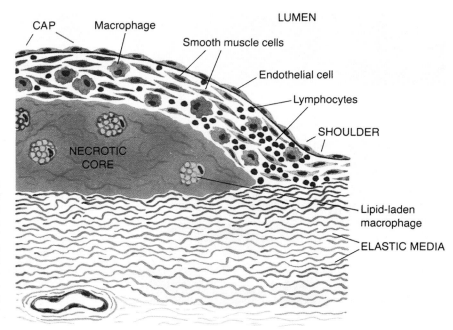

FIGURE 10-6

Fibrous plaque of atherosclerosis. In this fully developed fibrous plaque, the core contains lipid-filled macrophages and necrotic smooth muscle cell debris. The "fibrous" cap is composed largely of smooth muscle cells, which produce collagen, small amounts of elastin, and glycosaminoglycans. Also shown are infiltrating macrophages and lymphocytes. Note that the endothelium over the surface of the fibrous cap frequently appears to be intact.

sis. In any event, as illustrated in Figure 10-4, there is a general agreement that fat accumulation and monoclonal smooth muscle proliferation are the critical processes that lead to the characteristic lesion of atherosclerosis.

Characteristic Lesion of Atherosclerosis

The characteristic lesion of atherosclerosis is a fibrofatty plaque consisting of a fibrous cap and an atheroma (Fig. 10-6). The **fibrous cap** is a layer of fibrous connective tissue that is much thicker and less cellular than the normal intima. It contains fat-filled macrophages (foam cells) and smooth muscle cells. The **atheroma** is a necrotic mass of lipid that forms the middle part of the characteristic lesion of atherosclerosis.

Virtually all studies have shown some loss of endothelial continuity during progression to the characteristic lesion of atherosclerosis. In addition to monocytes, the characteristic lesion may contain other blood-borne cells. These cells have received little attention in experimental animals, but advanced lesions in humans show numerous activated T lymphocytes.

Complicated Plaques

The characteristic lesions described previously are of little clinical significance in impairing the flow of blood. **However, their distribution and similarity to more advanced lesions suggest a progression to the final and clinically significant lesion, namely the complicated plaque.** Certain critical changes characterize complicated plaques (Fig. 10-7):

- **Thrombosis,** on and within the fibrous cap
- **Neovascularization** of the cap and shoulders of the lesion
- **Thinning** of the underlying tunica media
- **Calcification** within the atheroma and fibrous cap
- **Ulceration** of the fibrous cap.

It is likely that thrombosis on the surface of the final complicated lesion leads to vascular occlusion and clinical cardiovascular disease. Progression from the simple characteristic lesion to the more complicated, clinically significant lesion can be found in some persons still in their twenties and, in our society, in virtually everyone by 50 or 60 years of age.

Mechanisms of Lesion Progression in Atherosclerosis

The sequence of events in the development of atherosclerosis possibly begins as early as the fetal stage, when intimal cell masses form, or perhaps shortly after birth, when fatty streaks evolve. **However, the characteristic lesion, which is not clinically significant, requires as long as 20 to 30 years to form. Moreover, the clinically important complicated plaques emerge only after several more decades of development** (Fig. 10-8). Some of the factors that may contribute to progression of the simple lesions to complicated ones are:

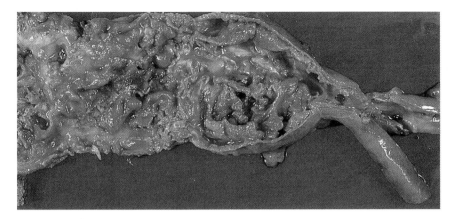

FIGURE *10-7*
Complicated lesions of atherosclerosis. The luminal surface of the abdominal aorta and the common iliac arteries show numerous fibrous plaques and raised, ulcerated lesions containing friable, atheromatous debris. The distal portion of the aorta displays a small, aneurysmal dilatation.

• **Cytokines.** A prominent factor in lesion progression may be the inflammatory role of the macrophage (Fig. 10-9). For example, the monocyte synthesizes PDGF, fibroblast growth factor, tumor necrosis factor (TNF), interleukin (IL)-1, interferon-α, and transforming growth factor (TGF)-β, each of which can modulate the growth of smooth muscle cells or endothelial cells. Interferon and TGF-β inhibit cell proliferation and could account for the failure of endothelial cells to maintain continuity over the lesion. IL-1 and TNF stimulate

the expressions of platelet-activating factor, tissue factor, and plasminogen-activator inhibitor by endothelial cells. **Thus, the combination of monocytes and endothelial cells may be capable of transforming the normal, anticoagulant vascular surface to a procoagulant surface.**
• **T Lymphocytes.** Atherosclerotic plaques also contain T lymphocytes. Expression of HLA-DR antigens on both endothelial cells and smooth muscle cells in plaques implies that they have undergone some kind of immunologic activation, perhaps in

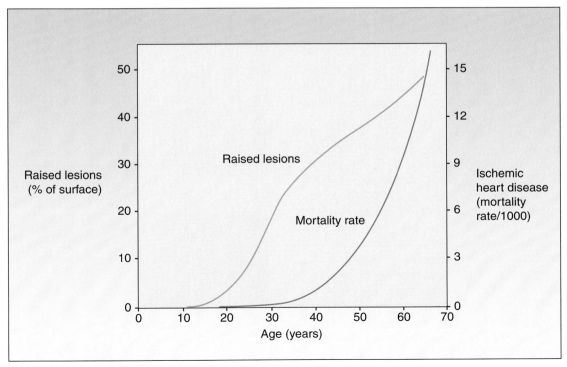

FIGURE *10-8*
Raised lesions in coronary arteries and mortality rate from ischemic heart disease as a function of age. There is a protracted incubation period of approximately 25 years between the appearance of raised lesions in the coronary vessels and their lethal complications.

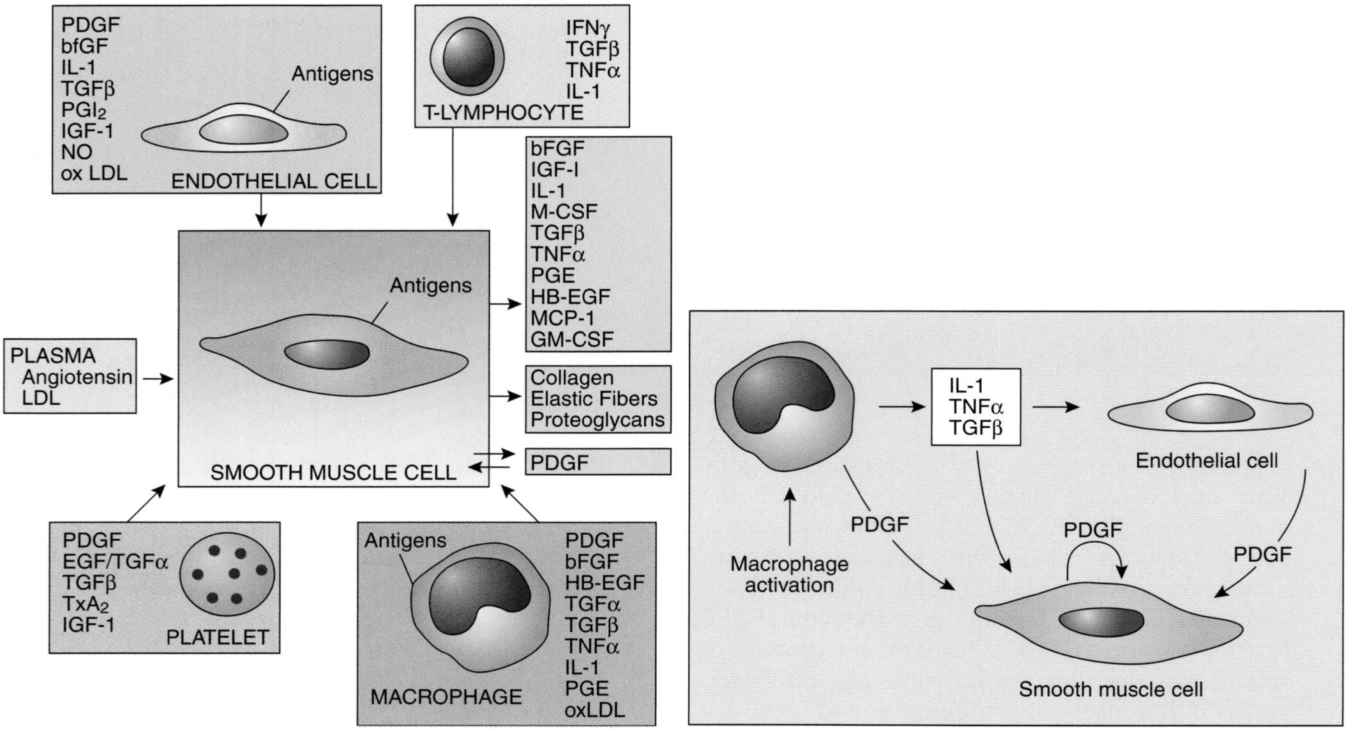

FIGURE 10-9
Cellular interactions in the progression of the atherosclerotic plaque. (A) Endothelium, platelets, macrophages, T lymphocytes, and smooth muscle cells elaborate a variety of cytokines, growth factors, and other substances. The scheme illustrated here emphasizes their influence on smooth muscle cells. (B) The cellular interactions that promote the proliferation of smooth cells.

response to interferon-γ released by activated T cells in the plaque. It is possible that these T cells reflect an autoimmune response important for the progression of atherosclerotic lesions.

- **Endothelium.** A loss of endothelial continuity on the luminal surface is another potential antecedent of plaque progression. Loss of endothelial continuity would (1) increase permeability of the wall to lipoproteins and, therefore, accelerate lipoprotein accumulation; (2) permit platelet interaction with the vessel wall and the subsequent release of growth factors, thereby resulting in more rapid lesion progression; and (3) allow formation of a thrombus on the surface of an atherosclerotic lesion. Endothelial-lined channels are found in many advanced plaques and are a potential source of hemorrhage into these lesions. Alternatively, blood may enter the plaque from the circulation through tears in its surface.
- **Thrombosis. Formation of a thrombus is the most common clinical event that leads to myocardial infarction** (Fig. 10-10).

Risk Factors

Any factor associated with a doubling in the incidence of ischemic heart disease is defined as being a risk factor.

- **Hypertension.** An increase in blood pressure is consistently associated with augmented risk of

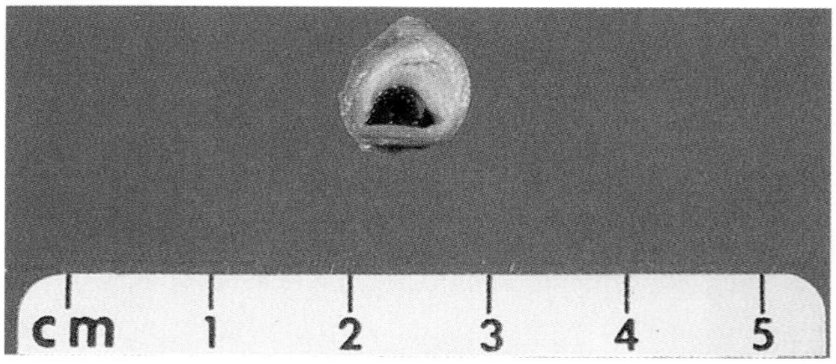

FIGURE 10-10
Coronary artery thrombosis. A cross-section of a coronary artery shows a fresh thrombus overlying an atherosclerotic plaque and occluding the lumen.

T A B L E *10-3.* Apolipoproteins

Apolipoprotein	Approximate Molecular Weight	Major Density Class[a]	Major Sites of Synthesis in Humans	Major Function in Lipoprotein Metabolism
AI	28,000	HDL	Liver, intestine	Activates lecithin: cholesterol acyltransferase
AII	18,000	HDL	Liver, intestine	
AIV	45,000	Chylomicrons	Intestine	
B-100	250,000	VLDL, IDL, LDL	Liver	Binds to LDL receptor
B-48	125,000	Chylomicrons VLDL, IDL	Intestine	
CI	6500	Chylomicrons VLDL, HDL	Liver	Activates lecithin: cholesterol acyltransferase
CII	10,000	Chylomicrons VLDL, HDL	Liver	Activates lipoprotein lipase
CIII	10,000	Chylomicrons	Liver	Inhibits lipoprotein uptake by the liver
D	20,000	HDL		Cholesteryl ester exchange protein
E	40,000	Chylomicrons, VLDL, HDL	Liver, macrophage	Binds to E receptor system

[a] *HDL*, high-density lipoprotein; *IDL*, intermediate-density lipoprotein; *LDL*, low-density lipoprotein; *VLDL*, very-low-density lipoprotein.

myocardial infarction. Men with systolic blood pressures greater than 160 mm Hg have almost threefold the incidence of myocardial infarction as those with pressures less than 120 mm Hg. Control of hypertension has resulted in a significant decrease in the incidence of myocardial infarction and stroke.

- **Blood Cholesterol Level.** Levels of serum cholesterol are directly correlated with the incidence of ischemic heart disease. Of all known risk factors, serum cholesterol seems to be the most important determinant of the geographic differences in the incidence of atherosclerotic coronary artery disease. In the absence of genetic disorders of lipid metabolism (discussed later), the amount of cholesterol in the blood is strongly related to the dietary intake of saturated fat.
- **Cigarette Smoking.** Atherosclerosis of the coronary arteries and the aorta is more severe and extensive among cigarette smokers than among nonsmokers. As a result, the incidence of myocardial infarction and abdominal aortic aneurysms is markedly increased among smokers.
- **Diabetes.** Diabetics have a substantially greater risk of occlusive atherosclerotic vascular disease in many organs. However, the relative contributions of carbohydrate intolerance itself and of the secondary changes in blood lipids are not well defined.
- **Increasing Age and Male Sex.** These factors are strong determinants for the risk of myocardial infarction.

- **Physical Inactivity and Stressful Life Patterns.** Both factors have been correlated with an increased risk of ischemic heart disease.

Lipid Metabolism and Atherosclerosis

The insolubility of cholesterol and other lipids (mainly triglycerides) necessitates a special transport system, which is subserved by a system of lipoprotein particles (Table 10-3). The major classes of particles are:

- Chylomicrons
- Very-low-density lipoproteins (VLDL)
- Low-density lipoproteins (LDL)
- High-density lipoproteins (HDL).

Each of these particles consists of a lipid core with associated proteins (apolipoproteins). A number of the latter have been described, and each is designated by a letter (frequently accompanied by a number), as indicated in Table 10-3. The metabolic pathways for lipoproteins containing the B apolipoproteins are two major lipoprotein cascades, with one originating from the intestine and the other from the liver (Fig. 10-11).

Exogenous Pathway. This metabolic route involves chylomicrons secreted by the intestine. These triglyceride-rich lipoproteins primarily transport lipid from the intestine to the liver. The triglycerides in the chylomicrons are hydrolyzed by lipoprotein lipase, which is attached to the endothelial cells of the capillary walls.

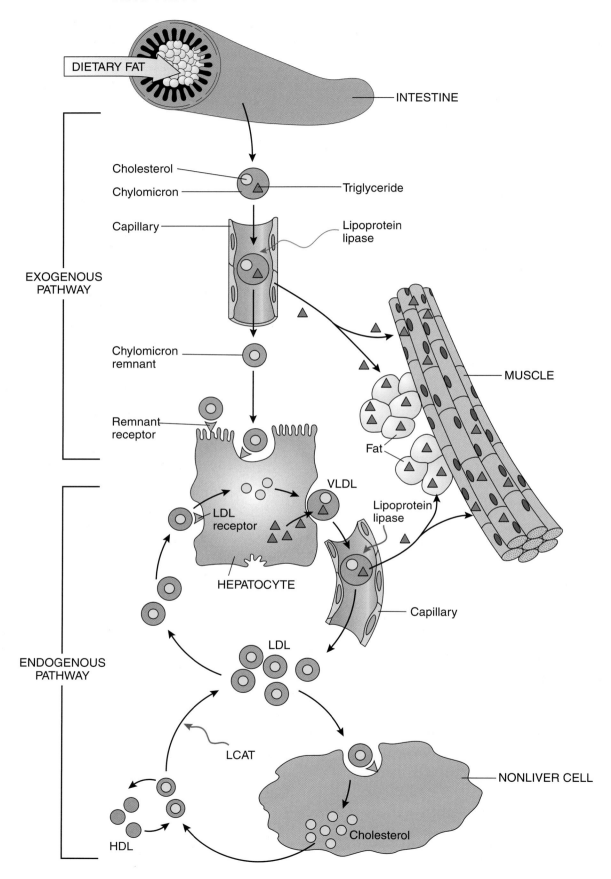

Chylomicrons are first converted to "remnants" and finally to intermediate-density lipoproteins (IDLs). The chylomicron remnants are removed by the hepatocytes.

Endogenous Pathway. This network of reactions involves triglyceride-rich VLDLs secreted by the liver. The triglycerides on the VLDLs undergo hydrolysis by lipoprotein lipase. The lipoproteins are first converted to IDLs and finally to LDLs, which interact with high-affinity receptors on the hepatocytes and the peripheral cells, including smooth muscle cells and fibroblasts (see Fig. 10-11). The interaction of LDL with its receptor initiates receptor-mediated endocytosis, which is followed by catabolism of LDL.

High-Density Lipoprotein. HDL is synthesized by several pathways, including direct secretion of HDL by the intestine and liver and transfer of the lipid and apolipoprotein constituents released during the lipolysis of lipoproteins. Two major functions have been proposed for HDL, namely a reservoir for apolipoproteins and an interaction with cells in the transport system to carry extrahepatic cholesterol to the liver for ultimate removal from the body. The latter function has been termed **reverse cholesterol transport.**

Cholesterol removed from the cells is principally free cholesterol, which rapidly undergoes esterification to cholesteryl esters. Defects in cholesteryl ester transfer and exchange lead to dyslipoproteinemias, increased intracellular cholesteryl esters, and premature atherosclerosis.

Oxidized Low-Density Lipoprotein. Macrophages recognize and ingest LDL that is modified by oxidation. Each cell type in atherosclerotic lesions (macrophages, endothelial cells, smooth muscle cells) is capable of oxidizing LDL. Oxidized LDL products are present in the macrophages of human atherosclerotic lesions, and evidence is emerging that they affect processes that may contribute to atherogenesis. These include regulation of vascular tone, activation of inflammatory and immune responses, and coagulation.

Hereditary Disorders of Lipid Metabolism and Atherosclerosis

Familial clustering of ischemic heart disease has been recognized for decades, and a number of genetic defects that produce dyslipoproteinemias have been identified as causes of heritable predisposition to atherosclerosis.

Familial Hypercholesterolemia. The LDL receptor is a cell surface glycoprotein that regulates plasma cholesterol by mediating the endocytosis and recycling of apolipoprotein E (ApoE), the major cholesterol transport protein in human plasma. Mutations in the LDL receptor gene are responsible for familial hypercholesterolemia, an autosomal dominant disease (see Chapter 6).

Homozygotes exhibit plasma cholesterol levels of between 600 and 1000 mg/dL, a value that is four- to sixfold higher than the mean value in most whites. The majority of untreated homozygotes die before 20 years of age from coronary artery disease. In heterozygotes, LDL cholesterol levels vary from 250 to 500 mg/dL, or roughly twice the normal range. These patients suffer from premature myocardial infarction, but at a later age than do the homozygotes (40–45 years in men).

FIGURE *10-11*

Exogenous and endogenous cholesterol transport pathway. In the exogenous pathway, cholesterol and fatty acids from food are absorbed through the intestinal mucosa. Fatty acid chains are linked to glycerol to form triglycerides. Triglycerides and cholesterol are packaged into chylomicrons that are returned via the lymph to the blood. The lipids are coupled to proteins by enzymes such as the microsomal transfer protein complex. In the capillaries (mainly of fat tissue and muscle, but also other tissues), the ester bonds holding the fatty acids in triglycerides are split by lipoprotein lipase. Fatty acids are removed, leaving cholesterol-rich lipoprotein remnants. These bind to special remnant receptors and are taken up by liver cells. The cholesterol of the remnant is either secreted into the intestine, largely as bile acids, or packaged as very low-density lipoprotein particles (VLDL), which are then secreted into the circulation. This is the first step in the endogenous cycle. In fat or muscle tissue the triglyceride is removed from the VLDL with the aid of lipoprotein lipase. The intermediate-density lipoprotein particles (IDL [*not shown*]) remain in the circulation. Some IDL is immediately taken up by the liver via the mediation of low-density lipoprotein (LDL) receptors for ApoB/E. The remaining IDL in the circulation is either taken up by nonliver cells or converted to LDL. Most of the LDL in the circulation bind to hepatocytes or other cells and are removed from the circulation. High-density lipoproteins (HDL) take up cholesterol from cells. This cholesterol is esterified by the enzyme lecithin: cholesterol acyltransferase (LCAT), after which the esters are transferred to LDL and taken up by cells.

Apolipoprotein E. ApoE is one of the main protein constituents of VLDL and of a subclass of HDL. The several polymorphic forms of ApoE have a significant influence on plasma cholesterol levels and lipoprotein variations. **In fact, 20% of the variability in serum cholesterol has been attributed to ApoE polymorphism.**

High-Density Lipoprotein: An inverse correlation between ischemic heart disease and HDL cholesterol levels has been established.

Lipoprotein(a). Some studies have correlated high circulating levels of lipoprotein(a) (Lp[a]) with a high risk of atherosclerotic disease, whereas others have failed to confirm this association. Lp(a) is an LDL-like lipoprotein particle to which the glycoprotein apo(a) is attached to apoB-100. It has been suggested that Lp(a) inhibits endothelial cell–induced fibrinolysis and also binds to plasmin-modified fibrin. These interactions might be a basis for the involvement of Lp(a) in atherosclerotic and thrombotic processes.

Homocysteine. Homocysteinuria, which is a rare, hereditary disease characterized by high concentrations of homocysteine in the blood, results in premature and severe atherosclerosis. It is now recognized that milder elevations of plasma homocysteine are common and represent an independent risk factor for atherosclerosis of the coronary arteries and other large vessels. The mechanism underlying this effect is unclear, but homocysteine is toxic to endothelial cells and inhibits several anticoagulant mechanisms.

C-Reactive Protein. The plasma level of this protein is a marker for systemic inflammation. Elevated concentrations of C-reactive protein have been associated with an increased risk of myocardial infarction and ischemic stroke.

Complications of Atherosclerosis

Complications of atherosclerosis vary with the location and size of the affected vessel and with the chronicity of the process (Fig. 10-12).

- **Acute Occlusion. The major clinical complication of atherosclerosis is occlusive coronary artery disease and the resulting myocardial infarction.** Thrombosis on an atherosclerotic plaque or hemorrhage into it abruptly occludes the lumen. The result is ischemic necrosis (infarction) of the tissue supplied by that vessel, which manifests clinically as myocardial infarction, stroke, or gangrene of the intestine or lower extremities.
- **Chronic Narrowing of the Lumen.** As an atherosclerotic plaque grows, it often impinges on

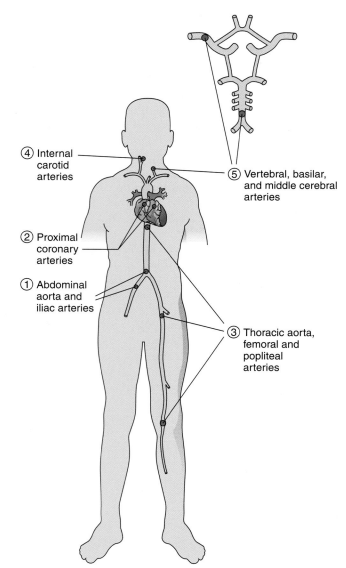

FIGURE *10-12*
Sites of severe atherosclerosis in order of frequency.

④ Internal carotid arteries
⑤ Vertebral, basilar, and middle cerebral arteries
② Proximal coronary arteries
① Abdominal aorta and iliac arteries
③ Thoracic aorta, femoral and popliteal arteries

the lumen, thereby progressively reducing the flow of blood to the distribution of the artery. Chronic ischemia of the affected tissue is evidenced by atrophy of the organ, as exemplified by unilateral renal artery stenosis with atrophy of a kidney, intestinal stricture in mesenteric artery atherosclerosis, or ischemic atrophy of the skin in a patient with diabetes and severe peripheral vascular disease.
- **Aneurysm Formation.** The complicated lesions of atherosclerosis may extend into the media of an elastic artery and sufficiently weaken the wall to allow formation of an aneurysm, typically in the abdominal aorta.
- **Embolism.** A thrombus formed over an atherosclerotic plaque may detach and lodge in a distal vessel as an embolus. For example, em-

bolization from a thrombus in an abdominal aortic aneurysm may acutely occlude the popliteal artery, with subsequent gangrene of the leg. Ulceration of an atherosclerotic plaque may also dislodge atheromatous debris and lead to the so-called **cholesterol crystal emboli,** which appear as needle-shaped spaces in the affected tissues, most commonly in the kidney but also in the lower extremities.

HYPERTENSIVE VASCULAR DISEASE

The World Health Organization has defined hypertension as being a systolic pressure greater than 160 mm Hg, a diastolic pressure greater than 90, or both. In the United States, hypertension, with its associated atherosclerotic vascular disease, is a common cause of death, especially among blacks. Most of the mortality and morbidity associated with hypertension is attributed to an increased risk for a variety of cardiovascular disorders. Hypertension occurs in more than half of patients with angina pectoris, sudden death, stroke, and atherothrombotic occlusion of the abdominal aorta or its branches. Three-fourths of patients with dissecting aortic aneurysm, intracerebral hemorrhage, or rupture of the myocardial wall also have an elevated blood pressure. Hypertension is a major risk factor for atherosclerosis as well.

The cause of most cases of hypertension remains unknown, and 95% of patients have no clearly identifiable pathogenesis. Thus, the large majority of persons with hypertension are described as having *essential* or *primary* hypertension.

☐ **Pathogenesis:** Primary hypertension is thought to result from an imbalance in the interactions between mechanisms for controlling cardiac output, renal function, peripheral resistance, and sodium homeostasis (Fig. 10-13). A complex endocrine axis centers on the renin-angiotensin system. Renal artery occlusion or dietary salt restriction leads to increased secretion of renin by the kidney. Renin is a protease that splits angiotensinogen to a decapeptide, termed *angiotensin I.* In turn, angiotensin I is converted to angiotensin II by angiotensin-converting enzyme, a protein found on the surface of the endothelial cell. Angiotensin II has major effects on centers in the central nervous system that control sympathetic outflow and that stimulate aldosterone release from the adrenal gland. Aldosterone acts on the renal tubules to increase sodium reabsorption. The net effect of all these actions is an increase in total body fluid volume. Thus, the renin-angiotensin system elevates blood pressure by three mechanisms: (1) increased sympathetic output, (2) increased mineralocorticoid secretion, and (3) direct vasoconstriction.

Atrial natriuretic factor (ANF) antagonizes the renin-angiotensin-aldosterone axis. ANF is a hormone secreted by specialized cells in the cardiac atria. It binds to specific receptors in the kidney and increases the urinary excretion of sodium, thereby opposing the vasoconstrictor effects of angiotensin II. Secretion of ANF may be controlled by atrial distention, which is a consequence of increased volume, or by as-yet-undefined endocrine interactions.

Despite these considerations, the role of the renin-angiotensin axis in the pathogenesis of essential hypertension remains elusive. **Nevertheless, the end result of the balance among the various autoregulatory mechanisms is always increased peripheral resistance.**

The causes of only a small proportion of all cases of hypertension are identifiable. These include renal artery stenosis, most forms of chronic renal disease, primary elevation of aldosterone (Conn syndrome), Cushing syndrome, neoplasms of the adrenal medulla (pheochromocytoma), thyrotoxicosis, coarctation of the aorta, and a few others.

☐ **Pathology:** The central lesion in most cases of hypertension is a decreased size of the lumen in small muscular arteries and arterioles. These are the resistance vessels that control the flow of blood through the capillary bed. The lumen may be restricted by active contraction of the vessel wall, increase in the structural mass of the vessel wall, or both.

Arteriosclerosis

■ *Arteriosclerosis refers to vascular changes characterized by thickening and loss of elasticity of arterial walls. When the disorder affects the arterioles, it is termed* arteriolosclerosis.

Benign Arteriosclerosis

■ *Benign arteriosclerosis reflects mild, chronic hypertension, and the major change is a variable increase in thickness of the vessel walls.* In the smallest arteries and arterioles, these changes are termed *hyaline arteriosclerosis.* "Hyaline" refers to the glassy, scarred appearance of the blood vessel walls as seen by light microscopy. The wall of the arteriole is thickened by the deposition of basement membrane material and the accumulation of plasma proteins. The small muscular arteries display new layers of elastin, presenting as reduplication of the intimal elastic lamina, and increased connective tissue. The vascular lesions subsumed under the *term benign arteriosclerosis* are particularly evident in the kidney, where they result in a loss of renal parenchyma, termed *benign nephrosclerosis.*

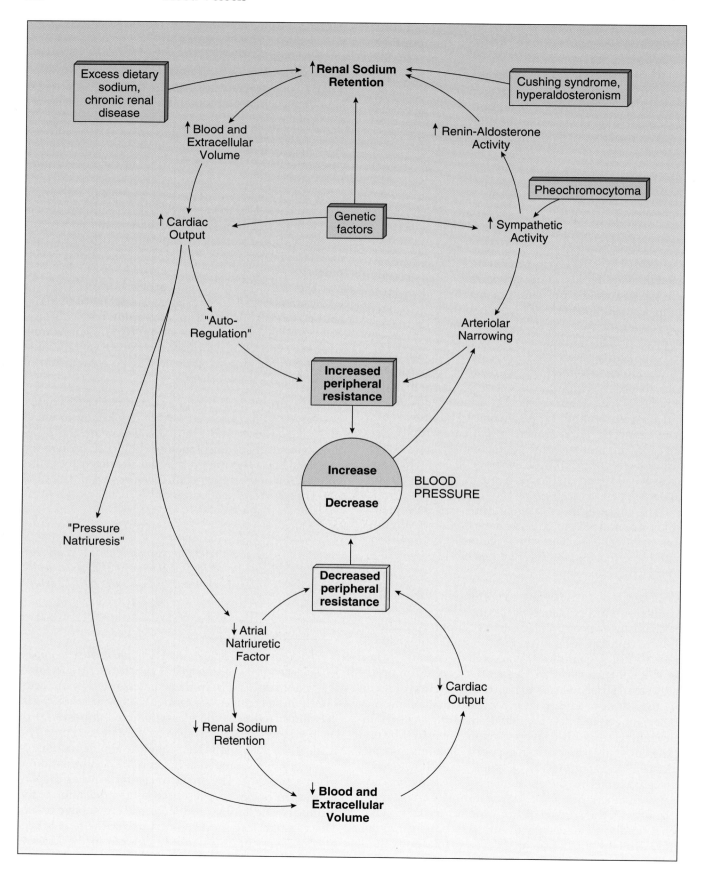

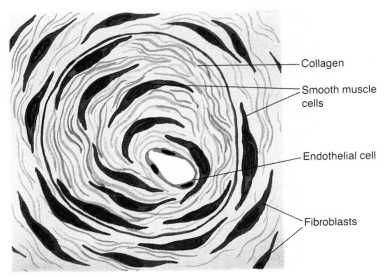

Collagen

Smooth muscle cells

Endothelial cell

Fibroblasts

F I G U R E   *10-14*
Arteriolosclerosis. In hypertension, the arterioles exhibit smooth muscle cell proliferation and increased amounts of intercellular collagen and glycosaminoglycans, resulting in an "onion-skin" appearance. The mass of smooth muscle and associated elements tends to fix the size of the lumen and to restrict the capacity of the arteriole to

Malignant (Accelerated) Hypertension

■ *Malignant (accelerated) hypertension refers to a situation in which elevated blood pressure results in rapidly progressive vascular compromise, with the onset of symptomatic disease of the brain, heart, or kidney.* Malignant hypertension is ordinarily not evident with pressures less than 160/110 mm Hg, and modern antihypertensive therapy has made malignant hypertension a rare disorder.

Malignant hypertension produces dramatic changes, particularly at the microvascular level. Retinal vessels display microaneurysms and focal hemorrhages, with resultant scarring of the retina. Necrosis of the smooth muscle and endothelial cells in small muscular arteries and arterioles leads to deposition of plasma proteins in the walls of these vessels, termed *fibrinoid necrosis.* The period of acute injury is rapidly followed by smooth muscle proliferation and a striking, concentric increase in the number of layers of smooth muscle cells, which yields the so-called "onion-skin appearance" (Fig. 10-14). Taken together, these changes are *termed malignant arteriosclerosis or malignant arteriolosclerosis,* depending on the size of the vessels affected. Lesions associated with malignant hypertension in the kidney are termed *malignant nephrosclerosis.*

Monckeberg Medial Sclerosis

■ *Monckeberg medial sclerosis refers to degenerative calcification of the media of large- and medium-size muscu-* lar arteries, which occurs principally in older persons. The cause of this medial calcification is unknown, but it is distinct from atherosclerosis and, ordinarily, does not lead to any clinical disorder. The vessels of the upper and lower extremities are most often involved. On gross examination, involved arteries are hard and dilated. Microscopically, the smooth muscle of the media is focally replaced by pale-staining, acellular, hyalinized fibrous tissue, which often exhibits concentric dystrophic calcification. Osseous metaplasia in calcified areas is occasionally observed.

Raynaud Phenomenon

■ *Raynaud phenomenon refers to intermittent, bilateral attacks of ischemia in the fingers or toes, and sometimes in the ears or nose, secondary to intense arterial vasospasm in the skin.* It is characterized by severe pallor (Fig. 10-15) and is often accompanied by paresthesias and pain. The symptoms are precipitated by cold or emotional stimuli, and they are relieved by heat.

Raynaud phenomenon may occur as an isolated disorder or as a prominent feature of a number of systemic diseases of the connective tissue (collagen vascular disorders), particularly scleroderma.

VASCULITIS

■ *Vasculitis refers to inflammation and necrosis of the blood vessels, including the arteries, veins, and capillaries*

F I G U R E   *10-13*
Factors contributing to hypertension and counterregulatory factors that lower blood pressure. An imbalance in these factors results in the increased peripheral resistance responsible for most cases of idiopathic (primary) hypertension. Note the central role of peripheral resistance.

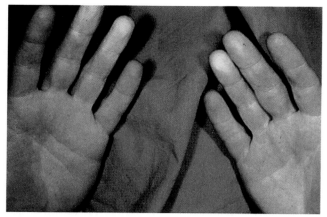

FIGURE   *10-15*
Raynaud phenomenon. The tips of the fingers show marked pallor.

(Box 10-2). Arteries or veins may be damaged by infectious agents, mechanical trauma, radiation, or toxins. However, in many cases of vasculitis, no specific cause is determined.

☐ **Pathogenesis:** Vasculitic syndromes are thought to involve immune mechanisms, including (1) deposition of immune complexes, (2) direct attack on vessels by circulating antibodies, and (3) various forms of cell-mediated immunity.

Serum sickness was one of the first human immunologic disorders to be associated with vasculitis. In animal models of serum sickness, immune complexes, together with complement, are found in the local tissue reaction (see Chapter 4). However, the search for immune complexes in human vascular lesions has yielded variable results, and firm evidence for immune complexes in the pathogenesis of many cases of vasculitis is lacking.

Viral antigens have been suspected as a cause of vasculitis in experimental animals and in humans. A case in point is chronic hepatitis B virus infection,

which is associated with some cases of polyarteritis nodosa. In this circumstance, circulating viral antigen-antibody complexes have been demonstrated, as well as the local deposition of such immune complexes in the vascular lesions. Vasculitis in humans has also been associated with a variety of other viral infections, including herpes simplex, cytomegalovirus, and human parvovirus. Several bacterial antigens have been identified in the lesions of some cases of vasculitis.

Some vasculitides, such as Wegener granulomatosis and microscopic polyarteritis (discussed later), are associated with antineutrophil cytoplasmic antibodies (ANCA), but the contribution of these autoantibodies to the vasculitis is not understood. Common morphologic patterns include a perinuclear immunofluorescence (P-ANCA, mainly against myeloperoxidase) and a more general, cytoplasmic immunofluorescence (C-ANCA, mainly against proteinase 3).

Polyarteritis Nodosa

■ *Polyarteritis nodosa is an acute, necrotizing vasculitis that affects medium-size and smaller muscular arteries and, occasionally, larger arteries.*

☐ **Pathology:** The characteristic lesion of polyarteritis nodosa is patchy and affects small- to medium-size muscular arteries. However, on occasion, it extends into larger arteries, such as the renal, splenic, or coronary arteries. Each lesion is no more than a millimeter in length and may involve either the entire circumference of the vessel or only a part of it. The most prominent morphologic feature of the affected artery is an area of fibrinoid necrosis, in which the medial muscle and adjacent tissues are fused into a structureless, eosinophilic mass that stains for fibrin. A vigorous acute inflammatory response envelops the area of necrosis, usually involving the entire adventitia (periarteritis), and extends through the other coats of the vessel (Fig. 10-16). Neutrophils, lymphocytes, plasma

B O X   *10-2*   **Inflammatory Disorders of Blood Vessels**

Polyarteritis nodosa group of systemic necrotizing vasculitis	Wegener granulomatosis
Classic polyarteritis nodosa	Lymphomatoid granulomatosis
Allergic angiitis and granulomatosis (Churg-Strauss variant)	Giant cell arteritis
"Overlap syndrome" of systemic angiitis	Temporal arteritis
Hypersensitivity vasculitis	Takayasu arteritis
Serum sickness and similar reactions	Central nervous system vasculitis
Henoch-Schönlein purpura	Vasculitis associated with cancer
Vasculitis associated with connective tissue disorders	Mucocutaneous lymph node syndrome (Kawasaki disease)
Vasculitis in cases of essential mixed cryoglobulinemia	Thromboangiitis obliterans (Buerger disease)
Vasculitis associated with other primary disorders	Behçet disease
	Miscellaneous vasculitis syndromes

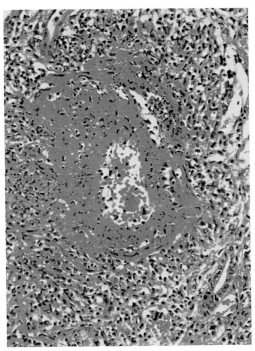

FIGURE   10-16
Polyarteritis nodosa. The intense inflammatory cell infiltrate in the arterial wall and surrounding connective tissue is associated with fibrinoid necrosis and disruption of the vessel wall.

cells, and macrophages are present in varying proportions, and eosinophils are often conspicuous. Polyarteritis nodosa affecting small vessels is frequently associated with P-ANCA.

As a result of thrombosis in the lumen of an affected segment, infarcts are commonly found in the involved organs. Injury to larger arteries results in formation of small aneurysms (diameter, <0.5 cm), particularly in branches of the renal, coronary, and cerebral arteries. An aneurysm may rupture and, if located in a critical area, be the source of fatal hemorrhage.

☐ **Clinical Features:** In polyarteritis nodosa, the kidneys, heart, skeletal muscle, skin, and mesentery are most frequently involved, but lesions may also occur in almost any organ of the body. Polyarteritis nodosa is, in most cases, fatal without treatment, but anti-inflammatory and immunosuppressive therapy in the form of corticosteroids and cyclophosphamide lead to remissions or cures in the large majority of patients.

Hypersensitivity Angiitis

■ *Hypersensitivity angiitis refers to a broad category of inflammatory vascular lesions thought to represent a re-*

sponse to exogenous substances, such as bacterial products or drugs. In the case of vascular lesions confined predominantly to the skin, the terms *leukocytoclastic vasculitis* (referring to the nuclear debris from disintegrating neutrophils), *cutaneous vasculitis*, or *cutaneous necrotizing venulitis* (emphasizing the predominant involvement of the venules) are applied. Systemic hypersensitivity angiitis, also referred to as microscopic polyarteritis, affects many of the same organs as polyarteritis nodosa, but it is restricted to the smallest arteries and arterioles.

Cutaneous vasculitis typically follows administration of a wide variety of drugs, including aspirin, penicillin, and thiazide diuretics. It also is commonly related to disparate infections, such as streptococcal and staphylococcal illnesses, viral hepatitis, tuberculosis, and bacterial endocarditis. The disease typically presents as palpable purpura, principally on the lower extremities. Microscopically, superficial cutaneous venules display fibrinoid necrosis and an acute inflammatory reaction. Cutaneous vasculitis is generally self-limited.

Systemic hypersensitivity angiitis may be an isolated entity or a feature of other conditions, including collagen vascular diseases (lupus erythematosus, rheumatoid arthritis, Sjögren syndrome), Henoch-Schönlein purpura, dysproteinemias, and a variety of malignant neoplasms. The most feared complication of microscopic polyarteritis is renal involvement, which is characterized by a rapidly progressive glomerulonephritis and renal failure. Hypersensitivity angiitis is strongly associated with ANCA (60% P-ANCA and 40% C-ANCA).

Allergic Granulomatosis and Angiitis

■ *Allergic granulomatosis and angiitis (also known as Churg-Strauss syndrome) refers to a systemic vasculitis with prominent eosinophilia that occurs in young persons with asthma.* Widespread, necrotizing vascular lesions of the small- and medium-size arteries, arterioles, and veins are found in the lungs, spleen, kidney, heart, liver, central nervous system, and other organs. Lesions are characterized by granulomas and an intense, eosinophilic infiltrate both in and around the blood vessels. The resulting fibrinoid necrosis, thrombosis, and aneurysm formation may simulate polyarteritis nodosa, although Churg-Strauss syndrome seems to be a distinct entity. Untreated persons with allergic granulomatosis and angiitis have a poor prognosis, but corticosteroids are almost always successful in treatment of the disease.

Giant Cell Arteritis

■ *Giant cell arteritis (also known as temporal arteritis or granulomatous arteritis) is a focal, chronic, granulomatous inflammation of the temporal arteries.* Today, it is perhaps the most common form of vasculitis. Although the disease most often affects the temporal artery, it can also involve additional cranial arteries, the aorta (giant cell aortitis) and its branches, and occasionally, other arteries. The average age at onset is 70 years, and the disease rarely occurs in those younger than 50. The incidence rises with age and may reach 1% by 80 years. The cause of giant cell arteritis is obscure, and no bacterial or viral cause has been found.

☐ **Pathology:** The affected artery is cord-like and exhibits nodular thickening. The lumen is either reduced to a slit or obliterated by a thrombus. Microscopic examination reveals granulomatous inflammation of the media and intima consisting of aggregates of macrophages, lymphocytes, and plasma cells, with varying admixtures of eosinophils and neutrophils (Fig. 10-17A). Giant cells usually are conspicuous but vary widely in number, and they tend to be distributed at the site of the internal elastic lamina (Fig. 10-17B). Both foreign body giant cells and Langhans giant cells may be found. Foci of necrosis are characterized by changes in the internal elastica, which becomes swollen, irregular, and fragmented and, in advanced lesions, may completely disappear. In the late stages, the intima is conspicuously thickened, and the media is fibrotic. Thrombosis may obliterate the lumen, after which organization and canalization occur.

☐ **Clinical Features:** Giant cell arteritis is usually benign and self-limited, the symptoms subsiding within 6 to 12 months. Patients present with headache and throbbing temporal pain, with tenderness and redness in the skin overlying the vessel. Visual symptoms occur in almost half of the patients and may proceed from transient to permanent blindness in one or both eyes. Response to corticosteroid therapy is usually dramatic, with symptoms subsiding in a matter of days.

Wegener Granulomatosis

■ *Wegener granulomatosis is a systemic, necrotizing vasculitis of unknown cause characterized by granulomatous lesions of the respiratory tract (nose, sinuses, and lungs) and renal glomerular disease.* Men are more often affected than women, usually during the fifth and sixth decades of life. The cause of the disease is unknown, and no infectious agent has been uncovered. It has been suggested that these antibodies activate circulating neutrophils to attack blood vessels.

☐ **Pathology:** Lesions of Wegener granulomatosis are characterized by parenchymal necrosis, vasculitis, and granulomatous inflammation composed of neutrophils, lymphocytes, plasma cells, macrophages, and eosinophils. The individual lesions in the lung may be as large as 5 cm across, and they must be distinguished from those of tuberculosis. Vasculitis involving small arteries and veins may be found anywhere but occurs most frequently in the respiratory tract (Fig. 10-18),

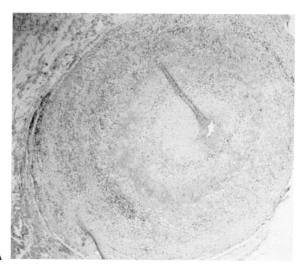
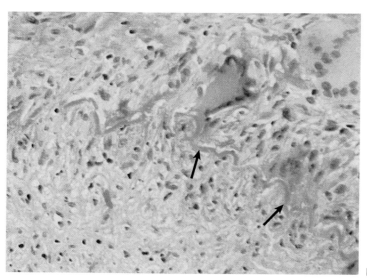

A   B

FIGURE *10-17*
Temporal (giant cell) arteritis. (A) A photomicrograph of a temporal artery shows chronic inflammation throughout the wall and a lumen severely narrowed by intimal thickening. (B) A higher-power view of *panel A* **shows giant cells adjacent to the fragmented internal elastic lamina (***arrows***).**

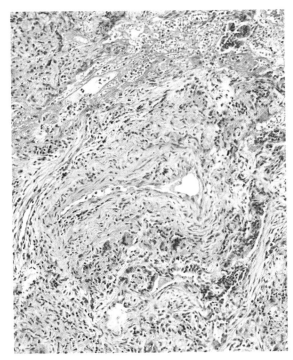

FIGURE 10-18
Wegener granulomatosis. A photomicrograph of the lung shows vasculitis of a pulmonary artery. There are chronic inflammatory cells and Langhans giant cells in the wall and thickening of the intima.

kidney, and spleen. The arteritis is characterized principally by chronic inflammation, although acute inflammation, necrotizing and nonnecrotizing granulomatous inflammation, and fibrinoid necrosis are frequently present. Medial thickening and intimal proliferation are common and often result in narrowing or obliteration of the lumen.

The most prominent pulmonary feature is a persistent bilateral pneumonitis, with nodular infiltrates that undergo cavitation in a manner similar to that of tuberculous lesions (although the mechanisms are clearly different). The kidney initially exhibits focal necrotizing glomerulonephritis, which progresses to crescentic glomerulonephritis. Chronic sinusitis and ulcerations of the nasopharyngeal mucosa are common.

☐ **Clinical Features:** The large majority of patients with Wegener granulomatosis present with symptoms referable to the respiratory tract, particularly pneumonitis and sinusitis. Radiologically, multiple pulmonary infiltrates, which are often cavitary, are prominent. Hematuria and proteinuria are common, and the glomerular disease can progress to renal failure. Rashes, muscular pains, joint involvement, and neurologic symptoms occur as well. Untreated Wegener

granulomatosis carries a very high mortality rate; most patients (80%) die within a year of onset, with a mean survival time of 5 to 6 months. Treatment with cyclophosphamide, however, produces a striking improvement in the prognosis, and both complete remissions and substantial disease-free intervals are induced in most patients.

Takayasu Arteritis

■ *Takayasu arteritis refers to an inflammatory disorder of large arteries, classically the aortic arch and its major branches.* This malady has a worldwide distribution and primarily affects young women (90%), the large majority of whom are younger than 30 years. The cause of Takayasu arteritis is unknown, but an autoimmune basis has been proposed.

☐ **Pathology:** On gross examination, the aorta is thickened, and the intima exhibits focal, raised plaques. Branches of the aorta often display localized stenosis or occlusion, which interferes with the flow of blood and accounts for the synonym "pulseless disease" when the subclavian arteries are affected. The aorta, particularly the distal thoracic and abdominal segments, commonly shows variably sized aneurysms. Early lesions of the aorta and its main branches consist of acute panarteritis, with infiltrates of neutrophils, mononuclear cells, and occasional Langhans giant cells. Late lesions display fibrosis and severe intimal proliferation, and secondary atherosclerotic changes may obscure the basic disease.

☐ **Clinical Features:** Patients with early Takayasu arteritis complain of constitutional symptoms, dizziness, visual disturbances, dyspnea, and occasionally, syncope. As the disease progresses, cardiac symptoms become more severe, and intermittent claudication of the arms or legs appears. Asymmetric differences in blood pressure may also develop, and the pulse in one extremity may actually disappear. Hypertension may reflect coarctation of the aorta or renal artery stenosis. The majority of patients eventually manifest congestive heart failure or loss of visual acuity, ranging from field defects to total blindness. Early lesions of Takayasu arteritis respond to corticosteroids, but later lesions require surgical reconstruction.

Kawasaki Disease

■ *Kawasaki disease (also known as mucocutaneous lymph node syndrome) is an acute disease of infancy and early childhood characterized clinically by high fever, rash, conjunctival and oral lesions, and lymphadenitis and pathologically by an acute necrotizing vasculitis.* The disease is similar to polyarteritis nodosa and affects the coronary arteries, with aneurysm formation in as many as 70%

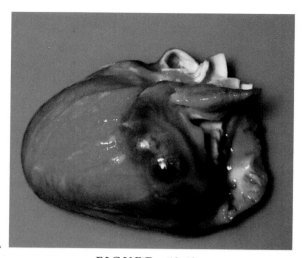

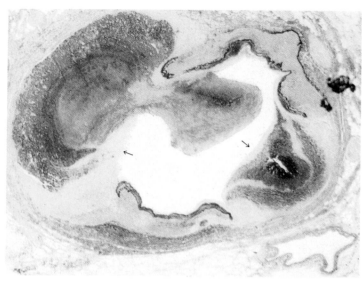

A   B

FIGURE   *10-19*
Kawasaki disease. (A) The heart of a child who died from Kawasaki disease shows conspicuous coronary artery aneurysms. (B) A microscopic section of a coronary artery from the same patient shows two large defects (*arrows*) in the internal elastic lamina, with two small aneurysms filled with thrombi.

of patients (Fig. 10-19). Kawasaki disease is fatal in 1% to 2% of cases.

Like many childhood viral illnesses, Kawasaki disease is usually self-limited, and although an infectious cause has been sought, none has been conclusively proved.

Thromboangiitis Obliterans

■ *Thromboangiitis obliterans or Buerger disease is an occlusive, inflammatory disease of the small- and medium-size arteries in the distal arms and legs.* Buerger disease occurs almost exclusively in young and middle-aged men who smoke heavily.

□ **Pathogenesis:** The causative role of smoking in Buerger disease is emphasized by the observation that cessation of smoking can be followed by a remission and resumption of smoking by an exacerbation. However, the mechanism of action by tobacco smoke is obscure.

□ **Pathology:** The earliest change in Buerger disease is an acute inflammation of small- and medium-size arteries. The neutrophilic infiltrate extends to involve neighboring veins and nerves, and involvement of the endothelium in the inflamed areas leads to thrombosis and obliteration of the lumen (Fig. 10-20). Early lesions often become severe enough to result in gangrene of the extremity, for which the only treatment is amputation. Late in the course of the disease, thrombi are completely organized and partly canalized.

□ **Clinical Features:** The symptoms of Buerger disease usually start between the ages of 25 and 40 years. They take the form of intermittent claudication (cramping pains in muscles following exercise, which are quickly relieved by rest). Patients often present

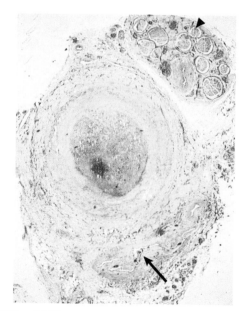

FIGURE   *10-20*
Buerger disease. Section of the upper extremity shows an organized arterial thrombus, which has occluded the lumen. Some inflammatory cells are evident in the adventitial fat. In this instance, the vein (*arrow*) and the adjacent nerve (*arrowhead*) show foci of chronic inflammation.

with painful ulceration of a digit, which often progresses to destruction of the involved tips. Persons with Buerger disease who continue to smoke may slowly lose both hands and feet.

ANEURYSMS

■ *Arterial aneurysms* are localized dilatations of blood vessels caused by a congenital or acquired weakness in the media. They are not rare, and their incidence tends to increase with age. In fact, aneurysms of the aorta and other arteries are found in as many as 10% of autopsies. The wall of an aneurysm is formed by the stretched remnants of the arterial wall.

Aneurysms are classified by location, configuration, and cause (Fig. 10-21). The location refers to the type of vessel involved—artery or vein—and the specific vessel affected, such as the aorta or popliteal artery. The classifications themselves are:

- **Fusiform Aneurysm.** An ovoid swelling parallel to the long axis of the vessel.
- **Saccular Aneurysm.** A bubble-like outpouching of the arterial wall at the site of weakened media.
- **Dissecting Aneurysm.** A dissecting hematoma in which hemorrhage into the media separates the layers of the vascular wall by a column of blood.
- **Arteriovenous Aneurysm.** A direct communication between an artery and a vein.

Atherosclerotic Aneurysms

Atherosclerotic aneurysms of the abdominal aorta and common iliac arteries are the most frequent aneurysms, usually developing after the age of 50 years. They occur much more often in men than in women, and half of these patients are hypertensive. Several studies have implicated genetic factors in the pathogenesis of aortic aneurysms.

□ **Pathology: Most atherosclerotic aneurysms of the aorta are distal to the renal arteries and proximal to the bifurcation** (Fig. 10-22). They are usually fusiform, although saccular varieties are occasionally encountered. Lesions may be of almost any size, but the majority of the symptomatic ones are more than 5 to 6 cm in diameter. Some of these aneurysms extend into the iliac arteries, which may also exhibit distinct aneurysms distal to the one in the aorta.

An atherosclerotic aneurysm, by definition, is lined by raised, ulcerated, and calcified (complicated) atherosclerotic lesions. Most contain a mural thrombus of varying degrees of organization. Portions of the thrombus may dislodge and be carried in the blood-

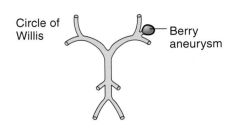

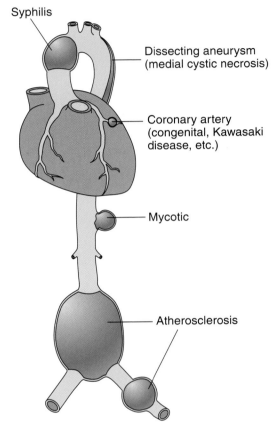

FIGURE   *10-21*
Locations of aneurysms. Syphilitic aneurysms are the common variety in the ascending aorta, which is usually spared by the atherosclerotic process. Atherosclerotic aneurysms can occur in the abdominal aorta or muscular arteries, including the coronary and popliteal arteries and other vessels. Berry aneurysms are seen in the circle of Willis, mainly at branch points; their rupture leads to subarachnoid hemorrhage. Mycotic aneurysms occur almost anywhere that bacteria can deposit on vessel walls.

stream as emboli to peripheral arteries, and the thrombus itself may enlarge sufficiently to compromise the lumen of the aorta.

Microscopic examination reveals destruction of the normal arterial wall and its replacement by fibrous tissue. Remnants of normal media are seen focally, and atheromatous lesions extend to variable depths. The adventitia is thickened and focally inflamed.

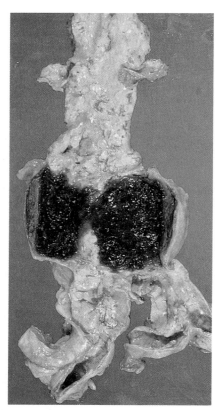

FIGURE   *10-22*
Atherosclerotic aneurysm of the abdominal aorta. The aneurysm has been opened longitudinally to reveal a large mural thrombus in the lumen. The aorta and common iliac arteries display complicated lesions of atherosclerosis.

□ **Clinical Features:** Many atherosclerotic aortic aneurysms are asymptomatic and are discovered only by palpation of a mass in the abdomen or radiologic examination for some other reason. In some cases, the condition is brought to medical attention by the onset of abdominal pain, which often reflects expansion of the aneurysm. Abrupt occlusion of a peripheral artery by an embolus from the mural thrombus presents as sudden ischemia of a lower limb. The most dreaded complication of aortic aneurysms is rupture and exsanguinating retroperitoneal (or thoracic) hemorrhage, in which the patient presents with pain, shock, and a pulsatile mass in the abdomen. Such a situation is an acute emergency, and even with prompt surgical intervention, half the patients die. Therefore, large aneurysms, even if entirely asymptomatic, are often replaced by, or bypassed with, prosthetic grafts.

Aneurysms of Cerebral Arteries

Aneurysms of cerebral arteries are particularly important, because they lead to fatal subarachnoid hemorrhage. The most common cerebral aneurysm is called a

berry aneurysm, because as a saccular aneurysm, it resembles a berry attached to a "twig" of the arterial tree. Berry aneurysms result from a congenital defect in a branch point of the arterial wall. They tend to arise at one of the branching angles of the circle of Willis or in one of the arterial branches. The most common sites are (1) between the anterior cerebral artery and anterior communicating artery, (2) between the internal carotid artery and posterior communicating artery, and (3) between the first main divisions of the middle cerebral artery and the bifurcation of the internal carotid artery. Berry aneurysms are discussed in detail in Chapter 28.

Dissecting Aneurysms

■ *Dissecting aneurysm refers to the entry of blood into the arterial wall and its extension along the length of the vessel* (Fig. 10-23). In effect, the blood is encompassed by a false lumen within the wall of the artery. **Although this lesion is conventionally termed an** *aneurysm,* **it is actually a form of hematoma.** Dissecting aneurysm most often affects the aorta and its major branches. Men are affected threefold as frequently as women. A dissecting aneurysm may occur at almost any age, but it is most common during the sixth and seventh decades of life. **The large majority of patients have a history of hypertension.**

□ **Pathogenesis:** The pathogenesis of dissecting aneurysm, in most instances, can be traced to weakening in the connective tissue of the aortic media. The changes were originally described as **cystic medial necrosis** (of Erdheim). Focal loss of elastic and muscle fibers in the media leads to "cystic" spaces filled with a metachromatic, myxoid material. The cause of the medial degeneration is not known, but some cases represent a complication of Marfan syndrome. More than 95% of dissecting aneurysms show a transverse tear in the intima and internal media, and many investigators hold that a spontaneous laceration of the intima allows blood from the lumen to enter and dissect the media.

□ **Pathology:** The majority of intimal tears are found in the ascending aorta, 1 or 2 cm above the aortic ring. Dissection in the media roughly separates the inner two-thirds of the aorta from the outer one-third. It can also involve the coronary arteries, great vessels of the neck, or the renal, mesenteric, or iliac arteries. Because the outer wall of the false channel of the dissecting aneurysm is thin, hemorrhage into the extravascular space, including the pericardium, mediastinum, pleural space, and retroperitoneum, is a frequent cause of death. In 5% to 10% of cases, blood within the dissecting aneurysm re-enters the lumen through a second, distal tear to form a "double-barreled aorta." In a comparable proportion, a re-entry

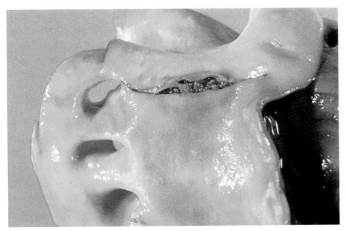
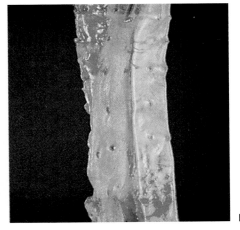
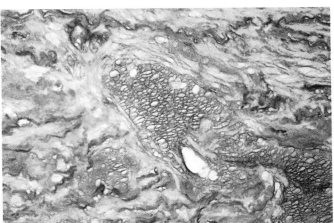

FIGURE *10-23*
Dissecting aneurysms of the aorta. (A) A transverse tear is present in the aortic arch. The orifices of the great vessels are on the left. (B) Blood dissected in the media of the thoracic aorta. The intimal aspect of the media (*right*) has been reflected to reveal the false lumen. (C) A section of the aortic wall stained with aldehyde fuchsin shows pools of metachromatic material characteristic of the degenerative process known as cystic medial necrosis.

site leads to communication of the aorta with a major artery (most often the iliac).

☐ **Clinical Features:** The typical patient with an aortic dissection is hypertensive and presents with acute onset of severe, "tearing" pain in the anterior chest, which is sometimes misdiagnosed as myocardial infarction. A loss of one or more arterial pulses is common, and a murmur of aortic regurgitation is often present. Whereas hypertension is a frequent finding, hypotension is an ominous sign, suggesting aortic rupture. Cardiac tamponade or congestive heart failure is diagnosed according to the usual criteria. Surgical intervention and control of hypertension have reduced the overall mortality rate to less than 20%.

Syphilitic Aneurysms

Syphilitic (luetic) aneurysms were once the most common form of aortic aneurysm, but the decline in the prevalence of syphilis has led to a marked decrease in syphilitic vascular disease, including aortitis and aneurysms. Microscopic examination shows endarteri-

tis and periarteritis of the vasa vasorum. These vessels ramify in the adventitia and penetrate the outer and middle thirds of the aorta, where they become encircled by lymphocytes, plasma cells, and macrophages. Obliterative changes in the vasa vasorum cause focal necrosis and scarring of the media, with disruption and disorganization of the elastic lamellae. Depressed medial scars lead to a roughened intimal surface, which imparts a "tree bark" appearance. Extensive atherosclerosis may be intermixed with syphilitic aortitis. The weakened wall of the ascending aorta and aortic arch eventually yields to the relentless pressure of the blood and balloons, thereby forming a fusiform aneurysm.

VEINS

Varicose Veins of the Legs

■ *Varicose veins are enlarged, tortuous blood vessels.* Superficial varicosities of the leg veins, usually in the saphenous system, are among the most common ailments of humans. They vary from a trivial knot of dilated veins to a disabling distention of the entire venous system of the leg, with secondary trophic disturbances. It has been estimated that as much as 10% to 20% of the population has some varicosities in the leg veins, but only a fraction of these persons develop symptoms.

☐ **Pathogenesis:** There are a number of risk factors for varicose veins:

- **Age.** The incidence of varicose veins rises with age, and it may reach 50% in persons older than 50 years.
- **Sex.** In the 30- to 50-year-old age group, women are affected by varicose veins more often than men, particularly women who have experienced the increased venous pressure associated with the weight of the pregnant uterus on the iliac veins.
- **Heredity.** There is a strong familial predisposition to varicose veins.
- **Posture.** The pressure in the leg veins is five- to 10-fold greater in the erect than in the recumbent position. As a result, the incidence of varicose veins is increased among persons whose occupations require them to stand in one place for long periods, such as dentists and sales clerks.
- **Obesity.** Excessive body weight increases the incidence of varicose veins.

Other factors that augment venous pressure in the legs can also cause varicose veins. These include pelvic tumors, congestive heart failure, and thrombotic obstruction of the main venous trunks of the thigh or pelvis.

In the pathogenesis of varicose veins, it is not clear whether incompetence of the valves or dilatation of the vessels comes first. Whatever the case, the two reinforce each other. The vein increases in both length and diameter, so that tortuosities develop. Once the process has begun, the varicosity extends progressively throughout the length of the affected vein, and as each valve becomes incompetent, a progressively increasing strain is thrown on the vessel and the valve below.

☐ **Pathology:** Microscopically, varicose veins exhibit variations in the thickness of the wall. Thinning by dilatation is present in some areas, whereas others are thickened by muscle hypertrophy, subintimal fibrosis, and the incorporation of mural thrombi into the wall. Valvular deformities consist of thickening, shortening, and rolling of the cusps.

☐ **Clinical Features:** Most varicose veins have no clinical effects and require no treatment. The principal symptom is aching in the legs, which is aggravated by standing and relieved by elevation. Severe varicosities may lead to trophic alterations in skin drained by the affected veins, termed **stasis dermatitis.** Surgical intervention is mandated in the presence of ulceration of the overlying skin, spontaneous bleeding, or extensive thrombosis (which may lead to pulmonary embolism).

Varicose Veins at Other Sites

Hemorrhoids. These dilatations of the veins of the rectum and anal canal may occur either inside or outside the anal sphincter. The condition is aggravated by constipation and pregnancy. It may also result from venous obstruction by rectal tumors. Hemorrhoids often bleed, a sign that can produce confusion with bleeding rectal cancers. Thrombosed hemorrhoids are exquisitely painful.

Esophageal Varices. These complications of portal hypertension are caused mainly by cirrhosis of the liver. High portal pressure leads to distention of the anastomoses between the portal system and the systemic veins at the lower end of the esophagus. Hemorrhage from esophageal varices is one of the most common causes of death in patients with cirrhosis.

Varicocele. A varicocele is a palpable mass in the scrotum formed by varicosities of the pampiniform plexus.

Deep Venous Thrombosis

Thrombophlebitis describes an inflammation and secondary thrombosis of small veins, and sometimes larger ones, commonly as part of a local reaction to bacterial infection. **Phlebothrombosis** is the term for venous thrombosis in the absence of an initiating infection or inflammation. Because the majority of cases of venous thrombosis are not associated with inflammation or infection, the term **deep venous thrombosis** now refers to both phlebothrombosis and thrombophlebitis. The condition is associated with prolonged bed rest or reduced cardiac output, and it frequently affects the deep leg veins. Such thrombi can be a major threat to life because of embolization to the lung (witness the well-known phenomenon of sudden death occurring on ambulation after surgery).

LYMPHATIC VESSELS

Lymphangitis

■ *Lymphangitis refers to inflammation of the lymphatic vessels caused by the entrance of bacteria and inflammatory cells from sites of drainage.* These elements are then conveyed to the regional lymph nodes, where they incite a lymphadenitis. The periphery of a focus of inflammation reveals dilated lymphatics filled with fluid exudate, cells, cellular debris, and bacteria.

Almost any virulent pathogen can cause acute lymphangitis, but group A β-hemolytic streptococci (*Streptococcus pyogenes*) are particularly notorious offenders. The draining lymph nodes are regularly enlarged and inflamed. Clinically, painful subcutaneous red streaks, often accompanied by painful regional lymph nodes, are characteristic of acute lymphangitis.

Lymphatic Obstruction

Lymphatics may be obstructed by scar tissue, intraluminal tumor cells, pressure from surrounding tumor tissue, or plugging with parasites. Because collateral lymphatic routes are abundant, **lymphedema** (distention of tissue by lymph) usually occurs only when major trunks are obstructed, especially in the axilla or groin. For example, when radical mastectomy for cancer of the breast was routine, dissection of the axillary lymph nodes frequently disrupted the lymphatic channels and led to lymphedema of the arm. Prolonged lymphatic obstruction causes progressive dilatation of the lymphatic vessels, called **lymphangiectasia,** and overgrowth of fibrous tissue. The term **elephantiasis** describes a lymphedematous limb that has become grossly enlarged. An important cause of elephantiasis in the tropics is filariasis, in which a parasitic worm invades the lymphatics. **Milroy disease** is an inherited type of lymphedema that is present at birth.

BENIGN TUMORS OF BLOOD VESSELS

Hemangiomas

■ *Hemangiomas are common, congenital vascular lesions formed by cavernous or capillary-type, endothelial-lined channels.* They usually occur in the skin but may also be found in the internal organs. Although hemangiomas are clearly benign, their true origin is uncertain, and they represent either true neoplasms or hamartomas. Hemangiomas are classified by histologic type and location.

Capillary Hemangioma. This lesion is composed of vascular channels that have both the size and the structure of normal capillaries. The most common sites are the skin, subcutaneous tissues, mucous membranes of the lips and mouth, and internal viscera, including the spleen, kidneys, and liver. Capillary hemangiomas vary from a few millimeters to several centimeters in diameter. Their color is bright red to blue, depending on the degree of oxygenation in the blood. In the skin, capillary hemangiomas are known as birthmarks or ruby spots. The only disability is cosmetic disfiguration.

Juvenile Hemangioma. Also called strawberry hemangiomas, these lesions are packed masses of capillaries on the skin of newborns. They grow rapidly during the first few months of life, begin to fade at 1 to 3 years of age, and completely regress in the majority of cases (80%) by 5 years. Histologically, juvenile hemangioma is composed of numerous endothelial-lined channels filled with blood and separated by connective tissue.

Cavernous Hemangioma. These lesions consist of large, vascular channels that are frequently interspersed with small, capillary-type vessels. Cavernous hemangiomas occur in the skin (Fig. 10-24), where they are termed **port wine stains.** They also appear on the mucosal surfaces and visceral organs, including the spleen, liver, and pancreas. Occasionally, they are found in the brain, where after long quiescent periods they may slowly enlarge and cause neurologic symptoms.

A cavernous hemangioma appears as a red-blue, soft, spongy mass, with a diameter of as much as several centimeters. Unlike the capillary hemangioma, a cavernous hemangioma does not regress spontaneously. Large endothelial-lined, blood-containing spaces are separated by sparse connective tissue.

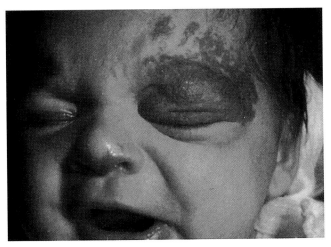

FIGURE *10-24*
Congenital cavernous hemangioma of the skin.

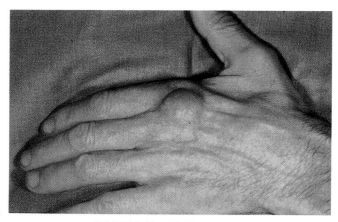
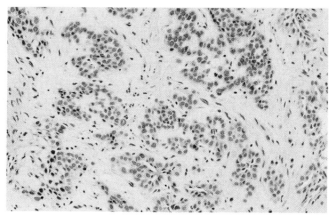

A   **B**

FIGURE   *10-25*
**Glomus tumor. (A) The dorsal surface of the hand displays a prominent tumor nodule on
the proximal third finger. (B) A photomicrograph of** *panel A* **reveals nests of glomus tumor cells embedded in a fibrovascular stroma.**

Multiple Hemangiomatous Syndromes. A number
of hemangiomas may be found in a single tissue. Two
or more tissues may be involved, such as the skin and
nervous system or the spleen and the liver. Eponym
enthusiasts have defined various combinations of sites.
For example, **von Hippel-Lindau syndrome** is a rare
entity in which cavernous hemangiomas occur within
the cerebellum or brainstem and the retina. **Sturge-
Weber syndrome** is characterized by a developmental
disturbance of blood vessels in the brain and skin.
Other closely related lesions are **plexiform** or **race-
mose angiomas, cirsoid aneurysms,** and **angiomatous
dilatation** of vessels of the central nervous system and
elsewhere.

Glomus Tumor (Glomangioma)

■ *Glomangioma is a benign, exquisitely painful tumor
of the glomus body, a convoluted arteriovenous anastomosis.*
Glomus bodies are normal neuromyoarterial receptors
that are sensitive to temperature and that regulate arteriolar flow. They are widely distributed in the skin
but are most frequent in the distal regions of the fingers
and toes. This pattern is reflected in the location of glomus tumors at these sites, typically in a subungual location.

The lesions are small, usually less than 1 cm in diameter; many are smaller than a few millimeters. In the
skin, they are slightly elevated, rounded, red-blue, and
firm (Fig. 10-25). The two main histologic components
are branching vascular channels in a connective tissue
stroma and aggregates or nests of specialized glomus
cells. The latter are regular, round to cuboidal cells that
by electron microscopy reveal typical features of
smooth muscle cells.

Hemangioendothelioma

■ *Hemangioendothelioma refers to a vascular tumor
composed of endothelial cells that is considered to be intermediate between a benign hemangioma and a frankly malignant angiosarcoma.*

The epithelioid, or histiocytoid, variant displays
endothelial cells with considerable eosinophilic, often
vacuolated, cytoplasm. Vascular lumina are evident,
and there is a paucity of mitoses. These tumors occur in
almost all locations. Surgical removal is generally curative, but approximately one-fifth of the patients develop metastases.

Spindle cell hemangioendothelioma occurs principally in males of any age, usually in the dermis and
subcutaneous tissue of the distal extremities. The tumor features vascular, endothelial-lined spaces, into
which papillary projections extend. Although the lesion may recur locally after excision, this variant of hemangioendothelioma rarely metastasizes.

MALIGNANT TUMORS OF BLOOD VESSELS

Angiosarcoma is a rare, highly malignant tumor composed of single or multiple masses of neoplastic endothelial cells. The lesions occur in either sex and at
any age. It begins as small, painless, sharply demarcated, red nodules. The most common locations are the
skin, soft tissue, breast, bone, liver, and spleen.
Eventually, most angiosarcomas enlarge to become
pale gray, fleshy masses without a capsule.

Angiosarcomas exhibit varying degrees of differentiation, ranging from those composed mainly of distinct vascular elements to undifferentiated tumors with few recognizable blood channels. The latter display frequent mitoses, pleomorphism, and giant cells, and they also tend to be more malignant. **Almost half of all patients with an angiosarcoma will die of the disease.**

Angiosarcoma of the liver is of special interest because of its association with environmental carcinogens, such as arsenic, and with thorium dioxide (Thorotrast), a material used by radiologists before 1950.

Hemangiopericytoma is a rare, malignant neoplasm that presumably arises from pericytes, the smooth muscle cells external to the walls of capillaries and arterioles. The tumor presents as small masses and consists of capillary-like channels surrounded by, and frequently enclosed within, nests and masses of round to spindle-shaped cells. The reported metastatic rate varies from 10% to 50%.

Kaposi sarcoma is a malignant tumor derived from endothelial cells. Whereas it was originally described as an uncommon, sporadic tumor, it has now appeared in epidemic form in association with acquired immunodeficiency syndrome (AIDS). This association suggests that an immune deficiency plays a role in pathogenesis of the tumor. The cause of this formerly rare disease is now clearer; its association with the current AIDS epidemic as a widespread, multifocal lesion suggests that it is related to the loss of immunity. A virus of the herpes family (HHV 8) is present in the endothelial and spindle cells of Kaposi sarcoma and is thought to contribute to the genesis of this tumor.

The tumor begins as painful, purple or brown nodules in the skin, varying from 1 mm to 1 cm in diameter. They occur most often on the hands or feet but may appear anywhere. The histologic appearance of Kaposi sarcoma is highly variable. One form resembles a simple hemangioma and is characterized by tightly packed clusters of capillaries and scattered, hemosiderin-laden macrophages. In other forms of the tumor, lesions are highly cellular, and vascular spaces are less prominent (Fig. 10-26). Although Kaposi sarcoma is considered to be a malignant lesion and may be widely disseminated in the body, it is only exceptionally a cause of death.

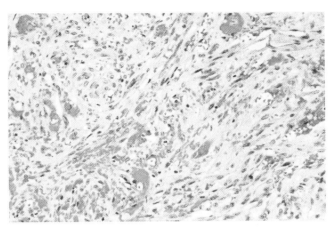

FIGURE *10-26*
Kaposi sarcoma. A photomicrograph of a vascular lesion from a patient with AIDS shows numerous poorly differentiated, spindle-shaped neoplastic cells and a vascular lesion filled with red blood cells.

CHAPTER 11

The Heart

Robert B. Jennings
Charles Steenbergen, Jr.

(continued)

Cardiac Tumors	**Diseases of the Pericardium**
Cardiac Myxoma	Pericardial Effusion
Rhabdomyoma	Acute Pericarditis
Metastatic Tumors	Constrictive Pericarditis

The heart is a fist-sized muscular pump that has a remarkable capacity to work unceasingly for the 70 to 80 years of a human lifetime. As demand requires, it can increase its output manyfold, in part because the coronary circulation can augment the flow of blood to a rate more than 10-fold greater than normal. The ventricles also respond to an acute increase in their workload by dilating, in accordance with Starling's law of the heart. Thus, dilatation of the ventricles at autopsy indicates that a patient died during heart failure. When increased workload is imposed for a longer period, such as in cases of essential hypertension, the left ventricle hypertrophies, which is an adaptation that increases its work capacity. However, when this compensatory mechanism reaches its limit, the heart no longer provides an adequate supply of blood to the peripheral tissues, with the result being congestive heart failure. Damage to the myocardium, caused mostly by ischemic heart disease, also limits the capacity of the left ventricle to pump blood and similarly results in heart failure.

CORONARY ARTERIES

The right and left main coronary arteries originate either in or immediately above the sinuses of Valsalva of the aortic valve. The left main coronary artery bifurcates within 1 cm of its origin into the left anterior descending (LAD) and the left circumflex coronary arteries. The left circumflex coronary artery supplies the lateral wall of the left ventricle (Fig. 11-1). The LAD coronary artery provides blood to (1) the anterior left ventricle, (2) the adjacent anterior right ventricle, and (3) the anterior two-thirds of the interventricular septum. In the apical region, the LAD coronary artery supplies the ventricles circumferentially.

The right coronary artery nourishes the remainder of the right ventricle and the posteroseptal region of the left ventricle, including the posterior one-third of the interventricular septum at the base of the heart (also referred to as the inferior or diaphragmatic wall). From these distributions, one can predict the location of the infarct that follows occlusion of any coronary artery branch.

Epicardial coronary arteries are usually arranged in the so-called right coronary dominant distribution. Dominance is determined by the coronary artery that contributes most of the blood to the posterior descending coronary artery. In 10% of human hearts, there is a left dominant pattern, with the left circumflex coronary artery supplying the posterior descending coronary artery.

MYOCARDIAL HYPERTROPHY AND HEART FAILURE

During systole, the normal ventricles contract vigorously and eject approximately 65% of the blood that is present in them at the end of diastole (ejection fraction). When the heart is injured, cardiac function is impaired. **If the initial impairment is severe, cardiac output is not maintained, and the result is acute, life-threatening, cardiogenic shock.** If the functional impairment is less extensive, compensatory mechanisms (discussed later) allow cardiac output to be maintained by increasing the diastolic ventricular filling pressure and the end-diastolic volume. This situation results in the characteristic signs and symptoms of congestive heart failure. **The most prominent feature of heart failure is the abnormally high atrial filling pressure relative to stroke volume.** Because of the heart's capacity to compensate, congestive heart failure often is tolerated for many years.

Myocardial hypertrophy provides another compensatory mechanism that requires time to develop. It is an adaptive process of the failing heart that augments the contractile strength of the myocytes.

PATHOLOGY OF HEART FAILURE

Almost anything that causes the heart to increase its workload for a prolonged period or that produces anatomic damage making it more difficult for the heart to function may eventuate in myocardial failure. **By far, the most common type of heart disease responsi-**

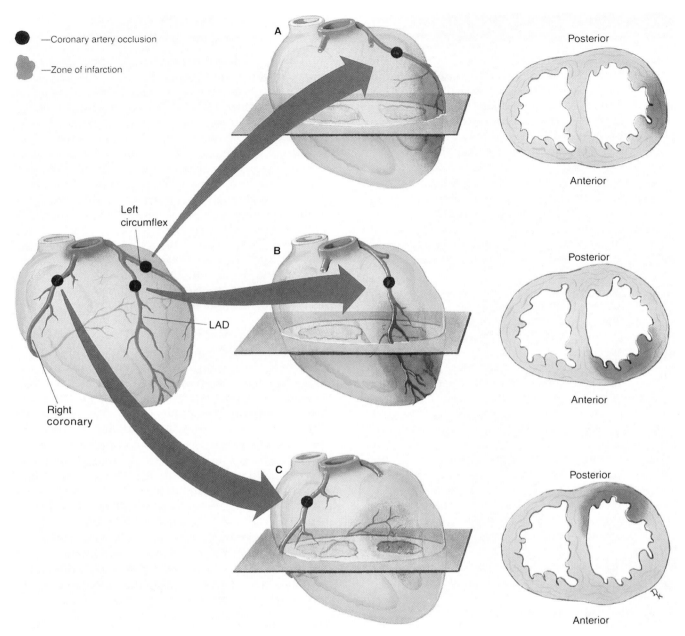

FIGURE *11-1*
Position of left ventricular infarcts resulting from occlusion of each of the three main coronary arteries. (A) Posterolateral infarct, which follows occlusion of the left circumflex artery and is present in the posterolateral wall. (B) Anterior infarct, which follows occlusion of the anterior descending branch (LAD) of the left coronary artery. The infarct is located in the anterior wall and adjacent two-thirds of the septum, in the apical three-quarters of the left ventricle. It involves the entire circumference of the wall near the apex. (C) Posterior ("inferior" or "diaphragmatic") infarct, which results from occlusion of the right coronary artery and involves the posterior wall, including the posterior one-third of the interventricular septum and the posterior papillary muscle in the basal half of the ventricle. Note the lateral displacement of the posterior papillary muscle caused by the expansion (stretching) of the infarct region of the left ventricle.

ble for cardiac failure is ischemic heart disease, which accounts for more than 80% of deaths from heart disease. Between 1% and 3% of cardiac deaths are caused by hypertensive heart disease and 1% by rheumatic heart disease. The remaining types of heart disease account for less than 1% of cardiac deaths each.

Virtually all organs of the body suffer the effects of heart failure. This subject is discussed in detail in Chapter 7, and only the salient features are reviewed here.

The ventricles are conspicuously dilated and, in cases of chronic failure, tend to be hypertrophied. The distribution of organ involvement depends on whether the heart failure is predominantly left- or right-sided.

Left-sided heart failure is the more common type of heart failure, because the most frequent causes of cardiac injury (ischemic heart disease, hypertension) primarily affect the left ventricle. As a compensatory response to left ventricular failure, both left atrial pressure and pulmonary venous pressure increase, thereby resulting in **passive pulmonary congestion.** The capillaries in the alveolar septa fill with blood, and the alveoli contain many hemosiderin-laden macrophages. Moreover, fluid leaks from the capillaries into the alveoli if the capillary hydrostatic pressure exceeds the plasma osmotic pressure. The resultant pulmonary edema may be massive, with alveoli being drowned in a transudate. Interstitial fibrosis results when congestion is present for an extended period of time.

Right-sided heart failure commonly complicates left-sided failure, but it can also develop independently secondary to intrinsic pulmonary disease and pulmonary hypertension. As a consequence of right ventricular failure, both right atrial pressure and systemic venous pressure rise, thereby resulting in jugular venous distention, edema of the lower extremities, and congestion of the liver and spleen.

Hepatic congestion in heart failure is characterized by distended central veins, which stand out as dark-red foci against the yellow of the cells in the periphery of the lobule. This imparts a gross appearance to the liver that has been compared to the cut surface of a nutmeg—hence the term **nutmeg liver** (see Chapter 14).

CONGENITAL HEART DISEASE

■ *Congenital heart disease (CHD) reflects faulty embryonic development, which is expressed either as misplaced structures (e.g., transposition of the great vessels) or as an arrested progression of a normal structure from an early stage to a more advanced one (e.g., atrial septal defect).*

The incidence of CHD is cited as being almost 1% of all live births. This figure does not include certain common defects that are not functionally significant,

however, such as an anatomically patent foramen ovale that is functionally closed by the right atrial flap that covers it. In this circumstance, the foramen ovale remains closed as long as the left atrial pressure is higher than the right atrial pressure. A bicuspid aortic valve is also common and, usually, is asymptomatic until adulthood. The reported incidence of particular cardiovascular anomalies varies depending on many factors. A range derived from several sources is shown in Box 11-1.

☐ **Pathogenesis:** Most CHDs reflect a combination of multifactorial genetic factors and environmental influences. As in other diseases with multifactorial inheritance (see Chapter 6), there is an increased risk of recurrence among the siblings of an affected child. Whereas the incidence of CHD in the general population is roughly 1%, it increases to as much as 6% for a second pregnancy after the birth of a child with a heart defect. The risk for a third affected child may be as high as 30%. Moreover, an infant born to a mother with CHD also has an increased risk of cardiac lesions.

Single-gene syndromes are only rare causes of CHD. A number of chromosomal abnormalities are associated with an increased incidence of congenital anomalies of the heart, most prominently Down syndrome (trisomy 21) but also other trisomies and Turner syndrome. However, these account for no more than 5% of all cases of CHD.

The best evidence for an intrauterine influence on the occurrence of congenital cardiac defects relates to maternal infection with rubella virus during the first trimester, especially during the first 4 weeks of gestation. An association with other viral infections is suspected, but this is not as well documented. Maternal use of drugs during early pregnancy is also linked to an increased number of cardiac defects in the offspring. For example, the thalidomide syndrome (phocomelia) was associated with a 10% incidence of CHD. Other drugs implicated in the pathogenesis of CHD include alcohol, phenytoin, amphetamines, lithium, and estrogenic steroids.

Initial Left-to-Right Shunt

The contemporary classification divides CHD into the groups shown in Box 11-2.

Ventricular Septal Defect (Roger Disease)

Ventricular septal defects are the most common of all congenital heart lesions (see Box 11-1). They occur as either isolated lesions or in combination with other malformations.

BOX *11-1* **Relative Incidence of Specific Anomalies in Patients with Congenital Heart Disease**

Ventricular septal defect	25–30%
Atrial septal defect	10–15%
Patent ductus arteriosus	10–20%
Tetralogy of Fallot	6–15%
Pulmonary stenosis	5–7%
Coarctation of the aorta	5–7%
Aortic stenosis	4–6%
Complete transposition of the great arteries	4–10%
Truncus arteriosus	2%
Tricuspid atresia	1%

☐ **Pathogenesis:** The fetal heart consists of a single chamber until the fifth week of gestation, after which it is divided by the development of the interatrial and interventricular septa and the formation of the atrioventricular valves from the endocardial cushions. A muscular interventricular septum grows upward from the apex toward the base of the heart (Fig. 11-2). The muscular septum is joined by the downgrowing membranous septum, thereby separating the right and left ventricles. **The most common ventricular septal defect is related to failure of the membranous portion of the septum to form, either in whole or in part.**

☐ **Pathology:** Defects in the muscular portion of the ventricular septum are more common anteriorly but can occur anywhere in the muscular septum. They vary in size from a small hole in the membranous septum to complete absence of the muscular septum (leaving a single ventricle).

BOX *11-2* **Classification of Congenital Heart Disease**

Initial Left-to-Right Shunt
Ventricular septal defect
Atrial septal defect
Patent ductus arteriosus
Persistent truncus arteriosus
Anomalous pulmonary venous drainage
Right-to-Left Shunt
Tetralogy of Fallot
No Shunt
Complete transposition of the great vessels
Coarctation of the aorta
Pulmonary stenosis
Aortic stenosis
Coronary artery origin from pulmonary artery
Ebstein malformation
Complete heart block
Endocardial fibroelastosis

☐ **Clinical Features:** A small septal defect may have little functional significance and actually close spontaneously as the child matures. In infants with large septal defects, the higher pressure in the left ventricle leads initially to a left-to-right shunt. Left ventricular hypertrophy and congestive heart failure are common complications of such shunts. If the defect is small enough to permit prolonged survival, the augmented pulmonary flow of blood caused by the higher left ventricular pressure eventually results in thickening of the pulmonary arteries and increased pulmonary vascular resistance. This increased vascular resistance may be so great that the direction of the shunt is reversed, thereby going from right to left (**Eisenmenger complex**). A patient with this condition displays a late onset of cyanosis (tardive cyanosis). These children develop right ventricular hypertrophy and right-sided congestive heart failure. Large ventricular septal defects are repaired surgically.

Atrial Septal Defect

☐ **Pathogenesis:** Embryologic development of the atrial septum occurs in a sequence that permits continued passage of oxygenated placental blood from the right to the left atrium through the valve of the inferior vena cava (eustachian valve). The developing atrial septum is programmed to permit this right-to-left shunt to continue until birth. Beginning at the fifth week of intrauterine life, the septum primum extends downward from the roof of the atrium to join with the endocardial cushions, thereby closing the incomplete segment, or ostium primum (see Fig. 11-2). Before this closure is complete, the midportion of the septum primum develops a defect, or ostium secundum, so that the right-to-left flow continues. During the sixth week, a second septum (septum secundum) develops to the right of the septum primum, passing from the roof of the atrium toward the endocardial cushions. This process leaves a patent foramen at approximately the midpoint of the septum, known as the **foramen ovale.** The defect persists after birth until it is sealed off by fusion of the septum primum and septum secundum, after which it is termed the **fossa ovalis.**

☐ **Pathology:** There are a number of sites at which the atrial septum may be defective:

- **Patent Foramen Ovale.** An incomplete seal of the foramen ovale, which can be detected with a probe, is found in 25% of normal adults and is not normally functional. However, it may become a true right-to-left shunt if circumstances elevate the right atrial pressure, as can happen with recurrent pulmonary thromboemboli. In such cases, thromboemboli from the right-sided circulation pass di-

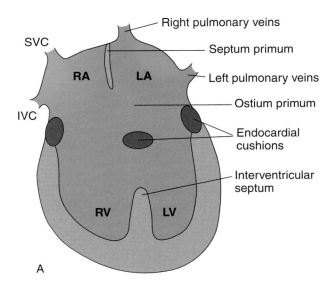

A

- Right pulmonary veins
- Septum primum
- Left pulmonary veins
- Ostium primum
- Endocardial cushions
- Interventricular septum

SVC

IVC

RA   LA

RV   LV

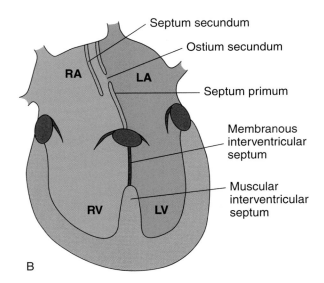

B

- Septum secundum
- Ostium secundum
- Septum primum
- Membranous interventricular septum
- Muscular interventricular septum

RA   LA

RV   LV

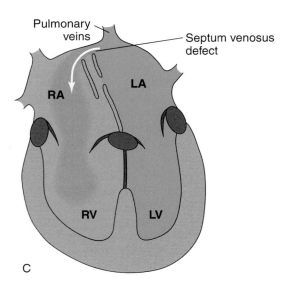

C

Pulmonary veins

Septum venosus defect

RA   LA

RV   LV

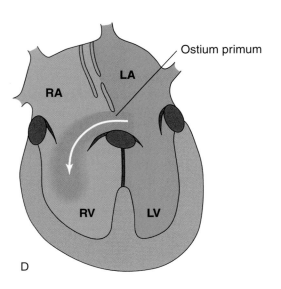

D

Ostium primum

RA   LA

RV   LV

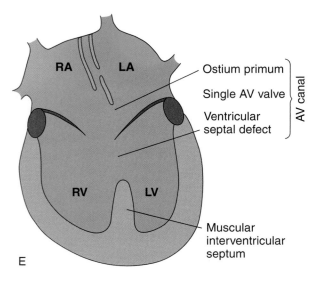

E

RA   LA

RV   LV

- Ostium primum
- Single AV valve   } AV canal
- Ventricular septal defect
- Muscular interventricular septum

rectly into the systemic circulation. These **paradoxical emboli** can produce infarcts in many parts of the arterial circulation but most commonly in the brain, heart, spleen, intestines, kidneys, and legs.

- **Atrial Septal Defect, Ostium Secundum Type.** This lesion is by far the most common, accounting for 90% of atrial septal defects. It reflects a true deficiency of the atrial septum and should not be confused with a patent foramen ovale. An ostium secundum defect occurs in the middle portion of the septum and varies in size, ranging from a trivial opening to a large defect of the entire fossa ovalis region. When the defect is small, it is not normally functional. When the defect is larger, it may result in sufficient shunting of blood from the left side to the right side of the heart to produce dilatation and hypertrophy of the right atrium and right ventricle. Under these circumstances, the pulmonary artery may become larger in diameter than the aorta.
- **Lutembacher syndrome** is a variant of the ostium secundum type of atrial septal defect. It is the combination of mitral stenosis (either congenital or as a result of rheumatic fever) and an ostium secundum type of atrial septal defect.
- **Sinus Venosus Defect.** This uncommon anomaly occurs in the upper portion of the atrial septum, above the fossa ovalis and near the entry of the superior vena cava. It is usually accompanied by drainage of the right pulmonary veins into the right atrium.
- **Atrial Septal Defect, Ostium Primum Type.** This infrequent condition involves the region adjacent to the endocardial cushion. There are usually clefts in the anterior leaflet of the mitral valve and the septal leaflet of the tricuspid valve, which may be accompanied by an associated defect in the adjacent interventricular septum.
- **Persistent Common Atrioventricular Canal.** This anomaly represents the fully developed, combined atrial and ventricular septal defects. Although ordinarily rare, this defect is common in patients with Down syndrome.

☐ **Clinical Features:** Young children with atrial septal defects are ordinarily asymptomatic, but later in life, usually during adolescence, changes in the pulmonary vasculature may reverse the flow of blood through the defect and create a right-to-left shunt. In such cases, cyanosis and clubbing of the fingers ensue. Complications of atrial septal defects include pulmonary hypertension, right ventricular hypertrophy, heart failure, paradoxical emboli, and bacterial endocarditis. Symptomatic cases are treated surgically.

Patent Ductus Arteriosus

The **ductus arteriosus** in the fetus connects the descending aortic arch with the pulmonary artery, conveying most of the pulmonary outflow into the aorta. After birth, the ductus contracts in response to the increased arterial oxygen content and becomes occluded by fibrosis (ligamentum arteriosus). **Persistent patent ductus arteriosus (PDA) is one of the most common congenital cardiac defects, and it is especially frequent in infants whose mothers were infected with rubella virus early during pregnancy.**

A large shunt leads to considerable diversion of blood from the aorta to the low-pressure pulmonary artery. As a result of the increased demand for cardiac output, left ventricular hypertrophy and failure ensue. In patients with a smaller but functional PDA, the increased volume and pressure of blood in the pul-

FIGURE *11-2*
Pathogenesis of ventricular and atrial septal defects. (A) The common atrial chamber is being separated into the right atrium (RA) and left atrium (LA) by the septum primum. Because the septum primum has not yet joined the endocardial cushion material, there is an open ostium primum. The ventricular cavity is being divided by a muscular interventricular septum into the right ventricle (RV) and left ventricle (LV). *IVC*, **inferior vena cava;** *SVC*, **superior vena cava. (B) The septum primum has joined the endocardial cushions but, at the same time, has developed an opening in its midportion (the ostium secundum). This opening is partly overlaid by the septum secundum, which has now grown down to cover, in part, the foramen ovale. Simultaneously, the membranous septum joins the muscular interventricular septum at the base of the heart, completely separating the ventricles. (C) The sinus venosus type of atrial septal defect is located in the most cephalad region and adjacent to the inflow of the right pulmonary veins, which tend, therefore, to open into the right atrium. (D) The ostium primum defect occurs just above the valve ring, sometimes in the presence of an intact valve ring. (E) The ostium primum defect may also, in conjunction with a defect of the valve ring and the ventricular septum, form an atrioventricular canal. This common opening allows free communication between the atria and the ventricles.**

monary circulation eventually lead to pulmonary hypertension and its cardiac complications. Infective endarteritis is a frequent complication in untreated patients with PDA.

A PDA can be corrected surgically, usually with complete success. The ductus can also be caused to contract and then close by inhibitors of prostaglandin synthesis (e.g., indomethacin).

Truncus Arteriosus

■ *Persistent truncus arteriosus refers to a common trunk for the origin of the aorta, pulmonary arteries, and coronary arteries.* It results from an absent or incomplete partitioning of the fetal truncus arteriosus by the spiral septum. Truncus arteriosus always overrides a ventricular septal defect and receives blood from both ventricles.

☐ **Clinical Features:** Most infants with truncus arteriosus have a torrential pulmonary blood flow and suffer from both heart failure and recurrent respiratory tract infections, often resulting in early death. In children with prolonged survival, pulmonary vascular disease develops, in which case cyanosis, polycythemia, and clubbing of the fingers appear. Open-heart surgery is effective treatment.

Tetralogy of Fallot (Dominant Right-to-Left Shunt)

■ *Tetralogy of Fallot is the most common cyanotic congenital heart disease in older children and adults, representing 10% of all congenital heart disease. The four anatomic changes that define the tetralogy of Fallot are* (Fig. 11-3):

- **Pulmonary stenosis**
- **Ventricular septal defect**
- **Dextroposition of the aorta,** so that it overrides the ventricular septal defect
- **Right ventricular hypertrophy**

The heart is hypertrophied in such a way as to give it a boot shape. Almost half of the patients with tetralogy of Fallot also display other cardiac anomalies. Patency of the ductus arteriosus is protective, because it provides a source of blood to the otherwise deprived pulmonary vascular bed.

☐ **Clinical Features:** In patients with pulmonary stenosis, right ventricular blood is shunted through the ventricular septal defect and into the aorta, thereby resulting in arterial desaturation and cyanosis. Dyspnea on exertion is particularly noticeable, and the affected child often assumes a squatting position to relieve the shortness of breath. Owing to marked polycythemia, cerebral thromboses may complicate the course of the

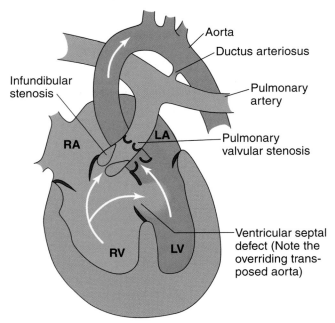

FIGURE *11-3*
Tetralogy of Fallot. Note the pulmonary stenosis, which results from infundibular hypertrophy as well as pulmonary valvular stenosis. The ventricular septal defect involves the membranous septum region. Dextroposition of the aorta and right ventricular hypertrophy are shown. Because of the pulmonary obstruction, the shunt is from right to left, and the patient is cyanotic.

disease. These patients are also at risk for bacterial endocarditis and brain abscesses, but heart failure is not a common complication.

Untreated tetralogy of Fallot carries a dismal prognosis, but following successful surgery, patients are asymptomatic and have an excellent long-term outlook.

Congenital Heart Diseases Without Shunts

Transposition of the Great Arteries

■ *Transposition of the great arteries (TGA) refers to a situation in which the aorta arises from the right ventricle and the pulmonary artery from the left ventricle.* It is responsible for more than half of the deaths in infants younger than 1 year with cyanotic heart disease.

Because venous blood from the right side of the heart flows to the aorta and oxygenated blood from the lungs returns to the pulmonary artery, there are, in effect, two independent and parallel blood circuits for the systemic and pulmonary circulations (Fig. 11-4). Thus, survival is possible only in the presence of a communication between the circuits. Virtually all infants with TGA have an atrial septal defect, half have a ven-

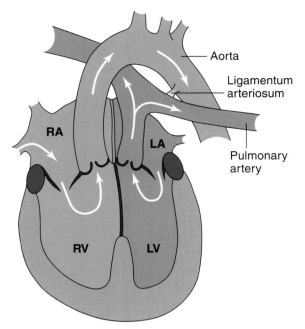

FIGURE *11-4*
Complete transposition of great arteries, regular type. The aorta is anterior to, and to the right of, the pulmonary artery "D-transposition") and arises from the right ventricle. Because there are no interatrial or interventricular connections and no patent ductus arteriosus, this anomaly is incompatible with life.

tricular septal defect, and two-thirds have a patent ductus arteriosus.

Before the advent of cardiac surgery, the outlook for infants born with TGA was hopeless, with 90% dying within the first year. However, it is now possible to correct the malformation within the first 2 weeks of life by an arterial switch operation, with an overall survival rate of 90%.

Coarctation of the Aorta

■ *Coarctation of the aorta is a local constriction of this vessel that almost always presents immediately below the origin of the left subclavian artery at the site of the ductus arteriosus* (Fig. 11-5). The condition is two- to fivefold more frequent in males than in females, and it is associated with a bicuspid aortic valve in two-thirds of the patients.

The clinical hallmark of coarctation of the aorta is a discrepancy between the blood pressure in the upper extremities and that in the lower ones. The pressure gradient produced by the coarctation causes hypertension proximal to the narrowed segment. In children older than 1 year, the mean systolic blood pressure measured in the arm is 145 mm Hg, compared with 70 mm Hg in the leg.

Hypertension in the upper body results in left ventricular hypertrophy. Hypotension below the coarcta-

tion leads to weakness, pallor, and coldness of the lower extremities. In an attempt to bridge the obstruction between the upper and the lower aortic segments, collateral vessels enlarge. Radiologic examination of the chest shows **notching of the inner surfaces of the ribs** owing to pressure from the markedly dilated intercostal arteries.

Most patients with coarctation of the aorta who remain untreated die by 40 years of age. Complications include (1) heart failure, (2) rupture of a dissecting aneurysm (secondary to cystic medial necrosis of the aorta), (3) infective endarteritis at the point of narrowing or the site of jet-stream impingement on the wall immediately distal to the coarctation, (4) cerebral hemorrhage, and (5) stenosis or infective endocarditis of a bicuspid aortic valve. Coarctation of the aorta is successfully treated by surgical excision of the narrowed segment, preferably between 2 and 4 years of age.

Congenital Aortic Stenosis

Valvular Aortic Stenosis. This is the most common type of congenital aortic stenosis and is considerably more frequent (4:1) in males than in females. It is associated with other cardiac anomalies (e.g., coarctation of the aorta) in 20% of the cases.

Congenital valvular aortic stenosis usually features the fusion of two of the three semilunar cusps (the right coronary cusp with one of the adjacent two cusps). Over the years that follow, the resulting bicuspid valve tends to become thickened and calcified.

Hypoplastic left heart syndrome is characterized by hypoplasia of the left ventricle, ascending aorta, and mitral valve. It is a condition in which severe aortic valvular stenosis or atresia is often the main defect.

Many children with valvular aortic stenosis are asymptomatic, but in severe cases, exertional dyspnea and angina pectoris may be prominent features. Sudden death poses a distinct threat to patients with severe obstruction, principally owing to ventricular arrhythmias. Bacterial endocarditis sometimes complicates the course of the disease. In symptomatic patients, aortic valvulotomy has had a high degree of success, although valve replacement is occasionally indicated. Hypoplastic left heart syndrome is treated surgically or by cardiac transplantation.

Subvalvular Aortic Stenosis. This type accounts for 10% of all cases of congenital aortic stenosis and results from abnormal development of a band of subvalvular fibroelastic tissue or a muscular ridge. The stenosis is caused by a membranous diaphragm or fibrous ring that surrounds the left ventricular outflow tract immediately below the aortic valve. It is twice as common in males as in females.

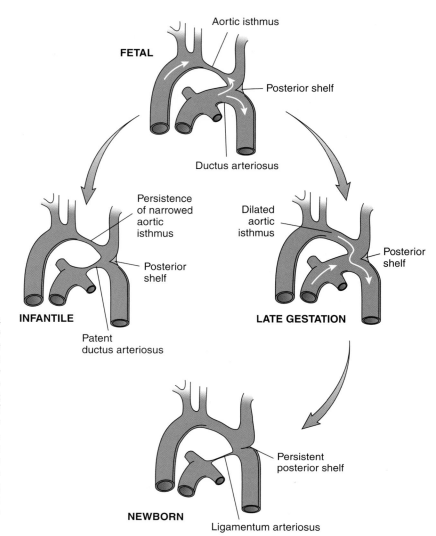

FIGURE 11-5
Pathogenesis of coarctation of the aorta. In the fetus, ductal blood is diverted into cephalad and descending streams by the posterior aortic shelf. In late fetal life, the isthmus dilates, and the increased descending blood flow is accommodated by the ductal orifice. After birth, if the shelf does not undergo normal involution, obliteration of the ductal orifice does not permit free flow around the persistent posterior shelf, thereby creating a juxtaductal obstruction to the flow of blood to the distal aorta. If the aortic isthmus does not dilate during late fetal life, it remains narrow, thereby resulting in an infantile or preductal coarctation. In this circumstance, the ductus arteriosus usually remains patent.

Many patients with subvalvular aortic stenosis develop thickening and immobility of the aortic cusps, with mild aortic regurgitation. Bacterial endocarditis carries its own risks and may also aggravate the regurgitation. Surgical treatment of subvalvular aortic stenosis is accomplished by excising the membrane or fibrous ridge.

Ebstein Malformation

■ *Ebstein malformation is a downward displacement of an abnormal tricuspid valve into an underdeveloped right ventricle.* One (or more) of the tricuspid valve leaflets is plastered to the right ventricular wall for a variable distance below the right atrioventricular annulus. The effective tricuspid valve orifice is displaced downward into the ventricle, thereby dividing it into two separate parts, namely the "atrialized" ventricle (proximal ventricle) and the functional right ventricle (distal ventricle). In approximately two-thirds of such cases, con-

spicuous dilatation of the functional ventricle hinders its ability to pump blood efficiently through the pulmonary arteries.

Ebstein malformation leads to heart failure, massive right ventricular dilatation, arrhythmias with palpitations and tachycardia, and sudden death. Surgical treatment of Ebstein malformation has met with variable success.

Endocardial Fibroelastosis

■ *Endocardial fibroelastosis* (EFE) *is a condition characterized by fibroelastic thickening of the endocardium of the left ventricle, which may also affect the valves.* The disorder is classified as either primary or secondary, with the latter being far more common.

Secondary EFE. This disorder occurs in association with underlying cardiovascular anomalies that lead to left ventricular hypertrophy during an inability to meet the increased oxygen demands of the myocardium. Thus, secondary EFE is a frequent complication of congenital aortic stenosis (including hypoplastic left ventricle syndrome) and coarctation of the aorta. On gross examination, the endocardium of the left ventricle displays irregular, white, opaque, and thickened patches, which may also be present on the cardiac valves. Microscopically, these plaques correspond to fibroelastic thickening, frequently accompanied by degeneration of the subendocardial myocytes. The valves may show collagenous thickening.

Primary EFE. Defined as the presence of fibroelastosis in the absence of any associated lesion, this disorder is a disease of unknown cause that afflicts infants, usually between 4 and 10 months of age. The left ventricle tends to be conspicuously dilated, but it is occasionally contracted and hypertrophic. Diffuse endocardial thickening involves most of the left ventricle (Fig. 11-6) as well as the aortic and the mitral valve leaflets. Infants suffering from primary EFE develop progressive heart failure, and their prognosis is dismal. Cardiac transplantation offers the only hope for a cure.

Dextrocardia

■ *Dextrocardia is an inverted position of the heart, which represents a mirror image of the normal, left-sided location and configuration.* When dextrocardia occurs without abnormal positioning of the visceral organs (situs inversus), the condition is invariably associated with severe cardiovascular anomalies. When it occurs in combination with situs inversus, the heart tends to be functionally normal.

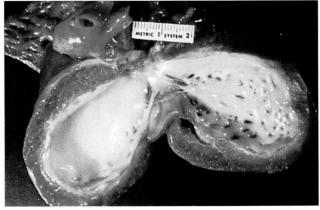

FIGURE *11-6*
Endocardial fibroelastosis. The left ventricle of an infant who died from endocardial fibroelastosis has been opened to reveal a thickened endocardium lining most of the cavity, which virtually obliterates the trabeculae carneae.

ISCHEMIC HEART DISEASE

■ *Ischemic heart disease is, in the vast majority of cases, a consequence of atherosclerosis of the coronary arteries and develops when the flow of blood is inadequate to provide for the oxygen demands of the heart.* **Ischemic heart disease is by far the most common type of heart disease in the United States and other industrialized countries, where it remains the leading cause of death and is responsible for at least 80% of all deaths from heart disease.** By contrast, atherosclerotic heart disease is far less frequent in less-developed countries, such as those of Africa and many parts of Asia. The pathogenesis of ischemic cell injury is discussed in detail in Chapter 1. The principal effects of ischemic heart disease are angina pectoris, myocardial infarction, and sudden death.

Angina Pectoris

■ *Angina pectoris, or pain in the chest, is the most common symptom of ischemic heart disease.* Coronary atherosclerosis usually becomes symptomatic only when the luminal cross-sectional area of the affected vessel is reduced by more than 75%. A patient with typical angina pectoris exhibits recurrent episodes of chest pain, usually brought on by increased physical activity or emotional excitement. The pain is of limited duration (1–15 min) and is relieved by reducing physical activity or by treatment with sublingual nitroglycerin, a potent vasodilator. Decreased coronary blood flow can also result from other conditions, including coronary vasospasm, aortic stenosis, or aortic insufficiency.

Unstable angina is a variety of chest pain that has a less predictable relationship than stable angina to exercise and that may occur during rest or sleep. It is related to development of nonocclusive thrombi over atherosclerotic plaques. Most of these patients ultimately progress to frank myocardial infarction, although in some cases, the symptoms may regress.

Myocardial Infarction

■ *Myocardial infarction refers to a discrete focus of ischemic necrosis in the heart.* Development of an infarct is related to the duration of ischemia and the metabolic rate of the ischemic tissue. In experimental coronary artery ligation, foci of necrosis result from as little as 20 minutes of ischemia, and they become more extensive as the period of ischemia is extended.

Sudden Death

The initial manifestation of ischemic heart disease may be unexpected ventricular fibrillation, which is an arrhythmia that results in sudden death. **Coronary atherosclerosis underlies most cases of sudden cardiac death, often occurring during the first hour after the onset of symptoms.**

Epidemiology

The major elements that predispose a person to coronary artery disease are an elevated blood cholesterol level, hypertension, and cigarette smoking. Any one of these factors significantly increases the risk of myocardial infarction (heart attacks), and the presence of all three augments the risk more than sevenfold (see Chapter 8).

In the United States, there has been a reversal in the trend toward progressively increasing mortality from ischemic heart disease, and a decrease of approximately 30% has occurred during the past 10 years. This shift may be due, at least in part, to a reduction in smoking, consumption of less saturated fat in the average diet, and effective control of hypertension.

Most populations in which men have a high mean serum cholesterol value exhibit a high rate of coronary artery disease; the usual diet of these persons is high in saturated fat. Correspondingly, the usual diet is low in saturated fat among most countries whose inhabitants have low serum cholesterol levels and low rates of coronary artery disease.

The risk of ischemic heart disease also rises with increasing blood pressure. A person with a blood pressure of 160/95 mm Hg has a twofold greater risk of ischemic heart disease compared to a person with a blood pressure of 140/75 mm Hg or lower.

Cigarette smoking is considered to be the major preventable cause of coronary artery disease, and the risk of ischemic heart disease increases in proportion to the number of cigarettes smoked. Passive exposure to environmental tobacco smoke also seems to increase the risk of coronary atherosclerosis.

Other risk factors for ischemic heart disease include:

- **Diabetes Mellitus.**
- **Obesity.** Higher rates of myocardial infarction may be only indirectly related to obesity considering that obese persons tend to have higher blood pressure and blood lipid levels.
- **Age.** The risk of infarction is greater with increasing age, up to age 80.
- **Sex.** Angina pectoris is considerably more frequent in men than in women, with the ratio below the age of 50 being 4:1 and that at the age of 60 being 2:1.
- **Family History.** Premature atherosclerosis in first-degree relatives is a risk factor for myocardial infarction.
- **Use of Oral Contraceptives.** Women older than the age of 35 who smoke cigarettes and use oral contraceptives have an increased incidence of myocardial infarction.
- **Sedentary Life Habits.** Regular exercise seems to reduce the risk of myocardial infarction, perhaps by increasing high-density lipoprotein levels.
- **Personality Features.** Early studies indicated that hard-driving, aggressive, time-conscious, executive-type persons (the "type A" personality) have a higher incidence of heart disease than more easygoing, relaxed persons (the "type B" personality). More recent studies, however, have failed to show the strong association that was previously reported.

Pathology of Myocardial Infarction

The causes of ischemic heart disease are listed in Box 11-3. It deserves emphasis that the large majority of cases of myocardial infarction are secondary to coronary atherosclerosis. The pathogenesis of atherosclerosis is described in detail in Chapter 10. Briefly, in advanced atherosclerotic lesions, much of the inner lining

BOX *11-3* **Causes of Ischemic Heart Disease**

Decreased Supply of Oxygen
Conditions Influencing the Supply of Blood
Atherosclerosis and thrombosis
Thromboemboli
Coronary artery spasm
Collateral blood vessels
Blood pressure, cardiac output, and heart rate
Miscellaneous: arteritis (e.g., periarteritis nodosa), dissecting aneurysm, luetic aortitis, anomalous origin of coronary artery, muscular bridging of coronary artery
Conditions Influencing the Availability of Oxygen in the Blood
Anemia
Shift in the hemoglobin-oxygen dissociation curve
Carbon monoxide
Cyanide
Increased Oxygen Demand (Increased Cardiac Work)
Hypertension
Valvular stenosis or insufficiency
Hyperthyroidism
Fever
Thiamine deficiency
Catecholamines

of the vessel is replaced by atherosclerotic plaque, and the lumen is greatly narrowed. Dystrophic calcification and cholesterol crystals are common in advanced lesions (Fig. 11-7). In many cases, the reduction in coronary blood flow becomes critical when the luminal cross-sectional area is decreased by 90% (70% reduction in luminal diameter). **Angiographic demonstration of thrombotic obstruction plus results from studies of experimental coronary occlusion establish that coronary artery thrombosis usually precipitates an acute myocardial infarction.** Frequently, the thrombus occluding the vessel can be lysed and the ischemia relieved by infusion of thrombolytic enzymes, such as streptokinase or tissue-plasminogen activator.

Location of Infarcts

Transmural infarcts conform to the distribution of one of the three major coronary arteries (see Fig. 11-2):

- **Right Coronary Artery:** An occlusion of the proximal portion of this vessel produces an infarct of the posterior basal region of the left ventricle and the posterior one-third of the interventricular septum ("inferior" infarct).
- **Left Anterior Descending Coronary Artery.** Blockage of the LAD artery produces an infarct of the apical, anterior, and anteroseptal walls of the left ventricle.
- **Left Circumflex Coronary Artery.** Obstruction of this vessel is the least common cause of a myocar-

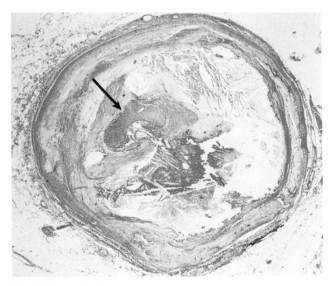

FIGURE *11-7*
Coronary atherosclerosis. This cross-section of an epicardial coronary artery shows severe atherosclerosis. The wall is thickened, and the lumen (*arrow*) is narrowed by an accumulation of atheromatous debris, including cholesterol crystals (*needle-like spaces*).

dial infarct but leads to an infarct of the lateral wall of the left ventricle.

Infarcts may predominantly involve the subendocardial portion of the myocardium, or they may be transmural. A subendocardial infarct affects the inner one-third to one-half of the left ventricle. It is commonly circumferential, so that it is not necessarily in the distribution of any one coronary artery. **Subendocardial infarction generally results from hypoperfusion of the heart in disorders such as aortic stenosis or hemorrhagic shock or from hypoperfusion during the course of cardiopulmonary bypass.**

Occlusion of a coronary artery often results in a transmural infarct (ischemic necrosis that extends from the endocardium to the epicardium). In fatal cases of acute myocardial infarction, transmural infarcts are more common than those restricted to the subendocardium. **Infarcts involve the left ventricle much more commonly and extensively than the right ventricle.**

Macroscopic Characteristics of Myocardial Infarcts

Total ischemia for 20 to 30 minutes produces reversible changes, but beyond that time, damaged myocytes progressively die. On gross examination, an acute myocardial infarct is not identifiable within the first 12 hours after onset.

- **By 24 hours,** the infarct can be recognized on the cut surface of the involved ventricle by its pallor.
- **After 3 to 5 days,** the infarct is mottled and more sharply outlined, with a central, pale, yellowish, and necrotic region bordered by a hyperemic zone (Fig. 11-8). Occasionally, the infarcted region is hemorrhagic.
- **By 2 to 3 weeks,** the infarcted region is depressed and soft, with a refractile, gelatinous appearance.
- **Older, healed infarcts** are firm and contracted, and they have the pale-gray appearance of scar tissue (Fig. 11-9).

Microscopic Characteristics of Myocardial Infarcts

The First 24 Hours. The noncontractile ischemic myocytes are stretched with each systole and become "wavy fibers." In longitudinal sections, the periphery of the infarct exhibits contraction bands. By 24 hours, the myocytes are deeply eosinophilic (Fig. 11-10) and show the characteristic changes of coagulation necrosis.

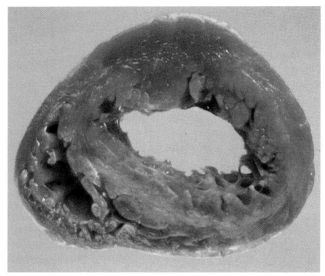

FIGURE   *11-8*
Acute myocardial infarct. This cross-section of the ventricles from a man who died a few days after the onset of severe chest pain shows a transmural infarct in both the posterior and septal regions of the left ventricle. The necrotic myocardium is soft, yellowish, and sharply demarcated.

Two to 3 Days. Polymorphonuclear leukocytes are attracted to the necrotic myocytes and reach their maximum concentration in infarcts after 2 days (see Figs. 11-10 and 11-11). Interstitial edema and areas of hemorrhage commonly appear. By 2 to 3 days, the muscle cells are more clearly necrotic, the nuclei disappear, and the striations become less prominent. Some of the polymorphonuclear leukocytes that were attracted to the area also begin to undergo karyorrhexis.

Five to 7 Days. The acute inflammatory leukocytic response has abated, so few (if any) polymorphonuclear leukocytes are now present. The periphery of the

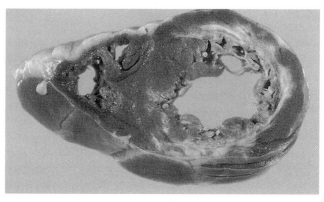

FIGURE   *11-9*
Healed myocardial infarct. This cross-section of the heart from a man who died after a long history of angina pectoris and several myocardial infarctions shows circumferential scarring of the left ventricle.

infarcted region shows phagocytosis of the dead muscle by macrophages. Fibroblasts begin to proliferate, and new collagen begins to form. Lymphocytes and pigment-laden macrophages are prominent. The process of repair is initiated at approximately 5 days, beginning at the periphery of the infarct and gradually extending toward the center.

One to 3 Weeks. Collagen deposition proceeds, the inflammatory infiltrate gradually recedes, and the newly sprouted capillaries are progressively obliterated.

More Than 4 Weeks. Considerable dense, fibrous tissue is present. The debris is progressively removed, and the scar becomes more solid and less cellular as it matures (Fig. 11-12).

Contraction band necrosis (Zenker necrosis) refers to the presence of thick, irregular, transverse bands across necrotic myocytes as a result of hypercontraction (Fig. 11-13). Contraction band necrosis is prominent in regions where the flow of blood persists, such as at the margins of an acute infarct. It is also seen during situations in which reflow occurs, such as in patients who have had coronary artery bypass grafts or been treated with thrombolytic agents to clear an obstructed coronary artery.

Clinical Diagnosis of Acute Myocardial Infarction

The onset of acute myocardial infarction is often sudden, with severe substernal or precordial, crushing pain. In some cases, acute myocardial infarction is preceded by unstable angina of several days' duration. **One-fourth to one-half of all nonfatal myocardial infarctions occur without any symptoms, and the infarcts are identified only later by electrocardiographic changes or at autopsy.**

The diagnosis of acute myocardial infarction is confirmed by electrocardiography and the appearance of increased levels of certain enzymes in the serum, particularly in the isoenzymes of lactic dehydrogenase and creatine kinase.

Complications of Myocardial Infarction

In some cases of acute myocardial infarction, the patient succumbs to pump failure (cardiogenic shock). However, in the majority of cases, the clinical course is dominated by a variety of other functional or mechanical complications of the infarct.

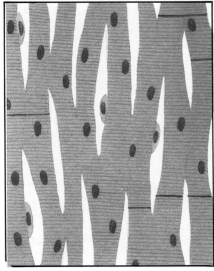
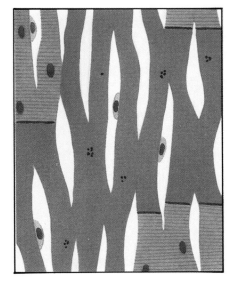
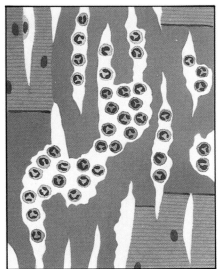

A, B

C

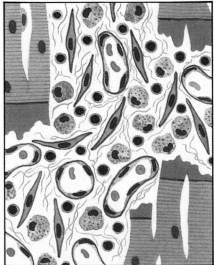
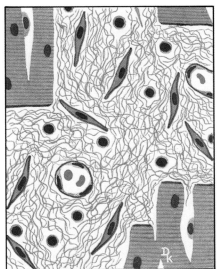

D

E

FIGURE *11-10*
Development of a myocardial infarct. (A) Normal myocardium. (B) After approximately 12 to 18 hours, the infarcted myocardium shows eosinophilia (*red*) in sections of the heart stained with hematoxylin-and-eosin. (C) After approximately 24 hours, polymorphonuclear neutrophils infiltrate around the necrotic myocytes. (D) After approximately 3 weeks, the infarct contains granulation tissue, with prominent capillaries, fibroblasts, lymphoid cells, and macrophages. The necrotic debris has been largely removed, and a small amount of collagen has been deposited. (E) After 3 months or longer, the infarcted region has been replaced by scar tissue.

Arrhythmias. Arrhythmias account for half of the deaths from ischemic heart disease. Premature ventricular beats, sinus bradycardia, ventricular tachycardia, ventricular fibrillation, paroxysmal atrial tachycardia, and partial or complete heart block can occur.

Left Ventricular Failure and Cardiogenic Shock. One of the most feared complications in patients with acute myocardial infarction is cardiogenic shock. It is most likely to occur early during the course of the illness, when the infarct involves more than 40% of the left ventricle, and the mortality rate in these cases is as high as 90%. The hemodynamic consequences of cardiogenic shock are discussed in Chapter 7.

Extension of the Infarct. Clinically recognizable extension of an acute myocardial infarct occurs during the first 1 to 2 weeks in as many as 10% of patients.

Significant infarct extension is associated with a twofold increase in the mortality rate.

Rupture of the Free Wall of the Myocardium. Myocardial rupture (Fig. 11-14) may occur at almost any time within the first 3 weeks of an acute myocardial infarction, but it is most common between the first and the fourth day, when the infarcted wall is weakest. After this time, the scar becomes progressively stronger and rupture, therefore, less likely. Rupture of the free wall is generally a complication of large transmural infarcts that involve at least 20% of the left ventricle.

Rupture of the infarcted myocardium most often results in hemopericardium and death from pericardial tamponade. Myocardial rupture accounts for 10% of the deaths from acute myocardial infarction in hospitalized patients.

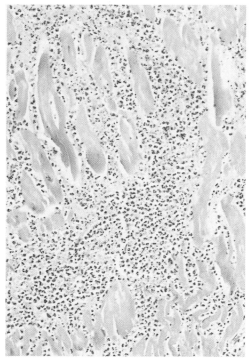

FIGURE   *11-11*
Acute myocardial infarct. The necrotic myocardial fibers, which are eosinophilic and devoid of cross-striations and nuclei, are immersed in a sea of acute inflammatory cells.

Other Forms of Myocardial Rupture. A few patients in whom a myocardial infarct involves the intraventricular septum develop a **septal perforation,** which may be 1 cm or greater in length. The magnitude of the resulting left-to-right shunt and, therefore, the prognosis varies with the size of the rupture.

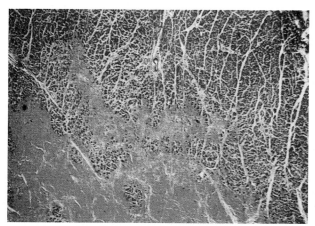

FIGURE   *11-12*
Healed myocardial infarct. A section of the scarred myocardium stained for collagen shows dense, acellular fibrosis that is sharply demarcated from the adjacent viable myocardium.

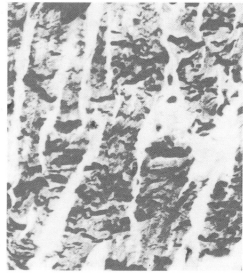

FIGURE   *11-13*
Contraction band necrosis. A section of infarcted myocardium shows prominent, thick, wavy, and transverse bands in the myofibers.

Uncommonly, **a portion of a papillary muscle ruptures**, thereby resulting in mitral regurgitation. In unusual cases, an entire papillary muscle is transected, in which case massive mitral valve incompetence is usually fatal.

Aneurysms: Left ventricular aneurysms complicate 10% to 15% of healed transmural myocardial infarcts. Following an acute transmural myocardial infarct, the affected ventricular wall tends to bulge outward during

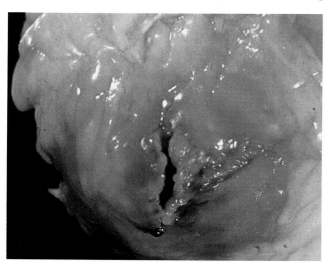

FIGURE   *11-14*
Rupture of an acute myocardial infarct. An elderly woman who had suffered a recent myocardial infarct died acutely from cardiac tamponade. The pericardium was filled with blood, and the external surface of the left ventricle shows a linear rupture of the necrotic myocardium.

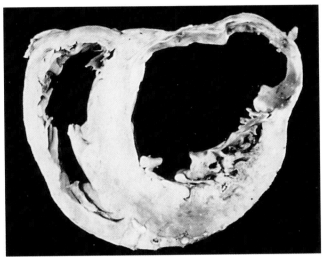

FIGURE   *11-15*
Ventricular aneurysm. This cross-section through the ventricles of a heart obtained at autopsy from a patient with a history of a posterior wall myocardial infarction shows thinning and aneurysmal dilatation of the left ventricular wall in the region of the healed infarct.

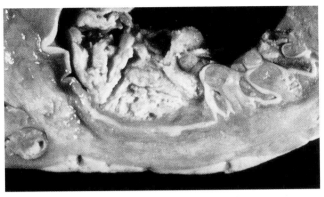

FIGURE   *11-16*
Mural thrombus overlying a healed myocardial infarct. This cross-section of a fixed heart shows an organized, friable, grayish-white mural thrombus that overlies a thickened endocardium situated over a scarred myocardium.

systole in one-third of the patients. As the infarct matures, the collagenous scar tissue is susceptible to further stretching. Localized thinning and stretching of the ventricular wall in the region of a healing myocardial infarct is termed **infarct expansion,** but it is actually an early aneurysm. It is composed of a thin layer of necrotic myocardium and collagenous tissue that expands with each contraction of the heart (Fig. 11-15).

As the aneurysm continues to dilate with each beat, it "steals" some of the left ventricular output and contributes to the workload of the heart. Patients with left ventricular aneurysms have an increased risk of myocardial rupture and a poorer prognosis. Mural thrombi develop within the aneurysm in half of these patients and are a source of systemic emboli.

False aneurysms result from rupture of a portion of the left ventricle that has been walled off by pericardial scar tissue. Thus, the wall of a false aneurysm is composed of pericardium and scar tissue and not of left ventricular myocardium.

Mural Thrombosis and Embolism. Almost half of all patients who die after myocardial infarction are discovered at autopsy to have mural thrombi overlying the infarct (Fig. 11-16), particularly when it involves the apex of the heart. In turn, half of these patients have some evidence of systemic embolization.

Pericarditis. A transmural myocardial infarct involves the epicardium and leads to inflammation of the pericardium in 10% to 20% of patients. This pericarditis is manifested clinically as chest pain and pericardial

friction rub. Patients with larger infarcts and congestive heart failure may develop a pericardial effusion, with or without pericarditis.

Postmyocardial infarction syndrome (Dressler syndrome) refers to a delayed pericarditis, which develops 2 to 10 weeks after infarction. A similar disorder may occur after cardiac surgery.

Therapeutic Interventions That Limit Infarct Size

Restoration of arterial blood flow remains the only way to salvage ischemic myocytes. There are several methods to restore the flow of blood to the area of myocardium supplied by an obstructed coronary artery:

- **Thrombolytic enzymes,** such as tissue-plasminogen activator or streptokinase, can be infused either intravenously or directly into an obstructed coronary artery.
- **Percutaneous transluminal coronary angioplasty** produces dilatation of a narrowed coronary artery by inflation of a balloon catheter.
- **Coronary artery bypass grafting** can restore the flow of blood to the distal segment of a coronary artery with a proximal occlusion.

Chronic Ischemic Heart Disease

Patients with severe coronary atherosclerosis follow a pattern of increasingly frequent episodes of angina pectoris, reflecting progressive narrowing of one or more coronary arteries. **In most patients with chronic ischemic heart disease, persistently depressed cardiac function reflects the presence of infarcts.**

In a minority of patients with severe coronary atherosclerosis, however, myocardial contractility is impaired globally in the absence of discrete infarcts, which is a situation that mimics dilated cardiomyopathy. In many cases, this condition reflects a combination of ischemic myocardial dysfunction, diffuse fibrosis, and multiple small, healed infarcts. However, there still remains a group of patients who present with left ventricular failure and in whom cardiac dysfunction occurs without tissue necrosis. These patients are said to have **ischemic cardiomyopathy.**

HYPERTENSIVE HEART DISEASE

Persistently elevated blood pressure leads to left ventricular hypertrophy and, eventually, to cardiac failure. Hypertension is not a primary disease of the heart and is described in detail in Chapter 10.

Systemic hypertension has been defined by the World Health Organization as being a persistent elevation of blood pressure to greater than 160 mm Hg systolic, greater than 90 mm Hg diastolic, or both. The term **hypertensive heart disease** is used when the heart is enlarged in the absence of a cause other than hypertension. Hypertension is common in the United States, having an overall prevalence rate of 20% to 35%. Both the prevalence and the severity of this disease are greater in blacks than in whites. The prevalence of hypertension is greater in women than in men, and it increases progressively with age. There has been a striking decrease in the number of deaths caused by hypertension during the past decade, however, similar to that seen in the case of coronary heart disease.

☐ **Pathology:** Hypertension causes compensatory left ventricular hypertrophy as a result of the increased workload imposed on the heart. The left ventricle is

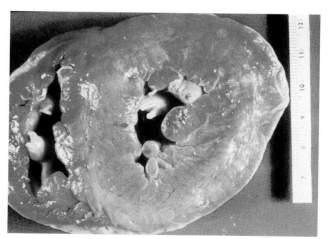

FIGURE   *11-17*
Hypertensive heart disease. This cross-section of a heart shows prominent hypertrophy of the left ventricular myocardium.

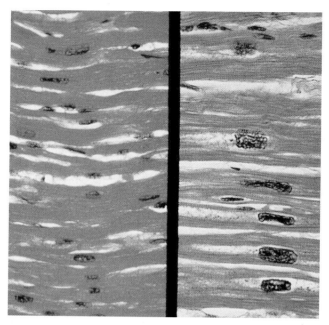

FIGURE   *11-18*
Hypertensive heart disease with myocardial hypertrophy. Compared with normal myocardium (*left*), hypertrophic myocardium (*right*) shows thicker fibers and enlarged, hyperchromatic, and rectangular nuclei.

thickened (Fig. 11-17), and the overall weight of the heart is increased, exceeding 375 g in men (normal, 300–350 g) and 350 g in women (normal, 250–300 g). Microscopically, the hypertrophic myocardial cells have an increased diameter with enlarged, hyperchromatic, and rectangular nuclei (Fig. 11-18). **Hypertension is also associated with an increased severity of atherosclerosis of the coronary arteries.** The combination of increased cardiac workload and narrowed coronary arteries leads to a greater risk of myocardial ischemia, infarction, and heart failure.

Congestive heart failure is the most common cause of death in patients with hypertension, accounting for 40% of all deaths from hypertension. Intracerebral hemorrhage is also a frequent fatal complication. In addition, death may occur as a result of coronary atherosclerosis, dissecting aneurysm of the aorta, or ruptured berry aneurysm of the cerebral circulation. Finally, death in patients with renal failure may occur when nephrosclerosis induced by hypertension becomes severe.

COR PULMONALE

■ *Cor pulmonale is right ventricular hypertrophy and dilatation secondary to pulmonary hypertension.* The latter may reflect a disorder of the pulmonary parenchyma or, more rarely, a primary disease of the vasculature (e.g., primary pulmonary hypertension, recurrent small pulmonary emboli).

Acute cor pulmonale refers to the sudden occurrence of pulmonary hypertension, most commonly as a result of sudden, massive pulmonary embolization. This condition often causes acute right-sided heart failure and is a medical emergency. At autopsy, the only cardiac findings are severe dilatation of the right ventricle and, sometimes, of the right atrium.

Chronic cor pulmonale is a common heart disease, accounting for 30% to 40% of all cases of heart failure in an English study and 10% to 30% in a series from the United States. This frequency reflects the prevalence of chronic pulmonary disease in these countries.

☐ **Pathogenesis:** Chronic cor pulmonale may be caused by any pulmonary disease that interferes with ventilatory mechanics or gas exchange or that obstructs the pulmonary vasculature (Box 11-4). The most common causes of chronic cor pulmonale are pulmonary fibrosis and chronic obstructive pulmonary disease.

Pulmonary hypertension secondary to recurrent pulmonary emboli is clearly a progressive, mechanical obstruction to the flow of blood. However, the situation in chronic parenchymal diseases of the lungs is more complicated. In these disorders, hypoxia, acidosis, and hypercapnia also lead to pulmonary arteriolar vasoconstriction, which reduces the effective cross-sectional area of the pulmonary vascular bed without destruction of the vessels.

☐ **Pathology:** Chronic cor pulmonale is characterized by conspicuous hypertrophy of the right ventricle

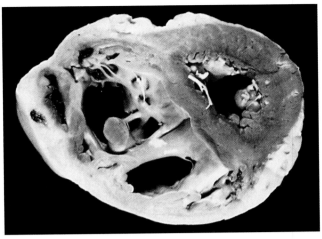

FIGURE *11-19*
Cor pulmonale. This cross-section of the heart from a patient with severe pulmonary fibrosis and pulmonary hypertension shows a hypertrophied right ventricle. The right ventricular cavity is dilated compared with the much smaller cavity of the left ventricle.

(Fig. 11-19), which measures more than 1.0 cm in thickness (normal, 0.3–0.5 cm). Hypertrophy of the trabeculae carneae and papillary muscles is also readily evident.

ACQUIRED VALVULAR AND ENDOCARDIAL DISEASES

A variety of inflammatory, infectious, and degenerative diseases damage the cardiac valves and impair their function. Cardiac valves normally consist of thin, flexible membranes that close tightly to prevent the backward flow of blood. When the valves become damaged, the leaflets or cusps may become so thickened as to obstruct the blood flow, a condition termed **valvular stenosis**. Diseases that destroy valve tissue may also allow retrograde blood flow, termed **valvular regurgitation or insufficiency**. In many instances, diseases involving the cardiac valves produce both stenosis and insufficiency, but generally one or the other predominates.

Pressure Overload. Stenosis of a cardiac valve results in hypertrophy secondary to pressure overload, with eventual myocardial failure and dilatation of the chamber proximal to the valve. Thus, mitral stenosis leads to left atrial hypertrophy and dilatation. As the left atrium decompensates and can no longer force the venous return through the stenotic mitral valve, signs of pulmonary congestion develop, followed by right ventricular hypertrophy and even cor pulmonale.

BOX *11-4*   **Causes of Cor Pulmonale**

Parenchymal Diseases of the Lung
Chronic bronchitis and emphysema
Pulmonary fibrosis (from any cause)
Cystic fibrosis
Pulmonary Vascular Diseases
Recurrent pulmonary emboli
Primary pulmonary hypertension
Peripheral pulmonary stenosis
Intravenous drug abuse
Residence at high altitude
Schistosomiasis
Congenital Heart Disease
Impaired Movement of the Thoracic Cage
Kyphoscoliosis
Pickwickian syndrome
Pleural fibrosis
Neuromuscular disorders
Idiopathic hypoventilation

Similarly, aortic stenosis causes left ventricular hypertrophy and heart failure.

Volume Overload. Valvular regurgitation or insufficiency also results in hypertrophy and dilatation of the cardiac chamber proximal to the valve owing to volume overload. In patients with aortic insufficiency, the left ventricle first hypertrophies and then dilates when it can no longer accommodate the regurgitant volume or provide adequate cardiac output. On the other hand, an incompetent mitral valve leads to hypertrophy and dilatation of both the left atrium and left ventricle, because both are subjected to volume overload.

Rheumatic Heart Disease

■ *Rheumatic heart disease encompasses myocarditis during acute rheumatic fever, which is a sequel of group A streptococcal infection, and residual chronic valvular deformities.*

Acute Rheumatic Fever

☐ **Epidemiology:** Rheumatic fever is a complication of an acute streptococcal infection, which is almost always a pharyngitis (see Chapter 9). **Despite its declining importance in the industrialized countries, rheumatic fever remains the leading cause of death from heart disease in persons between 5 and 25 years of age in less-developed regions.**

☐ **Pathogenesis:** The pathogenesis of rheumatic fever remains unclear, and with the exception of the link to streptococcal infection, no theory is generally accepted. Most theories relate rheumatic carditis to immunologic phenomena. In particular, some antibodies against streptococcal antigens cross-react with heart antigens, which raises the possibility of an autoimmune cause (Fig. 11-20).

☐ **Pathology:** Acute rheumatic heart disease is a pancarditis involving all three layers of the heart.

Myocarditis. In severe cases of rheumatic fever, the heart tends to be dilated, and a few patients die in the acute stage of the disease. At autopsy, the heart exhibits a nonspecific myocarditis, in which lymphocytes and macrophages predominate. Fibrinoid degeneration of collagen, in which the fibers become swollen and eosinophilic, is characteristic.

The **Aschoff body** is the typical lesion of rheumatic myocarditis (Fig. 11-21), developing several weeks after the onset of symptoms. This structure initially consists of a perivascular focus of swollen eosinophilic collagen surrounded by lymphocytes, plasma cells, and macrophages. In time, the Aschoff body assumes a granulomatous appearance, with a central fibrinoid focus being associated with a perimeter of lymphocytes, plasma cells, macrophages, and giant cells. Eventually, the Aschoff body is replaced by a nodule of scar tissue.

Pericarditis. Tenacious, irregular deposits of fibrin are found on both the visceral and parietal surfaces of the pericardium. These deposits resemble the shaggy surfaces of two slices of buttered bread that have been pulled apart ("bread-and-butter pericarditis"). The pericarditis may be recognized clinically by a friction rub, but it has little functional effect and, ordinarily, does not lead to constrictive pericarditis.

Endocarditis. During the acute stage of rheumatic carditis, an endocarditis involves mainly the mitral and aortic valves, which show a finely nodular, "verrucous" appearance at the line of closure. Areas of focal collagen degeneration in the valve are surrounded by inflammation, and ulceration of the valve surface as well as deposition of fibrin lead to the verrucous lesions.

☐ **Clinical Features:** The symptoms of rheumatic fever occur 2 to 3 weeks after infection with *Streptococcus pyogenes*. The major clinical manifestations of acute rheumatic fever include carditis (murmurs, cardiomegaly, pericarditis, and congestive heart failure), polyarthritis, chorea, erythema marginatum, and subcutaneous nodules.

FIGURE *11-20*
Biological factors in rheumatic heart disease. The upper portion illustrates the initiating β-hemolytic streptococcal infection of the throat, which introduces the streptococcal antigens into the body and may also activate cytotoxic T cells. These antigens lead to the production of antibodies to various antigenic components of the streptococcus, which can cross-react with certain cardiac antigens, including those from the myocyte sarcolemma and from the glycoproteins of the valves. This may be the mechanism for the production of the acute inflammation of the heart in acute rheumatic fever that involves all cardiac layers (endocarditis, myocarditis, and pericarditis). This inflammation becomes apparent after a latent period of 2 to 3 weeks. The insult may progress to chronic stenosis or insufficiency of the valves. These lesions involve the mitral, aortic, tricuspid, and pulmonary valves, in that order of frequency.

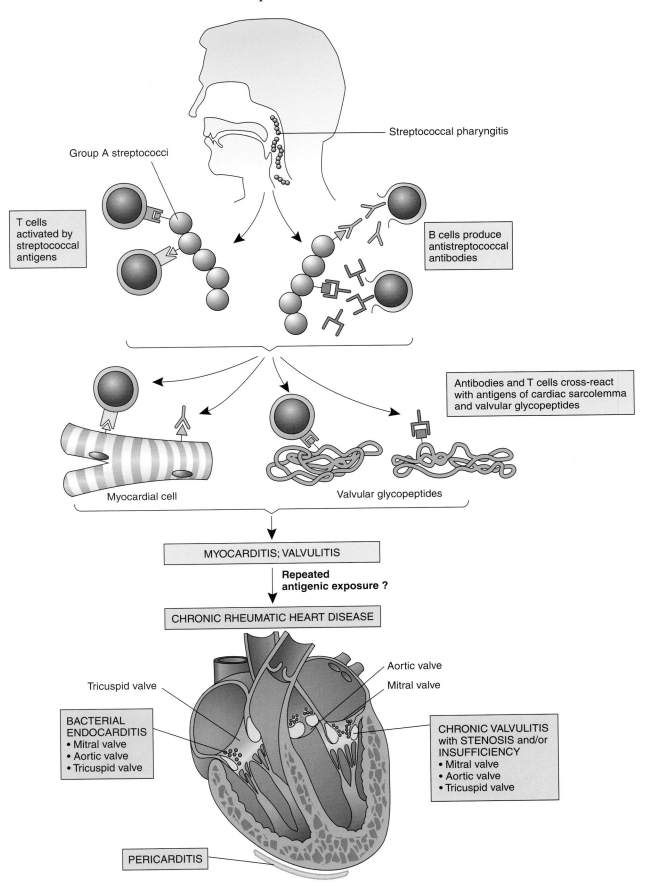

Streptococcal pharyngitis

Group A streptococci

T cells
activated by
streptococcal
antigens

B cells produce
antistreptococcal
antibodies

Antibodies and T cells cross-react
with antigens of cardiac sarcolemma
and valvular glycopeptides

Myocardial cell

Valvular glycopeptides

MYOCARDITIS; VALVULITIS

**Repeated
antigenic exposure ?**

CHRONIC RHEUMATIC HEART DISEASE

Tricuspid valve

Aortic valve

Mitral valve

BACTERIAL
ENDOCARDITIS
• Mitral valve
• Aortic valve
• Tricuspid valve

CHRONIC VALVULITIS
with STENOSIS and/or
INSUFFICIENCY
• Mitral valve
• Aortic valve
• Tricuspid valve

PERICARDITIS

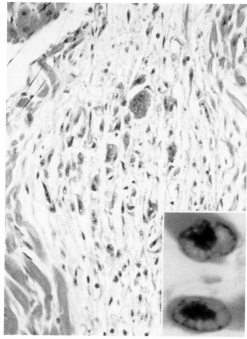

FIGURE   *11-21*
Acute rheumatic heart disease. A spindle-shaped Aschoff body is located interstitially in the myocardium. Collagen degeneration, lymphocytes, and a multinucleated giant cell (Aschoff myocyte) are noted. (Inset) The nuclei of Anitschkow myocytes show an "owl-eyed" appearance in cross-section and a "caterpillar" shape longitudinally.

The acute symptoms of rheumatic fever usually subside within 3 months, but in the presence of severe carditis, clinical activity may continue for 6 months or longer. The mortality rate of acute rheumatic carditis is low, and the main cause of death is heart failure from myocarditis. However, valvular dysfunction may also play a role. In patients with a history of a recent attack of rheumatic fever, the recurrence rate is as high as 65%, whereas after 10 years, a streptococcal infection is followed by an acute relapse in only 5%.

Treatment of streptococcal pharyngitis with penicillin prevents an initial attack of rheumatic fever and, less often, a recurrence of the disease. There is no specific treatment for acute rheumatic fever, but corticosteroids and salicylates are helpful in the management of symptoms.

Chronic Rheumatic Heart Disease

Severe valvular scarring may develop over a period of months or years after a single bout of acute rheumatic fever. On the other hand, recurrent episodes of acute rheumatic fever are common and result in repeated, progressively increasing damage to the heart valves. **The mitral valve is the most commonly and severely**

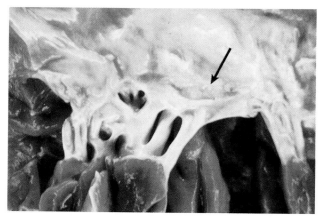

FIGURE   *11-22*
Chronic rheumatic valvulitis. The mitral valve leaflet is thickened and focally calcified (*arrow*). The chordae tendineae are short, thick, and fused.

affected valve in chronic rheumatic disease. Chronic mitral valvulitis is characterized by conspicuous, irregular thickening and calcification of the leaflets, often with fusion of the commissures and chordae tendineae (Fig. 11-22). As a result, the valve cannot close properly, and mitral regurgitation results. Varying degrees of mitral stenosis may also be present and, when severe, be the predominant functional lesion. When viewed from the atrial aspect, a severely stenotic mitral valve has a narrowed orifice, with the appearance of a "fish mouth" (Fig. 11-23).

The aortic valve is the second most commonly involved valve. It shows fused commissures and pronounced thickening of the cusps. This valve often becomes calcified as the patient ages, thereby resulting in stenosis and insufficiency, although either lesion may predominate.

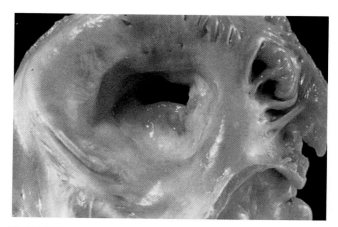

FIGURE   *11-23*
Chronic rheumatic valvulitis. This view of a mitral valve from the left atrium shows rigid, thickened, and fused leaflets with a narrow orifice, thereby creating the characteristic "fish mouth" appearance of rheumatic mitral stenosis.

Complications of Chronic Rheumatic Heart Disease

Bacterial endocarditis follows episodes of bacteremia, such as those that occur during dental procedures. The scarred valves of rheumatic heart disease provide an attractive environment for bacteria that would ordinarily bypass a normal valve. **Mural thrombi** form in the atrial or ventricular chambers in 40% of patients with rheumatic valvular disease, giving rise to thromboemboli, which produce infarcts in various organs. **Congestive heart failure** is associated with rheumatic disease of both the mitral and aortic valves. **Cor pulmonale** may develop as a result of secondary pulmonary hypertension.

The Heart in Collagen Vascular Diseases

Lupus Erythematosus

The heart is often involved in systemic lupus erythematosus (SLE), but the cardiac symptoms are usually less prominent than the other manifestations of this disease. The most common cardiac lesion is a fibrinous pericarditis, usually with an effusion. Myocarditis in patients with SLE, at least in the form of subclinical left ventricular dysfunction, is also common and reflects the severity of the disease in other organs. Microscopically, fibrinoid necrosis of small vessels and focal degeneration of interstitial tissue are seen.

Endocarditis is the most striking cardiac lesion of SLE. Verrucous vegetations, measuring as much as 4 mm across, occur on the endocardial surfaces and are termed **Libman-Sacks endocarditis.** They are most common on the surfaces of the mitral valve (Fig.

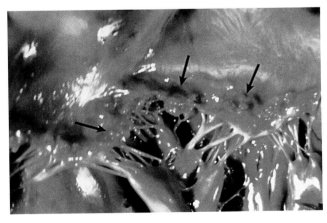

FIGURE *11-24*
Libman-Sacks endocarditis. This heart of a patient who died from complications of systemic lupus erythematosus displays verrucous vegetations on the leaflets of the mitral valve.

11-24). Libman-Sacks endocarditis ordinarily does not produce a functional deficit and heals without scarring.

Scleroderma

Involvement of the heart in patients with scleroderma is second only to renal disease as a cause of death in patients with this illness. The myocardium exhibits intimal sclerosis of the small arteries, which leads to small infarcts and patchy fibrosis. Cor pulmonale secondary to interstitial fibrosis of the lungs and hypertensive heart disease (caused by renal involvement) are also seen.

Bacterial Endocarditis

■ *Bacterial endocarditis is the colonization of cardiac valves by bacteria.* Before the antibiotic era, bacterial endocarditis was untreatable and, almost invariably, fatal. The infection was classified according to its clinical course as either acute or subacute endocarditis (Table 11-1).

Acute endocarditis was described as being an infection of a normal cardiac valve by suppurative organisms, typically *Staphylococcus aureus* and *Streptococcus pyogenes.* The affected valve was rapidly destroyed, and the patient died within 6 weeks from acute heart failure or overwhelming infection.

Subacute endocarditis was a less fulminant disease, in which less virulent organisms (e.g., *Streptococcus viridans* or *Staphylococcus epidermidis*) colonized deformed valves that usually had been damaged by rheumatic heart disease. In these cases, patients typically survived for 6 months or more, and infectious complications were uncommon.

The introduction of antimicrobial therapy has changed the clinical patterns of bacterial endocarditis, and the classic presentations just described are unusual today. **The disease is now classified according to the anatomic location and the offending organism.**

TABLE *11-1.* Comparison of Acute and Subacute Bacterial Endocarditis

	Acute	Subacute
Duration of clinical symptoms	<6 weeks	>6 weeks
Most common organisms	Staphylococcus aureus, β-Streptococci	α-Streptococci
Virulence of organism	Highly virulent	Less virulent
Condition of valves	Usually previously normal, perforations common	Usually previously damaged; perforations rare

☐ **Epidemiology:** The large majority of children who develop bacterial endocarditis have an underlying cardiac lesion. In the past, rheumatic heart disease accounted for one-third of such cases. However, with the declining incidence of rheumatic fever, less than 10% of cases of bacterial endocarditis in children are attributable to this disease today. **Now, the most common predisposing condition in children is by far congenital heart disease.**

The epidemiology of bacterial endocarditis has also changed in adults. Whereas rheumatic heart disease accounted for as many as three-fourths of these cases in the past, it now underlies only one-fourth. In addition, 25% to 50% have no predisposing cardiac lesion. **Mitral valve prolapse and congenital heart disease are today the most frequent basis for bacterial endocarditis in adults.**

Intravenous drug abusers inject pathogenic organisms along with their illicit drugs, and bacterial endocarditis is a notorious complication.

Prosthetic valves are the site of infection in 10% of all cases of endocarditis in adults, and as many as 4% of patients with prosthetic valves suffer this complication.

Transient bacteremia from any procedure may lead to infective endocarditis. Examples include dental procedures, urinary catheterization, gastrointestinal endoscopy, and obstetric procedures. Antibiotic prophylaxis is recommended for such maneuvers if the physician has reason to believe a patient is at increased risk for bacterial endocarditis (e.g., a history of rheumatic fever or the presence of a cardiac murmur).

☐ **Pathogenesis:** Virulent organisms, such as *Staphylococcus aureus*, can infect apparently normal valves, but the mechanism of such bacterial colonization is poorly understood. The pathogenesis of the infection of a damaged valve by less virulent organisms has been related to (1) hemodynamic factors, (2) formation of an initially sterile platelet and fibrin thrombus, and (3) adherence properties of the micro-organisms.

☐ **Pathology:** Bacterial endocarditis most commonly involves the mitral valve, the aortic valve, or both. In rheumatic heart disease, the mitral valve is affected in more than 85% of cases of bacterial endocarditis, and the aortic valve is infected in 50%. The most frequent congenital heart lesions that underlie bacterial endocarditis are patent ductus arteriosus, tetralogy of Fallot, and ventricular septal defect. Bicuspid aortic valve is an increasingly recognized risk factor, especially in men older than 60 years of age.

The vegetations, which are composed of platelets, fibrin, cell debris, and masses of organisms, form on

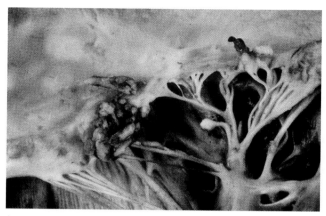

FIGURE *11-25*
Bacterial endocarditis. The mitral valve shows destructive vegetations, which have eroded through the free margin of the valve leaflet.

the valve surface at the point of closure of the leaflets or cusps (Fig. 11-25). The underlying valve is edematous and inflamed and, eventually, may be so damaged that it becomes insufficient. The lesions vary from a small, superficial deposit to exuberant vegetations.

Infected thromboemboli travel to multiple systemic sites, causing infarcts or abscesses in many organs, including the brain, kidneys, intestine, and spleen.

☐ **Clinical Features:** Many patients manifest the early symptoms of bacterial endocarditis within a week of the bacteremic episode, and almost all patients are symptomatic within 2 weeks. Heart murmurs almost invariably develop, often with a changing pattern during the course of the disease. **The most common serious complication of bacterial endocarditis is congestive heart failure, usually as a result of destruction of a valve.** In cases of more than 6 weeks' duration, splenomegaly, petechiae, and clubbing of the fingers are frequent. In one-third of the patients, systemic emboli are recognized at some point during the illness. One-third of the patients with bacterial endocarditis manifest some evidence of neurologic dysfunction owing to the frequency of embolization to the brain.

Antibacterial therapy is effective in limiting the morbidity and mortality of bacterial endocarditis, and most patients defervesce within a week of instituting such therapy. However, the prognosis depends, at least to some extent, on the offending organism and the stage at which the infection is treated. **As many as 25% to 40% of cases of endocarditis caused by *S. aureus* are still fatal.** Cardiac surgery with valve replacement is necessary for some cases in which the bacteria have been eliminated but structural damage remains.

Nonbacterial Thrombotic Endocarditis (Marantic Endocarditis)

■ *Nonbacterial thrombotic endocarditis (NBTE)* is *the presence of sterile vegetations on apparently normal cardiac valves, almost always in association with cancer or some other wasting disease.* NBTE affects the mitral (Fig. 11-26) and aortic valves equally, and it is similar in gross appearance to infective endocarditis. However, it does not destroy the affected valve, and on microscopic examination, neither inflammation nor microorganisms can be demonstrated.

The cause of NBTE is poorly understood, but it has been attributed to increased blood coagulability or immune complex deposition. It is commonly a paraneoplastic condition, usually complicating adenocarcinomas (particularly of the pancreas and lung) and hematologic malignancies. It may be part of the disseminated intravascular coagulation syndrome and accompany a variety of debilitating, nonneoplastic diseases, hence the synonym "marantic endocarditis" (Gr. *marantikos*, "wasting away"). The principal danger posed by NBTE is embolization to distant organs, which is manifested clinically as infarcts of the brain, kidneys, spleen, intestines, or extremities.

Calcific Aortic Stenosis

■ *Calcific aortic stenosis is a narrowing of the aortic valve lumen as a result of the deposition of calcium in the cusps and valve ring.* It occurs in a number of situations:

- Calcific stenosis develops in elderly patients as a degenerative process involving a normal aortic valve.

- Calcification may develop in an aortic valve scarred as a result of rheumatic fever.
- A congenital bicuspid aortic valve often becomes calcified with age (Fig. 11-27).
- Severe atherosclerosis of the aorta (e.g., in familial hypercholesterolemia) may be associated with calcific aortic stenosis.

The cause of isolated calcific aortic stenosis of both congenitally malformed valves and normal valves is thought to relate to the cumulative effect of years of trauma owing to turbulent blood flow around the valve. The dystrophic calcification produces nodules restricted to the base and lower half of the cusps and only rarely involves the free margins.

Severe aortic stenosis results in striking, concentric left ventricular hypertrophy, with the heart achieving a weight as great as 1000 g (cor bovinum). Eventually, the heart dilates and fails. The disease is treated with great success (5-year survival rate, 85%) by surgical valve replacement, after which the hypertrophic left ventricle is restored to a normal size.

Mitral Valve Prolapse

■ *Mitral valve prolapse (MVP) is a situation in which redundant mitral valve leaflets fail to approximate during systole, resulting in mitral regurgitation.* This abnormality is caused by a variety of conditions, all of which have in common excessive mobility of the mitral valve leaflets (Fig. 11-28), which allows them to billow or prolapse into the left atrium during systole. The condition is one of the most prevalent cardiac abnormalities, affecting 5% to 10% of the adult population. In fact,

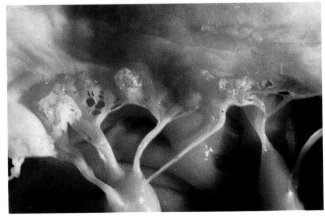

FIGURE *11-26*
Nonbacterial thrombotic endocarditis. Sterile vegetations are seen on the leaflets of an apparently normal mitral valve.

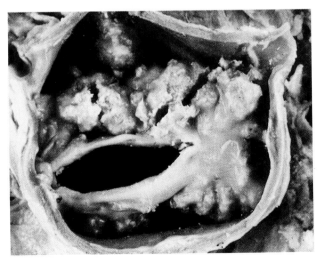

FIGURE *11-27*
Calcific aortic stenosis of a congenitally bicuspid, aortic semilunar valve.

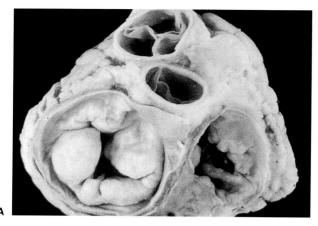
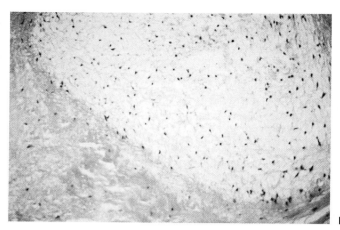

A   B

FIGURE *11-28*
Mitral valve prolapse. (A) This view of the mitral valve (*left*) from the left atrium shows redundant and deformed leaflets, which billow into the left atrial cavity. (B) This microscopic section of one of the mitral valve leaflets shows conspicuous myxomatous connective tissue in the center of the leaflet.

MVP is today the most frequent cause of mitral regurgitation that requires surgical replacement of the valve.

☐ **Pathogenesis:** MVP has an important hereditary component, and many cases appear to be transmitted as an autosomal dominant trait. Patients with primary MVP exhibit a striking accumulation of myxomatous connective tissue in the center of the valve leaflet (see Fig. 11-28*B*).

☐ **Pathology:** On gross examination, the mitral valve leaflets are redundant and deformed, and on cross-section, they have a gelatinous appearance. **Myxomatous proliferation** may involve not only the mitral valve leaflets but also the annulus and chordae tendineae. The damage to the chordae is often so severe that chordal rupture occurs, with a consequent flail valve that is totally incompetent. Myxomatous proliferation has also been described in the other cardiac valves, especially in patients with Marfan syndrome, 90% of whom have some clinical evidence of MVP.

☐ **Clinical Features:** The large majority of patients with MVP are entirely asymptomatic. Endocarditis, both infective and nonbacterial, is sometimes a serious complication, and cerebral emboli are common. In 15% of patients with MVP, significant mitral regurgitation develops in 10 to 15 years and often requires surgical intervention.

Carcinoid Heart Disease

Patients with carcinoid tumors that have metastasized to the liver often display changes in the endocardium of the right side of the heart. These alterations consist of deposits of pearly gray, uniform, fibrous tissue on the tricuspid (Fig. 11-29) and pulmonary valves and on the endocardial surface of the right ventricle. Microscopically, these patches appear to be "tacked on" to the endocardium and are without elastic fibers.

Carcinoid involvement of the endocardium can result in tricuspid insufficiency or stenosis and in pulmonary valve stenosis. The endocardial lesions are thought to result from high concentrations of tumor-produced serotonin and, perhaps, other tumor products, which are metabolized in the lung. As a result, the effects of high levels of carcinoid secretions affect almost exclusively the right side of the heart, whereas the left side tends to be spared.

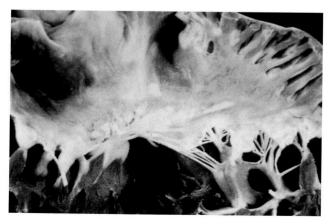

FIGURE *11-29*
Carcinoid heart disease. Pearly white deposits are seen on the tricuspid valve leaflets and adjacent endocardium.

MYOCARDITIS

■ *Myocarditis is a generalized inflammation of the myocardium associated with necrosis and degeneration of myocytes.* This definition specifically excludes ischemic heart disease. Myocarditis can occur at any age, and it is one of the few heart diseases that can produce acute heart failure in previously healthy adolescents or young adults. Numerous infectious agents can cause myocarditis, as can hypersensitivity reactions and some toxic injuries.

Most cases of myocarditis in North America occur without a demonstrable cause, but the majority are believed to be viral. The pathogenesis of viral myocarditis is thought to involve direct viral cytotoxicity or T cell-mediated immune reactions directed against infected myocytes. The most common viruses that cause myocarditis are listed in Box 11-5.

☐ **Pathology:** The hearts of symptomatic patients with myocarditis, during the active inflammatory phase, show biventricular dilatation and generalized hypokinesis of the myocardium. At autopsy, the hearts of patients dying acutely are flabby and dilated, whereas chronic myocarditis is associated with myocardial hypertrophy. The histologic changes of viral myocarditis vary with the clinical severity of the disease. Most cases involve a patchy or diffuse interstitial infiltrate, which is composed principally of T lymphocytes and macrophages (Fig. 11-30). The inflammatory cells often surround individual myocytes, and there is focal or patchy acute myocyte necrosis associated with the inflammatory cell infiltrate. During the early

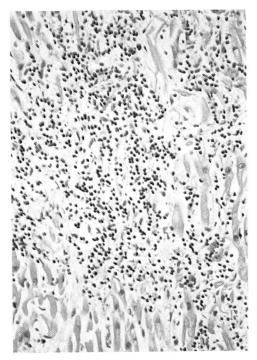

FIGURE   *11-30*
Viral myocarditis. The myocardial fibers are disrupted by a prominent interstitial infiltrate of lymphocytes and macrophages.

stages, necrosis and accumulation of interstitial proteinaceous material are prominent, whereas during the resolving phase, fibroblast proliferation and interstitial collagen deposition predominate.

☐ **Clinical Features:** In most patients with viral myocarditis, symptoms begin a few weeks after the initial infection. Despite extensive inflammation, most patients recover from acute myocarditis, although a few succumb to congestive heart failure or arrhythmias. During the resolving phase of the disease, subtle functional impairment may persist for years, and progression to overt cardiomyopathy has been observed in a few patients. There is no specific therapy for viral myocarditis, and supportive measures are the rule.

METABOLIC DISEASES OF THE HEART

Hyperthyroid Heart Disease

Hyperthyroidism causes conspicuous tachycardia and increased cardiac workload owing to lowered peripheral resistance and increased cardiac output. The disorder may eventually lead to angina pectoris and high output failure.

BOX   *11-5*   **Causes of Myocarditis**

Idiopathic
Infectious
Viral: Coxsackievirus, echovirus, influenza virus, human immunodeficiency virus, and many others
Rickettsial: Typhus, Rocky Mountain spotted fever
Bacterial: Diphtheria, staphylococcal, streptococcal, meningococcal, and leptospiral infections
Fungi and protozoan parasites: Chagas disease, toxoplasmosis, aspergillosis, cryptococcal, and candidal infections
Metazoan parasites: *Echinococcus, Trichina*
Noninfectious
Hypersensitivity and immunologically related diseases: Rheumatic fever, systemic lupus erythematosus, scleroderma, drug reaction (e.g., to penicillin or sulfonamide), rheumatoid arthritis
Radiation
Miscellaneous: Sarcoidosis, uremia

Hypothyroid Heart Disease

Patients with severe hypothyroidism (myxedema) have decreased cardiac output, reduced heart rate, and impaired myocardial contractility—that is, changes that are the reverse of those seen in patients with hyperthyroidism. The hearts of these patients are usually flabby and dilated. The myocardium exhibits myofiber swelling, and basophilic (mucinous) degeneration is common. Despite these changes, myxedema does not produce congestive heart failure in the absence of other cardiac disorders.

Thiamine Deficiency (Beriberi) Heart Disease

Beriberi heart disease has been seen in the Orient among persons who consume a diet that is inadequate in vitamin B_1 (thiamine) for at least 3 months (see Chapter 8). In the United States, thiamine deficiency is occasionally encountered in persons with alcoholism or who are neglected. Beriberi heart disease results in decreased peripheral vascular resistance and increased cardiac output, which is a combination similar to that produced by hyperthyroidism. The result is high output failure. At autopsy, the heart is dilated and shows only nonspecific microscopic changes.

CARDIOMYOPATHY

■ *Cardiomyopathy refers to primary disease of the myocardium and, in this sense, excludes myocardial disease caused by ischemia, hypertension, valvular dysfunction, congenital anomalies, or inflammatory disorders.*

Idiopathic Dilated Cardiomyopathy

☐ **Pathogenesis:** Numerous theories regarding the cause of idiopathic dilated cardiomyopathy (DCM) have been proposed, but none has been established. It has been suggested that the disease results from an autoimmune disorder that is precipitated by an asymptomatic episode of viral myocarditis. However, this attractive hypothesis is weakened by the observation that only 15% of patients with known myocarditis evolve into DCM. Circumstantial evidence favoring an autoimmune process includes (1) the common observation of a focal or mild lymphocytic infiltrate in the myocardium, (2) the presence of heart-specific autoantibodies in some patients, and (3) occasional abnormalities of cellular immunity.

Genetic factors now appear to be more important than was previously believed. Large families with idiopathic DCM have been documented and are believed to suffer from single-gene defects. A careful, prospective study of asymptomatic relatives of patients with idiopathic DCM demonstrated that at least 20% of the index cases were actually familial.

☐ **Pathology:** The pathologic changes in patients with DCM are, for the most part, similar whether the disorder is idiopathic or secondary. At autopsy, the heart is enlarged owing to both hypertrophy and dilatation. The weight of the heart may be as much as tripled (900 g). All chambers of the heart are dilated, although the ventricles are more severely affected than the atria (Fig. 11-31). The myocardium is flabby and pale, and small, subendocardial scars are occasionally evident. The endocardium of the left ventricle, especially at the apex, tends to be thickened, and adherent mural thrombi are often present in this area.

Microscopically, DCM is characterized by both atrophic and hypertrophic myocardial fibers. Interstitial and perivascular fibrosis of the myocardium is evident, especially in the subendocardial zone. Although scattered chronic inflammatory cells may be present, they are not prominent.

☐ **Clinical Features:** The clinical courses of idiopathic and secondary DCM are comparable. The disease begins insidiously, with asymptomatic left ventricular dilatation. Commonly, exercise intolerance progresses relentlessly to frank congestive heart failure, and 75% of the patients die within 5 years. Although supportive treatment is useful, cardiac transplantation offers the only hope of cure.

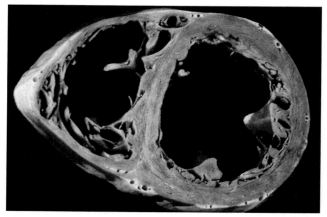

FIGURE *11-31*
Idiopathic dilated cardiomyopathy. This cross-section of the enlarged heart reveals conspicuous dilatation of both ventricles.

Secondary Dilated Cardiomyopathy

Almost 100 distinct myocardial diseases can result in the clinical features of DCM. Thus, secondary DCM is best viewed as being a final common pathway for the effects of virtually any toxic, metabolic, or infectious disorder causing widespread degenerative changes in the myocardium. In this context, alcohol abuse, hypertension, pregnancy, and viral myocarditis are thought to predispose to secondary DCM. Cigarette smoking has also been linked to an increased incidence of this disorder.

Toxic Cardiomyopathy

Numerous chemicals and drugs cause myocardial injury, but only a few of the more important chemicals that cause DCM are discussed here.

Ethanol. Alcoholic cardiomyopathy is the single most common identifiable cause of DCM in the United States and Europe, probably accounting for more than half of all cases in which the etiology can be ascertained. Ethanol abuse can lead to chronic, progressive cardiac dysfunction, which may be fatal. The typical patient has been drinking heavily for at least 10 years. The mechanism by which alcohol injures the heart remains obscure, but the degree of myocardial damage correlates with the total lifetime dose of ethanol.

Catecholamines. In high concentrations, catecholamines may cause focal myocyte necrosis. Toxic myocarditis may occur in patients with pheochromocytomas, in persons who require inotropic drugs to maintain blood pressure, and in accident victims who sustain massive head trauma.

Anthracyclines. Drugs such as doxorubicin (Adriamycin) and daunorubicin are potent chemotherapeutic agents, but their usefulness is limited by a cumulative, dose-dependent, cardiac toxicity. The major effect is a chronic, irreversible degeneration of cardiac myocytes, which is characterized pathologically by vacuolization and loss of myofibrils and functionally by depressed contractility. Intractable congestive heart failure develops, and the prognosis is grim.

Cocaine. Use of this illicit drug is frequently associated with chest pain and palpitations. True DCM is not a usual complication of cocaine abuse, but myocarditis, focal necrosis, and thickening of intramyocardial coronary arteries have been reported in some cases. A few instances of myocardial ischemia or infarction associated with cocaine use have been attributed to coronary vasoconstriction. Sudden death from ventricular arrhythmias has received a great deal of public attention. The mechanisms underlying these effects of cocaine are unclear, but they include vasoconstriction, sympathomimetic activity, hypersensitivity responses, and direct toxicity.

Cardiomyopathy of Pregnancy

A unique form of DCM develops during the last trimester of pregnancy or the first 6 months after delivery. The disorder is uncommon in the United States, but in some regions of black Africa, it is encountered in as many as 1% of pregnant women. The cause of this form of DCM is unknown, but there is increasing evidence of an underlying myocarditis in many patients.

Hypertrophic Cardiomyopathy

■ *Hypertrophic cardiomyopathy (HCM) is an uncommon condition in which cardiac hypertrophy is out of proportion to the hemodynamic load on the heart.* Myocardial hypertrophy develops progressively during the first two decades of life in the absence of an extrinsic stress. In roughly half of the cases, the disorder is transmitted as a single-gene, autosomal dominant trait. In the remainder, the disease arises spontaneously, without evidence of this disorder in relatives.

☐ **Pathogenesis:** In one-third to one-half of the cases, mutations are found in the cardiac β-myosin heavy-chain gene on chromosome 14. The remaining cases demonstrate mutations in the cardiac troponin T gene on chromosome 1, the β-tropomyosin gene on chromosome 15, and the myosin-binding protein C gene on chromosome 11. All these defects involve sarcomeric proteins, and it is thought that changes in protein conformation may affect sarcomere assembly and turnover.

☐ **Pathology:** The heart in patients with HCM is always enlarged, with an average weight of approximately 500 g. The wall of the left ventricle is thick, and its cavity is small, sometimes even being reduced to a slit. The papillary muscles and trabeculae carneae are prominent and encroach on the ventricular lumen. More than half of the cases exhibit asymmetric hypertrophy of the interventricular septum, with a ratio of the thickness of the septum to that of the left ventricular free wall of greater than 1.5 (Fig. 11-32).

The most notable histologic feature of HCM is myofiber disarray, which is most extensive in the interventricular septum. Instead of the usual, parallel arrangement of myocytes into muscle bundles, myofiber disarray is characterized by an oblique and often perpendicular orientation of adjacent hypertrophic myocytes (see Fig. 11-32).

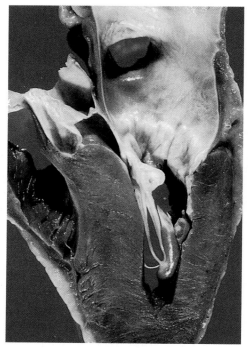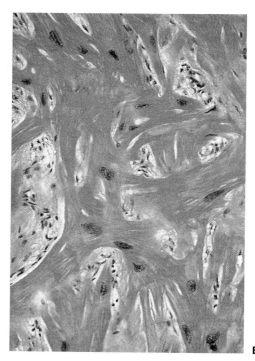

FIGURE   *11-32*
Hypertrophic cardiomyopathy. (A) The heart has been opened to show striking, asymmetric left ventricular hypertrophy. The interventricular septum is thicker than the free wall of the left ventricle and impinges on the outflow tract. (B) A section of the myocardium shows myofiber disarray characterized by an oblique and often perpendicular orientation of adjacent hypertrophic myocytes.

☐ **Clinical Features:** Most patients with HCM have few (if any) symptoms, and the diagnosis is commonly made at screening of the family of a patient with symptomatic HCM. Despite the absence of symptoms, such persons are at risk for sudden death, particularly during severe exertion. In fact, unsuspected HCM is the most common abnormality found at autopsy in young, competitive athletes who die suddenly. HCM is usually first diagnosed in the fourth and fifth decades of life, but the disorder is also encountered in elderly patients.

Some patients with HCM become incapacitated by cardiac symptoms, although the severity of the clinical disease bears little relation to the degree of cardiac hypertrophy. Dyspnea and angina pectoris eventually are followed by severe congestive heart failure.

Restrictive Cardiomyopathy

■ *Restrictive cardiomyopathy refers to a group of diseases in which myocardial or endocardial abnormalities limit diastolic filling while allowing contractile function to remain relatively normal.* It is the least common category of cardiomyopathy in Western countries, although in some less-developed regions (e.g., parts of equatorial Africa, South America, and Asia), endomyocardial disease leads to many cases of restrictive cardiomyopathy.

Restrictive cardiomyopathy is caused by (1) interstitial infiltration of amyloid, metastatic carcinoma, or sarcoid granulomas; (2) endomyocardial disease; (3) storage diseases, including hemochromatosis; and (4) a marked increase in interstitial fibrous tissue. Many cases are classified as being idiopathic, with interstitial fibrosis as the only histologic abnormality. Restrictive cardiomyopathy almost invariably progresses to congestive heart failure, and only 10% of the patients survive for 10 years. There is no specific treatment for the condition.

Amyloidosis

The heart is affected in most of the generalized forms of amyloidosis (see Chapter 23). In fact, restrictive cardiomyopathy is the most common cause of death in patients with the AL amyloidosis of plasma cell dyscrasias.

☐ **Pathology:** Amyloid infiltration of the heart results in cardiac enlargement without significant ventricular dilatation. The ventricular walls are thickened, firm, and rubbery. Microscopically, amyloid

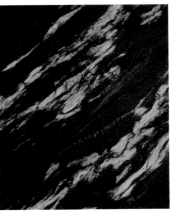

FIGURE   *11-33*
Cardiac amyloidosis. A section of myocardium stained with Congo red (*left*) shows interstitial, pink-staining deposits of amyloid. Under polarized light (*right*), the same section displays the characteristic green birefringence of amyloid fibrils.

deposits are interstitial, perivascular, or endocardial (Fig. 11-33).

☐ **Clinical Features:** Cardiac amyloidosis most often presents as a restrictive cardiomyopathy, with symptoms predominantly referable to the right side of the heart, particularly peripheral edema. Infiltration of the conduction system can result in arrhythmias, and sudden cardiac death is not unusual.

Senile Cardiac Amyloidosis

■ *Senile cardiac amyloidosis is the deposition of a protein closely related to prealbumin (transthyretin) in the hearts of elderly persons* (see Chapter 23). The disorder has been reported to be present in 25% of patients who are 80 years of age or older. The functional significance of senile cardiac amyloidosis is often minimal.

Endomyocardial Disease

■ *Endomyocardial disease (EMD) comprises two geographically separate disorders that are associated with restrictive cardiomyopathy and characterized by fibrosis of both the endocardium and myocardium.*

Endomyocardial Fibrosis. This disorder is particularly common in equatorial Africa, where it accounts for 10% to 20% of all deaths attributed to heart disease. It is most common in children and young adults, but it has been reported to occur in patients as old as 70 years. Endomyocardial fibrosis leads to progressive myocardial failure and has a poor prognosis.

Eosinophilic EMD (Löffler Endocarditis). This is a cardiac disorder of temperate regions and is characterized by hypereosinophilia. The disease is usually encountered in men during the fifth decade and is often accompanied by a rash. Peripheral eosinophil counts may attain levels as high as 50,000 cells/μL. Löffler endocarditis typically progresses to congestive heart failure and death, although corticosteroids may improve the survival rate.

☐ **Pathogenesis:** There is a growing consensus that endomyocardial fibrosis and Löffler endocarditis represent variants of the same underlying disease. EMD is suspected to result from myocardial injury produced by eosinophils, possibly mediated by cardiotoxic constituents of the granules. In tropical climates, transient high blood eosinophil counts often result from parasitic infestations, whereas in temperate climates, idiopathic hypereosinophilia is often persistent.

☐ **Pathology:** At autopsy, a grayish-white layer of thickened endocardium extends from the apex of the left ventricle over the posterior papillary muscles, to the posterior leaflet of the mitral valve, and a short distance into the left outflow tract. On a cut section of the ventricle, endocardial fibrosis spreads into the inner one-third to one-half of the wall. Mural thrombi at various stages of organization may be present. Microscopically, the fibrotic endocardium contains only a few elastic fibers. Myofibers trapped within the collagenous tissue display a variety of degenerative changes.

Storage Diseases

The various lysosomal storage diseases are discussed in detail in Chapter 6, and only the cardiac manifestations are reviewed here.

Glycogen Storage Diseases. The most common and severe cardiac involvement occurs with type II glycogen storage disease (Pompe disease). In infants with this condition, the heart is markedly enlarged, as much as sevenfold greater than normal, and endocardial fibroelastosis is seen in 20% of patients. The myocytes are vacuolated as a result of the large amounts of stored glycogen. The usual cause of death is cardiac failure.

Mucopolysaccharidoses. Several of the numerous mucopolysaccharidoses involve the heart. Cardiac disease results from the lysosomal accumulation of mucopolysaccharides (glycosaminoglycans) in various cells.

Sphingolipidoses. In **Fabry disease,** accumulation of glycosphingolipids in the heart results in functional and pathologic changes similar to those complicating the mucopolysaccharidoses.

Hemochromatosis. This multiorgan disease is associated with excessive iron deposition in many tissues and is caused by a genetic defect of iron metabolism (see Chapter 14). Involvement of the heart presents with features of both dilated and restrictive cardiomyopathy. **Congestive heart failure occurs in as many as one-third of patients with hemochromatosis.**

At autopsy, the heart is dilated and the ventricular walls are thickened. The brown color seen on gross examination correlates with the deposition of iron in cardiac myocytes. Interstitial fibrosis invariably occurs, but its extent does not correlate well with the degree of iron accumulation. The severity of myocardial dysfunction seems to be proportional to the quantity of iron deposited.

CARDIAC TUMORS

Primary cardiac tumors are rare, but when they occur, they can result in serious problems.

Cardiac Myxoma

The most common primary tumor of the heart is myxoma, accounting for 35% to 50% of all primary cardiac tumors. The tumor is usually sporadic but is occasionally associated with familial autosomal dominant syndromes. Most myxomas arise in the left atrium (75%), although they can occur in any cardiac chamber or on a valve. The tumor appears as a glistening, gelatinous, and polypoid mass, usually 5 to 6 cm in diameter, with a short stalk (Fig. 11-34). Sometimes, the tumor is sufficiently mobile to obstruct the mitral valve orifice. Microscopically, cardiac myxoma has a loose, myxoid matrix containing abundant proteoglycans. Polygonal stellate cells are found within the matrix, occurring either singly or in small clusters.

More than half of the patients with left atrial myxoma have clinical evidence of mitral valve dysfunction. One-third of those with a myxoma of the left atrium or left ventricle succumb to embolization of the tumor to the brain. Surgical removal of the tumor is successful in most patients.

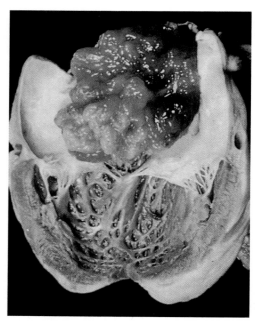

FIGURE *11-34*
Cardiac myxoma. The left atrium contains a large, polypoid tumor that protrudes into the mitral valve orifice.

Rhabdomyoma

Rhabdomyoma is the most common primary cardiac tumor in infants and children, forming nodular masses in the myocardium. There is reason to believe that cardiac rhabdomyoma may actually be a hamartoma rather than a true neoplasm, although the issue is still being debated. Almost all rhabdomyomas are multiple and involve both the left and right ventricles and, in one-third of the cases, the atria as well. In half of the cases, the tumor mass projects into the cardiac chamber and obstructs the lumen or the valve orifices.

On gross examination, cardiac rhabdomyomas are pale masses, varying from 1 mm to several centimeters in diameter. Microscopically, the cells show small, central nuclei and abundant glycogen-containing, clear cytoplasm, in which fibrillar processes radiate to the margin of the cell ("spider cell"). Rhabdomyomas often occur in association with tuberous sclerosis (one-third to one-half of the cases). A few cardiac rhabdomyomas have been successfully excised.

Metastatic Tumors

Metastases to the heart derive from cancer of the lung, breast, and gastrointestinal tract. Lymphomas and leukemia may also involve the heart, and for unknown reasons, many malignant melanomas metastasize to the heart. Metastatic cancer of the myocardium can result in manifestations of restrictive cardiomyopathy.

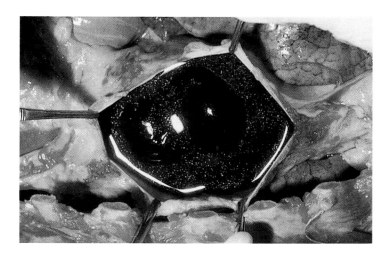

FIGURE *11-35*
Hemopericardium. The parietal pericardium has been opened to reveal the pericardial cavity, which has been distended with fresh blood. This patient had sustained a rupture of a myocardial infarct.

DISEASES OF THE PERICARDIUM

Pericardial Effusion

■ *Pericardial effusion is the accumulation of excess fluid, either in the form of a transudate or an exudate, within the pericardial cavity.* The pericardial sac normally contains no more than 50 mL of lubricating fluid. If the pericardium is slowly distended, it can stretch to accommodate as much as 2 L of fluid without notable hemodynamic consequences. However, the rapid appearance of as little as 150 to 200 mL of pericardial fluid or blood may significantly raise the intrapericardial pressure and, thereby, restrict diastolic filling.

Serous pericardial effusion is often a complication of an increased extracellular fluid volume, as occurs in patients with congestive heart failure or the nephrotic syndrome. The fluid has a low protein content and few cellular elements.

Chylous effusion (fluid-containing chylomicrons) results from a communication between the thoracic duct and the pericardial space secondary to lymphatic obstruction by tumor or infection.

Hemopericardium refers to bleeding directly into the pericardial cavity (Fig. 11-35). The most common cause is rupture of a myocardial infarct, although penetrating cardiac trauma, dissecting aneurysm of the aorta, vessel rupture by an infiltrating tumor, or a bleeding diathesis may also be responsible.

Cardiac tamponade is the syndrome produced by rapid accumulation of pericardial fluid, which restricts the filling of the heart. The hemodynamic consequences range from a minimally symptomatic condition to abrupt cardiovascular collapse and death.

Acute Pericarditis

■ *Pericarditis is an inflammation of the visceral or parietal pericardium.* The causes of pericarditis are similar to those of myocarditis (see Box 11-5). In most cases, the cause of acute pericarditis is obscure and, as in patients

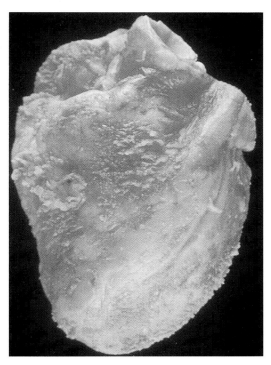

FIGURE *11-36*
Fibrinous pericarditis. This heart of a patient who died in uremia displays a shaggy, fibrinous exudate covering the visceral pericardium.

with myocarditis, is attributed to an undiagnosed viral infection. Metastatic neoplasms may also induce a serofibrinous or hemorrhagic exudate and inflammatory reaction when they involve the pericardium. Pericarditis associated with myocardial infarction and rheumatic fever was discussed earlier.

Acute pericarditis can be classified according to its gross morphologic characteristics. For example, it can be described as being **fibrinous, purulent,** or **hemorrhagic.** Uremia is frequently the cause of a fibrinous pericarditis (Fig. 11-36). Viral infection also produces a fibrinous pericarditis, as do myocardial infarcts. Bacterial infection leads to a purulent pericarditis.

The initial manifestation of acute pericarditis is sudden, severe, substernal chest pain. It is distinguished from the pain of angina pectoris or myocardial infarction by its failure to radiate down the left arm.

Constrictive Pericarditis

■ *Constrictive pericarditis is a chronic, fibrosing disease of the pericardium that compresses the heart and restricts inflow.* Today, the condition is infrequent and, in developed countries, is predominantly idiopathic. Previous radiation therapy to the mediastinum and cardiac surgery account for more than one-third of the cases, whereas in others, constrictive pericarditis follows a purulent or tuberculous infection. Although tuberculosis today accounts for less than 15% of cases of constrictive pericarditis in industrialized countries, it remains the major cause of this condition in underdeveloped regions.

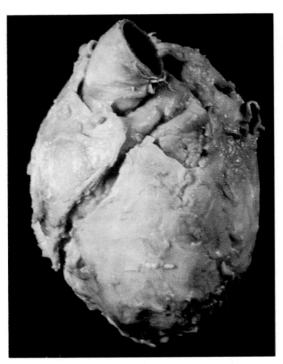

FIGURE   *11-37*
Constrictive pericarditis. The heart is encased in a fibrotic, thickened, and adherent pericardium.

The scarred pericardium may be so thick (as much as 3 cm) that it obliterates the pericardial space and presents as a rigid mass of fibrous tissue that narrows the orifices of the venae cavae (Fig. 11-37).

Patients with constrictive pericarditis have a small, quiet heart, in which venous inflow is restricted and the rigid pericardium determines the diastolic volume.

CHAPTER 12

The Respiratory System

William D. Travis
John L. Farber
Emanuel Rubin

(continued)

Pulmonary Hypertension	Bronchioloalveolar Carcinoma
Increased Flow	Small Cell Carcinoma
Precapillary Pulmonary Hypertension	Carcinoid Tumors
Cardiac Causes of Pulmonary Hypertension	Metastatic Tumors
Carcinoma of the Lung	**PLEURA**
Squamous Cell Carcinoma	Pneumothorax
Adenocarcinoma	Pleural Effusion
	Mesothelioma

Diseases of the lung are not only important problems for individual patients but also major public health concerns. Cancer of the lung causes more deaths—greater than 100,000 per year in the United States—than any other cancer. Chronic obstructive pulmonary disease represents the single greatest cost for the Veterans Administration. Adult respiratory distress syndrome is responsible for 75,000 deaths per year in the United States. Even humble respiratory tract infections, mostly benign and self-limited, are the most common cause of days lost from work.

Larynx

EPIGLOTTITIS

Epiglottitis is a serious condition and most commonly caused by *Haemophilus influenzae* type B. Occurring in infants and young children, it may be a life-threatening emergency. Swelling of the acutely inflamed epiglottis obstructs the flow of air. Inspiratory stridor (a loud wheezing sound on inspiration) occurs, and the onset of cyanosis may indicate airway obstruction so severe as to require tracheostomy.

SQUAMOUS CELL CARCINOMA

The large majority of laryngeal cancers are squamous cell carcinomas, which are tumors strongly related to cigarette smoking. Based on the location of the lesion, these cancers are divided into four groups that have relevance to treatment and prognosis:

- **Glottic carcinoma** is a tumor limited to one or both true vocal cords. This cancer is slow to metastasize

to the lymph nodes, and it has a good prognosis, at least during the early stage. Radiation therapy or voice-saving surgery is usually curative.
- **Transglottic carcinoma** involves the true and false vocal cords (Fig. 12-1). This tumor is likely to metastasize to the lymph nodes and often requires total laryngectomy.
- **Supraglottic carcinoma** arises in the ventricle, false vocal cords, or epiglottis. It does not involve the true cords. Nodal metastases are more common than in glottic tumors. Voice-saving surgical treatment is often possible.
- **Infraglottic carcinoma** is located below or involves the true vocal cords, with considerable infraglottic extension. Nodal metastases are common, and total laryngectomy is generally required.

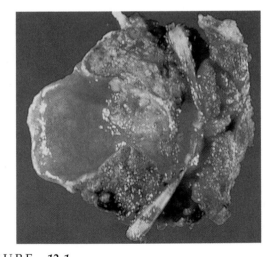

FIGURE   *12-1*
Carcinoma of the larynx. This transglottic carcinoma has an irregular, exophytic, indurated tan-white surface. It involves the right vocal cord and displays supraglottic extension.

Lungs

CONGENITAL ANOMALIES

Pulmonary Hypoplasia

■ *Pulmonary hypoplasia reflects incomplete or defective development of the lung.* The lung is smaller than normal owing to fewer acini or a decrease in their size. Pulmonary hypoplasia is the most common congenital lesion of the lung, being found in 10% of neonatal autopsies. In the large majority of cases (90%), it occurs in association with other congenital anomalies, most of which impinge on the thorax. Major factors that have been implicated as causes of pulmonary hypoplasia include (1) compression of the lung, usually secondary to a congenital diaphragmatic hernia; (2) oligohydramnios (an inadequate volume of amniotic fluid); and (3) decreased respiratory excursions in experimental models.

Congenital Cystic Adenomatoid Malformation

■ *Congenital cystic adenomatoid malformation is a common anomaly in which the lung parenchyma is converted into multiple gland-like spaces lined by bronchiolar epithelium and separated from each other by loose, fibrous tissue* (Fig. 12-2). This condition usually affects only one lobe of a lung, and it may be associated with other congenital abnormalities. With large symptomatic lesions, the infant presents with respiratory distress and cyanosis, and surgical resection is indicated.

Bronchogenic Cyst

■ *Bronchogenic cyst is a discrete, extrapulmonary, fluid-filled mass in the lung parenchyma and mediastinum.* The cyst is lined by respiratory epithelium and delimited by walls containing muscle and cartilage. In newborns, a bronchogenic cyst may compress a major airway and cause respiratory distress. Secondary infection of the cyst in older patients may lead to hemorrhage and perforation. Many bronchogenic cysts are asymptomatic and found on routine chest radiographs.

Extralobar Sequestration

■ *Extralobar sequestration is a mass of lung tissue that is not connected to the bronchial system and is located out-*

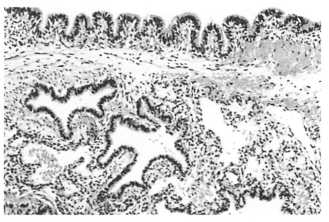

FIGURE *12-2*
Congenital cystic adenomatoid malformation. Multiple gland-like spaces are lined by bronchiolar epithelium.

side the visceral pleura. An abnormal artery, usually arising from the aorta, supplies the sequestered tissue. The lesion occurs three- to fourfold as often in boys as in girls, and in two-thirds of the patients, is associated with other anomalies.

On gross examination, extralobar sequestration appears as a pyramidal or round mass, covered by pleura, that ranges from 1 to 15 cm in greatest dimension. Microscopically, dilated bronchioles, alveolar ducts, and alveoli are noted.

In half of the cases, extralobar sequestration is recognized during the first month of life, and by 2 years, the diagnosis has been made in 75% of the patients. In the neonatal period, often during the first day of life, the disorder may present as dyspnea and cyanosis. In older children, the lesion frequently comes to medical attention because of recurrent bronchopulmonary infections. Surgical excision is curative.

Intralobar Sequestration

■ *Intralobar sequestration is an acquired lesion composed of a mass of lung tissue within the visceral pleura that is isolated from the tracheobronchial tree and supplied by a systemic artery.* This abnormality is only rarely identified in infants, and the large majority of cases follow repeated bouts of pneumonia. Intralobar sequestration is found in a lower lobe in almost all (98%) of the cases, and bilateral involvement is distinctly unusual. On gross examination, the sequestered pulmonary tissue contains fluid-filled cysts, as large as 5 cm in diameter, that lie in a dense, fibrous stroma. Microscopically, the lining of the cyst is cuboidal or columnar epithelium, and the lumen contains foamy macrophages and eosinophilic material. Symptoms of cough, sputum production, and recurrent pneumonia are noted in almost all patients, only one-fourth of whom are in the first decade of life. Surgical resection is often indicated.

DISEASES OF THE BRONCHI AND BRONCHIOLES

Infections

Influenza. Influenza is a characteristic example of tracheobronchitis, and an occasional patient dies with this infection.

Adenovirus. Infection with adenovirus produces extensive inflammation of bronchioles and subsequent healing by fibrosis.

Respiratory Syncytial Virus. This viral infection tends to occur as epidemics in nurseries and elsewhere. It is usually a self-limited illness, but rare, fatal cases can occur.

Bordetella pertussis. This bacterium is the cause of **whooping cough** and commonly produces a bacterial infection of the airways. After introduction of a pertussis vaccine, the disease became rare in the United States.

Bronchial Obstruction and Atelectasis

Atelectasis

■ *Atelectasis is the collapse of expanded lung tissue* (Fig. 12-3). If the supply of air is obstructed, the loss of gas from the alveoli to the blood leads to collapse of the affected region. Atelectasis is an important postoperative complication of abdominal surgery, occurring because of mucous obstruction of a bronchus and diminished respiratory movement, which, in turn, occurs because of postoperative pain. It is often asymptomatic, but when severe, it results in hypoxemia.

In patients with longstanding atelectasis, the collapsed lung becomes fibrotic, and the bronchi dilate, in part because of infection distal to the bronchus. Permanent bronchial dilatation (bronchiectasis) results.

Bronchiectasis

■ *Bronchiectasis is the irreversible dilatation of bronchi as a consequence of destruction of the muscular and elastic elements of their walls.*

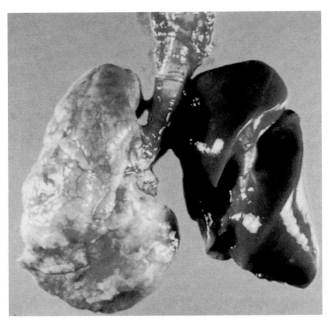

FIGURE   *12-3*
Atelectasis. The right lung of this infant is pale and expanded by air, whereas the left lung is collapsed.

☐ **Pathogenesis:** Bronchiectasis may result from mechanical obstruction of central bronchi by inhaled foreign bodies, tumors, mucous plugs in asthma, and compressive lymphadenopathy. More commonly, it is not obstructive in origin but, rather, a complication of respiratory infections or defects in the defense mechanisms that protect the airways from infection. Whereas obstructive bronchiectasis tends to be localized to the lung segment distal to the obstruction, nonobstructive bronchiectasis may be more widespread and involve many lobes of the lungs.

Localized, nonobstructive bronchiectasis was once a common disease, usually resulting from childhood bronchopulmonary infections such as measles, pertussis, or other bacterial infections. Although vaccines and antibiotics have reduced the frequency of bronchiectasis, one-half to two-thirds of all cases still follow a bronchopulmonary infection. At present, infections with adenovirus and respiratory syncytial virus are frequent causes of bronchiectasis in children.

Generalized bronchiectasis (nonobstructive) is, for the most part, secondary to inherited impairments in host defense mechanisms or acquired conditions that permit introduction of infectious organisms into the airways. Acquired disorders that predispose to bronchiectasis include (1) neurologic diseases that impair consciousness, swallowing, respiratory excursions, and the cough reflex; (2) incompetence of the lower esophageal sphincter; (3) nasogastric intubation; and (4) chronic bronchitis. The principal inherited conditions associated with generalized bronchiectasis are cystic fibrosis, the dyskinetic ciliary syndromes, hypogammaglobulinemias, and deficiencies of specific immunoglobulin (Ig) G subclasses.

☐ **Pathology:** Generalized bronchiectasis is usually bilateral and most common in the lower lobes (Fig. 12-4). Localized bronchiectasis may be situated wherever the obstruction or infection occurred. In both cases, the dilated bronchi contain thick, mucopurulent secretions. Microscopically, there is destruction of all components of the bronchial wall, chronic inflammation, a disproportionate number of goblet cells, and squamous metaplasia of the epithelium. The distal bronchi and bronchioles are scarred and often obliterated.

☐ **Clinical Features:** A patient with bronchiectasis has a chronic, productive cough, often with several hundred milliliters of mucopurulent sputum per day. Hemoptysis is a common symptom owing to rupture of the prominent bronchial arteries. Pneumonia is a common complication, and patients with longstanding bronchiectasis are at risk of chronic hypoxia and pul-

monary hypertension. Localized bronchiectasis can be treated surgically, but in patients with the generalized disease, surgical resection is more palliative than curative.

INFECTIONS

Bacterial Pneumonia

■ *Pneumonia is a generic term that refers to inflammation and consolidation (solidification) of the pulmonary parenchyma.* Traditionally, bacterial pneumonias were classified as either lobar pneumonia or bronchopneumonia, but these terms have little clinical relevance today. In general, the term **lobar pneumonia** refers to consolidation of an entire lobe (Fig. 12-5), whereas the term **bronchopneumonia** signifies scattered, solid foci in the same or several lobes (Fig. 12-6). Bronchopneumonia remains a common cause of death and typically develops in patients who are terminally ill.

Most bacteria that cause pneumonia are normal inhabitants of the oropharynx and nasopharynx, and they reach the alveoli by aspiration of secretions. A number of conditions predispose to infection by depressing host defenses, including cigarette smoking, chronic bronchitis, alcoholism, severe malnutrition, wasting diseases, and poorly controlled diabetes.

Pneumococcal Pneumonia

Despite the impact of antibiotic therapy, pneumonia caused by *Streptococcus pneumoniae* remains a significant problem.

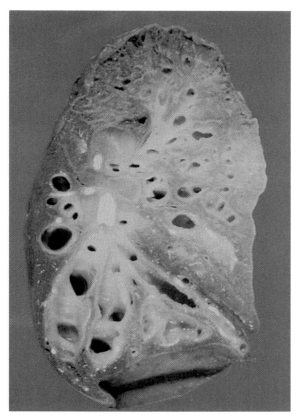

FIGURE *12-4*
Bronchiectasis. The resected upper lobe shows widely dilated bronchi, with thickening of the bronchial walls and collapse and fibrosis of the pulmonary parenchyma.

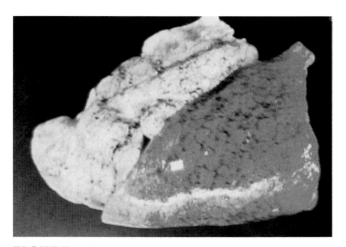

FIGURE *12-5*
Lobar pneumonia. The entire left lower lobe is consolidated and in the stage of red hepatization. The upper lobe is normally expanded.

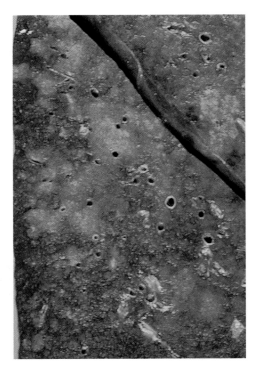

FIGURE   *12-6*
Bronchopneumonia. Scattered foci of consolidation are evident throughout.

☐ **Pathogenesis:** *S. pneumoniae* organisms, which are normal denizens of the nasopharynx, are carried into the alveoli, thereby initiating an inflammatory response. Pneumococcal pneumonia is mostly a consequence of altered defense barriers in the respiratory tract. Frequently, this pneumonia follows a viral infection of the upper respiratory tract (e.g., influenza).

☐ **Pathology:** During the earliest stage of pneumococcal pneumonia, protein-rich, edematous fluid containing numerous organisms fills the alveoli. Marked congestion of the capillaries is followed by massive outpouring of polymorphonuclear leukocytes, which is accompanied by intra-alveolar hemorrhage (Fig. 12-7). Because the firm consistency of the affected lung is

reminiscent of the liver, this stage has been aptly named **red hepatization.**

The next phase, occurring after 2 or more days, depending on the success of treatment, involves the lysis of polymorphonuclear leukocytes and the appearance of macrophages. At this stage, the congestion has diminished, but the lung still remains firm (**gray hepatization**). The alveolar exudate is then removed, and the lung gradually returns to normal.

A number of complications may follow pneumococcal pneumonia:

- **Pleuritis,** often painful, is common, because the pneumonia readily extends to the pleura.
- **Pleural effusion.**
- **Pyothorax.**
- **Empyema.**
- **Bacteremia** is present in more than 25% of patients in the early stages of pneumococcal pneumonia and may lead to endocarditis or meningitis.
- **Pulmonary fibrosis** is a rare complication.
- **Lung abscess** is an unusual complication.

☐ **Clinical Features:** The onset of pneumococcal pneumonia is acute, with fever and chills. Chest pain caused by pleural involvement is common, as is hemoptysis. The latter is derived from altered blood in the alveolar spaces and is characteristically rusty. Although the symptoms of pneumonia respond rapidly to antibiotic therapy, the lesion itself still takes several days to resolve radiologically.

Klebsiella Pneumonia

Other than *S. pneumoniae*, *Klebsiella pneumoniae* is the only other organism that causes lobar pneumonia with any frequency. However, it accounts for no more than 1% of all cases of community-acquired pneumonia. The disease is commonly associated with alcoholism and is seen most frequently in middle-aged men. Persons with diabetes and chronic pulmonary disease are also at risk.

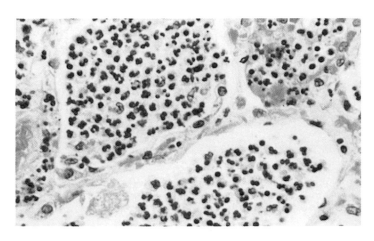

FIGURE   *12-7*
Pneumococcal pneumonia. The alveoli are packed with an exudate composed of polymorphonuclear leukocytes and occasional macrophages.

☐ **Pathology:** *K. pneumoniae* has a thick, gelatinous capsule. This feature is responsible for the characteristic **mucoid appearance** of the cut surface of the lung. There is a tendency toward tissue necrosis and abscess formation. A serious complication is **bronchopleural fistula,** which is a communication between the bronchial airway and the pleural space. Even with prompt antibiotic treatment, the mortality rate from *Klebsiella* pneumonia is still considerable.

Staphylococcal Pneumonia

Staphylococcal pneumonia is an uncommon community-acquired disease, accounting for only 1% of bacterial pneumonias. However, pulmonary infection with *Staphylococcus aureus* is common as a superinfection following influenza and other viral infections of the respiratory tract. Repeated episodes of staphylococcal pneumonia are encountered in patients with cystic fibrosis owing to colonization of the bronchiectatic airways. Similar to staphylococcal infection elsewhere, staphylococcal pneumonia is characterized by the development of pulmonary abscesses.

Legionella Pneumonia

In 1976, a mysterious respiratory ailment, which carried a high mortality rate, broke out at an American Legion convention in Philadelphia. The responsible organism, *Legionella pneumophila,* was soon identified as being a fastidious bacterium with special cultural characteristics. *Legionella* organisms thrive in aquatic environments, and outbreaks of pneumonia have been traced to contaminated water in air-conditioning cooling towers, evaporative condensers, and construction sites. Person-to-person spread does not occur, and there is no animal or human reservoir.

☐ **Pathology:** In fatal cases of *Legionella* pneumonia, multiple lobes exhibit bronchopneumonia, with large confluent areas. On microscopic examination, the alveoli contain fibrin and inflammatory cells, with either neutrophils or macrophages predominating. Necrosis of the inflammatory cells (leukocytoclasis) may be extensive. If the patient survives for several weeks, the exudate may show fibrous organization. One-third of the cases have been complicated by empyema. *Legionella* organisms are usually abundant both within and without the phagocytic cells.

☐ **Clinical Features:** The onset of *Legionella* pneumonia tends to be acute, with malaise, fever, muscle aches and pains, and curiously, abdominal pain. A productive cough is usual, and chest pain due to pleuritis occasionally occurs. The mortality rate has been high (10–20%), especially in immunocompromised patients. Erythromycin is the treatment of choice.

Psittacosis

Psittacosis is a pulmonary infection that results from inhalation of *Chlamydia psittaci* in dust contaminated by excreta from birds, usually pets (and often parrots). It is characterized by severe systemic symptoms, with fever, malaise, and muscle aches, but surprisingly few respiratory symptoms other than cough. Fatal cases involve varying degrees of diffuse alveolar damage, together with edema, intra-alveolar pneumonia, and necrosis.

Mycoplasma pneumoniae

Mycoplasma pneumoniae causes the syndrome of **atypical pneumonia.** The onset of this disease is insidious, and respiratory symptoms may be minimal. However, the course of this disease is prolonged. *Mycoplasma* pneumonia is only rarely fatal.

Tuberculosis

Tuberculosis, which is caused by infection with *Mycobacterium tuberculosis,* is divided into primary and secondary (or reactivation) tuberculosis.

Primary Tuberculosis

The disease is acquired from the initial exposure to *M. tuberculosis,* most commonly as a result of inhaling infected aerosols produced by the coughing of a person with cavitary tuberculosis. The inhaled organisms multiply in the alveoli, because the alveolar macrophages cannot readily kill the bacteria.

The **Ghon complex** is the first lesion of primary tuberculosis, consisting of a peripheral parenchymal granuloma, often in the lower lobes, and a prominent, infected mediastinal lymph node (Fig. 12-8). On gross examination, the healed, subpleural Ghon nodule is 1 to 2 cm in diameter, well circumscribed, and centrally necrotic. In later stages, the lesion is fibrotic and calcified. Microscopically, a granuloma with central, caseous necrosis shows varying degrees of fibrosis. The microscopic features of the draining hilar lymph nodes are similar to those of the peripheral parenchymal lesion.

The large majority (≥90%) of primary infections are asymptomatic, and the lesions remain localized and heal. However, less commonly, primary tuberculosis does not remain limited but, rather, spreads to other parts of the lung (**progressive primary tuberculosis**). This condition is usually seen in early childhood or in immunosuppressed adults. The initial lesion enlarges, producing necrotic areas as large as 6 cm or

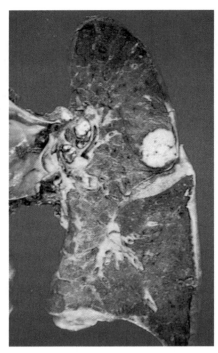

FIGURE   *12-8*
Primary tuberculosis. A healed Ghon complex is represented by a subpleural nodule and involved hilar lymph nodes.

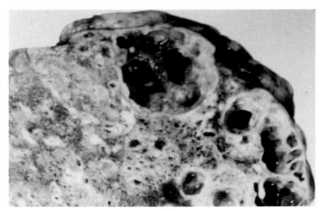

FIGURE   *12-9*
Cavitary tuberculosis. The apex of the left upper lobe shows tuberculous cavities surrounded by a consolidated and fibrotic pulmonary parenchyma, which contains small tubercles.

more in the greatest dimension. Central liquefaction results in cavities, which may expand to occupy most of the lower lobe. At the same time, the draining lymph nodes display similar histologic changes.

Secondary Tuberculosis

This stage represents either reactivation of primary pulmonary tuberculosis or new infection in a host previously sensitized by primary tuberculosis. The initial reaction to *M. tuberculosis* is different in patients with secondary tuberculosis. A cellular immune response occurs after a latent interval and leads to formation of many granulomas and extensive tissue necrosis. The apical and posterior segments of the upper lobes are most commonly involved. A diffuse, fibrotic, and poorly defined lesion develops that displays focal areas of caseous necrosis. Often, these foci heal and calcify, but some erode into a bronchus, after which drainage of infectious material creates a tuberculous cavity.

Tuberculous cavities range in size from less than 1 cm in diameter to large, cystic areas that occupy almost the entire lung. Most cavities measure from 3 to 10 cm in diameter, however, and tend to be situated in the apices of the upper lobes (Fig. 12-9), although they may occur anywhere in the lung. The wall of the cavity is composed of an inner, thin, gray membrane en-

compassing soft necrotic nodules, a middle zone of granulation tissue, and an outer collagenous border. The lumen is filled with caseous material containing acid-fast bacilli. The tuberculous cavity often communicates freely with a bronchus, and release of infectious material into the airways serves to disseminate the infection within the lung. The walls of healed tuberculous cavities eventually become fibrotic and calcified.

Secondary tuberculosis is associated with a number of complications:

- **Miliary tuberculosis** refers to the presence of multiple, small (size of millet seeds), tuberculous granulomas (Fig. 12-10) in many organs. It results from hematogenous dissemination of the organisms, usually from secondary pulmonary tuberculosis but occasionally from primary pulmonary tuberculosis or from other sites.
- **Hemoptysis** results from the erosion of small pulmonary arteries in the wall of a cavity. It may be severe enough to drown patients in their own blood.
- **Bronchopleural fistula** occurs when a subpleural cavity ruptures into the pleural space. In turn, **tuberculous empyema** and **pneumothorax** result.
- **Intestinal tuberculosis** may follow swallowing of the tuberculous material.

Fungal Infections

Histoplasmosis

Histoplasmosis is a disease of the midwestern and southeastern regions of the United States, particularly the Mississippi and Ohio river valleys. The disease is caused by inhalation of *Histoplasma capsulatum* in infected dust, commonly from bird droppings.

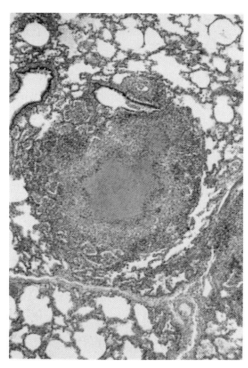

FIGURE   *12-10*
Miliary tuberculosis. A small tuberculous granuloma with conspicuous central caseation is present in the pulmonary parenchyma.

☐ **Pathology:** Histoplasmosis has many clinical and pathologic similarities with tuberculosis. The great majority of infections are asymptomatic and result in lesions similar to the Ghon complex, including a parenchymal granuloma and similar lesions in the draining lymph nodes. The granulomas are particularly prone to calcify, often with a concentric, laminar pattern. In a few cases, the pulmonary lesion progresses or reactivates, which leads to a progressive fibrotic and necrotic lesion that closely resembles reactivation tuberculosis.

Coccidioidomycosis

Coccidioidomycosis, which is caused by inhalation of the spores of *Coccidioides immitis,* is widely spread through the southwestern part of the United States, sharing many of the clinical and pathologic features of histoplasmosis and tuberculosis. In most instances, the lesions are limited to a peripheral parenchymal granuloma, with or without lymph node granulomas. In a few instances, however, the lesion is progressive, although the rate of progression is slow. Immunocompromised patients may experience rapid progression of the disease.

Cryptococcosis

Cryptococcosis results from inhalation of the spores of *Cryptococcus neoformans,* an organism that is frequently encountered in pigeon droppings. The pulmonary lesions range from small parenchymal granulomas to several large, granulomatous nodules, pneumonic consolidation, and even cavitation. Most serious cases of pulmonary cryptococcosis occur in those who are immunocompromised.

North American Blastomycosis

Blastomycosis is an uncommon condition caused by *Blastomyces dermatitidis.* It is concentrated in the basins of the Missouri, Mississippi, and Ohio rivers in the United States. The clinical and pathologic features resemble those associated with the fungi mentioned earlier. They may present as a lesion resembling a Ghon complex or as a progressive pneumonic condition.

Aspergillosis

Infection of the lungs by *Aspergillus* species, usually *A. niger* or *A. fumigatus,* can occur in a number of circumstances:

- **Invasive Pulmonary Aspergillosis.** This is the most serious manifestation of *Aspergillus* infection, occurring almost exclusively as an opportunistic infection in persons with compromised immunity, usually because of cytotoxic therapy or acquired immunodeficiency syndrome (AIDS). The lungs exhibit patchy, multifocal areas of consolidation and, occasionally, cavities. **Extensive blood vessel invasion** (usually arterial [Fig. 12-11]) results in occlusion, thrombosis, and infarction of lung tissue. Invasive aspergillosis is a fulminant pulmonary infection that is not amenable to therapy.
- **Aspergilloma.** *Aspergillus* species may grow in pre-existing cavities, such as those caused by tuberculosis or bronchiectasis. They proliferate to form an aspergilloma ("fungus ball" or mycetoma) within the cavities.
- **Allergic Bronchopulmonary Aspergillosis.** Certain persons with asthma demonstrate an unusual immunologic reaction to *Aspergillus* infection, which is characterized by (1) transient pulmonary infiltrates on chest radiographs, (2) eosinophilia of blood and sputum, (3) skin sensitivity and serum precipitins to *A. fumigatus,* and (4) elevated levels of serum IgE. The administration of systemic corticosteroids usually controls the acute episode.

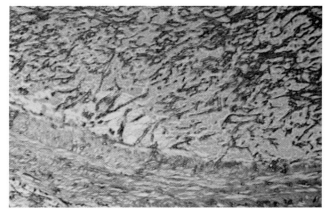

FIGURE   *12-11*
Invasive pulmonary aspergillosis. A branch of the pulmonary artery shows fungal hyphae in the wall and within the lumen.

Pneumocystis carinii Pneumonia

Infection with *Pneumocystis carinii* occurs in immunocompromised persons and is now one of the most frequent causes of death in patients with AIDS.

☐ **Pathology:** The classic lesion of *Pneumocystis* pneumonia comprises an interstitial infiltrate of plasma cells and lymphocytes, diffuse alveolar damage (discussed later), and hyperplasia of type II pneumocytes. The alveoli are filled with a characteristic, foamy exudate, with the organisms appearing as small bubbles against a background of proteinaceous exudate (Fig. 12-12). With silver impregnation, the cysts appear to be round or indented ("new moon") bodies approximately 5 μm in diameter.

☐ **Clinical   Features:** The   presentation   of *Pneumocystis* pneumonia is variable. At one extreme,

symptoms are minimal, whereas at the other, there is rapidly progressive respiratory failure. Treatment is with trimethoprim-sulfisoxazole or pentamidine.

Viral Pneumonia

Viral infections of the pulmonary parenchyma produce interstitial (rather than alveolar) pneumonia and diffuse alveolar damage. Initially, viral infection affects the alveolar epithelium and results in a mononuclear infiltrate in the interstitium of the lung (Fig. 12-13). There is necrosis of the type I epithelial cells and formation of hyaline membranes, an appearance that is indistinguishable from that of diffuse alveolar damage from other causes. In some instances, the alveolar damage may be indolent, in which case the disease is characterized by hyperplasia of type II pneumocytes and interstitial inflammation.

Cytomegalovirus produces a characteristic interstitial pneumonia. Initially described in infants, it is now well recognized in immunocompromised persons. This viral pneumonia features an intense. interstitial infiltrate of lymphocytes. The alveoli are lined by type II cells that have regenerated to cover the epithelial defect left by the necrosis of type I cells. The infected alveolar cells are very large and display the typical dark-blue nuclear inclusions.

Measles infection, which involves both the airways and parenchyma, is characterized by the presence of very large (diameter, 100 μm), multinucleated giant cells, which have nuclear inclusions. Although interstitial pneumonia is a well-recognized complication of measles, it is rarely fatal except in immunocompromised, previously unexposed people.

Varicella infection (both chickenpox and herpes zoster) produces disseminated, focally necrotic lesions

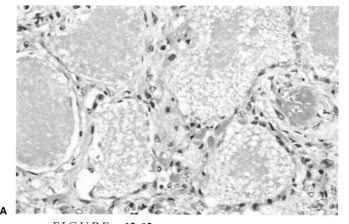

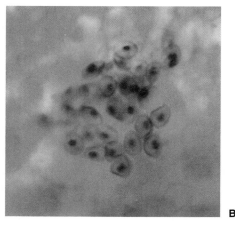

A   B

FIGURE   *12-12*
Pneumocystis carinii pneumonia. (*A*) The alveoli are filled with a foamy exudate, and the interstitium is thickened and contains a chronic inflammatory infiltrate. (*B*) A centrifuged bronchoalveolar lavage specimen impregnated with silver shows a cluster of *Pneumocystis* cysts.

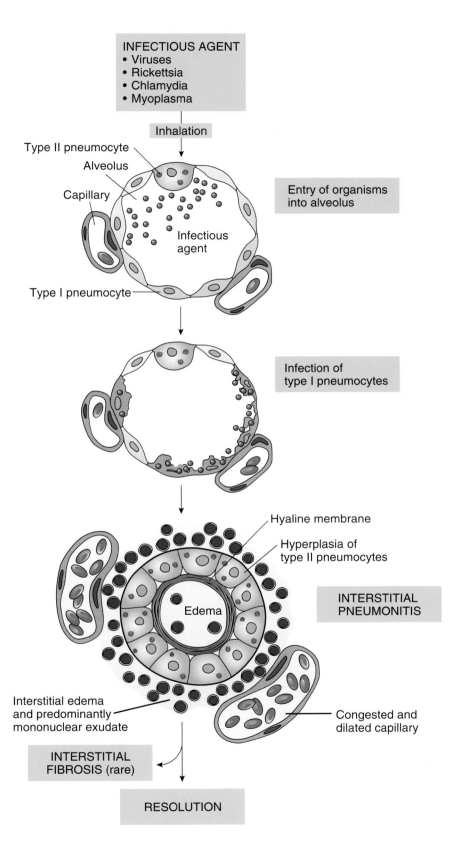

INFECTIOUS AGENT
• Viruses
• Rickettsia
• Chlamydia
• Myoplasma

Inhalation

Type II pneumocyte

Alveolus

Capillary

Infectious agent

Type I pneumocyte

Entry of organisms into alveolus

Infection of type I pneumocytes

Hyaline membrane

Hyperplasia of type II pneumocytes

Edema

INTERSTITIAL PNEUMONITIS

Interstitial edema and predominantly mononuclear exudate

Congested and dilated capillary

INTERSTITIAL FIBROSIS (rare)

RESOLUTION

FIGURE *12-13*
Pathogenesis of interstitial fibrosis. Although interstitial pneumonia is most commonly caused by viruses, other organisms may also cause significant interstitial inflammation. Type I cells are the most sensitive to damage, and loss of their integrity leads to intra-alveolar edema. The proteinaceous exudate and cell debris form hyaline membranes, and type II cells multiply to line the alveoli. Interstitial inflammation is characterized mainly by mononuclear cells. The disease generally resolves completely, but occasionally, it progresses to interstitial fibrosis.

in the lung as well as interstitial pneumonia. Pulmonary involvement is usually asymptomatic except in immunocompromised hosts, in whom it may be fatal.

Lung Abscess

■ *Lung abscess is a localized accumulation of pus that is accompanied by destruction of the pulmonary parenchyma, including the alveoli, airways, and blood vessels.*

□ **Pathogenesis:** The most common cause of pulmonary abscess is aspiration, often in the setting of altered consciousness. The large majority (>90%) of cases of lung abscess reflect aspiration of anaerobic bacteria from the oropharynx. The infections are typically polymicrobial, with fusiform bacteria and *Bacteroides* species often being isolated. Other organisms encountered in lung abscesses caused by aspiration include *S. aureus, K. pneumoniae, S. pneumoniae,* and *Nocardia.*

Alcoholism is the single most common condition predisposing to lung abscess. Persons suffering from drug overdosage, epilepsy, or neurologic impairment are also at risk. Other causes of lung abscess include necrotizing pneumonias, bronchial obstruction, infected pulmonary emboli, penetrating trauma, and extension of infection from tissues adjacent to the lung.

□ **Pathology:** Lung abscesses mostly range from 2 to 6 cm in diameter, and 10% to 20% have multiple cavities. They exhibit abundant polymorphonuclear leukocytes and, depending on the age of the lesion, variable numbers of macrophages. Debris derived from necrotic tissue may also be evident. The abscess is surrounded by hemorrhage, fibrin, and inflammatory cells. As the abscess ages, a fibrous wall forms around the margin. Lung abscesses differ from those in other locations by their capacity for spontaneous drainage. The cavity thus formed contains air, necrotic debris, and inflammatory exudate (Fig. 12-14), thereby creating a fluid level that is easily visualized radiographically.

□ **Clinical Features:** Almost all patients with a lung abscess present with cough and fever. One of the most characteristic symptoms is the production of large amounts of foul-smelling sputum. Many patients complain of pleuritic chest pain, and 20% develop hemoptysis. Complications of lung abscess include rupture into the pleural space, with resulting empyema, severe hemoptysis, and drainage of the abscess contents into a bronchus, which, in turn, leads to dissemination of the infection to other parts of the lung. Despite vigorous antimicrobial therapy, which is principally directed against anaerobic bacteria, the mortality rate among patients with a lung abscess remains in the range of 5% to 10%.

DIFFUSE ALVEOLAR DAMAGE (ADULT RESPIRATORY DISTRESS SYNDROME)

■ *Diffuse alveolar damage (DAD) is a nonspecific pattern of reaction by the distal pulmonary parenchyma to a variety of acute insults that is characterized by interstitial inflammation and accumulation of a proteinaceous alveolar exudate.* The clinical counterpart of severe DAD is adult respiratory distress syndrome (ARDS), in which a patient with apparently normal lungs sustains pulmonary damage and then develops rapidly progressive respiratory failure. The overall mortality rate of ARDS is more than 50%, and in patients older than 60 years, it is as high as 90%.

□ **Pathogenesis:** DAD is a final common pathway of pathologic changes caused by many different agents (Box 12-1). These include viral respiratory tract infections, sepsis, shock, aspiration of gastric contents, in-

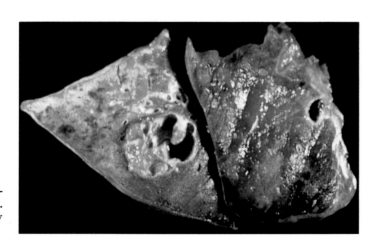

FIGURE *12-14*
Pulmonary abscess. A large, cystic abscess contains a purulent exudate and is contained by a fibrous wall. Pneumonia is present in the surrounding pulmonary parenchyma.

BOX *12-1* **Important Causes of the Adult Respiratory Distress Syndrome**

Nonthoracic Trauma
Shock due to any cause
Fat embolism
Infection
Gram-negative septicemia
Other bacterial infections
Viral infections
Aspiration
Near-drowning
Aspiration of gastric contents
Drugs and Therapeutic Agents
Heroin
Oxygen
Radiation
Paraquat
Cytotoxic agents

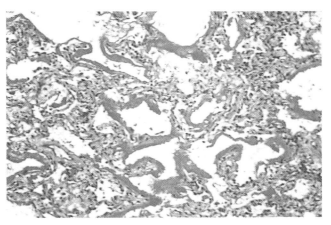

FIGURE *12-15*
Diffuse alveolar damage, acute (exudative) phase. The alveolar septa are thickened by edema and a sparse inflammatory infiltrate. The alveoli are lined by eosinophilic hyaline membranes.

halation of toxic gases, near-drowning, radiation pneumonitis, and a large assortment of drugs and other chemicals. **Despite the diversity of these conditions, all are capable of injuring the epithelial and endothelial cells of the alveoli, thereby producing DAD.**

Injury to the endothelial cells allows leakage of protein-rich fluid from the alveolar capillaries into the interstitial space. Destruction of type I pneumocytes permits exudation of fluid into the alveolar spaces, where the deposition of plasma proteins results in the formation of fibrin-containing precipitates (hyaline membranes) on the injured alveolar walls. Although it is denuded of type I pneumocytes, the alveolar basement membrane remains intact and functions as a scaffold for type II pneumocytes, the proliferation of which replaces the normal epithelial lining of the alveoli.

☐ **Pathology:** The evolution of DAD can be divided into two periods, namely the initial exudative phase and the organizing phase that follows.

The **exudative phase** develops during the first week following the pulmonary insult and features edema, exudation of plasma proteins, accumulation of inflammatory cells, and the appearance of hyaline membranes (Fig. 12-15). Hyaline membranes begin to appear by the second day and, after 4 to 5 days, are the most conspicuous morphologic feature of the exudative phase. These eosinophilic, glassy "membranes" consist of precipitated plasma proteins and the cytoplasmic and nuclear debris from sloughed epithelial cells. Mild interstitial inflammation, consisting of lymphocytes, plasma cells, and macrophages, is apparent early on and reaches its maximum in approximately 1 week. Toward the end of the first week, and persisting during the subsequent organizing stage, regularly

spaced, cuboidal type II pneumocytes become arrayed along the denuded alveolar septa.

The **organizing phase** of DAD, which begins approximately 1 week after the initial injury, is marked by proliferation of fibroblasts both within the interstitial space and focally within the alveolar spaces (Fig. 12-16). Whereas this fibrosis resolves in mild cases, it progresses to restructuring of the pulmonary parenchyma and cyst formation in severe ones.

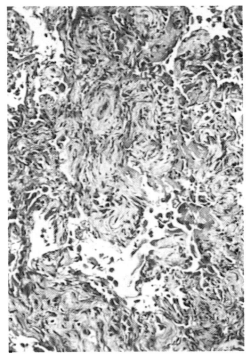

FIGURE *12-16*
Diffuse alveolar damage, organizing phase. Fibroblasts and nascent connective tissue are present within the septa and alveoli.

☐ **Clinical Features:** Patients destined to develop ARDS experience a symptom-free interval for a few hours following the initial insult, after which tachypnea and dyspnea mark the onset of the syndrome. At this time, arterial hypoxemia and a decreased Pco_2 are evident on measurement of blood gases. As ARDS progresses, the dyspnea worsens, and the patient becomes cyanotic. In fatal cases, the combination of increasing tachypnea and decreasing tidal volume eventuates in alveolar hypoventilation, progressive hypoxemia, and a rising Pco_2. Patients who survive ARDS may recover normal pulmonary function, but in severe cases, they are left with scarred lungs, respiratory dysfunction, and in some cases, pulmonary hypertension.

Specific Causes of Diffuse Alveolar Damage

Oxygen

Patients who are given high levels of oxygen (usually >60%) for respiratory problems may develop DAD. The mechanism of oxygen toxicity is thought to be related to an increased production of activated oxygen species in the lung.

Shock

Often, ARDS follows shock from any cause, including gram-negative sepsis, trauma, or blood loss, in which case the pulmonary condition is colloquially referred to as "shock lung." The pathogenesis of DAD associated with shock likely is multifactorial. Tissue necrosis in organs damaged by trauma or ischemia may lead to the release of vasoactive peptides into the circulation; these peptides enhance vascular permeability in the lung. Disseminated intravascular coagulation may damage the alveolar capillaries, and fat emboli from bone fractures may obstruct the distal capillary bed of the lung. The pathogenesis of endothelial cell injury in endotoxic shock is discussed in Chapter 7.

Drug-Induced Diffuse Alveolar Damage

The long list of drugs that cause DAD includes most chemotherapeutic agents. The best known is bleomycin, but other frequently used agents, such as BCNU (carmustine), methotrexate, 5-fluorouracil, busulfan, and cyclophosphamide, are also known causes.

Bizarre, atypical, and hyperchromatic nuclei in type II cells are particularly common in cases of alveolar damage from chemotherapeutic agents. The damage progresses despite withdrawal of the offending agent, although it may be modified by administration of corticosteroids. Progressive interstitial fibrosis occurs, usually with retention of the lung structure.

Radiation Pneumonitis

Radiation pneumonitis occurs in two forms, namely acute DAD and chronic pulmonary fibrosis. Alveolar injury is believed to result from generation of oxygen radicals through the radiolysis of water.

Acute radiation pneumonitis occurs in as many as 10% of patients who receive radiation therapy for cancer of the lung or breast or for mediastinal lymphoma. DAD caused by radiation is, for the most part, dose-related and appears 1 to 6 months after the radiation therapy. Most patients recover from acute radiation pneumonitis.

Chronic radiation pneumonitis is characterized by interstitial fibrosis and may follow acute DAD or develop insidiously. The disease remains asymptomatic unless a substantial volume of the lung is affected.

Respiratory Distress Syndrome of the Newborn

The counterpart of ARDS in neonates is termed *respiratory distress syndrome (RDS) of the newborn*. The disease is also associated with DAD, which, in this circumstance, is known as **hyaline membrane disease.** RDS of the newborn and bronchopulmonary dysplasia are discussed in further detail in Chapter 6.

GOODPASTURE SYNDROME

■ *Goodpasture syndrome is a triad of diffuse alveolar hemorrhage, glomerulonephritis, and a circulating, cytotoxic autoantibody to a component of basement membranes.* The cross-reactivity between the basement membrane of the alveolus and the glomerulus accounts for the simultaneous attack on the lung and kidney. The pathogenesis of Goodpasture syndrome is discussed in greater detail in Chapter 16.

☐ **Pathology:** Patients with Goodpasture syndrome suffer extensive intra-alveolar hemorrhage (Fig. 12-17). Histologically, erythrocytes and hemosiderin-laden macrophages fill the airspaces. By immunofluorescence, linear deposition of IgG and complement are demonstrated in the alveolar basement membranes.

☐ **Clinical Features:** Patients with Goodpasture syndrome are typically young men, although the disease may affect adults of either sex and of any age. The large majority (95%) of patients present initially with

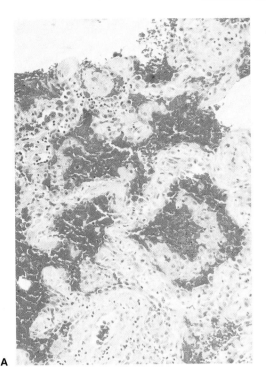
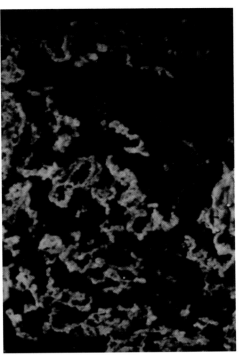

FIGURE   *12-17*
Goodpasture syndrome. (A) A section of the lung shows extensive intra-alveolar hemorrhage. The alveolar septa are thickened and evidence loose fibrosis. The alveoli are lined by hyperplastic type II pneumocytes. (B) Deposition of immunoglobulin G within the alveolar septa is demonstrated by immunofluorescence.

hemoptysis, often accompanied by dyspnea, weakness, and mild anemia. Evidence of glomerulonephritis follows the pulmonary manifestations in approximately 3 months (1 week to 1 year), but in some patients, renal disease does not develop. Hypoxemia and respiratory alkalosis are common, but respiratory function returns to normal as the hemorrhage resolves.

Goodpasture syndrome is treated by the administration of corticosteroids and cytotoxic drugs and by plasmapheresis. Before such aggressive treatment was instituted, the mortality rate of Goodpasture syndrome was 80%. Even with current treatment, however, the 2-year survival rate is only 50%, and the prognosis is considerably worse if renal failure is present.

CHRONIC OBSTRUCTIVE PULMONARY DISEASES

■ *Chronic obstructive pulmonary disease* (COPD) *is a nonspecific term that describes patients with chronic bronchitis or emphysema who show evidence for a decrease in forced expiratory volume as measured by spirometric pulmonary function tests.*

Chronic Bronchitis

■ *Chronic bronchitis is defined clinically as the presence of a chronic, productive cough without a discernible cause for more than half of a 2-year period.* **Chronic bronchitis is primarily a disease of cigarette smokers** (see Chapter 8). In fact, some 90% of all cases occur in smokers.

☐ **Pathology:** Chronic bronchitis is characterized by hyperplasia and hypertrophy of the mucus-secreting cells and an increased proportion of mucous to serous cells (Fig. 12-18). Other morphologic changes are variable and include (1) excess mucus in the central and peripheral airways; (2) thickening of the bronchial wall by mucous gland enlargement and edema, which, in turn, leads to encroachment on the bronchial lumen; (3) an increase in goblet cells; and (4) increased amounts of smooth muscle, which may indicate bronchial hyperreactivity.

☐ **Clinical Features:** Chronic bronchitis is often accompanied by emphysema (discussed later), and it is often difficult to separate the relative contribution of each disease to the clinical presentation. In general, patients who suffer predominantly from chronic bronchitis have had a productive cough for many years, particularly during the winter months. Exertional

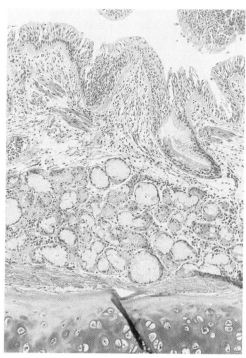

FIGURE   *12-18*
Chronic bronchitis. The bronchial wall is thickened by hypertrophy and hyperplasia of the mucus-secreting glands. The Reid index is greater than 0.5. The submucosa shows increased smooth muscle and mild chronic inflammation.

dyspnea and cyanosis supervene, and cor pulmonale may ensue. The combination of cyanosis and edema secondary to cor pulmonale has led to the label "blue bloater" for such patients.

Emphysema

■ *Emphysema is enlargement of the airspaces distal to the terminal bronchioles, with destruction of their walls but without fibrosis.* Emphysema is classified in anatomic terms, but the classification should not obscure the fact that the severity of emphysema is more important than the type.

☐ **Pathogenesis:** The major cause of emphysema is cigarette smoking, and moderate to severe emphysema is rare in nonsmokers (see Chapter 8). Increased numbers of neutrophils, which contain serine elastase and other proteases, are found in the bronchoalveolar lavage fluid of smokers. Smoking also reduces the α_1-antitrypsin (α_1-AT) activity (discussed later) in the lung owing to oxidation of methionine residues in the enzyme. In this way, unopposed and increased elastolytic activity leads to destruction of elastic tissue in the walls of the distal airspaces, thereby impairing elastic recoil.

α_1-Antitrypsin Deficiency. A hereditary deficiency in α_1-AT accounts for approximately 1% of all patients with a clinical diagnosis of COPD. A circulating glycoprotein produced in the liver, α_1-AT is a major inhibitor of a variety of proteases, including elastase, trypsin, chymotrypsin, thrombin, and bacterial proteases. In the lung, the most important action of α_1-AT is the inhibition of neutrophil elastase, which is an enzyme that digests elastin and other structural components of the alveolar septa.

☐ **Pathology:** Emphysema is morphologically classified according to the location of the lesions within the pulmonary acinus (Fig. 12-19).

Centrilobular Emphysema. This form of emphysema is the most frequently encountered variant and the one that is usually associated both with cigarette smoking and with clinical symptoms. Centrilobular emphysema is characterized by destruction of the cluster of terminal bronchioles near the end of the bronchiolar tree in the central pulmonary lobule (Fig. 12-20). The lobule is the smallest portion of the lung bounded by septa and includes several acini. The enlarged respiratory bronchioles form enlarged airspaces, which are separated from each other and from the lobular septa by normal alveolar ducts and alveoli. As centrilobular emphysema progresses, these distal structures may also be involved. The bronchioles proximal to the emphysematous spaces are inflamed and narrowed. Centrilobular emphysema is most severe in the upper zones of the lung, the upper lobe, and the superior segment of the lower lobe.

Panacinar Emphysema. In this type of emphysema, the acinus is uniformly involved, with destruction of the alveolar septa from the center to the periphery of the acinus (Fig. 12-21). In the final stage, panacinar emphysema leaves behind a lacy network of supporting tissue ("cotton-candy lung"). This variant occurs in several different situations, but is often found in cigarette smokers in association with centrilobular emphysema. In such cases, the panacinar pattern tends to occur in the lower zones of the lung, whereas centrilobular emphysema is seen in the upper zones. Diffuse panacinar emphysema is the lesion associated with α_1-AT deficiency.

Localized Emphysema. This condition, which was previously known as paraseptal emphysema, is characterized by the destruction of alveoli and resulting emphysema in only one or, at most, a few locations, with the remainder of the lungs being normal. Although it has no clinical significance itself, rupture

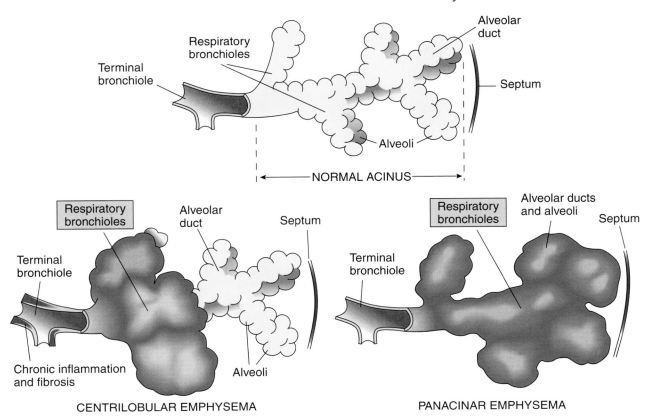

FIGURE 12-19
Types of emphysema. The acinus is the unit gas–exchanging structure of the lung distal to the terminal bronchiole. It consists of, in order, respiratory bronchioles, alveolar ducts, alveolar sacs, and alveoli. In centrilobular (proximal acinar) emphysema, the respiratory bronchioles are predominantly involved. In paraseptal (distal acinar) emphysema, the alveolar ducts are particularly affected. In panacinar (panlobular) emphysema, the acinus is uniformly damaged.

of an area of localized emphysema produces spontaneous pneumothorax (discussed later). Progression of localized emphysema can result in a large area of destruction, termed a **bulla.** Bullae range in size from as small as 2 cm to large lesions that occupy an entire hemithorax.

☐ **Clinical Features:** Most patients with symptomatic emphysema present at 60 years of age or older with a prolonged history of exertional dyspnea but with minimal, nonproductive cough. Tachypnea and a prolonged expiratory phase are typical. The most prominent radiologic abnormality is overinflation of the lung, as evidenced by enlarged lungs, depressed diaphragm, inversion of the convexity of the diaphragm, and increased posteroanterior diameter ("barrel chest"). Because these patients have a higher respiratory rate and increased minute volume, they can maintain arterial hemoglobin saturation at near-normal levels and, therefore, are referred to as "pink puffers." The clinical course of emphysema is marked

by an inexorable decline in respiratory function, manifested as progressive dyspnea, for which no treatment is adequate.

Asthma

■ *Asthma is characterized by variable obstruction to the flow of air and increased responsiveness of the airways to a variety of stimuli. It is characterized clinically by paroxysms of wheezing, dyspnea, and cough.* When severe acute asthma is unresponsive to therapy, it is referred to as **status asthmaticus.** In the United States, bronchial asthma is a common disorder, affecting as many as 10% of children and 5% of adults. Half of the cases appear in patients younger than 10 years of age, and the incidence is twice as great in boys as in girls.

☐ **Pathogenesis:** Asthma has been attributed to an increased airway responsiveness to an inflammatory reaction provoked by diverse stimuli. The best-studied situation associated with induction of asthma is the in-

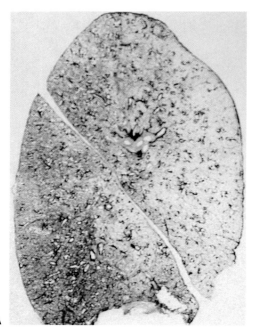
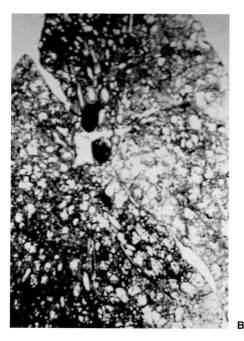

A

B

FIGURE   *12-20*
Centrilobular emphysema. (A) A whole mount of the left lung of a smoker with mild emphysema shows enlarged air spaces scattered throughout both lobes, which represent destruction of the terminal bronchioles in the central part of the pulmonary lobule. These abnormal spaces are surrounded by intact pulmonary parenchyma. (B) In a more advanced case of centrilobular emphysema, destruction of the lung has progressed to produce large, irregular air spaces.

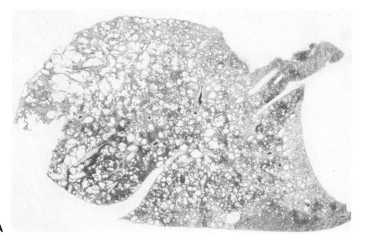
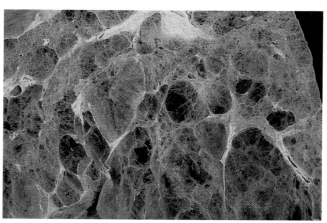

A

B

FIGURE   *12-21*
Panacinar emphysema. (*A*) A whole mount of the left lung from a patient with severe emphysema reveals widespread destruction of the pulmonary parenchyma, which in some areas leaves behind only a lacy network of supporting tissue. (*B*) The lung from this patient with α_1-antitrypsin deficiency shows a panacinar pattern of emphysema. The loss of alveolar walls has resulted in markedly enlarged air spaces.

halation of allergens (Fig. 12-22). An inhaled allergen in a sensitized person interacts with IgE antibody that is bound to the surface of mast cells interspersed among the epithelial cells of the bronchial mucosa. As a result, mast cells degranulate and release mediators of type I (immediate) hypersensitivity, including histamine, bradykinin, leukotrienes, prostaglandins, thromboxane A_2, and platelet-activating factor (PAF). These substances produce (1) smooth muscle contraction, (2) mucus secretion, and (3) increased vascular permeability and edema, each of which is a potent, albeit reversible, cause of airway obstruction. Chemotactic factors, including leukotriene B_4, as well as neutrophil and eosinophil chemotactic factors, attract neutrophils, eosinophils, and platelets to the bronchial wall. In turn, eosinophils release leukotriene B_4 and PAF, thereby aggravating bronchoconstriction and edema. Discharge of eosinophil granules containing eosinophil cationic protein and major basic protein into the bronchial lumen further impairs mucociliary function and damages the epithelial cells. Epithelial cell injury is suspected to stimulate nerve endings in the mucosa, thereby initiating an autonomic discharge that contributes to airway narrowing and mucus secretion. Moreover, leukotriene B_4 and PAF recruit more eosinophils and other effector cells, thereby augmenting the vicious circle that both prolongs and amplifies the asthmatic attack. Recent evidence suggests that activated T lymphocytes also contribute to the propagation of the inflammatory response through various cytokine networks.

Allergic Asthma. This is the most common form of asthma and is usually found in children. Common allergens include pollens, animal hair or fur, and contamination of house dust with mites.

Infections. A common precipitating factor in childhood asthma is a viral respiratory tract infection rather than allergic stimuli.

Exercise-Induced Asthma. Exercise can precipitate some degree of bronchospasm in the majority (65%) of all patients with asthma, and in some patients, exercise may be the only inciting factor. The more rapid the ventilation (severity of exercise) and the colder and drier the air that is breathed, the more likely it is that an attack of asthma will occur. The mechanism underlying exercise-induced asthma is unclear but may be the consequence of mediator release or vascular congestion in the bronchi secondary to rewarming of the airways after the exertion.

Occupational Asthma. More than 80 different occupational exposures have been linked to the development of asthma. In some instances, these substances provoke allergic asthma by IgE-related hypersensitivity mechanisms. Those affected include animal handlers, bakers, and workers exposed to wood and vegetable dusts, metal salts, pharmaceutical agents, and industrial chemicals.

Drug-Induced Asthma. Drug-induced bronchospasm occurs most commonly in patients with known asthma. The best known of these compounds is **aspirin,** but nonsteroidal anti-inflammatory agents have also been implicated.

Air Pollution. Massive air pollution, usually in association with temperature inversions, is associated with bronchospasm in patients with asthma and other pre-existing lung conditions.

Emotional Factors. Psychological stress can aggravate or precipitate an attack of bronchospasm in as many as half of all patients with asthma.

☐ **Pathology:** Most information regarding the pathology of asthma has been derived from autopsies of patients who died in status asthmaticus; thus, the most severe lesions are described. On gross examination, the lungs are remarkably distended with air, and the airways are filled with thick, tenacious, and adherent mucous plugs. Microscopically, the plugs (Fig. 12-23) contain strips of epithelium and many eosinophils, the extruded granules of which coalesce to form needle-like crystals (**Charcot-Leyden crystals**). In some cases, the mucoid exudate forms a cast of the airways (**Curschmann spirals**), which may be expelled with coughing.

The epithelium displays a loss of the normal, pseudostratified appearance and may be denuded, with only the basal cells remaining. The basal cells are hyperplastic, and squamous metaplasia is seen. An increase in the number of goblet cells is also apparent. Characteristically, the epithelial basement membrane is thickened owing to an increase in collagen deep to the true basal lamina. One of the most characteristic features of status asthmaticus is the prominence of bronchial smooth muscle, which reflects muscle hyperplasia. The submucosa is edematous and contains a mixed inflammatory infiltrate, including variable numbers of eosinophils.

☐ **Clinical Features:** In a typical attack of asthma, both inspiratory and expiratory wheezes appear, the respiratory rate increases, and the patient becomes dyspneic. Characteristically, the expiratory phase is particularly prolonged. The end of the attack is often heralded by severe coughing and expectoration. **Status asthmaticus** refers to an increasingly severe bronchoconstriction that does not respond to the drugs that

A IMMEDIATE RESPONSE

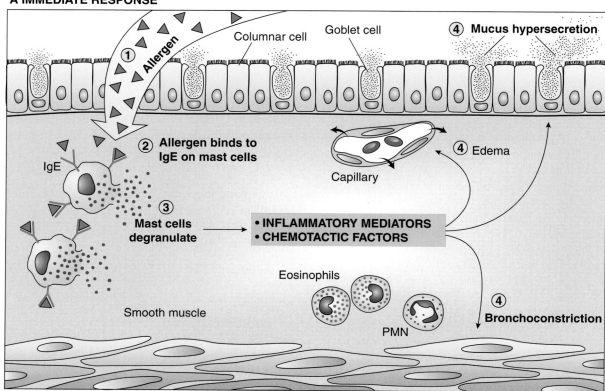

B DELAYED RESPONSE

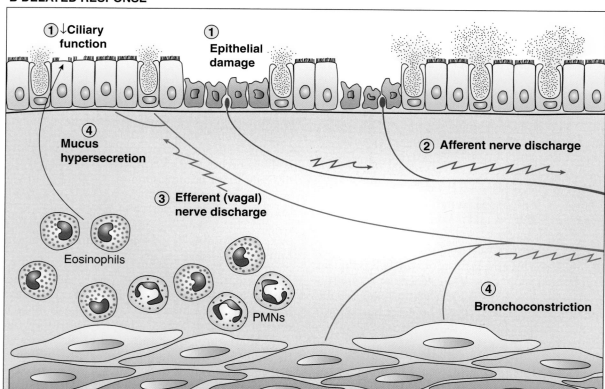

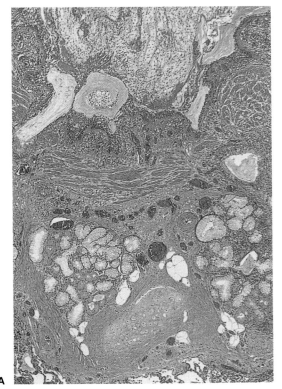
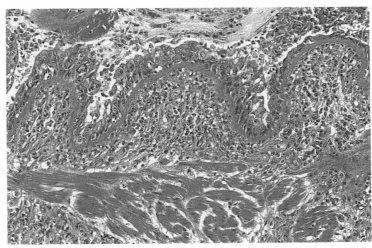

A   B

FIGURE   12-23

Asthma. (*A*) A section of lung from a patient who died in status asthmaticus reveals a bronchus containing a luminal mucous plug, submucosal gland hyperplasia, and smooth muscle hyperplasia. (*B*) Higher magnification shows hyaline thickening of the subepithelial basement membrane and marked inflammation of the bronchiolar wall, with numerous eosinophils. The mucosa exhibits an inflamed and metaplastic epithelium.

usually abort an acute attack. This situation is potentially serious and requires hospitalization.

The cornerstone of treatment in patients with asthma is pharmacologic and includes the administration of β-adrenergic agonists, inhaled corticosteroids, cromolyn sodium, methylxanthines, and anticholinergic agents. Systemic corticosteroids are reserved for status asthmaticus or resistant chronic asthma. Inhalation of bronchodilators often provides dramatic relief.

PNEUMOCONIOSES

■ *Pneumoconioses are pulmonary diseases caused by inhalation of inorganic dusts.* **The most important factor in the production of symptomatic pneumoconioses is the capacity of inhaled dusts to stimulate fibrosis** (Fig. 12-24). Thus, small amounts of silica or asbestos may produce extensive fibrosis, whereas coal and iron are weakly fibrogenic at best.

FIGURE   12-22

Pathogenesis of asthma. (A) Immunologically mediated asthma. Allergens interact with immunoglobulin E on mast cells, either on the surface of the epithelium or, when there is abnormal permeability of the epithelium, in the submucosa. Mediators are released and may react locally or by reflexes mediated through the vagus. (B) Discharge of eosinophilic granules further impairs mucociliary function and damages the epithelial cells. In turn, epithelial cell injury stimulates nerve endings in the mucosa, thereby initiating an autonomic discharge that contributes to airway narrowing and mucus secretion.

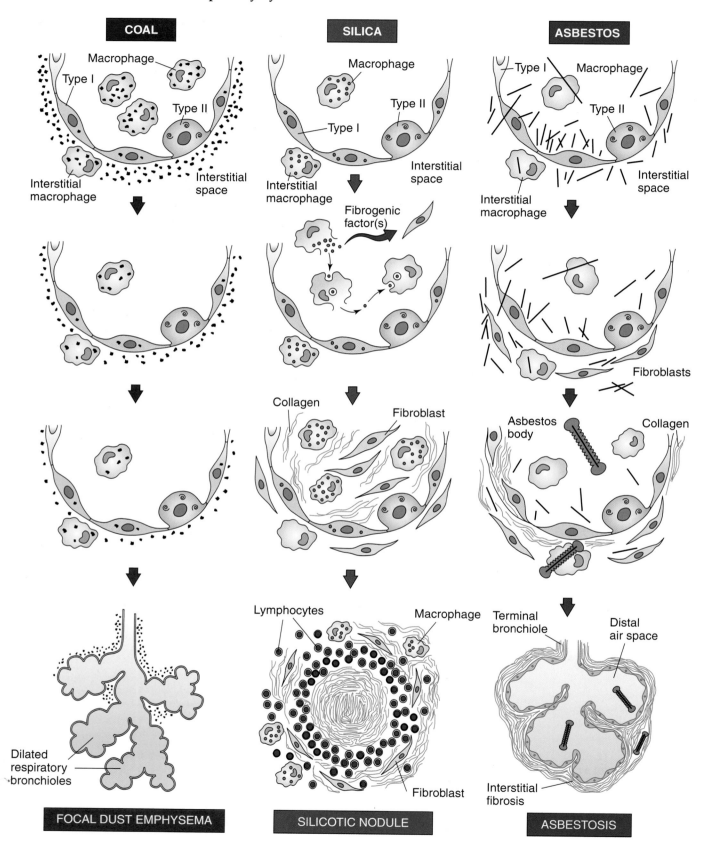

COAL

Macrophage

Type I

Type II

Interstitial
macrophage

Interstitial
space

SILICA

Macrophage

Type II

Type I

Interstitial
space

Interstitial
macrophage

Fibrogenic
factor(s)

Collagen

Fibroblast

ASBESTOS

Type I   Macrophage

Type II

Interstitial
space

Interstitial
macrophage

Fibroblasts

Asbestos
body

Collagen

Dilated
respiratory
bronchioles

Lymphocytes   Macrophage

Fibroblast

Terminal
bronchiole

Distal
air space

Interstitial
fibrosis

FOCAL DUST EMPHYSEMA

SILICOTIC NODULE

ASBESTOSIS

Silicosis

■ *Silicosis is a pneumoconiosis caused by inhalation of silicon dioxide (silica), usually in crystalline form (as quartz).* The disease was described historically in sandblasters. Mining also involves exposure to silica, as do numerous other occupations, including stone cutting, metal polishing and sharpening, ceramic manufacturing, foundry work, and cleaning of boilers. Use of air-handling equipment and masks, however, has substantially reduced the incidence of silicosis.

☐ **Pathogenesis:** Following their inhalation, silica particles are ingested by alveolar macrophages. Silicon hydroxide groups on the surface of the particles form hydrogen bonds with phospholipids and proteins, an interaction that is presumed to damage cellular membranes and, thereby, to kill the macrophage. The dead macrophages release free silica particles and fibrogenic factors. The released silica is then reingested by living macrophages, and the process is amplified.

☐ **Pathology**

Simple Nodular Silicosis. This is the most common form of silicosis and is almost inevitable in any worker with long-term exposure to silica. Twenty to 40 years after the initial exposure (but sometimes after only 10 years), the lungs contain **silicotic nodules.** These characteristic lesions of silicosis are less than 1 cm in diameter (usually 2–4 mm). On histologic examination, they have a characteristic, whorled appearance, with concentrically arranged collagen that forms the largest part of the nodule (Fig. 12-25). At the periphery are aggregates of mononuclear cells, mostly lymphocytes, and fibroblasts. Polarized light reveals doubly refractile silicates within the nodule. Simple silicosis is not ordinarily associated with significant respiratory dysfunction.

Progressive Massive Fibrosis. Progressive massive fibrosis is characterized by nodular masses more than 1 cm in diameter against a background of simple silicosis. These larger lesions represent the coalescence of smaller nodules. Most of the lesions are 5 to 10 cm across and are usually located bilaterally in the upper zones of the lungs (Fig. 12-26). They often exhibit central cavitation as well. Progressive massive fibrosis is related to the amount of silica in the lung.

☐ **Clinical Features:** The diagnosis of simple silicosis is usually established on the basis of radiologic results and without significant symptomatology. Dyspnea on exertion—and, later, at rest—suggests progressive massive fibrosis or other complications of silicosis. In acute silicosis, dyspnea may become rapidly disabling, and respiratory failure ensues. **It is well recognized that tuberculosis is much more common in patients with silicosis than in the general population.** There appears to be no increase in the rate of lung cancer among patients with silicosis.

Coal Workers' Pneumoconiosis

Coal dust is composed of amorphous carbon together with other constituents of the earth's surface, including variable amounts of silica. Amorphous carbon by itself is not fibrogenic, but inhalation of coal particles may lead to the lesions of anthracosilicosis.

☐ **Pathology:** The characteristic pulmonary lesions in coal workers are the coal dust macules, which appear as black areas, 1 to 4 mm across, scattered throughout the lungs. The pigmented appearance of the lungs accounts for the term **black lung disease,** also termed **simple coal workers' pneumoconiosis.** Microscopically, the coal dust macule exhibits numerous carbon-laden macrophages that surround the distal respiratory bronchioles, extend to fill adjacent alveolar spaces, and infiltrate the peribronchiolar interstitial space. There is an accompanying mild dilatation of respiratory bronchioles (**focal dust emphysema**) that probably results from the atrophy of smooth muscle.

Black lung disease causes, at worst, a minor impairment of pulmonary function. When coal miners have severe obstruction to the flow of air, it is usually due to smoking. The appearance of larger, nodular lesions in the lungs of coal workers suggests a change caused by silica in the inhaled dust, and the disease is then termed **anthracosilicosis.**

FIGURE **12-24**
Pathogenesis of pneumoconioses. The three most important pneumoconioses are illustrated. In simple coal pneumoconiosis, massive amounts of dust are inhaled and engulfed by macrophages. The macrophages pass into the interstitium of the lung and aggregate around the respiratory bronchioles. Subsequently, the bronchioles dilate. In silicosis, the silica particles are toxic to macrophages, which die and release a fibrogenic factor. In turn, the released silica is again phagocytosed by other macrophages. The result is a dense, fibrotic nodule (the silicotic nodule). Asbestosis is characterized by little dust and much interstitial fibrosis. Asbestos bodies are the classic feature.

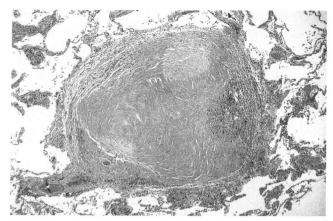

FIGURE *12-25*
Silicosis. A silicotic nodule is composed of concentric whorls of dense, sparsely cellular collagen.

Asbestos-Related Disease

■ *Asbestosis-related disease refers to the pneumoconiosis that results from inhalation of asbestos fibers.* The disease occurs as a result of the processing and handling of asbestos, rather than in mining; such processing and handling is a surface operation. Exposure starts with the baggers who package asbestos and continues with those who modify or use it, such as workers who make asbestos products (e.g., tiles, cement, and insulation material) and those in the construction and shipbuilding industries.

□ **Pathogenesis:** Asbestos fibers, which are composed of silicates, deposit in the distal airways and alveoli, particularly at the bifurcations of the alveolar ducts. The smallest particles are engulfed by macrophages, but many of the larger fibers penetrate the interstitial space. Release of inflammatory mediators by activated macrophages and the fibrogenic character of free asbestos fibers in the interstitium promote interstitial pulmonary fibrosis.

□ **Pathology: Asbestosis is an interstitial fibrosis of the lung.** In the early stages, fibrosis occurs both in and around the alveolar ducts and respiratory bronchioles as well as in the periphery of the acinus. As the disease becomes more advanced, gross examination of the lungs shows gray streaks of fibrous tissue and diffuse thickening of the visceral pleura. Rarely, the interstitial fibrosis proceeds to a "honeycomb" lung.

The **asbestos body** consists of an asbestos fiber (length, 10–50 μm) that has beaded aggregates of iron along its length. By light microscopy, it is golden brown (Fig. 12-27) and stains strongly for iron. The iron staining derives from hemoglobin that has been liberated from microhemorrhages. Asbestos bodies are

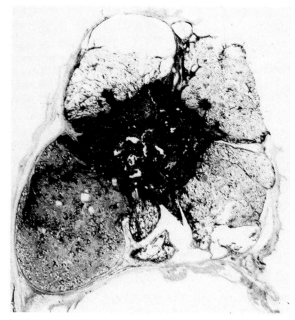

FIGURE *12-26*
Progressive, massive fibrosis. A whole mount of a silicotic lung from a coal miner shows a large area of dense fibrosis containing entrapped carbon particles.

found in the walls of bronchioles or within the alveolar spaces, often engulfed by alveolar macrophages. Exposure to asbestos also leads to a number of additional complications.

Pleural Plaques. During a period of many years, inhalation of asbestos fibers results in the appearance of plaques on the parietal pleura, most commonly in the posterolateral regions of the lower thorax and on the dome of the diaphragm. The interval between exposure and appearance of the plaques is from 10 to 20 years. On gross examination, these localized lesions are raised, white, and shiny, with the consistency of cartilage. They are 2 to 3 mm in thickness and vary

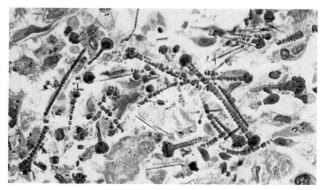

FIGURE *12-27*
Asbestos body. These structures are golden-brown, beaded bodies, which represent asbestos fibers that have been encrusted with protein and iron.

from a few millimeters to several centimeters across. Microscopically, pleural plaques are densely collagenous, hyalinized, and sometimes, calcified. Following digestion of the tissue, asbestos fibers can be demonstrated by electron microscopy.

Mesothelioma. A clear-cut relationship between asbestos exposure and malignant mesothelioma is firmly established. Sometimes, the exposure is slight, as in the wives of asbestos workers who wash their husbands' clothes. More often, mesothelioma is found in workers who are heavily exposed to asbestos, predominantly of the crocidolite variety. The clinical and pathologic features of this disease are discussed with diseases of the pleura.

Carcinoma of the Lung. Bronchogenic carcinoma has been reported to be approximately three- to fivefold more common in nonsmoking asbestos workers than in nonsmoking workers not exposed to asbestos, although this figure remains to be firmly established. **However, in asbestos workers who smoke, the incidence of lung carcinoma is vastly increased, being some 60-fold greater than that in the general nonsmoking population.** Development of the tumor occurs most often linked in the presence of asbestosis.

Berylliosis

■ *Berylliosis is the pulmonary disease that follows inhalation of beryllium.* Today, this metal is used principally in structural materials employed by the aerospace industries, in the manufacture of industrial ceramics, and in atomic reactors. Exposure to beryllium may also occur during the mining and extraction of beryllium ores.

Berylliosis occurs as an acute, chemical pneumonitis or a chronic pneumoconiosis. The pathologic findings are those of diffuse alveolar damage. Ten percent of persons with acute berylliosis progress to chronic disease, although chronic berylliosis is often encountered in workers without any history of acute illness.

The chronic disease differs from other pneumoconioses in that the amount and duration of exposure may be small, and the lesion is suspected to be a hypersensitivity phenomenon. On gross examination, the lungs are shrunken and fibrotic, and they may exhibit numerous cysts (honeycomb lung). Microscopically, granulomatous inflammation and interstitial fibrosis are conspicuous.

Patients with chronic berylliosis present with an insidious onset of dyspnea 15 or more years after the initial exposure. The disease must be distinguished from sarcoidosis, and it appears to be associated with an increased risk of lung cancer.

INTERSTITIAL LUNG DISEASES

A large number of pulmonary disorders are grouped as interstitial, infiltrative, or restrictive diseases, because they are characterized by inflammatory infiltrates in the interstitial space and have similar clinical and radiologic presentations.

Hypersensitivity Pneumonitis

■ *Hypersensitivity pneumonitis refers to a group of immunologically mediated conditions caused by exposure to organic dusts, in which the alveoli and distal airways are preferentially involved.*

□ **Pathogenesis:** More than 30 environmental antigens are known to produce hypersensitivity pneumonitis. Inhalation of these antigens leads to acute or chronic interstitial inflammation in the lung. Most of the responsible antigens are encountered in occupational settings, and the diseases are often labeled according to the specific occupation. For example, farmers exposed to moldy hay suffer from **farmer's lung**. Sugar cane workers exposed to moldy, pressed sugar cane (bagasse) acquire **bagassosis**; and bird breeders who come in contact with feathers, serum, and excrement of pigeons have **pigeon breeder's disease.**

Hypersensitivity pneumonitis represents a combination of immune complex–mediated (type III) and cell-mediated (type IV) hypersensitivity reactions, although the precise contribution of each is still being debated. Whereas acute hypersensitivity pneumonitis is characterized by a neutrophilic infiltrate in the alveoli and respiratory bronchioles, the more chronic lesions display mononuclear cells and granulomas, which are typical of delayed hypersensitivity.

□ **Pathology:** In the acute phase of hypersensitivity pneumonitis, bronchiolar necrosis, an eosinophilic infiltrate, vasculitis, and interstitial pneumonia are present. Chronic disease is characterized by extensive interstitial pneumonitis, with a dense infiltrate of lymphocytes and a few plasma cells in the alveolar walls. Mild, diffuse alveolar damage is usually present, with hyperplasia of type II pneumocytes. There is also a significant bronchiolar infiltrate, sometimes with bronchiolitis obliterans. **Most characteristic is the presence of scattered, poorly formed granulomas that contain foreign body giant cells** (Fig. 12-28). In the chronic end stage, the interstitial inflammation recedes. However, fibrosis is more apparent, the lung architecture is distorted, and honeycombing occurs.

□ **Clinical Features:** Hypersensitivity pneumonitis may present as acute, subacute, or chronic pulmonary

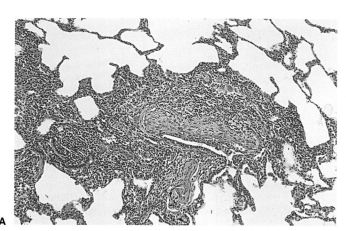
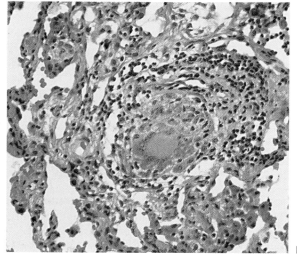

FIGURE 12-28
Hypersensitivity pneumonitis. (*A*) A lung biopsy shows a mild peribronchiolar chronic inflammatory interstitial infiltrate, with a focus of intraluminal organizing fibrosis. (*B*) Focal poorly formed granulomas were scattered in the lung biopsy.

disease, depending on the frequency and intensity of exposure to the offending antigen. The prototype of hypersensitivity pneumonitis is farmer's lung, which is caused by inhalation of thermophilic actinomycetes that grow in moldy hay. Typically, a farm worker enters a barn where hay has been stored for winter feeding. After a lag period of several hours, the worker rapidly develops dyspnea, cough, and mild fever. The symptoms remit within 24 to 48 hours but return on reexposure and, with time, become chronic.

Pulmonary function studies show a restrictive pattern, which is characterized by decreased compliance, reduced diffusion capacity, and hypoxemia. In the chronic stage of hypersensitivity pneumonitis, airway obstruction may become troublesome.

Sarcoidosis

■ *Sarcoidosis is a chronic disease of unknown cause in which noncaseating granulomas occur in almost any organ of the body.* The lung is most frequently involved, but the lymph nodes, skin, and eye are also common targets (Fig. 12-29).

☐ **Epidemiology:** Sarcoidosis is a worldwide disease affecting all races and both sexes. In North America, sarcoidosis occurs much more frequently in blacks than in whites, with the ratio being approximately 15 : 1. The disease is often encountered in the Scandinavian countries, where the prevalence is 64 per 100,000 persons(compared with 10 per 100,000 in France and 3 per 100,000 in Poland). It has been reported that the prevalence of sarcoidosis in Irish women in London is an astonishing 200 per 100,000 persons. Sarcoidosis is distinctly uncommon in China.

☐ **Pathogenesis:** There is a consensus that sarcoidosis represents an exaggerated cellular immune response on the part of helper/inducer T lymphocytes to unknown exogenous antigens or autoantigens. These cells accumulate in the affected organs, where they secrete lymphokines and recruit macrophages that participate in formation of noncaseating granulomas.

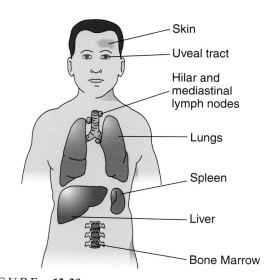

FIGURE 12-29
Organs commonly affected by sarcoidosis. Sarcoidosis involves many organs, most commonly the lymph nodes and lung.

Nonspecific polyclonal activation of B cells by T-helper cells leads to hyperglobulinemia, which is characteristic of active sarcoidosis.

☐ **Pathology:** Pulmonary sarcoidosis most commonly affects the lung and hilar lymph nodes. Histologically, multiple sarcoid granulomas are scattered in the interstitium of the lung (Fig. 12-30). The central part of the granuloma may be fibrotic and surrounded by palisaded histiocytes. Giant cells at the periphery resemble those of tuberculosis, but caseous necrosis is invariably absent. There is increased cellularity of the alveolar walls owing to an infiltrate of mononuclear cells. In two-thirds of the cases, granulomatous angiitis can be demonstrated in lung biopsy specimens.

☐ **Clinical Features:** Sarcoidosis often has an insidious onset over a period of a few weeks to a few months, presenting as fever, malaise, and weight loss. Cough and dyspnea, which not infrequently appear in the absence of constitutional symptoms, are the major respiratory complaints. Half of the patients develop some degree of permanent respiratory dysfunction, usually dyspnea on exertion, and as many as 15% demonstrate progressive pulmonary fibrosis. The other organs commonly involved by sarcoidosis include the skin, eye, heart, central nervous system, extrathoracic lymph nodes, spleen, and liver.

The prognosis in sarcoidosis is favorable, and most patients do not manifest clinically significant sequelae. The disease directly accounts for the death of the patient in only 10% of cases. Active sarcoidosis responds well to administration of corticosteroids.

Usual Interstitial Pneumonia

■ *Usual interstitial pneumonia (UIP) is the most common type of idiopathic interstitial pneumonitis and is characterized clinically by progressive respiratory insufficiency and pathologically by interstitial inflammation and fibrosis.* The disease affects persons of all ages, with a mean age at onset of 50 to 60 years.

☐ **Pathogenesis:** It is generally held that UIP has an immunologic basis. Approximately 20% of the cases are associated with collagen vascular diseases, including rheumatoid arthritis, systemic lupus erythematosus, and progressive systemic sclerosis. The disease also occurs in the context of other autoimmune disorders, such as Hashimoto thyroiditis, primary biliary cirrhosis, idiopathic thrombocytopenic purpura, and myasthenia gravis. Patients with UIP frequently exhibit circulating autoantibodies (e.g., antinuclear antibodies and rheumatoid factor). Immune complexes have been demonstrated in the circulation, inflamed alveolar walls, and bronchoalveolar lavage specimens, although the antigen has not been identified.

☐ **Pathology:** The hallmark of UIP is chronic inflammation in the interstitial space, together with widespread fibrosis of the alveolar septa (Fig. 12-31). Severe disease manifests as diffuse alveolar damage, with pronounced accumulation of lymphocytes and plasma cells in the alveolar walls and hyperplasia of type II pneumocytes. At the extreme end of the spectrum is honeycomb lung, which is characteristically most prominent in the subpleural areas of the lower zones of the lung. Extensive vascular changes, particularly intimal fibrosis and thickening of the media, are

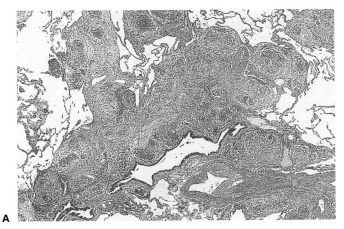
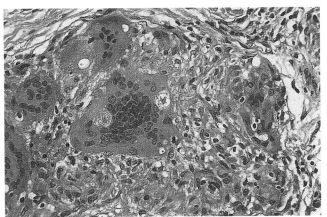

A B

FIGURE *12-30*
Sarcoidosis. (A) Multiple noncaseating granulomas are present along the bronchovascular interstitium. (B) Noncaseating granulomas consist of tight clusters of epithelioid macrophages and multinucleated giant cells.

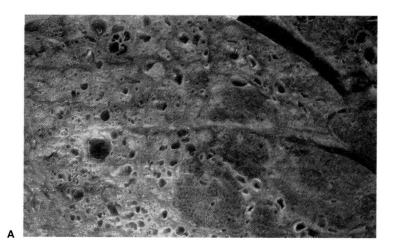

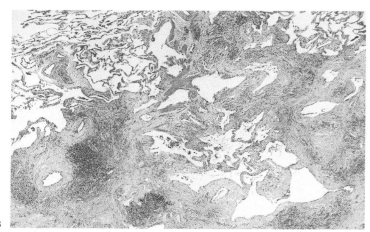

FIGURE *12-31*
Usual interstitial pneumonitis. (*A*) **A gross specimen of the lung shows patchy dense scarring with
extensive areas of honeycomb cystic change.** (*B*) **A
microscopic view discloses patchy interstitial
dense fibrosis and interstitial chronic inflammation. The areas of dense fibrosis display remodeling, with loss of the normal lung architecture.**

caused by inflammation, fibrosis, and pulmonary hypertension.

□ **Clinical Features:** UIP begins insidiously, with gradual onset of dyspnea on exertion and dry cough, often over a period of 5 to 10 years. Tachypnea at rest, cyanosis, and cor pulmonale eventually ensue. The prognosis is bleak, with an average survival time of 5 years. Patients are treated with corticosteroids and, sometimes, cyclophosphamide, but lung transplantation generally offers the only hope of cure.

Bronchiolitis Obliterans with Organizing Pneumonia

■ *Bronchiolitis obliterans with organizing pneumonia (BOOP) is a reaction of the peribronchiolar parenchyma to a variety of injuries and is characterized by a distinctive fibrosis that involves the distal airways and alveoli.* BOOP is associated with many respiratory tract infections, particularly viral bronchiolitis, inhalation of toxic materials, administration of a number of drugs, and several inflammatory processes, including colla-

gen vascular diseases. A substantial number of cases remain idiopathic.

□ **Pathology:** The typical histologic appearance of BOOP is patchy areas of loose fibrosis and chronic inflammatory cells in the distal airways. These assume the form of plugs that occlude the bronchioles (bronchiolitis obliterans), alveolar ducts, and surrounding alveoli (organizing pneumonia) (Fig. 12-32). Some of the fibrous plugs are lined by bronchiolar or type II alveolar lining cells and, thus, appear to represent interstitial fibrosis. Because of occlusion of the bronchioles, obstructive pneumonia may develop distal to the airways, which is characterized by the accumulation of foamy, lipid-laden macrophages. In addition to the prominent fibrosis in the airspaces, the alveolar septa are thickened and display chronic inflammatory cells and hyperplasia of type II pneumocytes.

□ **Clinical Features:** BOOP presents with the acute onset of fever, cough, and dyspnea. Most patients recover within weeks or months, even without therapy. Corticosteroid treatment is often instituted to hasten recovery.

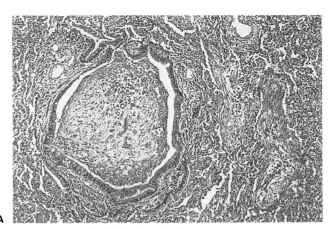
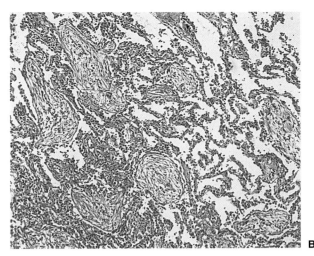

A   B

FIGURE   *12-32*
Bronchiolitis obliterans with organizing pneumonia (BOOP). (*A*) Polypoid plugs of loose fibrosis tissue are present in a bronchiole and the adjacent alveolar ducts and alveoli. (*B*) The alveolar spaces contain similar plugs of loose organizing connective tissue.

PULMONARY HYPERTENSION

During fetal life, the pulmonary arterial walls are thick, and the pulmonary arterial pressure is correspondingly high. Blood is oxygenated through the placenta rather than the lungs. Thus, the high fetal pulmonary arterial pressure shunts the output of the right ventricle through the ductus arteriosus and into the systemic circulation, effectively bypassing the lungs. After birth, the lungs assume the obligation of oxygenating the venous blood, and the ductus arteriosus closes. Under these circumstances, the lungs must adapt to accept the entire cardiac output, a situation that demands the high-volume and low-pressure system of the mature

lung. Accordingly, by the third day of life, the pulmonary arteries dilate, their walls become thin, and the pulmonary arterial pressure correspondingly declines.

In the child or adult, the pressure within the pulmonary arterial system may be increased either by augmented flow or by increased vascular resistance. Whatever the cause, characteristic morphologic abnormalities result from increased pulmonary artery pressure (Fig. 12-33). In order of increasing severity, the grades of pulmonary hypertension, reflecting the changes in the pulmonary arteries, are:

1. **Medial hypertrophy** of muscular pulmonary arteries and appearance of smooth muscle in the pulmonary arterioles.

SMALL PULMONARY ARTERIES

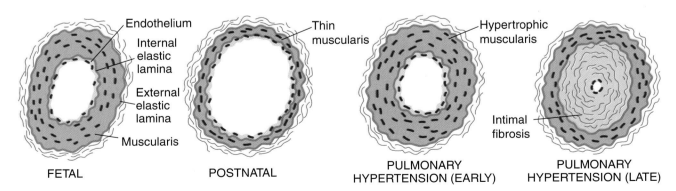

FETAL   POSTNATAL   PULMONARY   PULMONARY
                                                      HYPERTENSION (EARLY)   HYPERTENSION (LATE)

FIGURE   *12-33*
Histopathology of pulmonary hypertension. During late gestation, the pulmonary arteries have thick walls. After birth, the vessels dilate, and the walls become thin. Mild pulmonary hypertension is characterized by thickening of the media. As pulmonary hypertension becomes more severe, extensive intimal fibrosis and muscle thickening occur.

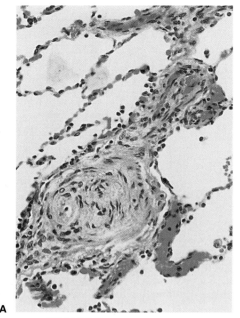
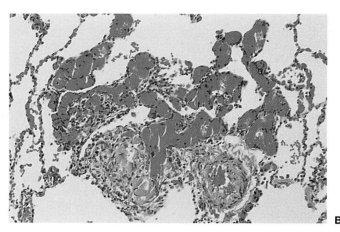

FIGURE *12-34*
Pulmonary arterial hypertension. (*A*) A small pulmonary artery is virtually occluded by concentric intimal fibrosis and thickening of the media. (*B*) A plexiform lesion is characterized by marked dilatation, congestion, and thinning of arterial walls, forming interconnected vascular channels adjacent to the small arteries. The latter show marked hypertensive changes of intimal fibrosis and medial thickening.

2. **Intimal proliferation,** with increasing medial hypertrophy (Fig. 12-34).
3. **Intimal fibrosis** of muscular pulmonary arteries and arterioles, which may be occlusive.
4. **Formation of plexiform lesions, together with dilatation and thinning of pulmonary arteries.** These nodular lesions are composed of irregular, interlacing blood channels and impose a further obstruction in the pulmonary circulation.
5. **Rupture of pulmonary arteries,** with parenchymal hemorrhage and hemosiderosis.
6. **Fibrinoid necrosis** of the arteries and arterioles.

With all grades of pulmonary hypertension, atherosclerosis is seen in the largest pulmonary arteries. In this respect, even mild degrees of atherosclerosis are uncommon when pulmonary arterial pressure is normal. As a result of the increased pressure in the lesser circulation, hypertrophy of the right ventricle of the heart occurs (cor pulmonale).

Increased Flow

An excess volume of blood presented to the lesser circulation may lead to pulmonary hypertension and its associated morphologic changes. This situation occurs principally in the case of patients with congenital left-to-right shunts.

Precapillary Pulmonary Hypertension

Increased resistance to flow may be caused by obstruction proximal to the lung capillary bed (precapillary hypertension), destruction of the capillary bed, or obstruction distal to the capillary bed (postcapillary hypertension).

Primary Pulmonary Hypertension

■ *Pulmonary hypertension of unknown cause (primary or idiopathic) is a rare condition caused by increased tone within the pulmonary arteries.* It occurs at all ages but is most common among young women in their twenties and thirties. Severe morphologic changes of pulmonary hypertension eventually ensue, and the patients die of cor pulmonale. Medical treatment is ineffective, and the disease is an indication for heart–lung transplantation.

Recurrent Pulmonary Emboli

Multiple thromboemboli in the smaller pulmonary vessels, often the result of asymptomatic, episodic showers of small emboli from the periphery, gradually restrict the pulmonary circulation. The presenting symptoms are the same as in primary pulmonary hypertension, but some patients have evidence of peripheral venous thrombosis, usually in the leg veins, or a history of circumstances predisposing to peripheral venous thrombosis. If the condition is diagnosed during life, placement of a filter in the inferior vena cava prevents further embolization.

Functional Resistance to Arterial Flow (Vasoconstriction)

Any disorder that produces hypoxemia results in pulmonary hypertension. This is the most common circumstance underlying pulmonary hypertension, and it includes chronic obstruction to the flow of air (chronic bronchitis), infiltrative lung disease, and living at high altitude. Severe kyphoscoliosis or extreme obesity (pickwickian syndrome) may interfere with the mechanics of ventilation and cause hypoxemia and pulmonary hypertension. Hypoxemia leads to constriction of small pulmonary arteries and consequent hypertension.

Cardiac Causes of Pulmonary Hypertension

Left ventricular failure from any cause increases pulmonary venous pressure and, to some extent, pulmonary arterial pressure. By contrast, mitral stenosis produces severe venous hypertension and significant pulmonary artery hypertension.

CARCINOMA OF THE LUNG

Carcinoma of the lung is the most common cause of death from cancer in the United States. **The large majority (90%) of lung cancers are a consequence of cigarette smoking** (see Chapter 8).

Squamous Cell Carcinoma

Squamous cell carcinoma accounts for 30% of all invasive lung cancers in the United States.

☐ **Pathology:** Most squamous cell carcinomas arise in the central portion of the lung, from the major or segmental bronchi. On gross examination, they tend to be firm, gray-white, and ulcerated lesions that extend through the bronchial wall into the adjacent parenchyma (Fig. 12-35). The microscopic appearance of squamous cell carcinoma is highly variable. The range of differentiation extends from mature squamous cells with keratin pearls to an anaplastic lesion recognized as being of squamous cell origin only by electron microscopy and immunohistochemical examination. In well-differentiated tumors, keratin often occurs as "pearls," which appear as central, brightly eosinophilic aggregates of keratin surrounded by "onion skin" layers of squamous cells.

Carcinomas of the lung, of all histologic types, metastasize most frequently to the regional lymph nodes, particularly the hilar and mediastinal nodes. The most common site of extranodal metastasis is the

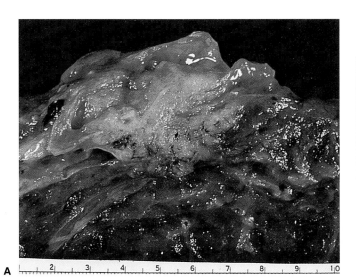
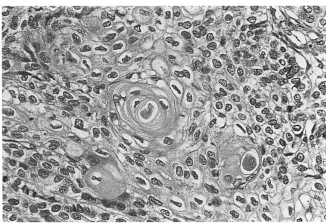

A   B

FIGURE *12-35*
Squamous cell carcinoma of the lung. (A) The tumor grows within the lumen of a bronchus and invades the adjacent intrapulmonary lymph node. (B) A photomicrograph shows well-differentiated squamous cell carcinoma, with a keratin pearl composed of cells with brightly eosinophilic cytoplasm.

adrenal gland, although adrenal insufficiency is distinctly uncommon. Lung cancer not infrequently presents initially as metastatic disease, with the brain, bone, and liver all being common sites.

☐ **Clinical Features:** Most squamous cell carcinomas present with symptoms related to their bronchial origin, including persistent cough, hemoptysis, or bronchial obstruction, with the last being accompanied by pulmonary infections (recurrent pneumonias, lung abscesses) or atelectasis. Extension of the tumor may cause compression of the superior vena cava, thereby resulting in severe venous and lymphatic congestion of the upper body (**superior vena cava syndrome**). Growth of a lung cancer (usually squamous) in the apex of the lung (**Pancoast tumor**) may extend to involve the eighth cervical and the first and second thoracic nerves, thereby resulting in shoulder pain radiating in an ulnar distribution down the arm (**Pancoast syndrome**). A Pancoast tumor may also paralyze the cervical sympathetic nerves and cause **Horner syndrome,** which is characterized by depression of the eyeball (enophthalmos), ptosis of the upper eyelid, constriction of the pupil (miosis), and absence of sweating (anhidrosis) on the affected side. Pleural effusion is common and leads to dyspnea. Lymphangitic spread of the tumor within the lung may impair oxygenation. Invasion of the pericardium by cancer results in pericardial effusion and, sometimes, cardiac tamponade.

The median survival time for patients with untreated squamous cell carcinoma of the lung is less than 1 year. At the time of diagnosis, approximately 60% of all squamous carcinomas are deemed to be resectable, and the overall 5-year survival rate after surgery is 37%.

Adenocarcinoma

Adenocarcinoma of the lung comprises one-third of all invasive lung cancers. The tumor tends to arise in the periphery, usually in the upper lobes, with puckering of the overlying pleura (Fig. 12-36). Most of these tumors occur in smokers. In the past, many of these cancers were thought to arise in scars secondary to old tuberculosis, healed infarcts, and so on, but it is now recognized that most of these scars represent a desmoplastic response to the tumor.

☐ **Pathology:** At the initial presentation, adenocarcinomas of the lung appear as irregular masses from 2 to 5 cm in diameter, although many are larger. On cut section, the tumor is grayish-white and often glistening, owing to the production of mucus. Histologically, adenocarcinomas of the lung present a wide variety of morphologic patterns. The neoplastic cells may resem-

ble ciliated or nonciliated columnar epithelial cells, goblet cells, cells of the bronchial glands, or Clara cells. In the most common pattern, well-differentiated acinar carcinomas form regular glands, which are lined by columnar cells with basal nuclei (see Fig. 12-36). Papillary adenocarcinomas exhibit columnar to cuboidal cells and form a single layer on a core of fibrous connective tissue. Solid adenocarcinomas are poorly differentiated tumors, although in some cases, there is a suggestion of gland formation. Mucus production in all varieties of adenocarcinoma varies from scant to abundant.

Adenocarcinomas readily metastasize to the same sites as squamous cell carcinomas, but they tend to grow more rapidly and frequently invade the pleura. Less than 40% of adenocarcinomas can be resected, and the 5-year survival rate for these patients is only 25%.

Bronchioloalveolar Carcinoma

■ *Bronchioloalveolar carcinoma is a distinctive subtype of adenocarcinoma that grows along pre-existing alveolar walls.* These cancers account for 1% to 5% of all invasive lung tumors. The tumor shows little or no relationship to tobacco smoking. Most of these cancers originate from Clara cells, although a minority are composed principally of type II pneumocytes.

On gross examination, bronchioloalveolar carcinoma presents as a single peripheral nodule, as multiple nodules, or as a diffuse infiltrate that resembles pneumonia. The cut section of the tumor is often mucoid and may not even be recognized macroscopically as being a tumor (Fig. 12-37). On microscopic examination, well-differentiated, mucin-containing columnar cells line the alveolar spaces without invading the stroma. However, tumors composed of neoplastic type II pneumocytes do not contain mucin.

In cases involving a single lesion, the prognosis for patients with bronchioloalveolar carcinoma is good. In the absence of lymph node metastases, the cure rate is more than 50%.

Small Cell Carcinoma

■ *Small cell carcinoma is a highly malignant lung cancer that is characterized by sheets of small tumor cells that differentiate in the direction of the neuroendocrine cells.* This variant accounts for 20% of all lung cancers. The male:female ratio is 2:1, and 90% of the patients are cigarette smokers. Small cell carcinoma is believed to arise from the pluripotential basal cells of the bronchial epithelium.

In the majority of cases, small cell carcinoma originates near the hilum of the lung. On cut section, the tumor is soft, glistening, and grayish-white, often with

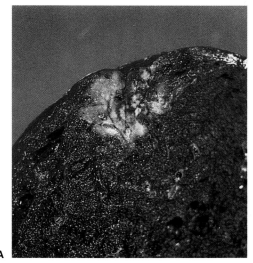

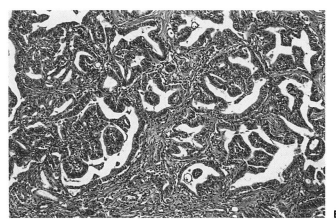

FIGURE 12-36
Adenocarcinoma of the lung. (A) A peripheral tumor in the right upper lobe puckers the pleural surface. (B) A papillary adenocarcinoma consists of malignant epithelial cells growing along thin fibrovascular cores.

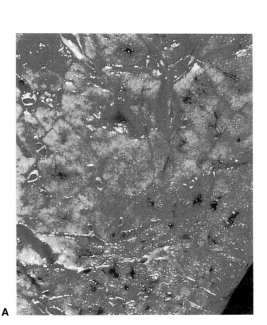

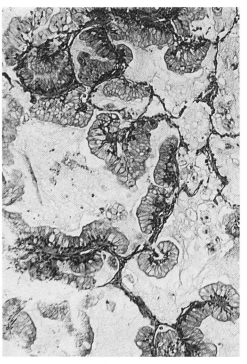

FIGURE 12-37
Bronchioloalveolar carcinoma. (A) The cut surface of the lung is solid, glistening, and mucoid, an appearance that reflects a diffusely infiltrating tumor. (B) A microscopic view shows alveoli lined by columnar, mucus-producing tumor cells and filled with mucus.

areas of necrosis. Microscopically, in half of the cases the tumor cells are small and round or oval (Fig. 12-38), with dense, hyperchromatic nuclei and scanty cytoplasm. The appearance is similar to that of lymphocytes (oat cells). One-fourth of the tumors display fusiform or elongated cells, and another one-fourth exhibit medium-size, polygonal cells with abundant cytoplasm (intermediate cell variants).

The majority of patients with small cell carcinoma are symptomatic at the time of diagnosis, and two-thirds of the tumors have already metastasized to bone, liver, brain, and other organs. Chemotherapy is the common treatment for disseminated small cell carcinoma, and recent advances have led to a dramatic improvement in prognosis. Tumors limited to the lung are treated by radiation. However, the overall cure rate remains low.

Carcinoid Tumors

■ *Carcinoid tumors are a group of neuroendocrine, pulmonary neoplasms derived from the pluripotential basal layer of the respiratory epithelium.* They comprise less than 5% of primary lung tumors, show no sex predilection, and do not relate to cigarette smoking. Although neuropeptides are readily demonstrated in the tumor cells, the large majority are endocrinologically silent. The tumor is of low-grade malignancy, but 5% to 10% metastasize to the regional lymph nodes.

Metastatic Tumors

The most common malignant neoplasm of the lung is metastatic tumor. Typically, metastatic tumors in the

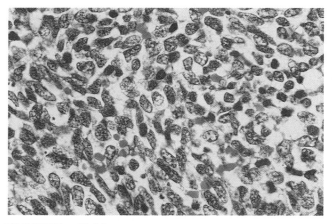

FIGURE   *12-38*
Small cell carcinoma of the lung. This tumor consists of small oval to spindle-shaped cells with scant cytoplasm, finely granular nuclear chromatin, and conspicuous mitoses.

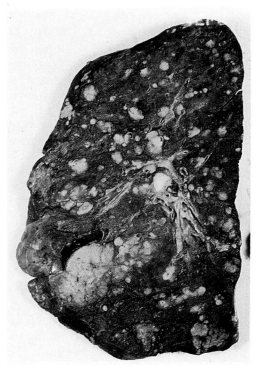

FIGURE   *12-39*
Metastatic carcinoma of the lung. A section through the lung shows numerous nodules of metastatic carcinoma, which correspond to the "cannon ball" metastases seen radiologically.

lung are multiple and circumscribed (Fig. 12-39), and are viewed radiologically as "cannon ball" metastases. The common primary sites are the breast, stomach, pancreas, and colon.

Lymphangitic carcinoma is a condition in which the metastatic tumor spreads widely through the pulmonary lymphatic channels, forming a sheath of tumor around the bronchovascular tree and the veins.

Pleura

PNEUMOTHORAX

■ *Pneumothorax is the presence of air in the pleural cavity.* It may result from traumatic perforation of the pleura or may be spontaneous. Traumatic causes include penetrating wounds of the chest wall, such as a stab wound or rib fracture. Actually, traumatic pneumothorax is most commonly iatrogenic and seen after aspiration of fluid from the pleura (thoracocentesis), pleural or lung biopsies, transbronchial biopsy, and positive pressure–assisted ventilation.

Spontaneous pneumothorax is typically encountered in young adults. For example, while exercising vigorously, a tall young man develops acute chest pain and shortness of breath. A chest radiograph reveals collapse of the lung on the side of the pain and a large collection of air in the pleural space. The condition is due to the rupture of subpleural emphysematous blebs. In most cases, spontaneous pneumothorax subsides by itself, but in some patients, withdrawal of the air is required.

Tension pneumothorax refers to a unilateral pneumothorax sufficiently extensive to shift the mediastinum to the opposite side, with compression of the opposite lung. The condition may be life-threatening and must be relieved by immediate drainage.

PLEURAL EFFUSION

■ *Pleural effusion is the accumulation of excess fluid in the pleural cavity.* The severity varies from a few milliliters of fluid, which is detected only radiologically as obliteration of the costophrenic angle, to a massive accumulation that shifts the mediastinum and trachea to the opposite side.

Hydrothorax is an effusion that resembles water and, if it occurred elsewhere, would be regarded as edema. It may be due to increased hydrostatic pressure within the capillaries, as occurs in patients with heart failure or any condition that produces systemic or pulmonary edema.

Pyothorax is a turbid effusion containing many polymorphonuclear leukocytes that results from infections of the pleura. It commonly occurs as a complication of bacterial pneumonia that extends to the pleural surface, the classic example of which is pneumococcal pneumonia.

Empyema is a variant of pyothorax in which thick pus accumulates within the pleural cavity, often with loculation and fibrosis.

Hemothorax is the accumulation of blood in the pleural cavity as a result of trauma or rupture of a vessel (e.g., a dissecting aneurysm of the aorta).

Chylothorax is the accumulation of a milky, lipid-rich fluid (chyle) in the pleural cavity caused by lymphatic obstruction. It has an ominous portent, because obstruction of the lymphatics suggests disease of the lymph nodes in the posterior mediastinum.

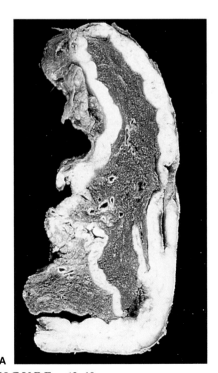 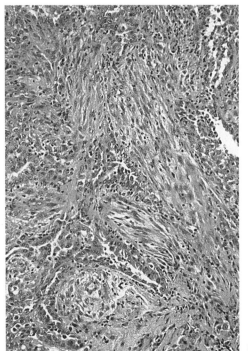

A   B

FIGURE *12-40*
Pleural mesothelioma. (A) The lung is encased by a dense pleural tumor that extends into the fissures. (B) A microscopic view shows the sarcomatous and epithelial components of the tumor.

MESOTHELIOMA

■ *Mesothelioma is a malignant tumor of mesothelial cells that is most common in the pleura but also occurs in the peritoneum and tunica vaginalis of the testis.* **Most pleural and peritoneal mesotheliomas are related to asbestos exposure** (see the earlier discussion on asbestos-related disease), although some patients deny contact with this mineral. The tumors are typically encountered in middle-age men who are occupationally exposed to asbestos, even for a short time.

☐ Pathology: On gross examination, pleural mesothelioma characteristically encases and compresses the lung, extending into the fissures and interlobar septa (Fig. 12-40). Microscopically, classic mesothelioma exhibits a biphasic appearance, namely epithelial and sarcomatous patterns. Glands and tubules that resemble adenocarcinoma are admixed with sheets of spindle cells that are similar to a fibrosarcoma.

☐ Clinical Features: Patients with pleural mesothelioma present with a pleural effusion or with a pleural mass, chest pain, and dyspnea. The lesion may be limited to the thorax, but in approximately one-fourth of the cases, metastases appear elsewhere. Treatment is ineffective, and the prognosis is hopeless.

CHAPTER 13

The Gastrointestinal Tract

Stanley R. Hamilton
John L. Farber
Emanuel Rubin

SMALL INTESTINE

Congenital Disorders

Atresia and Stenosis

Meckel Diverticulum

Meconium Ileus

Infections

Bacterial Diarrhea

Viral Gastroenteritis

Tuberculosis

Vascular Diseases

Acute Intestinal Ischemia

Chronic Intestinal Ischemia

Malabsorption

Causes of Luminal-Phase Malabsorption

Causes of Intestinal-Phase Malabsorption

Lactase Deficiency

Celiac Disease (Celiac Sprue)

Whipple Disease

Tropical Sprue

Mechanical Obstruction

Intussusception

Volvulus

Adhesions

Hernias

Neoplasms

Benign Tumors

Malignant Tumors

LARGE INTESTINE

Congenital Disorders

Congenital Megacolon (Hirschsprung Disease)

Anorectal Malformations

Infections

Pseudomembranous Colitis

Neonatal Necrotizing Enterocolitis

Diverticular Disease

Diverticulosis

Diverticulitis

Inflammatory Bowel Disease

Crohn's Disease

Ulcerative Colitis

Vascular Diseases

Ischemic Colitis

Angiodysplasia (Vascular Ectasia)

Hemorrhoids

Polyps of the Colon

Adenomatous Polyps

Inherited Adenomatous Polyposis Syndromes

Nonneoplastic Polyps

Adenocarcinoma of the Colon and Rectum

Risk Factors

Cancer of the Anal Canal

APPENDIX

Acute Appendicitis

Neoplasms

Mucocele

Carcinoid Tumor

Esophagus

TRACHEOESOPHAGEAL FISTULA

■ *Tracheoesophageal fistula is a communication between the trachea and esophagus* (Fig. 13-1). It is the most common esophageal anomaly and is frequently combined with some form of **esophageal atresia**. Esophageal atresia and fistulas are often associated with congenital heart disease.

In the most common variety of tracheoesophageal fistula, which accounts for approximately 90% of all such fistulas, the upper portion of the esophagus ends in a blind pouch, and the upper end of the lower segment communicates with the trachea. In this type of atresia, the upper blind sac soon fills with mucus, which the infant then aspirates.

Among the remaining 10% of cases, the most common fistula involves a communication between the proximal esophagus and trachea, and the lower esophageal pouch communicates with the stomach. Infants with this condition develop aspiration immediately after birth. In another variant, termed *H-type fistula*, a communication exists between an intact esophagus and intact trachea.

RINGS AND WEBS

Esophageal Webs. Occasionally, a thin mucosal membrane projects into the lumen of the esophagus. Usually single, the webs are sometimes multiple and can be found anywhere in the esophagus.

Plummer-Vinson (Paterson-Kelly) Syndrome. *This disorder is characterized by (1) a cervical esophageal web, (2) mucosal lesions of the mouth and pharynx, and (3) iron-deficiency anemia.* Dysphagia, which is often associated with aspiration of swallowed food, is the most common clinical manifestation. Ninety percent of cases occur in women. The prevalence of this syndrome has significantly declined in recent years, possibly owing to improved nutrition and addition of supplemental nutrients to food. **Carcinoma of the oropharynx and upper esophagus is a recognized complication of Plummer-Vinson syndrome.**

Schatzki Ring. *This lower esophageal narrowing is seen at the junction of the squamous and columnar epithelium.* Although it has been noted in as many as 14% of barium meal examinations, a Schatzki ring is only uncommonly symptomatic.

ESOPHAGEAL DIVERTICULA

■ *Esophageal diverticulum is an outpouching of the wall that contains all layers of the esophagus. When the sac lacks a muscular layer, it is known as a false diverticulum.* Esophageal diverticula occur in the hypopharyngeal area above the upper esophageal sphincter, in the middle esophagus, and immediately proximal to the lower esophageal sphincter.

Zenker Diverticulum

■ *Zenker diverticulum is an uncommon outpouching that appears high in the esophagus.* It affects men more than women and usually occurs in patients older than 60 years. A Zenker diverticulum can accumulate a large amount of food, and the typical symptom is regurgitation of previously eaten food. Recurrent aspiration pneumonia may be a serious complication.

Traction Diverticula

■ *Traction diverticula are outpouchings that occur principally in the midportion of the esophagus.* They were so named because of their attachment to adjacent mediastinal lymph nodes, usually associated with tuberculous lymphadenitis. However, fibrous adhesions between midesophageal diverticula and diseased mediastinal nodes are uncommon today.

Epiphrenic Diverticula

■ *Epiphrenic diverticula are located immediately above the diaphragm.* Motor disturbances of the esophagus (e.g., achalasia, diffuse esophageal spasm) are found in two-thirds of patients with this true diverticulum. In addition, it has been speculated that reflux esophagitis plays a role in the pathogenesis of epiphrenic diverticula.

Unlike other types, epiphrenic diverticula are encountered in young persons. Nocturnal regurgitation of large amounts of fluid stored in the diverticulum during the day is typical.

MOTOR DISORDERS

Any failure of proper muscular function is included in the concept of motor disorders of the esophagus. The hallmark of motor disorders is difficulty in swallowing, which is termed **dysphagia.** Pain on swallowing is termed **odynophagia.**

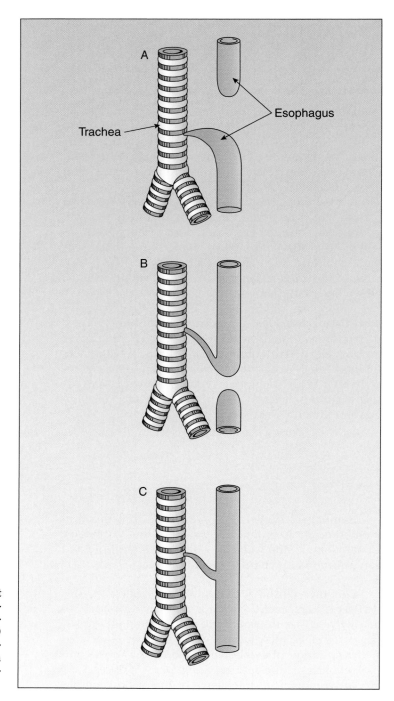

FIGURE   *13-1*
Congenital tracheoesophageal fistulas. (A) The most common type is a communication between the trachea and the lower portion of the esophagus. The upper segment of the esophagus ends in a blind sac. (B) In a few cases, the proximal esophagus communicates with the trachea. (C) The least common anomaly, the H type, is a fistula between a continuous esophagus and the trachea.

Achalasia

■ *Achalasia, which was at one time termed car-diospasm, is a disease characterized by the absence of peristalsis in the body of the esophagus and failure of the lower esophageal sphincter to relax in response to swallowing.* As a result of these defects in both the outflow tract and the pumping mechanisms of the esophagus, food is retained within the esophagus, and the organ hypertrophies and dilates conspicuously (Fig. 13-2).

Although the cause of achalasia is not precisely understood, there is a consensus that loss or absence of ganglion cells in the myenteric plexus of the esophagus is involved. In Latin America, achalasia is a common complication of **Chagas disease,** in which the ganglion cells are destroyed by *Trypanosoma cruzi.* Dysphagia, occasionally odynophagia, and regurgitation of material retained in the esophagus are common symptoms of achalasia.

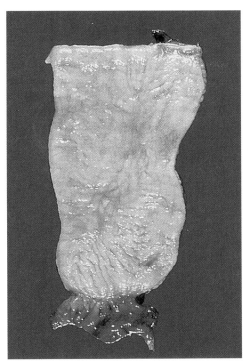

FIGURE *13-2*
Esophagus and upper stomach of a patient with advanced achalasia. The esophagus is markedly dilated above the esophagogastric junction, where the lower esophageal sphincter is located. The esophageal mucosa is redundant and has hyperplastic squamous epithelium.

Scleroderma (Progressive Systemic Sclerosis)

Scleroderma causes fibrosis in many organs and produces a severe abnormality of esophageal muscle function. The disease affects principally the lower esophageal sphincter, which may become so impaired that the lower esophagus and upper stomach are no longer distinct functional entities and are visualized as a common cavity. In addition, there may be a lack of peristalsis in the entire esophagus.

Microscopically, fibrosis of the esophageal smooth muscle and submucosa as well as nonspecific inflammatory changes are seen. Intimal fibrosis of the small arteries and arterioles is common and may play a role in the pathogenesis of the fibrosis. Clinically, patients suffer dysphagia and heartburn caused by peptic esophagitis, owing to reflux of acid from the stomach.

HIATAL HERNIA

■ *Hiatal hernia is a herniation of the stomach through an enlarged esophageal hiatus in the diaphragm* (Fig. 13-3). A

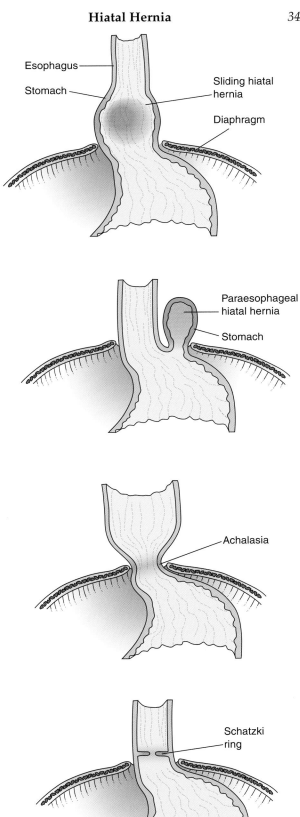

FIGURE *13-3*
Disorders of the esophageal outlet.

common acquired condition, hiatal hernia is, in most cases, of unknown cause.

Sliding Hernia

■ *Sliding hernia is an enlargement of the diaphragmatic hiatus and a laxity of the circumferential connective tissue that allows a cap of gastric cardia to move upward to a position above the diaphragm.* Sliding hiatal hernia is asymptomatic in the large majority of patients, and only 5% of those diagnosed radiologically complain of symptoms referable to gastroesophageal reflux.

Paraesophageal Hernia

■ *Paraesophageal hernia is characterized by herniation of a portion of the gastric fundus beside the esophagus through a defect in the diaphragmatic connective tissue membrane that defines the esophageal hiatus.* With time, the hernia enlarges, and the hiatus progressively widens.

☐ **Clinical Features:** Symptoms of hiatal hernia, particularly heartburn and regurgitation, are attributed to gastroesophageal reflux. Classically, symptoms are exacerbated when the affected person is in the recumbent position, which facilitates acid reflux.

ESOPHAGITIS

Reflux Esophagitis

■ *Reflux esophagitis is an esophageal injury caused by the regurgitation of gastric contents into the lower esophagus.* By far the most common type of esophagitis, it is usually found in conjunction with a sliding hiatal hernia, although it may occur through an incompetent lower esophageal sphincter without any demonstrable anatomic lesion.

☐ **Pathogenesis:** The principal barrier to reflux of gastric contents into the esophagus is the lower esophageal sphincter. Transient reflux is a normal event, particularly after a meal. When these episodes become more frequent and are prolonged, however, esophagitis results. Although acid is damaging to the esophageal mucosa, the combination of acid and pepsin may be particularly injurious. Moreover, gastric fluid often contains refluxed bile from the duodenum, which is believed to be harmful to the esophageal mucosa.

☐ **Pathology:** If reflux is chronic, then thickening of the epithelium, traditionally termed **leukoplakia,** is occasionally seen as irregular, grayish-white patches.

Areas affected by reflux are susceptible to superficial mucosal ulcerations, which appear as vertical linear streaks. Microscopically, the basal layer of the epithelium is thickened, and the papillae of the lamina propria are elongated and extend toward the surface. A modest increase in the number of lymphocytes is seen in the lamina propria, and neutrophils and eosinophils may be present within the squamous epithelium.

Esophageal stricture may eventuate among those cases in which the ulcer persists and damages the esophageal wall deep to the lamina propria. In this circumstance, fibrosis is stimulated and, in turn, narrows the esophageal lumen.

Barrett Esophagus

■ *Barrett epithelium is replacement of the squamous epithelium of the esophagus by columnar epithelium secondary to chronic gastroesophageal reflux.* The majority of patients with Barrett esophagus drink alcoholic beverages regularly and smoke tobacco. This disorder occurs most commonly in the lower one-third of the esophagus, but it may extend higher. **Barrett epithelium represents columnar metaplasia of the squamous epithelium in response to the injury produced by chronic gastroesophageal reflux.**

☐ **Pathology:** The metaplastic Barrett epithelium may occur in patches or line the entire lower esophagus (Fig. 13-4). Histologically, the lesion is characterized by three types of metaplasia: (1) cardiac-like mucous glands, resembling those ordinarily seen at the gastroesophageal junction, with no parietal or chief cells being present; (2) an epithelium similar to that of the fundus of the stomach, with short glands containing parietal and chief cells; and (3) a distinctive, intestinal-like epithelium composed of goblet cells and surface cells similar to those of the gastric mucosa (see Fig. 13-4). Inflammatory changes are usually superimposed on the epithelial alterations, and in some cases, ulceration and even a stricture are found above the metaplastic epithelium. **As might be expected with a metaplastic epithelium, Barrett esophagus carries a serious risk of malignant transformation to adenocarcinoma.**

Infectious Esophagitis

Primary infections of the esophagus are rare, with the exceptions of candidiasis and herpes simplex.

Candida **Esophagitis:** This fungal infection has become common because of an increasing number of immunocompromised persons who (1) receive chemotherapy for malignant disease, (2) are treated with immunosuppressive drugs after organ transplan-

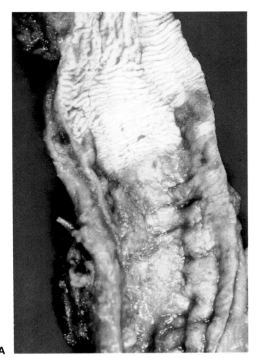
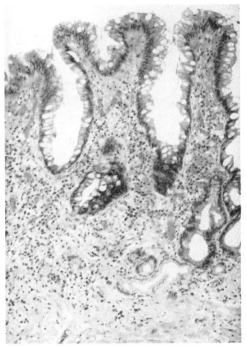

A

B

FIGURE 13-4

Barrett esophagus. (A) The white, squamous mucosa of the proximal esophagus (*top*) is contrasted with the columnar lining of the distal Barrett esophagus (*bottom*). (B) A microscopic section of the metaplastic epithelium in *panel A* shows a villiform surface with numerous goblet cells.

tation, or (3) have contracted acquired immunodeficiency syndrome. Dysphagia and severe pain on swallowing are usual, and bleeding from the infected site is common and, sometimes, severe.

In mild cases of candidiasis, a few small, elevated white plaques surrounded by a hyperemic zone are present on the mucosa of the middle or lower one-third of the esophagus. In severe cases, confluent pseudomembranes lie on a hyperemic and edematous mucosa. Microscopically, the candidal pseudomembrane contains fungal mycelia, necrotic debris, and fibrin.

Herpetic Esophagitis. Esophageal infection with herpesvirus type I is most frequently associated with lymphomas and leukemias. Indeed, the esophagus is the most common viscus that is involved with herpesvirus in those diseases. The well-developed lesions of herpetic esophagitis are grossly similar to those of candidiasis. In early cases, small ulcers or plaques are noted, and, as the infection progresses, these may coalesce to form larger lesions. Microscopically, the lesions are superficial, and the epithelial cells exhibit typical herpetic inclusions in their nuclei.

Chemical Esophagitis

Chemical injury to the esophagus is usually the result of accidental poisoning in children or attempted suicide in adults. It is produced by the intake of strong alkaline agents (e.g., lye) or strong acids (e.g., sulfuric or hydrochloric acid), both of which are used in various cleaning solutions.

□ **Pathology:** Histologically, alkali-induced liquefactive necrosis is accompanied by conspicuous inflammation and saponification of the membrane lipids in the epithelium, submucosa, and muscularis of the esophagus and stomach. Thrombosis of small vessels adds ischemic necrosis to the injury. Severe injury is the rule with liquid alkali, but less than 25% of those who ingest granular preparations have severe complications.

Strong acids produce immediate coagulation necrosis, which results in a protective eschar that, in turn, prevents injury and limits penetration. Nevertheless, half of the patients who ingest concentrated hydrochloric or sulfuric acid suffer severe esophageal injury.

ESOPHAGEAL VARICES

■ *Esophageal varices are dilated veins immediately beneath the mucosa, which are prone to rupture and hemor-*

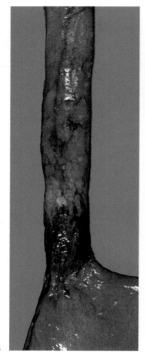
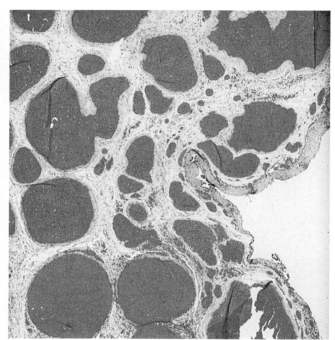

A   B

FIGURE   *13-5*
**Esophageal varices. (A) Numerous prominent, blue venous channels are seen beneath the
mucosa of the everted esophagus, particularly above the gastroesophageal junction. (B)
A section of the esophagus reveals numerous dilated submucosal veins.**

rhage (Fig. 13-5). They arise in the lower one-third of
the esophagus, virtually always in the setting of portal
hypertension secondary to cirrhosis of the liver. When
the varices reach a diameter greater than 5 mm, they
are likely to burst, in which case life-threatening hemorrhage ensues. See Chapter 14 for a further discussion
of esophageal varices.

CANCER OF THE ESOPHAGUS

Squamous Carcinoma

Worldwide, the majority of cancers of the esophagus
are squamous cell carcinomas. However, adenocarcinoma is now common in the United States.

☐ **Epidemiology:** The incidence of squamous carcinoma of the esophagus in the United States is low, accounting for only 7% of all gastrointestinal cancers.
However, worldwide geographic variations in the incidence of esophageal carcinoma are striking, and areas of high incidence are located adjacent to areas of
low incidence. There is an esophageal cancer "belt" extending across Asia from the Caspian Sea region of
northern Iran and the former Soviet Union through
Central Asia and Mongolia to northern China. In parts

of China, the mortality rate from esophageal cancer in
men is reported to be some 70-fold greater than that in
the United States. By contrast, a Chinese province near
one of these areas has a mortality rate comparable to
that in the United States. Similarly, the Caspian region
of Iran has an incidence of esophageal carcinoma approximately 30-fold greater than that in the United
States, whereas more southern zones of Iran have a low
incidence. In the United States, blacks have a considerably greater incidence than whites, and urban dwellers
are at greater risk than those in rural areas. Cancer of
the esophagus is also common in certain regions of
France, Finland, Switzerland, Chile, Japan, India, and
Africa. By contrast, other Scandinavian countries,
Holland, and Austria have low frequencies. In the
United States, there is a male predominance of approximately 3:1.

☐ **Pathogenesis:** The geographic variation in the
rates of esophageal cancer, even in relatively homogeneous populations, suggests that environmental factors contribute strongly to the development of this disease. However, no single factor can be incriminated as
being the cause of esophageal cancer.

- **Excessive consumption of alcohol** may be a risk
  factor in the United States, even when cigarette
  smoking and degree of urbanization are taken into
  account.

- **Cigarette smoking** is associated with a two- to fourfold increase in the risk of esophageal cancer.
- **Nitrosamines** and aniline dyes produce esophageal cancer in animals. Direct evidence for their contribution to human esophageal cancer, however, is lacking.
- **Diets lacking in fresh fruits, vegetables, and animal protein** have been described in areas endemic for esophageal cancer. In some hyperendemic areas, deficiencies of various vitamins and minerals have been claimed. However, the close proximity of endemic and nonendemic areas renders a causative role for these dietary factors unlikely.
- **Plummer-Vinson syndrome and celiac sprue** are both associated with an increased incidence of esophageal cancer.
- **Achalasia** is a well-known predisposing factor for esophageal carcinoma.
- **Esophageal stricture** is a risk factor. Five percent of persons with an esophageal stricture after ingesting lye develop cancer 20 to 40 years later.
- **Webs, rings, and diverticula** are sometimes associated with esophageal cancer.

Although the pathogenesis of esophageal cancer is not understood, it is tempting to speculate that irritation of the mucosa by gastric contents or other agents may stimulate cell proliferation and, thereby, act as a promoter for cells initiated by exposure to environmental carcinogens, such as those contained in tobacco smoke.

☐ **Pathology:** Approximately half of the cases of esophageal cancer involve the lower one-third of the esophagus; the middle and upper one-thirds account for the remainder. Grossly, the tumors are of three types: (1) **polypoid,** which projects into the lumen (Fig. 13-6); (2) **ulcerating,** which is usually smaller than polypoid; and (3) **infiltrating,** for which the principal plane of growth is in the wall. Usually, these features overlap. The bulky polypoid tumors tend to obstruct early, whereas the ulcerated ones are more likely to bleed. Infiltrating tumors gradually narrow the lumen by circumferential compression. Local extension of the tumor is commonly a major problem. Microscopically, the neoplastic squamous cells range from well differentiated, with epithelial "pearls," to poorly differentiated.

☐ **Clinical Features:** The most common presenting complaint is dysphagia, which is usually not recognized until the diameter of the esophageal lumen is reduced by 30% to 50%. By this time, most tumors are unresectable. Esophageal cancer spreads to the regional lymph nodes and, occasionally, to the lungs and liver.

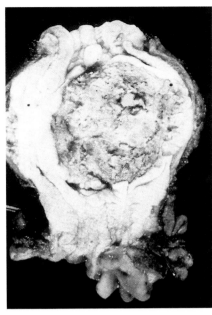

FIGURE *13-6*
Carcinoma of the esophagus. A large, fungating, ulcerated squamous carcinoma of the esophagus is surrounded by apparently normal mucosa.

Patients with esophageal cancer are almost invariably cachectic owing to the remote effects of a malignant tumor, anorexia, and difficulty in eating. Surgery and radiation therapy are useful for palliation, but the prognosis remains dismal.

Adenocarcinoma

The incidence of adenocarcinoma of the esophagus has been increasing in recent years and may now be greater than 50% in the United States. **Virtually all adenocarcinomas arise in Barrett epithelium**. The symptoms and clinical course of adenocarcinoma are similar to those of squamous cell carcinoma of the esophagus, but a 5-year survival rate of 20% following radical surgery has been reported.

Stomach

CONGENITAL PYLORIC STENOSIS

■ *Congenital pyloric stenosis is a concentric enlargement of the pylorus and narrowing of the pyloric canal that obstructs the outlet of the stomach.* The disorder is the most common indication for abdominal surgery during the initial 6 months of life. It is fourfold more common in males than in females, and it affects first-born children more often than subsequent ones.

☐ **Pathogenesis:** Congenital pyloric stenosis may have a genetic basis. There is a familial tendency, and the condition is more common in identical than in fraternal twins. Pyloric stenosis has also been recorded in the context of other developmental abnormalities, such as Turner syndrome, trisomy 18, and esophageal atresia. Embryopathies associated with rubella infection and maternal intake of thalidomide have been associated with congenital pyloric stenosis. In general, the disorder has been attributed to multifactorial inheritance. Evidence has been presented that, at least in some cases, congenital pyloric stenosis is associated with a deficiency of nitric oxide synthase in the nerves of pyloric smooth muscle (nitric oxide mediates relaxation of smooth muscle).

☐ **Pathology:** Gross examination of the stomach shows concentric enlargement of the pylorus and narrowing of the pyloric canal. The only consistent microscopic abnormality is extreme hypertrophy of the circular muscle coat. After pyloromyotomy, the "tumor" disappears, although occasionally. a small, symptomatic mass remains.

☐ **Clinical Features:** Symptoms of pyloric stenosis usually become apparent within the first month of life, when the infant manifests **projectile vomiting**. A palpable pyloric "tumor" and visible peristalsis are characteristic of the disorder. Surgical incision of the hypertrophied pyloric muscle is curative.

GASTRITIS

The terms **acute gastritis** and **chronic gastritis** may be confusing, because to the pathologist, they refer only to the morphologic appearance of gastric injury and do not connote a temporal difference. Yet, acute gastritis is ordinarily a self-limited disorder, whereas chronic gastritis is typically present for many years. Therefore, it seems preferable to use the terms **erosive** for acute gastritis and **nonerosive** for chronic gastritis.

Acute Hemorrhagic (Erosive Gastritis)

■ *Acute hemorrhagic gastritis is the presence of focal necrosis of the mucosa in an otherwise normal stomach.* Erosion of the mucosa may extend into the deeper tissues to form an acute ulcer. The necrosis is accompanied by an acute inflammatory response and, often, by hemorrhage as well. In fact, hemorrhage may be so severe as to result in exsanguination.

☐ **Pathogenesis:** Today, acute hemorrhagic gastritis is most commonly associated with the intake of aspirin, other nonsteroidal anti-inflammatory agents, and excess alcohol. These agents are directly injurious to the gastric mucosa, and they exert their effects topically. Oral administration of corticosteroids also is occasionally complicated by hemorrhagic gastritis. Uncommonly, accidental or suicidal ingestion of corrosive substances, such as those that produce erosive esophagitis, produces acute gastric injury.

Any serious illness that is accompanied by profound physiologic alterations that require substantial medical or surgical intervention renders the gastric mucosa more vulnerable to acute hemorrhagic gastritis. The one factor common to all such situations is generally believed to be "stress." Stress ulcers, long known to occur in severely burned persons **(Curling ulcer)**, commonly result in bleeding, which is occasionally severe.

Trauma to the central nervous system, either accidental or surgical **(Cushing ulcer)**, is another cause of stress ulcers. These ulcers may also occur in the esophagus or duodenum. They are characteristically deep, and they carry a substantial risk of perforation. **Severe trauma,** especially if accompanied by **shock, prolonged sepsis,** and **incapacitation** from many debilitating chronic diseases, also predispose patients to the development of hemorrhagic gastritis.

Hypersecretion of gastric acid has been incriminated in the pathogenesis of hemorrhagic gastritis, but its role is not clear. Gastric acid may play a permissive role, because inhibition of gastric acid secretion (e.g., with histamine receptor antagonists) protects against the development of stress ulcers.

Microcirculatory changes in the stomach induced by shock or sepsis suggest that ischemic injury may contribute to the development of hemorrhagic gastritis.

Impaired protective mechanisms of the gastric mucosa have been demonstrated, including decreased mucus production, prostaglandin deficiency, interference with renewal of gastric epithelial cells, and lowered intramural pH of the gastric mucosa.

☐ **Pathology:** The typical case of acute hemorrhagic gastritis is characterized grossly by widespread petechial hemorrhages in any portion of the stomach (Fig. 13-7). Erosions vary in size from 1 to 25 mm across and, occasionally, appear as sharply punched-out ulcers. Microscopically, patchy mucosal necrosis extending to the submucosa is visualized adjacent to normal mucosa. The necrotic epithelium is eventually sloughed, and deeper erosions and hemorrhage may be present. Depending on the age of the process, there may be mild inflammation, which is initially neutrophilic and

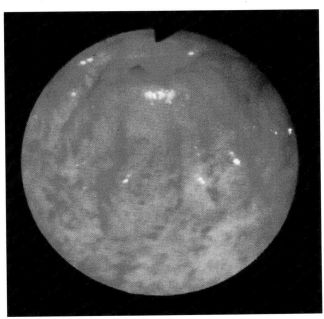

FIGURE *13-7*
Erosive gastritis. This endoscopic view of the stomach in a patient who was ingesting aspirin reveals acute hemorrhagic lesions.

then mononuclear. Healing is usually complete within a few days.

☐ **Clinical Features:** The symptoms of acute hemorrhagic gastritis range from vague abdominal discomfort to massive, life-threatening hemorrhage or clinical manifestations of gastric perforation. Patients with acute gastritis induced by aspirin and other nonsteroidal anti-inflammatory agents may present with hypochromic, microcytic anemia caused by undetected, chronic bleeding. In patients with a severe underlying illness, the first sign of stress ulcers may be exsanguinating hemorrhage. In critically ill patients, the overall mortality rate of hemorrhagic gastritis may reach 40% to 50%. Treatment with antacids and histamine receptor antagonists has proved to be useful, particularly when these agents are given prophylactically.

Chronic Gastritis

■ *Chronic gastritis refers to chronic inflammatory diseases of the stomach, which range from mild, superficial involvement of the gastric mucosa to severe atrophy.*

Autoimmune Gastritis and Pernicious Anemia

■ *Autoimmune gastritis is a chronic, diffuse inflammatory disease of the stomach that is restricted to the body and fundus and is associated with autoimmune phenomena.* This disorder typically exhibits:

- Diffuse atrophic gastritis in the body and fundus of the stomach, with lack of or only minimal involvement of the antrum.
- Antibodies to parietal cells and intrinsic factor.
- Significant reduction in or absence of gastric secretion, including acid.
- Increased serum gastrin because of G-cell hyperplasia of the antral mucosa.
- Enterochromaffin-like cell hyperplasia in atrophic oxyntic mucosa due to gastrin stimulation.

■ *Pernicious anemia is a megaloblastic anemia that is associated with complete achlorhydria and is caused by malabsorption of vitamin B_{12}, which, in turn, is occasioned by a deficiency of intrinsic factor.* **In the large majority of cases, pernicious anemia is a complication of autoimmune gastritis.**

☐ **Pathogenesis:** Autoimmune gastritis is so named because of the presence of autoantibodies and the association with other diseases believed to have a similar pathogenesis. Autoantibodies include cytotoxic antibodies to parietal cells, intrinsic factor antibodies, and antibodies to other tissues (e.g., thyroid). Although these phenomena are conspicuous in patients with pernicious anemia, it remains to be established whether they cause the chronic gastritis or represent reactive epiphenomena. Genetic factors may also play a role, because pernicious anemia shows a familial tendency.

Multifocal Atrophic Gastritis (Environmental Metaplastic Atrophic Gastritis)

■ *Multifocal atrophic gastritis is an inflammatory disease of the stomach with an uncertain cause that typically involves the antrum and adjacent areas of the body.* This form of chronic gastritis has the following features:

- It is considerably more common than the autoimmune variety of chronic gastritis and is, perhaps, fourfold as frequent in whites as in other races.
- It is not linked to autoimmune phenomena.
- Similar to autoimmune gastritis, it is often associated with reduced acid secretion (hypochlorhydria).
- Complete absence of gastric secretion (achlorhydria) and pernicious anemia are uncommon.

☐ **Epidemiology and Pathogenesis:** The age and geographic distribution of environmental metaplastic gastritis parallel that of carcinoma of the stomach, and this type of gastritis is believed to be a precursor of this cancer. The disease exhibits a striking localization to certain populations, being particularly common in Asia, Scandinavia, and parts of Europe and Latin America. It also demonstrates an increasing incidence with age in all populations in which it is prevalent. In asymptomatic Japanese, chronic idiopathic gastritis was found in 90% of men and women older than 60 years. Approximately half of the adult population of Finland, Italy, and Hungary has been reported to show evidence of chronic gastritis. Environmental factors in its etiology include infection with *Helicobacter pylori* infection (discussed later) and diet.

☐ **Pathology:** The pathologic features of autoimmune and multifocal atrophic gastritis are virtually identical, except for the localization of the autoimmune type to the fundus and body and of the multifocal variety mainly to the antrum.

Superficial Gastritis. This is the mildest form of nonerosive gastritis. Although superficial gastritis may occasionally revert to normal, it is estimated that it proceeds to atrophic gastritis in nearly half of the cases. Superficial gastritis typically shows lymphocytes and plasma cells and, occasionally, neutrophils, in the lamina propria of the mucosa of the antrum and body of the stomach.

Atrophic Gastritis. This condition may evolve from superficial gastritis, but there is no sharp distinction between the two. Like superficial gastritis, active atrophic gastritis is characterized by prominent chronic inflammation in the lamina propria. However, lymphocytes and plasma cells extend into the deepest reaches of the mucosa, as far as the muscularis mucosae. Occasionally, lymphoid cells are arranged as follicles, which is an appearance that can lead to an erroneous diagnosis of lymphoma or pseudolymphoma. Involvement of the gastric glands proceeds to degenerative changes in their epithelial cells and, ultimately, a conspicuous reduction in the number of glands, hence the name atrophic gastritis (Fig. 13-8). Eventually, the inflammatory process may abate, leaving only a thin, atrophic mucosa, in which case the term **gastric atrophy** is applied.

Intestinal Metaplasia. This lesion is a common and important histologic feature of both autoimmune and multifocal atrophic chronic gastritis. In this response of the injured gastric mucosa, the normal epithelium is replaced by one that is composed of intestinal-type cells (Fig. 13-9). Numerous mucin-containing goblet cells and enterocytes line crypt-like glands, and many Paneth cells, which are not normal inhabitants of the

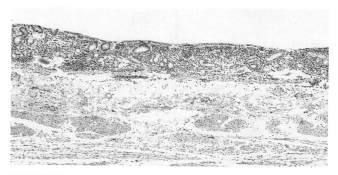

FIGURE *13-8*
Atrophic gastritis. The gastric mucosa is thinned and displays a conspicuous, chronic inflammatory infiltrate that separates the atrophic glands.

gastric mucosa, are present. However, intestinal villi do not usually form.

Atrophic Gastritis and Stomach Cancer

Persons with atrophic gastritis of the autoimmune or multifocal type have a high incidence of carcinoma of the stomach. Patients with pernicious anemia, who invariably suffer from atrophic gastritis, have a three- to fourfold increased risk of developing gastric cancer. Cancer arises in the antrum several times more frequently than in the body of the stomach. Results of epidemiologic studies—particularly from Japan, where gastric cancer is common—suggest that antral gastritis is related to the development of carcinoma of the stomach. However, direct evidence for a causal connection has not been firmly established. **Intestinal metaplasia of the stomach in particular has been identified as being a preneoplastic lesion.**

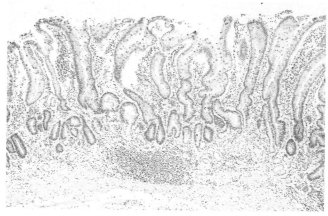

FIGURE *13-9*
Chronic gastritis with intestinal metaplasia. The glands are of the intestinal type, with an evident villous pattern. Chronic inflammation and atrophic gastric glands are seen immediately above the muscularis mucosae.

Helicobacter pylori Gastritis

***Helicobacter pylori* gastritis** *is a chronic inflammatory disease of the antrum and body of the stomach caused by infection with* H. pylori. It is the most common type of chronic gastritis in the United States, and the organism causes one of the most frequent chronic infections among humans. In the United States, it is estimated that approximately one-third of all asymptomatic adults have histologic evidence of *H. pylori* gastritis. *H. pylori* **infection is also strongly associated with peptic ulcer disease of the stomach and duodenum** (discussed later).

□ **Pathogenesis:** The prevalence of infection with *H. pylori* increases with age, and by 60 years, it is estimated that as much as half the population has serologic evidence of infection. Approximately two-thirds of those infected with *H. pylori* manifest histologic evidence of chronic gastritis. ***H. pylori* infection has been found only in association with gastric-type epithelium and does not occur in other tissues.** Although the bacterium is clearly associated with chronic gastritis, it is found only on the epithelial surface and does not invade the gastric mucosa.

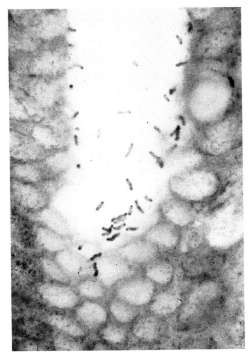

FIGURE **13-10**
Helicobacter pylori **gastritis.** *Helicobacter pylori* **appears on silver staining as small, curved rods on the surface of the gastric mucosa.**

□ **Pathology:** The curved rods of *H. pylori* are found in the surface mucus of the epithelial cells and in the gastric foveolae (Fig. 13-10). Active gastritis features polymorphonuclear leukocytes in the neck glands and increased numbers of plasma cells and lymphocytes in the lamina propria. It has been claimed that chronic infectious gastritis caused by *H. pylori* can lead to gastric atrophy and intestinal metaplasia. In addition, infection with *H. pylori* has been linked to the development of gastric adenocarcinoma (discussed later).

□ **Clinical Features of Chronic Gastritis:** The predominant symptom ascribed to chronic gastritis has been dyspepsia. However, gastritis is so common—and such symptomatic complaints are so nonspecific—that any association with specific symptoms remains suspect. Among populations in whom chronic idiopathic gastritis is endemic, the disease is commonly discovered in asymptomatic persons undergoing routine endoscopic screening.

PEPTIC ULCER DISEASE

■ *Peptic ulcer disease refers to breaks in the mucosa of the stomach and small intestine, principally the proximal duodenum, that are produced by the action of gastric secretions.* Peptic ulcers of the stomach and duodenum are estimated to afflict 10% of the population in Western industrialized countries at some time during their lives. It remains unknown why ulcers develop—and also why they heal. Although peptic ulceration can occur as high as the Barrett esophagus and as low as Meckel diverticulum of the ileum, for practical purposes **peptic ulcer disease affects the distal stomach and the proximal duodenum.** Many clinical and epidemiologic features distinguish gastric from duodenal ulcers; the common factor that unites them is gastric secretion of hydrochloric acid. **With rare exceptions, a person who does not secrete acid will not develop a peptic ulcer anywhere.**

□ **Epidemiology:** The peak incidence of duodenal ulcer disease is between the ages of 30 and 60 years, although the disorder may occur in persons of any age (even infants). Gastric ulcers afflict the middle-aged and elderly more than young persons. The incidence of gastric ulcers is the same for men and women.

□ **Pathogenesis:**

Environmental Factors. It does not appear that consumption of alcohol, caffeine, or spicy foods is linked to either gastric or duodenal ulcers. However, cirrhosis from any cause is associated with an increased incidence of peptic ulcers. Aspirin and other nonsteroidal anti-inflammatory agents are important contributing factors in the genesis of duodenal and, especially, gastric ulcers. Cigarette smoking is a definite risk factor for duodenal and gastric ulcers, particularly gastric ulcers.

Genetic Factors. First-degree relatives of patients with duodenal ulcers have a threefold increased risk of developing a duodenal ulcer themselves, but they do not have a similar increase in risk for gastric ulcer. Patients with gastric ulcers similarly "breed true." These data are confirmed by the finding of a considerably higher concordance for these ulcers in monozygotic than in dizygotic twins. That identical twins show only a 50% concordance indicates that genetic factors alone are not sufficient to produce an ulcer; environmental factors must also be involved.

Blood-group antigens provide further evidence for the role of genetic factors. The risk of duodenal ulcer is approximately 30% higher in persons with type O blood than in those with types A, B, or AB. Interestingly, patients with gastric ulcers do not exhibit a greater frequency of blood group O. The one-fourth of the population that does not secrete blood-group antigens in the saliva and gastric juice is at a 50% increased risk of developing a duodenal ulcer. The risk of duodenal ulceration is more conspicuously increased (2.5 : 1) when nonsecretory status is combined with blood group O, which is a combination that occurs in 10% of the white population.

Pepsinogen I is secreted by the chief and mucous neck cells of the gastric mucosa, and it appears in the gastric juice, blood, and urine. Serum levels of this proenzyme correlate with the gastric capacity for acid secretion and are considered to be a measure of parietal cell mass. A person with high circulating levels of pepsinogen I is at fivefold the normal risk of developing a duodenal ulcer.

Psychological Factors

"Stress" has been anecdotally related to peptic ulcers for at least a century, and repressed stress has been considered to be particularly ulcerogenic. The common stereotype of the patient with a peptic ulcer is that of a highly motivated executive operating in a stressful environment. However, results of careful epidemiologic surveys in both the United States and Great Britain have actually suggested an inverse relationship between duodenal ulcers and socioeconomic status and education, although the trends are not marked. Whatever the final outcome of this debate may be, there is no need to incriminate stress in the pathogenesis of peptic ulcers.

Hydrochloric Acid

The formation and persistence of peptic ulcers in both the stomach and duodenum require the gastric secretion of acid. Gastric secretion of pepsin, which may also play a role in production of peptic ulcers, parallels that of hydrochloric acid.

Physiological Factors in Duodenal Ulcers

The maximal capacity for acid production by the stomach is a reflection of the total parietal cell mass. Both parietal cell mass and maximal acid secretion are increased as much as twofold in patients with duodenal ulcers. However, there is a large overlap with normal values, and **only one-third of these patients secrete excess acid.** The increase in the number of parietal cells is paralleled by a comparable increase in chief cells, a situation that is consistent with the increased prevalence of hyperpepsinogenemia in patients with ulcers.

Accelerated gastric emptying, which is a condition that might lead to excessive acidification of the duodenum, has been noted in patients with duodenal ulcers. However, as with other factors, there is substantial overlap with normal rates.

The pH of the duodenal bulb reflects the balance between the delivery of gastric juice and its neutralization by biliary, pancreatic, and duodenal secretions. The production of duodenal ulcers requires an acidic pH in the bulb—that is, an excess of acid over neutralizing secretions.

Impaired mucosal defenses have been invoked as contributing to peptic ulceration. The mucosal factors, including the function of prostaglandins, may or may not be similar to those protecting the gastric mucosa.

Physiological Factors in Gastric Ulcers

Gastric ulcers almost invariably arise in the soil of chronic, nonerosive antral gastritis. Most patients with gastric ulcers secrete less acid than those with duodenal ulcers—and even less than normal persons. The occurrence of gastric ulcers in the presence of gastric hyposecretion implies the following possibilities: (1) the gastric mucosa is, in some way, particularly sensitive to low concentrations of acid; (2) some material other than acid damages the mucosa; or (3) the gastric mucosa is exposed to potentially injurious agents for an unusually long period of time.

Role of *Helicobacter pylori*

***H. pylori* has been isolated from the gastric antrum of virtually all patients with duodenal ulcers.** It is important to emphasize that the converse is *not* true—that is, only a small minority of persons infected with *H. pylori* suffer from duodenal ulcer disease. Thus, *H. pylori* infection may be accepted as a necessary, but not sufficient, condition for development of peptic ulcer disease of the duodenum.

The mechanism by which *H. pylori* infection predisposes to duodenal ulcers is unknown. Infection with *H. pylori* may stimulate acid secretion by promoting gastrin release and suppressing somatostatin secretion. The release of histamine metabolites by the organism may increase basal acid secretion. Acidification of the duodenal bulb leads to islands of metaplastic gastric mucosa, which show the same colonization with *H. pylori* as the gastric mucosa. It has been theorized that infection of the metaplastic epithelium by

H. pylori may render the mucosa more susceptible to peptic injury (Fig. 13-11).

Infection with *H. pylori* is probably also important in the pathogenesis of gastric ulcers, because this organism is responsible for most cases of chronic gastritis that underlies this disease. It is estimated that three-quarters of patients with gastric ulcers harbor *H. pylori*.

The various gastric and duodenal factors that have been implicated as possible mechanisms in the pathogenesis of duodenal ulceration are summarized in Figure 13-12.

Diseases Associated with Peptic Ulcers

Cirrhosis. The incidence of duodenal ulcers in patients with cirrhosis is tenfold greater than in normal persons.

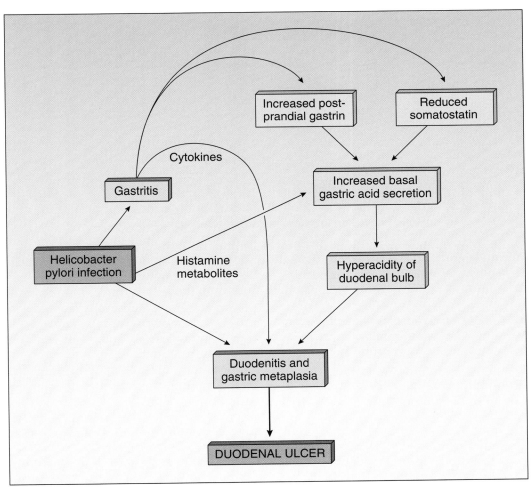

FIGURE   *13-11*
Possible mechanisms in the pathogenesis of duodenal ulcer disease associated with *Helicobacter pylori* **infection.**

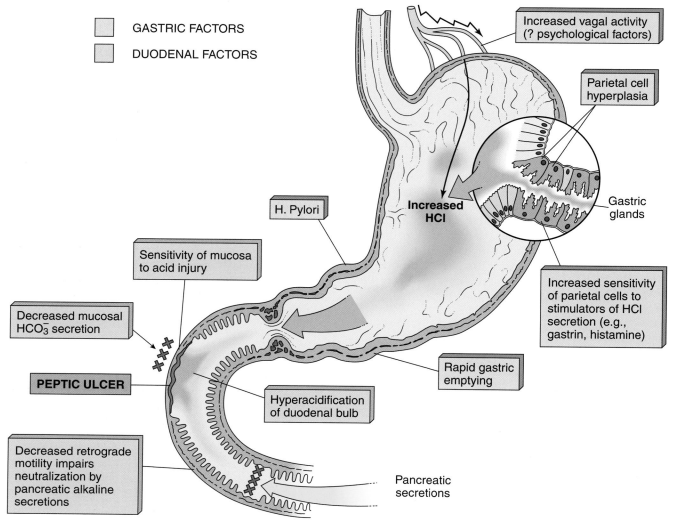

GASTRIC FACTORS

DUODENAL FACTORS

Increased vagal activity
(? psychological factors)

Parietal cell
hyperplasia

H. Pylori

Sensitivity of mucosa
to acid injury

Increased
HCl

Gastric
glands

Decreased mucosal
HCO$_3^-$ secretion

Increased sensitivity
of parietal cells to
stimulators of HCl
secretion (e.g.,
gastrin, histamine)

PEPTIC ULCER

Hyperacidification
of duodenal bulb

Rapid gastric
emptying

Decreased retrograde
motility impairs
neutralization by
pancreatic alkaline
secretions

Pancreatic
secretions

FIGURE 13-12
Gastric and duodenal factors in the pathogenesis of duodenal peptic ulcers.

Chronic Renal Failure. Patients subjected to renal transplantation show a substantially increased incidence of peptic ulceration.

Hereditary Endocrine Syndromes. Multiple endocrine neoplasia type I (Zollinger-Ellison syndrome; see Chapter 15) is a cause of severe peptic ulceration.

Chronic Pulmonary Disease. Fully one-fourth of the patients with longstanding pulmonary dysfunction suffer from peptic ulcer disease.

☐ **Pathology:** A peptic ulcer should be considered chronic when it does not heal readily and when scarring at its base precludes complete restoration of the normal submucosa and muscularis. Most peptic ulcers arise in the lesser curvature of the stomach, in the antral and prepyloric regions, and in the first part of the duodenum.

Gastric ulcers (Fig. 13-13) are usually single and less than 2 cm in diameter, although occasionally they reach a diameter of 10 cm or more, particularly if they are on the lesser curvature. The edges are sharply punched out, with overhanging margins. The flat base is gray and indurated, and it may exhibit clotted blood or an eroded vessel.

Duodenal ulcers (Fig. 13-14) are ordinarily located on the anterior or posterior wall of the first part of the duodenum, within a short distance of the pylorus. The lesion is usually solitary, but it is not uncommon to find paired ulcers on both walls (so-called "kissing ulcers").

Microscopically, gastric and duodenal ulcers have a similar appearance (Fig. 13-15). From the lumen outward, the following are noted: (1) a superficial zone of fibrinopurulent exudate, (2) necrotic tissue, (3) granulation tissue, and (4) fibrotic tissue at the base of the ulcer, which exhibits variable degrees of chronic inflam-

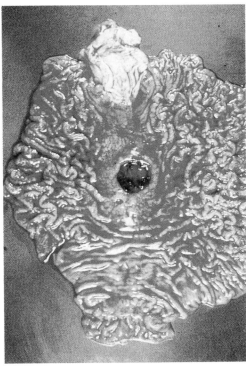

FIGURE   *13-13*
Gastric ulcer. The stomach has been opened to reveal a sharply demarcated, deep peptic ulcer on the lesser curvature.

mation. The ulceration typically penetrates the muscle layers, thereby causing them to be interrupted by scar tissue.

☐ **Clinical Features:** The symptomatologies of gastric and duodenal ulcers are sufficiently similar that the two conditions are generally not distinguishable by history or physical examination. The "classic" case of duodenal ulcer is characterized by burning epigastric pain that is experienced 1 to 3 hours after a meal or that awakens the patient at night. Both alkali and food are

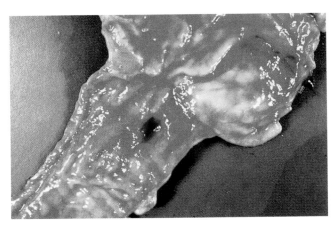

FIGURE   *13-14*
Duodenal ulcer. A sharply punched-out peptic ulcer of the duodenum situated immediately below the pylorus.

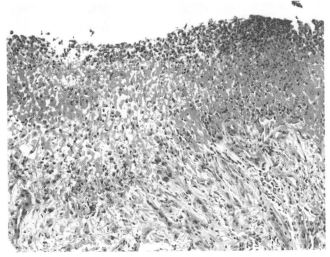

FIGURE   *13-15*
Peptic ulcer of the stomach. A photomicrograph of the ulcer shows the mucosa to be denuded. The surface is covered with a fibrinous exudate containing neutrophils, below which is inflamed granulation tissue.

said to relieve the symptoms. However, detailed studies have demonstrated that the majority of patients do not conform to the "classic" presentation. Half do not describe their pain as being related to meals, and fewer than half report that the pain is relieved by food or alkali.

Hemorrhage. The most common complication of peptic ulcers is bleeding, which occurs in as many as 20% of these patients. In many cases, bleeding is occult and, in an otherwise asymptomatic ulcer, may be manifested as iron-deficiency anemia or occult blood in the stools. **Massive, life-threatening hemorrhage is a well-recognized danger in patients with active peptic ulcers.**

Perforation. Perforation is a serious complication of peptic ulcer disease, occurring in approximately 5% of these patients. Perforations present more commonly with duodenal than with gastric ulcers, and the large majority occur on the anterior wall of the duodenum. **Perforated ulcers continue to be associated with a high mortality rate.** The overall mortality rate for patients with perforated gastric ulcers is 10% to 40%, which is two- to threefold greater than that for patients with duodenal ulcers (5–13%).

Malignant Transformation of a Benign Gastric Ulcer. It is extremely difficult to distinguish a cancer arising in a pre-existing gastric ulcer from an ulcerated primary carcinoma. This difficulty does not complicate the study of duodenal ulcers, however, because **malignant transformation of a duodenal ulcer is virtually unknown.** Cancers originating in well-recognized, benign peptic ulcers probably account for considerably less than 1% of all malignant tumors in the stomach, but such cancers have been documented.

BENIGN NEOPLASMS

Leiomyoma

Leiomyoma, which is a benign tumor of smooth muscle cells, is the most common tumor of the stomach, occurring in 25% to 50% of the population older than 50 years. The tumors range in size from barely detectable nubbins to large masses with a diameter of more than 20 cm. Large tumors may ulcerate and bleed or cause pain.

☐ Pathology: Leiomyomas are submucosal and covered by intact mucosa or, when they project externally, by peritoneum. The cut surface has a whorled appearance and often shows cystic spaces. Microscopically, gastric leiomyomas show variable cellularity and are composed of spindle-shaped smooth muscle cells that are embedded in a collagenous stroma, which is similar to their appearance elsewhere.

Epithelial Polyps

Epithelial polyps of the stomach, which are classified as either hyperplastic or adenomatous, account for almost half of all benign gastric tumors. The large majority of gastric polyps are found in patients with achlorhydria, and both types occur in association with atrophic gastritis and pernicious anemia, as well as in stomachs that harbor carcinoma.

Hyperplastic Polyps. These tumors represent the large majority of polyps. They may be single or multiple and may present as small pedunculated or sessile lesions. Hyperplastic polyps are not true neoplasms, and their origin is uncertain. It is suspected that they result from chronic inflammation and regenerative hyperplasia of the mucosa. Microscopically, the polyps consist of elongated, branched crypts that are lined by normal foveolar epithelium, beneath which pyloric or gastric glands mingle with collagen and smooth muscle fibers. Cystic dilatation of the glands and chronic inflammation may be conspicuous. **Hyperplastic polyps have no malignant potential.**

Adenomatous Polyps. These are true neoplasms, which occur most commonly in the antrum. The polyps range from less than 1 cm in diameter to a considerable size, with the average being approximately 4 cm. Most adenomatous polyps are sessile and are more often single than multiple. Microscopically, adenomas are composed of villous structures or a combination of tubular and villous glands (usually lined by intestinal or superficial gastric epithelium).

Adenomatous polyps manifest a malignant potential, which is variably reported as being from 5% to 75%. This danger increases with the size of the polyp, however, and is greatest for lesions larger than 2 cm in diameter. As in the colon, villous adenomas seem to undergo malignant transformation more frequently than tubular adenomas.

CARCINOMA OF THE STOMACH

As recently as the mid-twentieth century, carcinoma of the stomach was the most common cause of death from cancer among men in the United States. For reasons that have not yet been explained, the incidence of gastric carcinoma has steadily decreased.

☐ Epidemiology: Gastric cancer accounts for 3% of all deaths from cancer in the United States. The incidence of stomach cancer remains exceedingly high in countries such as Japan and Chile, where the rates are seven- to eightfold that in the United States. Although the cause of gastric cancer is unknown, as discussed in Chapter 5, emigrants from high-risk to low-risk areas show a decline in the incidence of this cancer, which strongly implicates environmental factors in its pathogenesis.

☐ Pathogenesis:

Dietary Factors. Carcinoma of the stomach is more common among persons who eat large amounts of starch, smoked fish and meat, and pickled vegetables. Benzo[α]pyrene, which is a potent carcinogen, has been detected in smoked foods.

Nitrosamines. Attention has been focused on the possible role of nitrosamines, which are powerful animal carcinogens, in the pathogenesis of cancer of the stomach. The stomach may be exposed to nitrosamines derived from the soil. Alternatively, nitrates or nitrites may be converted by bacterial action to nitrosamines in poorly preserved food or within the gastrointestinal tract.

The decreased incidence of gastric cancer in the United States has paralleled the increased use of refrigeration, which inhibits the conversion of nitrates to nitrites and also obviates the addition such compounds for food preservation. Consumption of whole milk and fresh vegetables rich in vitamin C is inversely related to the occurrence of stomach cancer. Vitamin C has been shown to inhibit the nitrosation of secondary amines in vivo.

Genetic Factors. Hereditary traits have not been identified in most cases of carcinoma of the stomach. Blood type A is found in 38% of the general population, whereas half of the patients with gastric cancer display this type.

Age and Sex. Gastric cancer is uncommon in persons younger than 30 years; it shows a sharp peak in incidence among persons older than 50 years. However, the age at onset seems to be somewhat lower in Japan, where the disease is endemic. In the United States, there is only a slight male predominance, but in countries with a high incidence of this tumor, the male:female ratio is approximately 2:1.

Helicobacter pylori. Serologic studies have demonstrated a high prevalence of gastric infection with *H. pylori* many years before the appearance of stomach cancer. Populations at high risk for this tumor exhibit a high prevalence of infection with *H. pylori* in children, whereas those populations at low risk do not. However, it is probable that the other environmental factors discussed earlier also play an important role.

Atrophic gastritis, pernicious anemia, subtotal gastrectomy, and gastric adenomatous polyps have been discussed earlier as factors being associated with a high risk of stomach cancer. **It is generally accepted that many gastric cancers originate from epithelium that has undergone intestinal metaplasia.**

☐ **Pathology:** Adenocarcinoma of the stomach accounts for more than 95% of all malignant gastric tumors. It originates primarily from mucous cells of the normal superficial epithelium or from areas of intestinal metaplasia. The tumors are most common in the distal stomach, on the lesser curvature of the antrum, and in the prepyloric region. Adenocarcinoma is rare in the fundus, but it may occur in any location.

Advanced Gastric Cancer. By the time most gastric cancers in the Western world are detected, they are advanced—that is, they have penetrated beyond the submucosa into the muscularis and may extend through the serosa. Advanced gastric cancers are divided into three major macroscopic types:

- **Polypoid (fungating) adenocarcinoma** accounts for approximately one-third of advanced cancers. It is a solid mass, as much as 10 cm in diameter, that projects into the lumen of the stomach. The surface may be partly ulcerated, and the deeper tissues may or may not be infiltrated.
- **Ulcerating adenocarcinoma** constitutes another one-third of all gastric cancers. Visualized as a shallow ulcer, it varies in size from 1 to 10 cm in diameter (Fig. 13-16). The surrounding tissue is firm, raised, and nodular. Characteristically, the lateral margins of the ulcer are irregular, and the base is ragged. This is in contrast to the benign peptic ul-

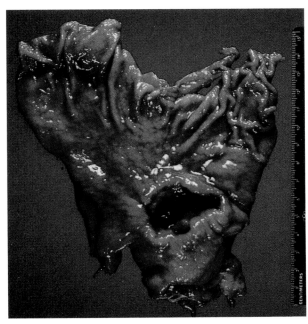

FIGURE *13-16*
Ulcerating carcinoma of the stomach. The stomach has been opened along the greater curvature to reveal a large, centrally ulcerated adenocarcinoma in the antrum, which is characterized by raised, indurated margins.

cer, which exhibits punched-out margins and a smooth base.
- **Diffuse or infiltrating adenocarcinoma** makes up one-tenth of all stomach cancers. No true tumor is seen macroscopically; instead, the wall of the stomach is conspicuously thickened and firm (Fig. 13-17). When the entire stomach is involved, the

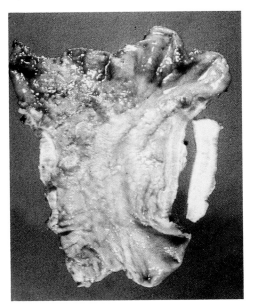

FIGURE *13-17*
Infiltrating gastric carcinoma (linitis plastica). The wall of the stomach is thickened and indurated by diffusely infiltrating cancer.

term **linitis plastica** ("leather-bottle stomach") is applied. In the diffuse type of gastric carcinoma, invading tumor cells induce extensive fibrosis in the submucosa and muscularis. As a result, the wall is stiff and may be more than 2 cm in thickness. Whereas the normal stomach has a volume greater than 1 L, the leather-bottle stomach contains as little as 150 mL.

Microscopically, the histologic pattern of advanced gastric cancer varies from a well-differentiated adenocarcinoma to a totally anaplastic tumor. The tumor cells may contain clear mucin that displaces the nucleus to the periphery of the cell, thereby resulting in the so-called **signet ring cell** (Fig. 13-18).

Early Gastric Cancer. Early gastric cancer is a tumor that is confined to the mucosa or submucosa (Fig. 13-19). A previous term, superficial spreading carcinoma, is synonymous with early gastric cancer. In Japan, early gastric cancer accounts for fully one-third of all stomach cancers, whereas in the United States and Europe, it constitutes only approximately 5% of diagnosed cancers.

Early gastric cancer is strictly a pathologic diagnosis; the term does not refer to the duration of the malignant tumor, its size, the presence of symptoms, the absence of metastases, or the curability. In fact, 5% to 20% of early gastric cancers are already metastatic to the lymph nodes at the time of detection. Similar to advanced cancer, most early gastric cancers are found in the distal stomach.

Gastric cancer metastasizes principally by the lymphatic route to the regional lymph nodes of the lesser and greater curvature, the porta hepatis, and the sub-

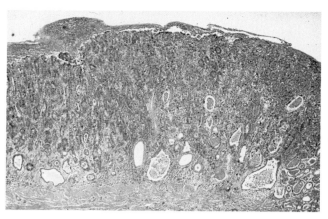

FIGURE   *13-19*
Early gastric cancer. Irregular neoplastic glands are seen in the mucosa superficial to the muscularis mucosae.

pyloric region. Distant lymphatic metastases also occur, with the most common being an enlarged supraclavicular node, called a **Virchow node** or a **sentinel node.** Hematogenous spread may seed any organ, including the liver, lung, or brain. Direct extension to nearby organs is often encountered. Carcinoma of the stomach can also spread to the ovary, where it commonly elicits a desmoplastic response, in which case it is termed a **Krukenberg tumor.**

☐ **Clinical Features:** In the United States and Europe, most patients with gastric cancer have metastases by the time they present for examination. Thus, the symptoms and course are usually those of advanced cancer. Obstruction of the gastric outlet may occur with large tumors of the antrum or prepyloric region. Chronic bleeding is often reflected in the finding of occult blood in the stools and anemia. Two-thirds of patients with stomach cancer have **fasting achlorhydria,** compared with less than 25% of normal persons at the same age.

The level of **carcinoembryonic antigen** is increased in the blood of one-fourth of patients with advanced gastric cancer. This test has little value in establishing the diagnosis of stomach cancer, but it may be helpful in monitoring the course of metastatic disease or of postoperative recurrence.

Even in the presence of lymph node metastases, early gastric cancer has a considerably better prognosis than advanced cancer. The 10-year survival rate for patients with surgically treated advanced gastric cancer is approximately 20%, compared with 95% for early gastric cancer.

Gastric Lymphoma

Primary lymphoma of the stomach accounts for approximately 5% of all malignant stomach tumors, but it

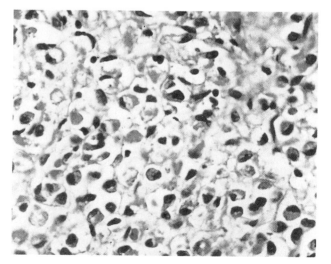

FIGURE   *13-18*
Signet ring cells of gastric adenocarcinoma. Intracellular mucin (*red*) displaces the nuclei to the periphery of the tumor cells (mucicarmine stain).

is the most common of all extranodal lymphomas, constituting 20% of such neoplasms. **Clinically and radiologically, gastric lymphoma mimics gastric adenocarcinoma.** The histologic varieties are similar to those in primary nodal lymphomas, as described in Chapter 20.

The prognosis for gastric lymphoma is considerably better than that for adenocarcinoma. The overall 5-year survival rate for these patients is approximately 50%, depending on the extent of disease at the time of diagnosis.

Small Intestine

CONGENITAL DISORDERS

Atresia and Stenosis

Intestinal atresia and stenosis, although rare, are the most frequent causes of neonatal intestinal obstruction.

Atresia is a complete occlusion of the intestinal lumen, which may be manifested as (1) a thin intraluminal diaphragm, (2) blind proximal and distal sacs joined by a cord, or (3) disconnected blind ends. **Stenosis** is an incomplete stricture of the small intestine, which narrows, but does not occlude, the lumen.

Intestinal atresia or stenosis is diagnosed on the basis of persistent vomiting of bile-containing fluid within the first day of life. Meconium is not passed. Surgical correction is usually successful, but coexistent anomalies often complicate the course.

Meckel Diverticulum

■ *Meckel diverticulum is a congenital sacculation on the antimesenteric border of the ileum caused by persistence of the vitelline duct.* It is the most common and most clinically significant congenital anomaly of the small intestine (Fig. 13-20). At the time of diagnosis, two-thirds of the patients are younger than 2 years.

☐ **Pathology:** The diverticulum occurs 60 to 100 cm from the ileocecal valve in adults. It is approximately 5 cm in length and has a diameter slightly less than that of the ileum but considerably larger than that of the appendix. Meckel diverticulum is a true diverticulum, in that it possesses all the coats of the normal intestine and the mucosa is similar to that of the adjoining ileum. Of the minority of Meckel diverticula that become symptomatic, approximately half contain ectopic gastric, duodenal, pancreatic, biliary, or colonic tissue.

☐ **Clinical Features:** Meckel diverticulum may be complicated by (1) hemorrhage secondary to peptic ulceration, (2) intestinal obstruction caused by intussus-

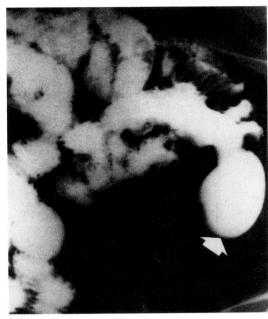

FIGURE   *13-20*
Meckel diverticulum. A contrast radiograph of the small intestine shows a barium-filled diverticulum of the ileum (*arrow*).

ception, (3) diverticulitis mimicking appendicitis, and (4) perforation from peptic ulceration.

Meconium Ileus

The earliest manifestation of **cystic fibrosis** is often neonatal intestinal obstruction caused by accumulation of tenacious meconium in the small intestine. In half of the affected infants, meconium ileus is complicated by (1) volvulus, (2) perforation with a meconium peritonitis, or (3) intestinal atresia.

INFECTIONS

Bacterial Diarrhea

Bacterial diarrhea has plagued humans since the dawn of recorded history, and it continues to be an important clinical problem. **The most significant factor in infectious diarrhea is increased intestinal secretion stimulated by bacterial toxins and enteric hormones.**

Toxigenic Diarrhea

■ *Toxigenic diarrhea refers to frequent, watery stools caused by infection with toxin-producing bacteria.* The prototypic organisms that produce diarrhea by secreting toxins are *Vibrio cholerae* and toxigenic strains of

Escherichia coli. Toxigenic diarrhea is characterized by the following:

- Damage to the intestinal mucosa is minimal or absent.
- The organism remains on the mucosal surface, where it secretes its toxin.
- Fluid secreted into the small intestine causes watery diarrhea, which can lead to dehydration, particularly in the case of cholera.

Although many organisms have been isolated in so-called **travelers' diarrhea,** the most common pathogen found in almost all studies is toxigenic *E. coli.*

Diarrhea Caused by Invasive Bacteria

■ *Invasive bacteria, as their name implies, cause diarrhea by directly injuring the intestinal mucosa.* Among these organisms, *Shigella, Salmonella,* and certain strains of *E. coli, Yersinia,* and *Campylobacter* are the most widely recognized. Invasive organisms tend to infect the distal ileum and colon, whereas toxigenic bacteria mainly infect the upper intestinal tract.

Shigellosis. Shigellosis principally affects the colon, although the terminal ileum is occasionally involved. Microscopically, a granular and hemorrhagic mucosa exhibits numerous shallow, serpiginous ulcers. The inflammation, which is especially severe in the sigmoid colon and rectum, is usually superficial. During the early stage, the accumulation of neutrophils in damaged crypts (crypt abscesses) is similar to that in ulcerative colitis, and the lymphoid follicles of the mucosa break down to form ulcers. As the infection recedes, the ulcers heal, and the mucosa returns to normal.

Typhoid Fever. Typhoid fever (*Salmonella* enteritis) is uncommon in industrialized countries today but still presents a problem in underdeveloped countries. Infection of Peyer's patches results in oval ulcers, in which the longer dimension follows the long axis of the intestine. The base of the ulcer is composed of black necrotic tissue mixed with fibrin.

Microscopically, the early lesions of typhoid fever contain large, basophilic macrophages filled with typhoid bacilli, erythrocytes, and necrotic debris. Necrosis of the lymphoid follicles becomes confluent, and mucosal ulceration follows. Healing of the ulcers is complete within 1 week of the acute symptoms and leaves little fibrosis or other sequelae. **Intestinal hemorrhage and perforation**, principally in the ileum, are the most feared complications of typhoid fever, tend-

ing to occur in the third week and during convalescence.

Nontyphoidal Salmonellosis. Formerly known as "paratyphoid fever," this enteritis is caused by *Salmonella* strains other than *S. typhi* and is generally a far less serious illness than typhoid fever. The organisms invade the mucosa, which shows mild ulceration, edema, and infiltration with neutrophils.

Enteroinvasive and Enterohemorrhagic Strains of *E. Coli.* These organisms are uncommon causes of a bloody diarrhea that resembles shigellosis. Certain strains of *E. coli,* particularly serotype 0157:H7, produce Shiga-like toxins, but the role of these proteins in the pathogenesis of the enterocolitis is not understood. Serotype 0157:H7 has also been implicated in the pathogenesis of hemolytic-uremic syndrome in children.

Yersinia Enterocolitis. *Yersinia* organisms are transmitted by pets or contaminated food, and infection is most common in young children. *Yersinia* infection causes diarrhea, cramps, and fever, lasting from 1 to 3 weeks. The disease is characterized by hyperplasia of Peyer's patches, with acute ulceration of the overlying mucosa.

Campylobacter jejuni. Infection with *C. jejuni* is now recognized as being one of the most important causes of bacterial diarrhea. Humans are involved mainly by contact with infected domestic animals or by ingestion of poorly cooked or contaminated food. Adults usually recover from the diarrheal illness in less than 1 week.

Food Poisoning

Infectious agents can produce gastroenteritis not only by infecting the bowel directly but also by elaborating enterotoxins in contaminated food, which is then ingested.

Staphylococcus aureus. This widespread bacterium is a common cause of food poisoning, which results from ingestion of food contaminated with strains of *Staphylococcus* that produce an exotoxin. Within 6 hours of the ingestion of tainted food, severe vomiting and abdominal cramps occur, which are often followed by diarrhea. Most victims recover in 1 to 2 days.

Clostridium perfringens. This anaerobe elaborates an enterotoxin that causes vomiting and diarrhea. In most cases, watery diarrhea and severe abdominal pain, which begin 8 to 24 hours after ingestion of the contaminated food, only last for approximately 1 day.

Viral Gastroenteritis

Rotavirus. Infection with rotavirus is a common cause of infantile diarrhea, accounting for half of the cases of acute diarrhea in hospitalized children younger than 2 years.

Norwalk Viruses. These agents cause one-third of the epidemics of viral gastroenteritis in the United States. The virus targets the upper small intestine, where it produces patchy mucosal lesions and malabsorption. Vomiting and diarrhea are usual, but the symptoms resolve within 2 days.

Tuberculosis

Virtually all cases of intestinal tuberculosis in Western countries are caused by *Mycobacterium tuberculosis*. Most of these cases result from ingestion of bacteria in food or swallowing of infectious sputum. The bacterium then establishes a locus of infection, usually (90% of patients) in the ileocecal region. Infection can also occur in the colon, jejunum, appendix, rectum, and duodenum, in that order of frequency. As many as half of the patients with intestinal tuberculosis do not have radiologic evidence of pulmonary involvement.

In more than half of the patients with intestinal tuberculosis, the small intestine shows one or more circular or oval ulcers of varying size. As the ulcers heal, reactive fibrosis may cause a circumferential ("napkin ring") stricture of the bowel lumen. In 10% of patients, the ileocecal region or colon exhibits an exuberant inflammatory and fibroblastic reaction throughout the thickness of the wall. Approximately one-third of the patients combine the features of the ulcerative and the hypertrophic forms. Microscopically, typical tuberculous granulomas are found in all layers of the bowel wall, particularly in Peyer's patches and lymphoid follicles, and in the mesenteric lymph nodes.

☐ **Clinical Features:** Almost all patients with intestinal tuberculosis complain of chronic abdominal pain, and two-thirds have a palpable abdominal mass, usually in the right lower quadrant. Complications of intestinal tuberculosis include obstruction, fistulas, perforation, and abscess.

VASCULAR DISEASES

Decreased blood flow to the intestines from any cause can lead to ischemic bowel disease.

Acute Intestinal Ischemia

Arterial Occlusion. Sudden occlusion of an artery by thrombosis or embolization leads to infarction of the small bowel before collateral circulation comes into play. Depending on the size of the vessel, the infarction may be segmental or produce gangrene of virtually the entire small bowel. Occlusive intestinal infarction is most often caused by embolic or thrombotic occlusion of the superior mesenteric artery. A lesser number are secondary to inferior mesenteric artery occlusion, mesenteric venous thrombosis, or arteritis. In addition to intrinsic vascular lesions, volvulus (Fig. 13-21), intussusception, and incarceration of the intestine in a hernial sac may all lead to bowel infarction.

Nonocclusive Intestinal Ischemia. Intestinal infarction in which no acute vascular occlusion is evident is more common today than the occlusive type. Nonocclusive intestinal infarction may be extensive and is seen in patients with hypoxia and reduced cardiac output from shock or acute myocardial infarction.

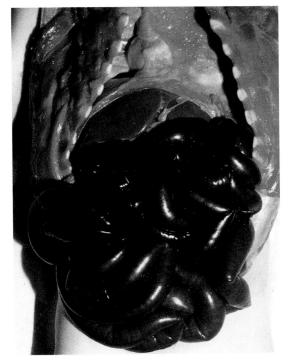

FIGURE   *13-21*
Infarct of the small bowel. This young boy died after an episode of intense abdominal pain and shock. Autopsy demonstrated volvulus of the small bowel, which had occluded the superior mesenteric artery. The entire small bowel is dilated, gangrenous, and hemorrhagic.

Thrombosis of the Mesenteric Veins. This cause of intestinal ischemia occurs in a variety of conditions, including hypercoagulable states, stasis, and inflammation. The large majority of thromboses affect the superior mesenteric vein.

☐ **Pathology:** The infarcted bowel is edematous and diffusely purple. The demarcation between the infarcted bowel and normal tissue is usually sharp, although venous occlusion may lead to a more diffuse appearance. Extensive hemorrhage is seen in the mucosa and submucosa, with the former becoming necrotic. Although the deep muscle layers are initially preserved, they eventually become necrotic as well. The mucosal surface shows irregular white sloughs, the wall becomes thin and distended, and bubbles of gas may be present in the mesenteric veins. The serosal surface is cloudy and covered by fibrin.

The death of smooth muscle interferes with peristalsis and leads to **adynamic ileus,** a condition in which the bowel proximal to the lesion is dilated and filled with fluid. Intestinal organisms may pass through the damaged wall and cause **peritonitis** or **septicemia.**

☐ **Clinical Features:** In occlusion of the mesenteric artery, an abrupt onset of abdominal pain is virtually invariable. Bloody diarrhea, hematemesis, and shock are common, and in untreated cases, perforation is frequent. **As the infarction progresses, systemic manifestations become more severe, and death is inevitable without surgical intervention.** In extensive infarction, resulting from occlusion in the proximal portion of the superior mesenteric artery, almost the entire small bowel must be resected, a condition that is also not compatible with ultimate survival.

Chronic Intestinal Ischemia

Atherosclerotic narrowing of the major splanchnic arteries leads to chronic intestinal ischemia. As in the heart, the result is intermittent abdominal pain, termed **intestinal (abdominal) angina.** Chronic ischemia of the small bowel may lead to fibrosis and formation of a stricture. Ischemic strictures of the small bowel, which may be single or multiple, produce intestinal obstruction or, occasionally, malabsorption secondary to stasis and bacterial overgrowth.

MALABSORPTION

■ *Malabsorption is a general term used to describe a number of clinical conditions in which one or more important nutrients are inadequately absorbed from the small intestine.*

Normal intestinal absorption is characterized by a luminal phase and an intestinal phase (Fig. 13-22). The **luminal phase,** which consists of those processes that occur within the lumen of the small intestine, alters the physicochemical state of the various nutrients so they can be taken up by the absorptive cells in the small bowel epithelium. The **intestinal phase** includes those events that occur in the cells and transport channels of the intestinal wall.

Causes of Luminal-Phase Malabsorption

Interruption of the normal continuity of the distal stomach and duodenum occurs after gastroduodenal surgery (gastrectomy, antrectomy, pyloroplasty).

Pancreatic dysfunction is a result of chronic pancreatitis, pancreatic carcinoma, or cystic fibrosis.

Deficient or ineffective bile salts may result from three possible causes:

- **Impaired excretion of bile** is secondary to liver disease.
- **Bacterial overgrowth** occurs from a disturbance in motility of the gut. It is seen in such conditions as blind loop syndrome, multiple diverticula of the small bowel, and muscular or neurogenic defects of the intestinal wall (e.g., amyloidosis, scleroderma, diabetic enteropathy). When gastrointestinal motility is defective, bile salts are deconjugated by the excess small bowel bacteria and rendered ineffective for micelle formation.
- **Deficient bile salts** reflect the absence or bypass of the distal ileum, which, in turn, results from surgical excision, surgical anastomoses, fistulas, or ileal disease (e.g., Crohn disease, lymphoma).

Causes of Intestinal-Phase Malabsorption

Microvilli. Intestinal disaccharidases are integrally bound to the microvillous membranes. Disaccharidases are essential for sugar absorption, because only monosaccharides can be absorbed by the intestinal epithelial cells. Abnormal function of the microvilli may be primary, such as in primary disaccharidase deficiencies, or secondary, as occurs with damage to the villi, as in celiac disease (sprue). The various enzyme deficiencies (e.g., that of lactase) are characterized by intolerance for the corresponding disaccharides.

Absorptive Area. The surface area of the small intestine that is available for absorption may be diminished by (1) small bowel resection (short bowel syn-

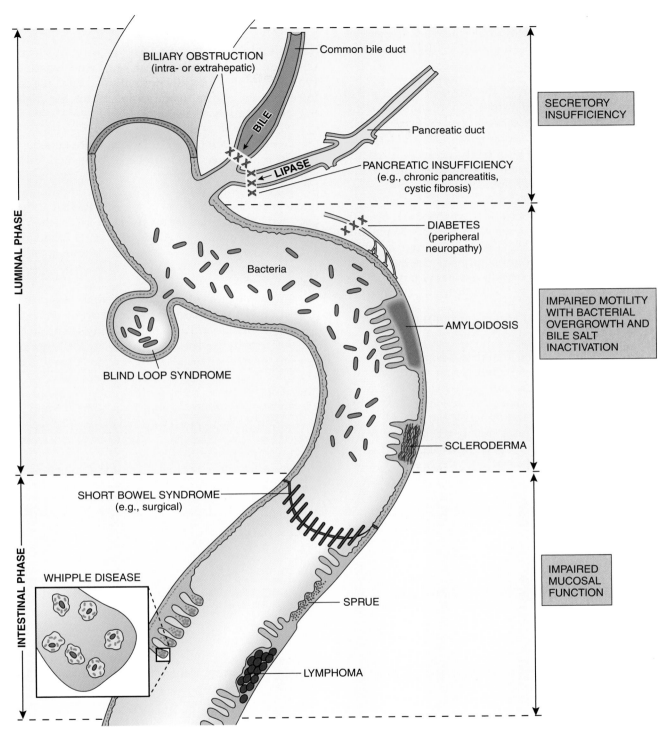

FIGURE   13-22
Causes of malabsorption.

drome), (2) gastrocolic fistula (bypassing the small intestine), or (3) a number of small intestinal diseases associated with mucosal damage (celiac disease, tropical sprue, Whipple disease).

Metabolic Function of the Absorptive Cells. For their subsequent transport to the circulation, nutrients within the absorptive cells depend on their metabolism within these cells. There, monoglycerides and free fatty acids are reassembled into triglycerides and coated with proteins (apoproteins) to form chylomicrons and lipoprotein particles. Nonspecific damage to the small intestinal epithelial cells occurs in celiac disease, tropical sprue, Whipple disease, and gastrinoma. Specific metabolic dysfunction is seen in abetalipoproteinemia (associated with acanthocytosis), a disorder in which the absorptive cells cannot synthesize the apoprotein required for the assembly of lipoproteins and chylomicrons.

☐ **Clinical Features:** Malabsorption may be either specific or generalized.

- **Specific or isolated malabsorption** refers to an identifiable molecular defect that causes malabsorption of a single nutrient. Examples of this group are the disaccharidase deficiencies (notably lactase deficiency) and deficiency of gastric intrinsic factor, which causes malabsorption of vitamin B_{12} and, consequently, pernicious anemia.
- **Generalized malabsorption,** which is defined as the inadequate absorption of all major nutrients (proteins, carbohydrates, and fats), leads to malnutrition.

Lactase Deficiency

As a prominent constituent of milk and many other dairy products, lactose is one of the most common disaccharides in the diet. Acquired lactase deficiency is a widespread disorder of carbohydrate absorption. In fact, two-thirds of Asian and African adults manifest evidence of this deficiency. Typically, symptoms of the disease begin during adolescence. Patients complain of abdominal distention, flatulence, and diarrhea after the ingestion of dairy products. These symptoms are relieved by eliminating milk from the diet.

Celiac Disease (Celiac Sprue)

■ *Celiac disease (gluten-sensitive enteropathy, nontropical sprue) is characterized by (1) generalized malabsorption; (2) a typical, but nonspecific, small intestinal mucosal lesion; and (3) a prompt clinical, but slower histologic, response to the withdrawal of gluten-containing foods from the diet.*

☐ **Pathogenesis:**

Role of Cereal Proteins. The ingestion or instillation of gluten-containing cereals (e.g., wheat, barley, or rye) into the histologically normal small intestine is followed by the clinical features and histologic changes that are typical of celiac sprue.

Genetic Factors. Although a definite genetic pattern of inheritance has not been established, 80% to 90% of the patients with celiac disease carry the class I histocompatibility antigen HLA-B8. A comparable frequency has been reported for the class II HLA antigens DR3 and DQw2. These antigens occur in less than 20% of the adult population and are frequently found in patients having other diseases associated with an altered immune response.

Immunologic Factors. The intestinal lesion in patients with celiac disease is characterized by damage to the epithelial cells and a markedly increased number of plasma cells in the lamina propria and of T lymphocytes in the epithelial cell layer. A region of amino acid sequence homology has been found between α-gliadin (the active component of gluten) and a protein of an adenovirus (serotype 12) that infects the human gastrointestinal tract. The large majority (90%) of untreated patients with celiac disease have evidence of previous infection with this virus.

One attractive hypothesis holds that infection with adenovirus 12 sensitizes T cells to an antigenic determinant that is shared with gliadin. Subsequent exposure to gluten-containing cereals in a genetically susceptible person stimulates an immunologic reaction to gliadin that is bound to the surface of intestinal epithelial cells.

Association with Dermatitis Herpetiformis. Celiac disease is occasionally associated with dermatitis herpetiformis, which is a vesicular skin disease that typically affects the extensor surfaces and exposed parts of the body.

A hypothetical mechanism for the pathogenesis of celiac disease is presented in Figure 13-23.

☐ **Pathology:** The hallmark of celiac disease is a flat, small, intestinal mucosa with (1) blunting or total disappearance of villi, (2) damaged epithelial cells on the mucosal surface, and (3) increased cellularity of the lamina propria but not of the deeper layers (Fig. 13-24). The most severe histologic abnormalities in patients with untreated celiac disease usually occur in the duodenum and proximal jejunum.

The villi are short and blunt or entirely absent, and the crypts are deeper than normal. The absorptive cells are flattened and more basophilic than normal, and the basal polarity of their nuclei is lost. The crypts, which are longer than usual, contain numerous mitotic figures. Numbers of lymphocytes and plasma cells in the lamina propria are markedly increased (see Fig. 13-24).

☐ **Clinical Features:** Celiac disease is characterized by a generalized malabsorption. Typically, a child comes to medical attention because he or she ceases to thrive soon after the introduction of cereals into the diet. Systemic manifestations of celiac disease are related to the various deficiency states that result from the generalized malabsorption. Late complications in some cases include lymphoma of the small bowel or other malignant diseases of the gastrointestinal tract. Treatment with a strict, gluten-free diet is usually followed by a complete and prolonged clinical and histologic remission.

Whipple Disease

■ *Whipple disease is a rare intestinal infection characterized clinically by malabsorption and pathologically by bacilli-laden macrophages in the mucosa.* It most commonly affects white men in their thirties and forties. Other clinical findings include fever, increased skin pigmentation, anemia, lymphadenopathy, arthritis, pericarditis, pleurisy, endocarditis, and involvement of the central nervous system.

☐ **Pathogenesis:** Whipple disease typically shows infiltration of the lamina propria of the small bowel mucosa by large macrophages packed with small, rod-shaped bacilli. Dramatic clinical remissions occur with antibiotic therapy. The causative organism has recently been identified as being a previously uncharacterized Actinomycete, which has been named *Tropheryma whippelii.*

☐ **Pathology:** The bowel wall is both thickened and edematous, and the mesenteric lymph nodes are usually enlarged. Histologic examination of the small intestine reveals flat, thickened villi and extensive infiltration of the lamina propria with large macrophages (Fig. 13-25). The cytoplasm of these macrophages is filled with large glycoprotein granules that stain strongly with periodic acid-Schiff. Electron microscopic examination reveals numerous small bacilli in the macrophages and free in the lamina propria. Lymphatic vessels in the mucosa and submucosa are dilated, and large lipid droplets abound within the

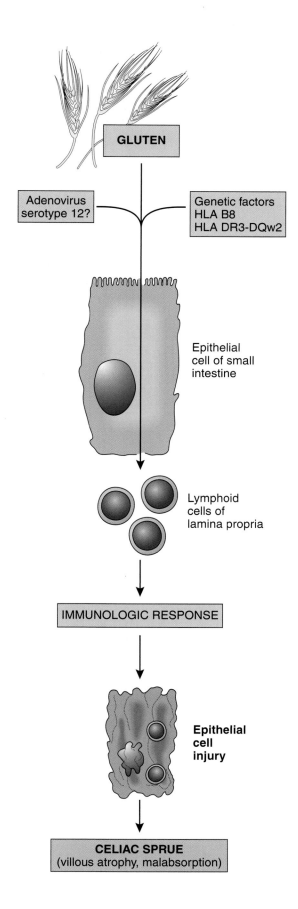

GLUTEN

Adenovirus serotype 12?

Genetic factors
HLA B8
HLA DR3-DQw2

Epithelial cell of small intestine

Lymphoid cells of lamina propria

IMMUNOLOGIC RESPONSE

Epithelial cell injury

CELIAC SPRUE
(villous atrophy, malabsorption)

FIGURE   *13-23*
Hypothetical mechanisms in the pathogenesis of celiac disease.

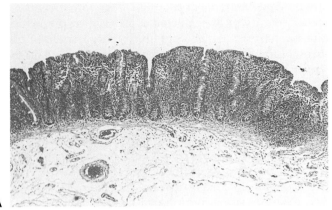

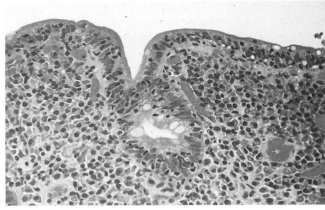

FIGURE 13-24

Celiac disease. (A) Villous atrophy with a flat surface, elongation of the crypts, and chronic inflammation of the lamina propria are characteristic of longstanding disease. (B) A higher-power view shows the flattened surface mucosa to be infiltrated predominantly by plasma cells.

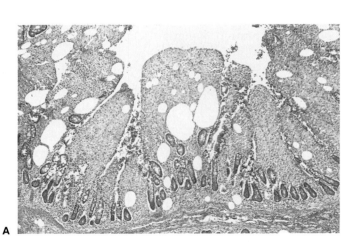

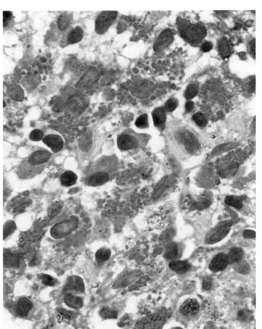

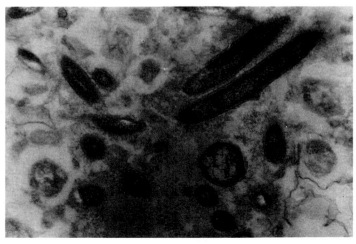

FIGURE 13-25

Whipple disease. (A) A photomicrograph of a section of jejunal mucosa shows distortion of the villi. The lamina propria is packed with large, pale-staining macrophages. Dilated mucosal lymphatics are prominent. (B) A periodic acid-Schiff reaction shows abundant, large macrophages filled with granular cytoplasmic material. (C) An electron micrograph demonstrates small bacilli in a macrophage.

lymphatics and in the extracellular spaces, a finding that suggests obstruction of the lymphatics.

The mesenteric lymph nodes draining affected segments of the small bowel reveal similar microscopic changes. A characteristic infiltration by macrophages containing bacilli may also be found in other organs, notably the lung, heart, spleen, liver, endocrine glands, brain, bone, and synovial membranes.

Tropical Sprue

■ *Tropical sprue is a poorly understood disease of obscure cause that is acquired in certain endemic tropical areas and is characterized by progressively severe malabsorption and nutritional deficiency.* Cure, or at least amelioration of the symptoms, usually follows treatment with oral tetracycline and folic acid. The disease is endemic to Puerto Rico, Cuba, the Dominican Republic, and Haiti. It also occurs in the northern parts of South America and in many Far Eastern countries. The cause of tropical sprue is not known. Results of some studies suggest that longstanding contamination of the bowel with bacteria (perhaps toxigenic strains of *E. coli*) may be important, and that folate deficiency may play a role in perpetuating the intestinal lesion.

Histologic findings are variable, ranging from a mild widening and blunting of the villi to a completely flat mucosa, which is indistinguishable from that seen in patients with celiac sprue. Typically, steatorrhea, anemia, and weight loss are followed by progressively severe manifestations of folic acid and vitamin B_{12} deficiencies and hypoalbuminemia.

MECHANICAL OBSTRUCTION

Mechanical obstruction of the passage of intestinal contents can be caused by (1) a luminal mass, (2) an intrinsic lesion of the bowel wall, or (3) extrinsic compression.

Intussusception

■ *Intussusception is a form of intraluminal small bowel obstruction in which a segment of bowel (intussusceptum) protrudes distally into a surrounding outer portion (intussuscipiens), much in the same way that a segment of a telescope inserts into the adjacent one.* This condition is usually a disorder of infants or young children, in whom it occurs without a known cause. In adults, the leading point of an intussusception is commonly a lesion in the bowel wall, such as a Meckel diverticulum or polypoid tumor. Once the leading point is entrapped in the in-

tussuscipiens, peristalsis drives the intussusceptum forward. In addition to acute intestinal obstruction, intussusception compresses the blood supply to the intussusceptum, which may then become infarcted. If the obstruction is not relieved spontaneously, treatment requires surgery.

Volvulus

■ *Volvulus is a cause of an acute abdomen and an example of an intestinal obstruction in which a segment of gut twists on its mesentery, thereby kinking the bowel and usually interrupting the blood supply.* Volvulus is virtually always a consequence of an underlying congenital abnormality. Malrotation of the bowel permits undue mobility of the bowel loops, predisposing it to volvulus.

Adhesions

Fibrous scars caused by previous surgery or peritonitis may cause obstruction, either by kinking or angulating the bowel or by directly compressing the lumen.

Hernias

Loops of small bowel may be incarcerated in an inguinal or a femoral hernia, in which case the lumen may become obstructed and the vascular supply compromised.

NEOPLASMS

The small intestine is curiously resistant to neoplasia, despite the fact that it is the longest portion of the alimentary tract. Tumors of the small intestine constitute less than 5% of all gastrointestinal tumors.

Benign Tumors

The most common benign tumors of the small intestine are adenomas, leiomyomas, and lipomas. As in other portions of the gastrointestinal tract, neurogenic tumors, fibromas, angiomas, and hamartomas may also be encountered. Benign tumors of the small intestine rarely become malignant.

Adenomas

Adenomas of the small intestine resemble those of the colon (discussed later). As in the colon, adenomatous polyps in the small intestine may be tubular, villous, or a mixture of these types. Although most adenomas remain benign, some, especially the villous type, undergo malignant transformation. Benign adenomas are ordinarily asymptomatic, but bleeding and intussusception are occasional complications.

Peutz-Jeghers Syndrome

■ *Peutz-Jeghers syndrome is an autosomal dominant, hereditary disorder characterized by intestinal polyps and mucocutaneous melanin pigmentation, which is particularly evident on the face, buccal mucosa, hands, feet, and perianal regions, as well as genital areas.* The polyps occur most commonly in the proximal regions, portions of the small intestine, but they are sometimes seen in the stomach and colon. Patients usually present with symptoms of obstruction or intussusception. Acute upper gastrointestinal tract hemorrhage and occult bleeding with anemia may complicate the course.

Peutz-Jeghers syndrome apparently results from inactivating mutations of a gene (*LKB1*) on chromosome 19p, which encodes a protein kinase. Carriers of the defective gene also have an increased risk for cancers of the breast, pancreas, testis, and ovary.

Polyps in Peutz-Jeghers syndrome are not true neoplasms but, rather, are hamartomas. Histologically, a branching network of smooth muscle fibers, which is continuous with the muscularis mucosae, supports the glandular epithelium of the polyp (Fig. 13-26). Peutz-Jeghers polyps are benign. However, 2% to 3% of patients develop adenocarcinoma, although not necessarily in the hamartomatous polyps.

Malignant Tumors

Adenocarcinoma

☐ **Epidemiology:** Although adenocarcinoma of the small intestine accounts for only a minute proportion of all gastrointestinal tumors, it constitutes half of all malignant small bowel tumors. The large majority of adenocarcinomas are located in the duodenum and jejunum. Most occur in middle-aged persons, and there is a moderate male predominance. Patients with Crohn's disease have a significantly increased risk of adenocarcinoma of the small bowel, perhaps as high as 100-fold.

☐ **Pathology and Clinical Features:** Adenocarcinoma of the small intestine may be polypoid or ulcerative, or it may simply be annular and stenosing. In addition to causing intestinal obstruction directly, a polypoid tumor may be the lead point of an intussusception. Microscopically, adenocarcinomas, which originate from the epithelium of the crypts rather than the villi, resemble colon cancer.

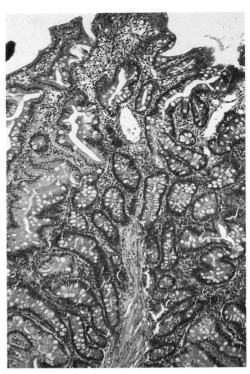

FIGURE　*13-26*
Peutz-Jeghers polyp. In this hamartomatous polyp, the glandular epithelium, which is composed of both goblet cells and absorptive cells, is supported by a network of smooth muscle.

Adenocarcinoma of the small intestine is usually annular; therefore, the symptoms are commonly those of progressive intestinal obstruction. Occult bleeding is common and often leads to iron-deficiency anemia. By the time the patient becomes symptomatic, most adenocarcinomas have metastasized to the local lymph nodes, and the overall 5-year survival rate is less than 20%.

Primary Lymphoma

Primary lymphoma originates in nodules of lymphoid tissue within the bowel wall. It represents the second most common malignant tumor of the small intestine in industrialized countries, where it accounts for approximately 15% of small bowel cancers. By contrast, another type of primary lymphoma accounts for more than two-thirds of all cancers of the small intestine in underdeveloped countries. This latter type of intestinal lymphoma was originally described in Mediterranean populations, but it is clearly distributed throughout the poorer parts of the world. Because these two types of lymphoma have distinct epidemiologic, clinical, and pathologic features, they are labeled, respectively, the Western type and the Mediterranean variety.

The cause of primary lymphoma of the small bowel is unknown, but an association with celiac disease is well documented, occurring in as many as one-tenth of the patients with primary lymphoma. The risk of intestinal lymphoma is also increased in patients with conditions favoring the development of nodal lymphoma, particularly immunodeficiency following treatment with immunosuppressive drugs.

Mediterranean Lymphoma. Mediterranean lymphoma typically occurs in poor countries among young men of low socioeconomic status. **This neoplasm has been associated with α-chain disease, a proliferative disorder of intestinal B lymphocytes that secrete immunoglobulin A.** Mediterranean lymphoma and α-chain disease are believed by some to be the same disorder, termed **immunoproliferative small intestinal disease.**

Mediterranean intestinal lymphoma typically affects men younger than 30 years of age, predominantly involving the duodenum and proximal jejunum. The lymphoma usually presents as a diffuse infiltration of the mucosa and submucosa by plasmacytoid lymphocytes or plasma cells. Lymphomatous infiltration of the mucosa leads to mucosal atrophy and severe malabsorption.

Western-Type Intestinal Lymphoma. The Western type of intestinal lymphoma usually affects adults older than 40 years of age and children younger than 10 years. It is most common in the ileum, where it presents as (1) a fungating mass that projects into the lumen; (2) an elevated, ulcerated lesion; (3) a diffuse, segmental thickening of the bowel wall; or (4) plaque-like mucosal nodules. As a result, intestinal obstruction, intussusception, and perforation are important complications. Occult bleeding is common, although massive acute hemorrhage may also occur. Microscopically, all varieties of malignant lymphoma are encountered. When the disease is localized and confined to the small intestine, it does not recur after surgical removal in more than half of the patients. When extraintestinal spread is present, however, the 5-year survival rate is less than 10%.

Carcinoid Tumor

Carcinoid tumors of the gastrointestinal tract arise from cells of the neuroendocrine system of the gut, at the base of the mucosal crypts. The most commonly secreted hormone is serotonin. Whereas carcinoid tumors constitute less than 1% of all gastrointestinal tumors, they account for 20% of all malignant tumors. The majority of carcinoid tumors are found incidentally in the appendix; most of the remainder occur in the ileum.

The malignant potential of intestinal carcinoid tumors appears to relate to their size. Tumors smaller

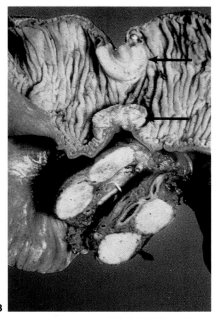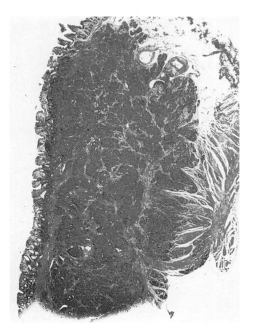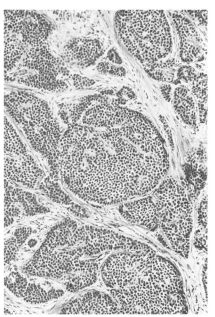

A, B   C

FIGURE   *13-27*
Carcinoid tumor of the small intestine. (A) A bisected annular carcinoid tumor (*arrows*) constricts the lumen of the small intestine. Lymph node metastases are evident. (B) A photomicrograph of the lesion in *panel A* shows an intact mucosa (*left*) and the predominant submucosal location of the malignant tumor. (C) A higher-power photomicrograph demonstrates nests and cords of uniform, small, round cells.

than 1 cm in diameter are rarely malignant. Fifty percent of those between 1 and 2 cm in diameter metastasize, and 80% of those larger than 2 cm in diameter metastasize. **However, for practical purposes, carcinoid tumors of the appendix that are smaller than 2 cm across do not metastasize.**

☐ **Pathology:** Macroscopically, small carcinoid tumors present as submucosal nodules covered by intact mucosa. Large tumors may grow in a polypoid, intramural, or annular pattern (Fig. 13-27) and often undergo secondary ulceration. The cut surface is firm and white to yellow in color. Microscopically, the neoplasms appear as nests, cords, and rosettes of uniform, small, and round cells. Occasional gland-like structures are also encountered. By electron microscopy, typical neurosecretory granules are noted. The nuclei exhibit a remarkable regularity, and mitoses are rare.

As they enlarge, carcinoid tumors invade the muscular coat and penetrate the serosa. These neoplasms metastasize first to the regional lymph nodes. Subsequently, hematogenous spread produces metastases at distant sites, particularly the liver.

☐ **Clinical Features:** Carcinoid syndrome is a unique clinical condition that marks carcinoid tumors. The disorder is caused by the release of a variety of active tumor products. Although most carcinoids are functional to some extent, this syndrome ordinarily occurs only in cases with extensive hepatic metastases. The classic symptoms of the carcinoid syndrome include diarrhea (often the most distressing symptom), episodic flushing, bronchospasm, cyanosis, telangiectasia, and skin lesions. Approximately half of the patients also suffer from right-sided cardiac valvular disease (see Chapter 11). Diarrhea is thought to be caused

by serotonin, but the tumor secretory products involved in the other symptoms have not been clearly identified. Surgical resection, which is the only current therapy for the primary tumor, accomplishes a 5-year cure in half of the patients of small bowel carcinoid tumors.

Large Intestine

CONGENITAL DISORDERS

Congenital Megacolon (Hirschsprung Disease)

■ *Hirschsprung disease is an uncommon familial disorder in which colonic dilatation results from defective innervation of the rectum.* The lesion is a congenital absence of ganglion cells in the wall of the rectum (Fig. 13-28). Most cases of Hirschsprung disease are sporadic, but 10% are familial. Half of the familial cases and 15% of the sporadic ones are associated with inactivating gene mutations of the RET receptor tyrosine kinase on chromosome 10q 11.2 (see the discussion of MEN-2 syndrome in Chapter 21). A few cases are linked to mutations in the genes encoding the ligands of the RET receptor and the endothelin-B receptor. The incidence of congenital megacolon is also 10-fold greater than normal in infants with Down syndrome.

☐ **Pathology:** The rectum in patients with Hirschsprung disease reveals a constricted and spastic segment that corresponds to the aganglionic zone. Proximal to this area, the bowel is conspicuously di-

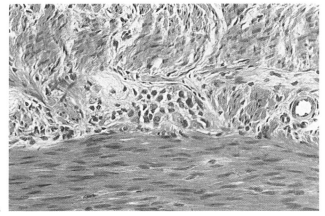
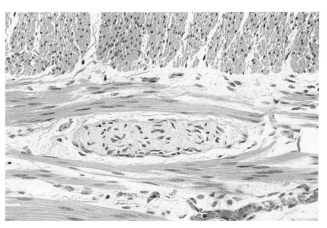

A   B

FIGURE   *13-28*
Hirschsprung disease. (A) A photomicrograph of ganglion cells in the wall of the normal rectum. (B) A rectal biopsy specimen from a patient with Hirschsprung disease shows a nonmyelinated nerve fiber but an absence of ganglion cells.

lated. The definitive diagnosis of Hirschsprung disease is made on the basis of the absence of ganglion cells in a rectal biopsy specimen.

☐ **Clinical Features:** Congenital megacolon is marked by the delayed passage of meconium in the newborn and the development of vomiting in 2 to 3 days. In some cases, complete intestinal obstruction requires immediate surgical relief. In others, repeated enemas ameliorate the obstruction. The most serious complication of congenital megacolon is an enterocolitis, in which necrosis and ulceration affect the dilated proximal segment of the colon and may extend into the small intestine. The cure for Hirschsprung disease is surgical removal of the aganglionic segment.

Anorectal Malformations

Anorectal malformations are among the most common developmental defects, varying from minor narrowing to serious and complex anomalies. These include anorectal agenesis or stenosis and imperforate anus. Fistulas between the malformation and the bladder, urethra, vagina, or skin may occur with all types of anorectal anomalies.

Pilonidal cyst, which is an acquired lesion in the gluteal cleft superior to the anus, consists of cysts or sinus tracts containing hair. It is thought to be initiated by the penetration of hair beneath the skin.

INFECTIONS

Pseudomembranous Colitis

■ *Pseudomembranous colitis is an inflammatory disease of the colon characterized by exudative plaques superimposed on a congested and edematous mucosa.*

☐ **Pathogenesis:** *Clostridium difficile,* which has also been implicated in neonatal necrotizing enterocolitis, is the offending organism in patients with pseudomembranous colitis. The organism is not invasive, but it produces toxins that damage the colonic mucosa. Most cases of pseudomembranous colitis are today associated with antibiotic therapy, although gastrointestinal surgery remains an important risk factor.

☐ **Pathology:** Macroscopically, the colon, particularly the rectosigmoid region, exhibits raised, yellowish plaques as much as 2 cm in diameter that adhere to the underlying mucosa (Fig. 13-29). The intervening mucosa appears congested and edematous, but it is not ulcerated. In severe cases, the plaques coalesce to form extensive pseudomembranes. Microscopic examina-

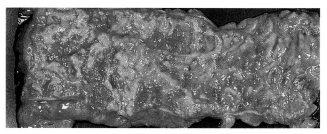

FIGURE **13-29**
Pseudomembranous colitis. The mucosal surface of the colon is covered by raised, irregular plaques, which are composed of necrotic debris and an acute inflammatory exudate.

tion of the lesions discloses necrosis of the superficial epithelium, which is believed to be the initial pathologic event. Subsequently, the crypts become disrupted and are expanded by mucin and neutrophils, an appearance similar to that of the crypt abscesses of ulcerative colitis. The pseudomembrane consists of the debris of necrotic epithelial cells, mucus, fibrin, and neutrophils.

☐ **Clinical Features:** In patients who develop pseudomembranous colitis, fever, leukocytosis, and abdominal cramps are superimposed on diarrhea. Pseudomembranous colitis, although still a serious disease, is usually controlled with oral vancomycin or metronidazole therapy.

Neonatal Necrotizing Enterocolitis

■ *Neonatal necrotizing enterocolitis is an intestinal infection in which lesions vary from those of typical pseudomembranous enterocolitis to gangrene and perforation of the bowel.* It is one of the most common acquired surgical emergencies in the neonate, and it is particularly common in premature infants. The disease is believed to relate principally to an ischemic event involving the intestinal mucosa, which is then followed by bacterial colonization, usually with *C. difficile.*

DIVERTICULAR DISEASE

Diverticular disease refers to two entities, namely a bland, asymptomatic condition termed **diverticulosis** and an inflammatory complication termed **diverticulitis.**

Diverticulosis

■ *Diverticulosis is an acquired herniation (diverticulum) of the mucosa and submucosa through the muscular layers of the colon.*

☐ **Epidemiology:** Diverticulosis shows a striking geographic variation, being common in Western societies but infrequent in Asia, Africa, and underdeveloped countries. The disorder is unusual in persons younger than 40 years of age and increases in frequency with age. Approximately 10% of persons in Western countries are afflicted by diverticulosis, which has been demonstrated in one-third to one-half of persons older than 60 years of age.

☐ **Pathogenesis:** The striking variation in the prevalence of diverticulosis implies that environmental factors are primarily responsible for the disease. Western populations consume a diet in which refined carbohydrates and meat have replaced crude cereal grains, and it is widely assumed that this lack of indigestible fibers, in some way, predisposes to the formation of diverticula in susceptible persons. According to the fiber hypothesis, a lack of dietary residue in the Western diet leads to sustained bowel contractions and a consequent increase in the intraluminal pressure. Such prolonged elevated pressure is believed to result in herniation of the superficial coats of the colon through the muscular layers into the serosa. It is probable that, in addition to pressure, defects in the wall of the colon are also required for the formation of a diverticulum.

☐ **Pathology:** The abnormal structures that characterize diverticulosis are not true diverticula, which contain all layers of the intestinal wall, but, rather, **pseudodiverticula,** in which only the mucosa and submucosa are herniated through the muscle layers. **The sigmoid colon is affected in 95% of the cases,** but diverticulosis can affect any segment of the colon, including the cecum.

Diverticula vary in number from a few to several hundred. Most appear in parallel rows between the mesenteric and lateral taeniae. The diverticula, which measure as much as 1 cm in greatest dimension, are connected to the intestinal lumen by necks of varying length and caliber. Hardened fecal material (fecalith) is frequently present in the diverticula, but this does not signify diverticulitis.

Microscopically, a diverticulum characteristically presents as a flask-like structure that extends from the lumen through the muscle layers (Fig. 13-30). The wall of the diverticulum is in continuity with the surface mucosa and, therefore, displays an epithelium and a submucosa. The base of the diverticulum is formed by serosal connective tissue.

☐ **Clinical Features:** Diverticulosis is generally asymptomatic, and 80% of affected persons remain free of symptoms. However, a significant number of

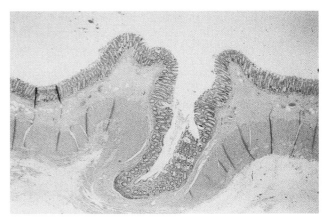

FIGURE   *13-30*
Diverticulosis of the colon. A low-power photomicrograph shows a diverticulum, which extends through the muscle layers.

those with diverticulosis complain of episodic, colicky abdominal pain. Both constipation and diarrhea, sometimes alternating, may occur, and flatulence is common. Sudden, painless, and severe bleeding from colonic diverticula is a cause of serious lower gastrointestinal hemorrhage in elderly persons, occurring in as many as 5% of persons with diverticulosis. Chronic blood loss may lead to anemia.

Diverticulitis

■ *Diverticulitis refers to inflammation at the base of a diverticulum, presumably in response to irritation caused by retained fecal material.* The large majority of persons with diverticulosis remain asymptomatic, but in 10% to 20%, diverticulitis supervenes at some time during their lives.

☐ **Pathology:** Diverticulitis produces necrosis of the wall of the diverticulum, which, in turn, results in perforation and release of fecal contents containing bacteria into the peridiverticular tissues. The resulting abscess is usually contained by the appendices epiploicae, the pericolonic fat, the mesentery, or adjacent organs, but infrequently, free perforation leads to generalized peritonitis. Fibrosis in response to repeated episodes of diverticulitis may constrict the lumen of the bowel, thereby causing intestinal obstruction. Fistulas may form between the colon and adjacent organs, including the bladder, vagina, small intestine, and skin of the abdomen.

☐ **Clinical Features:** The most common symptoms of diverticulitis, usually following microscopic or gross perforation of the diverticulum, are persistent lower abdominal pain and fever. Tenderness in the left lower quadrant is exhibited by most patients, and a mass in that area is not infrequently palpated. Leukocytosis is the rule. Antibiotic treatment and supportive measures are usually successful in alleviating acute diverticulitis, but approximately 20% of patients eventually require surgical intervention.

INFLAMMATORY BOWEL DISEASE

Crohn's Disease

■ *Crohn's disease is a chronic, granulomatous, inflammatory disease of the bowel wall of unknown cause.* The disease occurs principally in the small intestine and, occasionally, in the colon, but it may affect any part of the digestive tract. Although infectious, immunologic, dietary, and genetic causes have been invoked in the pathogenesis of Crohn's disease, none of these causes has been proved.

☐ **Epidemiology:** Crohn's disease occurs throughout the world, and the incidence of this disease seems to have risen dramatically during the past 30 years. The disease usually appears in adolescents or young adults and is most common among persons of European origin. A family history of either Crohn's disease or ulcerative colitis has been found in as many as 40% of cases.

☐ **Pathology:** The inflammation of Crohn's disease usually involves **all** layers of the bowel wall and, therefore, is referred to as transmural inflammatory disease. The inflammation of the intestine is discontinuous—that is, segments of inflamed tissue are separated by apparently normal intestine. Crohn's disease involves (1) mainly the ileum and cecum in 50% of cases, (2) only the small intestine in 15%, (3) only the colon in 20%, and (4) principally the anorectal region in 15%.

On gross examination, the affected bowel appears thickened and edematous, as does the adjacent mesentery. Mesenteric lymph nodes are frequently enlarged, firm, and matted together. The lumen is narrowed by edema in early cases and by a combination of edema and fibrosis in longstanding disease. Nodular swelling, fibrosis, and ulceration of the mucosa lead to a "cobblestone" appearance (Fig. 13-31). In early cases, ulcers have a superficial or a serpiginous appearance; later, they become deeper and appear as linear clefts or fissures.

The cut surface of the bowel wall shows the transmural nature of the disease, with thickening, edema, and fibrosis of all layers. Involved bowel loops often

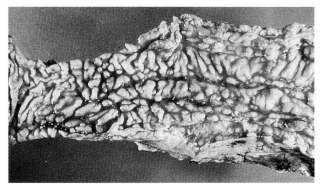

FIGURE *13-31*
Crohn's disease. The mucosal surface of the colon displays a "cobblestone" appearance owing to linear ulcerations, as well as edema and inflammation of the intervening tissue.

become adherent, and fistulas between such segments are frequent. These fistulas, which are presumably a late result of the deep mural ulcers, may also penetrate from the bowel into other organs, including the bladder, uterus, vagina, and skin. Most fistulas end blindly,

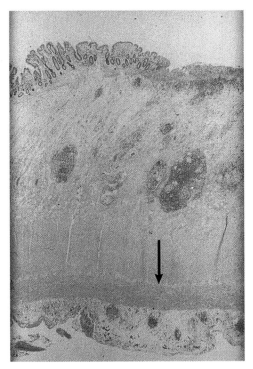

FIGURE *13-32*
Crohn's disease. A section of the colon shows mucosal ulceration (*right*), a submucosa thickened by edema and nodular aggregates of chronic inflammatory cells, prominence of the myenteric plexus (*arrow*), and an expanded and congested serosa.

forming abscess cavities within the peritoneal cavity, mesentery, or retroperitoneal structures. Lesions in the distal rectum may create perianal fistulas, a well-known presenting feature of Crohn's disease.

Microscopically, Crohn's disease appears as a chronic inflammatory process that typically extends through all layers of the bowel wall (Fig. 13-32). During the early phases of this disease, inflammation may be confined to the mucosa and submucosa. Small, superficial mucosal ulcerations (aphthous ulcers) are seen, together with mucosal and submucosal edema and increased numbers of lymphocytes, plasma cells, and macrophages. Later, long and deep, fissure-like ulcers are noted, and vascular hyalinization and fibrosis become apparent.

The microscopic hallmark of Crohn's disease is transmural nodular lymphoid aggregates, which are accompanied by proliferative changes of the muscularis mucosae and nerves of the submucosal and myenteric plexuses. Discrete, noncaseating granulomas, mostly in the submucosa, are often present as well. Although the presence of discrete granulomas is strong evidence in favor of the diagnosis of Crohn's disease, the absence of granulomas by no means excludes this diagnosis.

Pathologic features of Crohn's disease are summarized in Figure 13-33.

□ **Clinical Features:** The most frequent symptoms of Crohn's disease are abdominal pain and diarrhea, which occur in more than 75% of the patients, and recurrent fever, which is evident in 50%. In cases of diffuse small intestinal involvement, malabsorption and malnutrition may be the major features. Crohn's disease of the colon leads to diarrhea and, sometimes, colonic bleeding. In a few patients, the major site of involvement is the anorectal region, and recurrent anorectal fistulas are the presenting sign. Intestinal obstruction and fistulas are the most common intestinal complications of Crohn's disease. Occasionally, free perforation of the bowel occurs. **The risk of intestinal cancer is at least threefold greater in patients with Crohn's disease.**

No curative treatment is available for patients with Crohn's disease, but several medications are effective in suppressing the inflammatory reaction. Surgical resection of the obstructed areas or of severely involved portions of intestine and drainage of abscesses caused by fistulas are required in some cases.

Ulcerative Colitis

■ *Ulcerative colitis is a disease of the large intestine characterized by chronic diarrhea and rectal bleeding, with a pattern of exacerbations and remissions and the possibility of serious local and systemic complications.* The disorder oc-

curs principally, but not exclusively, in young adults, although it also afflicts children and elderly persons. In the United States, whites are affected more commonly than blacks.

The cause of ulcerative colitis is not known. The possibility that an abnormal immune response may play a role in the pathogenesis of ulcerative colitis has been extensively studied, but immune features may be merely epiphenomena—that is, they may be the result, rather than the cause, of the mucosal damage.

□ **Pathology:** Three major pathologic features characterize ulcerative colitis and help to differentiate it from other inflammatory conditions:

- **Ulcerative colitis is a diffuse disease.** It usually extends from the most distal part of the rectum for a variable distance proximally (Fig. 13-34). Sparing of the rectum or involvement of the right side of the colon alone is rare and, when present, suggests the possibility of another disorder (e.g., Crohn's disease).
- **The inflammatory process of ulcerative colitis is limited to the colon.**
- **Ulcerative colitis is essentially a disease of the mucosa.** Involvement of the deeper layers is uncommon, occurring only in fulminant cases and usually in association with toxic megacolon.

Early Colitis. Early in the evolution of ulcerative colitis, the mucosal surface appears raw, red, and granular. Later, small and superficial ulcers appear. These ulcers coalesce to form irregular, shallow, ulcerated areas that appear to surround islands of intact mucosa. In cases of **toxic megacolon,** the lumen is widely dilated, and the wall is thin and friable. Single or multiple perforations are common in patients with toxic megacolon, and the serosal surface is often covered by a fibrinopurulent exudate.

Early microscopic features of ulcerative colitis are (1) mucosal congestion; (2) edema; (3) microscopic hemorrhages; (4) diffuse, inflammatory infiltrate in the lamina propria; (5) variable loss of the surface epithelium; and (6) damage to the intestinal crypts, which are often surrounded and infiltrated by neutrophils (Fig. 13-35). Suppurative necrosis of the crypt epithelium gives rise to the characteristic crypt abscess, which appears as a dilated, degenerated crypt filled with neutrophils.

Progressive Colitis. As the disease progresses, lateral extension and coalescence of crypt abscesses undermine the mucosa, thereby leaving areas of ulceration adjacent to hanging fragments of mucosa. Such mucosal excrescences, surrounded by ulceration, are

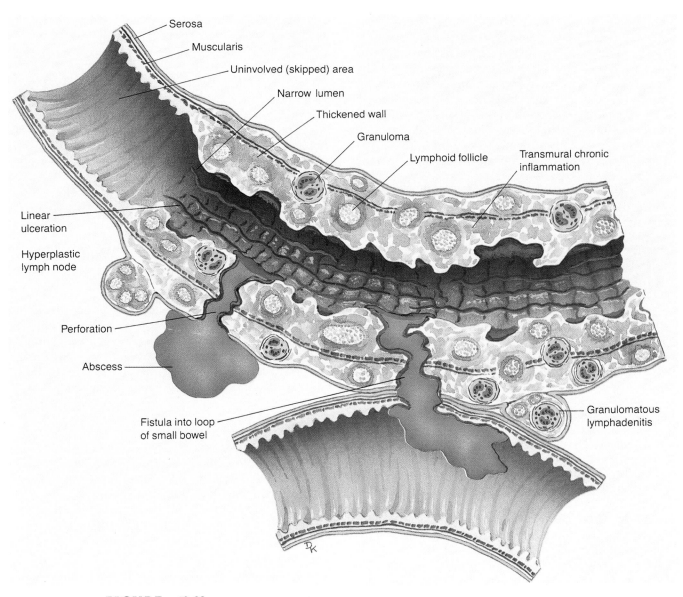

FIGURE 13-33
Crohn's disease. A schematic representation of the major features of Crohn's disease in the small intestine.

seen by endoscopy or roentgenographic examination as **inflammatory polyps** (Fig. 13-36). Microscopically, the intestinal crypts may appear tortuous, branched, and shortened during the late stages, or the mucosa may be diffusely atrophic.

Advanced Colitis. In longstanding cases, the large bowel is almost invariably shortened, especially in the left side. Microscopically, advanced ulcerative colitis is characterized by mucosal atrophy and a chronic inflammatory infiltrate in the mucosa and submucosa.

☐ **Clinical Features:** The clinical course and manifestations of ulcerative colitis are highly variable. Most patients (70%) have intermittent attacks, with partial or complete remission between them. A small number (<10%) have a very long remission (several years) following their first attack. The remaining 20% have continuous symptoms without remission. The major symptoms are recurrent diarrhea, rectal bleeding, crampy abdominal pain, and frequently, low-grade fever (lasting days or weeks). Moderate anemia is a common result of chronic fecal blood loss.

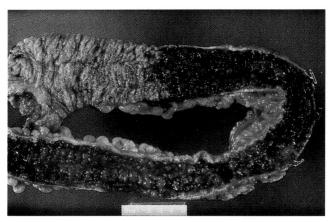

FIGURE   *13-34*
Ulcerative colitis. Prominent erythema and ulceration of the colon begin in the ascending colon and are most severe in the rectosigmoid area.

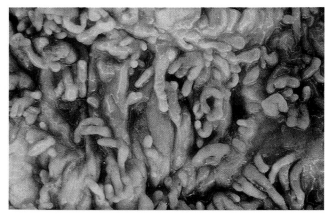

FIGURE   *13-36*
Inflammatory polyps of the colon in ulcerative colitis. Islands of regenerative mucosa surrounded by denuded areas provide a polypoid appearance.

A small minority (10%) of patients have severe or fulminant ulcerative colitis. They have more than six—and sometimes more than 20—bloody bowel movements a day, frequently accompanied by fever and other systemic manifestations. The loss of blood and fluids rapidly leads to anemia, dehydration, and electrolyte depletion. Massive hemorrhage is occasionally life-threatening. A particularly dangerous complication is toxic megacolon, which is characterized by extreme

dilatation of the colon. Patients with this condition are at high risk for perforation of the colon. Fulminant ulcerative colitis is a medical emergency requiring immediate, intensive medical therapy and, in some cases, prompt colectomy. Approximately 15% of patients with fulminant ulcerative colitis die from the disease.

Extraintestinal Manifestations

Arthritis is seen in 25% of patients with ulcerative colitis. Eye inflammation (mostly uveitis) develops in approximately 10%, and skin lesions occur in approximately the same number. The most common cutaneous lesions are erythema nodosum and pyoderma gangrenosum, with the latter being a serious, noninfective disorder characterized by deep, purulent, and necrotic ulcers in the skin.

Liver disease occurs in as many as 3% of patients, with the most common pathologic findings being pericholangitis and fatty liver. Chronic active hepatitis is occasionally encountered in conjunction with ulcerative colitis, and sclerosing cholangitis and carcinoma of the bile ducts are both associated with the intestinal disease. Thromboembolic phenomena, mostly deep vein thromboses of the lower extremities, occur in approximately 6% of patients with ulcerative colitis. The various complications of ulcerative colitis are shown in Figure 13-37, and the features that distinguish it from Crohn's disease are listed in Table 13-1.

Treatment is aimed at improving the general condition of the patient, suppressing the inflammatory response with corticosteroids and other anti-inflammatory agents, and maintaining remission for as long as possible. Selected patients benefit from a total colectomy.

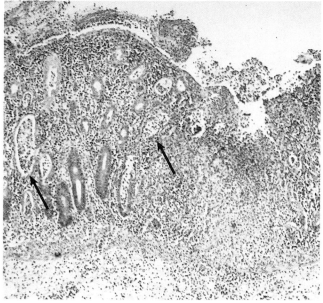

FIGURE   *13-35*
Ulcerative colitis. A section of the colonic mucosa from a patient with active ulcerative colitis shows purulent exudate on the surface, ulceration (*center*), diffuse inflammation superficial to the muscularis mucosae, and numerous crypt abscesses (*arrows*).

LOCAL COMPLICATIONS

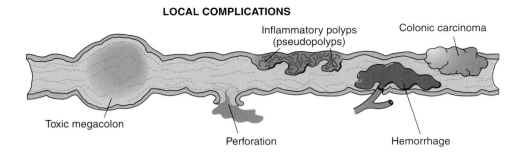

SYSTEMIC COMPLICATIONS

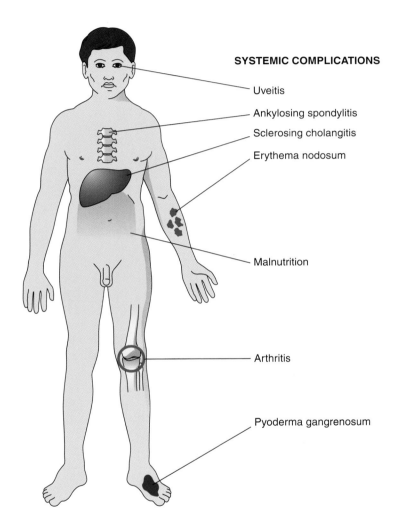

FIGURE *13-37*
Complications of ulcerative colitis.

Ulcerative Colitis and Colon Cancer

Persons with longstanding, extensive ulcerative colitis have a higher risk of colon cancer than the general population. A recent study in the United States places the cumulative risk of colon cancer after 25 years of ulcerative colitis at approximately 12%.

Epithelial dysplasia is a common finding in the colon and rectum of patients with longstanding ulcerative colitis (Fig. 13-38). Severe epithelial dysplasia is thought to reflect a high probability of cancer elsewhere in the colon or an increased risk of developing such cancer.

T A B L E   *13-1.*   Pathologic Features in the Colon of Crohn's Disease and Ulcerative Colitis

Lesion	Crohn's Disease	Ulcerative Colitis
Macroscopic		
Thickened bowel wall	Typical	Uncommon
Luminal narrowing	Typical	Uncommon
"Skip" lesions	Common	Absent
Right colon predominance	Typical	Absent
Fissures and fistulas	Common	Absent
Circumscribed ulcers	Common	Absent
Confluent linear ulcers	Common	Absent
Pseudopolyps	Absent	Common
Microscopic		
Transmural inflammation	Typical	Uncommon
Submucosal fibrosis	Typical	Absent
Fissures	Typical	Rare
Granulomas	Common	Absent
Crypt abscesses	Uncommon	Typical

VASCULAR DISEASES

Ischemic Colitis

The colon is subject to the same types of ischemic injury as the small intestine. Unlike the small bowel, however, extensive infarction of the colon is uncommon, and chronic segmental disease is the rule. Because most cases of ischemic colitis are caused by atherosclerosis, the intestinal disease usually occurs in persons older than 50 years of age.

☐ **Pathology:** Some patients present with symptoms and complications of bowel infarction and require immediate surgical intervention. However, in the majority of patients, the acute signs stabilize.

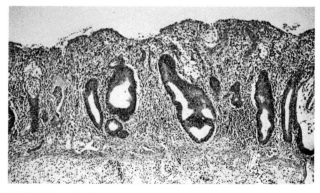

FIGURE   *13-38*
Epithelial dysplasia in ulcerative colitis. The colonic mucosa exhibits severe inflammation and irregular crypts lined by dysplastic epithelial cells. The epithelial cells exhibit hyperchromatic nuclei and basophilic cytoplasm and are focally stratified.

Biopsy specimens reveal the characteristic changes of ischemic necrosis of the bowel: mucosal ulcerations, crypt abscesses, and submucosal inflammation and fibrosis. Such patients may recover completely or develop a colonic stricture.

☐ **Clinical Features:** Ischemic disease of the rectosigmoid area is typically manifested as abdominal pain, rectal bleeding, and change in bowel habits. On clinical grounds alone, ischemic colitis often cannot be distinguished from nonspecific ulcerative colitis, Crohn disease of the colon, or certain forms of infectious colitis.

Angiodysplasia (Vascular Ectasia)

■ *Angiodysplasia, an established cause of lower intestinal bleeding, is characterized by localized arteriovenous malformations, predominantly in the cecum and ascending colon.* The mean age at presentation is 60 years. Surgical removal of the affected segment is curative.

The resected specimen displays small and often multiple hemangiomatous lesions, usually less than 0.5 cm in diameter. Microscopically, the veins and capillaries of the submucosa are tortuous, thin-walled, and dilated.

Hemorrhoids

■ *Hemorrhoids are dilated venous channels of the hemorrhoidal plexuses that result from downward displacement of the anal cushions.* These cushions are composed of submucosal connective tissue and are believed to aid in anal continence. **Internal hemorrhoids** arise from the superior hemorrhoidal plexus above the pectinate line, whereas **external hemorrhoids** originate from the inferior hemorrhoidal plexus below that line. That bleeding from hemorrhoids is bright red (arterial) suggests that these vessels are not truly varicose veins but, rather, a form of arteriovenous shunt, similar to those of the corpus cavernosum of the genitalia.

Hemorrhoids are common, to some degree afflicting at least half of the population older than 50 years in Western countries. By contrast, they are infrequent in populations who consume high-fiber diets. Hemorrhoids are common during pregnancy, presumably because of the increased abdominal pressure.

☐ **Pathology:** Microscopic examination of hemorrhoidectomy specimens discloses dilated vascular spaces with excess smooth muscle in their walls. Hemorrhage and thrombosis of varying severity are common. As a result of thrombosis and organization in an internal hemorrhoid, a fibrous polyp of the anal canal may develop. A similar process in an external hemorrhoid results in an anal tag.

□ **Clinical Features:** The salient clinical feature of hemorrhoids is bleeding, and chronic blood loss may lead to iron-deficiency anemia. Prolapsed hemorrhoids may become irreducible, which is a situation that leads to painful, "strangulated" hemorrhoids. Thrombosis of external hemorrhoids is exquisitely painful and requires evacuation of the intravascular clot.

POLYPS OF THE COLON

■ *Gastrointestinal polyp is defined as a mass that protrudes into the lumen of the gut.*

Adenomatous Polyps

■ *Adenomatous polyps of the colon are benign neoplasms that arise from the mucosal epithelium.* They are composed of crypt cells that have migrated to the surface and accumulated beyond the needs for replacement of the cells sloughed into the lumen.

□ **Epidemiology:** The prevalence of adenomatous polyps of the colon is highest in Western countries. As in diverticular disease, the only consistent environmental difference that has been identified between high-risk and low-risk populations is the diet (see the section on adenocarcinoma of the colon). In the United

States, it appears that at least one adenomatous polyp is present in half of the adult population, a figure that rises to more than two-thirds among persons older than 65 years of age.

□ **Pathology:** Almost half of all adenomatous polyps of the colon are located in the rectosigmoid region and, therefore, can be detected by digital examination or sigmoidoscopy. The remaining half is evenly distributed throughout the rest of the colon. The macroscopic appearance of an adenoma varies from a barely visible nodule or small, pedunculated tubular adenoma to a large, sessile villous adenoma. Many adenomatous polyps share features of both, in which case they are referred to as tubulovillous adenomas.

Tubular Adenoma: This polyp constitutes two-thirds of benign, large bowel adenomas. Tubular adenomas are typically smooth-surfaced spheres, usually less than 2 cm in diameter, and attached to the mucosa by a stalk (Fig. 13-39). Some 4% are reported to be larger than 2 cm in diameter.

Microscopically, a tubular adenoma exhibits closely packed epithelial tubules, which may be uniform or irregular and excessively branched. The stalk of a pedunculated tubular adenoma is lined by normal colonic mucosa, and its interior is composed of fibrovascular tissue, which is continuous with the normal submucosa.

Although the majority of tubular adenomas display little epithelial atypia, one-fifth, particularly the

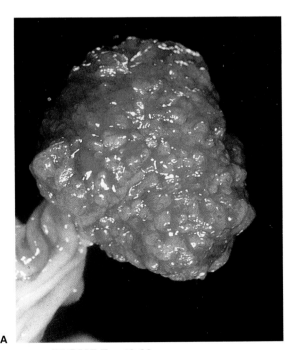
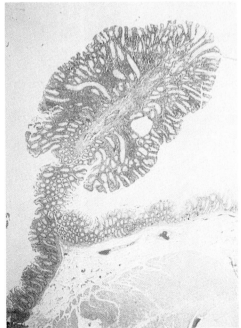

A   **B**

FIGURE   *13-39*
Tubular adenoma of the colon. (A) A pedunculated tubular adenoma. (B) A low-power photomicrograph of a tubular adenoma of the colon shows closely packed epithelial tubules. The fibrous stalk is vascular and covered by normal colonic epithelium.

larger tumors, show a range of more pronounced dysplastic features, which vary from mild nuclear pleomorphism to frank invasive carcinoma (Fig. 13-40). Intramucosal lesions that are severely dysplastic are classed by some pathologists as being carcinoma in situ. **As long as the dysplastic focus remains superficial to the muscularis mucosae, the lesion is invariably cured by resection of the polyp.**

The risk of invasive carcinoma correlates with the size of the tubular adenoma. Only 1% of tubular adenomas smaller than 1 cm in diameter contain invasive carcinoma at the time of resection. Among those between 1 and 2 cm in diameter, 10% are found to be malignant, and among those greater than 2 cm, 35% are malignant. Given that only few tubular adenomas are more than 2 cm in diameter, the overall risk of invasive carcinoma in these growths remains small.

Villous Adenoma. This polyp accounts for one-tenth of colonic adenomas and is found predominantly in the rectosigmoid region. It is typically a large, broad-based, and elevated lesion that grossly displays a shaggy, cauliflower-like surface (Fig. 13-41). More than half of villous adenomas are larger than 2 cm in diameter, and on occasion, they reach a diameter of 10 to 15 cm. Microscopically, villous adenomas are composed of thin, tall, finger-like processes that superficially resemble the villi of the small intestine. They are lined ex-

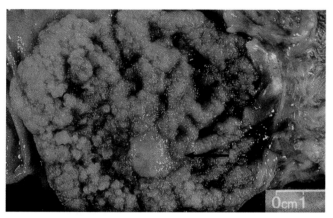

FIGURE　*13-41*
Villous adenoma of the colon. The colon contains a large, broad-based, elevated lesion that has a cauliflower-like surface. A firm area near the center of the lesion (*arrow*) proved on histologic examination to be an adenocarcinoma.

ternally by epithelial cells and are supported by a core of fibrovascular connective tissue corresponding to the normal lamina propria.

In contrast to tubular adenomas, villous adenomas commonly contain foci of carcinoma. In polyps less than 1 cm in diameter, the risk is 10-fold greater than that for comparably sized tubular adenomas. Of greater importance is the observation that villous adenomas greater than 2 cm in diameter have a 50% incidence of invasive carcinoma at the time of resection. **Given that 60% of villous adenomas measure more than 2 cm in greatest dimension, more than one-third of all resected villous adenomas contain invasive cancer.**

Adenomatous Polyps and Colorectal Cancer. It is now generally accepted that most colon cancers arise in pre-existing polyps. It is, therefore, common practice to remove all clinically detected polyps through a colonoscope.

Inherited Adenomatous Polyposis Syndromes

Familial Adenomatous Polyposis

■ *Familial adenomatous polyposis (APC), also termed adenomatous polyposis, is inherited as an autosomal dominant trait and is characterized by progressive development of innumerable adenomatous polyps of the colon, particularly in the rectosigmoid region.* Although young patients with APC have only few polyps, in a matter of a few years the colonic mucosa becomes carpeted, sometimes throughout its length, with thousands of adenomas (Fig. 13-42). These are mostly of the tubular vari-

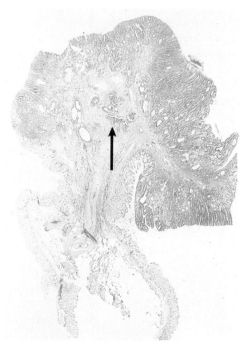

FIGURE　*13-40*
Adenocarcinoma arising in a pedunculated adenomatous polyp. A low-power photomicrograph shows irregular neoplastic glands (*arrow*) invading the stalk.

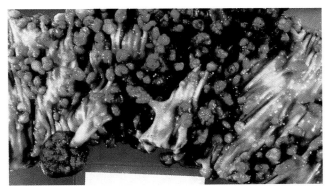

FIGURE   *13-42*
Familial polyposis. The mucosal surface of the colon is carpeted by innumerable adenomatous polyps.

ety, although tubulovillous and villous adenomas are also present. **Carcinoma of the colon is inevitable, nearly always by 40 years of age, unless a total colectomy is performed.**

Children of an afflicted parent have an even chance of developing polyposis; other relatives exhibit a 10% risk of manifesting the disease. **The *APC* gene has been mapped to the long arm of chromosome 5 (5q21).**

Gardner Syndrome

■ *Gardner syndrome is an autosomal dominant, familial disorder characterized by (1) gastrointestinal polyposis, principally in the colon but commonly in the stomach and the vicinity of the ampulla of Vater; (2) osteomas of the skull, mandible, and long bones; and (3) soft-tissue tumors of the skin.* **Gardner syndrome ultimately progresses to cancer of the colon.**

Nonneoplastic Polyps

Hyperplastic Polyps (Metaplastic Polyps)

■ *Hyperplastic polyps are small, sessile mucosal excrescences that display an exaggerated crypt architecture.* They are the most common polypoid lesions of the colon and are particularly frequent in the rectum.

Hyperplastic polyps are remarkably common, being present in 40% of rectal specimens from persons younger than 40 years of age and in 75% of older persons. The association of hyperplastic polyps with rectal cancer is striking: 90% of rectal specimens removed for cancer contain such polyps. Thus, although these asymptomatic lesions are not themselves preneoplastic, they reflect an increased risk of colon cancer. The pathogenesis of the hyperplastic polyp is believed to involve a maturation defect of the normal mucosal epithelium.

□ **Pathology:** Hyperplastic polyps present macroscopically as small, sessile, raised mucosal nodules that are as much as 0.5 cm in diameter (and occasionally larger). They are almost always multiple, and they have even been mistaken for familial polyposis coli. Histologically, the crypts of the hyperplastic polyp are elongated (Fig. 13-43) and may exhibit cystic dilatation. The overall appearance is superficially similar to that of a villous adenoma. The epithelium is composed of well-differentiated goblet cells and absorptive cells, without any atypical features.

Juvenile Polyps (Retention Polyps)

■ *Juvenile polyps are hamartomas of the colonic mucosa.* They are most common in children younger than 10 years of age, but approximately one-third occur in adults.

□ **Pathology:** Juvenile polyps may be single or multiple. They occur most commonly in the rectum, although they may be seen anywhere in the small or large bowel. Grossly, most polyps are pedunculated lesions as much as 2 cm in diameter. They have a smooth, rounded surface, which is in contrast to the fissured surface of an adenomatous polyp. Histologically, dilated and cystic epithelial tubules are embedded in a fibrovascular lamina propria (Fig. 13-44). The cells lining the tubules are regular and show no atypical features. The polyps usually slough by autoamputation or regress spontaneously. **Juvenile polyps do not progress to cancer.**

Inflammatory Polyps

Inflammatory polyps are not neoplasms but, rather, elevated masses of chronically inflamed and regenerat-

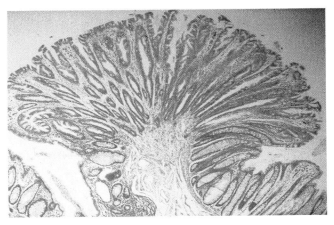

FIGURE   *13-43*
Hyperplastic polyp of the colon. A low-power photomicrograph shows elongated crypts, which create an appearance somewhat similar to that of a villous adenoma.

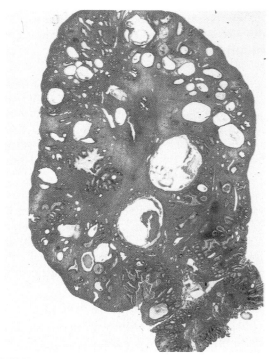

FIGURE *13-44*
Juvenile polyp of the colon. A low-power photomicrograph shows cystic epithelial tubules embedded in a fibrovascular stroma.

ing epithelium over ulcerations caused by an inflammatory disease of the colon. Such polyps are commonly found in association with ulcerative colitis and Crohn disease. They are also encountered in cases of amebic colitis and bacterial dysentery. Microscopically, inflammatory polyps are composed of distorted and inflamed mucosal glands, which may be intermixed with regenerating, large, basophilic epithelial cells. When the surface of the polyp is ulcerated, granulation tissue may be prominent.

ADENOCARCINOMA OF THE COLON AND RECTUM

In Western industrialized societies, colorectal cancer is second in incidence only to carcinoma of the lung in men, and it is third in incidence (after breast and lung cancer) in women. Overall, in the United States, one-third of large bowel cancers occur in the rectum and rectosigmoid regions, and an additional one-fourth develop in the sigmoid colon.

☐ **Pathogenesis:** Cancer of the colon arises in adenomatous polyps. Therefore, factors associated with development of such polyps are probably relevant to the genesis of colorectal cancer.

Dietary Fiber. A diet low in indigestible fiber has been suggested as being a causative factor in cancer of the colon and other colonic diseases, including diverticulosis, adenomatous polyps, appendicitis, and ulcerative colitis. However, a recent report from the National Research Council Committee on Diet, Nutrition, and Cancer stated that there is "no conclusive evidence to indicate that dietary fiber exerts a protective effect against colorectal cancer in humans."

Dietary Fat. An increase in the consumption of animal fats (e.g., that associated with the recent change in dietary habits in Japan) is paralleled by an increased incidence of colon cancer.

Other Dietary Factors. A low prevalence of colon cancer has been correlated with high levels of selenium in the soil and plants of certain geographic areas. Exogenous antioxidants (e.g., butylated hydroxytoluene and vitamin E) and a reducing agent such as ascorbic acid have protected animals against experimental production of colon cancer. Diets rich in cruciferous vegetables (e.g., cauliflower, brussels sprouts, and cabbage) and those that provide vitamin A are said to be associated with a lower incidence of colon cancer.

Anaerobic Bacteria. Feces of persons in high-risk populations have a higher content of anaerobic bacteria than those of persons in low-risk populations.

Molecular Biology of Colon Cancer. It is now believed that sequential alterations of at least one proto-oncogene and several suppressor genes are required for development of colorectal cancers:

- *APC* **gene.** As previously noted, germline mutations in the *APC* gene, a putative tumor suppressor gene, are responsible for familial adenomatous polyposis. Colorectal cancers also contain a mutation in this gene. Some tumors display a mutation in the gene for β-catenin, whose product binds to the APC protein.
- *ras* **Oncogene.** Many colorectal cancers and adenomas demonstrate point mutations that activate the *ras* proto-oncogene.
- **p53 Tumor suppressor gene.** The *p53* gene is mutated, or even deleted, in many cases of colorectal cancer.
- *DCC* **gene.** A putative tumor suppressor gene, labeled "deleted in colon cancer" (DCC), is located on chromosome 18 and is often missing in colorectal cancers.
- **Mismatch repair genes.** In approximately 15% of patients with colorectal cancer, mutations in a group of genes involved in mismatch repair are

found. Such alterations lead to DNA replication errors and other mutations.

It has been estimated that a minimum of eight to 10 mutagenic events must accumulate to produce an invasive colon cancer. Figure 13-45 presents a model of the genetic events that accompany development of colon cancer.

Risk Factors

Age. Increasing age is probably the single most important risk factor for colorectal cancer in the general population. The risk is low before the age of 40 years but then increases steadily to age 50, after which it doubles with each decade of life, finally reaching a maximum at age 75.

Previous Colorectal Cancer. Patients who previously had colorectal cancer have an increased risk of a subsequent tumor.

Ulcerative Colitis. This chronic disease increases the risk of colorectal cancer in proportion to its duration and its extent within the colon.

Hereditary Polyposis Syndromes. These genetic disorders, with the exception of the Peutz-Jeghers syndrome, are inevitably complicated by colon cancer.

Even Peutz-Jeghers syndrome is not a true exception, however. Its hamartomatous lesions are associated with a higher-than-normal incidence of adenomatous polyps and, therefore, of colon cancer.

Genetic Factors. Colon cancer shows a modest increase in frequency among relatives of patients with the disease. Familial kindreds with colorectal cancer have also been described. A previous history of cancer at other sites, particularly breast or genital cancer in women, is associated with a higher-than-normal frequency of colorectal cancer.

Diet. As previously noted, prospective studies involving large populations in various countries have reported that daily consumption of red meat and animal fat is associated with a 2.5-fold increase in the risk of colon cancer compared with persons who eat little or no meat.

☐ **Pathology:** The gross appearance of colorectal cancers is similar to that of adenocarcinomas elsewhere in the gastrointestinal tract. They may be polypoid, ulcerating, or infiltrative, being in the last case customarily annular and constrictive (Fig. 13-46). Polypoid cancers are most common on the right side of the colon, particularly in the cecum, where the large caliber of the colon allows unimpeded intraluminal growth. Annular constricting tumors occur most often

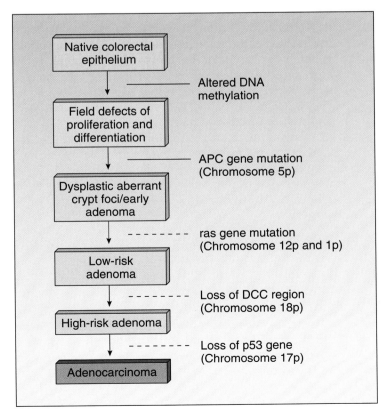

FIGURE *13-45*
Model of some of the genetic alterations involved in sporadic colorectal carcinogenesis.

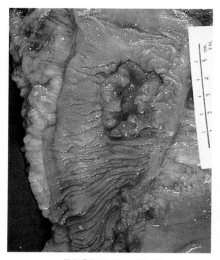
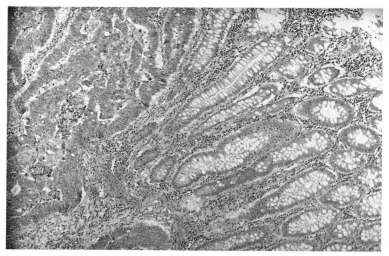

A   **B**

FIGURE   *13-46*
Adenocarcinoma of the colon. (A) The opened colon contains an elevated, centrally ulcerated, infiltrating mass. (B) A section taken at the margin of the tumor shows infiltrating adenocarcinoma (*left*) adjacent to normal colonic mucosa.

in the distal portions of the colon. Ulceration of tumors, irrespective of the growth pattern, is usual.

The vast majority of colorectal cancers are adenocarcinomas, which are similar microscopically to their counterparts in other portions of the gastrointestinal tract. Most are well differentiated and secrete small amounts of mucin.

The prognosis of a patient with colon cancer is more closely related to the extension of the tumor through the wall of the colon than to its histologic characteristics. Colorectal cancers are staged according to the original Dukes classification of 1932 or the modification proposed by Astler and Coller:

- **Stage A.** Tumor confined to the mucosa.
- **Stage B$_1$.** Tumor invading the muscularis propria but not penetrating to the serosa.
- **Stage B$_2$.** Tumor invading the serosa but without lymph node metastases.
- **Stage C$_1$.** B$_1$ tumors with metastases to the regional lymph nodes.
- **Stage C$_2$.** B$_2$ tumors with metastases to the regional lymph nodes.
- **Stage D.** Distant metastases.

Colorectal cancer invades the lymphatic channels and, initially, involves the lymph nodes immediately underlying the tumor. Venous invasion leads to blood-borne metastases, which involve the liver in 75% of patients with metastatic disease. The lungs, bones, and brain are not uncommon sites of metastases.

☐ **Clinical Features:** During its initial stages, colorectal cancer is clinically silent. As the tumor grows,

the most common sign is occult intestinal bleeding (when the tumor is in the proximal portions of the colon) or bright-red blood (when the lesion is in the rectum). In the right side of the colon, particularly in the cecum, where the diameter of the lumen is large and the fecal contents are liquid, tumors grow to a large size without causing symptoms of obstruction. Chronic asymptomatic bleeding from such tumors typically causes severe anemia, which thus is often the first indication of colon cancer. By contrast, cancers on the left side of the colon, where the caliber of the lumen is small and the fecal contents are more solid, often constrict the lumen, thereby producing obstructive symptoms. These symptoms are manifested as changes in bowel habits, gaseousness, abdominal pain, and reduced caliber of the stools.

Patients with stage A colon cancer are almost invariably cured by surgical resection. The 5-year survival rate of patients with stage B tumors is 70%, whereas that of patients with stage C disease is 50%. The only curative treatment for colorectal cancer is surgery.

CANCER OF THE ANAL CANAL

Carcinomas of the anal canal, which constitute 2% of all cancers of the colon, may arise either at or above the dentate line. These tumors occur in both sexes but are more common in women, who usually are older than 50 years of age.

☐ **Pathology:** Although anal cancers have various histologic patterns, such as squamous, basaloid (cloacogenic), or mucoepidermoid, there are few clinical differences in behavior among the different tumor types, and they can be conveniently classed as epidermoid carcinoma. Anal cancers penetrate directly into the surrounding tissues, including the internal and external sphincters, perianal soft tissues, prostate, and vagina. Lymphatic spread carries the tumor to the pelvic and the inguinal nodes, and hematogenous dissemination may lead to distant metastases.

☐ **Clinical Features:** Chronic inflammatory disease of the anus (e.g., venereal disease), fissures, and trauma produced by anal intercourse predispose to anal cancer. In fact, receptive anal intercourse among male homosexuals is associated with a 30-fold increase in the risk of anal cancer.

Usual symptoms include bleeding, pain, and an anal or rectal mass. Abdominal-perineal resection, with or without radiation therapy, is the customary treatment for large lesions. More than half of the patients survive for at least 5 years.

Appendix

ACUTE APPENDICITIS

■ *Acute appendicitis is an inflammatory disease affecting the wall of the vermiform appendix that often results in transmural necrosis and perforation, with subsequent localized or generalized peritonitis.* This condition, which is by far the most common disease of the appendix, is the most frequent cause of an abdominal emergency. Although the incidence peaks during the second and third decades of life, acute appendicitis may occur in persons of any age.

☐ **Pathogenesis:** The pathogenesis of acute appendicitis is believed to relate to obstruction of its orifice, with secondary distention of the lumen and bacterial invasion of the wall. Mechanical obstruction by fecaliths or solid fecal material in the cecum is often demonstrated. However, no obstruction is demonstrated in as many as half of the patients with appendicitis, and in these cases, the factor that precipitates the disease is unknown.

☐ **Pathology:** Macroscopically, the resected appendix is congested, tense, and covered by a fibrinous exudate. The lumen often contains purulent material, and a fecalith may be evident (Fig. 13-47).

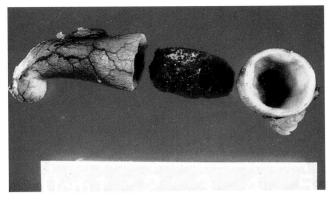

FIGURE   *13-47*
Acute appendicitis. The lumen of this acutely inflamed appendix is dilated and contains a large fecalith.

Microscopically, early cases show mucosal microabscesses and a purulent exudate in the lumen. As the infection progresses, the entire wall becomes infiltrated with neutrophils, which eventually reach the serosa. In turn, necrosis of the wall leads to perforation and release of the luminal contents into the peritoneal cavity. The inflammatory process may subside, leaving a narrow, scarred appendix in which the lumen is obliterated.

Complications of appendicitis principally relate to perforation, which is reported to occur in approximately one-third of children and young adults:

- **Periappendiceal abscesses** are common.
- **Fistulous tracts** may appear between the perforated appendix and adjacent structures.
- **Pylephlebitis** (thrombophlebitis of the intrahepatic portal vein radicals) and **secondary hepatic abscesses** may occur, because venous blood from the appendix drains into the superior mesenteric vein.
- **Diffuse peritonitis** and **septicemia** are dangerous sequelae.
- **Wound infection** is the most common complication of acute appendicitis following surgery.

☐ **Clinical Features:** Acute appendicitis is typically manifested as epigastric or periumbilical cramping pain. Shortly thereafter, nausea and vomiting occur, and the patient develops a low-grade fever and moderate leukocytosis. The pain shifts to the right lower quadrant, where point tenderness is the rule. Treatment of acute appendicitis is surgical in the vast majority of cases.

NEOPLASMS

Mucocele

■ *Mucocele is a dilated, mucus-filled appendix.* The pathogenesis may be neoplastic or nonneoplastic. In the nonneoplastic variety, the mucosa of the appendix is often hyperplastic, resembling hyperplastic polyps of the colon. It is thought that hyperplasia of the mucosa obstructs the lumen and that chronic obstruction leads to retention of mucus in the appendiceal lumen.

A more common cause of mucocele of the appendix is the presence of a cystadenoma or cystadenocarcinoma. These tumors are usually lined by a villous adenomatous mucosa or, in the case of cystadenocarcinoma, may exhibit infiltrating neoplastic glands. Perforation may lead to seeding of the peritoneum by malignant, mucus-secreting tumor cells, a condition known as **pseudomyxoma peritonei.**

Carcinoid Tumor

The most common neoplasm of the appendix is the carcinoid tumor, which, in this location, rarely metastasizes.

CHAPTER 14

The Liver and Biliary System

Emanuel Rubin
John L. Farber

(continued)

Wilson Disease (Hepatolenticular Degeneration)

Cystic Fibrosis

α_1-Antitrypsin Deficiency

Inborn Errors of Carbohydrate Metabolism

Portal Hypertension

Intrahepatic Portal Hypertension

Prehepatic Portal Hypertension

Posthepatic Portal Hypertension

Budd-Chiari Syndrome

Complications of Portal Hypertension

Toxic Liver Injury

Zonal Hepatocellular Necrosis

Fatty Liver

Intrahepatic Cholestasis

Lesions Resembling Viral Hepatitis

Chronic Active Hepatitis

Vascular Lesions

Hyperplastic and Neoplastic Lesions

Circulatory Disorders

Congestive Heart Failure (Chronic Passive Congestion)

Shock

Infarction

Bacterial Infections

Neonatal Hepatitis

Biliary Atresia

Benign Tumors and Tumor-Like Lesions

Hepatic Adenoma

Focal Nodular Hyperplasia

Hemangioma

Hepatocellular Carcinoma

Cholangiocarcinoma (Bile Duct Carcinoma)

Metastatic Cancer

GALLBLADDER AND EXTRAHEPATIC BILE DUCTS

Cholelithiasis

Cholesterol Stones

Pigment Stones

Acute Cholecystitis

Chronic Cholecystitis

Carcinoma of the Gallbladder

Carcinoma of the Bile Duct and Ampulla of Vater

Liver

The liver subserves a wide variety of functions. These functions can be broadly categorized as metabolic, synthetic, storage, catabolic, and excretory.

Metabolic Functions. As the central organ of glucose homeostasis, the liver maintains blood glucose levels by glycogenolysis and gluconeogenesis.

Synthetic Functions. The liver produces albumin, blood coagulation factors, complement and other acute-phase reactants, and numerous specific binding proteins (e.g., for iron, copper, and vitamin A).

Storage Capacity. The liver is an important storage site for glycogen, triglycerides, iron, copper, and lipid-soluble vitamins.

Catabolic Processes. Endogenous substances, including hormones and serum proteins, are catabolized by the liver to maintain a balance between their production and elimination.

Excretory Function. The principal excretory product of the liver is bile, which not only provides a repository for the products of heme catabolism but is vital for the absorption of fat in the small intestine.

BILIRUBIN METABOLISM AND MECHANISMS OF JAUNDICE

Normal Bilirubin Metabolism

Bilirubin, which is the major end product of heme catabolism, has no known physiologic function. As much as 85% of bilirubin is derived from senescent **erythrocytes,** which are removed from the circulation by mononuclear phagocytes of the spleen, bone marrow, and liver. Most of the remaining bilirubin arises from the degradation of heme produced by other sources, the most important of which is the premature breakdown of hemoglobin in developing erythroid cells of the bone marrow.

Bilirubin is released from phagocytes and other cells into the circulation, where it is bound to albumin for transport to the liver. On reaching the sinusoidal plasma membrane of the hepatocyte, the albumin/bilirubin complex is dissociated. Transfer of bilirubin from the blood to the bile involves (1) **uptake** of bilirubin by a plasma membrane receptor, (2) **binding** to specific proteins, (3) **conjugation** with glucuronic acid, and (4) **excretion** into the bile canaliculus, where it is then excreted into the bile.

■ *Hyperbilirubinemia refers to an increased concentration of bilirubin in the blood (>1.0 mg/dL).*

■ *Jaundice or icterus describes yellow skin and sclerae* (Fig. 14-1), which become apparent when the circulating bilirubin concentration attains a level of greater than 2.0 to 2.5 mg/dL.

■ *Cholestasis is the presence of plugs of inspissated bile in dilated bile canaliculi and visible bile pigment in hepatocytes.*

■ *Cholestatic jaundice is characterized by histologic cholestasis and hyperbilirubinemia.*

Conditions associated with hyperbilirubinemia are shown in Figure 14-2.

Overproduction of Bilirubin

Increased production of bilirubin results from increased destruction of erythrocytes (hemolytic anemia) or ineffective erythropoiesis (dyserythropoiesis). The hyperbilirubinemia of uncomplicated hemolytic disease principally involves unconjugated bilirubin, whereas in parenchymal liver disease, both conjugated and unconjugated bilirubin participate. The unconjugated hyperbilirubinemia of hemolytic disease has little clinical significance in adults, but in newborns, it may be catastrophic. As discussed in Chapter 6, hemolytic disease of the newborn may result in concentrations of unconjugated bilirubin that are high enough to cause damage to the brain (**kernicterus**). Kernicterus has generally been associated with bilirubin concentrations of greater than 20 mg/dL, but subtle degrees of psychomotor retardation may follow the presence of considerably lower concentrations.

Decreased Hepatic Uptake of Bilirubin

Hyperbilirubinemia can result from impaired hepatic uptake of unconjugated bilirubin. Such a situation occurs in generalized liver cell injury, as exemplified by viral hepatitis. Certain drugs (e.g., rifampin and probenecid) interfere with the net uptake of bilirubin by the liver cell and may produce a mild unconjugated hyperbilirubinemia.

Decreased Bilirubin Conjugation

Crigler-Najjar Disease

■ *Crigler-Najjar disease is a recessively inherited malady in which little or no bilirubin is conjugated in the hepatocyte and patients suffer unremitting unconjugated hyperbilirubinemia.* The hereditary defect resides in a complete absence of uridine diphosphoglucuronyl transferase activity. The morphologic appearance of the liver is normal by both light and electron microscopy. Infants with Crigler-Najjar disease invariably develop bilirubin encephalopathy and usually die during the first year of life. The condition can be treated with liver transplantation.

Gilbert Syndrome

■ *Gilbert syndrome is an inherited, autosomal dominant, mild, chronic, unconjugated hyperbilirubinemia (<6 mg/dL) caused by impaired clearance of bilirubin in the absence of any detectable functional or structural liver disease.* Gilbert syndrome is exceptionally common, occurring in 5% to 10% of the population. It is seen more often in men than in women and is usually recognized after puberty. The coding region of the uridine diphosphoglucuronyl transferase (UGT) gene is normal, but mutations in the promoter region lead to reduced transcription of the gene and, consequently, inadequate synthesis of the enzyme. Gilbert syndrome is, for the most part, asymptomatic, although vague symptoms of lassitude and weakness are common.

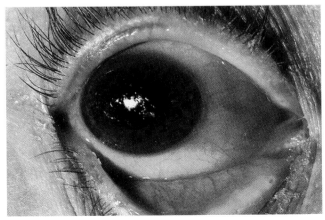

FIGURE **14-1**
Jaundice. A patient in hepatic failure displays yellow sclera.

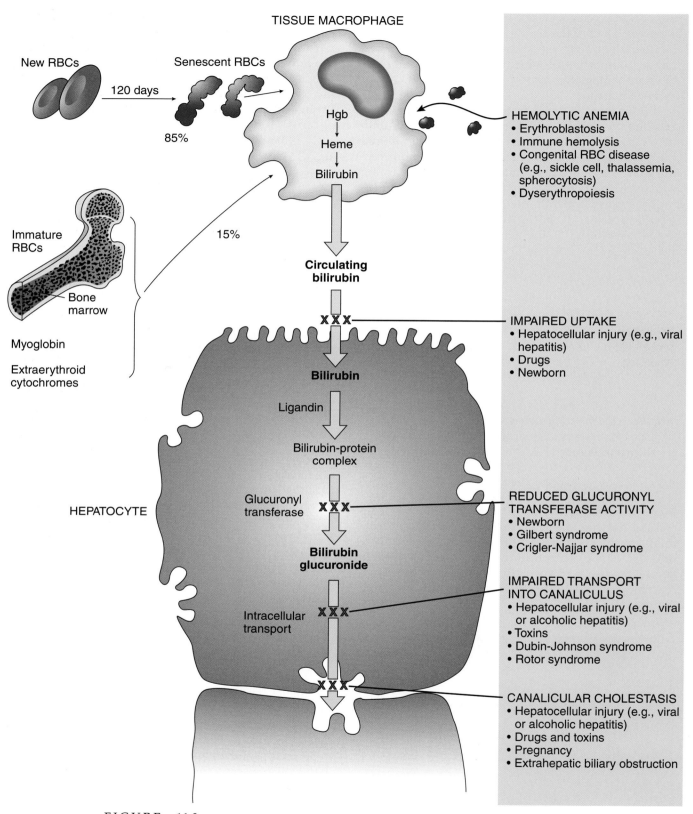

F I G U R E   *14-2*
Mechanisms of jaundice at the level of the hepatocyte. Bilirubin is derived principally from the senescence of circulating red blood cells, with a smaller contribution being derived from the degradation of erythropoietic elements in the bone marrow, myoglobin, and extraerythroid cytochromes. Jaundice results from overproduction of bilirubin (hemolytic anemia) or from defects in its hepatic metabolism. The locations of specific blocks in the metabolic pathway of bilirubin in the hepatocyte are illustrated.

Decreased Intracellular Transport of Conjugated Bilirubin

Dubin-Johnson Syndrome

■ *Dubin-Johnson syndrome is an autosomal recessive, familial disease that is recognized by chronic or intermittent conjugated hyperbilirubinemia and is accompanied by a "black" liver.* The hereditary defect resides in an impaired transport of conjugated bilirubin from the hepatocyte to the canalicular lumen.

☐ **Pathology:** The microscopic appearance of the liver is entirely normal, except for the accumulation of coarse, iron-free, dark-brown granules in the hepatocytes and Kupffer cells, primarily in the centrilobular zone (Fig. 14-3). By electron microscopy, the pigment is seen in enlarged lysosomes.

☐ **Clinical Features:** Except for mild intermittent jaundice, most patients with Dubin-Johnson syndrome do not complain of any symptoms. The serum bilirubin concentration varies from 2 to 5 mg/dL, although it may be much higher transiently.

Neonatal (Physiologic) Jaundice

Almost 70% of full-term, normal newborns exhibit hyperbilirubinemia. The large majority of these newborns are entirely healthy and are said to manifest "physiologic jaundice." However, in a few, this jaundice is the initial manifestation of a pathologic process that requires further investigation.

☐ **Pathogenesis:** The liver of the newborn assumes the responsibility for bilirubin clearance before its conjugating and excretory capacities are fully developed. **As a consequence, normal newborns, and particularly premature infants, exhibit a transient, physiologic unconjugated hyperbilirubinemia.** The hepatic bilirubin-conjugating capacity reaches adult levels approximately 2 weeks after birth, and serum bilirubin levels then rapidly decline to adult values.

Impairment of Canalicular Bile Flow

Secretion of bile into the canaliculus and its passage into the biliary collecting system is an active process that depends on a number of factors. Interference with any of these results in **cholestasis**, which is defined by three distinct criteria: (1) morphologic, (2) clinical, and (3) functional:

- The pathologist defines cholestasis as the morphologic demonstration of visible biliary pigment within bile canaliculi and hepatocytes (Fig. 14-4).
- The clinical diagnosis is based on the accumulation in the blood of materials normally transferred to the bile, including bilirubin, cholesterol, and bile acids, and the presence in the blood of elevated activities of certain enzymes, typically alkaline phosphatase.
- Functionally, cholestasis represents a decrease in bile flow through the canaliculus and a reduction in the secretion of water, bilirubin, and bile acids by the hepatocyte.

Cholestasis may be produced by intrinsic liver disease, in which case the term **intrahepatic cholestasis** is used, or by obstruction of the large bile ducts, when the label **extrahepatic cholestasis** is applied. Whatever the

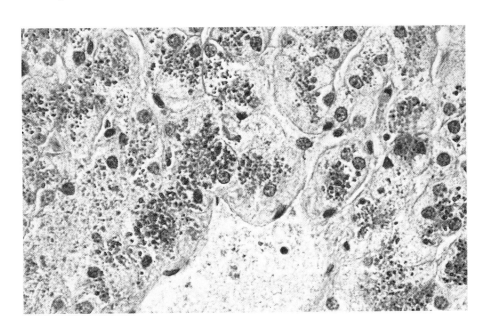

FIGURE *14-3*
Dubin-Johnson syndrome. The hepatocytes contain coarse, iron-free, dark-brown granules.

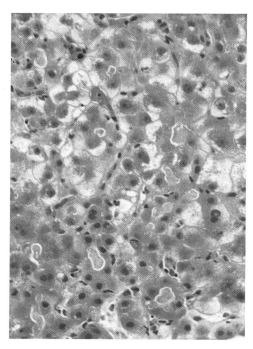

FIGURE 14-4
Bile stasis. A photomicrograph of the liver shows prominent bile plugs in dilated bile canaliculi.

biochemical basis of cholestasis, there is a centrilobular predilection for the appearance of canalicular bile plugs. The invariable presence of bile constituents in the blood of persons with cholestasis implies regurgitation from the hepatocyte into the bloodstream.

Morphology of Cholestasis

The morphologic hallmark of cholestasis is the presence of brownish bile pigment within dilated canaliculi and in hepatocytes (see Fig. 14-4). By electron microscopy, the canaliculus is enlarged, and the microvilli are usually blunted and decreased in number (or even absent). When cholestasis persists, secondary morphologic abnormalities develop. Scattered necrotic hepatocytes probably reflect a toxic effect of excess intracellular bile. Within the sinusoids, macrophages and lymphoid cells appear. The macrophages and resident Kupffer cells contain bile pigment and cellular debris. Whereas early cholestasis is restricted almost exclusively to the central zone, chronic cholestasis is marked by the appearance of bile plugs in the periphery of the lobule as well.

In patients with longstanding cholestasis (usually the result of extrahepatic biliary obstruction), groups of hepatocytes manifest hydropic swelling, diffuse impregnation with bile pigment, and reticulated appearance, thereby forming a triad termed **feathery degeneration.** The necrosis of such cells, together with the

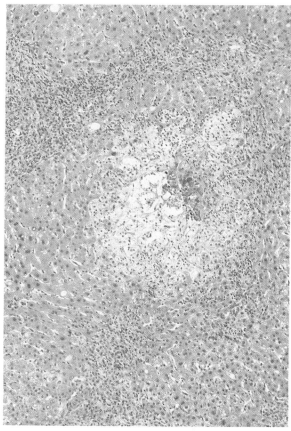

FIGURE 14-5
Bile infarct (bile lake). A photomicrograph of the liver in a patient with extrahepatic biliary obstruction shows an area of necrosis and accumulation of extravasated bile.

accumulation of extravasated bile in the area, results in a golden-yellow focus of extracellular pigment and debris known as a **bile infarct** or **bile lake** (Fig. 14-5).

Sites of obstruction to the flow of bile in the liver are depicted in Figure 14-6.

HEPATIC FAILURE

■ *Hepatic failure is a clinical syndrome characterized by jaundice, encephalopathy, and other metabolic derangements that occur when the mass of liver cells is sufficiently diminished or their function is impaired.* Consequences of acute and chronic hepatic failure are depicted in Figure 14-7.

Jaundice

Hepatic failure is always associated with jaundice as a result of an inadequate clearance of bilirubin by the diseased liver. The hyperbilirubinemia is, for the most part, conjugated, but on occasion, increased erythro-

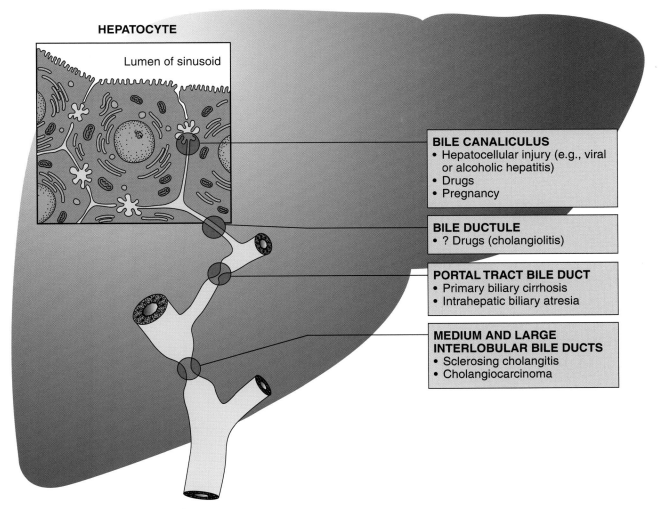

HEPATOCYTE

Lumen of sinusoid

BILE CANALICULUS
• Hepatocellular injury (e.g., viral or alcoholic hepatitis)
• Drugs
• Pregnancy

BILE DUCTULE
• ? Drugs (cholangiolitis)

PORTAL TRACT BILE DUCT
• Primary biliary cirrhosis
• Intrahepatic biliary atresia

MEDIUM AND LARGE INTERLOBULAR BILE DUCTS
• Sclerosing cholangitis
• Cholangiocarcinoma

FIGURE *14-6*
Sites of intrahepatic cholestasis.

cyte turnover may lead to unconjugated hyperbilirubinemia, thereby aggravating the jaundice.

Hepatic Encephalopathy

■ *Hepatic encephalopathy refers to a variety of neurologic signs and symptoms in patients who suffer chronic liver failure or in whom the portal circulation is diverted.* With unrelenting liver failure, hepatic encephalopathy progresses from lethargy to deep somnolence and, eventually, to coma.

□ **Pathogenesis:** The pathogenesis of hepatic encephalopathy remains elusive. The encephalopathy is probably caused, at least in part, by toxic compounds absorbed from the intestine that have escaped hepatic detoxification because of hepatocyte dysfunction or the existence of structural or functional vascular shunts. The latter mechanism is particularly evident after surgical construction of a portal/systemic anastomosis (portal vein to inferior vena cava or its equivalent) for the relief of portal hypertension, which accounts for the synonym **portasystemic encephalopathy.**

Substances that have been proposed to account for hepatic encephalopathy include:

• **Ammonia.** Most of the body's ammonia is of dietary origin, coming from the ingestion of ammonia in foods, digestion of proteins in the small intestine, bacterial catabolism of dietary protein, and urea secreted into the intestine.

• **γ-Aminobutyric acid.** The γ-aminobutyric acid (GABA)/benzodiazepine receptor complex may play an important role in hepatic encephalopathy. There is now substantial evidence that endogenous benzodiazepine-like substances contribute to the encephalopathy of liver failure by stimulating GABA-ergic neurotransmission.

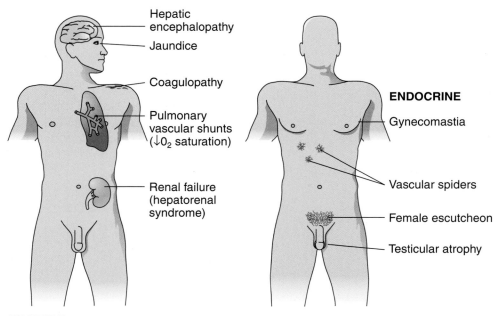

FIGURE   *14-7*
Complications of hepatic failure.

- **Mercaptans.** These compounds result from the breakdown of sulfur-containing amino acids in the colon.
- **False Neurotransmitters.** These include substances such as octopamine.

☐ Pathology: In patients who have died with chronic liver disease and hepatic coma, the most striking changes are found in the cerebral astrocytes. These cells are increased in number and size, and they show the swelling, nuclear enlargement, and nuclear inclusions characteristic of **Alzheimer type II astrocytes.**

Hepatorenal Syndrome

Acute hepatic failure is commonly marked by an associated renal failure, which is characterized by azotemia and oliguria or anuria. The major determinant of hepatorenal syndrome seems to be decreased renal blood flow and consequent reduction in the glomerular filtration rate.

☐ Pathology: In patients with hepatorenal syndrome, no intrinsic renal disease can be demonstrated morphologically. At autopsy, patients with jaundice and hepatorenal syndrome show bile staining of the renal tubular cells and bile casts in the lumina (so-called biliary nephrosis). However, these morphologic alterations are not believed to contribute to the renal dysfunction.

Defects of Coagulation

Bleeding often accompanies hepatic failure, in part because of defects in hemostasis that parallel the severity of the liver disease. Reduced hepatic synthesis of coagulation factors and thrombocytopenia are the principal causes of the impaired hemostasis. A low platelet count ($<80,000$ cells$/\mu$L) occurs commonly in patients with hepatic failure and is accompanied by qualitative abnormalities in platelet function. The thrombocytopenia may result from hypersplenism, bone marrow depression, or consumption of circulating platelets by intravascular coagulation.

Hypoalbuminemia

Decreased levels of circulating albumin almost invariably complicate hepatic failure. Hypoalbuminemia is an important factor in the pathogenesis of the edema often noted in patients with chronic liver disease. Impaired synthesis of albumin by the injured liver is the most common cause of hypoalbuminemia.

Endocrine Complications

In assessing endocrine changes associated with chronic hepatic failure, it is important to distinguish between the direct effects of alcohol abuse, which is a common cause of liver disease, and the changes that are better attributed to hepatic dysfunction. Chronic liver failure always leads to gynecomastia, female body habitus, and female distribution of pubic hair (female escutcheon). In addition, vascular manifestations of hyperestrogenism are common and include **spider angiomas** in the territory drained by the superior vena cava (upper trunk and face) and palmar erythema. Feminization is attributed to a reduction in the hepatic catabolism of estrogens and weak androgens, such as androstenedione and dehydroepiandrosterone.

In addition to feminization, the large majority of men with chronic alcoholism also suffer hypogonadism, which is manifested by testicular atrophy, impotence, and loss of libido. Women with alcoholism also exhibit gonadal failure, presenting as oligomenorrhea, amenorrhea, infertility, ovarian atrophy, and loss of secondary sex characteristics. These effects on gonadal function in both sexes reflect a direct, toxic action of alcohol independent of chronic liver disease.

ACUTE VIRAL HEPATITIS

■ *Viral hepatitis is a viral infection of the hepatocytes that produces necrosis and inflammation of the liver.* Many viruses and other infectious agents are capable of producing hepatitis and jaundice (Box 14-1), but in the industrialized world, more than 95% of the cases of viral hepatitis involve a limited number of hepatotropic viruses. Still, there remain patients who apparently suffer from viral hepatitis, both clinically and by liver biopsy, but who do not display any marker for the aforementioned viruses. It appears that several hepatotropic viruses remain to be identified.

BOX   *14-1*   **Infectious Agents That Cause Hepatitis**

Hepatitis A virus
Hepatitis B virus
Hepatitis C virus
Hepatitis E virus
Yellow fever virus
Epstein-Barr virus (infectious mononucleosis)
Lassa, Marburg, and Ebola viruses
Rubella virus
Herpes simplex virus
Cytomegalovirus
Enteroviruses other than hepatitis A virus
Leptospires (leptospirosis)
Entamoeba histolytica (amebic hepatitis)

Hepatitis A

■ *Hepatitis A virus* (HAV) *is a small, RNA-containing enterovirus of the picornavirus group that is spread by the fecal-oral route.* The hepatocyte is the sole site of viral replication. Presumably, shedding of progeny virus into the bile accounts for the appearance of HAV in the feces.

☐ **Epidemiology:** Less than 5% of persons with serologic evidence of previous hepatitis caused by HAV recall a previous episode of jaundice or other liver ailment. **This circumstance indicates that the large majority of infections with HAV are anicteric.** Among hospitalized patients, a population clearly selected for more severe disease, hepatitis A accounts for 10% to 25% of all cases of viral hepatitis. By contrast, in less-developed countries, hepatitis A is hyperendemic, and rates of inapparent infection among children are extremely high. As a result, adult cases of hepatitis A are unusual in those regions. In the United States childhood hepatitis A is also common among those in institutions for the mentally retarded and in day-care centers.

For hepatitis A, as for other viral diseases that do not lead to a chronic carrier state, the only reservoir for the disease seems to be the acutely infected person. **Transmission depends primarily on serial transmission from person to person by the fecal-oral route.** Epidemics of hepatitis A also depend on person-to-person spread and occur under crowded and unsanitary conditions, such as exist in warfare, or by fecal contamination of water and food. Edible shellfish concentrate the virus in contaminated waters and may also transmit the infection if eaten after being inadequately cooked. Although hepatitis A is not ordinarily a sexually transmitted disease, the infection rate is particularly high among male homosexuals (as a result of oral-anal contact).

☐ **Clinical Features:** Following an incubation period of 3 to 6 weeks (mean period, ≈4 weeks), patients infected with HAV develop nonspecific symptoms, including fever, malaise, and anorexia. Concomitantly, liver injury is evidenced by a rise in serum aminotransferase activity (Fig. 14-8). As the activity of aminotransferase begins to decline, usually 5 to 10 days later, jaundice may appear. Jaundice remains evident for an average of 10 days but may persist for more than a month. **Hepatitis A never pursues a chronic course. There is no carrier state, and infection provides lifelong immunity.** Fatal fulminant hepatitis occurs only rarely. Vaccines for hepatitis A are available.

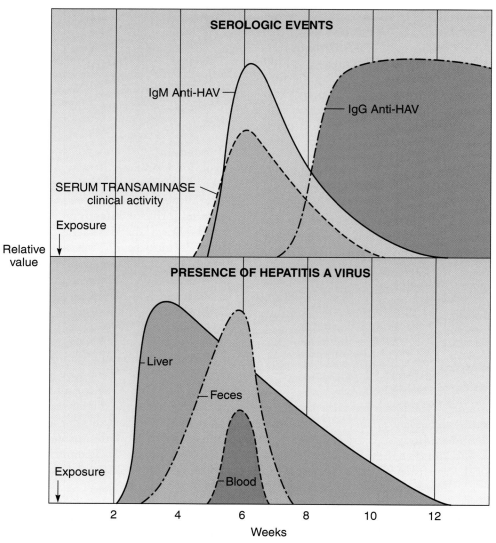

FIGURE   *14-8*
Typical serologic events associated with hepatitis A.

Hepatitis B

■ *Hepatitis B virus (HBV) is a hepatotropic DNA virus that causes acute and chronic liver disease.* The DNA is predominantly double-stranded, with a variable, single-stranded segment (Fig. 14-9). The core of the virus contains a DNA polymerase, the core antigen (HBcAg), and the e antigen (HBeAg).

The core of HBV is enclosed in a coat that contains lipid, protein, and carbohydrate and that expresses an antigen termed *hepatitis B surface antigen (HBsAg)*. The surface coat is synthesized by the infected hepatocyte independently from the viral core and is secreted into the blood in vast amounts. This material is visualized by electron microscopy in centrifuged serum as two distinct particles (see Fig. 14-9), namely a sphere, which is 22 nm in diameter, and a tubular structure, which is 22 nm in diameter and 40 to 400 nm in length. **HBsAg**

particles are immunogenic but not infectious. The intact and infectious virus is also found in the serum as a 42-nm sphere (Dane particle), consisting of an inner core of 27 nm and an outer shell of 7 nm in thickness.

□ **Epidemiology:** It is estimated that approximately 300 million persons worldwide are chronic carriers of HBV, constituting an enormous reservoir of infection. Depending on the incidence of primary infection with HBV, the carrier rates vary from as little as 0.3% (United States and Western Europe) to 20% (Southeast Asia, sub-Saharan Africa, and Oceania). In the latter populations, an important avenue by which the high carrier rate is sustained is vertical transmission of the virus from a carrier mother to her newborn.

The threat of HBV-positive posttransfusion hepatitis has been largely eliminated by routine screening for HBsAg, although 5% to 10% of posttransfusion hepati-

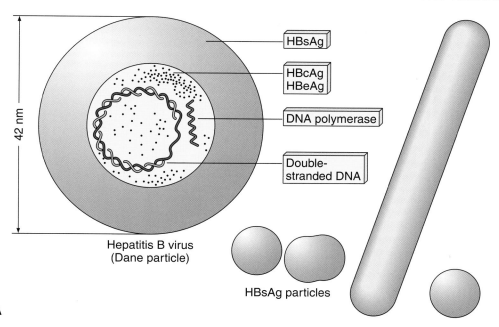

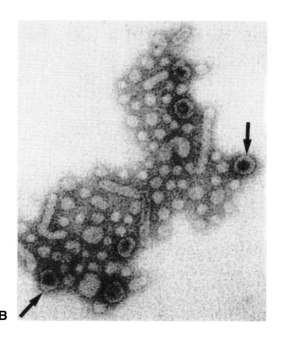

FIGURE *14-9.*
(A) Schematic representation of the hepatitis B virus (HBV) and serum particles associated with HBV infection. (B) Electron micrograph of particles from centrifuged serum in a case of hepatitis B. Rod-like and spherical particles containing HBsAg are evident. The complete virion, which is composed of the viral core and its surrounding envelope, is represented by Dane particles (*arrows*).

tis is still attributed to hepatitis B. Whereas no more than 10% of adults infected with HBV become carriers, neonatal hepatitis B is, as a rule, followed by persistent infection. Males exhibit an increased tendency to become carriers. It has been suggested that immunosuppressed persons are more susceptible to persistent HBV infection, and the carrier state is more common in patients undergoing renal dialysis and in persons afflicted with Down syndrome, leprosy, and chronic lymphocytic leukemia. In the United States, chronic HBV carriers are particularly common among male homosexuals, drug addicts, certain health-care workers, and mentally retarded children who are institutionalized. Of particular public health concern is that paid blood donors are far more likely than the general population to harbor HBV.

Humans are the only significant reservoir of HBV. Unlike hepatitis A, hepatitis B is not transmitted by the fecal-oral route, nor does HBV contaminate food and water supplies. **Although HBsAg is found in most secretions, infectious virus has been demonstrated only in blood, saliva, and semen.** Historically, transmission of hepatitis B was believed to be limited to direct transfer of blood products, either by transfusion or use of contaminated needles. However, it is now clear that the large majority of cases of hepatitis B result from transmission associated with intimate contact. The routes by which contact transmission occurs are not

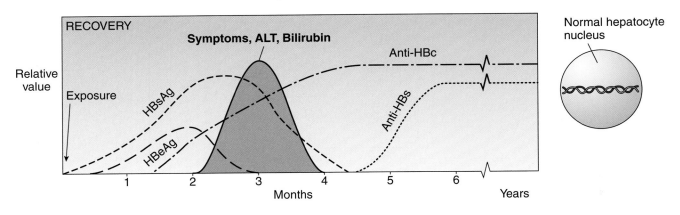

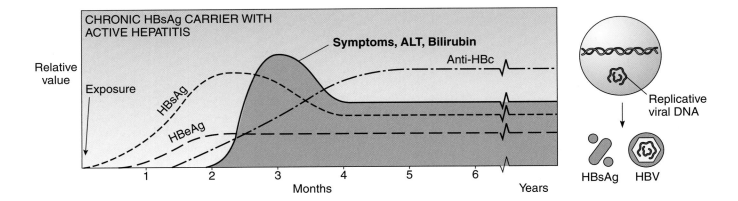

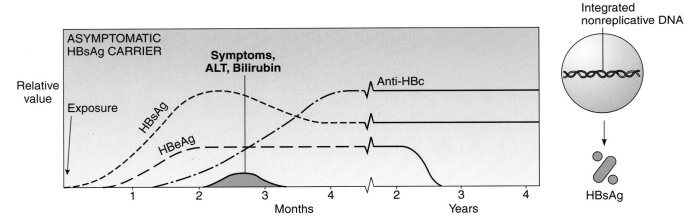

FIGURE   *14-10*
Typical serological events in three distinct outcomes of hepatitis B.

(Top) In most cases, the appearance of anti-HBs ensures complete recovery. Viral DNA disappears from the nucleus of the hepatocyte.

(Middle) In approximately 10% of cases of hepatitis B, HBs antigenemia is sustained for longer than 6 months owing to the absence of anti-HBs. Patients in whom viral replication remains active, as evidenced by sustained high levels of HBeAg in the blood, develop active hepatitis. In such cases, the viral genome persists in the nucleus but is not integrated into host DNA.

(Lower) Patients in whom active viral replication ceases or is attenuated, as reflected in the disappearance of HBeAg from the blood, become asymptomatic carriers. In these individuals, fragments of the HBV genome are integrated into the host DNA, but episomal DNA is absent.

entirely defined, but a direct transfer of the virus through breaks in the skin or mucous membranes is probably the most common. In this respect, sexual contact (heterosexual but particularly homosexual) is an important mode of transmission.

☐ **Clinical Features:** In contrast to hepatitis A, three well-recognized clinical courses are associated with HBV infection (Fig. 14-10):

- Acute, self-limited hepatitis
- Fulminant hepatitis
- Chronic hepatitis

Acute, Self-Limited Hepatitis B. The large majority of patients have acute, self-limited hepatitis; complete recovery and lifelong immunity are the rule. Typically, symptoms do not appear for 2 to 3 months after exposure, but incubation periods of less than 6 weeks and as long as 6 months are occasionally encountered. Many cases, including virtually all infections among infants and children, are anicteric and, therefore, are not clinically apparent. **The presence of HBeAg in the serum correlates with a period of intense viral replication and, hence, maximal infectivity of the patient.**

Circulating HBsAg–anti-HBsAg immune complexes cause a variety of extrahepatic ailments. These include arthritis, polyarteritis, glomerulonephritis, rash, urticaria, pancreatitis, and cryoglobulinemia.

Fulminant Hepatitis B. More often than hepatitis A, but still only rarely, acute hepatitis B pursues a fulminant course, which is characterized by massive liver cell necrosis, hepatic failure, and a high mortality rate.

Chronic Carrier State. In 5% to 10% of cases of hepatitis B, the patients do not develop anti-HBs and, consequently, do not resolve HBs antigenemia. Accordingly, the infection persists, the patients do not recover, and the disease progresses to chronic hepatitis B. **Clinically, HBsAg antigenemia that is sustained for longer than 6 months and is accompanied by hepatic dysfunction indicates chronic hepatitis.** A few of these patients eventually develop anti-HBs (often after many years), clear the virus, and are restored to full health. Others (≤3% of patients with hepatitis B) never develop anti-HBs and suffer a relentless and progressive chronic hepatitis, which may lead to cirrhosis. **All patients with persistent HBV infection develop anti-HBc, and chronic hepatitis B is characterized by the presence of anti-HBc and HBsAg.** Hepatitis associated with persistent HBsAg antigenemia is often accompanied by the continued presence of HBeAg. The possible outcomes of infection with the hepatitis B virus are summarized in Figure 14-11.

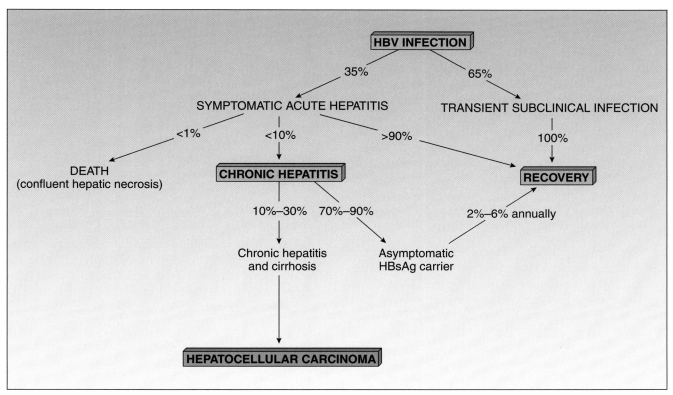

FIGURE **14-11**
Possible outcomes of infection with the hepatitis B virus.

Effective vaccines have been developed against HBV infection. Worldwide use of these vaccines should eventually reduce the prevalence of HBV infection and prevent the major cause of hepatocellular carcinoma in the world.

Hepatitis D

■ *Hepatitis D virus (HDV, delta agent), a distinct hepatotropic RNA virus, is associated exclusively with HBV infection. HDV is a defective virus for which HBV is the helper.* Assembly of HDV in the liver requires synthesis of HBsAg; therefore, infection with this virus is limited to persons (and subhuman primates) infected with HBV.

In these patients, HDV and HBsAg are cleared together, and the clinical course is generally no different from that of the usual acute hepatitis B. **Superinfection of an HBV carrier with HDV typically increases the severity of an existing chronic hepatitis.** Such a combination accounts for a large proportion (30–60%) of cases of fulminant HBsAg-positive hepatitis.

Hepatitis C

■ *Hepatitis C virus (HCV), which contains a single strand of RNA and is believed to resemble a flavivirus or togavirus, is a major cause of acute and chronic liver disease.* Testing blood for anti-HCV substantially diminishes, but does not eliminate, the risk of posttransfusion hepatitis.

□ **Epidemiology: In the United States, owing to the screening of blood for HBV, HCV accounts for more than 90% of hepatitis cases that develop after blood transfusion.** Transmission of hepatitis C is similar to that of hepatitis B. Only 5% to 10% of patients with documented hepatitis C have a history of blood transfusion, and at least 40% of patients in the United States are intravenous drug abusers. In the general population, hepatitis C is responsible for half of the cases of sporadic acute viral hepatitis. Almost half of the patients with hepatitis C report no recognizable source of infection.

□ **Clinical Features:** The clinical course of most cases of hepatitis C is similar to that of hepatitis B (Fig. 14-12). The acute illness tends to be less severe than that in hepatitis B, and fulminant hepatitis occurs only rarely or not at all. **Chronic liver disease is also a more frequent complication in patients with hepatitis C than in those with hepatitis B** (Fig. 14-13). Approximately 25% of these chronic carriers of HCV eventually develop cirrhosis. **Of those who develop cirrhosis, as many as 20% (depending on the population) of HCV**

carriers will develop hepatocellular carcinoma.** Hepatitis C is also associated with an immune complex glomerulonephritis (see Chapter 16).

Hepatitis E

Major epidemics of hepatitis in underdeveloped countries have been attributed to an RNA virus that is transmitted by the fecal-oral route and is now labeled hepatitis E. Large outbreaks have been reported in India, Nepal, Burma, Pakistan, the former Soviet Union, Africa, and Mexico. No chronic disease or carrier state has been identified.

CHRONIC HEPATITIS

■ *Chronic hepatitis refers to the presence of inflammation and necrosis in the liver for more than 6 months.* Only 15% of patients with chronic hepatitis in the United States display HBsAg antigenemia. The prevalence in Italy is 50%, and in parts of Asia, it may be even higher. HBsAg-negative chronic hepatitis is caused, in large part, by hepatitis C, but it may also result from the use of drugs such as isoniazid and methyldopa. Chronic hepatitis may also be a feature of certain systemic diseases, including Wilson disease and α_1-antitrypsin deficiency.

Chronic Hepatitis B and C

Ninety percent of patients with chronic hepatitis B are male, whereas chronic hepatitis of unknown cause that has "autoimmune" features shows a female predominance. Chronic hepatitis C does not seem to show a sex predilection. Chronic active hepatitis B or hepatitis C carries a high risk for development of cirrhosis. Furthermore, chronic hepatitis B and hepatitis C are the major predisposing causes of primary hepatocellular carcinoma worldwide.

□ **Pathogenesis:** It appears that, at least in part, the severity of chronic hepatitis B is related to the degree of viral replication, as indicated by the presence of HBeAg, HBV DNA, and HBV DNA polymerase in the blood. Considering that HBV is not directly cytopathic to hepatocytes, it is thought that cell-mediated immunity underlies the pathogenesis of chronic hepatitis B.

□ **Clinical Features:** Patients with chronic hepatitis B display variable degrees of jaundice and hepatosplenomegaly, and in severe cases, hepatic encephalopathy may develop. Extrahepatic manifestations are similar to those in patients with acute hepatitis

ACUTE RESOLVING HEPATITIS C

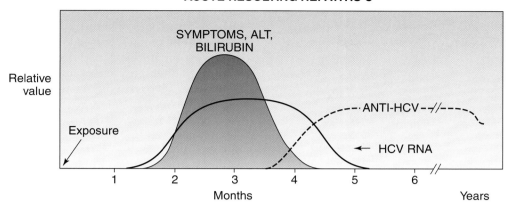

CHRONIC HEPATITIS C

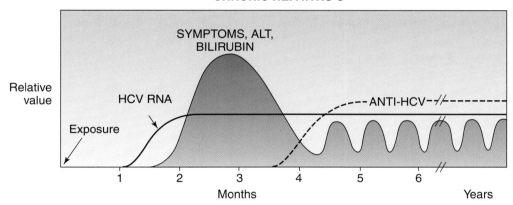

FIGURE **14-12**
Clinical course of hepatitis C. Typical serologic events in two distinct outcomes of infection with hepatitis C virus (HCV). (Top) Approximately half of the patients with acute hepatitis C have a self-limited infection, which resolves in a few months. Anti-HCV appears at the end of the clinical course and persists. (Bottom) The other half of the patients with hepatitis C develop chronic illness, with exacerbations and remissions of clinical symptoms. The development of anti-HCV does not affect the clinical outcome. Chronic active hepatitis often eventuates in cirrhosis.

B. No specific therapy is available for chronic viral hepatitis, but promising results have been obtained with recombinant interferon-α in the treatment of chronic hepatitis C and, to some extent, of chronic hepatitis B.

Autoimmune Hepatitis

■ *Autoimmune hepatitis is a clinically distinct form of chronic hepatitis that occurs in young and middle-age women.* It is accompanied by (1) hypergammaglobu-linemia, (2) autoantibodies, (3) the lupus erythematosus cell phenomenon, and (4) multisystemic involvement of other organs, of a kind commonly attributed to autoimmune mechanisms. Whereas the response to corticosteroid therapy in other forms of chronic hepatitis is generally unsatisfactory, patients with "autoimmune" hepatitis often respond favorably to such treatment. Patients who are untreated or refractory to therapy have a high risk of developing liver failure and cirrhosis.

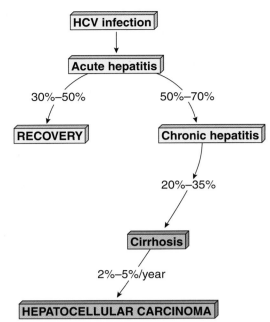

FIGURE *14-13*
Possible outcomes of infection with the hepatitis C virus.

PATHOLOGY OF ACUTE AND CHRONIC HEPATITIS

Acute Viral Hepatitis

The morphologic appearance of the liver in patients with acute viral hepatitis is similar in hepatitis A, B, and C. The hallmark of viral hepatitis is liver cell injury and necrosis (Fig. 14-14). Within the hepatic lobule, scattered necrosis of single cells or small clusters of hepatocytes are seen. A few necrotic liver cells appear as small, deeply eosinophilic bodies (Councilman or acidophilic bodies), sometimes containing pyknotic nuclear material, that have been extruded from the liver cell plate into the sinusoid (see Fig. 14-14). In acute viral hepatitis many liver cells appear to be normal, but others show varying degrees of hydropic swelling (balloon cells) and differences in size, shape, and staining qualities. Concomitantly, regenerative liver cells, which display a larger nucleus and expanded basophilic cytoplasm, are also seen. The resulting irregularity of the liver cell plates is termed **lobular disarray.**

Chronic inflammatory cells (principally lymphoid) infiltrate the lobule diffusely, surround individual necrotic liver cells, and accumulate in areas of focal necrosis. In addition to lymphoid cells, macrophages may be prominent, and eosinophils and polymorphonuclear leukocytes are not uncommon. Characteristically, lymphoid cells infiltrate between the wall of the central vein and the liver cell plates, an appearance termed **central phlebitis.** Swelling and proliferation of

the endothelial cells of the central vein (**endophlebitis**) often develop. The Kupffer cells are enlarged, project into the lumen of the sinusoid, and contain lipofuscin pigment and phagocytosed debris (particularly evident with the periodic acid-Schiff [PAS] reaction), including fragments of acidophilic bodies. Cholestasis is sometimes seen, in which case the term **cholestatic hepatitis** is applied.

The portal tracts are almost always enlarged and edematous. As a rule, chronic inflammatory cells accumulate within the portal tracts, but the severity of this inflammatory reaction varies from mild to pronounced. All of the pathologic changes are gradually reversed, and the normal hepatic architecture is completely restored.

Confluent Hepatic Necrosis

■ *Confluent hepatic necrosis refers to a severe variant of acute hepatitis characterized by the death of many hepatocytes and, in extreme cases, of almost all the liver cells.* In contrast to the most common form of acute viral hepatitis described earlier, in which the necrosis of hepatocytes appears to be random and patchy, **confluent hepatic necrosis typically affects whole regions of the**

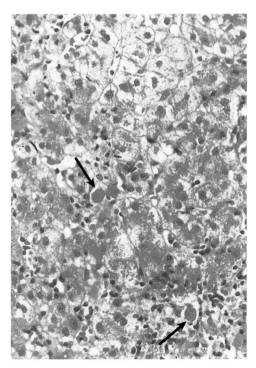

FIGURE *14-14*
Acute viral hepatitis. A photomicrograph shows disarray of liver cell plates, swollen (ballooned) hepatocytes, and an infiltrate of lymphocytes and scattered mononuclear inflammatory cells. The remnants of necrotic hepatocytes have been extruded into the sinusoids, where they appear as acidophilic, or Councilman, bodies (*arrows*).

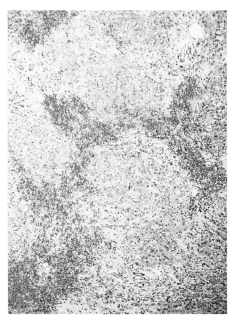

FIGURE *14-15*
Confluent hepatic necrosis. Hemorrhagic zones of necrosis bridge adjacent portal tracts (bridging necrosis).

lobule (Fig. 14-15). The lesions of confluent hepatic necrosis, in order of increasing severity, are bridging necrosis, submassive necrosis, and massive necrosis.

Bridging Necrosis. At the milder end of the spectrum of lesions constituting confluent hepatic necrosis are bands of necrosis (bridging necrosis) that stretch between adjacent portal tracts, adjacent central veins, and portal tracts and central veins. Curiously, the lobular inflammatory infiltrate is often scanty, although the portal tracts are generally inflamed and often contain an appreciable number of polymorphonuclear leukocytes. In younger persons (<30 years), bridging necrosis has no adverse prognostic significance. However, when this lesion occurs in patients older than 40 years, as many as half eventually die in hepatic failure.

Submassive Confluent Necrosis. This form of acute hepatitis defines an even more severe injury involving necrosis of entire lobules or groups of adjacent lobules. Clinically, these patients manifest severe hepatitis that may rapidly proceed to hepatic failure, in which case the disease is classed as **fulminant hepatitis.** In one-fifth of the cases that eventually prove to be fatal, the course is protracted, with death from hepatic failure occurring in 2 to 5 months.

Massive Hepatic Necrosis (Acute Yellow Atrophy). Although uncommon, massive hepatic necrosis is the most feared variant of acute hepatitis, because this form of fulminant hepatitis is almost invariably fatal. Grossly, the liver is shrunken to as little as 500 g (one-third of the normal weight). The capsule is wrinkled, and the mottled red parenchyma is soft and flabby. Microscopic examination reveals that virtually all of the hepatocytes are dead (Fig. 14-16), and the hepatic lobule is represented only by the reticulin framework, which in many areas has collapsed. Often, the only viable hepatocytes are disposed as a thin rim surrounding the portal tracts. Macrophages, erythrocytes, and necrotic debris fill the sinusoids and impinge on the necrotic remnants of the liver cell plates. For unknown reasons, the massive necrosis does not elicit a vigorous inflammatory response in either the parenchyma or the portal tracts.

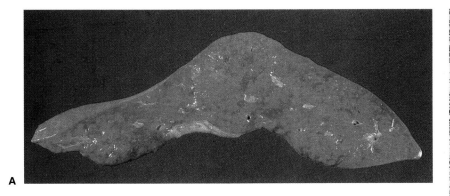
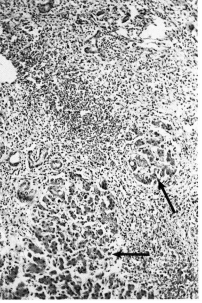

FIGURE *14-16*
Massive hepatic necrosis. (A) The liver is soft and reduced in size, and it shows mottled, irregularly hemorrhagic cut surfaces. (B) A photomicrograph shows the loss of most of the hepatocytes. The reticulin framework has collapsed, and the area in the center of the field is hemorrhagic. A sparse, chronic inflammatory infiltrate is evident throughout. Islands of regenerating hepatocytes (*arrows*) are evident.

Young patients who survive submassive or massive confluent hepatic necrosis generally do not develop cirrhosis and, in the case of hepatitis B, do not become HBsAg carriers. By contrast, older persons who recover from fulminant hepatitis are more likely to progress to chronic hepatitis and cirrhosis.

Chronic Hepatitis

The lesions of chronic hepatitis are not necessarily static; mild lesions can progress to severe ones, and vice versa. The spectrum of chronic viral hepatitis (B and C) ranges from mild portal inflammation, with little or no evidence of liver cell necrosis (Fig. 14-17), to a widespread inflammatory, necrotizing, and fibrosing condition (Fig. 14-18). The pathologic features of chronic hepatitis are common to both HBV and HCV infections and include piecemeal necrosis, portal inflammation, and periportal fibrosis. The lobules may display inflammation, necrosis, and regeneration.

Piecemeal Necrosis. This periportal lesion refers to focal destruction of the limiting plate of hepatocytes. A chronic inflammatory infiltrate creates an irregular border between the portal tracts and the lobular parenchyma (see Fig. 14-18).

Portal Tract Lesions. Chronic hepatitis is characterized by variable infiltration of the portal tracts by lymphocytes, plasma cells, and macrophages (see Fig. 14-18). Mild to severe proliferation of bile ductules represents a nonspecific response to chronic liver injury.

Intralobular Lesions. Focal necrosis and inflammation within the parenchyma are typical of chronic hepatitis. Scattered acidophilic bodies are common.

Periportal Fibrosis. The progressive erosion of periportal hepatocytes by piecemeal necrosis leads to deposition of collagen, which gives the portal tract a

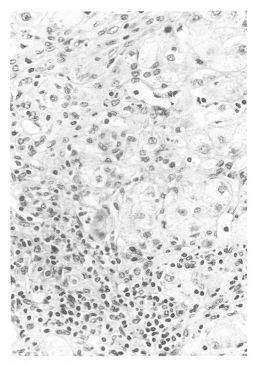

FIGURE   *14-18*
Severe chronic hepatitis. A photomicrograph discloses a mononuclear inflammatory infiltrate in an expanded portal tract. The inflammation penetrates the limiting plate and surrounds groups of hepatocytes on the border of the portal tract.

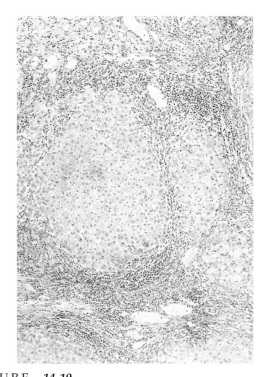

FIGURE   *14-19*
Cirrhosis in chronic active hepatitis. A photomicrograph of the liver from a patient with longstanding chronic active hepatitis B shows hepatocellular nodules and chronically inflamed fibrous septa.

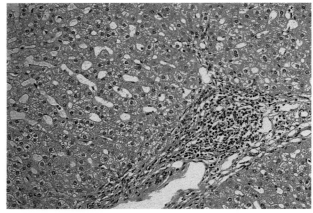

FIGURE   *14-17*
Mild chronic hepatitis. A photomicrograph shows a portal tract infiltrated by mononuclear inflammatory cells. The lobular parenchyma is intact.

TABLE 14-1. Comparative Features of the Common Forms of Viral Hepatitis

Feature	Hepatitis A	Hepatitis B	Hepatitis C
Genome	RNA	DNA	RNA
Incubation period	3–6 weeks	6 weeks to 6 months	7–8 weeks
Transmission	Oral	Parenteral	Parenteral
Blood	No	Yes	Yes
Feces	Yes	No	No
Vertical	No	Yes	?
Fulminant hepatic necrosis	Very rare	Yes	Yes
Chronic hepatitis	No	10%	50%
Carrier state	No	Yes	Yes
Liver cancer	No	Yes	Yes

stellate (star-shaped) appearance. Fibrosis may extend to adjacent portal tracts or toward the central vein. The end stage of chronic hepatitis is characterized by dense collagenous septa that destroy the lobular architecture and divide the liver into hepatocellular nodules, which is an appearance termed *cirrhosis* (Fig. 14-19).

Table 14-1 compares major features of the common forms of viral hepatitis.

ALCOHOLIC LIVER DISEASE

It has been known since Biblical times that excess consumption of alcoholic beverages leads to chronic liver disease. Although alcoholic liver injury was attributed to nutritional deficiencies a few decades ago, it is now generally accepted that ethanol per se is a hepatotoxin.

☐ **Epidemiology:** Excess alcohol consumption and chronic liver disease are related regardless of the specific nature of the preferred beverage (e.g., wine in France, beer in Australia, and spirits in Scandinavia). Only a minority of patients with chronic alcoholism develop cirrhosis, but a dose-response relationship between the lifetime dose of alcohol (duration of exposure in years and daily amount of alcohol consumed) and the appearance of cirrhosis has been established.

It is estimated that some 7% of the total U.S. population is alcoholic. However, when one considers only the population at risk, thereby eliminating children, the aged, institutionalized persons, and ethnic or religious groups that abjure the use of alcohol, the prevalence of alcoholism is then considerably higher. **Approximately 15% of persons with alcoholism can be expected to develop cirrhosis, and many of these persons die in hepatic failure or from extrahepatic complications of cirrhosis.** In fact, in many urban areas of the United States with high rates of alcoholism, cirrho-

sis of the liver, approximately 70% of which is associated with alcoholism, is now the third- or fourth-leading cause of death in men younger than 45 years of age.

The daily amount of alcohol in patients with established cirrhosis usually ranges from 160 to 220 g. In general, more than 10 years of alcoholism are required to produce cirrhosis, although a few patients with cirrhosis give shorter histories of heavy alcohol use. It has been suggested that, for practical purposes, a pint of whiskey a day (or its equivalent in other beverages) for 15 years is the threshold for development of cirrhosis.

Liver Diseases Produced by Alcohol Consumption

The spectrum of alcoholic liver disease spans three major morphologic and clinical entities: (1) **fatty liver,** (2) **alcoholic hepatitis,** and (3) **cirrhosis.** Although these lesions usually occur sequentially, they may coexist in any combination and may, indeed, be independent entities.

Fatty Liver and Associated Lesions

☐ **Pathogenesis:** Virtually all patients with chronic alcoholism accumulate fat in hepatocytes (steatosis). Most of the fat deposited in the liver after chronic alcohol consumption is derived from the diet. Ethanol increases lipolysis and, thus, delivery of free fatty acids to the liver. Within the hepatocyte, ethanol (1) increases fatty acid synthesis, (2) decreases mitochon-

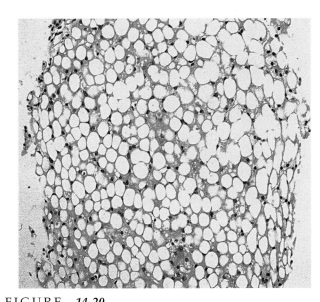

FIGURE 14-20
Alcoholic fatty liver. A photomicrograph shows the cytoplasm of almost all the hepatocytes to be distended by fat, which displaces the nucleus to the periphery. Note the absence of inflammation and fibrosis.

drial oxidation of fatty acids, (3) increases production of triglycerides, and (4) impairs release of lipoproteins. Collectively, these metabolic consequences produce a fatty liver.

☐ **Pathology:** In the patient with alcoholism, the liver becomes yellow and enlarged, sometimes massively, to as much as threefold the normal weight. Microscopically, the extent of visible fat accumulation varies from minute droplets scattered in the cytoplasm of a few hepatocytes to distention of the entire cytoplasm of most cells by coalesced droplets (Fig. 14-20). The cytoplasm is represented by a distended clear area, and the nucleus is both flattened and displaced to the periphery of the cell.

☐ **Clinical Features:** Patients with uncomplicated alcoholic fatty liver have surprisingly few symptoms of liver disease. It is a fully reversible lesion and does

not, by itself, progress to more severe disease, notably cirrhosis.

Alcoholic Hepatitis

■ *Alcoholic hepatitis is an acute, necrotizing lesion characterized by (1) necrosis of hepatocytes, predominantly in the central zone; (2) cytoplasmic hyaline inclusions within hepatocytes; (3) a neutrophilic inflammatory response; and (4) perivenular fibrosis* (Fig. 14-21). The pathogenesis of alcoholic hepatitis is mysterious. Patients with alcoholism may have mild fatty liver for many years and, without any change in drinking habits, suddenly develop acute alcoholic hepatitis.

☐ **Pathology:** The hepatic architecture is basically intact, with a normal relationship of the portal tracts to the central venules. The hepatocytes show variable hy-

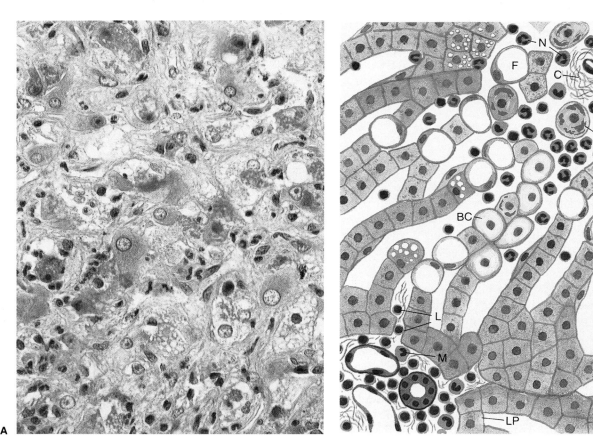

A   **B**

FIGURE *14-21*
Alcoholic hepatitis. (A) A photomicrograph shows necrosis and degeneration of hepatocytes, Mallory bodies (eosinophilic inclusions) in the cytoplasm of injured hepatocytes, and infiltration by neutrophils. (B) Schematic representation of the major pathologic features of alcoholic hepatitis. The lesions are predominantly centrilobular and include necrosis and loss of hepatocytes, ballooned cells (BC), and Mallory bodies (MB) in the cytoplasm of damaged hepatocytes. The inflammatory infiltrate consists predominantly of neutrophils (N), although a few lymphocytes (L) and macrophages (M) are also present. The central vein, or terminal hepatic venule (THV), is encased in connective tissue (C) (central sclerosis). Fat-laden hepatocytes (F) are evident in the lobule. The portal tract displays moderate chronic inflammation, and the limiting plate (LP) is focally breached.

dropic swelling, which gives them a heterogeneous appearance. Isolated necrotic liver cells, or clusters of them, exhibit pyknotic nuclei and karyorrhexis. Scattered hepatocytes contain **Mallory bodies** (so-called alcoholic hyaline; see Fig. 14-21). These cytoplasmic inclusions, which are more common in visibly damaged, swollen hepatocytes, are visualized as irregular skeins of eosinophilic material or as solid eosinophilic masses, often in a perinuclear location. Ultrastructurally, they are composed of aggregates of intermediate (cytokeratin) filaments. The damaged, ballooned hepatocytes, particularly those containing Mallory bodies, are surrounded by neutrophils, although a more diffuse, intralobular inflammatory infiltrate is also present. Cholestasis, which varies from mild to severe, is present in as many as one-third of the cases. **An important point is that alcoholic hepatitis is usually superimposed on an existing fatty liver, although no evidence suggests that fat accumulation predisposes or contributes to development of alcoholic hepatitis.**

Collagen deposition is a constant feature of alcoholic hepatitis, especially around the central vein (terminal hepatic venule). In severe cases, the venule and perivenular sinusoids are obliterated and surrounded by dense fibrous tissue, in which case the lesion is termed **central hyaline sclerosis** (Fig. 14-22).

The appearance of the portal tracts is highly variable. In some instances, they appear to be virtually normal, whereas in others, they are enlarged and contain a mononuclear infiltrate and proliferated bile ductules.

☐ **Clinical Features:** The classic clinical features associated with alcoholic hepatitis are malaise and anorexia, fever, right upper quadrant abdominal pain, and jaundice. A mild leukocytosis is common. The serum aminotransferase activity, particularly that of aspartate aminotransferase, is moderately elevated, but not to the levels often noted in viral hepatitis. Serum alkaline phosphatase activity is usually increased.

The prognosis in patients with alcoholic hepatitis correlates with the severity of the liver cell injury. In some patients, the disease rapidly progresses to hepatic failure and death, with the mortality rate ranging from 10% to 30%. If the patient survives and continues to drink, the acute stage may be followed by persistent alcoholic hepatitis, and more than a one-third of such patients progress to cirrhosis in only 1 or 2 years. Among those who abstain from alcohol after recovery from acute alcoholic hepatitis, only one-fourth have no morphologic residuals by 6 months, and one-fifth progress to cirrhosis. Recovery in the remaining patients who abstain is slow, and most show histologic lesions more than 1 year after the initial episode.

Alcoholic Cirrhosis

In 15% of persons with alcoholism, hepatocellular necrosis, fibrosis, and regeneration eventually lead to the formation of fibrous septa surrounding the hepatocellular nodules, which are the two features that define cirrhosis (Fig. 14-23). The other lesions of alcoholic liver disease—fatty liver and acute or persistent alcoholic hepatitis—are often seen in conjunction with cirrhosis. Patients with alcoholic cirrhosis often die from bleeding esophageal varices (portal hypertension), hepatic failure, or both.

PRIMARY BILIARY CIRRHOSIS

■ *Primary biliary cirrhosis is a chronic, cholestatic liver disease characterized by destruction of the intrahepatic bile ducts (nonsuppurative, destructive cholangitis).* It occurs principally in middle-aged women, and the clinical course is characterized by progressive cholestasis. Use of the term **cirrhosis** for this malady is misleading, however, in that cirrhosis is actually a late complication of the disease.

☐ **Pathogenesis:** Primary biliary cirrhosis is associated with many immunologic abnormalities and, therefore, is widely held to be an autoimmune disease. The large majority (85%) of patients with primary

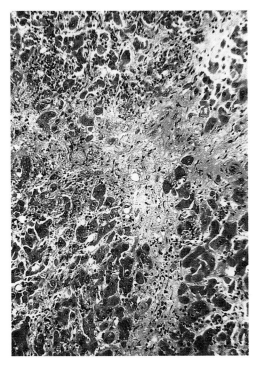

FIGURE *14-22*
Central hyaline sclerosis. This photomicrograph from the liver of a patient with alcoholic liver disease shows the central terminal venule to be obliterated by fibrous tissue.

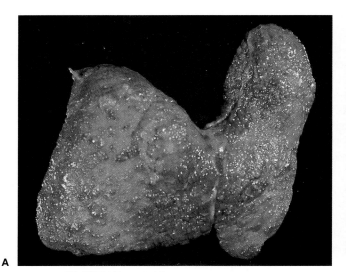

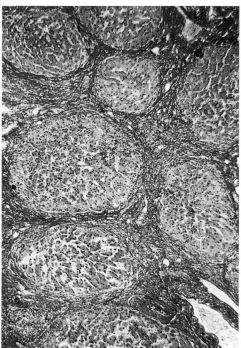

A   B

FIGURE   *14-23*
Alcoholic cirrhosis. (A) The surface of the liver displays innumerable small, regular nodules. (B) A photomicrograph shows small, regular nodules surrounded by uniform fibrous septa.

biliary cirrhosis have at least one other disease that is usually classed as being autoimmune, and almost half (40%) have two or more such ailments. Among these disorders are chronic thyroiditis, rheumatoid arthritis, scleroderma, Sjögren syndrome, and systemic lupus erythematosus. **More than 95% of the patients have circulating antimitochondrial antibodies, which is a finding commonly used in establishing the diagnosis of primary biliary cirrhosis.** Despite the specificity of antimitochondrial antibodies, they have no inhibitory effect on mitochondrial function, and they play no known role in the pathogenesis or progression of the disease. Other circulating autoantibodies are antinuclear, antithyroid, antiplatelet, antiacetylcholine receptor, and antiribonucleoprotein antibodies.

The most attractive explanation for the initial destruction of bile ducts in primary biliary cirrhosis is an attack on the biliary epithelial cells by cytotoxic T lymphocytes.

☐ Pathology: Three major pathologic stages in the evolution of primary biliary cirrhosis are recognized.

Stage I: Duct Lesion. Early stage I primary biliary cirrhosis is characterized by a unique lesion, namely a **chronic destructive cholangitis** affecting the intrahepatic small- and medium-size bile ducts (Fig. 14-24). The bile ducts are surrounded principally by lymphocytes, but plasma cells and macrophages are

also seen. Characteristically, the bile duct epithelium is irregular and hyperplastic, with stratification of epithelial cells and occasional papillary ingrowths. Foci of necrotic epithelial cells and ulceration of the epithelium are not uncommon. In some portal tracts, lymphoid follicles, occasionally containing germinal centers, are conspicuous. Discrete epithelioid granulomas often occur in the portal tracts and may impinge on the bile ducts. In patients with stage I primary biliary cirrhosis, the lobular parenchyma tends to be normal, but in a minority of patients, mild central cholestasis is present.

Stage II: Scarring. Because of the destructive inflammatory process characteristic of stage I primary biliary cirrhosis, **the small bile ducts virtually disappear,** and scarring of the medium-size bile ducts is common. Proliferation of bile ductules within the portal tracts is usual and may be florid. Relatively acellular collagenous septa extend from the portal tracts into the lobular parenchyma and begin to encircle some lobules. Cholestasis, when present, may be severe and is now located at the periphery of the portal tracts.

Stage III: Cirrhosis. The disease terminates as end-stage liver disease—namely, cirrhosis—characterized by fibrous septa that encompass regenerative nodules. Grossly, the bile-stained liver is dark green and exhibits a fine nodularity. Microscopically, small bile

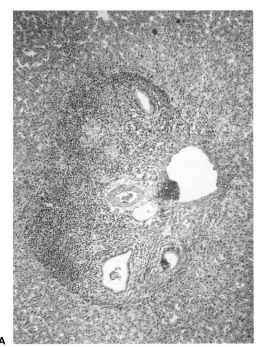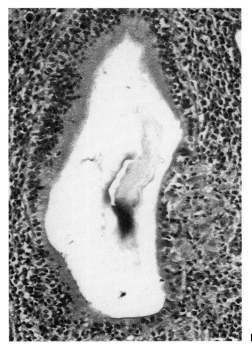

A   B

FIGURE   *14-24*
Primary biliary cirrhosis, stage 1. (A) A photomicrograph shows that a large portal tract containing three bile ducts is expanded by a lymphocytic infiltrate. (B) A higher-power view of the same patient shows a dense infiltrate of lymphoid cells surrounding a damaged interlobular bile duct and an adjacent granuloma. The bile duct epithelium shows both atrophy and hyperplasia.

ducts are scarce, and medium-size ducts are conspicuously reduced in number.

☐ **Clinical Features: Women, usually between 30 and 65 years of age, account for 90% to 95% of those afflicted with primary biliary cirrhosis.** In many patients, the initial symptoms are fatigue and pruritus without jaundice, although one-fifth of patients have jaundice when first seen.

In a typical case, a high serum alkaline phosphatase activity is accompanied by a normal, or only slightly elevated, serum bilirubin level. As the disease advances, most patients have a progressive increase in serum bilirubin level. The serum cholesterol level is strikingly increased, and an abnormal lipoprotein, known as lipoprotein X, which is found in many forms of chronic cholestasis, appears. Cholesterol-laden macrophages accumulate in the subcutaneous tissues, where they appear as localized lesions termed **xanthomas.** Impairment in the excretion of bile into the intestine often leads to severe **steatorrhea** owing to fat malabsorption. Because of associated malabsorption of vitamin D and calcium, **osteomalacia** and **osteoporosis** are important complications of primary biliary cirrhosis. Those patients who eventually develop cirrhosis die from hepatic failure or the complications of **portal hypertension.**

Primary biliary cirrhosis generally pursues an indolent course. Patients who develop cirrhosis tend to survive for 10 to 15 years, whereas in those without symptoms, life expectancy may not be curtailed. Treatment with methotrexate seems to be promising. Liver transplantation is highly effective in patients with end-stage disease, with a 1-year survival rate of 75% and a projected 5-year survival rate of more than 65%.

PRIMARY SCLEROSING CHOLANGITIS

■ *Primary sclerosing cholangitis* is an inflammatory and fibrosing process that narrows and, eventually, obstructs the intrahepatic and extrahepatic bile ducts. The majority of patients are men younger than 40 years of age. Progressive biliary obstruction typically leads to persistent obstructive jaundice and, eventually, to secondary biliary cirrhosis. The cause of primary sclerosing cholangitis is unknown, but two-thirds of the patients also have ulcerative colitis.

☐ **Pathology:** The liver disease associated with primary sclerosing cholangitis can be divided into four histologic stages:

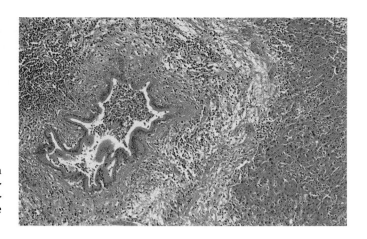

FIGURE *14-25*
Primary sclerosing cholangitis. A photomicrograph of a liver removed for hepatic transplantation shows an edematous, fibrotic, and chronically inflamed portal tract. Inflammatory debris is present within the lumen of the bile duct.

- **Stage I.** The initial lesion is periductal inflammation and fibrosis in the portal tracts.
- **Stage II.** Connective tissue extends into the periportal parenchyma, and chronic periductal inflammation is still present (Fig. 14-25).
- **Stage III.** Many bile ducts become obliterated, and fibrous septa extend further into the parenchyma.
- **Stage IV.** Secondary biliary cirrhosis eventually develops.

Primary sclerosing cholangitis has a poor prognosis; the mean survival time after the appearance of symptoms is 6 years. **Cholangiocarcinoma** has been reported to develop in as many as 10% of patients with primary sclerosing cholangitis. Liver transplantation is curative.

CIRRHOSIS

■ *Cirrhosis, which is the end stage of chronic liver disease, is the destruction of the normal hepatic architecture by fibrous septa that encompass regenerative nodules of hepatocytes.*

Morphologic Classification

Micronodular Cirrhosis. This form of cirrhosis was previously termed **Laennec, portal, or septal cirrhosis.** Micronodular cirrhosis exhibits nodules that are scarcely larger than a lobule, measuring less than 3 mm in diameter (see Fig. 14-23). The micronodules show no landmarks of lobular architecture in the form of portal tracts or central venules. The connective tissue septa separating the nodules are usually thin, but irregular focal collapse of parenchyma may lead to wider septa. During the active stages of the cirrhotic process, numerous mononuclear inflammatory cells and proliferated bile ductules inhabit the septa. The prototype of micronodular cirrhosis is alcoholic cirrhosis, but this pattern may also be observed in primary and secondary biliary cirrhosis, hemochromatosis, Wilson disease, and certain inherited metabolic disorders.

Macronodular Cirrhosis. This morphologic variety of cirrhosis was formerly labeled **postnecrotic, posthepatic, or multilobular cirrhosis.** The large, irregular nodules often contain portal tracts and efferent venous channels, thereby providing evidence that the original process was characterized by multilobular necrosis that healed with the formation of large scars surrounding more than a single lobule (Fig. 14-26). **However, it is now recognized that the micronodular pattern can be converted into a macronodular one by continued regeneration and expansion of existing nodules.** This is particularly the case in persons with alcoholism who abstain from drinking after the diagnosis of cirrhosis has been made. Given sufficient time, almost all (90%) of the cases of micronodular cirrhosis, even in those who continue to drink, will be converted to the macronodular pattern, usually within 2 to 3 years. The connective tissue septa in macronodular cirrhosis are characteristically broad and contain elements of preexisting portal tracts, mononuclear inflammatory cells, and proliferated bile ductules. Macronodular cirrhosis is classically associated with chronic active hepatitis. It is also occasionally a result of submassive hepatic necrosis, in which case the liver may be grossly misshapen.

☐ **Pathogenesis:** Diseases associated with cirrhosis are listed in Box 14-2. Clearly, they have little in common, except that they are all accompanied by persistent liver cell necrosis. Most cases of cirrhosis are attributable to alcoholism and chronic viral hepatitis, although a significant contribution from unexplained chronic active hepatitis is also a factor.

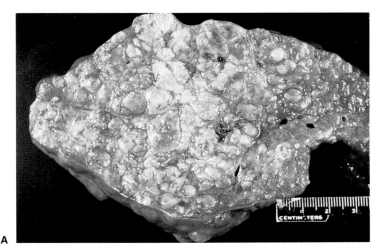

A

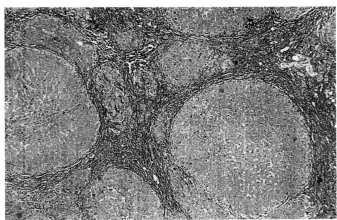

B

FIGURE *14-26*
Macronodular cirrhosis. (A) The liver is misshapen, and the cut surface reveals irregular nodules and connective tissue septa of varying width. (B) A photomicrograph shows nodules of varying size and irregular fibrous septa.

BOX *14-2* **Causes of Cirrhosis**

Alcoholic liver disease
Chronic active hepatitis
Primary biliary cirrhosis
Extrahepatic biliary obstruction
Hemochromatosis
Wilson disease
Cystic fibrosis
α_1-Antitrypsin deficiency
Glycogen storage disease, types III and IV
Galactosemia
Hereditary fructose intolerance
Tyrosinemia
Hereditary storage diseases (Gaucher, Niemann-Pick, Wolman, mucopolysaccharidoses)
Zellweger syndrome
Indian childhood cirrhosis

EXTRAHEPATIC BILIARY OBSTRUCTION (SECONDARY BILIARY CIRRHOSIS)

The extrahepatic biliary system may be obstructed by a number of lesions. These include (1) gallstones passing through the cystic duct to lodge in the common bile duct, (2) cancer of the bile duct or surrounding tissues (pancreas or ampulla of Vater), (3) external compression by enlarged neoplastic lymph nodes in the porta hepatis (as in Hodgkin's disease), (4) benign strictures (postoperative or primary sclerosing cholangitis), and (5) congenital biliary atresia (Fig. 14-27).

□ **Pathology:** Early during the precirrhotic stage of extrahepatic biliary obstruction, the liver is swollen and bile-stained. As obstruction proceeds, the initial polymorphonuclear inflammatory infiltrate in the portal tracts is replaced by a mononuclear one. Tortuous and distended bile ductules, which are characterized by a high cuboidal epithelium, proliferate. Cholestasis

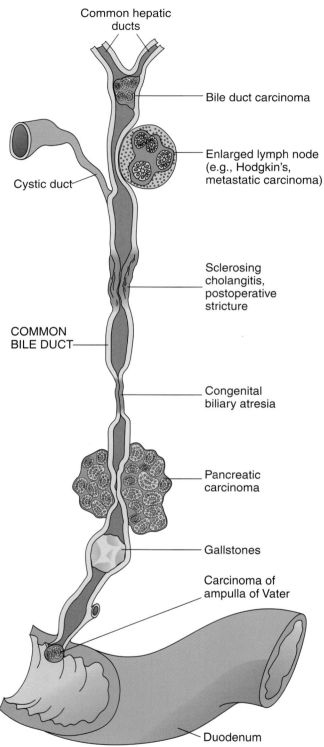

FIGURE   *14-27*
Major causes of extrahepatic biliary obstruction.

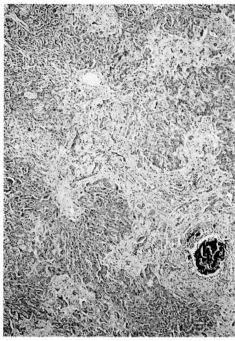

FIGURE   *14-28*
Secondary biliary cirrhosis. A photomicrograph of the liver from a patient with a pancreatic carcinoma that obstructed the common bile duct. Irregular fibrous septa extend from an enlarged portal tract (*lower right*), containing a dilated interlobular bile duct that encloses a dense biliary concretion. Numerous proliferated bile ductules are seen within the septa.

eventually extends to the periphery of the lobule. Dilated bile ducts may rupture, thereby leading to the formation of **bile lakes,** a feature that is diagnostic of extrahepatic biliary obstruction. Bile lakes appear as focal, golden-yellow deposits that are surrounded by degenerating hepatocytes. Leakage of bile into the portal tracts also causes the appearance of foamy, lipid-laden macrophages, which are often aggregated as **granulomas.** Damaged hepatocytes containing large amounts of bile show a characteristic reticulated cytoplasm, termed **feathery degeneration.** Within bile ducts and proliferated ductules, biliary concretions may be conspicuous, which is again a diagnostic feature of extrahepatic biliary obstruction.

With time, the portal tracts become enlarged and fibrotic (Fig. 14-28). Typically, **periductal fibrosis** is concentric, thereby giving rise to the term **onion-skin fibrosis.** As in other forms of cirrhosis characterized by periportal necrosis, 10% of the cases of prolonged extrahepatic biliary obstruction eventually show septa extending between the portal tracts of contiguous lobules and forming a micronodular cirrhosis (secondary biliary cirrhosis).

IRON-OVERLOAD SYNDROME

A number of conditions are characterized by excessive accumulation of iron in the body (siderosis). Iron overload results from inordinate intestinal absorption of iron or from its parenteral administration. Iron overload is divided into two major categories based on the cause of the increased body iron. **Hereditary hemochromatosis** is caused by a common genetic alteration in control of the intestinal absorption of iron. **Secondary iron overload** is a condition that (1) complicates certain hematologic disorders; (2) is associated with parenteral iron overload, in which the iron is obtained from multiple blood transfusions or parenteral administration of iron itself; or (3) is caused by an enormous dietary intake of iron.

Hereditary Hemochromatosis

■ *Hereditary hemochromatosis is a common inherited disorder of iron metabolism that is characterized by excessive iron absorption and toxic accumulation of iron in the parenchymal cells.* In this disease, 20 to 40 g of iron (as much as 10-fold the normal content) accumulates in the body. The excess iron in hereditary hemochromatosis is located exclusively within the storage compartment; thus, iron stores are increased as much as 50-fold over the normal value. **The clinical hallmarks of advanced hemochromatosis are cirrhosis, diabetes, skin pigmentation, and cardiac failure** (Fig. 14-29). The disease most often manifests clinically in patients between 40 and 60 years of age, and men are afflicted 10-fold as often as women. This striking male predilec-

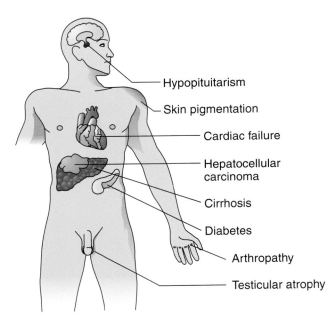

Hypopituitarism

Skin pigmentation

Cardiac failure

Hepatocellular carcinoma

Cirrhosis

Diabetes

Arthropathy

Testicular atrophy

FIGURE *14-29*
Complications of hemochromatosis.

tion may be attributed to the increased loss of iron in women during the reproductive years. However, given sufficient time to absorb additional iron, postmenopausal women also seem to be at risk for development of hemochromatosis. Because maximum daily iron absorption is approximately 4 mg, hemochromatosis clearly takes years to develop.

☐ **Pathogenesis:** Hereditary hemochromatosis is inherited as an **autosomal recessive** disorder. Although only a few families have been reported in which more than one member has hemochromatosis, lesser degrees of iron overload are often found in relatives of those with the disease.

The hemochromatosis gene is located on the short arm of chromosome 6. There is a linkage between this gene and the HLA locus of the human major histocompatibility complex. The HLA-A3 antigen is present in 70% of persons with hereditary hemochromatosis but in only 25% of the normal population. In white populations, approximately 11% are heterozygous, and one person in every 220 is homozygous. However, only one in five homozygotes develops clinically apparent hemochromatosis.

The mechanisms underlying the increased deposition of iron in parenchymal organs among patients with hereditary hemochromatosis are obscure, but an increased uptake of iron by the duodenal mucosa has been documented.

☐ **Pathology:** Hereditary hemochromatosis is characterized pathologically by the accumulation of very large amounts of iron in the parenchymal cells of a variety of organs and tissues.

Liver. The liver contains more than 0.5 g of iron per 100 g of wet weight, and it is usually cirrhotic. The organ is enlarged and reddish-brown, and exhibits a uniform micronodular cirrhosis. The hepatocytes and bile duct epithelium are filled with iron granules (Fig. 14-30). The excess cellular iron is stored predominantly in lysosomes and in the ferric form. Late in the disease, many Kupffer cells contain large deposits of iron derived from the phagocytosis of necrotic hepatocytes. Within the fibrous septa, iron is conspicuous in proliferated bile ductules and macrophages.

Skin. The skin in patients with primary hemochromatosis is typically pigmented, but only half of the patients exhibit increased iron deposition in the skin. Most patients display increased melanin in the basal melanocytes.

Pancreas. Diabetes, which is a common complication of hemochromatosis, results from the deposition of iron in the pancreas. Grossly, the organ appears rust-colored and firm, thereby reflecting the underlying fi-

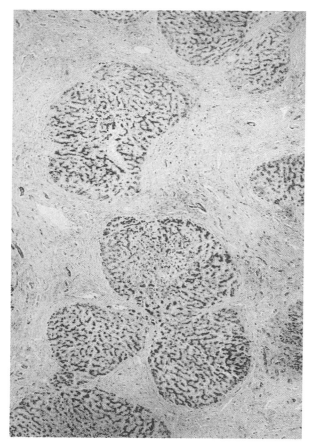

FIGURE *14-30*
Hemochromatosis. A Prussian blue stain for iron demonstrates considerable iron in a cirrhotic liver.

brosis. Both exocrine and endocrine cells are affected, particularly the former. Frequently, there is degeneration of acinar cells and a reduction in the number of islets of Langerhans. The combination of pigmented skin and glucose intolerance in patients with hemochromatosis is often referred to as **bronze diabetes.**

Heart. Congestive heart failure is a common cause of death in patients with hemochromatosis. The heart is often enlarged, sometimes weighing more than twice the normal value. Microscopically, the myocardial fibers contain iron pigment. Necrosis of cardiac myocytes and accompanying interstitial fibrosis are common.

Endocrine System. Numerous endocrine glands are typically involved in hemochromatosis. Iron is deposited in the pituitary, adrenal, thyroid, and parathyroid glands. However, tissue damage is not a usual feature in these organs, except for the pituitary gland, in which the release of gonadotropins is impaired. As a result, testicular atrophy is seen in one-fourth of the male patients.

Joints. Arthropathy, most severe in the fingers and hands, occurs in half of patients with hemochromatosis.

☐ **Clinical Features:** The liver disease in hemochromatosis generally pursues an indolent and prolonged course, but one-fourth of the patients eventually die in hepatic coma or as a result of bleeding from esophageal varices. **Hepatocellular carcinoma is a significant late complication of hemochromatosis, occurring in as many as 15% of cases.**

Treatment of hemochromatosis is based on removal of iron from the body, which is accomplished most effectively by repeated phlebotomy. The 10-year survival rate of untreated patients with hemochromatosis is a mere 6%, whereas in those treated by phlebotomy, it is more than fivefold as great.

Secondary Iron-Overload Syndromes

Many features of hereditary hemochromatosis may also occur in persons who do not carry the gene for that disease.

☐ **Pathogenesis:** Within certain limits, the amount of iron absorbed relates to the amount of iron ingested. Many patients with secondary iron overload (≤40%) have a long history of alcohol abuse, and it is thought that alcohol may enhance both the accumulation of iron and its associated cell injury.

Massive iron overload occurs in patients with certain anemias such as thalassemia major, sideroblastic anemias, and other anemias associated with ineffective erythropoiesis. The source of the excess iron is the patient's diet or transfused blood. Increased iron absorption occurs despite the saturation of transferrin, and the release of iron by intravascular hemolysis adds a further burden. The causes of iron overload are summarized in Box 14-3.

B O X *14-3* **Causes of Iron Overload**

Increased Iron Absorption
Hereditary hemochromatosis
Chronic liver disease
Iron-loading anemias
Porphyria cutanea tarda
Congenital diseases (e.g., atransferrinemia)
Dietary iron overload (Bantu siderosis)
Excess medicinal iron
Parenteral Iron Overload
Multiple blood transfusions
Injectable medicinal iron
Focal Iron Overload
Idiopathic pulmonary hemosiderosis
Renal hemosiderosis

☐ **Pathology:** Cirrhosis with secondary iron overload shows varying degrees of iron accumulation, but the iron deposition is generally less extensive than that in hereditary hemochromatosis and is often restricted to the periphery of the nodules. Transfusional and other types of siderosis are characterized initially by the uniform deposition of iron in Kupffer cells, with eventual spillover into hepatocytes.

HERITABLE DISORDERS ASSOCIATED WITH CIRRHOSIS

Wilson Disease (Hepatolenticular Degeneration)

■ *Wilson disease is a hereditary disorder of copper metabolism in which injury to the liver and brain is associated with deposition of excess copper.* The disease is transmitted by an autosomal recessive gene (*WD* gene) located on chromosome 13.

☐ **Pathogenesis:** Unlike iron absorption, body copper homeostasis is not regulated at the level of the intestine. Biliary excretion of copper is the primary mechanism by which body copper balance is maintained, because negligible amounts of copper are reabsorbed by the intestine. Up to 95% of circulating copper is bound to ceruloplasmin, from which it is made available to peripheral tissues as well as returned to the liver.

Wilson disease is characterized by a striking reduction in serum ceruloplasmin levels. Intestinal absorption of copper is unaltered. However, biliary and, therefore, fecal excretion of copper is reduced to approximately one-fourth of the normal rate. Although the primary lesion in Wilson disease is probably related to defective biliary excretion of copper, the exact pathogenesis remains obscure.

The primacy of the liver as the seat of Wilson disease is attested to by its cure with liver transplantation. The mechanism by which excess copper injures the liver cells, however, remains elusive. Like iron, copper may catalyze the formation of potent oxidizing species from superoxide anions and hydrogen peroxide produced by normal oxygen metabolism.

☐ **Pathology:** Wilson disease progresses from mild to severe **chronic active hepatitis,** with all of the typical histologic features of that disease. The periportal hepatocytes often contain Mallory bodies, and cholestasis with bile casts in proliferated bile ductules is not infrequent. **Cirrhosis may develop rapidly, even during childhood.**

In the **brain,** the corpus striatum and, occasionally, the subthalamic nuclei display a reddish-brown discoloration. The central white matter of the cerebral or cerebellar hemispheres may manifest spongy softening or cavitation, in which case the overlying cortex is atrophic. The astrocytes proliferate in the putamen, and the number of neurons is decreased.

☐ **Clinical Features:** Half of the patients with Wilson disease display some symptoms by adolescence, and the remainder become ill in their early adult years. The presenting symptoms are referable to chronic liver disease in half of the patients, whereas one-third initially present with neurologic complaints and one-tenth with psychiatric manifestations. One-fourth of the patients show symptoms related both to the liver and to the central nervous system.

Liver. Chronic hepatitis and cirrhosis result in jaundice, portal hypertension, and hepatic failure. Unlike hemochromatosis, Wilson disease is not associated with an increased risk of primary hepatocellular carcinoma.

Brain. Progressive behavioral abnormalities and dementia may lead to the institutionalization of patients before the diagnosis of Wilson disease becomes evident. In untreated cases, dysarthria and dysphagia appear, and during the late stages of the disease, disabling dystonia and spasticity occur.

Eye. Kayser-Fleischer ring is a golden-brown, bilateral discoloration of the cornea that encircles the periphery of the iris and obscures its muscular pattern.

Kidney. Renal glomerular and tubular dysfunction, manifested by proteinuria, lowered glomerular filtration, aminoaciduria, and phosphaturia, is common in patients with Wilson disease.

Wilson disease is treated with D-penicillamine, a copper-chelating agent that augments the excretion of copper in the urine. In severe cases, liver transplantation has been successful.

Cystic Fibrosis

Newborns with cystic fibrosis may present with obstructive jaundice caused by mucous plugs in the intrahepatic biliary tree. Secondary biliary cirrhosis is found in 10% of the patients who survive beyond 25 years of age. Cystic fibrosis is discussed in detail in Chapter 6.

α_1-Antitrypsin Deficiency

Liver disease associated with α_1-antitrypsin deficiency is characterized by accumulation of the mutant α_1-antitrypsin in the hepatocytes and the development of chronic hepatitis and cirrhosis during early childhood. α_1-Antitrypsin deficiency is inherited as an autosomal recessive trait and was initially described as a cause of emphysema (see Chapter 12). Thereafter, cases of liver disease without pulmonary involvement were reported, and concurrent disease of both organs has also been recognized.

☐ **Pathogenesis:** α_1-Antitrypsin is synthesized in the liver, and both the pulmonary and hepatic disorders result from a defect in secretion of the mutant protein from the liver. The abnormal protein accumulates as an insoluble aggregate within the lumen of the endoplasmic reticulum of the hepatocyte.

☐ **Pathology:** The characteristic feature in the liver of patients with α_1-antitrypsin deficiency is the presence of faintly eosinophilic, PAS-positive cytoplasmic droplets (Fig. 14-31). By electron microscopy, these inclusions are visualized as amorphous material within dilated cisternae of the endoplasmic reticulum. α_1-Antitrypsin deficiency is an important cause of neonatal hepatitis and cannot be distinguished morphologically from other forms of neonatal hepatitis or from chronic active hepatitis.

Clinical Features. The clinical expression of liver disease in α_1-antitrypsin deficiency is highly variable, ranging from a rapidly fatal neonatal hepatitis to an absence of any hepatic dysfunction. Most infants recover within 6 months, but a few progress to cirrhosis within 1 or 2 years. Children with cirrhosis usually die before the age of 10 years, either from hepatic failure or from other complications of α_1-antitrypsin deficiency. Cirrhosis of α_1-antitrypsin deficiency is complicated by a very high incidence of hepatocellular carcinoma.

Inborn Errors of Carbohydrate Metabolism

Glycogen Storage Diseases

The biochemical basis of glycogen storage diseases is discussed in Chapter 6. These disorders are inherited as autosomal recessive traits. **Only glycogenosis type IV (brancher deficiency, Andersen disease) is always complicated by cirrhosis.** A slowly developing cirrhosis may occur in glycogenosis type III (debrancher deficiency, Cori disease), but this is not inevitable. Glycogenosis type I (glucose-6-phosphatase deficiency, von Gierke disease) is associated with striking hepatomegaly, and glycogenosis type II (acid-glucosidase deficiency, Pompe disease) features mild hepatomegaly. Neither of those two disorders, however, is complicated by cirrhosis.

Galactosemia

■ *Galactosemia, which is inherited as an autosomal recessive trait, results from a deficiency of galactose-1-phosphate uridyl transferase, the enzyme that catalyzes the second step in the conversion of galactose to glucose.* As a result of this metabolic defect, galactose and its metabolites accumulate in the liver and other organs. Milk-fed infants with this disorder rapidly develop **hepatosplenomegaly, jaundice,** and **hypoglycemia.** Cataracts and mental retardation are also common.

Microscopically, within 2 weeks of birth, the liver shows extensive and uniform fat accumulation and striking proliferation of bile ductules both in and around the portal tracts. At approximately 6 weeks of age, fibrosis begins to extend from the portal tracts into the lobule and, within 6 months, progresses to cirrhosis. Institution of a galactose-free diet has been re-

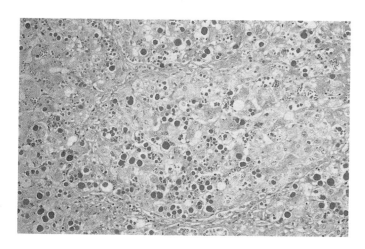

FIGURE *14-31*
α_1-**Antitrypsin deficiency. A photomicrograph of a section of liver stained by the periodic acid-Schiff reaction shows numerous cytoplasmic granules in the hepatocytes.**

ported to ameliorate the disease and to reverse many of the morphologic alterations.

Hereditary Fructose Intolerance

■ *Hereditary fructose intolerance is an autosomal recessive disease caused by a deficiency of fructose-1-phosphate aldolase.* When fructose is fed early during infancy, hepatomegaly, jaundice, and ascites develop. However, feeding of fructose after the age of 6 months results in far less severe disease. Progressive fibrosis culminates in cirrhosis.

Tyrosinemia

■ *Tyrosinemia is an autosomal recessive trait in which the catabolism of tyrosine to fumarate and acetoacetate is impaired owing to a deficiency of fumarylacetoacetate hydrolase.*

Acute tyrosinemia, which begins within a few weeks or months of birth, is characterized by hepatosplenomegaly and is associated with liver failure and death, usually before the age of 12 months. The appearance of the liver is remarkably similar to that in patients with galactosemia, including progression to cirrhosis.

Chronic tyrosinemia begins during the first year of life and is characterized by growth retardation, renal disease, and hepatic failure. Death usually supervenes before the age of 10 years. **The incidence of hepatocellular carcinoma associated with chronic tyrosinemia is extraordinarily high.**

PORTAL HYPERTENSION

■ *Portal hypertension is a sustained increase in portal venous pressure and is almost always the result of obstruction to flow of blood somewhere in the portal circuit* (Fig. 14-

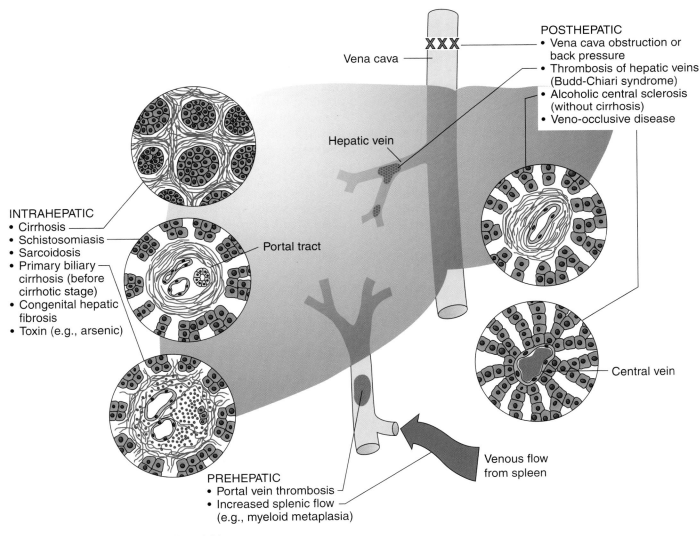

POSTHEPATIC
- Vena cava obstruction or back pressure
- Thrombosis of hepatic veins (Budd-Chiari syndrome)
- Alcoholic central sclerosis (without cirrhosis)
- Veno-occlusive disease

Vena cava

Hepatic vein

INTRAHEPATIC
- Cirrhosis
- Schistosomiasis
- Sarcoidosis
- Primary biliary cirrhosis (before cirrhotic stage)
- Congenital hepatic fibrosis
- Toxin (e.g., arsenic)

Portal tract

Central vein

Venous flow from spleen

PREHEPATIC
- Portal vein thrombosis
- Increased splenic flow (e.g., myeloid metaplasia)

FIGURE **14-32**
Causes of portal hypertension.

32). Complications of portal hypertension arise from the increased pressure and dilatation of the venous bed behind the obstruction. Major complications of this increased pressure and the opening of collateral channels are bleeding from gastroesophageal varices, ascites, and splenomegaly.

Intrahepatic Portal Hypertension

By far, the most common cause of portal hypertension is cirrhosis. Regenerative nodules impinge on and deform the hepatic veins, thereby obstructing the flow of blood distal to the lobules. The small portal veins and venules are trapped, narrowed, and often obliterated by scarring of the portal tracts. Moreover, blood flow through the hepatic artery is increased, and small arteriovenous communications become functional. In this way, portal hypertension caused by obstruction to the flow of blood distal to the sinusoid is augmented by an increase in the arterial blood flow. Moreover, an increase in splanchnic arterial blood flow, the cause of which is unclear, is an important factor in the maintenance of portal hypertension. Central vein sclerosis and sinusoidal fibrosis also contribute to the development of portal hypertension in alcoholic liver disease.

Worldwide, hepatic schistosomiasis (*Schistosoma mansoni* and *S. japonicum*) is a major cause of portal hypertension. The schistosomal ova released from the intestinal veins traverse the portal system and lodge in the intrahepatic portal venules, where they elicit a granulomatous reaction that heals by scarring. Because the obstruction within the liver occurs predominantly before the portal blood enters the hepatic sinusoids, hepatic schistosomiasis is functionally similar to prehepatic portal hypertension.

Prehepatic Portal Hypertension

■ *Prehepatic portal hypertension* results from an obstruction to the flow of portal blood before its entrance into the portal tracts. The classic example of prehepatic portal hypertension is **portal vein thrombosis,** commonly in association with cirrhosis. Other causes of portal vein thrombosis include tumors, infections, hypercoagulability states associated with oral contraceptive use and pregnancy, pancreatitis, and surgical trauma. Some cases are of unknown cause.

Posthepatic Portal Hypertension

■ *Posthepatic portal hypertension* is any obstruction to the flow of blood through the hepatic veins beyond the liver lobules, either within or distal to the liver.

Budd-Chiari Syndrome

■ *Budd-Chiari syndrome* refers to occlusion of the hepatic veins occurring in venous tributaries of any size, including the central hepatic venules.

□ **Pathogenesis:** The principal cause of Budd-Chiari syndrome is thrombosis of the hepatic veins in association with such diverse conditions as polycythemia vera, hepatocellular carcinoma, tumor metastases from the adrenals and kidneys, bacterial infections, use of oral contraceptives, pregnancy, and trauma. However, in more than half of the cases, no specific cause for Budd-Chiari syndrome is evident. Thrombosis is most common in the large hepatic veins close to their exit from the liver and in the intrahepatic portion of the inferior vena cava.

Hepatic veno-occlusive disease is a variant of Budd-Chiari syndrome and is caused by occlusion of the central venules and small branches of the hepatic veins. Most commonly, this disorder is traced to the ingestion of toxic pyrrolizidine alkaloids in plants of the *Crotalaria* and *Senecio* families, which are used in the formulation of "bush teas" among primitive societies. It is also seen in patients treated with certain antineoplastic chemotherapeutic agents, after hepatic irradiation, and in association with bone marrow transplantation (possibly as a manifestation of graft-versus-host disease).

□ **Pathology:** During the early acute stage of hepatic vein thrombosis, the liver is swollen and tense, and the cut surface exhibits a mottled appearance and oozes blood. During the chronic stage, the cut surface is paler, and the liver is firm owing to an increase in connective tissue.

Microscopic examination during the acute phase reveals hepatic veins that display thrombi in varying stages of evolution, from recent clots to well-organized, canalized thrombi. The sinusoids of the central zone are dilated and packed with erythrocytes. The liver cell plates are compressed, and necrosis of centrilobular hepatocytes is accompanied by the deposition of fibrin. In patients with longstanding venous congestion, fibrosis of the central zone, radiating into the more peripheral portions of the lobules, is conspicuous. The sinusoids are dilated, and the central to midzonal hepatocytes show pressure atrophy. Eventually, connective tissue septa link adjacent central zones to form nodules with a single portal tract in the center, which is a process known as reverse lobulation; the fibrosis is usually not severe enough to justify a label of cirrhosis.

□ **Clinical Features:** Thrombosis of the hepatic veins, when total, presents as an acute illness that is characterized by abdominal pain, enlargement of the liver, ascites, and mild jaundice. Often, acute hepatic failure and death rapidly occur. The more usual course, in which obstruction of the hepatic venous circulation is incomplete, is marked by similar symptoms but may pursue a protracted course over periods ranging from a month to a few years. More than 90% of these patients develop ascites, which is usually severe, and splenomegaly is seen in more than 30%. The liver is usually enlarged. Most patients eventually die in hepatic failure or from complications of portal hypertension. Liver transplantation has been successful in curing the disease.

Complications of Portal Hypertension

Portal hypertension leads to several systemic complications (Fig. 14-33), especially esophageal varices, splenomegaly, and ascites.

Esophageal Varices

Esophageal varices arise from the opening of portal-systemic collaterals as an adaptation to decompress the portal venous system. One of the most common causes of death in patients with portal hypertension is exsanguinating upper gastrointestinal tract hemorrhage from bleeding esophageal varices. Permanent decompression of the portal circulation can be achieved by surgically constructed portasystemic shunts. Liver transplantation is now increasingly being considered as an alternative to shunt surgery.

Fibrocongestive Splenomegaly

The spleen in portal hypertension enlarges progressively. This enlarged spleen often gives rise to the syndrome of **hypersplenism**—that is, a decrease in the life span of all of the formed elements of the blood and, therefore, a reduction in their circulating numbers. Hypersplenism is attributed to an increased rate of removal of erythrocytes, leukocytes, and platelets because of the prolonged transit time through the hyperplastic spleen.

On gross examination, the spleen is firm and enlarged, weighing as much as 1000 g, and its cut surface is uniformly deep red, with an inapparent white pulp. Microscopically, the sinusoids are dilated, and their walls are thickened by fibrous tissue and lined by hyperplastic monocytes/macrophages.

Ascites

■ *Ascites is the accumulation of fluid in the peritoneal cavity.* It often accompanies portal hypertension, most commonly in patients with decompensated cirrhosis. The amount of fluid may be so great (frequently many liters) that it not only distends the abdomen but also interferes with breathing. The onset of ascites in patients with cirrhosis is associated with a poor prognosis.

☐ **Pathogenesis:** There is a consensus that, in addition to portal hypertension itself, sodium and water retention in patients with cirrhosis is clearly important to the pathogenesis of ascites (Fig. 14-34). Other factors also contribute to the formation of ascites in cirrhosis. Portal hypertension increases the hydrostatic pressure in the mesenteric capillaries, whereas, at the same time, the low serum albumin level, which is characteristic of cirrhosis, is associated with decreased plasma oncotic pressure and transudation of fluid into the peritoneal cavity. Finally, the formation rate of hepatic lymph exceeds the capacity of the lymphatics to remove it, and the liver "weeps" lymph into the abdomen.

Spontaneous Bacterial Peritonitis

Spontaneous bacterial peritonitis is an important complication in patients with both cirrhosis and ascites. The infection is extremely dangerous and carries a very high mortality rate even when treated with antibiotics.

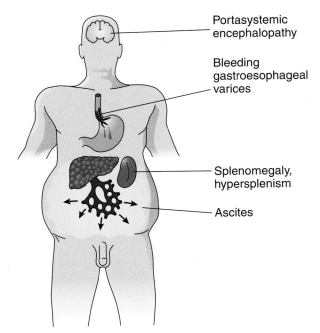

Portasystemic encephalopathy

Bleeding gastroesophageal varices

Splenomegaly, hypersplenism

Ascites

FIGURE *14-33*
Complications of portal hypertension.

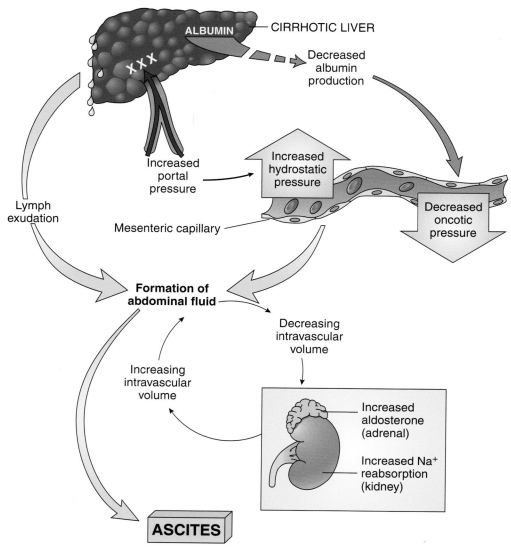

FIGURE   *14-34*

Traditional concept (hypovolemic hypothesis) of the pathogenesis of ascites. In addition to the other factors depicted, the traditional concept holds that renal retention of sodium is a response to a decreased "effective" blood volume. It should be noted that an alternative view (overflow hypothesis) considers the increased renal reabsorption of sodium to be a primary effect of cirrhosis that precedes the formation of ascites. Peripheral vasodilatation is an additional factor to be considered.

TOXIC LIVER INJURY

The diversity of acute, chemically induced hepatic injury is so broad that it spans the entire spectrum of liver disease, from clinically trivial, transient cholestasis to fatal, fulminant hepatitis. Chronic toxic injury to the liver is equally diverse, being expressed at one extreme as a mild, persistent hepatitis and at the other as an active cirrhosis. Although hepatic injury caused by drugs accounts for less than 5% of all cases of jaundice, it comprises as much as 25% of the cases of fulminant hepatic necrosis.

Certain hepatotoxic chemicals invariably produce liver cell necrosis—that is, their action is entirely **predictable**. Among such agents are substances as diverse as yellow phosphorus, the organic solvent carbon tetrachloride, the mushroom poison phalloidin, and the analgesic acetaminophen. The defining characteristics of liver injury produced by "predictable" hepatotoxins are:

- The agent, in sufficiently high doses, always produces liver cell necrosis.
- The extent of hepatic injury is dose-dependent.
- These compounds produce the same lesions in different species.

- Liver necrosis is characteristically zonal and often, but not exclusively, centrilobular.
- The period between administration of the toxin and development of liver cell necrosis is brief.

Chapter 1 discusses the possible mechanisms by which these toxins produce liver necrosis.

In contrast to the aforementioned classic poisons, **most reactions to drugs are unpredictable** and seem to represent idiosyncratic events or manifestations of unusual sensitivity to a dose-related side effect.

Zonal Hepatocellular Necrosis

Drugs and chemicals that are predictable hepatotoxins and act through their metabolites typically cause centrilobular necrosis. Examples of such agents are carbon tetrachloride, acetaminophen, and toxins of the mushroom *Amanita phalloides* (Fig. 14-35).

In the affected zones, hepatocytes show coagulative necrosis, hydropic swelling, and variable amounts of fat. Inflammation is often sparse, but if the patient survives, a secondary inflammatory response becomes more conspicuous. Patients die in acute hepatic failure or recover without sequelae.

Long-term administration of hepatotoxins that cause zonal necrosis, exemplified by carbon tetrachlo-

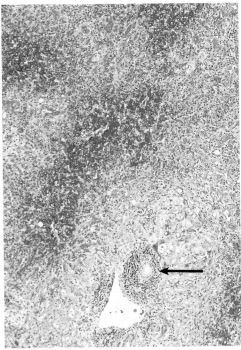

FIGURE *14-35*
Toxic centrilobular necrosis. This autopsy specimen in a case of mushroom poisoning shows hemorrhagic necrosis in the central zones of the liver lobules. (The *arrow* indicates the portal tract.)

ride, produces cirrhosis in experimental animals. However, this is generally not a problem in humans, because the acute toxic injury is almost always recognized and measures are taken to preclude re-exposure to the offending agent.

Fatty Liver

Accumulation of triglycerides within the hepatocytes (hepatic steatosis or fatty liver) occurs in response to a variety of hepatotoxins and generally in a predictable fashion. Although substantial overlap may exist, two morphologic patterns occur, namely macrovesicular steatosis and microvesicular steatosis.

Macrovesicular Steatosis

In macrovesicular steatosis, light microscopy shows the cytoplasm of the liver cell to be occupied by fat, which is seen as a large, clear area that distends the cell and displaces the nucleus to the periphery. In addition to its association with chronic ethanol ingestion, macrovesicular fat results from experimental administration of, or accidental exposure to, such direct hepatotoxins as carbon tetrachloride and poisonous constituents of certain mushrooms. Corticosteroids and some antimetabolites (e.g., methotrexate) may also cause macrovesicular steatosis.

Microvesicular Steatosis

In the microvesicular fatty liver, small fat vacuoles are dispersed throughout the cytoplasm, and the nucleus retains its central position. In contrast to macrovesicular steatosis, which by itself is, in general, clinically inconsequential, the microvesicular variety is commonly associated with severe and, sometimes, fatal liver disease, although milder forms are recognized.

Reye syndrome is an acute disease of children that is characterized by hepatic failure and encephalopathy. Symptoms usually begin after a febrile illness, commonly influenza or varicella infection, and have been claimed to correlate with the administration of **aspirin.** Clearly, Reye syndrome is more complex than simple aspirin toxicity, because it almost always occurs after a febrile illness. In addition, the doses of aspirin consumed are far too small to produce liver injury in otherwise normal children.

On light microscopy, the liver in a patient with Reye syndrome displays a typical microvesicular steatosis, without accompanying hepatocellular necrosis or inflammation (Fig. 14-36). Cerebral edema and fat accumulation are reported in the brain. Mitochondrial dysfunction is thought to play a role in the pathogenesis of this disease.

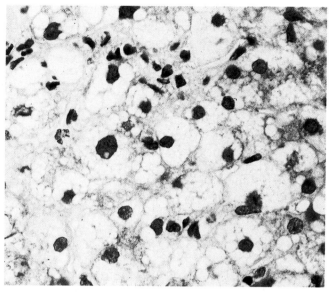

FIGURE *14-36*
Microvesicular fatty liver. A liver biopsy specimen in a case of Reye syndrome shows small droplet fat in hepatocytes and centrally located nuclei.

Intrahepatic Cholestasis

Acute intrahepatic cholestasis is one of the most frequent manifestations of the idiosyncratic types of drug-induced liver disease.

Bland centrilobular cholestasis, with virtually no hepatocellular necrosis or inflammation, is caused by a few drugs, principally sex steroids of the contraceptive or the anabolic type. Except for mild jaundice, pruritus, and an elevated serum alkaline phosphatase level, the patients feel well.

Centrilobular cholestasis with slight to moderate inflammation and mild hepatocellular injury is associated with many other drugs, of which chlorpromazine is the prototype.

Lesions Resembling Viral Hepatitis

All of the typical clinical and morphologic features of acute viral hepatitis can be seen after administration of drugs that cause idiosyncratic (unpredictable) liver injury. The most widely appreciated examples are the inhalation anesthetic halothane, the antituberculosis agent isoniazid, and the antihypertensive drug methyldopa. Although the incidence of these viral hepatitis–like reactions is low, they are far more dangerous than viral hepatitis itself, causing more severe disease and carrying a much higher mortality rate. The entire range of acute liver injury, from mild anicteric hepatitis to rapidly fatal fulminant hepatic necrosis, is encountered. It deserves repetition that, for practical purposes, **the pattern of liver injury is morphologi-**cally indistinguishable from that of documented acute viral hepatitis. As in viral hepatitis, when the offending agent is removed (when the virus is cleared or the drug withdrawn), complete recovery is the rule.

That hepatitis caused by halothane is typically more severe after a second or third exposure suggests that an allergic or immunologic mechanism mediates the injury. The frequent occurrence of peripheral eosinophilia and of eosinophils in the liver in patients with halothane hepatitis supports this concept. However, it has not been definitively established that an immunologic mechanism produces halothane hepatitis.

Chronic Active Hepatitis

Persistent intake of hepatotoxic drugs can lead to a syndrome that is indistinguishable from chronic active hepatitis. Like chronic active hepatitis caused by persistent viral infection, drug-induced chronic active hepatitis may progress to cirrhosis. On discontinuation of drug administration, the lesion usually resolves, although this may require many months. Among the drugs incriminated in the production of chronic active hepatitis are the laxative oxyphenisatin, the antihypertensive agent methyldopa, the antituberculosis drug isoniazid, and certain sulfonamides.

Vascular Lesions

As noted in the discussion of portal hypertension, occlusion of the hepatic veins (Budd-Chiari syndrome and veno-occlusive disease) has been reported to follow the use of drugs and chemicals.

Peliosis hepatis is a peculiar hepatic lesion that is characterized by cystic, blood-filled cavities that are not lined by endothelial cells (Fig. 14-37). Anabolic sex steroids and, occasionally, contraceptive steroids sometimes produce this lesion.

Hyperplastic and Neoplastic Lesions

Hepatic adenomas are recognized as a complication of oral contraceptive use and, uncommonly, of anabolic steroids. These tumors of hepatocytes are benign, and their greatest danger lies in their propensity to rupture and then bleed profusely.

Hemangiosarcomas of the liver appeared many years after the intravenous administration of thorium dioxide (Thorotrast), a radioactive compound used in the past to visualize the liver. This particulate isotope is engulfed by Kupffer cells, where it remains inert indefinitely and emits local radiant energy, thereby producing neoplastic transformation. Long-term exposure

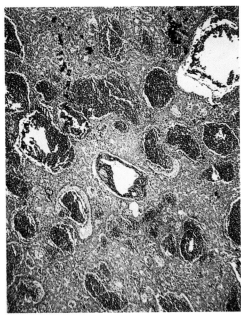

FIGURE   14-37
Peliosis hepatis. The liver contains numerous large, irregular, blood-filled spaces.

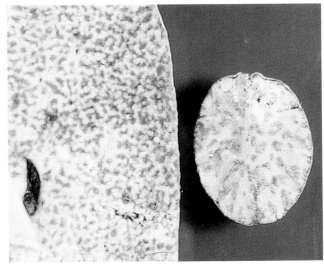

FIGURE   14-38
Chronic passive congestion of the liver. The surface of this fixed liver exhibits an accentuated lobular pattern, with an appearance resembling that of a nutmeg (*right*).

to inorganic arsenic, usually in the form of insecticides, and inhalation of vinyl chloride in an industrial setting have also been linked to the development of hemangiosarcoma of the liver.

CIRCULATORY DISORDERS

Congestive Heart Failure (Chronic Passive Congestion)

In the face of persistent congestive heart failure, pressure in the peripheral venous circulation increases, thereby impeding venous outflow from the liver and producing chronic passive congestion of that organ. Unlike acute congestion, however, in which the congested liver is somewhat enlarged, the chronically congested liver is often reduced in size. On gross examination, the cut surface exhibits an accentuated lobular pattern, with a mottled appearance of alternating light and dark areas (Fig. 14-38). Because this pattern is reminiscent of a cut nutmeg, it has been termed **nutmeg liver**. In severe cases, the centrilobular terminal venules and adjacent sinusoids are conspicuously dilated and filled with erythrocytes. The liver cell plates in this zone are thinned by pressure atrophy and may even be absent, leaving a collapsed reticulin framework. Chronic passive congestion of the liver is of more pathologic than clinical interest, because the condition has little effect on hepatic function.

Cardiac Fibrosis of the Liver

In cases of particularly severe and longstanding **right-sided heart failure** (e.g., tricuspid valvular disease or constrictive pericarditis), chronic passive congestion progresses to varying degrees of hepatic fibrosis. Delicate fibrous strands envelop the terminal venules, and septa radiate from the centrilobular zones. The older term **cardiac cirrhosis** is inappropriate, because the complete septa and regenerative nodules of true cirrhosis are rarely encountered.

Shock

Shock from any cause results in decreased perfusion of the liver and often leads to ischemic necrosis of the centrilobular hepatocytes. Microscopically, coagulative necrosis of centrilobular hepatocytes is accompanied by frank hemorrhage.

Infarction

Infarcts of the liver are uncommon because of the organ's dual blood supply and the anastomotic structure of the hepatic sinusoids. Acute occlusion of the hepatic artery or its branches is unusual but can occur as a result of embolism, polyarteritis nodosa, or accidental ligation during surgery. Under such circumstances, irregular, pale areas, which are often surrounded by a hyperemic zone, reflect the underlying ischemic necrosis.

BACTERIAL INFECTIONS

Pyogenic liver abscesses are produced by staphylococci, streptococci, and gram-negative enterobacteria. It is being increasingly recognized that anaerobic inhabitants of the gastrointestinal tract, particularly *Bacteroides* species and microaerophilic streptococci, are also common causes of liver abscesses. Organisms reach the liver in the arterial or portal blood or through the biliary tract.

Pylephlebitic abscesses (Fig. 14-39) result from intra-abdominal suppuration, as in peritonitis or diverticulitis, with the organism being transmitted to the liver in the portal blood.

Cholangitic abscesses in the liver are today the most common form of hepatic abscess in Western countries. Biliary obstruction from any cause is often complicated by bacterial infection of the biliary tree, which is termed **ascending cholangitis**. The retrograde biliary dissemination of organisms (usually *Escherichia coli*) then leads to the formation of cholangitic abscesses. Nevertheless, in half of all cases of hepatic abscess, the source of infection cannot be demonstrated.

☐ **Clinical Features:** Patients with a hepatic abscess typically present with high fever, rapid weight loss, right upper quadrant abdominal pain, and hepatomegaly. Jaundice occurs in one-fourth of the cases, but the serum alkaline phosphatase level is almost always elevated. Solitary abscesses are treated with surgical drainage and antibiotics, but multiple abscesses present a difficult therapeutic problem. The mortality rate from hepatic abscess, even among treated cases, remains high, ranging from 40% to 80%.

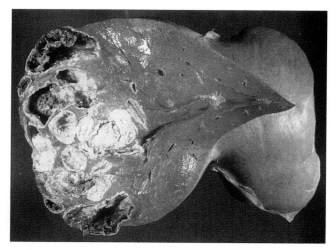

FIGURE   *14-39*
Pylephlebitic abscesses of the liver. The cut surface of the liver shows large, confluent, and irregular abscess cavities.

Parasitic infestations of the liver are a serious public health problem worldwide, although they are uncommon in industrialized countries. These diseases are discussed in Chapter 9.

NEONATAL HEPATITIS

■ *Neonatal hepatitis is a poorly defined clinical and pathologic entity of multiple causes, which have in common prolonged cholestasis, morphologic evidence of liver cell injury, and inflammation.*

☐ **Pathogenesis:** In half of all cases of neonatal hepatitis, the cause is discernible (Box 14-4), and 30% of the cases are assigned to α_1-antitrypsin deficiency alone. Most of the other cases with known causes can be attributed to viral hepatitis B and infectious agents such

BOX   *14-4*   **Causes of Neonatal Hepatitis**

Idiopathic
Idiopathic neonatal hepatitis
Prolonged intrahepatic cholestasis
    Arteriohepatic dysplasia (Alagille syndrome)
    Paucity of intrahepatic bile ducts not associated with
        specific syndromes
    Zellweger syndrome (cerebrohepatorenal syndrome)
    Byler disease
Mechanical Obstruction of the Intrahepatic Bile Ducts
Congenital hepatic fibrosis
Caroli disease (cystic dilatation of intrahepatic ducts)
Metabolic Disorders
Defects of carbohydrate metabolism
    Galactosemia
    Hereditary fructose intolerance
    Glycogenosis type IV
Defects of lipid metabolism
    Gaucher disease
    Niemann-Pick disease
    Wolman disease
Tyrosinemia (defect of amino acid metabolism)
α_1-Antitrypsin deficiency
Cystic fibrosis
Parenteral nutrition
Hepatitis
Hepatitis B
TORCH agents
Varicella
Syphilis
ECHO viruses
Neonatal sepsis
Chromosomal Abnormalities
Down syndrome
Trisomy 18
Extrahepatic Biliary Atresia

as the TORCH group (toxoplasmosis, rubella, cytomegalovirus, and herpes simplex).

☐ **Pathology:** The characteristic hepatic lesion of neonatal hepatitis is giant cell transformation of hepatocytes, hence the former term *giant cell hepatitis* (Fig. 14-40). Bile pigment is often prominent within the canaliculi and hepatocytes. Ballooned hepatocytes, acinar transformation, and acidophilic bodies are also typical of neonatal hepatitis, and extramedullary hemopoiesis is often conspicuous. Chronic inflammatory infiltrates are seen in the portal tracts as well as in the lobular parenchyma. Pericellular fibrosis around degenerating hepatocytes, either singly or in groups, is common, and fibrous tissue septa extend from the portal tracts.

Biliary Atresia

■ *Biliary atresia refers to the absence or hypoplasia of intrahepatic biliary radicals or the extrahepatic bile ducts.*

☐ **Pathogenesis:** It has been suggested that biliary atresia in the newborn, whether intrahepatic or extrahepatic, is secondary to neonatal hepatitis. Alternatively, the causative agent of neonatal hepatitis may independently result in biliary atresia. At one end of the

spectrum are cases in which a striking paucity of intrahepatic bile ducts is seen in a liver that exhibits little cellular injury and inflammation. At the other extreme, a comparable scarcity of bile ducts is accompanied by severe neonatal hepatitis. **It is thought that neonatal hepatitis, intrahepatic biliary atresia, and extrahepatic biliary atresia all result from a common inflammatory process ("infantile obstructive cholangiopathy"), and that they are not true congenital anomalies.**

☐ **Pathology:** Both intrahepatic and extrahepatic biliary atresia lead to a proliferation of bile ductules in the portal tracts (more severe in extrahepatic atresia). Such proliferation may be inconspicuous in patients with classic neonatal hepatitis.

☐ **Clinical Features:** Most patients who have uncomplicated neonatal hepatitis recover without sequelae. Intrahepatic biliary atresia associated with neonatal hepatitis carries a much poorer prognosis, however, and in many children progresses to biliary cirrhosis. Uncorrected extrahepatic biliary atresia invariably results in progressive secondary biliary cirrhosis and is incompatible with survival. The majority of cases of extrahepatic and intrahepatic biliary atresia can be cured only by liver transplantation.

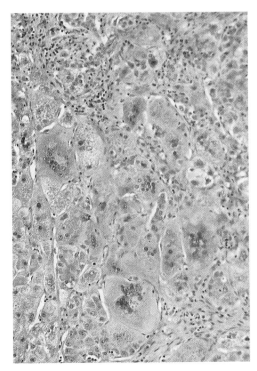

FIGURE *14-40*
Neonatal hepatitis. A photomicrograph shows multinucleated giant hepatocytes, liver cell injury, and a mild chronic inflammatory infiltrate.

BENIGN TUMORS AND TUMOR-LIKE LESIONS

Hepatic Adenoma

■ *Hepatic adenomas are benign tumors of hepatocytes that almost always occur in women during the reproductive years.* These tumors were exceedingly rare before the availability of oral contraceptives, but since their introduction, many such neoplasms have been reported. Today, hepatic adenomas are a well-recognized, although uncommon, complication of the use of oral contraceptives.

☐ **Pathology:** Hepatic adenomas usually occur as solitary, sharply demarcated masses of as much as 40 cm in diameter and 3 kg in weight (Fig. 14-41). In one-fourth of the cases, multiple smaller adenomas are present. On gross examination, the tumor is encapsulated and paler than the surrounding parenchyma. Occasionally, hemorrhage and necrosis are present in the center of the tumor.

Microscopically, the neoplastic hepatocytes resemble their normal counterparts, except that they are not arranged in a lobular architecture (see Fig. 14-41). Portal tracts and central venules are not present. Cells composing the adenoma may be very large and

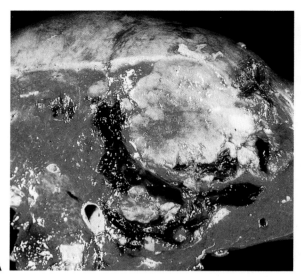
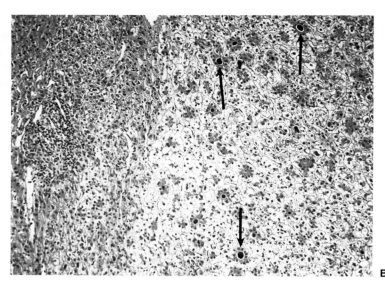

A   B

FIGURE   *14-41*
Hepatic adenoma. (A) A surgically resected portion of liver shows a tan, lobulated mass beneath the liver capsule. Hemorrhage into the tumor has broken through the capsule and into the surrounding liver parenchyma. The patient was a woman who had taken birth control pills for a number of years and presented with sudden intraperitoneal hemorrhage. (B) There is a clear border between the normal liver (*left*) and the adenoma. The adenomatous hepatocytes exhibit no discernible lobular architecture and show a clear cytoplasm filled with glycogen. Occasional cells are arranged in acini, which contain inspissated bile (*arrows*).

eosinophilic or filled with glycogen, which makes the cytoplasm appear to be clear. The tumor is circumscribed by a fibrous capsule of variable thickness, and the adjacent hepatocytes appear to be compressed. Large, thick-walled arteries are often seen in the vicinity of the capsule, and arteries and veins traverse the tumor.

☐ **Clinical Features:** In one-third of patients with hepatic adenomas (particularly pregnant women who have used oral contraceptives), the tumors bleed into the peritoneal cavity and require treatment as a surgical emergency. Even large adenomas have been reported to disappear after discontinuation of oral contraceptives, and they do not progress to cancer.

Focal Nodular Hyperplasia

■ *Focal nodular hyperplasia is a liver mass composed of fibrous septa and hepatocytic nodules, varying in size from 5 to 15 cm in diameter and weighing as much as 700 g.* The cut surface exhibits a characteristic central scar, from which fibrous septa radiate. Microscopically, hepatocytic nodules are circumscribed by fibrous septa (Fig. 14-42), which contain numerous tortuous bile ducts and mononuclear inflammatory cells. Within the nodules, lobular architecture is absent. The lesion exhibits large arteries and veins in the septa, but hemor-

rhage is uncommon. Focal nodular hyperplasia does not progress to cancer.

Hemangioma

Hemangiomas are the most common benign tumor of the liver, being found in as many as 7% of autopsy specimens. They are ordinarily small and asymp-

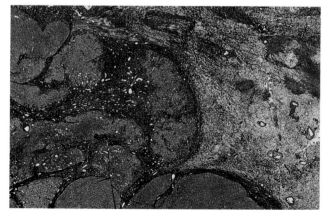

FIGURE   **14-42**
Focal nodular hyperplasia. A photomicrograph of a resected mass from the liver demonstrates a vascular central scar. Irregular fibrous septa dissect the hepatic parenchyma, accounting for the resemblance to cirrhosis.

tomatic, although larger tumors have been reported to cause abdominal symptoms and even hemorrhage into the peritoneal cavity. Grossly, the tumor is usually solitary and less than 5 cm in diameter, but multiple hemangiomas and giant forms have also been described. Microscopically, liver hemangiomas are similar to the cavernous hemangiomas found elsewhere.

HEPATOCELLULAR CARCINOMA

Hepatocellular carcinoma refers to malignant tumors that derive from hepatocytes or their precursors.

☐ **Epidemiology and Pathogenesis:** Hepatocellular carcinoma is probably the most common malignant visceral tumor of humans. It occurs in all parts of the world, but its incidence shows a striking geographic variability. In Western industrialized countries, the tumor is uncommon; in sub-Saharan Africa, Southeast Asia, and Japan, the rates are as much as 50-fold greater. For example, in Mozambique, which seems to have the highest incidence in the world, two-thirds of all cancers in men and one-third in women are hepatocellular carcinomas.

Hepatitis B. An association between hepatocellular carcinoma and infection with HBV is clearly established. In areas of high incidence, HBV infection has been documented in 80% to 90% of patients with hepatocellular carcinoma. Most patients have had chronic HBV infection for many years, with the disease often being transmitted from an infected mother to her newborn child perinatally. The carrier state is indeed dangerous, because such persons are estimated to have as much as a 200-fold increased risk of developing hepatocellular carcinoma. One-fourth of those with chronic hepatitis B acquired either at or near birth ultimately develop hepatocellular carcinoma.

Evidence that HBV has an important role in the development of hepatocellular carcinoma comes from the demonstration that **the genome of HBV is integrated into the host DNA of both the non-neoplastic liver cells and the tumor cells.** The role of HBV itself in the pathogenesis of liver cancer is discussed in Chapter 5.

Hepatitis C. It has recently been demonstrated that two-thirds to three-fourths of patients with primary hepatocellular carcinoma in areas not endemic for HBV demonstrate antibodies to HCV. **Thus, hepatitis C must also be considered as an important risk factor for hepatocellular carcinoma.** In fact, the pattern in Japan has changed, and two-thirds of all patients with hepatocellular carcinoma in that country are now positive for HCV markers but negative for HBV markers.

Cirrhosis occurring in conjunction with hemochromatosis and α_1-antitrypsin deficiency also carries a substantial risk of hepatocellular carcinoma.

☐ **Pathology:** On gross examination, hepatocellular carcinomas appear as soft and hemorrhagic, tan masses in the liver (Fig. 14-43). Occasionally, a green color is present, indicating bile staining. In some cases, a large, solitary tumor occupies a portion of the liver, whereas in others, many smaller tumors are found. The tumor has a tendency to grow into the portal veins and may extend to the vena cava (and even to the right atrium) through the hepatic veins.

Although a number of histologic patterns are recognized, no prognostic significance can be attributed to any of them. Most hepatocellular carcinomas exhibit a **trabecular pattern**—that is, the tumor cells are arranged in trabeculae or plates that resemble the normal liver (see Fig. 14-43). A second histologic variant is termed the **pseudoglandular (adenoid, acinar) pattern.** In this variety, malignant hepatocytes are arranged around a lumen and, thus, resemble glands.

A distinctive histologic appearance has been noted in hepatocellular carcinomas arising in an apparently normal liver, principally among adolescents and young adults. Termed **fibrolamellar hepatocellular carcinoma,** the tumor is composed of large, eosinophilic, and neoplastic hepatocytes arranged in clusters and surrounded by delicate collagen fibers. The prognosis is said to be better than that in other varieties of hepatocellular carcinoma.

Metastases from liver cancer occur widely, but the most common sites are the lungs and portal lymph nodes.

☐ **Clinical Features:** Hepatocellular carcinoma usually presents as a painful and enlarging mass in the liver. Ascites, portal vein thrombosis, occlusion of hepatic veins, and hemorrhage from esophageal varices are common. The prognosis is dismal, and patients die of (1) malignant cachexia; (2) rupture of the tumor, with catastrophic bleeding into the peritoneal cavity; or (3) hepatic failure.

Cholangiocarcinomas (Bile Duct Carcinomas)

■ *Cholangiocarcinomas are malignant hepatic tumors of the biliary epithelium.* They arise anywhere from the large intrahepatic bile ducts at the porta hepatis to the smallest bile ductules at the periphery of the hepatic lobule.

☐ **Pathology:** Cholangiocarcinomas are composed of small, cuboidal cells arranged in a ductular or glan-

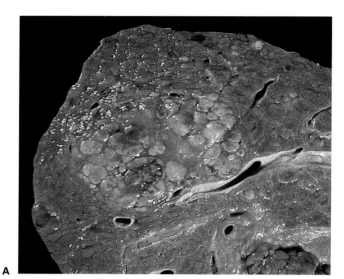

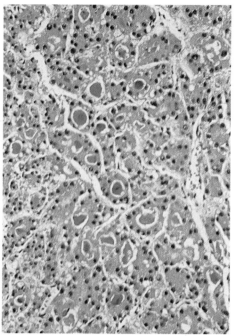

FIGURE 14-43
Hepatocellular carcinoma. (A) This cross-section of a cirrhotic liver shows a poorly circumscribed, nodular area of yellow, partially hemorrhagic hepatocellular carcinoma. (B) A photomicrograph of the tumor shows a trabecular pattern of malignant hepatocytes. Many are arranged in an acinar pattern and surround concretions of inspissated bile.

dular configuration (Fig. 14-44). Characteristically, they show substantial fibrosis, and on liver biopsy may be confused with metastatic scirrhous carcinoma of the breast or pancreas. Cholangiocarcinomas metastasize to a wide variety of extrahepatic sites but show a distinct predilection for the portal lymph nodes.

Metastatic Cancer

Metastatic cancers are by far the most common malignant neoplasms of the liver. The liver is involved in one-third of all metastatic cancers, including half of those of the gastrointestinal tract, breast, and lung. Other tumors that characteristically metastasize to the liver are pancreatic carcinoma and malignant melanoma.

☐ **Pathology:** The liver may show only a single nodule of tumor or be virtually replaced by metastases (Fig. 14-45), and liver weights of 5 kg or more are not uncommon. In fact, **liver metastases are the most common cause of massive hepatomegaly.** The metastatic deposits are often histologically similar to the primary tumor, but on occasion, they are so undifferentiated that the primary site cannot be determined.

☐ **Clinical Features:** Weight loss is a common early finding among patients with metastatic cancer in the

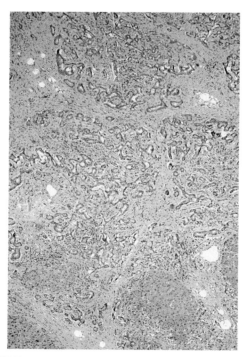

FIGURE 14-44
Cholangiocarcinoma. Well-differentiated neoplastic glands are embedded in a dense, fibrous stroma. A few islands of hepatocytes are present.

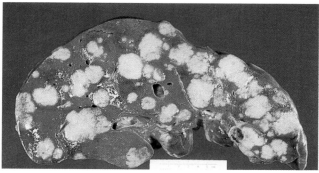

FIGURE   *14-45*
Metastatic carcinoma in the liver. The cut surface of the liver shows many firm, pale masses of metastatic colon cancer.

liver. Portal hypertension with splenomegaly, ascites, and gastrointestinal bleeding may occur. Obstruction of the major bile ducts or replacement of most of the liver parenchyma leads to jaundice. If the patient lives long enough, hepatic failure may ensue. The majority of patients die within 1 year of the diagnosis of liver metastases.

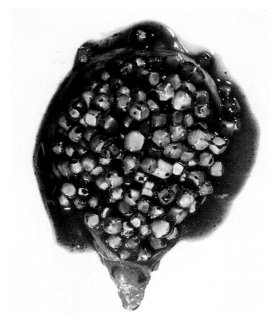

FIGURE   *14-46*
Cholesterol gallstones. The gallbladder has been opened to reveal numerous yellow cholesterol gallstones.

Gallbladder and Extrahepatic Bile Ducts

CHOLELITHIASIS

■ *Cholelithiasis is the presence of stones within the gallbladder lumen or the extrahepatic biliary tree.* Three-fourths of gallstones among patients in industrialized countries consist primarily of cholesterol, and the remainder consist of calcium bilirubinate and other calcium salts (pigment gallstones). However, pigment stones predominate among patients in tropical areas and the Orient.

Cholesterol Stones

■ *Cholesterol stones are round or faceted, yellow to tan, and single or multiple, varying from 1 to 4 cm in greatest dimension* (Fig. 14-46). More than 50% of the stone is composed of cholesterol; the rest is composed of calcium salts and mucin.

☐ **Epidemiology:** Cholesterol gallstones are common in the United States: 20% of American men and 35% of American women older than 75 years of age have gallstones at autopsy. **However, during their re-**

productive period, women are threefold more likely than men to develop cholesterol gallstones.

☐ **Pathogenesis:** The pathogenesis of cholesterol stones relates principally to the composition of the bile (Fig. 14-47). Normally, cholesterol is secreted by hepatocytes into the bile, where it is held in solution by the combined action of bile acids and lecithin. If the bile contains excess cholesterol or is deficient in bile acids, the bile becomes supersaturated, and under some circumstances, the cholesterol then precipitates as solid crystals. **The bile of persons afflicted with cholesterol gallstones has more cholesterol than that of normal persons, thus pointing to the liver rather than to the gallbladder as being the culprit in the genesis of cholesterol stones.** The hepatocytes of patients with cholesterol gallstones are deficient in 7-hydroxylase, the enzyme involved in the rate-limiting step by which bile salts are formed from cholesterol. As a result, the total size of the bile salt pool is reduced. The resulting decrease in bile salt secretion contributes to the stone-forming (lithogenic) properties of the bile. Additionally, in obese persons, cholesterol secretion by the liver is augmented, further adding to the supersaturation of bile with cholesterol. It is thought that mucinous glycoproteins secreted by the gallbladder epithelium provide the necessary nidus for crystallization.

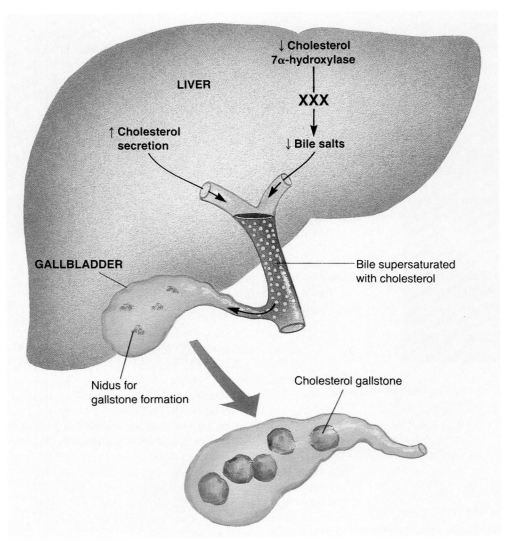

FIGURE   *14-47*
Pathogenesis of cholesterol gallstones.

Risk Factors

The higher prevalence of gallstones in premenopausal women has been attributed to estrogens stimulating formation of lithogenic bile by the liver. Estrogens increase the hepatic secretion of cholesterol and may decrease the secretion of bile acids. Additional risk factors for cholelithiasis include:

- Increasing age
- Obesity
- Membership in certain ethnic groups (e.g., Chilean women, some northern European groups, Pima Indians)
- Familial predisposition
- Diets high in calories and cholesterol

- Certain metabolic abnormalities associated with high blood levels of cholesterol (e.g., diabetes, some genetic hyperlipoproteinemias, primary biliary cirrhosis)

Pigment Stones

Pigment stones are classed as either black or brown stones, each of which has different characteristics.

Black Pigment Stones

■ *Black pigment stones contain calcium bilirubinate, bilirubin polymers, calcium salts, and mucin.* They are irregular and measure less than 1 cm across. On cross-section, the surface appears glassy (Fig. 14-48).

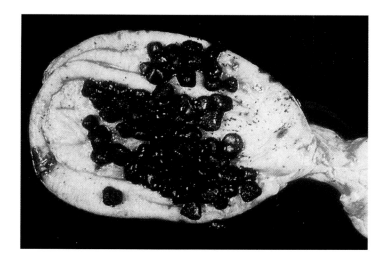

FIGURE *14-48*
Pigment gallstones. The gallbladder has been opened to reveal numerous small, dark stones composed of calcium bilirubinate.

☐ **Pathogenesis:** The incidence of black stones is increased in old and undernourished persons, but no correlations with gender, ethnicity, or obesity have been made. Chronic hemolysis, such as occurs in patients with sickle cell anemia and thalassemia, predisposes to development of black pigment stones. Cirrhosis, either because it leads to increased hemolysis or because of damage to liver cells, is also associated with a high incidence of black stones. **However, in most instances, no predisposing cause for the formation of black pigment stones is evident.**

The pathogenesis of black pigment stones is related to an increased concentration of unconjugated bilirubin in the bile. Unconjugated bilirubin is insoluble in bile and is usually present in only trace amounts. When increased amounts are secreted by the hepatocyte, the unconjugated bilirubin precipitates as calcium bilirubinate, probably around a nidus of mucinous glycoproteins. For reasons still unexplained, patients without known predisposing factors who develop black pigment stones have increased bile concentrations of unconjugated bilirubin.

Brown Pigment Stones

■ *Brown pigment stones are spongy and laminated, and contain principally calcium bilirubinate mixed with cholesterol and calcium soaps of fatty acids.* In contrast to other types of gallstones, brown pigment stones are found more frequently in the intrahepatic and extrahepatic bile ducts than in the gallbladder.

☐ **Pathogenesis:** Brown stones are almost always associated with bacterial cholangitis, in which *Escherichia coli* is the predominant organism. Rare or uncommon in Western countries, brown stones are not infrequent in Asia, where they are almost entirely restricted to persons infested with *Ascaris lumbricoides*

or *Clonorchis sinensis*, which are helminths that may invade the biliary tract. In the rare cases occurring in Western countries, these stones are found only in patients with chronic mechanical obstruction to the flow of bile, as in sclerosing cholangitis, or as a result of a catheter in the common bile duct after common bile duct surgery.

The pathogenesis of brown pigment stones also relates to an increased concentration of unconjugated bilirubin in the bile. It has been proposed that conjugated bilirubin is hydrolyzed to unconjugated bilirubin by the action of bacterial β-glucuronidase or other hydrolytic enzymes.

☐ **Clinical Features:** Gallstones may remain silent in the gallbladder for many years, and few patients ever die of cholelithiasis itself. The 15-year cumulative probability that asymptomatic stones will lead to biliary pain or other complications is less than 20%.

Medical treatment of gallstones is now possible. Oral intake of a bile acid, chenodeoxycholic acid (and, more recently, ursodeoxycholate), has dissolved radiologically documented gallstones. Development of laparoscopic cholecystectomy, which is far less traumatic than laparotomy, has changed the approach to cholecystectomy and may also influence the choice of therapy.

Most complications of cholelithiasis relate to obstruction of the cystic duct or common bile duct by gallstones. Passage of a stone into the cystic duct often, but not invariably, causes severe biliary colic and may lead to acute cholecystitis. Repeated episodes of acute cholecystitis then produce chronic cholecystitis. The latter condition can also result from the presence of stones alone. Gallstones may pass into the common duct (choledocholithiasis), where they may lead to obstructive jaundice, cholangitis, and pancreatitis. In fact, among populations in whom alcoholism is not a factor, gallstones are the most common correlate of acute pancreatitis. In patients with obstruction of the cystic duct, with or without acute cholecystitis, the bile in the gallbladder is reabsorbed and replaced by a clear, mucinous fluid secreted by the gallbladder epithelium. The term **hydrops of the gallbladder (mucocele)** is applied to the distended and palpable gallbladder, which may become secondarily infected.

ACUTE CHOLECYSTITIS

■ *Acute cholecystitis is a diffuse inflammation of the gallbladder that usually occurs secondary to obstruction of the gallbladder outlet.* The pathogenesis of acute cholecystitis relates to the presence of concentrated bile and gallstones within the gallbladder. In fact, 95% of the cases are associated with the presence of gallstones.

☐ **Pathology:** The external surface of the gallbladder in patients with acute cholecystitis is congested and layered with a fibrinous exudate. The wall is remarkably thickened by edema, and opening the viscus reveals a fiery-red or purple mucosa. Gallstones are usually found within the lumen, and a stone is often seen obstructing the cystic duct. Microscopically, edema and hemorrhage in the wall are striking, but neutrophilic infiltration is ordinarily only modest (Fig. 14-49). The mucosa shows focal ulcerations or, in severe cases, widespread necrosis, in which case the term **gangrenous cholecystitis** is applied.

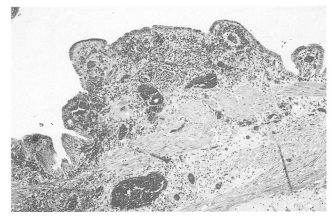

FIGURE *14-49*
Acute cholecystitis. The gallbladder is congested and edematous, and the mucosa is infiltrated by neutrophils.

Perforation is a feared complication in severe cases of acute cholecystitis and may occur after secondary bacterial infection, most commonly of the fundus. Discharge of bile into the abdominal cavity results in **bile peritonitis.** More commonly, the contents of the perforated gallbladder are localized by inflammatory adhesions.

☐ **Clinical Features:** The initial symptom of acute cholecystitis is abdominal pain in the right upper quadrant, and most patients have already experienced episodes of biliary colic. Mild jaundice, caused by stones in or edema of the common bile duct, is evident in 20% of the patients. In most cases, the acute illness subsides within a week, but persistent pain, fever, leukocytosis, and shaking chills indicate progression of the acute cholecystitis and the need for cholecystectomy. As the inflammatory process resolves, the gallbladder wall becomes fibrotic, and the mucosa heals. The function of the gallbladder, however, usually remains impaired.

CHRONIC CHOLECYSTITIS

■ *Chronic cholecystitis, which is almost invariably associated with gallstones, is the most common disease of the gallbladder.* It may result from repeated attacks of acute cholecystitis or, more often, from longstanding gallstones. In the latter case, the pathogenesis probably relates to chronic irritation and chemical injury to the gallbladder epithelium.

☐ **Pathology:** Grossly, the wall of the gallbladder is thickened and firm (Fig. 14-50). Gallstones are usually found within the lumen, and the bile often contains "gravel" (fine precipitates of calculous material). The bile is infected with coliform organisms in half of the cases. The mucosa may be focally ulcerated and atrophic, or it may appear to be intact. Microscopically, the wall is fibrotic and often penetrated by sinuses of Rokitansky-Aschoff. Chronic inflammation of varying degree may be seen in all layers. In longstanding chronic cholecystitis, the wall of the gallbladder may become calcified, in which case the term **porcelain gallbladder** is used.

☐ **Clinical Features:** Pain in the right hypochondrium is typical and often episodic. The diagnosis is best made on the basis of ultrasound examination, which demonstrates gallstones in a thick, contracted gallbladder. Cholecystectomy is the definitive treatment.

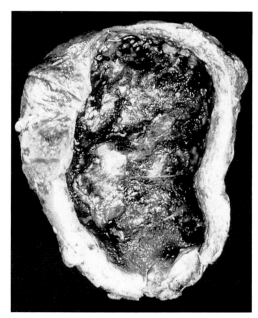

FIGURE   *14-50*
Chronic cholecystitis.

CARCINOMA OF THE GALLBLADDER

The most common tumor of the gallbladder is adenocarcinoma. This neoplasm is found incidentally in 2% of patients who undergo gallbladder surgery. **Because this cancer is usually associated with cholelithiasis and chronic cholecystitis, it is considerably more common in women than in men.** The calcified gallbladder (porcelain gallbladder), which represents an extreme variant of chronic cholecystitis, is particularly prone to the development of gallbladder cancer.

☐ **Pathology:** Gallbladder carcinoma is characteristically an infiltrative, well-differentiated adenocarcinoma. It is usually desmoplastic; thus, the wall of the gallbladder becomes thickened and leathery. The rich lymphatic plexus of the gallbladder provides the most common route of metastasis, but vascular dissemination and direct spread into the liver and contiguous structures also can occur.

☐ **Clinical Features:** Symptoms produced by carcinoma of the gallbladder are similar to those encountered in patients with gallstone disease. However, by the time the tumor becomes symptomatic, it is almost invariably incurable, with the 5-year survival rate being less than 3%.

CARCINOMA OF THE BILE DUCT AND AMPULLA OF VATER

Cancer of the extrahepatic bile ducts (almost always adenocarcinoma) typically presents as obstructive jaundice. It may occur anywhere along the length of the bile duct, including the location where the right and left hepatic ducts join to form the common hepatic duct. The tumor is less common than gallbladder cancer, and the female predominance of gallbladder cancer is not evident. The prognosis is poor. However, because symptoms arise early during the course of the disease, the outcome is somewhat better than that of gallbladder carcinoma.

The bile duct may also be obstructed by **adenocarcinoma of the ampulla of Vater.** The initial symptom is, again, obstructive jaundice, although a few patients present with pancreatitis. In contrast to bile duct carcinoma, surgical treatment of cancer of the ampulla of Vater leads to a 5-year survival rate of 35%.

The Pancreas

Dante G. Scarpelli

The pancreas comprises two functionally and anatomically distinct "organs," namely the exocrine and the endocrine pancreas. The exocrine pancreas secretes digestive enzymes, whereas the endocrine pancreas releases a variety of important hormones that participate in glucose homeostasis and other metabolic activities. Clinically important diseases of the exocrine pancreas are acute and chronic pancreatitis as well as cancer. Dysfunction of beta cells in the islets of Langerhans results in diabetes mellitus (see Chapter 22). The islets are also the site of origin for a variety of functional neoplasms.

CONGENITAL ANOMALIES

Developmental defects of the pancreas include:

- **Aberrant or Accessory Pancreas.** Pancreatic tissue is present outside its normal location.
- **Annular Pancreas.** The duodenum is encircled by pancreatic tissue and, less frequently, by the bile duct or portal vein.
- **Pancreas Divisum.** Failure of fusion by the two pancreatic anlagen, including the ducts, results in separation of the gland into two parts.
- **Absence of the Parts of the Adult Gland.** The parts of the adult gland derived from the dorsal pancreas, namely the body and tail, are missing.
- **Congenital Cysts.**

PANCREATITIS

■ *Pancreatitis is an inflammatory condition of the exocrine pancreas that results from injury to acinar cells.* At one end of the spectrum of **acute pancreatitis** is a mild, self-limited disease consisting of acute inflammation and edema of the stroma, with little or no acinar cell necrosis. At the other extreme is a severe, and sometimes fatal, acute hemorrhagic pancreatitis, with massive necrosis. In some cases, repeated episodes of acute pancreatitis lead to **chronic pancreatitis**, which is characterized by recurrent attacks of severe abdominal pain and progressive fibrosis, ultimately leading to pancreatic insufficiency. However, in approximately half the cases of chronic pancreatitis, no acute episodes are recognized.

Acute Pancreatitis

Interstitial or edematous pancreatitis is the mild and, presumably, reversible form of acute pancreatitis. An infiltrate of polymorphonuclear leukocytes and edema of the connective tissue between the lobules of acinar cells constitute the initial lesion. There is no necrosis of acinar cells, fat necrosis, or hemorrhage.

Acute hemorrhagic pancreatitis is a condition of middle age, with a peak incidence at 60 years. It is often associated with alcoholism (more commonly in men) or chronic biliary disease (more often in women). Acute pancreatitis occurs abruptly, usually following a heavy meal or excessive alcohol intake.

☐ Pathogenesis: **Acute pancreatitis results from the inappropriate activation of pancreatic digestive enzymes and the consequent autodigestion of pancreatic tissue.**

Secretion Against Obstruction. Any condition that narrows the lumen of the pancreatic ducts or impairs the easy outflow of exocrine secretions can raise the intraductal pressure and exacerbate backdiffusion across the ducts. This effect has been postulated to result in an inappropriate activation of digestive proenzymes. Although gallstones may cause pancreatic duct obstruction, fewer than 5% of patients with acute pancreatitis have an impacted stone at the ampulla of Vater. Moreover, neither ligation of the pancreatic duct nor occlusion of it by tumor results in acute pancreatitis.

Bile Reflux. The association of acute pancreatitis with cholelithiasis has also led to the suggestion that reflux of bile into the pancreatic duct is a pathogenetic factor. However, the association more likely reflects transient pancreatic duct obstruction rather than bile reflux.

Reflux of Duodenal Contents. Retrograde injection of a mixture of bile and activated pancreatic enzymes into the pancreatic duct has been shown experimentally to produce acute pancreatitis.

Intracellular Activation of Proteases. A block in the secretion of zymogen granules by the acinar cells seems to be an early event in certain types of experimental toxic pancreatic injury. Intracellular activation of potent digestive enzymes may then lyse the cell or result in secretion of prematurely activated enzymes.

Activated Pancreatic Enzymes. Activated trypsin, by itself, does not produce cell necrosis and pancreatitis, but it does activate other pancreatic proenzymes, including prophospholipase A_2 and proelastase. Phospholipase A_2 can attack membrane phospholipids, thereby leading to necrosis, and elastase digests the walls of blood vessels, thereby resulting in hemorrhage. Moreover, liberation of pancreatic lipase into the interstitium contributes to fat necrosis.

Protease Inhibitors. The various inhibitors of proteolytic enzymes present in many body fluids and tissues constitute a defense against inappropriate activation of the digestive proenzymes of the pancreas. On activation of trypsin, the balance between activated proteases and protease inhibitors determines the extent of pancreatic injury. Importantly, the protection that these inhibitors render is less than complete. Because activated trypsin can also activate other pancreatic proenzymes, such as chymotrypsinogen, proelastase, prophospholipase, and procarboxypeptidase, its incomplete inhibition in pancreatic juice and plasma poses a hazard.

Ethanol. As many as two-thirds of all cases of acute pancreatitis are associated with alcohol abuse, but the pathogenesis remains obscure.

Gallstones. Between one-third and one-half of all patients with acute pancreatitis also have cholelithiasis, and the risk of developing acute pancreatitis in patients with gallstones is 25-fold higher than that in the general population.

Other Causes of Pancreatitis. Other factors that cause pancreatitis, albeit uncommonly, include viruses, endotoxemia, ischemia, drugs (e.g., corticosteroids, estrogens, azathioprine), trauma, hypertriglyceridemia, and hypercalcemia. After a careful search for known risk factors, 10% to 20% of cases of pancreatitis cannot be attributed to a specific cause.

Factors involved in the pathogenesis of acute hemorrhagic pancreatitis are depicted in Figure 15-1.

☐ **Pathology:** In patients with acute hemorrhagic pancreatitis, the pancreas is initially edematous and hyperemic. Within a day, pale and gray foci appear, which rapidly become friable and hemorrhagic (Fig. 15-2). **As the disease progresses, hemorrhagic foci enlarge and become so numerous that most of the pancreas is converted into a large, retroperitoneal hematoma, in which the pancreatic tissue is barely recognizable.** Yellow-white areas of fat necrosis appear at the interface between necrotic foci and fat tissue both in and around the pancreas, including the adjacent mesentery (see Fig. 15-2). These nodules of necrotic fat have a pasty consistency, which becomes firmer and chalk-like as more calcium and magnesium soaps are produced.

Microscopically, the most prominent tissue alterations in acute pancreatitis are acinar cell necrosis, an intense and acute inflammatory reaction, and foci of necrotic fat cells (Fig. 15-3). Irregular fibrosis of the pancreas and, occasionally, calcification are the residuals of healed acute pancreatitis.

Pancreatic Pseudocyst. Pancreatic pseudocysts exhibit large spaces, limited by connective tissue, that contain degraded blood, debris of necrotic pancreatic tissue, and fluid rich in pancreatic enzymes. Patients who survive acute pancreatitis are at risk for development of pancreatic abscesses and pseudocysts (Fig. 15-4), with the latter having an incidence of as high as 50%. Pseudocysts may enlarge to compress, and even obstruct, the duodenum. They may also become secondarily infected and form an abscess.

☐ **Clinical Features:** The patient with acute pancreatitis presents with severe epigastric pain referred to the upper back and accompanied by nausea and vomiting. Within a matter of hours, catastrophic peripheral vascular collapse and shock ensue. Early in the disease, pancreatic digestive enzymes are released from injured acinar cells into the blood and abdominal cavity. Elevation of serum amylase and lipase levels as early as 24 to 72 hours after onset is diagnostic for acute pancreatitis.

Chronic Pancreatitis

■ *Chronic pancreatitis is characterized by progressive destruction of the pancreas, with accompanying irregular fibrosis and chronic inflammation.* Clinically, the disorder presents as recurrent or persistent abdominal pain or as evidence of pancreatic exocrine or endocrine insufficiency in the absence of pain.

☐ **Pathogenesis: Longstanding alcohol abuse is the major cause of chronic pancreatitis, being responsible for more than 90% of adult cases today.** In almost half of patients with alcoholism who had no symptoms of chronic pancreatitis during life, autopsy reveals evidence of this disease.

The earliest morphologic abnormality in alcoholic chronic pancreatitis is generally precipitation of protein plugs in the ducts, which serve as the nidus for subsequent calculi. It is speculated that these stones chronically obstruct the ductal system. Cholelithiasis does not seem to be an causative factor in chronic pancreatitis. In populations with a high prevalence of alcoholism, only 5% to 10% of cases of chronic pancreatitis are idiopathic, whereas this figure may reach as high as 50% among populations in which alcoholism is infrequent.

Functional obstruction of the pancreatic duct caused by pancreas divisum or mechanical obstruction by cancer or the inspissated mucus of cystic fibrosis leads to chronic pancreatitis. Chronic injury to the acinar cells (e.g., in hemochromatosis) is also associated with fibrosis and atrophy of the pancreas. That chronic pancreatitis is often characterized by intermittent, "acute" attacks followed by periods of quiescence sug-

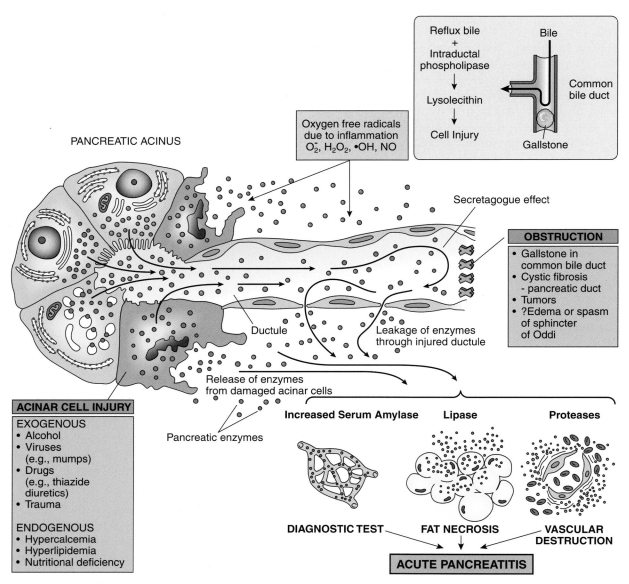

PANCREATIC ACINUS

Reflux bile
+
Intraductal
phospholipase
↓
Lysolecithin
↓
Cell Injury

Bile

Common
bile duct

Gallstone

Oxygen free radicals
due to inflammation
O_2^-, H_2O_2, •OH, NO

Secretagogue effect

OBSTRUCTION
- Gallstone in
  common bile duct
- Cystic fibrosis
  - pancreatic duct
- Tumors
- ?Edema or spasm
  of sphincter
  of Oddi

Ductule

Leakage of enzymes
through injured ductule

Release of enzymes
from damaged acinar cells

ACINAR CELL INJURY

EXOGENOUS
- Alcohol
- Viruses
  (e.g., mumps)
- Drugs
  (e.g., thiazide
  diuretics)
- Trauma

ENDOGENOUS
- Hypercalcemia
- Hyperlipidemia
- Nutritional deficiency

Pancreatic enzymes

Increased Serum Amylase   **Lipase**   **Proteases**

DIAGNOSTIC TEST   **FAT NECROSIS**   **VASCULAR
DESTRUCTION**

ACUTE PANCREATITIS

FIGURE   15-1
Pathogenesis of acute pancreatitis. Injury to the ductules or acinar cells leads to the release of pancreatic enzymes. Lipase and proteases destroy tissue, thereby causing acute
pancreatitis. Release of amylase is the basis of a test for acute pancreatitis.

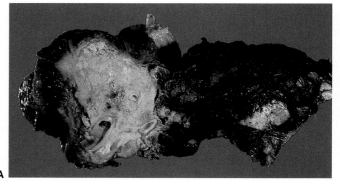
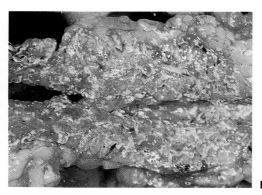

FIGURE   15-2
Acute hemorrhagic pancreatitis. (A) Large areas of the pancreas are intensely hemorrhagic. (B) The cut surface of the pancreas in a less severe case of acute pancreatitis, and
at a somewhat later stage than in *panel A*, shows numerous, yellow-white foci of fat
necrosis.

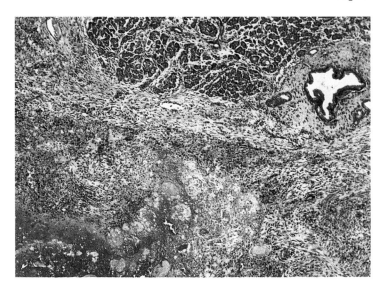

FIGURE 15-3
Acute hemorrhagic pancreatitis. A photomicrograph of the pancreas shows areas of acinar cell necrosis and hemorrhage. An intact lobule is also seen (*top*).

gests that in many patients, the pathogenesis involves repeated bouts of acute pancreatitis followed by scarring. However, in patients without a history of acute episodes, the pathogenesis of chronic pancreatitis may relate to persistent necrosis and insidious scarring, similar to the progression of cirrhosis of the liver.

☐ **Pathology:** Chronic calcifying pancreatitis is the most common type of chronic pancreatitis. On gross examination, the pancreas is firm, and the cut surface lacks the usual, lobular appearance (Fig. 15-5). Often, the pancreatic duct is dilated owing to obstruction by intraductal stones or strictures. True cysts and poorly defined pseudocysts (Fig. 15-6) are common and, presumably, have formed distal-to-ductal obstructions.

Microscopically, large regions of the pancreas display irregular areas of fibrosis, and the exocrine and endocrine elements are reduced in both number and size (see Fig. 15-5). Fibrotic areas exhibit activated fibroblasts, lymphocytes, and plasma cells, particularly around surviving pancreatic lobules. Pancreatic ducts of all sizes contain variably calcified proteinaceous material.

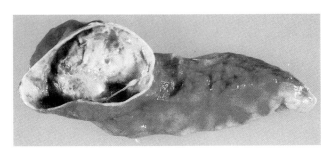

FIGURE 15-4
Pancreatic pseudocyst. A cystic cavity arises from the head of the pancreas.

☐ **Clinical Features:** Half of the patients with chronic pancreatitis suffer repeated episodes of acute pancreatitis. One-third of the cases are characterized by gradual onset of continuous or intermittent pain, without any acute attacks. In a few patients, chronic pancreatitis is initially painless but heralded by the appearance of diabetes or malabsorption. Conspicuous weight loss is common, and unrelenting epigastric pain, radiating to the back, may cripple the patient. The mortality rate in patients with chronic pancreatitis is 3% to 4% per year, although many of these deaths are secondary to other causes owing to the large majority of the patients having alcoholism as well.

Cystic Fibrosis

Cystic fibrosis manifests as a form of chronic pancreatitis. A full discussion of this disorder is presented in Chapter 6.

NEOPLASMS OF THE EXOCRINE PANCREAS

Cystadenoma

■ *Cystadenomas of the pancreas are large, multiloculated, cystic tumors, usually localized in the body or tail.* They occur most frequently in women between the ages of 50 and 70 years, and they constitute 10% of cystic lesions of the pancreas. These neoplasms are of two types, depending on whether they are lined by serous or mucinous epithelium.

Mucinous cystadenoma accounts for 1% of all pancreatic exocrine tumors and features multilocu-

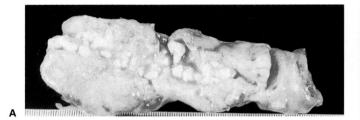

A

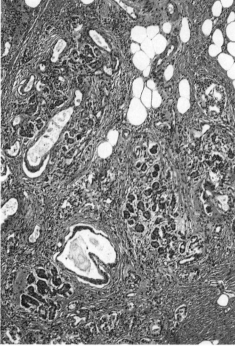

B

FIGURE *15-5*
Chronic calcifying pancreatitis. (A) The pancreas is shrunken and fibrotic, and the dilated duct contains numerous stones. (B) Atrophic lobules of acinar cells are surrounded by dense, fibrous tissue infiltrated by lymphocytes. The pancreatic ducts are dilated and contain inspissated proteinaceous material.

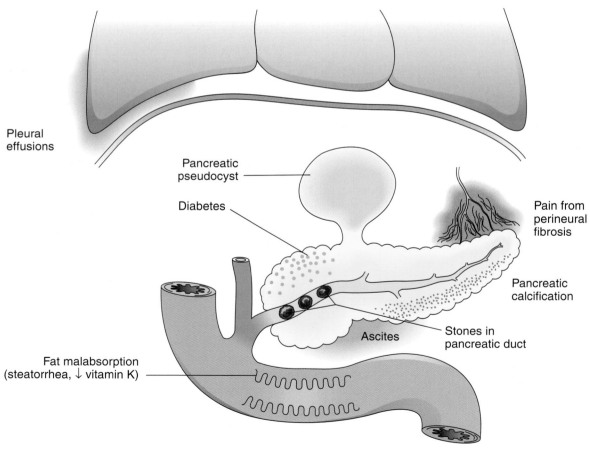

Pleural effusions

Pancreatic pseudocyst

Diabetes

Pain from perineural fibrosis

Pancreatic calcification

Stones in pancreatic duct

Ascites

Fat malabsorption (steatorrhea, ↓ vitamin K)

FIGURE *15-6*
Complications of chronic pancreatitis.

lated cysts lined by a highly mucin-producing, columnar epithelium.

Serous cystadenoma, the rarer of the two types and the one with malignant potential, is composed of variably sized cysts lined by cuboidal epithelial cells with clear, glycogen-rich cytoplasm.

Carcinoma

Carcinoma of the pancreas, a virtually incurable malignancy, is the fourth most common cause of death from cancer in men and the fifth most common in women. The incidence of pancreatic cancer seems to be increasing in all countries studied and, in the United States, has tripled during the past 50 years. Ductal adenocarcinoma accounts for 90% of all pancreatic cancers.

☐ **Epidemiology:** The distribution of pancreatic adenocarcinoma is worldwide, with the highest incidence (twice that in the United States) occurring among male Maoris of New Zealand and female natives of Hawaii. Cancer of the pancreas shows a significant male predominance (as much as 3:1) in younger age groups but an almost equal distribution among older people. In the United States, the disease is more common in Native Americans and blacks than in whites. Pancreatic carcinoma is a disease of late life, with the greatest frequency being found in persons older than 60 years, although its appearance as early as the third decade is not rare.

☐ **Pathogenesis:** Factors involved in the causation of pancreatic cancer are obscure. Epidemiologic studies have implicated both host and environmental factors as being of possible causative significance.

Smoking. There is a significant increase (two- to threefold) in the risk of pancreatic cancer among cigarette smokers.

Chemical Carcinogens. Results of experimental studies in animals lend support to a role for chemical carcinogenesis in pancreatic cancer.

Dietary Factors. Results of epidemiologic studies suggest that dietary factors may be involved in the development of pancreatic cancer. A high intake of meat and fat, but especially the latter, may be of particular significance. Consumption of both alcohol and coffee as risk factors, however, is controversial.

Diabetes Mellitus. Patients, especially women, with diabetes may be at increased risk for development of pancreatic carcinoma, although the relationship is not firmly established.

Chronic Pancreatitis. Chronic pancreatitis is a risk factor for development of pancreatic adenocarcinoma, but it accounts for only a few cases.

Molecular Genetics. Mutational activation of K-*ras* and overexpression of *erb* B2 are common. Mutational inactivation or deletion in a number of tumor suppressor genes, including DPC-4 (deleted in pancreatic cancer, locus 4), is often present.

☐ **Pathology:** Adenocarcinoma arises anywhere in the pancreas, with the most frequent focus being found in the head (60%), followed by the body (10%) and the tail (5%). In the remaining 25% of cases, the pancreas is diffusely involved, which suggests either a late diagnosis or a multicentric origin. Carcinomas of the pancreatic head tend to be smaller than those of the body and tail, and they show more limited spread to the regional lymph nodes and more distant sites. In large part, these differences reflect earlier diagnosis of cancer of the pancreatic head, which causes early biliary obstruction and jaundice by compressing the ampulla of Vater and the common bile duct.

On gross examination, pancreatic carcinoma is a firm, gray, poorly demarcated, multinodular mass (Fig. 15-7), often embedded in a dense connective tissue stroma. Tumors of the pancreatic head may invade the common duct and the duodenal wall. When they penetrate the duodenum, they often compress or invade the ampulla of Vater.

Microscopically, more than 75% of ductal adenocarcinomas of the pancreas are well differentiated, secrete mucin, and stimulate a florid deposition of collagen (desmoplastic reaction). Pancreatic cancer metastasizes most commonly to the regional lymph nodes and liver. Other frequent metastatic locations include the peritoneum, lungs, adrenals, and bones. Perineural infiltration by tumor is characteristic of pancreatic cancer and accounts for the early and persistent pain of this disease.

☐ **Clinical Features:** Early diagnosis of pancreatic cancer is unusual, because the tumor does not ordinarily give rise to characteristic signs and symptoms until it is well advanced. Patients with pancreatic carcinoma present with anorexia, conspicuous weight loss, and gnawing pain in the epigastrium, which often radiates to the back. Jaundice is present in approximately half of all patients with cancer localized to the pancreatic head and in fewer than 10% of those in whom the body or tail is the site of the tumor. Progressive deterioration almost invariably ensues, with intractable pain, cachexia, and death.

Courvoisier sign refers to an acute, painless dilatation of the gallbladder, which is accompanied by

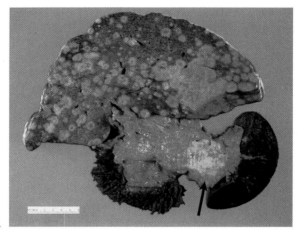
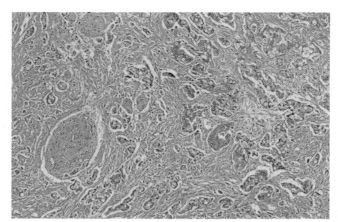

A

B

FIGURE *15-7*
Carcinoma of the pancreas. (A) An autopsy specimen shows a large tumor in the tail of the pancreas (*arrow*) and extensive metastases in the liver. (B) A section of the tumor reveals malignant glands embedded in a dense fibrous stroma. A nerve (*left*) shows peripheral invasion.

jaundice owing to obstruction of the common bile duct by tumor. It may be the first indication of pancreatic cancer in approximately one-third of patients.

Migratory thrombophlebitis develops in 10% of patients with pancreatic cancer, especially when the tumor involves the body and the tail of the pancreas.

The outlook for patients with pancreatic carcinoma is bleak. Half die within a few months of the onset of symptoms. The 1-year survival rate is 8% to 10%, and the 5-year survival rate is only 2%.

Complications of pancreatic ductal adenocarcinoma are summarized in Figure 15-8.

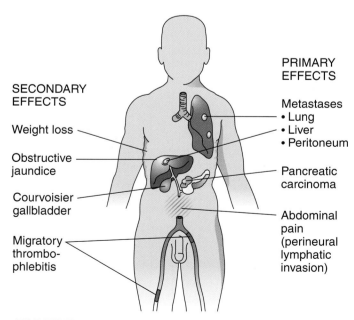

FIGURE *15-8*
Complications of pancreatic carcinoma.

Acinar Cell Carcinoma

Acinar cell carcinoma is principally a disease of mature adults in their fifth to eighth decades of life. The tumors are usually large and show foci of necrosis. They tend to metastasize locally to the regional lymph nodes and liver and more distantly to the lungs and other body sites.

NEOPLASMS OF THE ENDOCRINE PANCREAS

Islet cell tumors are rare, accounting for less than 10% of all pancreatic neoplasms. Of these, many are nonfunctional and discovered only as incidental findings at autopsy. Functional islet cell tumors may occur either alone or as part of the multiple endocrine neoplasia syndrome type I.

Beta Cell Tumors (Insulinomas)

■ *Beta cell tumors, the most common of the islet cell neoplasms (75%), may release sufficient insulin to induce severe hypoglycemia.* Neoplastic beta cells, unlike their normal counterparts, are not regulated by the blood glucose level and continue to secrete insulin autonomously, even when the blood level of glucose is very low.

□ **Pathology:** Most beta cell tumors are benign lesions in the body or tail of the pancreas (Fig. 15-9). They are generally less than 3 cm in diameter, and occasionally, they are as small as 1 mm. The large majority (90%) are solitary and can be surgically excised. Only a minority (5–15%) demonstrate malignant be-

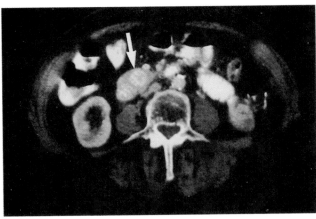
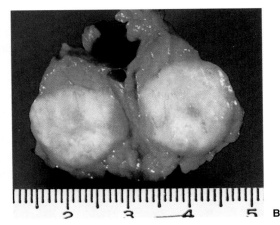

FIGURE *15-9*
Insulinoma. (A) A computed tomographic scan of the abdomen shows a solitary insulinoma (*arrow*). (B) An insulinoma is embedded in tan, lobular pancreatic tissue.

havior. Histologically, insulinoma cells resemble normal beta cells but are dispersed in trabecular or solid patterns (Fig. 15-10*A*). A reliable distinction between benign and malignant insulinomas is usually not possible on histologic grounds and, in most cases, awaits the appearance of metastases.

☐ **Clinical Features:** A low blood sugar level produces a syndrome of sweating, nervousness, and hunger, which may progress to confusion, lethargy, and coma. Most cases are characterized by only a mild

hypoglycemia, and in some, the tumor is not functional at all. The diagnosis is established by demonstration of high insulin levels in the blood and in the tumor cells (Fig. 15-10*B*).

Pancreatic Gastrinoma (Zollinger-Ellison Syndrome)

■ *Pancreatic gastrinoma is an islet cell tumor consisting of so-called G cells, which secrete gastrin, a potent hor-*

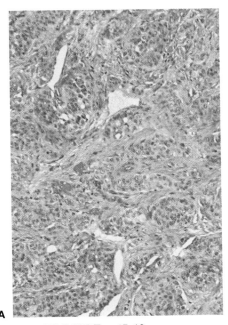
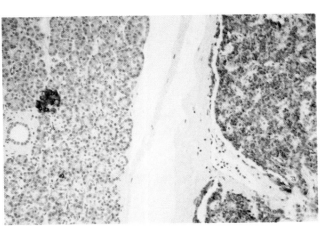

FIGURE *15-10*
A functional insulinoma. (A) Nests of tumor cells are surrounded by numerous capillaries. (B) Immunochemical localization of insulin in an insulinoma (*right*) and an islet in the adjacent normal pancreas.

monal stimulus for the secretion of acid by the stomach. Pancreatic gastrinoma is the cause of Zollinger-Ellison syndrome, which is a disorder characterized by (1) intractable gastric hypersecretion, (2) severe peptic ulceration of the duodenum and jejunum, and (3) high levels of gastrin in the blood. The location of this tumor in the pancreas is curious, because gastrin-containing cells have not been demonstrated in normal islets.

Among islet cell tumors, pancreatic gastrinomas are second in frequency only to insulinomas and account for one-fourth of islet cell tumors. They are most common between the ages of 30 and 50 years, with a slight male predominance. Fifteen percent of cases of the Zollinger-Ellison syndrome result from gastrinomas outside the pancreas, particularly in the duodenum. The majority of gastrinomas are malignant (70–90%). The tumor may be solitary or multiple, with the latter usually occurring in the context of multiple endocrine neoplasia type I. Histologically, gastrinomas are remarkably similar to intestinal carcinoid tumors. Metastases to the regional lymph nodes and the liver are often functional.

Alpha Cell Tumors (Glucagonomas)

■ *Alpha cell tumors (glucagonomas), which are glucagon-secreting tumors of the alpha cells, are associated with a syndrome consisting of (1) mild diabetes; (2) a necrotizing, migratory, erythematous rash; (3) anemia; (4) venous thromboses; and (5) severe infections.* These tumors are rare (1% of functional islet cell tumors) and occur between the ages of 40 and 70 years, with a slight female predominance. Two-thirds of symptomatic glucagonomas are malignant.

Functional glucagonomas are usually large tumors that invade surrounding structures. Microscopically, they resemble the trabecular and solid patterns of insulinomas.

Delta Cell Tumors (Somatostatinomas)

■ *Delta cell tumors are rare and produce a syndrome consisting of mild diabetes mellitus, gallstones, steatorrhea, and hypochlorhydria.* These effects result from the inhibitory actions of somatostatin on other cells of the pancreatic islets and neuroendocrine cells of the gastrointestinal tract, which secrete insulin, cholecystokinin, glucagon, and gastrin. The tumor is usually solitary, and the majority are malignant, with metastases already being present at the time of diagnosis.

D₁ Tumors (VIPomas, Verner-Morrison Syndrome)

■ *D_1 tumors secrete vasoactive intestinal polypeptide (VIP) and give rise to the Verner-Morrison syndrome, which is characterized by explosive, profuse, and watery diarrhea accompanied by hypokalemia and hypochlorhydria.* This disorder has also been referred to as pancreatic cholera. VIPomas are rare tumors (<5% of all islet tumors), are usually large and solitary, and in most cases, are malignant.

Multiple Endocrine Neoplasia Syndrome Type I

■ *Multiple endocrine neoplasia syndrome type I is an infrequent, familial disorder characterized by multiple adenomas of the pituitary, parathyroids, and pancreas.* Multiple endocrine neoplasia syndromes are described in detail in Chapter 21.

CHAPTER *16*

The Kidney

J. Charles Jennette
Benjamin H. Spargo

Acute Tubular Necrosis	**Hydronephrosis**
Drug-Induced (Hypersensitivity) Acute Interstitial Nephritis	**Renal Stones (Nephrolithiasis and Urolithiasis)**
Analgesic Nephropathy	**Wilms Tumor (Nephroblastoma)**
Multiple Myeloma Cast Nephropathy	**Renal Cell Carcinoma**
Urate Nephropathy	

The kidney serves as the principal regulator of the fluid and electrolyte content of the body. This task is accomplished by the complex filtering mechanism of the glomerulus and the selective tubular reabsorption of solutes from the filtrate. The kidney is also an endocrine organ, secreting renin, which regulates sodium metabolism and blood pressure, and erythropoietin, a hormone that stimulates production of red blood cells by the bone marrow.

rara interna; and (3) a lamina rara externa. The glomerular basement membrane has a strong negative charge owing to the presence of the polyanionic proteoglycan heparan sulfate. This property allows charge-selective filtration of electrically neutral and cationic molecules. In addition, the basement mem-

GLOMERULUS

The glomerulus is a specialized tuft of capillaries with an arteriole at either end (Figs. 16-1 to 16-3).

Glomerular Basement Membrane. The glomerular basement membrane is functionally and chemically distinct. It is approximately 300 nm in thickness and has three definable layers by electron microscopy: (1) a central dense zone, the lamina densa; (2) a paler lamina

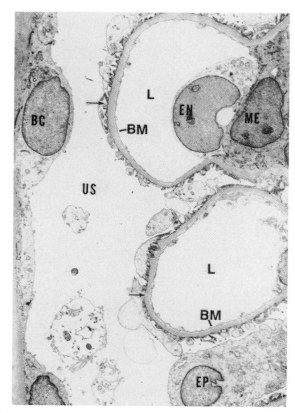

FIGURE   *16-2*
Electron micrograph of a normal glomerulus. The normal glomerular capillary is covered by epithelial cells (EP), with foot processes (*arrows*) in contact with the basement membrane (BM). The endothelial cell (EN) has large pores and surrounds the capillary lumen (L). The mesangial cell (ME) is bordered by the endothelial cell on the luminal surface and by the stalk basement membrane on the lateral areas. *BC*, Bowman capsule; *US*, urinary space.

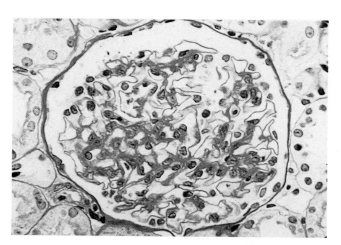

FIGURE   *16-1*
Light micrograph of a normal glomerulus. The periodic acid-Schiff stain highlights the delicate basement membranes and mesangial matrix.

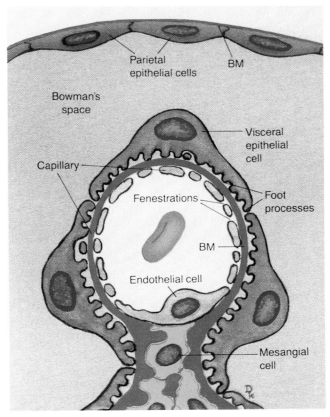

FIGURE *16-3*
Normal glomerulus. The relation of the different glomerular cell types to the stroma is illustrated using a single glomerular loop. The entire outer aspect of the glomerular basement membrane (BM; peripheral loop and stalk) is covered by the epithelial cell foot processes. The outer portions of the endothelial cell, which surrounds the capillary lumen, are in contact with the inner surface of the basement membrane, whereas the central part is in contact with the mesangial cell of the stalk. The relationship of the mesangial cell to its stroma is unique to the glomerulus and has not yet been entirely clarified.

brane also discriminates between molecules on the basis of size.

Endothelial Cells. Glomerular capillaries have a fenestrated endothelial layer. The fenestrae are too large to influence capillary permeability, however, and the endothelium probably plays a largely passive role in filtration.

Epithelial Cells. Glomerular epithelial cells line Bowman's space. The visceral epithelial cells rest on the basement membrane and send cytoplasmic projections, termed *foot processes*, onto it.

Mesangium. The glomerulus is supported by a mixed cellular and stromal network that is collectively termed the *mesangium*. Important functions of the mesangium include (1) endocytosis and processing of plasma proteins, (2) modulation of glomerular filtration by the contractility of mesangial cells, and (3) generation of vasoactive agents (e.g., prostaglandins and cytokines).

CONGENITAL ANOMALIES

Renal Agenesis. Renal agenesis is the complete absence of renal tissue. Clearly, the absence of both kidneys is not compatible with life. The majority of infants born with this anomaly are stillborn, and in most cases, the mother suffers from oligohydramnios (insufficient amniotic fluid). Bilateral renal agenesis is often associated with other congenital anomalies, including low-set ears, receding chin, beak-like nose, and pulmonary hypoplasia. Congenital anomalies of the genitalia are also common, as are lower-limb anomalies. The pattern of malformations associated with oligohydramnios is known as **Potter syndrome.**

Unilateral renal agenesis is not a serious matter if there are no associated anomalies, because the single kidney undergoes sufficient hypertrophy to maintain normal renal function.

Horseshoe Kidney. Horseshoe kidney is a single, large, and midline organ that results from failure of the renal anlage to divide. The infant is born with fusion of the two kidneys, usually at the lower poles.

Ectopic Kidney. Renal ectopia is an abnormal location of the kidney, usually in the pelvis. Most commonly, this condition results from failure of the fetal kidney to migrate from the pelvis to the flank.

RENAL DYSPLASIA

■ *Cystic renal dysplasia is characterized by the presence of numerous cysts in all or part of a kidney together with the persistence of abnormal structures, such as cartilage and undifferentiated mesenchyme.*

Unilateral renal dysplasia is the most common cystic disorder in children, and it is the most frequent cause of an abdominal mass in newborns. Malformations of other organs (e.g., ventricular septal defects, tracheoesophageal fistulas, and lumbosacral

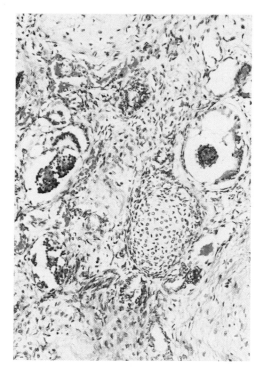

FIGURE *16-4*
Renal dysplasia. A light micrograph shows immature glomeruli, tubules, and cartilage surrounded by loose, undifferentiated mesenchymal tissue.

meningomyeloceles) occasionally occur in conjunction with renal dysplasia.

☐ **Pathology:** The dysplastic kidney is enlarged and reveals a disorderly mass of cysts that vary in size from microscopic to several centimeters in diameter. An associated ureteral malformation, which is often obstructive, is usually found. Histologically, dysplasia is recognized by focally dilated ducts that are lined by a cuboidal or columnar epithelium. These are surrounded by mantles of undifferentiated mesenchyme (Fig. 16-4), which sometimes contain smooth muscle and islands of hyaline cartilage.

☐ **Clinical Features:** In most cases of cystic renal dysplasia, a palpable flank mass is discovered shortly after birth, although small, multicystic kidneys may not become apparent until many years later. Unilateral dysplasia is adequately treated by removal of the affected kidney.

POLYCYSTIC KIDNEY DISEASES

■ *Polycystic kidney diseases are a heterogeneous group of congenital and acquired disorders that are charac-*

terized by distortion of the renal parenchyma because of numerous cysts (Fig. 16-5).

Autosomal Dominant (Adult) Polycystic Kidney Disease

■ *Adult polycystic kidney disease is an autosomal dominant trait that is characterized by progressively expanding cysts.* The disorder is responsible for 10% of all end-stage kidney disease. The pathogenesis of adult polycystic kidney disease is not understood, although a defective gene (*AKPKD-1*) has been localized to the short arm of chromosome 16.

☐ **Pathology:** The kidneys in patients with polycystic kidney disease are markedly enlarged bilaterally, each kidney weighing as much as 4500 g (Fig. 16-6).

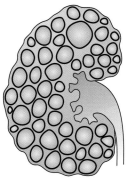

Adult polycystic
disease

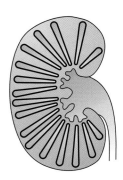

Infantile polycystic
disease

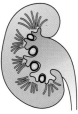

Medullary
sponge kidney

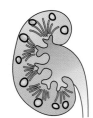

Medullary cystic
disease complex

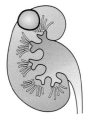

Simple cyst

FIGURE   *16-5*
Cystic diseases of the kidney.

The external contour of the kidney is distorted by the presence of numerous cysts, which can be as large as 5 cm in diameter. These cysts are usually filled with a clear to straw-yellow fluid. Microscopically, the cysts are lined by a nondescript cuboidal and columnar epithelium. As the cysts progressively expand, they exert pressure on the normal areas, thereby leading to an increasing loss of renal parenchyma.

One-third of the patients with adult polycystic kidney disease also have hepatic cysts lined by biliary epithelium. Fifteen percent of the patients have an associated cerebral aneurysm, and subarachnoid hemorrhage is the cause of death in many of these patients.

☐ **Clinical Features:** Patients typically present with symptoms by the fourth decade of life. These include bilateral flank masses and passage of blood clots in the urine. Azotemia (elevated blood urea nitrogen level) is common and, in half of the patients, progresses to uremia (clinical renal failure) over a period of several years. Therapy consists of long-term dialysis or renal transplantation.

Autosomal Recessive (Infantile) Polycystic Kidney Disease

■ *Infantile polycystic kidney disease is an uncommon autosomal recessive condition in which dilatation of cortical and medullary collecting ducts leads to a cystic kidney.*

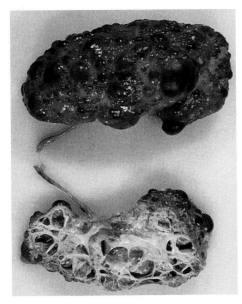

FIGURE *16-6*
Adult polycystic disease. The kidney is enlarged, and the parenchyma is almost entirely replaced by cysts of varying size.

☐ **Pathology:** In contrast to patients with adult polycystic kidney disease, the external surface of the kidney in patients with the infantile disorder is smooth, and the involvement is invariably bilateral. The fusiform cysts are dilatations of cortical and medullary collecting ducts, which have a striking radial arrangement (see Fig. 16-5). Interstitial fibrosis and tubular atrophy are common. There are usually associated liver changes, termed *congenital hepatic fibrosis*, that are characterized by the enlargement of portal areas, an increase in connective tissue, and a proliferation of bile ducts. A candidate gene has been proposed to reside on the short arm of chromosome 6.

☐ **Clinical Features:** Two clinical presentations occur in this condition. The more frequent is in newborns, who suffer from congenitally enlarged, spongy kidneys and renal insufficiency. Less frequently, older children present with enlarged kidneys that have small cysts, tubular atrophy, and interstitial fibrosis. Most infants with severe polycystic kidney disease die in the perinatal period, often because the large kidneys compromise expansion of the lungs.

Nephronophthisis–Medullary Cystic Disease Complex

■ *Nephronophthisis, the medullary cystic disease complex, is a group of related, autosomal recessive diseases that are characterized by renal medullary cysts, sclerotic kidneys, and renal failure.* Eighty-five percent of the cases are familial. Most of the patients are in the first or second decade of life, and the disease complex accounts for 10% to 20% of the cases of renal insufficiency during childhood.

☐ **Pathology:** The kidneys are small, and when they are sectioned, multiple, variable-size cysts (diameter, ≤1 cm) are seen at the corticomedullary junction (see Fig. 16-5). These cysts arise from the distal portions of the nephron. Eventually, the corticomedullary cysts accumulate, and the remainder of the parenchyma becomes increasingly atrophic. Secondary glomerular sclerosis, interstitial fibrosis, and a nonspecific inflammatory infiltrate dominate the histologic picture.

☐ **Clinical Features:** These patients present with evidence of deteriorating tubular function. A defect in the concentrating ability of the tubules is reflected in polyuria, polydipsia, and enuresis (bed-wetting). Progressive azotemia and renal failure then follow, usually within 5 years of the onset of symptoms.

Simple Renal Cysts

Simple renal cysts are very common acquired lesions and are found in approximately half of the population older than 50 years. They rarely produce clinical symptoms unless they are very large. These cysts, which may be solitary or multiple, are found in the outer cortex, bulging the capsule, or less commonly, in the medulla (see Fig. 16-5). Microscopically, they are lined by a nondescript, flat epithelium.

RENAL FAILURE

Acute renal failure refers to an acute decline in the glomerular filtration rate, with a resultant increase in blood urea nitrogen and serum creatinine values. It may result from damage to any portion of the kidney, including the glomeruli, tubules and interstitium (e.g., with acute tubular necrosis or acute allergic interstitial nephritis), or blood vessels (e.g., in some forms of vasculitis). Acute renal failure may also result from extrarenal lesions (e.g., bilateral lower urinary tract obstruction) and is a frequent complication of hypotensive shock.

Chronic renal failure refers to end-stage renal disease, which is characterized clinically by uremia—that is, the clinical syndrome associated with a severe and chronically elevated level of blood urea nitrogen (azotemia). It results from a large variety of renal diseases, including glomerular, tubulointerstitial, and vascular diseases. Pathologically, end-stage renal disease is characterized by marked sclerosis of both glomeruli and the interstitium and by tubular atrophy.

GLOMERULAR SYNDROMES

■ *Nephrotic syndrome is characterized principally by heavy proteinuria (>3.5 g of protein per 24 hours) together with hypoproteinemia (hypoalbuminemia), peripheral edema, and hyperlipidemia* (Fig. 16-7). Box 16-1 lists the major causes of nephrotic syndrome in both adults and children. The vast majority of the cases of "pure" nephrotic syndrome (those without features of the nephritic syndrome) result from glomerular diseases within the category of noninflammatory glomerulopathies.

■ *Nephritic syndrome* (Box 16-2) *is characterized by (1) hematuria, (2) proteinuria (<3.5 g/d), (3) oliguria, and (4) decreased glomerular filtration rate (with resulting elevations in blood urea nitrogen and serum creatinine values).* Salt and water retention often results in hypertension and edema. In clear contrast to the nephrotic syn-

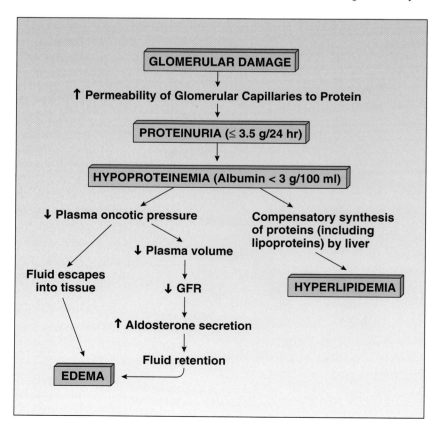

FIGURE 16-7
Pathophysiology of the nephrotic syndrome.

BOX *16-1*   Major Causes of the Nephrotic Syndrome

Adults
Membranous nephropathy (30%)
Glomerulopathies associated with systemic diseases (20–30%)[a]
Epithelial cell (minimal change) disease (20%)
Focal segmental glomerulosclerosis (10–20%)
Membranoproliferative glomerulonephritis (5%)[b]
Other primary glomerulopathies (5%)

Children
Epithelial cell (minimal change) disease (70%)
Focal segmental glomerulosclerosis (≈10%)
Membranous nephropathy (5–10%)
Glomerulopathies associated with systemic diseases (5–10%)[a]
Other primary glomerulopathies (5%)

[a] Includes diabetes, systemic amyloidosis, systemic lupus erythematosus, and others.
[b] Also frequently associated with nephritic syndrome.

BOX *16-2*   Signs and Symptoms of Nephritic Syndrome

Hematuria (gross or microscopic)
Decreased urine output (oliguria)
Elevated blood urea nitrogen and serum creatinine levels
Hypertension
Proteinuria ($\leq$ 3.5 g per 24 hours), with or without edema

drome, the nephritic syndrome is most often associated with inflammatory glomerular diseases (glomerulonephritis).

NONINFLAMMATORY GLOMERULOPATHIES

Minimal Change Glomerulopathy

■ *Minimal change glomerulopathy is a glomerular disorder that is characterized clinically by the nephrotic syn-* drome and pathologically by fusion of the visceral epithelial foot processes.

Minimal change nephrotic syndrome (also known as epithelial cell disease or lipoid nephrosis) is largely a disorder of children, in whom it is the major cause of nephrotic syndrome. However, the disease also occurs in adults with a significant frequency (20% of adults with nephrotic syndrome). Most children with the disease are boys who initially present before the age of 6 years.

☐ **Pathogenesis:** Neither the cause nor the pathogenesis of minimal change nephrotic syndrome is understood. Because of the association between the onset of nephrotic syndrome and an allergic history, and also because the disease sometimes follows infection or exposure to allergens, involvement of the immune system has been postulated. In experimental models, heavy proteinuria has been related to a loss of polyanionic sites on the glomerular basement membrane. The loss of these sites allows anionic proteins, particularly albumin, to pass easily through the normal barrier.

☐ **Pathology:** By definition, the light microscopic appearance of glomeruli in patients with minimal

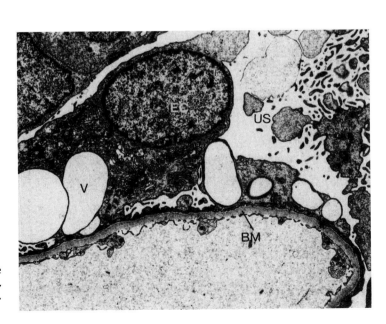

FIGURE *16-8*
Epithelial cell disease. In this electron micrograph, the epithelial cells (EC) display foot process effacement, "villous" hyperplasia, and numerous vacuoles (V). *BM,* basement membrane; *US,* urinary space.

change nephrotic syndrome (epithelial cell disease) is essentially normal. However, there is often some irregular prominence of the epithelial cells, and minor degrees of mesangial enlargement are common.

Electron microscopic examination of the glomeruli reveals total effacement of the epithelial cell foot processes, with the basement membrane being covered by a sheet of cytoplasm (Fig. 16-8). Scanning electron microscopy shows that loss of foot processes results from their retraction into the parent epithelial cell bodies rather than from actual fusion. Numerous microvilli protrude from the surface of the epithelial cells (Fig. 16-8). No electron-dense deposits are seen, and immunofluorescence studies for antibodies or complement in patients with epithelial cell disease most often are negative. Because all of these changes are completely reversible during remission, the diagnosis of epithelial cell disease can be made only when there is significant proteinuria.

☐ **Clinical Features:** Most patients with epithelial cell disease show complete remission of proteinuria within 8 weeks of the initiation of corticosteroid therapy. However, after the withdrawal of corticosteroids, approximately half of these patients suffer intermittent relapses for as long as 10 years. Each relapse is responsive to corticosteroid therapy, however, and **there is no tendency to progress into chronic renal failure.** A few patients achieve complete remission without any therapy.

Death from infection was frequent before antibiotics and corticosteroids became readily available. A fatal outcome or progression to renal failure is now exceptional. Thus, in the absence of complications, the long-term outlook for patients with epithelial cell disease today is probably no different from that of the general population.

Focal Segmental Glomerulosclerosis

■ *Focal segmental glomerulosclerosis refers to a malady in which some (focal) glomeruli exhibit segmental areas of sclerosis in the capillary tufts whereas others appear to be normal.* The majority of these cases occur in the context of nephrotic syndrome in children, accounting for 10% of such cases. In adults, 10% to 20% of the cases of nephrotic syndrome also exhibit focal segmental glomerulosclerosis.

☐ **Pathogenesis:** Focal segmental glomerulosclerosis represents a morphologic pattern that is common to at least three circumstances:

- **Idiopathic.** The majority of the cases of focal segmental glomerulosclerosis are of unknown cause.

Major features that distinguish idiopathic focal segmental glomerulosclerosis from the typical case of epithelial cell disease are (1) the poor response to corticosteroids, (2) the poorly selective nature of the proteinuria, (3) the presence of focal sclerosing lesions early in the disease, and (4) an unfavorable clinical course.

- **Decreased Renal Mass.** Focal segmental glomerulosclerosis occurs in conditions characterized by a decrease in functional renal mass (e.g., unilateral nephrectomy or agenesis) or in various types of acquired renal disease. The ratio of renal mass to body mass is also decreased in patients with morbid obesity, a condition in which the most frequent cause of nephrotic syndrome is focal segmental glomerulosclerosis. In all such situations, the total capillary surface area that is available for glomerular filtration is selectively reduced. As a result, increased glomerular capillary pressure and filtration injure the cells of the glomerulus and lead to capillary thrombosis, microaneurysms, mesangial enlargement, and subendothelial hyaline deposits. These lesions cause focal segmental glomerulosclerosis which may progress to sclerotic obliteration of the affected glomeruli. Low-protein diets and certain drugs that ameliorate the hemodynamic disturbances in the kidney protect, at least to some extent, against the development and progression of glomerular injury.

- **Healed Focal Glomerular Lesions.** The separation of focal segmental glomerulosclerosis from healed lesions of other focal glomerular disorders (e.g., focal glomerulonephritis, microscopic polyarteritis, malignant hypertension) on morphologic grounds alone is difficult.

☐ **Pathology:** By light microscopy, varying numbers of glomeruli show segmental areas of capillary loop obliteration, initially in the juxtamedullary glomeruli (Fig. 16-9). Adhesions to the Bowman capsule are seen adjacent to these lesions. The mesangium is hypercellular, and lipid-containing foam cells are often found within it. The frequent accumulation of a periodic acid-Schiff (PAS)–positive material in the affected areas produces a lesion referred to as **hyalinosis.** Uninvolved glomeruli appear to be entirely normal, although on occasion, a diffuse, global mesangial hypercellularity is superimposed on all the glomeruli.

By electron microscopy, diffuse effacement of the epithelial cell foot processes is identical to the lesion of epithelial cell disease. In addition, folding and thickening of the basement membrane (Fig. 16-10) and capillary collapse are present in sclerotic glomeruli. In more advanced lesions, an extensive accumulation of granu-

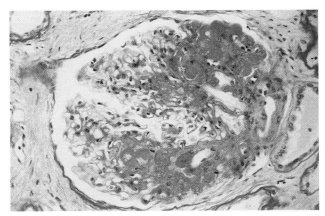

FIGURE   *16-9*
Focal segmental glomerulosclerosis. A periodic acid-Schiff stain shows perihilar areas of segmental sclerosis and adjacent adhesions to the Bowman capsule.

lar, electron-dense material throughout the affected segments represents insudative trapping of plasma proteins, which manifests as hyalinosis by light microscopy. Discrete, well-defined deposits of immune complexes are not found.

Immunofluorescence studies show trapping of immunoglobulin (Ig) M and C3 in the segmental areas of sclerosis and hyalinosis. IgG, C4, and C1q are less frequently found. This trapping of immune proteins is nonspecific and, presumably, is not related to the pathogenesis of this disease.

☐ **Clinical Features:** Most patients with the diagnosis of focal segmental glomerulosclerosis present with the insidious onset of proteinuria and the nephrotic syndrome. Many of these patients are hypertensive, and microscopic hematuria is frequent.

When focal segmental glomerulosclerosis is detected soon after the onset of nephrotic syndrome, it is probably progressive at all ages. Most patients suffer an uninterrupted decline in renal function for a period of as long as 10 years. In severe cases, progression to end-stage renal failure occurs in less than 3 years. Corticosteroids are rarely of benefit in adults with focal segmental glomerulosclerosis, and their effect in children is variable. Renal transplantation has been successful in many cases, but the disease recurs in as many as half of these patients.

Membranous Glomerulopathy

■ *Membranous glomerulopathy is a frequent cause of nephrotic syndrome in adults and results from the accumulation of immune complexes in the subepithelial zone of glomerular capillaries.* In fact, this condition is the most frequent cause of nephrotic syndrome in adults (30% of

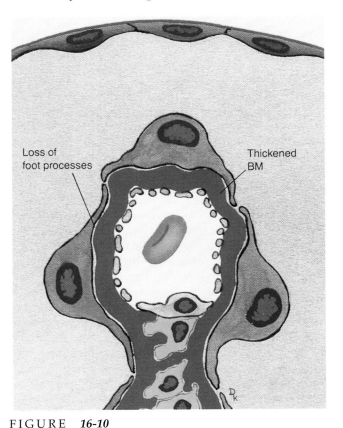

FIGURE   *16-10*
Focal segmental glomerulosclerosis. This disorder typically displays epithelial cell change and basement membrane thickening. Epithelial cells show effacement of the foot processes and distention of the cytoplasm. The basement membrane is thickened and folded. The glomeruli located deep within the cortex are the earliest to demonstrate these pathognomonic changes, at a time when other glomeruli may show only the minimal change described in Figure 16-8.

cases). Although the disease has been associated with many precipitating factors, most cases are idiopathic.

☐ **Pathogenesis:** Membranous nephropathy is believed to result from the deposition of immune complexes from the circulation or the formation in situ of immune complexes within the capillary walls. Electron-dense immune complex deposits have been demonstrated by electron microscopy, and immunoglobulins and complement have been shown by immunofluorescence.

Most patients have the primary, idiopathic form of membranous nephropathy. However, a number of associated conditions predispose to the development of "secondary" membranous nephropathy. In such cases, the immune complexes within the glomerular capillary walls may contain endogenous antigens (e.g., tumor antigens) or antigens derived from an infectious agent. **In adults, one of the most frequent associations of** membranous nephropathy is with carcinomas, being found in as many as 10% of these patients. Certain drugs, such as gold and penicillamine, used in the treatment of rheumatoid arthritis, can cause the lesion. Membranous nephropathy has been seen in association with various systemic infections, most frequently **hepatitis B.** As many as 10% of patients with **systemic lupus erythematosus** present with a lesion of membranous nephropathy. When these predisposing conditions are recognized, their treatment often results in eradication of the membranous lesion and clinical remission of the nephrotic syndrome.

☐ **Pathology:** By light microscopy, the glomeruli are slightly enlarged yet normocellular (Fig. 16-11). Depending on the duration of the disease, the capillary walls are normal or thickened. During the early stages, silver stains, which demonstrate basement membrane material, reveal multiple projections, or spikes, of argyrophilic material on the epithelial surface of the basement membrane. Such spikes represent projections of basement membrane material that is deposited around the immune complexes (Fig. 16-12), which do not stain with silver. As the disease progresses, the capillary lumina are encroached on, and glomerular obsolescence eventually ensues. Membranous nephropathy is classified as being noninflammatory, because no cellular proliferation occurs. If the lesion heals, the basement membrane is reconstituted and assumes an essentially normal appearance, except for the increased thickness.

Immunofluorescence studies reveal diffuse, granular deposition of IgG and C3 in the glomerular capillary loops (Fig. 16-13). Mesangial deposits are not typically seen in patients with the idiopathic variety of membranous nephropathy, but they are frequently seen in the membranous lesion of systemic lupus erythematosus.

☐ **Clinical Features:** At one end of the clinical spectrum, patients have spontaneous remissions, whereas at the severe end, progressive renal failure ensues within 10 to 15 years. In the middle of these extremes, many patients have persistent proteinuria, with normal renal function, for many years. The benefits of corticosteroids in the treatment of patients with idiopathic membranous nephropathy remain controversial. Overall, the prognosis is better in children.

Diabetic Glomerulosclerosis

■ *Diabetic glomerulosclerosis (Kimmelstiel-Wilson disease) embraces the glomerular changes seen in patients with diabetes, which result in proteinuria and progressive renal failure.* Only the glomerular lesion of diabetes mellitus is discussed here; a more general discussion of diabetes is found in Chapter 22.

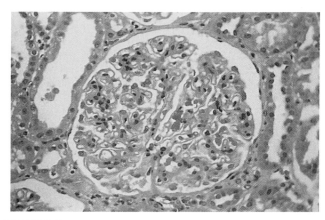

FIGURE   *16-11*
Membranous glomerulopathy. The glomerulus is slightly enlarged and shows diffuse thickening of the capillary walls. There is no hypercellularity.

☐ **Pathogenesis:** The alterations in diabetic glomerulosclerosis are an expression of the diabetic microangiopathy that occurs in many systemic small arteries, arterioles, and capillaries. As in the systemic vessels, glomerulosclerosis results from progressive accumulation of basement membrane material, a process that, in turn, produces enlargement of the glomeruli. The pathogenesis appears to be related to the severity and duration of hyperglycemia.

The reasons for proteinuria in patients with diabetic glomerulopathy are not clear, but they may relate, in part, to nonenzymatic glycosylation of proteins making up the glomerular filtration barrier, including the basement membrane components. This chemical reaction leads to changes in the charge of these proteins and in the filtration properties of the glomerulus.

☐ **Pathology:** Early thickening of the glomerular basement membrane is followed by a diffuse widening of the mesangial areas, with the accumulation of a PAS-positive matrix (Fig. 16-14). The glomerulus becomes enlarged and may appear hypercellular.

Diffuse glomerulosclerosis refers to enlarged glomeruli with expanded mesangial areas and diffusely thickened basement membranes.

Nodular glomerulosclerosis describes single or multiple nodules in the glomeruli. These are rounded, homogeneous, and eosinophilic masses in centrilobular areas (see Fig. 16-14). With time, the nodules become acellular, in which case only a rim of peripheral mesangial nuclei is visible.

Insudative changes occur in both the adjacent arterioles and the glomerular tufts. **These are manifested by hyaline arteriolosclerosis, which in patients with diabetes uniquely involves both the afferent and efferent arterioles.**

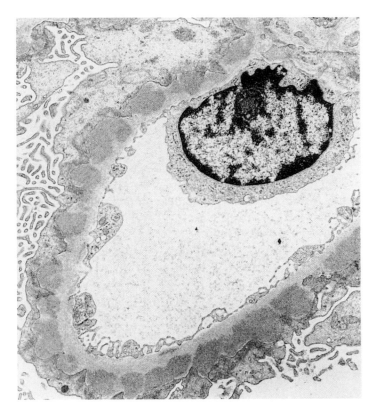

FIGURE *16-12*
Stage II membranous glomerulopathy. An electron micrograph shows deposits of electron-dense material, with intervening delicate projections of basement membrane material.

Electron microscopy reveals widening of the basement membrane lamina densa, which may be many times its normal width. Accumulation of basement membrane–like stroma in the mesangium parallels diffuse widening of the basement membrane and may become nodular and acellular. The insudative lesions consist of granular, electron-dense masses, which often contain lipid material and debris. There are no deposits of immune complexes.

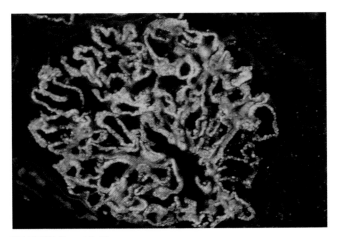

FIGURE *16-13*
Membranous glomerulopathy. Immunofluorescent microscopy shows granular deposits of immunoglobulin G outlining the glomerular capillary loops.

☐ **Clinical Features:** Diabetic glomerulosclerosis is the leading cause of end-stage renal disease in the United States, accounting for one-third of all patients with chronic renal failure. Proteinuria in patients with diabetic glomerulosclerosis is initially mild and may remain so, although patients with nephrotic-range proteinuria usually progress to renal failure within 6 years. Hematuria is usually not present. Significant proteinuria is usually accompanied by other signs of advanced microangiopathy, such as diabetic retinopathy.

Renal Amyloidosis

■ *Renal amyloidosis refers to the deposition in the kidneys of diverse extracellular proteins that have common morphologic properties, stain with specific dyes, and have a characteristic appearance under polarized light when stained with certain dyes.* Amyloidosis is associated with many different diseases, and the protein material (amyloid) may be deposited in a variety of tissues, as described in detail in Chapter 23.

Glomerular involvement is a prominent feature in most cases of systemic amyloidosis. In 60% of the patients, proteinuria is severe enough to produce nephrotic syndrome. Severe infiltration of the glomeruli and blood vessels by amyloid results in renal failure.

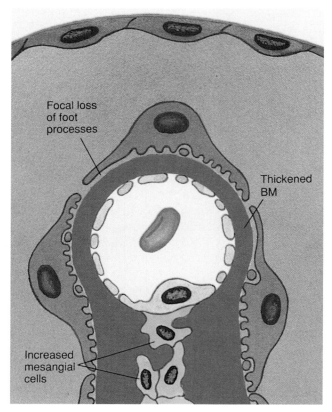

FIGURE **16-14**
Diabetic glomerulosclerosis. The glomerular tuft is enlarged and displays a thickened basement membrane that retains a normal texture and density, with smooth inner and outer contours. Focal effacement of the epithelial cell foot processes is common. Accumulation of basement membrane–line stroma in the mesangium parallels diffuse widening of the basement membrane.

□ **Pathology:** Amyloid deposition initially tends to be mesangial, thereby producing diffuse mesangial widening without hypercellularity (Fig. 16-15). However, it progressively spreads to obliterate capillary lumina.

Hereditary Nephritis (Alport Syndrome)

■ *Alport syndrome is a proliferative and sclerosing glomerular disease that is often accompanied by defects of the ears or, occasionally, the eyes and that is caused by a genetic abnormality in type IV collagen.*

□ **Pathogenesis:** The most common genetic abnormality leading to molecular defects in the glomerular basement membrane is X-linked and is caused by a mutation in the gene (*COL4A5*) that codes for type IV collagen. Glomerular basement membranes from patients with Alport syndrome lack the 28-kd, noncol-

lagenous (globular) domain of type IV collagen. Many patients with hereditary nephritis have defective expression of the target antigen in antiglomerular basement membrane (anti-GBM) antibody disease (e.g., Goodpasture syndrome).

□ **Pathology:** By light microscopy, there is no diagnostic renal lesion of Alport syndrome. Histologic severity of the glomerular lesion varies from only mild, focal, and segmental mesangial widening to, in rare cases, a full-blown crescentic glomerulonephritis. By electron microscopy, an irregularly thickened glomerular capillary basement membrane shows splitting of the lamina densa into interlacing lamellae surrounding electron-lucent areas.

□ **Clinical Features:** Patients with Alport syndrome typically present with recurrent hematuria before 20 years of age. Proteinuria and hypertension tend to develop later during the course of disease. One-third to one-half of the patients exhibit a progressive hearing impairment, which initially manifests as deafness to high frequencies. A smaller proportion of patients suffer ocular defects, most often involving the lens. Renal failure eventually ensues.

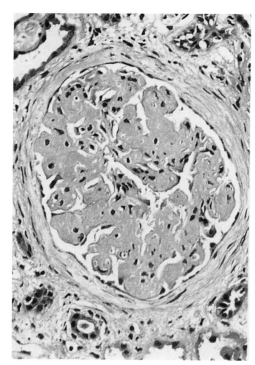

FIGURE **16-15**
Amyloid nephropathy. The mesangial areas are expanded and the glomerular capillaries obstructed by amorphous acellular material. Deposits of amyloid may take on a nodular appearance, somewhat resembling those of diabetic glomerulosclerosis. However, amyloid deposits are not positive on staining with periodic acid-Schiff but are identifiable on staining with Congo red.

Thin Glomerular Basement Membrane Nephropathy

■ *Thin basement membrane nephropathy, which is also termed benign familial hematuria, is a hereditary, noninflammatory disorder that typically presents as recurrent hematuria in childhood or young adulthood and is characterized by reduced thickness of the glomerular capillary basement.* Unlike patients with Alport syndrome, patients with benign familial hematuria do not progress to renal failure. The glomeruli of these patients are usually unremarkable by light microscopy.

Thin basement membrane disease is now recognized as being one of the most frequent causes of asymptomatic hematuria, even in patients with no family history of renal disease. In fact, both this disorder and IgA nephropathy are the two major diagnostic considerations in patients with asymptomatic hematuria.

GLOMERULONEPHRITIS

■ *Glomerulonephritis refers to inflammatory lesions of the glomerulus that are characterized histologically by hypercellularity of the glomeruli and clinically by nephritic syndrome.* Occasionally, proteinuria may predominate. Box 16-3 lists the diagnostic features of glomerular diseases.

Pathogenetic Mechanisms

Because of their importance in both experimental and human glomerular disease, immunologically mediated processes have been studied extensively. Immunologic injury can be divided into four basic types:

- Trapping of circulating immune complexes
- In situ immune complex formation
- Activation of the alternative pathway of complement
- Cell-mediated processes

Circulating Immune Complex Nephritis

Circulating immune complex nephritis results from the glomerular trapping of circulating antigen/antibody complexes (Fig. 16-16). In such disorders, the glomerulus can be considered an innocent bystander, involved only because of filtration by glomerular capillaries. Aggregates of immune complexes may penetrate the glomerular basement membrane and are then

---

BOX 16-3 Diagnostic Features of Glomerular Diseases

I. Light Microscopic Features
 A. Increased cellularity
  Infiltration by leukocytes (e.g., neutrophils, monocytes, macrophages)
  Proliferation of "endocapillary" cells (endothelial and mesangial cells)
  Proliferation of "extracapillary" cells (epithelial cells, crescent formation)
 B. Increased extracellular material
  Localization of immune complexes
   Thickening or replication of glomerular basement membrane (GBM)
   Increases in collagenous matrix (sclerosis)
   Insudation of plasma proteins (hyalinosis)
   Fibrinoid necrosis
   Deposition of amyloid

II. Immunofluorescence Features
 A. Linear staining of GBM
  Anti-GBM antibodies
  Multiple plasma proteins (e.g., in diabetic glomerulosclerosis)
  Monoclonal light chains
 B. Granular immune complex staining
  Mesangium (e.g., immunoglobulin [Ig] A nephropathy)
  Capillary wall (e.g., membranous glomerulopathy)
  Mesangium and capillary wall (e.g., lupus glomerulonephritis)
 C. Irregular (fluffy) staining
  Monoclonal light chains (AL amyloidosis)
  AA protein (AA amyloidosis)

III. Electron Microscopic Features
 A. Electron-dense immune complex deposits
  Mesangial (e.g., IgA nephropathy)
  Subendothelial (e.g., lupus glomerulonephritis)
  Subepithelial (e.g., membranous glomerulopathy)
 B. GBM thickening (e.g., diabetic glomerulosclerosis)
 C. GBM replication (e.g., membranoproliferative glomerulonephritis)
 D. Collagenous matrix expansion (e.g., focal segmental glomerulosclerosis)
 E. Fibrillary deposits (e.g., amyloidosis)

---

trapped in a subepithelial location. Their presence is confirmed on electron microscopy by the presence of subepithelial "humps." With immunofluorescence, a peripheral and granular staining with antisera directed against IgG and C3 is noted. Alternatively, circulating immune complexes usually do not penetrate the glomerular basement membrane and often localize in the subendothelial zone or mesangium.

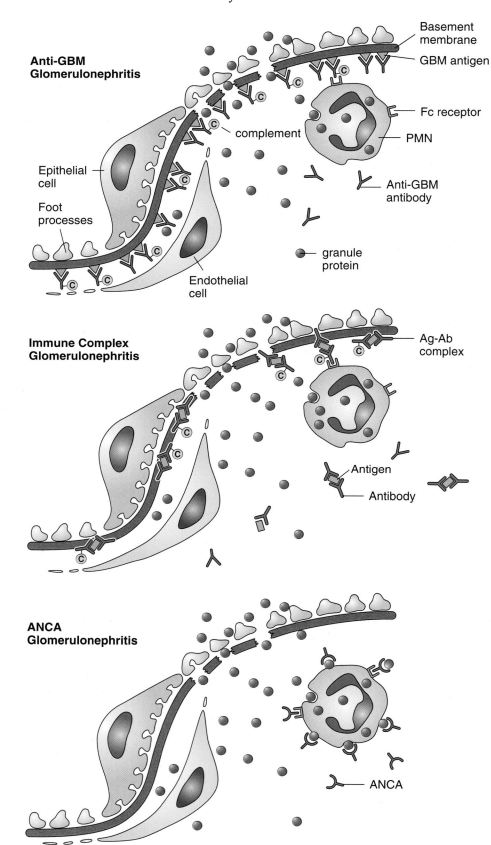

Anti-GBM Glomerulonephritis

Basement membrane
GBM antigen
Fc receptor
PMN
complement
Anti-GBM antibody
Epithelial cell
Foot processes
granule protein
Endothelial cell

Immune Complex Glomerulonephritis

Ag-Ab complex
Antigen
Antibody

ANCA Glomerulonephritis

ANCA

F I G U R E   *16-16*
Antibody-mediated glomerulo-nephritis. (Top) Antiglomerular basement membrane (GBM) anti-bodies cause glomerulonephritis by binding in situ to basement membrane antigens. This acti-vates complement and recruits in-flammatory cells. (Middle) Im-mune complexes that deposit from the circulation also activate com-plement and recruit inflammatory cells. (Bottom) Antineutrophil cytoplasmic antibodies (ANCA) are thought to cause inflammation by activating leukocytes through direct binding of the antibodies to the leukocytes, by Fc receptor engagement, or by both.

Antigens in clinically important forms of circulating immune complex nephritis may be either exogenous or endogenous. Examples of immune complex nephritis induced by exogenous antigens include bacterial antigens in glomerulonephritis associated with streptococcal infections and bacterial endocarditis and viral antigens in glomerulonephritis induced by hepatitis B. By contrast, DNA is an endogenous antigen in the pathogenesis of lupus nephritis. Tumor-associated antigens have also been implicated in some cases of glomerulonephritis.

In Situ Immune Complex Formation

The glomerulus may be damaged by the binding in situ of circulating antibody to an antigen already deposited in the glomerular basement membrane. The best-known example of this is **Goodpasture syndrome,** in which a subunit of the globular domain of type IV collagen in the glomerular basement membrane acts as an endogenous antigen to which circulating antibodies bind. Immunofluorescence shows a linear localization of IgG along the basement membrane. The combination of antigen with antibody results in activation of complement, and a rapidly progressive glomerulonephritis usually ensues.

Alternative Complement Pathway

The alternative complement pathway is important in the pathogenesis of a form of membranoproliferative glomerulonephritis. The alternative pathway for complement activation is also thought to be important in focal glomerulonephritis caused by deposition of IgA.

Cell-Mediated Immunity

Although there is no direct evidence that cell-mediated processes cause any specific form of human glomerulonephritis, occasional cases of immunologically mediated disease occur in which the accumulation of mononuclear cells and the absence of immunoglobulins suggest a delayed-type (cell-mediated) reaction.

Once immune complexes have localized within a glomerulus, a number of secondary pathogenetic mechanisms appear to play a role in effecting immunologic injury:

- **Complement** may produce glomerular injury through two distinct mechanisms. The terminal components of complement (C5b-9) form the membrane-attack complex that directly produces cell injury at the level of the plasma membrane.
- **Neutrophils** are attracted to the glomerulus in exudative forms of glomerulonephritis, such as in acute postinfectious glomerulonephritis and anti-GBM antibody disease. The chemotactic actions of specific complement components, particularly C5a, are responsible (see Fig. 16-16).
- **Monocytes and macrophages** infiltrate the glomerulus in many forms of renal disease and contribute to the cellularity of glomerular tufts and the surrounding crescents. Activated macrophages release a number of cytokines and growth factors that are probably important in tissue damage.
- **Activation of the coagulation cascade** is important in some forms of glomerular injury. Fibrin can usually be demonstrated in Bowman's space early during the formation of crescents and is probably responsible, in part, for the subsequent epithelial cell proliferation and crescent formation.
- **Platelets** may be activated by sensitized mast cells and basophils on exposure to antigen or immune complexes. Growing evidence suggests that platelet-derived, polycationic proteins disturb the anionic charge of the glomerular wall and contribute to its damage. Platelets also contribute to glomerular injury through the release of inflammatory mediators.

Acute Postinfectious Glomerulonephritis

■ *Acute postinfectious glomerulonephritis* is characterized clinically by the sudden onset of nephritic syndrome and morphologically by diffuse hypercellularity of glomeruli. The disease is a sequel to infection with a variety of agents (e.g., staphylococci, pneumococci, spirochetes, and viruses), but the most frequent association is with certain strains of **group A β-hemolytic streptococci** (*S. pyogenes*). Acute glomerulonephritis most commonly affects children, and although it is not seen as frequently in developed countries now as in the past, it remains one of the most common renal diseases of childhood.

☐ **Pathogenesis:** The exact mechanism by which streptococcal infection produces the characteristic proliferative changes in the glomeruli is still not completely characterized, although the similarities with the experimental model of acute serum sickness suggest that the disease is caused by glomerular localization of immune complexes generated by an antibody response to circulating antigens. Circulating immune complexes are demonstrable in half of the patients with acute poststreptococcal glomerulonephritis. Evidence also suggests the formation of glomerular immune complexes in situ, between trapped bacterial antigens and circulating antibodies. Immune complexes within glomeruli initiate inflammation by activating complement as well as other humoral and cellular inflammatory mediator systems. These effects result in the marked glomerular hypercellularity that defines acute diffuse proliferative glomerulonephritis.

☐ **Pathology:** By light microscopy, diffuse enlargement and hypercellularity of the glomeruli are present during the first 3 weeks after the onset of acute glomerulonephritis (Fig. 16-17). The hypercellularity is caused by the proliferation of both endothelial and mesangial cells (Fig. 16-18) and the infiltration of neutrophils and monocytes. Crescents may be present but are usually sporadic and segmental. Tubulointerstitial damage and inflammation occur in parallel with the glomerular changes.

The characteristic ultrastructural features of acute postinfectious glomerulonephritis are subepithelial humps, and these deposits are invariably accompanied by mesangial and subendothelial deposits. The humps are variably sized, dome-shaped deposits that are situated on the epithelial aspect of the basement membrane (see Fig. 16-18). Immunofluorescence typically reveals granular peripheral reactions for IgG and C3 along the basement membrane, in locations corresponding to the humps.

The characteristic morphologic features of acute inflammation usually resolve by 8 weeks after the onset of nephritis. Generally, those patients who recover completely do so both clinically and histologically by 3 years after onset. A small number of patients develop an unusually severe lesion, however, that displays many crescents and progresses quickly to renal failure.

☐ **Clinical Features:** The primary infections may be in the pharynx or, especially in hot and humid

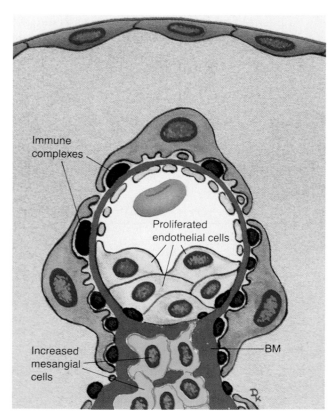

FIGURE   *16-18*
Postinfectious glomerulonephritis. Trapping of immune complexes in a subepithelial pattern ("lumpy-bumpy") is seen together with focal effacement of the foot processes. Less prominent subendothelial immune complexes are associated with endothelial cell proliferation and are related to increased capillary permeability and narrowing of the lumen. Frequently, proliferation of mesangial cells and a thickened mesangial basement membrane result in widening of the stalk and conspicuous trapping of immune complexes.

environments, the skin. The nephritic syndrome typically begins abruptly, with oliguria, hematuria, facial edema, and hypertension. Usually, there is a depression of the serum C3 level during the acute syndrome. This returns to normal within 1 to 2 weeks, however, as does the clinical condition of most patients. However, in a minority of patients, an abnormal urinary sediment persists for years after the acute episode. Complete recovery, particularly in children, is the rule, although some adults with initially severe disease manifest persistent renal dysfunction.

Membranoproliferative Glomerulonephritis

■ *Membranoproliferative lesions* are characterized by the combination of glomerular basement membrane thicken-

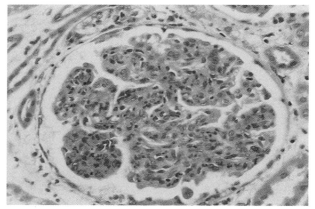

FIGURE   *16-17*
Acute poststreptococcal glomerulonephritis. The glomerulus of a patient who developed glomerulonephritis after a streptococcal infection is hypercellular because of the proliferation of endothelial and mesangial cells and infiltration by neutrophils.

ing ("membrano") and mesangial cell proliferation ("proliferative"). Although such lesions may present initially as nephrotic syndrome (see Box 16-1), the prominent glomerular hypercellularity in membranoproliferative lesions clearly distinguishes them from the previously discussed, noninflammatory primary glomerular lesions that cause nephrotic syndrome. By light microscopy, the glomeruli are hypercellular, mainly because of mesangial cell proliferation. Variable infiltration by leukocytes is noted, and the glomeruli show prominent lobulation (Fig. 16-19).

Type I Membranoproliferative Glomerulonephritis

Type I membranoproliferative glomerulonephritis (Fig. 16-20) has been associated with a number of conditions, including hepatitis B and hepatitis C antigenemia, infection of ventriculoatrial shunts (for treatment of hydrocephalus), bacterial endocarditis, streptococcal infections, and cancer. However, the great majority of cases are idiopathic. Circulating immune complexes have been found in some patients with this disease, and there is evidence that they may play a role in the activation of complement through the classical pathway.

☐ **Pathology:** By light microscopy, diffusely enlarged glomeruli show a marked mesangial cell proliferation that produces a lobular distortion of the glomeruli (see Fig. 16-19). Owing to inflammatory expansion of the mesangial area, the cells and matrix of the mesangium are forced peripherally, into

the capillary loops, and insinuate themselves between the endothelial cells and the basement membrane (see Fig. 16-20). Electron microscopy reveals a continuous layer of mesangial cytoplasm around the entire capillary. Subendothelial and mesangial electron-dense deposits are present in patients with type I disease. Subepithelial humps may also be seen. Immunofluorescence typically demonstrates granular deposition of immunoglobulins (IgG, IgM) and

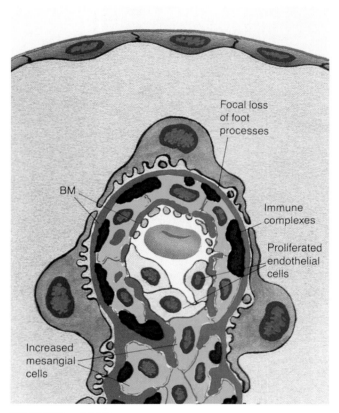

FIGURE 16-20
Type I membranoproliferative glomerulonephritis. In this disease, the glomeruli are enlarged. Hypercellular tufts and narrowing or obstruction of the capillary lumen are seen, and large subendothelial deposits of immune complexes extend along the inner border of the basement membrane. The mesangial cells proliferate and migrate peripherally into the capillary. Basement membrane material accumulates in a linear fashion, parallel to the basement membrane in a subendothelial position. Interposition of mesangial cells and basement membrane between the endothelial cells and the original basement membrane creates a double-contour effect. Accumulation of mesangial cells and stroma in the tufts narrows the capillary lumen. The stalk is also widened by the proliferation of mesangial cells and the accumulation of basement membrane stroma. The entire process leads progressively to lobulation of the glomerulus, consolidation of the lobules, and eventually, a "cannonball" effect. Note the proliferation of endothelial cells and focal effacement of foot processes.

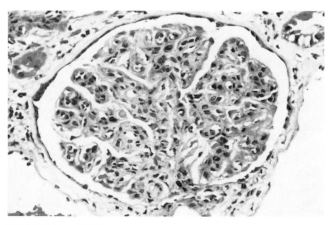

FIGURE 16-19.
Membranoproliferative glomerulonephritis. Light microscopy of this type I lesion shows markedly accentuated glomerular lobulation as well as the accumulation of cells and matrix in the mesangium. The increased mesangial cells and matrix obstruct the capillary lumina and widen their walls.

complement in the glomerular capillary loops and mesangium.

Type II Membranoproliferative Glomerulonephritis

☐ **Pathogenesis:** The clinical presentation and course of type II membranoproliferative glomerulonephritis are similar to those of type I disease. Circulating immune complexes are found only infrequently in patients with type II disease. Most patients with type II disease, however, do have a circulating IgG autoantibody, termed *C3 nephritic factor.*

☐ **Pathology:** The light microscopic appearance of type II disease is similar to that of type I. By electron microscopy, the pathognomonic feature of type II disease is the characteristic, ribbon-like zone of increased density located centrally within the thickened basement membrane (Fig. 16-21), hence the name **dense deposit disease.** In contrast to type I disease,

immunofluorescence shows only pseudolinear, often discontinuous staining of the glomerular capillary loops for complement.

☐ **Clinical Features:** Membranoproliferative lesions occur primarily in older children and young adults, although they may also be seen in older adults. The clinical presentation may be the nephrotic syndrome, nephritic syndrome, or a combination of both. Patients frequently have low levels of C3, and most patients with membranoproliferative glomerulonephritis progress to end-stage renal failure, regardless of treatment.

Systemic Lupus Erythematosus

As many as 70% of patients with systemic lupus erythematosus (SLE; see Chapter 4) will develop clinically significant renal disease. The variety of renal lesions in patients with SLE is reflected by a wide spectrum of clinical manifestations, including the nephritic and nephrotic syndromes.

☐ **Pathogenesis:** SLE is the prototypical example of a human immune complex disease. Trapping of circulating immune complexes, probably those containing double-stranded DNA, is responsible for much of the renal damage in SLE. In situ formation of immune complexes, subsequent to binding of DNA to the glomerular basement membrane and extracellular matrix, may also play a role.

☐ **Pathology:** In the glomeruli, cellular proliferation is typically mesangial and often irregular. Mild involvement is characterized by diffuse mesangial expansion, with or without hypercellularity, and there is often a superimposed, segmental endothelial cell proliferation (Fig. 16-22). More severe inflammation is

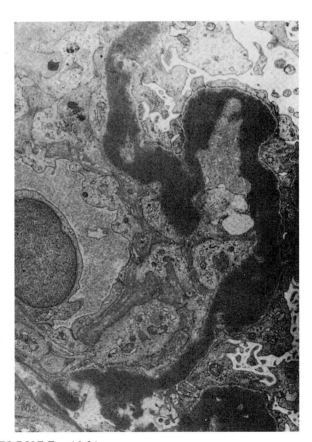

FIGURE *16-21*
Type II membranoproliferative glomerulonephritis (dense deposit disease). An electron micrograph demonstrates thickening of the basement membrane and increased density of the lamina densa.

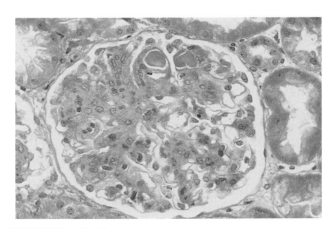

FIGURE *16-22*
Proliferative lupus glomerulonephritis. Segmental endocapillary hypercellularity and thickening of capillary walls are present.

manifested by enlarged, hypercellular glomeruli, enhanced lobulation, segmental areas of tuft necrosis, karyorrhexis, polymorphonuclear leukocyte infiltration, and crescent formation.

Heavy subendothelial deposits can usually be recognized by light microscopy as a marked thickening of the involved capillary wall, which, in turn, results in a characteristic formation termed a **wire loop** (Fig. 16-23). Hyaline thrombi are also seen as eosinophilic plugs of material that seem to occlude the lumina of involved capillary loops. In areas of segmental necrosis, hematoxylin bodies (lilac-tinged, fragmented nuclei) may be found. Hematoxylin bodies are considered to be the only pathognomonic light microscopic feature of tissue damage from SLE in the kidney and other organs.

By electron microscopy, immune complexes, which are particularly prominent in this disease and may display unusual crystalline patterns, localize in the mesangial, subendothelial, or subepithelial areas. IgG is the most frequently demonstrated immunoglobulin, although IgA and IgM are also usually present. Both early and late complement components are commonly seen, and staining for C1q is often especially intense. Frequently, IgG, IgA, IgM, C3, C4, and C1q are present in the same glomerulus (the so-called "full house" pattern).

The World Health Organization system recognizes the following five classes of lupus nephritis:

- **Class I: Histologically Normal.**
- **Class II: Pure Mesangial Lesion.** Immune complexes confined to the mesangial areas.
- **Class III: Focal and Segmental Glomerulonephritis.** These lesions are noted in less than 50% of the glomeruli (focal). They also tend to involve no more than 50% of the area of the affected glomeruli (segmental).
- **Class IV: Diffuse Proliferative Glomerulonephritis.** Proliferative lesions are seen in 50% or more of the glomeruli. These lesions also tend to involve a greater fraction of the glomerular area.
- **Class V: Diffuse Membranous Nephropathy.** In 10% of the patients with lupus nephritis, the appearance of the lesion is similar to that of idiopathic membranous nephropathy. A "full house" of immunoglobulin (IgG, IgA, and IgM) is frequently encountered.

Renal disease is one of the major prognostic determinants in patients with SLE, and renal failure is the cause of death in more than one-third of the patients. Generally, the mesangial (class II) and membranous (class V) nephropathies have a more benign course than do proliferative glomerulonephritis (classes III and IV).

IgA Nephropathy

IgA nephropathy (Berger disease) is a glomerulonephritis caused by accumulation of immune complexes, composed predominantly of IgA. It is the most common form of primary glomerulonephritis in several parts of the world. In France, Italy, Austria, Japan, and Singapore, IgA nephropathy accounts for more than 20% of the cases of primary glomerulonephritis in adults. In the United States, the proportion is reported to be lower but still significant (3–10%).

☐ **Pathogenesis:** The pathogenesis of IgA nephropathy is not understood, but a number of findings suggest a role for circulating IgA-containing immune complexes. Aggregates of IgA and fibronectin in the blood are found in the majority (70%) of patients with IgA nephropathy, and IgA autoantibodies to nuclear antigens and glomerular components have also been reported. There is a known association between IgA nephropathy and patients with chronic liver disease, who have an impaired capacity to remove circulating immune complexes. IgA may also combine with antigens trapped in the glomerular mesangium to form immune complexes in situ. Antigens hypothesized as being involved in the pathogenesis of IgA nephropa-

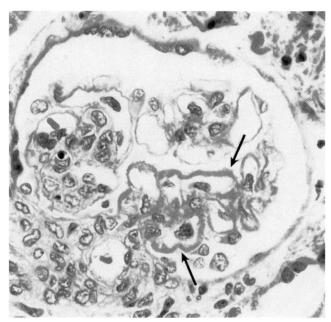

FIGURE   *16-23*
Lupus nephritis, focal proliferative type (World Health Organization class III). The glomerulus shows segmental areas of hypercellularity and some markedly thickened capillary loops or "wire loops" (*arrows*), which reflect the subendothelial deposition of immune complexes.

thy include viral, bacterial, and dietary antigens. By immunofluorescence, C3 and properdin are frequently present together with IgA, whereas C1q and C4 (indicative of classical pathway activation) are typically absent.

Genetic susceptibility may also play a role in the development of IgA nephropathy among some patients. Study results suggest an increased frequency of certain HLA class II antigens (DR4 in France and Japan, and gene[s] in the DQ region in Great Britain).

☐ **Pathology:** IgA nephropathy is a mesangial proliferative lesion, meaning that mesangial cell proliferation and widening of the matrix are the sole, or predominant, light microscopic abnormalities in many of these cases. The involvement is usually focal, but it may also be diffuse (Fig. 16-24). Biopsy specimens from those patients destined to progress to renal failure often exhibit segmental necrosis of the glomerular tufts, crescents, and scarring. Particularly in such specimens, hyaline material (representing immune deposits) may be seen in the mesangium. Ultrastructural examination shows a variable amount of granular, electron-dense deposits, which are located primarily in the mesangium and typically immediately beneath the

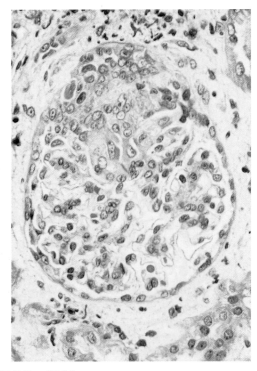

FIGURE   *16-24*
Immunoglobulin A nephropathy. A light micrograph shows segmental mesangial cell proliferation and areas of increased mesangial matrix.

paramesangial basement membrane. Immunofluorescence microscopy is essential in establishing the diagnosis of IgA nephropathy; it reliably demonstrates granular mesangial deposition of IgA, usually accompanied by C3 and sometimes by IgG, IgM, or both. IgA deposition in the glomerular capillary wall (in addition to the mesangium) may be present in more severe cases and suggests a less favorable prognosis.

☐ **Clinical Features:** IgA nephropathy is most common in young men, with a peak incidence occurring from 15 to 30 years of age. It usually presents as macroscopic (gross) or microscopic hematuria. As many as 20% of patients with IgA nephropathy progress to end-stage renal failure. Furthermore, the lesion does not spontaneously resolve, and it is not responsive to therapy.

Crescentic Glomerulonephritis

■ *Crescentic (or rapidly progressive) glomerulonephritis is an ominous morphologic pattern in which the majority of glomeruli are surrounded by an accumulation of cells in the Bowman space.* The crescent is an expression of fulminant glomerular damage and always leaves severe residual scarring. Clinically, most patients with a substantial number of crescents suffer a rapid and progressive decline in renal function. Irreversible renal failure with severe oliguria or anuria occurs within weeks unless adequate therapy is administered.

☐ **Pathogenesis:** Escape of fibrin into the Bowman space seems to be important for the formation of glomerular crescents. Fibrin can invariably be demonstrated by immunofluorescence in active crescentic glomerulonephritis. Fibrin and other plasma proteins presumably gain access to the Bowman space through breaks in the inflamed glomerular capillaries. In this regard, crescents are often associated with areas of segmental necrosis within glomeruli. Fibrin and fibrin products may also stimulate the migration of macrophages into glomeruli. Such macrophages, together with proliferating visceral and parietal epithelial cells as well as variable numbers of infiltrating polymorphonuclear cells, comprise the cellular component of acute or "cellular" crescents. In older "fibrocellular" or "fibroepithelial" crescents, many of the cells have the appearance of fibroblasts.

☐ **Pathology:** Crescents range from groups of cells filling only a segment of the Bowman space to circumferential masses of cells that completely surround the glomerulus (Fig. 16-25). They evolve from a cellular to a fibrocellular form, and they eventually scar, thereby creating a fibrous crescent. The cells in a cellular cres-

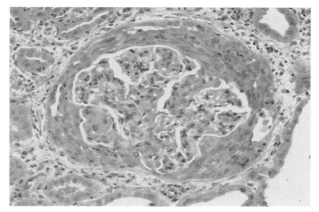

FIGURE   *16-25*
Crescentic antiglomerular basement membrane glomerulonephritis. A crescent that surrounds the periphery of the glomerulus is composed of cells contiguous with the lining of Bowman's capsule.

cent, which range in shape from spindle to ovoid, are often intermingled with neutrophils and fibrin.

Anti-GBM Antibody Disease

■ *Antiglomerular basement membrane antibody disease is a rare condition in which renal disease is mediated by an autoantibody directed against a component of the glomerular basement membrane* (see Fig. 16-17). The antigenic site within the basement membrane against which the antibody is directed has been localized to a subunit of the globular or noncollagenous domain of type IV collagen. This immune attack results in a rapidly progressive, crescentic glomerulonephritis. Eighty percent of these patients are male, and the average age at the onset of disease is 29 years. Because of cross-reactivity of the antibodies with the alveolar basement membranes, many patients simultaneously suffer pulmonary hemorrhages and recurrent hemoptysis, which are sometimes severe enough to be life-threatening. When both the lungs and the kidneys are involved, the eponym **Goodpasture syndrome** is used.

☐ **Pathology:** In patients with anti-GBM antibody disease, immunofluorescence microscopy shows linear deposits of IgG and C3 in glomerular capillary loops (Fig. 16-26). The patient's serum reacts with normal human glomerular basement membranes or with the globular domain of type IV collagen.

☐ **Clinical Features:** Many patients with anti-GBM antibody disease initially respond to immunosuppressive therapy and plasma exchange. However, later progression to end-stage renal failure is not uncommon. Renal transplantation is frequently successful.

Antineutrophil Cytoplasmic Autoantibody Glomerulonephritis

■ *Antineutrophil cytoplasmic autoantibody (ANCA) glomerulonephritis is an aggressive, neutrophil-mediated disease that is characterized by necrosis in glomerular crescents but not immunoglobulin deposits.*

☐ **Pathogenesis:** This category of glomerulonephritis was once called *idiopathic crescentic glomerulonephritis*, because immunofluorescence microscopy did not demonstrate glomerular deposition of anti-GBM antibodies or immune complexes. The discovery that 90% of the patients with this pattern of glomerular injury have circulating ANCAs, however, prompted the hypothesis that these autoantibodies cause the disease. ANCAs are specific for proteins in the cytoplasm of neutrophils and monocytes, usually myeloperoxidase or proteinase 3. However, there is no proof that ANCAs are actually pathogenic.

☐ **Pathology:** ANCA glomerulonephritis features focal glomerular necrosis and crescent formation. Immunoglobulins and complement are not demonstrated, and this feature distinguishes ANCA glomerulonephritis from anti-GBM glomerulonephritis and immune complex glomerulonephritis.

☐ **Clinical Features:** The most common clinical presentation for ANCA glomerulonephritis is rapidly progressive renal failure, with nephritic signs and symptoms. In fact, this disease accounts for 75% of rapidly progressive (crescentic) glomerulonephritis in

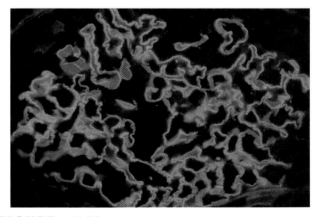

FIGURE   *16-26*
Anti-GBM glomerulonephritis. Linear immunofluorescence for immunoglobulin is seen along the glomerular basement membrane. Contrast this linear pattern of staining with the granular pattern of immunofluorescence typical for most types of immune complex deposition within capillary walls.

patients older than 60 years of age, 45% of that in middle-aged patients, and 30% of that in patients who are young adults and children. Importantly, three-quarters of patients with ANCA glomerulonephritis have systemic small vessel vasculitis, which has many extrarenal manifestations, including pulmonary hemorrhage. As a result, ANCA glomerulonephritis with pulmonary vasculitis can cause a pulmonary-renal vasculitic syndrome identical to that of Goodpasture syndrome. Without treatment, more than 80% of patients with ANCA glomerulonephritis develop end-stage renal disease within 5 years. Immunosuppressive therapy, however, decreases the incidence of this complication to less than 25%.

VASCULAR DISEASES

Benign Nephrosclerosis (Hypertensive Nephrosclerosis)

■ *Benign nephrosclerosis refers to renal vascular and glomerular sclerosis that occurs with mild to moderate hy-pertension.* No definition is completely accepted for hypertension, but a systolic blood pressure of 160 mm Hg and a diastolic blood pressure of 90 mm Hg are generally considered to represent unequivocal hypertension. The pathogenesis of hypertension is discussed in Chapter 10.

☐ **Pathology:** Benign nephrosclerosis is a consequence of renal ischemia. The kidneys are smaller than normal and are affected bilaterally. The cortical surface exhibits a fine granularity (Fig. 16-27), but coarser scars are also encountered. On cut section, the cortex is thinned. Microscopically, many glomeruli appear to be normal, whereas others show varying degrees of ischemic change, which is distinctly different from the lesions of intrinsic glomerular disease (e.g., glomerulonephritis). Initially, the glomerular capillaries are thickened and shriveled. Cells of the glomerular tuft are progressively lost, and both collagen and matrix material are deposited within the Bowman space opposite the hilus. Eventually, the glomerular tuft is obliterated by a dense, eosinophilic globular mass that is enclosed in a scar, all within Bowman's capsule. Tubular atrophy, which is a consequence of the obsolescence of the glomerulus, is associated with fibrosis of the related interstitium.

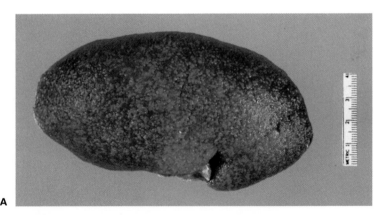

A

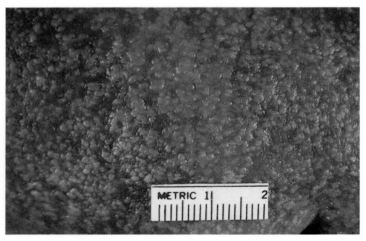

B

FIGURE   *16-27*
Benign nephrosclerosis. (A) The kidney is reduced in size, and the cortical surface exhibits fine granularity. (B) Higher magnification of the surface.

The pattern of change in the blood vessels of the kidney depends on the size of the vessel involved. Large arteries, down to the size of the arcuate arteries, exhibit arteriosclerotic changes of the intima, replication of the internal elastic lamina, and partial replacement of the muscular coat with fibrous tissue. Interlobular arteries show medial hypertrophy in addition to the changes just described. Arterioles display hyaline thickening of the entire wall (**arteriolosclerosis**).

☐ **Clinical Features:** Benign nephrosclerosis is not ordinarily associated with marked abnormalities of renal function, but a few of the many persons with "benign" hypertension do progress to end-stage renal disease. Because "benign" hypertension has such a high prevalence, even the small proportion of these patients who develop renal insufficiency amounts to approximately one-third of all patients with end-stage renal disease and includes most blacks with this complication. In fact, among blacks in the United States, hypertension without any evidence of a malignant phase is the single leading cause of end-stage renal disease.

Malignant Nephrosclerosis

■ *Malignant nephrosclerosis refers to the renal changes associated with malignant hypertension, including a diastolic blood pressure of greater than 125 mm Hg, the presence of retinal changes and papilledema, and functional impairment of the kidney.* Approximately half of the patients with malignant hypertension have an antecedent history of benign hypertension. The remainder include patients with intrinsic renal diseases (e.g., pyelonephritis or chronic glomerulonephritis) and various systemic disorders (e.g., lupus erythematosus, scleroderma, and polyarteritis). Occasionally, malignant hypertension arises de novo in apparently healthy persons, particularly young black men. Malignant hypertension occurs more frequently in men than in women, typically around the age of 40 years.

☐ **Pathology:** The size of the kidneys in patients with malignant hypertension varies from small to enlarged, depending on the duration of the pre-existing benign hypertension. The cortical surface characteristically displays petechiae, thereby accounting for the name "flea-bitten" kidney. The cut surface is mottled red and yellow and, occasionally, exhibits small cortical infarcts. Microscopically, malignant nephrosclerosis shows many of the changes of benign nephrosclerosis, but in addition, the glomeruli frequently show fibrinoid necrosis, sometimes in continuity with the same process in the afferent arterioles. Whereas the arterioles exhibit fibrinoid necrosis, the larger arteries reveal a lumen that is markedly reduced in size because of profuse intimal thickening, owing to cellular proliferation and accumulation of a myxoid matrix (Fig. 16-28).

☐ **Clinical Features:** Patients with malignant hypertension typically suffer headache, dizziness, and visual disturbances. Gross and microscopic hematuria is frequent, and proteinuria is virtually invariable. Progressive deterioration of renal function eventually leads to uremia. The outlook for patients with malignant hypertension was previously dismal, but today, antihypertensive therapy usually controls the disease.

Renal Vasculitis

Vasculitis is a general descriptive term that, like glomerulonephritis, is used in both a clinical and a pathologic sense. The diagnosis of renal vasculitis is generally established on the basis of identifying renal impairment in the context of a systemic vasculitis syndrome.

☐ **Pathology:** Morphologic features that aid in the classification of vasculitis emphasize the size and type of the vessels involved:

- **Small Vessel Vasculitis.** This process affects the small arteries, arterioles, capillaries, and venules. Glomerulonephritis is a frequent component of small vessel vasculitides. The disease may also lead to purpura, arthralgias, myalgias, peripheral neuropathy, and pulmonary hemorrhage. It can be caused by immune complexes, anti-basement membrane antibodies, or ANCAs.
- **Henoch-Schönlein purpura.** This is the most common type of childhood vasculitis and is caused by vascular localization of immune complexes, containing predominantly IgA. In 75% of the patients

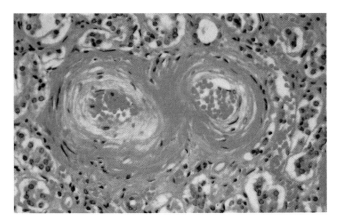

FIGURE *16-28*
Malignant nephrosclerosis. The kidney of a patient with malignant hypertension shows narrowing of the arterial lumina by concentric intimal thickening.

with ANCA glomerulonephritis, the kidney disease is a component of a systemic small vessel vasculitis (e.g., Wegener granulomatosis or Churg-Strauss syndrome).

- **Medium-Size Vessel Vasculitis.** This condition involves the arteries but not the arterioles, capillaries, or venules. **Polyarteritis nodosa**, which occurs mainly in adults, and **Kawasaki disease**, which principally affects children, are rare causes of renal dysfunction.

- **Large Vessel Vasculitis.** Large vessel vasculitides, such as **giant cell arteritis** and **Takayasu arteritis**, affect the aorta and its major branches. These disorders may cause renovascular hypertension by involving the renal arteries or aorta at the origin of the renal arteries.

Thrombotic Microangiopathy

■ *Thrombotic microangiopathy refers to a group of diseases sharing similar renal microvascular lesions, including thrombosis, arterial intimal expansion, arteriolar fibrinoid necrosis, and glomerular consolidation.* This systemic condition often affects the kidney, in which microvascular thrombi produce injury that may progress to acute renal failure. The major diseases included under the rubric of thrombotic microangiopathy are the hemolytic-uremic syndrome and thrombotic thrombocytopenic purpura.

Hemolytic-Uremic Syndrome

■ *Hemolytic-uremic syndrome describes a combination of acute renal failure, thrombocytopenia, and hemolytic anemia.*

□ **Pathogenesis:** **Hemolytic-uremic syndrome seems to result from glomerular injury produced by toxins elaborated by a virulent serotype of** *Escherichia coli.* The toxin injures endothelial cells, thereby setting in motion the sequence of events that produces thrombotic microangiopathy.

□ **Pathology:** The glomerulus displays prominent endothelial swelling. Foci of epithelial cell proliferation and even crescents may appear, and thrombi are variably present in the glomeruli. Afferent arterioles display focal damage, with insudation of fibrin (fibrinoid necrosis), accumulation of erythrocytes, and thrombosis.

□ **Clinical Features:** The infantile and childhood types of hemolytic-uremic syndrome, which frequently have only glomerular lesions, are associated with complete recovery in the large majority of cases, with a mortality rate of less than 5%. The prognosis in adult and postpartum cases is more guarded, however, and the disease is fatal in half of these patients.

Thrombotic Thrombocytopenic Purpura

■ *Thrombotic thrombocytopenic purpura is a microangiopathic disease that differs from adult hemolytic-uremic syndrome in that it (1) generally occurs among an older age group; (2) has a lesser involvement of the kidney; (3) affects many organs, particularly the central nervous system; and (4) has a worse prognosis.* The characteristic clinical features of thrombotic thrombocytopenic purpura include a low platelet count, generalized bleeding (skin, gastrointestinal tract, genitourinary tract, and retina), hemolytic anemia, neurologic abnormalities, fever, and renal disease. As in the adult hemolytic-uremic syndrome, women are more commonly affected than men. Thrombotic thrombocytopenic purpura is usually fatal, but an occasional patient survives.

Scleroderma (Progressive Systemic Sclerosis)

■ *Scleroderma is a disease in which excess collagen is deposited, typically in the skin but also in other organs such as the gastrointestinal tract, lungs, and heart* (see Chapter 4). Vascular changes, particularly in the fingers (Raynaud phenomenon) and the kidney, virtually always develop.

□ **Pathology:** The smaller arterial vessels of the kidney, namely the interlobular arteries and afferent arterioles, are the sites of the characteristic lesions. In the interlobular arteries, the lumen is narrowed by loose, fibrous tissue, in which nuclei are disposed in a concentric fashion. Fibrin is deposited within the thickened intima, and small fibrin thrombi are occasionally seen in the lumen. The afferent arterioles exhibit fibrinoid necrosis. These vascular changes may result in small infarcts.

In patients with scleroderma complicated by renal involvement, microangiopathic hemolytic anemia is related to vascular changes in the kidney. Azotemia, severe hypertension, and renal failure are common and indicate a grave prognosis.

Renovascular Hypertension

■ *Renovascular hypertension refers to elevated systemic blood pressure secondary to renal ischemia caused by narrowing of a renal artery.* Stenosis or total occlusion of a main renal artery produces a type of hypertension that, potentially, is curable by reconstitution of the arterial lumen. The majority (90–95%) of the cases are caused by lesions of atherosclerosis, which explains why this disorder is twice as common in men as in women and is seen primarily among older age groups (average age, 55 years). Most of the remaining cases re-

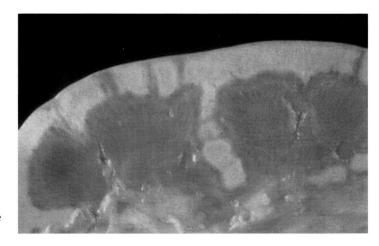

FIGURE   *16-29*
Renal cortical necrosis. The cortex of the kidney is pale yellow and soft owing to diffuse cortical necrosis.

flect **fibromuscular dysplasia**, a disorder that is characterized by fibrous and muscular stenosis of the renal artery.

☐ **Pathogenesis:** The pathogenesis of hypertension in cases of renal artery stenosis relates to hyperplasia of the juxtaglomerular apparatus and the resulting increase in the production of renin, angiotensin II, and aldosterone. Whereas plasma renin activity is conspicuously increased in the renal vein from the ischemic kidney, the renin content of the venous blood from the contralateral kidney is reduced. Hypertension is reversible on reconstitution of the blood supply to the ischemic kidney, and in approximately half of the cases, hypertension is cured by surgical revascularization, angioplasty, or nephrectomy.

☐ **Pathology:** When vascular stenosis is related to atherosclerosis, aortic plaques impinge on the ostium and narrow the proximal portion of the renal artery. This occurs more frequently on the left than on the right, and typically, the size of the involved kidney is reduced only slightly. The glomeruli, arteries, and arterioles all appear to be normal. Focal tubular atrophy is often noted. The juxtaglomerular apparatus is prominent and demonstrates hyperplasia, increased granularity, and a greater length.

Bilateral Cortical Necrosis

■ *Bilateral cortical necrosis refers to necrosis of part, or all, of the renal cortex, with sparing of the medulla.* Historically, the most common clinical circumstance associated with renal cortical necrosis was premature separation of the placenta (abruptio placentae), which is a complication of the third trimester of pregnancy. Renal cortical necrosis can also complicate any clinical condition that is associated with hypovolemic or endotoxic shock.

☐ **Pathogenesis:** The lesion of cortical necrosis is ischemic in origin. The vasa recta that supply arterial blood to the medulla arise from the arcuate and juxtamedullary interlobular arteries, proximal to the vessels supplying the outer cortex. Thus, occlusion of the outer cortical vessels by vasospasm or fibrin thrombi leads to cortical necrosis, with sparing of the medulla.

☐ **Pathology:** The extent of necrosis varies from focal to patchy to confluent. In the mildest variety, scattered areas of cortical necrosis less than 1 mm in diameter are seen. Within these foci, necrosis of some of the glomeruli, with thrombosis of the vascular pole, occurs. The proximal convoluted tubules are invariably necrotic, as are most of the distal tubules. In the viable portions of the cortex, the glomeruli and distal convoluted tubules are unaffected, but many of the proximal convoluted tubules are necrotic.

With more extensive necrosis, the cortex shows a marked pallor on gross examination (Fig. 16-29), and larger areas of necrosis involving both glomeruli and tubules are seen on microscopic examination. In those cases in which necrosis is confluent, the cortex is diffusely necrotic bilaterally, except for thin rims of viable tissue immediately beneath the capsule and at the corticomedullary junction.

Clinically, severe cortical necrosis leads to acute renal failure, which is indistinguishable from that produced by acute tubular necrosis.

DISEASES OF THE TUBULES AND INTERSTITIUM

■ *Tubulointerstitial diseases are characterized by injury to the renal tubules and an inflammatory infiltrate in the interstitium.* These disorders are caused by many different agents. Patients often demonstrate defects in tubular function, including (1) an inability to concentrate urine, (2) salt wasting, and (3) metabolic acidosis.

Pyelonephritis and Urinary Tract Infection

■ *Pyelonephritis is a combined inflammation of the parenchyma, calyces, and renal pelvis that is caused by a bacterial infection.*

Acute Pyelonephritis

☐ **Pathogenesis:** Development of ascending acute pyelonephritis depends on four factors:

- A source of pathogenic micro-organisms
- Infection of the urine
- Reflux of the infected urine up the ureters and into the renal pelvis and calyces
- Entry of the bacteria through the papillae and into the renal parenchyma

Normally, the urine is sterile. In some women who seem to be unusually vulnerable to recurrent attacks of acute pyelonephritis, however, fecal organisms gain entry to the urethra from the perineum and vestibule of the vagina. Thus, the most common offending organism is *E. coli.* The higher incidence of bladder infections in women may be related, in part, to the short urethra. In some cases, catheterization of the urinary bladder carries organisms into the bladder.

Increased Residual Urine. During micturition, the bladder normally empties completely, except for 2 to 3 mL of residual urine. The subsequent addition of sterile urine from the kidneys ordinarily dilutes any bacteria that may have found their way into the bladder. However, under some circumstances, the residual urine volume is increased—for example, in cases of prostatic obstruction or of an atonic bladder caused by neurogenic disorders (e.g., paraplegia or diabetic neuropathy). As a result, the bladder contents are not sufficiently diluted with sterile urine from the kidneys to prevent the accumulation of bacteria. The glycosuria of diabetes further predisposes to infection by providing a rich medium for bacterial growth. Asymptomatic bacteriuria occurs in as many as 10% of pregnant women, and one-fourth of these women develop acute pyelonephritis, presumably because of an increased residual urine volume.

Bladder Reflux. Bacteria in the bladder urine usually do not gain access to the kidneys. The ureter commonly inserts into the bladder wall at a steep angle (Fig. 16-30) and, in its most distal portion, courses parallel to the bladder wall, between the mucosa and the muscu-

laris. The intravesicular pressure produced by micturition occludes the distal lumen of the ureter, thereby preventing the reflux of urine. In many persons who are particularly susceptible to ascending pyelonephritis, an abnormally short passage of the ureter within the bladder wall is associated with an angle of insertion that is more perpendicular to the mucosal surface of the bladder. Thus, on micturition, rather than occluding the lumen, intravesicular pressure instead forces urine into the patent ureter. This reflux is sufficiently powerful to force the urine into the renal pelvis and calyces.

Interstitial Infection. Even when present in the calyces, bacteria are not necessarily carried into the renal parenchyma by the reflux pressure. The simple papillae of the central calyces are convex and do not readily admit reflux urine (see Fig. 16-30). By contrast, the concave shape of the peripheral compound papillae allows easier access to the collecting system. However, if the pressure is prolonged, as in obstructive uropathy, even the simple papillae are eventually rendered vulnerable to the retrograde entry of urine. Then, from the collecting tubules, the bacteria gain access to the interstitial tissue of the kidney.

Hematogenous Pyelonephritis. The majority of the cases of acute pyelonephritis stem from ascending infection, but under some circumstances, and with certain organisms, blood-borne pathogens can become resident in the kidney. For example, gram-positive organisms (e.g., staphylococci) can disseminate from an infected valve in patients with bacterial endocarditis and establish a focus of infection in the kidney. In such cases, the cortex is more commonly the site of infection rather than the medulla and pyramids.

☐ **Pathology:** On gross examination, the kidneys of acute pyelonephritis may have small abscesses on the subcapsular surface. In areas where there has been severe reflux or obstruction, the cortex is thinned, and the papillae are blunted. Most infections involve only one or two papillary systems. Microscopically, the parenchyma, particularly the cortex, may be extensively destroyed by the acute inflammatory process, although vessels and glomeruli often show some resistance to infection. Collecting ducts, extending from the cortex into the medulla, are often filled with neutrophils (Fig. 16-31). Fewer neutrophils, together with lymphocytes and plasma cells, are typically present in the interstitium.

In severe cases of acute pyelonephritis, necrosis of the papillary tips may occur (Fig. 16-32). **Papillary necrosis** is most common in elderly patients with diabetes and acute pyelonephritis secondary to urinary obstruction. Acute pyelonephritis is a focal disease, and much of the kidney often appears to be normal.

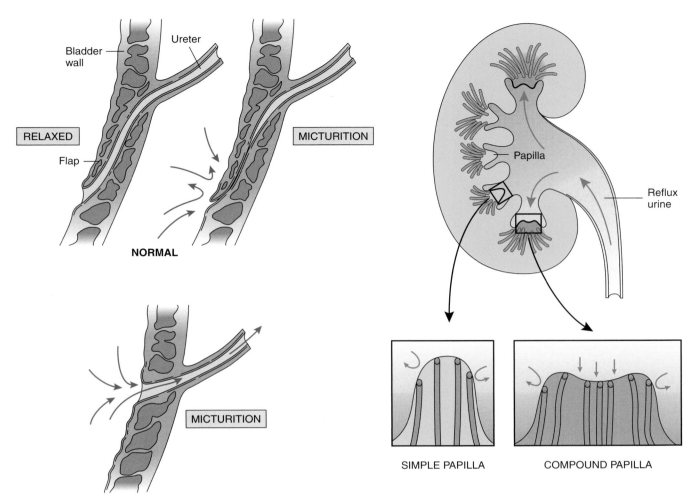

Bladder wall
Ureter
RELAXED
Flap
MICTURITION
NORMAL

Papilla

Reflux urine

MICTURITION

SHORT INTRAVESICAL URETER

SIMPLE PAPILLA   COMPOUND PAPILLA

FIGURE *16-30*
Anatomical features of the bladder and kidney in pyelonephritis caused by ureterovesical reflux. In the normal bladder, the distal portion of the intravesical ureter courses between the mucosa and the muscularis, forming a mucosal flap. On micturition, the elevated intravesicular pressure compresses the flap against the bladder wall, thereby occluding the lumen. Persons with a congenitally short intravesical ureter have no mucosal flap, because the angle of entry of the ureter into the bladder approaches a right angle. Thus, micturition forces urine into the ureter. In the renal pelvis, simple papillae of the central calyces are convex and do not readily allow reflux of urine. By contrast, the peripheral compound papillae are concave and permit entry of refluxed urine.

◻ **Clinical Features:** Symptoms of acute pyelonephritis include costovertebral angle tenderness and systemic evidence of infection, such as fever and malaise. The peripheral leukocyte count is often elevated. The finding of leukocyte casts in the urine is diagnostic of pyelonephritis.

Chronic Pyelonephritis

■ *Chronic pyelonephritis is a chronic tubulointerstitial disorder with gross, irregular, and often asymmetric scarring together with deformation of the calyces and the overly-*

ing parenchyma. It often progresses to so-called end-stage kidney—that is, a shrunken and fibrotic kidney that is insufficient to maintain renal function. In fact, 15% of patients referred for renal dialysis or transplantation suffer from chronic pyelonephritis.

◻ **Pathogenesis:** The relationship of tubulointerstitial damage to the calyx in patients with chronic pyelonephritis cannot be overemphasized. Tubular atrophy and interstitial fibrosis can result from a number of conditions, but only chronic pyelonephritis and analgesic nephropathy produce calyceal deformity

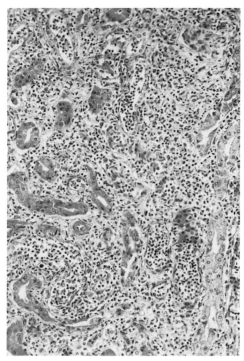

FIGURE *16-31*
Acute pyelonephritis. A light micrograph shows an extensive infiltrate of neutrophils in the collecting tubules and interstitial tissue.

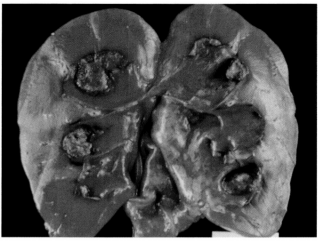

FIGURE *16-32*
Papillary necrosis. This bisected kidney shows a dilated renal pelvis and calyces secondary to urinary tract obstruction. The papillae are all necrotic and appear as sharply demarcated, ragged, and yellowish areas.

with overlying corticomedullary scarring. Chronic pyelonephritis is caused by recurrent and persistent bacterial infection secondary to obstruction of the urinary tract obstruction, reflux of urine, or both (Fig. 16-30).

Chronic pyelonephritis is divided into those cases with some form of obstruction and those cases without (Fig. 16-33). The large majority of cases without obstruction are associated with vesicoureteral reflux (so-called **reflux nephropathy**). In cases with mechanical obstruction, the pathologic changes result from a combination of obstruction and infection.

☐ **Pathology:** In obstructive uropathy, all of the calyces and the renal pelvis are dilated, and the parenchyma is uniformly thinned, a condition termed **hydronephrosis.** In cases associated with vesicoureteral reflux, calyces at the poles of the kidney are preferentially expanded and associated with overlying discrete, coarse scars, which cause an indentation of the renal surface. Microscopically, the scars are composed of atrophic dilated tubules that are surrounded by interstitial fibrous tissue (Fig. 16-34). The glomeruli may be completely uninvolved, have periglomerular fibrosis, or be sclerotic. The most characteristic tubular change is severe atrophy of the epithelium, with diffuse, eosinophilic, hyaline casts. Such tubules, which

are pinched-off spherical segments, resemble colloid-containing thyroid follicles, a pattern termed *thyroidization.* A mixed inflammatory infiltrate of lymphocytes and macrophages is seen, especially early during the course of the disease.

Acute Tubular Necrosis

■ *Acute tubular necrosis (ATN) is a severe, but potentially reversible, impairment of tubular epithelial function that is caused by ischemia or toxic injury and that results in acute renal failure.* As noted earlier, **acute renal failure** is a clinical term that defines an acute decline in the glomerular filtration rate, oliguria, and sometimes, anuria, with a rise in the blood urea nitrogen and serum creatinine levels.

Acute renal failure has three general types:

- **Prerenal** acute renal failure most often results from a fall in renal blood flow caused by systemic hypotension or hypovolemia, such as occurs with bacterial sepsis, severe trauma, extensive burns, or any situation that produces shock.
- **Postrenal** acute renal failure relates to urinary tract obstruction (e.g., tumors, benign prostatic hyperplasia, blood clots), which must involve both ureters or the common lower urinary outflow tract to produce acute renal failure.
- **Intrarenal** acute renal failure may result from a lesion in any part of the kidney, including (1) glomeruli (rapidly progressive glomerulonephritis), (2) blood vessels (e.g., malignant hypertension, disseminated intravascular coagulation,

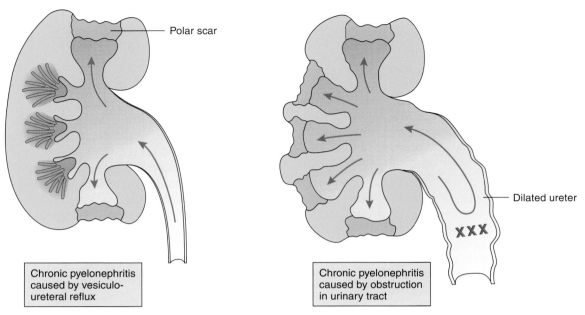

Polar scar

Dilated ureter

Chronic pyelonephritis
caused by vesiculo-
ureteral reflux

Chronic pyelonephritis
caused by obstruction
in urinary tract

FIGURE   16-33
The two major types of chronic pyelonephritis. (Left) Vesicoureteral reflux causes infection of the peripheral compound papillae and, therefore, scars in the poles of the kidney. (Right) Obstruction of the urinary tract leads to high-pressure backflow of urine, which causes infection of all papillae, diffuse scarring of the kidney, and thinning of the cortex.

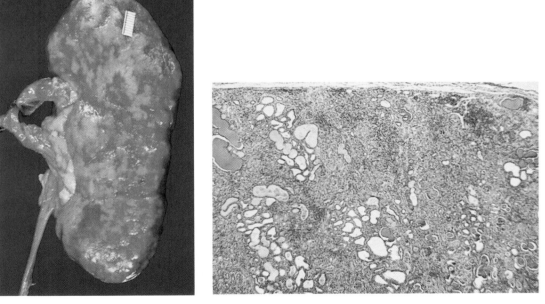

A

B

FIGURE   16-34
Chronic pyelonephritis. (A) The cortical surface contains many irregular, depressed scars (*reddish areas*). (B) A light micrograph shows tubular dilatation and atrophy, with many tubules containing eosinophilic hyaline casts that resemble the colloid of thyroid follicles (so-called "thyroidization"). The interstitium is scarred and contains a chronic inflammatory cell infiltrate.

hemolytic-uremic syndrome), and (3) interstitium and tubules (e.g., acute tubular necrosis, allergic acute interstitial nephritis).

Ischemic Acute Tubular Necrosis

Ischemic acute tubular necrosis (ATN) occurs most often in response to shock or dehydration, but it may also result from other causes, including hepatorenal syndrome and sepsis. The renal tubules are injured, and renal function does not quickly return to normal when the circulatory problem is corrected.

☐ **Pathogenesis:** The main factor responsible for the increased blood urea nitrogen and serum creatinine levels in patients with ischemic ATN is a reduction in the glomerular filtration rate (Fig. 16-35) owing to tubular obstruction and arteriolar vasoconstriction. Arteriolar vasoconstriction may also reduce the pressure difference that drives filtration and, thus, the glomerular filtration rate.

☐ **Pathology:** On gross examination, the kidneys in patients with ischemic ATN are swollen and reveal a pale cortex and congested medulla. By light microscopy, there are no pathologic changes in the glomeruli and vessels. Tubules typically show the following changes:

- **"Distalization" (Simplification) of Proximal Tubules.** The proximal tubules are dilated, with flattening of the epithelium and loss of the brush border. It is, therefore, difficult to distinguish proximal from distal tubules.
- **Single Cell Necrosis with Denudation of the Basement Membrane.** "Necrosis" is subtle and is reflected in individual necrotic cells within some proximal or distal tubules that are shed into the tubular lumen. As a result, focal denudation of the tubular basement membrane occurs.
- **Granular Casts.** Tubules, particularly distal tubules, are dilated and frequently contain granular casts.
- **Nucleated Cells in the Vasa Recta.** Capillaries (vasa recta) of the outer medulla frequently contain mononuclear leukocytes.

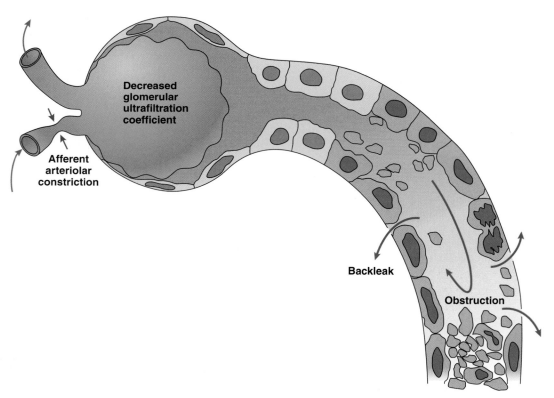

FIGURE *16-35*
Pathogenesis of acute tubular necrosis. Sloughing and necrosis of epithelial cells result in cast formation. The presence of casts leads to obstruction and increased intraluminal pressure, which reduce glomerular filtration. Afferent arteriolar vasoconstriction, caused in part by tubuloglomerular feedback, results in decreased glomerular capillary filtration pressure. Tubular injury and increased intraluminal pressure cause fluid backleak from the lumen into the interstitium.

- **Regenerative Changes of the Tubular Epithelium.** During the recovery phase of ATN, tubular epithelium regenerates, thereby leading to the appearance of mitoses, increased size of cells and nuclei, and cell crowding.

Toxic Acute Tubular Necrosis

Toxins known to cause ATN include heavy metals, antibiotics, certain radiolabeled contrast agents, organic solvents, and cyclosporin A.

Drug-Induced (Hypersensitivity) Acute Tubulointerstitial Nephritis

■ *Drug-induced acute nephritis is an acute inflammation of the tubules and interstitium that is characterized by infiltrating lymphocytes and eosinophils.* Unlike toxic mechanisms, hypersensitivity reactions are not dose-dependent. Drug-induced acute interstitial nephritis also differs from toxic ATN by showing considerably more interstitial inflammation. Drugs most commonly implicated in producing acute interstitial nephritis include nonsteroidal anti-inflammatory agents and certain antibiotics (synthetic penicillins, cephalosporins, sulfonamides).

☐ **Pathogenesis:** Acute drug-induced tubulointerstitial nephritis is characterized histologically by infiltrates of activated T lymphocytes and admixed eosinophils, a pattern that indicates a type IV cell-mediated immune response. The immunogen could be the drug itself, the drug bound to a certain tissue component, a drug metabolite, or a tissue component altered in response to the drug.

☐ **Pathology:** Microscopically, the interstitial inflammatory cell infiltrate is composed mainly of lymphocytes, with a small yet significant number of eosinophils. Neutrophils are rare. Foci of granulomatous inflammation may be present, generally without multinucleated giant cells, except in the case of sulfonamides. The inflammatory infiltrate may be patchy and is often prominent at the corticomedullary junction, with little or no involvement of the medulla itself. Proximal and distal tubules are focally invaded by leukocytes ("tubulitis"), but glomeruli are generally not involved.

☐ **Clinical Features:** Drug-induced acute interstitial nephritis usually presents as acute renal failure, frequently with low-grade (below the nephrotic range) proteinuria. The urine contains erythrocytes, leukocytes, and sometimes, leukocyte casts. Renal symptoms typically begin approximately 2 weeks after drug administration is started. Symptoms of systemic hypersensitivity (e.g., fever and rash) may also be present. Eventually, most patients recover fully if the lesion is recognized early and the drug is discontinued.

Analgesic Nephropathy

■ *Analgesic nephropathy is chronic inflammation and scarring of the renal parenchyma caused by the use of analgesic drugs.* **It is most commonly caused by heavy use of analgesic compounds that contain phenacetin.** The minimal requirement for the development of renal damage is the consumption of 2 to 3 kg of phenacetin over a period of 3 years. The pathogenesis of analgesic nephropathy is not clear. Possibilities include a direct nephrotoxicity of phenacetin ingestion or ischemic damage as a result of drug-induced vascular changes.

☐ **Pathology:** During the advanced stages of chronic tubulointerstitial disease caused by analgesic abuse, both kidneys are shrunken equally. Retracted cortical scars overlie necrotic papillae. Nearly all the papillae exhibit variable firmness and brownish discoloration, which are evidence of different stages of necrosis. Early microscopic changes are confined to the papillae and the inner medulla and consist of patchy necrosis of the loops of Henle and focal widening of the interstitium. These necrotic areas eventually become confluent and extend to the corticomedullary junction, after which the collecting ducts become involved. There are characteristically few inflammatory cells around the necrotic foci. Eventually, the entire papilla becomes necrotic, often remaining in place as a structureless mass.

Multiple Myeloma Cast Nephropathy

■ *Multiple myeloma cast nephropathy refers to renal injury caused by monoclonal immunoglobulin-like chains in the urine that produce tubular epithelial injury and numerous tubular casts.*

Circulating light chains filtered by the glomeruli are believed to cause the illness. At the acidic pH typical of urine, light chains are likely to precipitate and cause tubular damage and obstruction.

☐ **Pathology:** Microscopically, the characteristic tubular lesion associated with multiple myeloma consists of numerous dense, lamellated, and fractured casts in the distal and collecting tubules (Fig. 16-36). These casts are brightly eosinophilic and refractile, and are sometimes surrounded by multinucleated giant cells. Immunohistochemical staining shows that the casts contain light-chain material, usually κ light chains. Interstitial infiltrates of chronic inflammatory cells, as well as interstitial edema, typically accompany the tubular lesions.

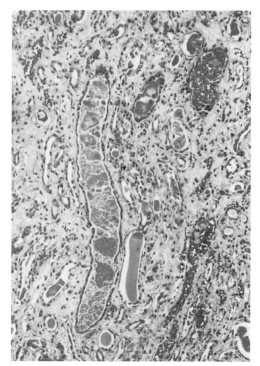

FIGURE   *16-36*
Light-chain cast nephropathy. A light micrograph shows the broad, dense, and fractured casts that are typical of this entity.

Myeloma cast nephropathy may present as either acute or chronic renal failure. Proteinuria is present, although usually not in the nephrotic range, and most often consists predominantly of immunoglobulin light chains.

Urate Nephropathy

■ *Urate nephropathy refers to renal disease caused by the deposition of uric acid crystals in the tubules and interstitium.* Any condition associated with elevated levels of uric acid in the blood may lead to urate nephropathy. The classic disease in this category is primary gout (see Chapter 26), but disorders in which hyperuricemia results from increased cell turnover (e.g., leukemia or polycythemia) are at least as common today. Chemotherapy for malignant tumors can result in a sudden increase in the blood uric acid level owing to the massive necrosis of cancer cells.

Acute urate nephropathy is often associated with the treatment of malignant diseases using cytotoxic agents. Hepatic catabolism of large amounts of purines released from the DNA of necrotic cells leads to hyperuricemia. Acute renal failure reflects obstruction of the collecting ducts by uric acid crystals, whose precipitation is promoted by the acidic pH of the urine.

Chronic tubulointerstitial urate nephropathy is associated with chronic gout and is caused by the tubular and interstitial deposition of crystalline monosodium urate.

□ **Pathology:** In patients with acute urate nephropathy, the precipitated uric acid in the collecting ducts is seen grossly as yellow streaks in the papillae. Histologically, the tubular deposits appear to be amorphic, but in frozen sections, the crystalline structure is apparent (Fig. 16-37). The tubules proximal to the obstruction are dilated.

The basic disease process of chronic urate nephropathy is similar to that of the acute form, but the prolonged course results in more substantial deposition of urate crystals in the interstitium, interstitial fibrosis, and cortical atrophy. Although renal lesions are found in most persons with chronic gout, significantly compromised renal function is seen in fewer than half of such cases.

HYDRONEPHROSIS

■ *Hydronephrosis is defined as dilatation of the renal pelvis and calyces, flattening of the papillae, and in chronic cases, atrophy of the renal cortex* (Fig. 16-38). Hydronephrosis is always the result of urinary tract obstruction, whether from tumors, stones, or some other cause. The causes of urinary tract obstruction are discussed in detail in Chapter 17.

In early hydronephrosis, the most prominent microscopic finding is dilatation of the collecting ducts, followed by dilatation of the proximal and the distal convoluted tubules. Eventually, the proximal tubules

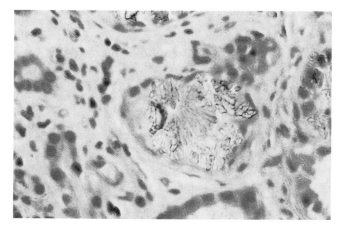

FIGURE   *16-37*
Urate nephropathy. A frozen section demonstrates tubular deposits of uric acid crystals.

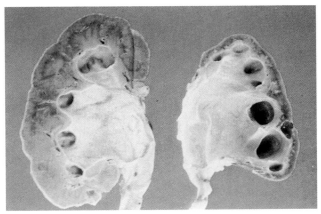

FIGURE   16-38
Hydronephrosis. Bilateral urinary tract obstruction has led to a conspicuous dilatation of the ureters, pelves, and calyces. The kidney on the right shows severe cortical atrophy.

become widely dilated, and loss of tubules is common. Interestingly, the glomeruli are usually spared. In patients who are left untreated, atrophy of an obstructed kidney is inevitable. In the case of bilateral obstruction, chronic renal failure ensues.

RENAL STONES (NEPHROLITHIASIS AND UROLITHIASIS)

■ *Nephrolithiasis and urolithiasis refer to stones within the collecting system of the kidney (nephrolithiasis) or elsewhere in the collecting system of the urinary tract (urolithiasis).* The pelvis and calyces of the kidney are common sites for the formation and accumulation of calculi. For reasons still unknown, renal stones are more common in men than in women. They vary in size from gravel (diameter, <1 mm) to a large stone that dilates the entire renal pelvis.

- **Calcium Stones.** The most common stone contains calcium complexed with oxalate, phosphate, or a mixture of these anions.
- **Magnesium Ammonium Phosphate Stones.** In the presence of infection with urea-splitting bacteria, the resulting alkaline urine favors precipitation of magnesium ammonium phosphate (struvite) stones. These stones vary in consistency from hard to soft and friable and, occasionally, fill the pelvis and calyces to form a cast of these spaces (**staghorn calculi**) (Fig. 16-39).
- **Uric Acid Stones.** These stones occur in 25% of patients with gout. The stones are smooth, hard, and yellow, and are usually less than 2 cm in diameter.

☐ **Pathogenesis:** In most cases, a renal stone is associated with an increased blood level and increased urinary excretion of its principal component. This is clearly the case with uric acid. In many patients with calcium stones, however, hypercalciuria is found in the absence of hypercalcemia. The mechanism underlying **idiopathic hypercalciuria** is not firmly established, but it has been linked to increased intestinal absorption of calcium and decreased reabsorption of calcium in the proximal tubules.

☐ **Clinical Features:** Kidney stones may be well tolerated, but in some cases, they lead to severe hydronephrosis and pyelonephritis. Moreover, they can erode the mucosa of the renal pelvis and cause hematuria. Passage of a stone into the ureter causes excruciating flank pain, termed **renal colic.** Until recently, most kidney stones required surgical methods for their removal, but today, ultrasonic disintegration (lithotripsy) and endoscopic removal are often effective alternatives.

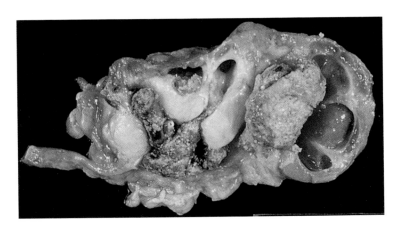

FIGURE   16-39
Staghorn calculi. The kidney shows hydronephrosis and stones, which are casts of the dilated calyces.

WILMS TUMOR (NEPHROBLASTOMA)

■ *Wilms tumor (nephroblastoma) is a malignant neoplasm of embryonal nephrogenic elements that is composed of mixtures of blastemal, stromal, and epithelial tissues.* It is one of the most common solid tumors in very young children and usually presents before the age of 4 years, although it is occasionally seen in adults. The large majority (99%) of all cases are sporadic, and the few familial cases exhibit autosomal dominant inheritance. Approximately 10% of sporadic Wilms tumors seem to be related to loss of suppressor gene activity. The gene (*WT-1*) is located on chromosome 11 (11p13). Another gene (*WT-2*), which is located close to *WT-1*, has also been found to be muted in cases of sporadic tumors.

☐ **Pathology:** A Wilms tumor is usually large, with a bulging, pale-tan, cut surface enclosed within a thin rim of renal cortex and capsule (Fig. 16-40). Histologically, the tumor is composed of elements that resemble three types of normal tissue: (1) metanephric blastema, (2) immature stroma (mesenchymal tissue), and (3) immature epithelial elements (Fig. 16-41). The component corresponding to blastema is composed of small ovoid cells, with a scanty cytoplasm and growing in nests and trabeculae. The epithelial component presents as small tubular structures, and occasionally, immature elements resembling glomeruli are found. The stroma between the other elements is composed of undifferentiated spindle cells. Bone, cartilage, adipocytes, and striated muscle cells are occasionally encountered as well.

☐ **Clinical Features:** Most children with Wilms tumor present with a large abdominal mass that is occa-sionally accompanied by abdominal pain or intestinal obstruction. Patients younger than 2 years of age tend to have a better prognosis. Chemotherapy and radiation therapy, combined with surgical resection, have dramatically improved the outlook for patients with this tumor. Many centers now report an overall long-term survival rate of 90%.

RENAL CELL CARCINOMA

■ *Renal cell adenocarcinoma, the most important neoplasm of the kidney, is a malignant tumor derived from the epithelial cells of the renal tubules.* This tumor accounts for 90% of all renal cancers in adults. The incidence of renal cell carcinoma peaks during the sixth decade of life and is twice as frequent in men as in women.

☐ **Pathogenesis:** Cigarette smoking is associated with an increased risk of renal cell carcinoma, and it is estimated that one-fourth to one-third of these tumors are directly caused by smoking. Obesity, particularly in women, has been associated with an increased risk of kidney cancer. Renal cell carcinoma has also been linked to analgesic nephropathy. Both inherited and acquired cystic diseases of the kidney may be complicated by development of a renal cell carcinoma.

Renal cell carcinoma is also associated with von Hippel-Lindau disease, an autosomal dominant, hereditary disorder that is characterized by retinal angiomas and hemangioblastomas in the brain. In both conditions, deletion of a gene (*VHL*) on chromosome 3 has been found.

☐ **Pathology:** Renal cell carcinomas are typically yellow-orange and often show conspicuous focal hem-

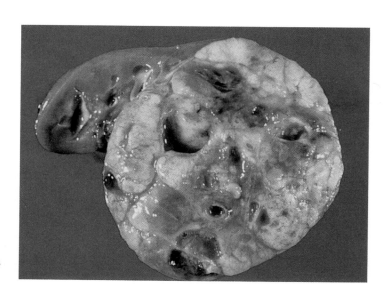

FIGURE *16-40*
Wilms tumor. A cross-section of a pale-tan neoplasm is attached to a residual portion of the kidney.

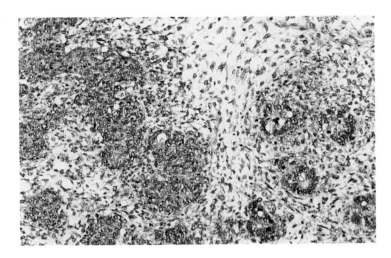

FIGURE *16-41*
Wilms tumor (nephroblastoma). This photomicrograph of the tumor depicted in Figure 16-41 shows highly cellular areas composed of undifferentiated blastema, loose stroma containing undifferentiated mesenchymal cells, and immature tubules.

orrhage and necrosis (Fig. 16-42). The tumors are solid or focally cystic. Histologic patterns are variable, and solid, alveolar, and tubular patterns of growth are common. The most frequent and characteristic neoplastic cell has an unusually clear cytoplasm (Fig. 16-43) owing to the removal of glycogen and lipids by the water and organic solvents used in preparation of the tissue. Frequently, there is little cellular or nuclear pleomorphism, although anaplastic sarcomatoid variants do occur.

Small tumors that appear microscopically to be well-differentiated renal cell carcinomas are often specifically referred to as **renal cell adenomas.** Because distant metastases have been documented from tumors with a diameter as small as 1 cm, it is generally believed that all such tumors, regardless of their size, should be considered as potentially malignant.

☐ **Clinical Features:** Hematuria is the single most common presenting sign; the classic triad of hematuria, flank pain, and palpable abdominal mass is found in less than 10% of patients. Renal cell carcinoma is a potential source of ectopic hormone production and is frequently associated with paraneoplastic syndromes.

The overall survival rate in of patients with renal cell carcinoma is 40% at 5 years. Distant metastases are found most frequently in the lung and in bone. Treatment is essentially limited to complete operative removal.

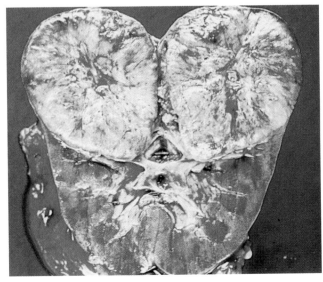

FIGURE   *16-42*
Renal cell carcinoma. This bisected kidney discloses a circumscribed, tannish-yellow tumor in the upper pole.

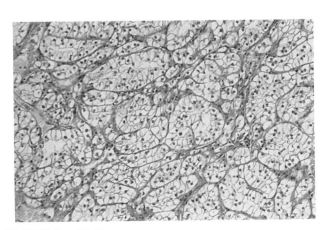

FIGURE   *16-43*
Renal cell carcinoma. Photomicrograph showing rounded collections of neoplastic cells with abundant clear cytoplasm.

CHAPTER 17

The Urinary Tract and Male Reproductive System

Robert O. Petersen

Nodular Hyperplasia (Benign Prostatic Hyperplasia)	Phimosis
Prostatic Adenocarcinoma	**Condyloma Acuminatum (Venereal Warts)**
Treatment	**Squamous Cell Carcinoma In Situ**
PENIS	**Verrucous Carcinoma**
Congenital Disorders	**Squamous Cell Carcinoma**

Renal Pelvis and Ureter

CONGENITAL DISORDERS

Ectopic Ureter. A ureter may have a distal terminus that is located somewhere other than the normal posterolateral wall of the urinary bladder, including the proximal urethra, ejaculatory duct, seminal vesicle, and vas deferens.

Ureteropelvic Junction Obstruction. The most common cause of hydronephrosis in both infants and children is ureteropelvic junction obstruction. Abnormal smooth muscle function of the ureteral wall or mechanical factors (e.g., unusual insertion of the ureter into the renal pelvis or aberrant renal vessels) have been documented in some cases.

Congenital Megaureter. The markedly enlarged ureter is associated with hydronephrosis and, if the structural defect is not corrected, eventual functional impairment of the kidney.

URETERAL OBSTRUCTION

Obstruction to the flow of urine in the ureter results in hydroureter, hydronephrosis, and functional impairment of the kidney. The causes of ureteral obstruction are either intrinsic or extrinsic to the ureter (Fig. 17-1). Proximal causes tend to be unilateral, whereas more distal causes, such as prostatic hyperplasia, tend to cause bilateral hydronephrosis, with the possibility of renal failure in untreated cases.

TRANSITIONAL CELL CARCINOMA

Tumors arising in the upper urinary tract (renal pelvis and ureter) are uncommon and most frequently (90%) transitional cell carcinoma. Patients, usually in their sixth and seventh decades of life, present with flank pain and hematuria. Transitional cell carcinoma of the ureter or renal pelvis requires radical nephroureterectomy.

Urinary Bladder

EXSTROPHY

■ *Exstrophy of the bladder is a developmental abnormality characterized by the absence of a portion of the lower abdominal wall and the anterior wall of the bladder.* This anomaly allows eversion of the posterior wall of the bladder through the defect.

☐ **Pathology:** Abrasion by clothing and the continuous escape of urine result in chronic infection of the bladder mucosa. The externalized mucosa exhibits both acute and chronic inflammation and metaplastic changes, most frequently squamous and glandular metaplasia. Although the congenital defect may be surgically repaired, the inflammation and the established metaplastic changes in the bladder mucosa tend to persist.

☐ **Clinical Features:** The condition of the patient with an uncorrected exstrophic bladder is lamentable. There is continuous leakage of urine, persistent or recurrent local infection, and increased risk of ascending urinary tract infection. Moreover, there is a substantial incidence of neoplastic transformation of the metaplastic urothelium, with resultant adenocarcinoma, squamous cell carcinoma, and least frequently, transitional cell carcinoma.

CYSTITIS

Acute and Chronic Cystitis

■ *Cystitis refers to inflammation of the urinary bladder and is the most commonly encountered clinical disorder of this organ.*

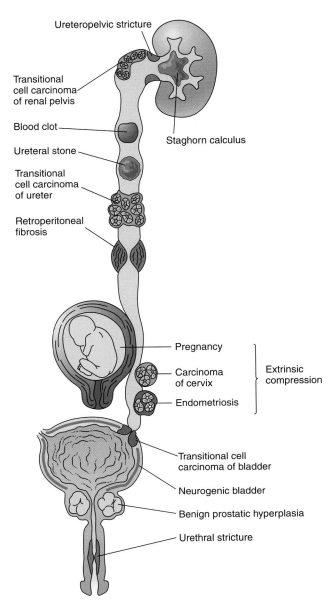

FIGURE **17-1**
Causes of ureteral obstruction.

□ **Pathogenesis:** In most cases, cystitis is secondary to infection of the bladder. Factors related to bladder infection and development of cystitis include the age and sex of the patient, the presence of bladder calculi, bladder outlet obstruction, diabetes mellitus, immunodeficiency, previous instrumentation or catheterization, and radiation therapy or chemotherapy. The risk of cystitis in females is increased because of the short urethra, especially during pregnancy. Bladder outlet obstruction associated with prostatic hyperplasia predisposes men to cystitis. Introduction of pathogens into the bladder may also occur during instrumentation (cystoscopy) and is particularly common among patients in whom indwelling catheters remain for prolonged periods. In the large majority of cases, coliform

bacteria, most frequently *Escherichia coli*, *Proteus*, *Pseudomonas*, and *Enterobacter*, are the cause of cystitis.

□ **Pathology:** Stromal edema and a neutrophilic infiltrate of variable intensity are typical of acute cystitis. Lack of resolution of the inflammatory reaction is associated with the hallmarks of chronic inflammation, including a predominance of lymphocytes and fibrosis of the lamina propria.

□ **Clinical Features:** Virtually all patients with acute or chronic cystitis complain of an excessive frequency of urination, pain on urination (dysuria), and lower abdominal or pelvic discomfort. Examination of the urine usually reveals inflammatory cells, and culture identifies the causative agent. Most cases of cystitis are treated with antimicrobial agents.

Chronic Interstitial Cystitis (Hunner Ulcer)

■ *Chronic interstitial cystitis is a disorder of unknown cause, typically affecting middle-aged women, that is characterized by transmural inflammation of the bladder wall and is occasionally associated with mucosal ulceration (Hunner ulcer).* The disease is typically persistent and refractory to all forms of therapy. Chronic inflammation and fibrosis are commonly observed within the muscularis. When present, a Hunner ulcer displays an intense, acute inflammatory reaction.

The most common symptoms of chronic interstitial cystitis are longstanding suprapubic pain, frequency, and urgency, with or without hematuria. Urine cultures are usually negative.

Malakoplakia

■ *Malakoplakia is an uncommon inflammatory disorder of unknown cause that features macrophage-containing mucosal plaques.* There is a marked preponderance of cases in women, mostly in their fifth to seventh decades of life. Malakoplakia is often associated with an infection of the urinary tract by *E. coli*, although a direct causal relationship is dubious. A clinical background of immunosuppression, chronic infections, or cancer is common.

□ **Pathology:** Malakoplakia is characterized by soft, yellow plaques on the mucosal surface of the bladder, measuring as large as 4 cm in diameter. Histologic examination reveals a chronic inflammatory cell infiltrate composed predominantly of large macrophages with abundant, eosinophilic cytoplasm containing periodic acid-Schiff–positive granules (von Hansemann cells). Some of these macrophages exhibit laminated, basophilic calcospherites termed **Michaelis-Gutmann bodies** (Fig. 17-2).

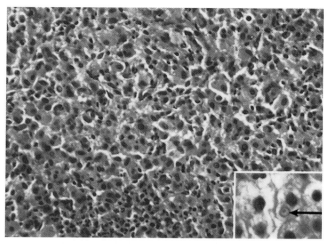

FIGURE *17-2*
Malakoplakia. Numerous Michaelis-Gutmann bodies are seen as well-defined, spherical structures in the cytoplasm. The background inflammatory cells are composed principally of macrophages, with fewer lymphocytes. (Inset) Michaelis-Gutmann body (*arrow*) is seen at high magnification.

The urinary bladder is the most common site of malakoplakia, with half of these cases occurring in this organ. This enigmatic disorder has also been reported in other regions of the genitourinary system, including the kidney, renal pelvis, ureter, testis, epididymis, and prostate. The clinical symptomatology of malakoplakia is nonspecific and suggests cystitis.

BLADDER OBSTRUCTION

Obstruction to the flow of urine from the bladder, most commonly as a result of prostatic hyperplasia in men and cystocele in women, is a far more common cause of hydronephrosis than obstruction of the upper urinary tract. Regardless of the cause of the obstruction, the bladder reacts in a similar manner, with dilatation, muscular hypertrophy, diverticula, and on gross examination, trabeculation of the mucosal surface.

BENIGN PROLIFERATIVE AND METAPLASTIC LESIONS

A spectrum of hyperplastic and metaplastic changes of the urothelium is observed throughout the urinary tract, from the renal pelvis to the urethra. These non-neoplastic lesions of the urothelium are characterized by either hyperplasia or combined hyperplasia and metaplasia (Fig. 17-3).

Simple hyperplasia refers to an increased number of cell layers in the mucosal transitional epithelium.

This change has a flat configuration, with neither papillary features nor invaginations into the lamina propria.

Brunn's buds are bulbous invaginations of the surface urothelium into the lamina propria.

Brunn's nests are similar to Brunn buds, but in this case, the urothelial cells have detached from the surface and are seen within the lamina propria.

Cystic lesions of the urinary tract (e.g., pyelitis cystica, ureteritis cystica, cystitis cystica) are characterized by small slits or round spaces in otherwise solid Brunn nests. Cystitis cystica is actually very common, occurring in 60% of otherwise normal adult bladders.

Cystitis glandularis refers to a lesion of the bladder mucosa characterized by metaplastic glandular structures lined by mucin-secreting columnar epithelial cells.

Squamous Metaplasia

The urinary tract may react to chronic injury and inflammation with squamous metaplasia, particularly when associated with calculi.

Nephrogenic Metaplasia

Nephrogenic metaplasia, which occurs most frequently in the urinary bladder, consists of a papillary exophytic nodule containing numerous small tubules clustered in the lamina propria. Nephrogenic metaplasia is often associated with chronic cystitis. It has no age predilection and is reported from infancy to the eighth decade of life. There is a pronounced male predominance (3 : 1). Transurethral resection is the most common form of therapy, but recurrences are not uncommon.

Patients with proliferative and metaplastic lesions of the urothelium have a significantly increased risk for the development of transitional cell carcinoma of the bladder and, in the case of cystitis glandularis, of adenocarcinoma as well. However, there is no evidence to suggest that these lesions are preneoplastic. Rather, persistence of the injury related to the development of proliferative and metaplastic urothelial lesions is more likely the important factor in the pathogenesis of bladder cancer.

TRANSITIONAL CELL CARCINOMA

Neoplastic transitional cell epithelial lesions arising from the bladder mucosa constitute a spectrum that be-

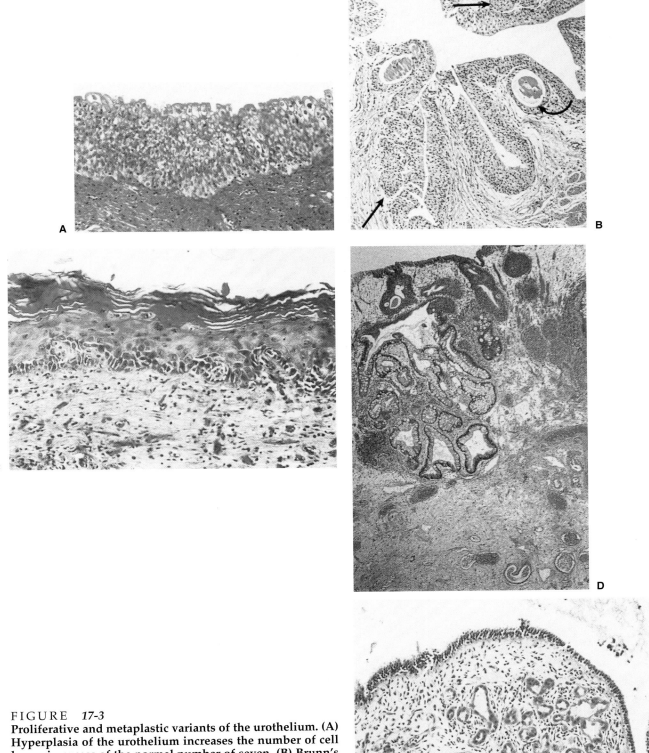

FIGURE 17-3
Proliferative and metaplastic variants of the urothelium. (A) Hyperplasia of the urothelium increases the number of cell layers in excess of the normal number of seven. (B) Brunn's nests (*straight arrows*) and ureteritis cystica (*curved arrow*) protrude into the lamina propria. (C) Squamous metaplasia has replaced the normal urothelium of the bladder. (D) Cystitis glandularis. (E) Nephrogenic metaplasia is characterized by clustered simple tubular structures lined by epithelium similar to that of the renal tubular epithelium.

gins with benign papillomatous lesions and extends through carcinoma in situ to invasive and metastatic transitional cell carcinomas. Any epithelial tumor in the bladder indicates a general propensity for further neoplastic transformation in other areas of the bladder mucosa. In other words, bladder tumors seem to arise against the background of an unstable urothelium.

The term **carcinoma in situ** is reserved for full-thickness, malignant changes confined to a flat (non-papillary) urothelium. The lesion is characterized by a urothelium of variable thickness that exhibits cellular atypia of the entire mucosa, from the basal layer to the surface (Fig. 17-4). In the absence of papillary carcinoma, carcinoma in situ of the bladder is associated with subsequent development of invasive carcinoma in one-third of the cases.

□ **Epidemiology:** The highest frequencies of bladder cancer are recorded among urban whites in the United States and Western Europe, whereas a low prevalence is recorded in Japan and among American blacks. Men are affected three- to fourfold as often as women. Bladder cancer may be encountered at any age, but most patients (80%) are between 50 and 80 years old.

□ **Pathogenesis:** The association of bladder cancer with occupational exposure to certain organic chemicals among workers in the German aniline dye industry was described in 1895, and it was subsequently confirmed among similar workers in the United States. Later, an increased risk of bladder cancer was identified among workers in the leather, rubber, paint, and organic chemical industries. Smoking has also been as-

sociated with a doubling of the incidence of bladder carcinoma. Transitional cell cancers of the bladder, ureters, and renal pelvis have been reported in the setting of analgesic abuse, particularly with phenacetin. Most cases, however, are not associated with known risk factors.

□ **Pathology:** Bladder cancer arises most frequently from the lateral walls and less often from the posterior wall. The tumors vary from small, delicate, and low-grade papillary lesions that are limited to the mucosal surface to larger, higher-grade, solid, and invasive masses that are often ulcerated (Fig. 17-5). Papillary and exophytic cancers tend to be more differentiated, whereas infiltrating tumors are usually more anaplastic. Histologically, transitional cell carcinomas are graded according to their degree of differentiation (Fig. 17-6).

□ **Clinical Features:** Transitional cell carcinoma of the bladder typically presents as sudden hematuria and, less frequently, as dysuria. Cystoscopy usually reveals single or multiple tumors. Noninvasive or superficially invasive transitional cell tumors are generally treated conservatively, even though as many as 30% of such patients eventually exhibit extension of the tumor. Patients with invasion of muscle or perivesical adipose tissue at the time of initial diagnosis often have regional lymph node metastases, with a median survival time of 1 year. In order of decreasing frequency, metastases of bladder cancer occur in the regional and periaortic lymph nodes, liver, lung, and bone. The most common causes of death are ureteral obstruction with uremia and carcinomatosis.

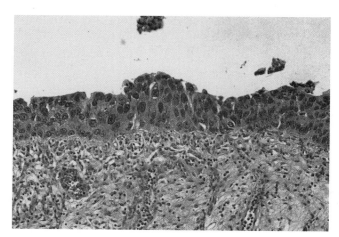

FIGURE **17-4**
Transitional cell carcinoma in situ. The urothelial mucosa shows nuclear pleomorphism and lack of polarity from the basal layer to the surface, without evidence of maturation.

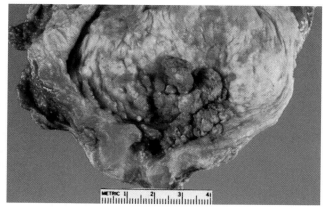

FIGURE **17-5**
Transitional cell carcinoma of the urinary bladder. A large exophytic tumor is situated above the bladder neck.

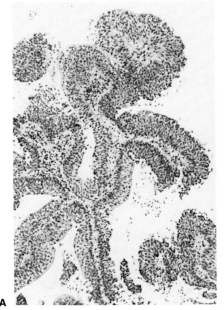

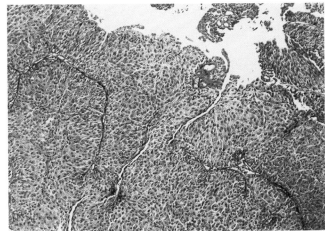

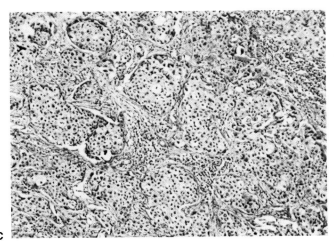

FIGURE 17-6
Transitional cell carcinoma, grades 1 through 3. (A) Grade 1: The papillary structures are covered by a thickened urothelium demonstrating only mild nuclear atypism. (B) Grade 2: This papillary neoplasm is characterized by nuclear pleomorphism and uncommon mitoses. (C) Grade 3: Marked nuclear pleomorphism and frequent mitoses, associated with blunting and fusing of the papillae, are present.

SQUAMOUS CELL CARCINOMA

Squamous cell carcinoma of the urinary bladder is distinctly uncommon in the Western world, whereas it is frequent in Egypt and other areas of the Middle East where schistosomiasis is endemic. Virtually all patients with squamous cell carcinoma demonstrate invasion of the bladder wall at the time of initial presentation and, thus, have a worse prognosis than the majority of patients with transitional cell carcinoma.

Urethra

URETHRITIS

The classic cause of urethritis is infection with *Neisseria gonorrhoeae*. However, urethritis today results more commonly from infection with *Chlamydia* sp., *E. coli*, or *Mycoplasma*. In males, urethritis typically complicates prostatitis, whereas in females, it follows cystitis. In many cases, no organisms can be identified. A complex of unknown cause is characterized by urethritis, arthritis, and conjunctivitis and is known as **Reiter syndrome.** Urinary frequency, dysuria, and urethral discharge characterize urethral inflammation regardless of the cause.

URETHRAL CARUNCLE

■ *Urethral caruncle is an inflammatory lesion near the female urethral meatus that produces pain and bleeding.* It occurs exclusively in women and most frequently after menopause. A urethral caruncle typically presents as an exophytic and often ulcerated polypoid mass, 1 to 2 cm in diameter, either at or near the urethral meatus. Histologically, caruncles exhibit acutely and chronically inflamed granulation tissue as well as ulceration

and hyperplasia of the transitional cell or squamous epithelium. Treatment is surgical excision.

Testis

CRYPTORCHIDISM

■ *Cryptorchidism refers to the failure of a testis to descend completely into its normal position within the scrotum.* Descent of the testis may be arrested at any point from the abdomen to the upper scrotum (Fig. 17-7). At term, 4% of male newborns are cryptorchid. In the large majority of these infants, however, the testis descends within the first year of life. Cryptorchidism is most commonly unilateral, but is bilateral in one-fourth of the cases.

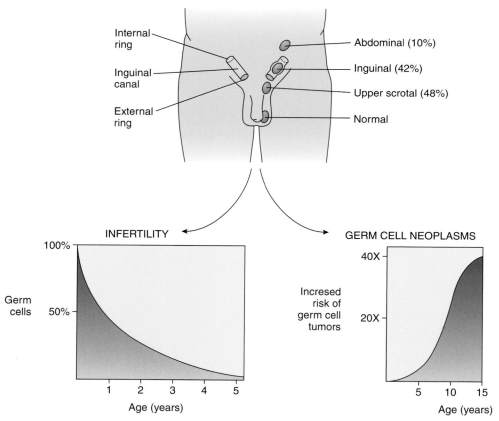

FIGURE *17-7*
Cryptorchidism and associated complications. There is a 50% reduction in germ cell number after the first year of life and a virtually complete loss by 4 to 5 years of age. After age 5, the risk of germ cell tumors increases steeply.

☐ **Pathology:** Histologic changes in the cryptorchid testis are related to age. From birth to 5 years, the earliest changes are reduced diameters of the seminiferous tubules and decreased numbers of germ cells. If surgical repositioning of the testis (orchiopexy) is delayed beyond puberty, a decreased number of germ cells, hyaline thickening of the tubular basement membrane, and stromal fibrosis are observed. Eventually, the tubules are reduced to hyalinized cords of connective tissue.

☐ **Clinical Features:** The risk of developing germ cell tumors in patients with untreated cryptorchidism, most commonly seminomas and embryonal carcinomas, is increased 35-fold. Germ cell tumors have not been reported among patients in whom orchiopexy was performed before 5 years of age; therefore, it is crucial to treat this disorder early. Adult men with untreated bilateral cryptorchidism are infertile. Orchiopexy before 2 years of age generally prevents this complication, but if surgery is postponed, only one-fourth of such patients will be fertile.

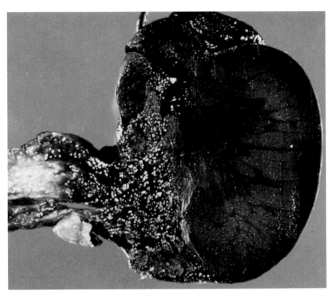

FIGURE   *17-8*

Testicular torsion. A cut section of the testicle from a man who experienced sudden, excruciating scrotal pain shows diffuse hemorrhage and necrosis of the testis and adnexal structures.

ORCHITIS

■ *Orchitis refers to acute or chronic inflammation of the testis, frequently in association with inflammation of the epididymis.* **Gram-negative bacterial orchitis** is the most common form of the disease, and it is often secondary to urinary tract infections. Syphilis and mumps can produce orchitis. **Granulomatous orchitis** of unknown cause is an infrequent disorder of middle-age men that presents as painful enlargement of the testis or insidiously with testicular induration.

TORSION OF THE TESTIS

Torsion of the spermatic cord, if complete, produces severe pain and infarction of the testicular germ cells within a few hours. Most commonly, torsion presents shortly after vigorous physical exercise, although such a history is not always obtained. Torsion of the spermatic cord is often associated with congenital abnormalities that contribute to increased mobility of the testis and epididymis (e.g., high attachment of the tunica vaginalis on the spermatic cord, incomplete descent of the testis, or absence of the scrotal ligaments).

An abrupt onset of scrotal pain followed by swelling heralds testicular torsion. The swollen, firm testis shows the gross and microscopic features of hemorrhagic infarction (Fig. 17-8).

GERM CELL TUMORS

Tumors of the testes are divided into two major histogenetic categories, namely germ cell tumors and gonadal stromal/sex cord tumors (Fig. 17-9). Tumors of germ cell origin constitute more than 90% of testicular tumors, and most of the remaining ones are of gonadal stromal/sex cord origin.

Germ cell tumors originate from the neoplastic transformation of germ cells and reflect their capacity to differentiate along many histogenetic lines. Thus, germ cell tumors are characterized by somatic differentiation, extraembryonic differentiation, or both. Alternatively, there is an absence of identifiable differentiation in some germ cell tumors.

☐ **Epidemiology:** High rates of testicular germ cell tumors are observed in the United States, in contrast to a low incidence in Japan. The frequency is consistently reported to be higher in whites than in blacks at all geographic locations. The incidence of germ cell tumors peaks in infants and children (teratomas, yolk sac tumors) and in adults during the third and fourth decades of life (principally seminomas). The frequency of these tumors declines after 40 years of age, although a modest increase occurs after the age of 50.

☐ **Histogenesis:** Neoplastic transformation of a germ cell gives rise to seminoma, undifferentiated tu-

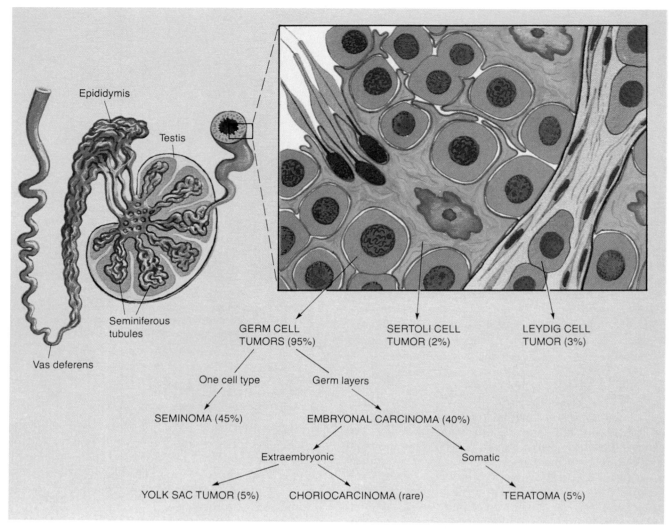

FIGURE   *17-9*
Histogenesis of testicular neoplasms.

mor, or embryonal carcinoma, which consists of totipotential cells. In turn, embryonal carcinoma may undergo somatic differentiation and become a teratoma. Alternatively, extraembryonic differentiation of an embryonal tumor results in a yolk sac tumor (endodermal sinus tumor) or a choriocarcinoma. Not uncommonly, germ cell tumors exhibit more than one type of differentiation, both within the primary testicular tumor and the metastatic sites. In addition, metastases of germ cell tumors may show a form of differentiation not present in the primary testicular tumor.

Germ cell tumors similar to those arising in the testis may occur in extragonadal sites, primarily in midaxial locations, such as the mediastinum and sacrococcygeal region. Such tumors are thought to reflect the neoplastic transformation of germ cells that mi-

grated from their endodermal yolk sac origin to these extragonadal sites.

Seminoma

Seminoma accounts for half of all germ cell tumors. This type of tumor is not found before puberty, and most patients are between 25 and 55 years of age. The peak incidence is in the fourth decade of life. Most seminomas are the so-called classic type, but two other, less common variants are also encountered.

On gross examination, classic seminoma is a solid, gray-white, poorly demarcated growth that tends to bulge from the cut surface of the testis (Fig. 17-10). Histologically, seminomas display solid nests of proliferating tumor cells between randomly scattered, thin,

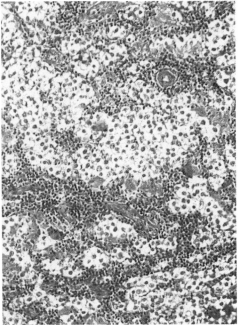
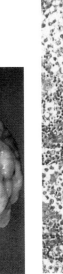

FIGURE   *17-10*
Classic seminoma. (A) The cut surface of the nodular tumor is tan and shows punctate hemorrhages in an otherwise solid mass. (B) Nests of tumor cells are confined by fibrous septa containing numerous lymphocytes.

fibrovascular trabeculae. The tumor cells have well-defined borders and clear cytoplasm, and the nuclei show limited pleomorphism and coarse granular chromatin. Typically, a lymphocytic infiltrate is present in the fibrovascular trabeculae. Classic seminomas are exquisitely sensitive to radiation, and in patients with localized tumors, radiation therapy has resulted in 5-year survival rates of 85% to 95%. Even in patients with more advanced cases, chemotherapy is curative in 90%.

Embryonal Carcinoma

Embryonal carcinoma is the second most common testicular germ cell tumor. As a rule, they do not occur before puberty, and most are found in persons between 20 and 35 years of age. The cut surface of the tumor discloses a gray-white, bulging, and poorly demarcated mass, with variable degrees of necrosis and hemorrhage. The tunica albuginea and epididymis are extensively invaded in 20% of the cases.

Embryonal carcinomas show variable histologic patterns. In many cases, they form sheets of cells, with clefts, acini, and papillary structures (Fig. 17-11). The cell borders are ill-defined, and the nuclei have prominent nucleoli and coarse chromatin. Cellular pleomorphism and mitoses are more prominent than in classic seminomas. Chemotherapy results in cure rates of 95% to 98% for localized embryonal carcinomas. Half of the

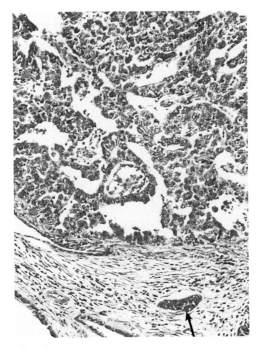

FIGURE   *17-11*
Embryonal carcinoma. A cystic space contains neoplastic cells that lack distinct cell membranes. A cluster of tumor cells is seen in a lymphatic (*arrow*).

patients with metastatic disease can expect a permanent cure.

Teratoma

■ *Testicular teratomas are germ cell tumors characterized by tissues from all three germ layers: (1) the ectoderm, (2) the endoderm, and (3) the mesoderm* (Fig. 17-12). They comprise almost half the germ cell tumors in infants and children but less than 5% of all germ cell tumors in adults.

- **Mature Teratoma.** This tumor is characteristically a solid, multicystic lesion that enlarges the testis. The cut surface displays mucinous cysts, and the solid foci often exhibit cartilaginous foci or, less frequently, bone formation. Mature teratomas are characterized by haphazard juxtaposition of a bewildering variety of cells and organoid structures, including neural elements, skeletal muscle, thyroid follicles, respiratory epithelium, cartilage, nests of squamous cells, and other tissues. The teratomatous elements are dispersed in a fibrous or myxoid stroma.

- **Immature Teratoma.** This tumor is much more common in adults than in children. The component tissues are less differentiated and more primitive than in mature teratomas.

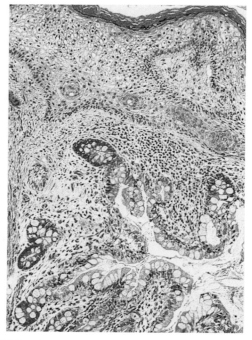

FIGURE 17-12
Teratoma. A cyst lined by well-differentiated squamous epithelium (*top*) is in proximity to a focus of endodermal glands that resembles colonic mucosa.

- **Teratoma with Malignant Transformation.** The presence of squamous cell carcinoma or a sarcomatous mesenchymal component identifies the malignant transformation of a teratoma.

The most important predictor for the biologic behavior of a testicular teratoma is the age of the patient. In adult men, mature teratomas that ordinarily would be interpreted as benign are commonly malignant and metastasize. In fact, all such tumors in the adult should be considered as potentially malignant. By contrast, teratomas in infants and children, even those with foci of immature cells, are invariably benign.

Yolk Sac Tumor (Endodermal Sinus Tumor)

Yolk sac tumors are the most common germ cell tumors in infants. The *terms endodermal sinus tumor* and *yolk sac tumor* reflect the histologic similarity of this tumor with normal structures of the rat placenta. These tumors enlarge the testis and appear grossly as poorly defined, lobulated masses. On cut section, the lesions tend to be yellow-gray, focally cystic, and solid masses of variable consistency. Focal areas of hemorrhage are common. Yolk sac tumors display a reticulated pattern of tumor cells, with multiple microcysts and papillary clusters, all against the background of a myxoid stroma. The tumor cells surround a characteristic structure, the Schiller-Duval body, which consists of a microcyst containing a glomerulus-like structure with a central fibrovascular core (Fig. 17-13). α-Fetoprotein and α_1-antitrypsin can be demonstrated in the cytoplasm. Yolk sac tumors in infants are removed by orchiectomy and ordinarily do not metastasize.

Testicular Choriocarcinoma

■ *Choriocarcinoma is a highly malignant testicular tumor that represents germ cell extraembryonic differentiation to the components of the placenta, namely syncytiotrophoblast and cytotrophoblast* (Fig. 17-14). The tumor is comparable to those arising from the placental tissue in pregnant women (see Chapter 18). Testicular choriocarcinoma often presents as a small, painless nodule in the testis, although on occasion, large, bulky tumors are encountered. The cut surface is typically necrotic and hemorrhagic.

Microscopically, the neoplastic syncytiotrophoblasts and cytotrophoblasts are usually found in the areas of hemorrhage. Syncytiotrophoblasts are large, multinucleated giant cells of irregular configuration, with abundant vacuolated cytoplasm that contains human chorionic gonadotropin. Cytotrophoblasts are polygonal cells, with round,

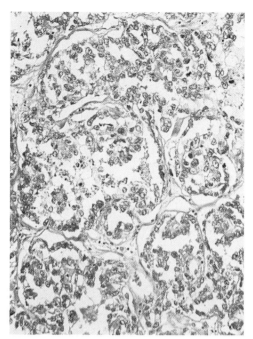

FIGURE   17-13
Yolk sac endodermal sinus tumor. The tumor is composed of dilated tubular spaces lined by flattened cells with an edematous stroma.

hyperchromatic nuclei and sparse cytoplasm, and are clustered with the syncytiotrophoblasts. The tumor is most frequently observed as a component of a mixed germ cell tumor.

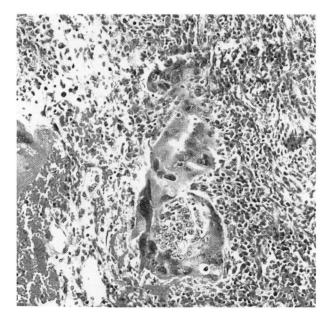

FIGURE   17-14
Testicular choriocarcinoma. The syncytiotrophoblast cell surrounds a cluster of cytotrophoblast cells. Hemorrhage is evident in the adjacent tissue.

Mixed Germ Cell Tumors

Approximately half of testicular germ cell tumors exhibit more than one type of neoplastic germ cell and, therefore, are referred to as mixed germ cell tumors. There are more than a dozen possible combinations, but the most frequent patterns are (1) teratoma with embryonal carcinoma (teratocarcinoma); (2) teratoma, embryonal carcinoma, and seminoma; and (3) embryonal carcinoma and seminoma. A surprisingly high frequency of yolk sac tumor components has been noted in these tumors. Twenty percent of patients with teratocarcinoma initially present with metastases, most frequently in the form of embryonal carcinoma.

Testicular Adnexae

DISORDERS OF THE TESTICULAR TUNICS

Hydrocele

■ *Hydrocele is a collection of serous fluid in the scrotal sac and the most common cause of scrotal swelling* (Fig. 17-15). Hydroceles are either congenital and associated with a patent processus vaginalis or acquired secondary to an inflammatory disorder of the epididymis or testis. Uncomplicated hydroceles present as unilateral scrotal swelling, with fluid accumulation in the tunica vaginalis.

Spermatocele

■ *Spermatocele is a cystic enlargement of the efferent ducts or the ducts of the rete testis and is clinically indistinguishable from a hydrocele.* The presence of sperm in the fluid of a spermatocele differentiates this cystic enlargement from a hydrocele.

Varicocele

■ *Varicocele is a dilatation of the testicular vein and is usually asymptomatic.* It may be accompanied by testicular atrophy and result in infertility. Varicoceles are treated by surgical ligation of the internal spermatic vein.

EPIDIDYMITIS

Most cases of acute epididymitis—that is, of inflammation of the epididymis—in young men are due to infection with *N. gonorrhoeae* and *Chlamydia trachomatis*. In

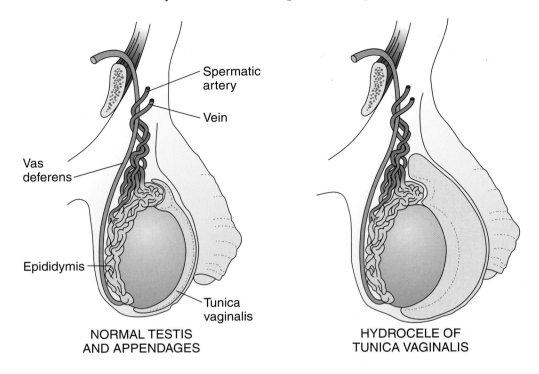

NORMAL TESTIS
AND APPENDAGES

HYDROCELE OF
TUNICA VAGINALIS

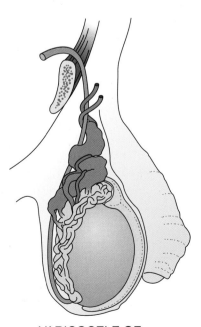

VARICOCELE OF
SPERMATIC CORD VEINS

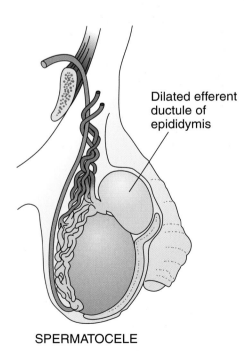

SPERMATOCELE

FIGURE *17-15*
Hydrocele, varicocele, and spermatocele.

older men, *E. coli* from associated urinary tract infections is the most common causative agent. Patients present with intrascrotal pain and tenderness, with or without associated fever. Epididymal inflammation caused by *N. gonorrhoeae* is a common cause of male infertility.

Prostate

PROSTATITIS

Bacterial Prostatitis

Infections of the prostate usually follow lower urinary tract infections and result from the reflux of infected urine into the prostate.

Acute bacterial prostatitis is most commonly caused by gram-negative bacteria, especially *E. coli*, although gram-positive cocci are not infrequent. An acute inflammatory infiltrate in the prostatic acini and stroma is observed. The disorder presents as intense discomfort on urination and is associated with fever, chills, and perineal pain.

Chronic bacterial prostatitis may be preceded by an episode of acute prostatitis, but many patients do not recall a previous infection of the prostate. Most patients with chronic prostatitis complain of suprapubic, perineal, and low back discomfort, and experience dysuria and nocturia. Their urine usually contains bacteria. In addition to the reflux of urine, additional factors, such as prostatic calculi and local prostatic duct obstruction, may contribute to the development of chronic bacterial prostatitis. In contrast to acute prostatitis, lymphocytes, plasma cells, and macrophages are the rule, and the inflammation tends to be more focal and less intense. Prolonged antibiotic therapy is often, but not necessarily, curative.

Nonbacterial Prostatitis

In the majority of cases of chronic prostatitis, no causative agent is identified. Nonbacterial prostatitis is most common in men older than 50 years of age, but it has been reported in virtually all age groups. The most common histologic pattern consists of dilated glands filled with neutrophils and foamy macrophages and surrounded by chronic inflammatory cells. The symptoms are similar to those of chronic bacterial prostatitis.

NODULAR HYPERPLASIA (BENIGN PROSTATIC HYPERPLASIA)

■ *Nodular hyperplasia of the prostate* is a common disorder characterized clinically by enlargement of the gland, with obstruction of the flow of urine through the bladder outlet, and pathologically by proliferation of glands and stroma.

☐ **Epidemiology:** Three epidemiologic factors—geography, race, and age—are related to the incidence of prostatic hyperplasia. The disorder is least frequent in the Orient and most frequent in Western Europe and the United States. The prevalence of prostatic hyperplasia in the United States is higher among blacks than among whites. Clinical prostatism—that is, nodular prostatic hyperplasia of sufficient degree to interfere with urination—peaks in the seventh decade of life. In fact, 75% of men aged 80 years or older have some degree of prostatic hyperplasia.

☐ **Pathogenesis:** Prepubertal castration prevents subsequent development of nodular hyperplasia of the prostrate. However, exogenous testosterone has no observable effect either on the histologic appearance of the hyperplastic nodules or on the areas of the prostate that provide evidence of senile atrophy. There is evidence that growth of prostatic tissue is stimulated by dihydrotestosterone (DHT), the metabolic product of testosterone. Indeed, administration of a drug (finasteride) that inhibits production of DHT by blocking 5α-reductase has reduced the size of the prostate in men with clinical prostatism.

☐ **Pathology:** Early nodular hyperplasia of the prostate begins in the submucosa of the proximal urethra. The developing prostatic nodules compress both the centrally located urethral lumen and the more peripherally located normal prostate (Figs. 17-16 and 17-17). The secondary changes that result from nodular prostatic hyperplasia are related to bladder outlet obstruction (Fig. 17-18).

Histologically, nodular hyperplasia reflects the proliferation of epithelial cells of the acini and ductules, smooth muscle cells, and stromal fibroblasts, all in variable proportions. Accordingly, five types of nodules have been described: (1) stromal (fibrous), (2) fibromuscular, (3) muscular, (4) fibroadenomatous, and (5) fibromyoadenomatous (the most common type).

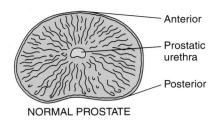

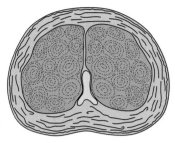

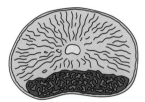

FIGURE *17-16*
Normal prostate, nodular hyperplasia, and adenocarcinoma. In prostatic hyperplasia, the nodules distort and compress the urethra and exert pressure on the surrounding normal prostatic tissue. Prostatic carcinoma usually arises from peripheral glands, in which case it does not compress the urethra.

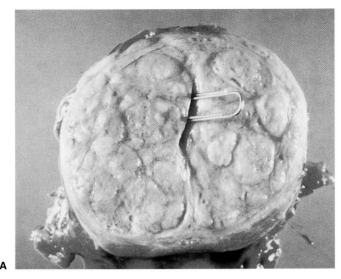

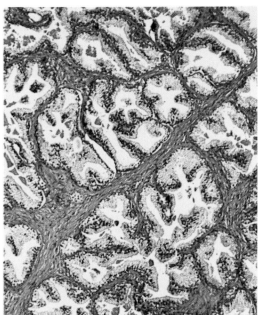

FIGURE *17-17*
Nodular hyperplasia of the prostate. (A) The cut surface of a prostate enlarged by nodular hyperplasia shows numerous, well-circumscribed nodules of prostatic tissue. The prostatic urethra (paper clip) has been compressed to a narrow slit. (B) The columnar epithelium lining the acini is composed of two cell layers. Numerous papillary projections are present in the enlarged acini.

The epithelial (adenomatous) component of a nodule is composed of a double layer of cells, with tall columnar cells overlying the basal layer. Papillary hyperplasia of the glandular epithelium is characteristic. Hyperplastic nodules often contain chronic inflammatory cells, and corpora amylaceae (eosinophilic, laminated concretions) are frequently seen within the acini. Immunoperoxidase staining of the hyperplastic epithelium is consistently positive for prostate-specific antigen (PSA) and prostatic acid phosphatase (PAP). Incidental foci of prostatic adenocarcinoma are found in 10% of surgical specimens submitted with the preoperative diagnosis of prostatic hyperplasia.

☐ **Clinical Features:** Clinical symptoms of nodular hyperplasia of the prostate result from compression of the prostatic urethra and consequent obstruction of the bladder outlet. A history of decreased vigor of the urinary stream and increased urinary frequency is typical. Rectal examination reveals a firm, enlarged, and nodular prostate. If the duration of severe obstruction is prolonged, backpressure results in hydroureter, hydronephrosis, and ultimately, renal failure and death.

The classic treatment of prostatic hyperplasia is surgical. Transurethral resection of the prostate or, less

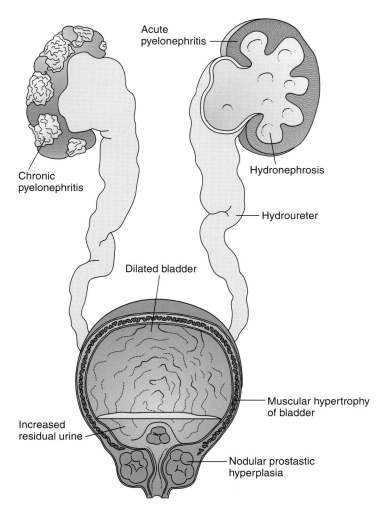

FIGURE *17-18*
Complications of nodular prostatic hyperplasia.

commonly, suprapubic enucleation of the hyperplastic tissue alleviates the symptoms of prostatism. Medical treatment with inhibitors of α-reductase in the prostate, which converts testosterone to DHT, seems to have therapeutic value.

PROSTATIC ADENOCARCINOMA

In 1990, cancer of the prostate became the most frequently diagnosed malignancy in American men, surpassing the incidence of lung cancer for the first time. Although 30,000 American men die annually of this tumor, far more still die from lung cancer.

☐ **Epidemiology:** Prostatic cancer is a disease of elderly men, and of all patients with this diagnosis, 75% are 60 to 80 years of age. The true frequency of prostatic carcinoma is considerably higher than its clinical incidence. Most cases (70–90%) are incidental microscopic findings at autopsy or are discovered in a specimen re-sected for prostatic hyperplasia. The prevalence of prostatic carcinoma at autopsy progressively increases with age, rising from less than 10% among men 40 to 50 years of age to between one-third and one-half of those older than 80 years of age.

The highest frequencies are reported in the United States and the Scandinavian countries, whereas the lowest are reported in Mexico, Greece, and Japan. The highest incidence in the world is recorded in American blacks, who exhibit a rate twice as high as that of American whites.

☐ **Pathogenesis:** The cause of prostatic adenocarcinoma is unknown, but the principal focus of current research is directed toward endocrine influences. The androgenic control of normal prostatic growth and the responsiveness of prostatic cancer to castration and exogenous estrogens support a role for male hormones in the pathogenesis of this neoplasm. However, higher levels of serum androgens have not been demonstrated consistently in patients with prostatic cancer.

☐ **Pathology:** Prostatic adenocarcinomas, which account for 98% of all primary prostatic tumors, are commonly multicentric and usually located in the peripheral zones. The cut surface of the prostate shows irregular, yellow-white, and indurated subcapsular nodules.

Histologic Features. The majority of prostatic adenocarcinomas are of acinar origin and characterized by small- to medium-size glands that lack organization and infiltrate the stroma. Well-differentiated tumors are lined by a single layer of uniform, neoplastic epithelial cells. **In fact, a single layer of cuboidal cells lining neoplastic acini is, from a practical standpoint, the most frequently employed criterion to establish the diagnosis of prostatic adenocarcinoma.** Progressive loss of differentiation of prostatic adenocarcinomas is characterized by (1) increasing variability of gland size and configuration, (2) papillary and cribriform patterns, and (3) rudimentary (or no) gland formation, with only solid cords of infiltrating tumor cells.

Grading. The spectrum of differentiation of prostatic adenocarcinomas has been formalized into several grading systems. The most widely employed is the **Gleason grading system** (Fig. 17-19), which is based on five histologic patterns of tumor gland formation and infiltration. Recognizing the high frequency of mixed tumor patterns, the final Gleason score (grade) is the sum of the grade attributed to the most prominent pattern and of the grade attributed to the minority pattern. The best-differentiated tumors have a Gleason score of 2 (1+1), whereas the poorest-differentiated tumors yield a Gleason score of 10 (5+5). The majority of prostatic cancers have Gleason scores of 4 to 7 (2+2 to 3+4 or 4+3). When combined with the tumor stage, the Gleason grading system has prognostic value: the lower the score, the better the outlook.

Invasion and Metastasis. The high frequency of invasion of the prostatic capsule by adenocarcinoma relates to the subcapsular location of the tumor. Perineural tumor invasion within the prostate and adjacent tissues is usual, and contiguous invasion of the

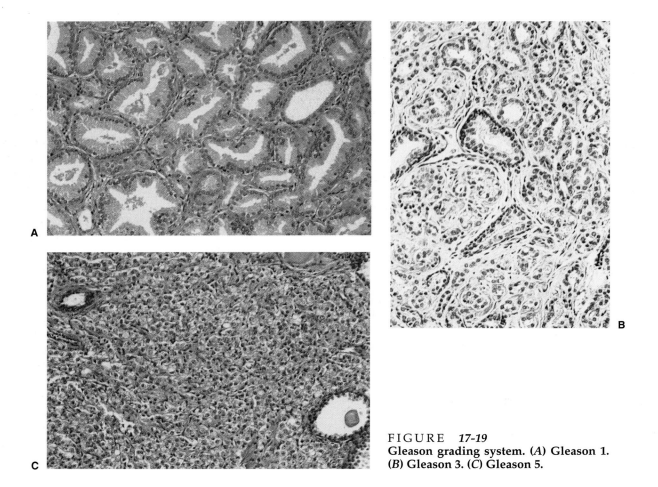

FIGURE   *17-19*
Gleason grading system. (*A*) Gleason 1.
(*B*) Gleason 3. (*C*) Gleason 5.

seminal vesicles by direct extension of prostatic cancer almost always occurs. Wide dissemination of prostatic carcinoma is characteristic at the time of death. Bony metastases, particularly to the vertebral column, ribs, and pelvic bones, occur in almost all patients who eventually die of prostatic carcinoma and present a thorny clinical problem.

☐ **Clinical Features:** In many patients, prostatic cancer is discovered in the tissue fragments obtained at the time of transurethral resection for prostatic hyperplasia. In others, a routine rectal examination reveals a hard nodule in the prostate or a diffusely indurated gland. Bladder obstruction may be the presenting complaint, and some patients are identified by the onset of symptoms attributable to metastases, such as weight loss, bone pain, and anemia.

Both PSA and PAP are detectable in the serum of patients with prostatic cancer. They serve as both useful screening tests for the disease and indicators of the response to treatment of metastatic disease, although false-negative results are well known. Serum PAP levels are elevated only in patients with metastatic prostatic cancer, especially those with osteoblastic bony metastases.

Treatment

Cancers localized to the prostate are most frequently treated by radical prostatectomy or radiation therapy. For those patients in whom tumors progress clinically, and for all patients judged to have regional or distant metastases at initial presentation, the principal form of therapy is hormonal. Whether hormonal therapy takes the form of orchiectomy or the administration of antagonists of pituitary luteinizing hormone-releasing hormone, the goal is androgen deprivation. Inhibition of luteinizing hormone release decreases testosterone production by the testis and results in pharmacologic castration.

Penis

CONGENITAL DISORDERS

Phimosis

■ *Phimosis refers to congenital or acquired inability to retract the prepuce.* Some cases are congenital, but most are residual to previous infections and scarring of the prepuce. Phimosis increases the risk of further inflammation of the glans and prepuce (balanoposthitis). Circumcision is effective therapy for phimosis.

Urethral Meatus. Anomalies of the urethral meatus are uncommon but of great clinical significance. **Epispadias** refers to opening of the urethra on the dorsal surface of the penis, and **hypospadias** signifies opening of the urethra on the ventral surface. Both anomalies are associated with recurrent urinary tract infections and other genitourinary anomalies (e.g., exstrophy of the bladder or cryptorchidism).

CONDYLOMA ACUMINATUM (VENEREAL WARTS)

Condylomata acuminata of the penis are circumscribed, exophytic, cauliflower-like lesions that usually occur on the glans but occasionally are found on the shaft as well. They tend to spread to involve other sites of the anogenital region. Venereal warts are caused by sexually transmitted infection with human papillomavirus (HPV), most commonly types 6 and 11. Histologically, the lesions are papillomatous and exhibit conspicuous acanthosis and parakeratosis.

SQUAMOUS CELL CARCINOMA IN SITU

Dysplastic epidermal lesions on the shaft of the penis are referred to as Bowen disease, whereas those on the glans and prepuce are called erythroplasia of Queyrat. **Bowen disease** appears as a sharply demarcated, erythematous plaque, usually occurring in middle-age or elderly men. **Erythroplasia of Queyrat** occurs in uncircumcised men who are younger than those with Bowen disease. It presents as shiny, soft, erythematous plaques on the glans and foreskin. Both of these conditions are characterized histologically by squamous cell carcinoma in situ, similar to that in other sites. They progress to invasive squamous cell carcinoma in less than 10% of cases.

Bowenoid papulosis is another disease of the penile skin associated with squamous carcinoma in situ. It presents clinically as multiple violaceous papules on the shaft of the penis. Microscopically, the disorder resembles other variants of carcinoma in situ but typically exhibits lesser cytologic atypia. HPV type 16 (but not type 18) antigens have been demonstrated in the majority of lesions. Virtually all lesions of bowenoid papulosis regress spontaneously or after topical therapy. The potential invasiveness of bowenoid papulosis is not established.

VERRUCOUS CARCINOMA

Verrucous carcinoma of the penis (giant condyloma of Buschke-Löwenstein) is a cytologically benign, but clinically malignant, exophytic squamous cell cancer. It is similar to condyloma acuminatum, but unlike the latter, it shows deep local invasion. The lesion is today recognized as a low-grade squamous cell carcinoma. It does not usually metastasize, although a few such cases have been reported.

Verrucous carcinoma of the penis occurs only in uncircumcised men. The tumor may enlarge to form a substantial warty mass, which destroys the end of the penis. Surgical removal of a verrucous carcinoma is usually curative.

SQUAMOUS CELL CARCINOMA

In the United States, invasive squamous cell carcinoma of the penis is an uncommon tumor, accounting for less than 0.5% of all cancers in male patients.

☐ **Epidemiology:** The average age of patients with invasive squamous cell carcinoma is 60 years. Penile cancer is much more common in less-developed countries, and in some parts of Africa and Asia comprises 10% of cancers in men. Because this tumor is virtually unknown in men who are circumcised at birth, these geographic variations have been attributed to differences in the frequency of circumcision.

More than half of the patients with cancer of the penis have phimosis since an early age, suggesting that prolonged contact between smegma and the penile epithelium may play a role. HPV types 16 and 18 have also been suggested as being factors in the pathogenesis of penile cancer.

☐ **Pathology:** Squamous cell carcinoma of the penis is most commonly found on the glans or the prepuce, and it usually presents as an ulcerated and hemorrhagic mass. An occasional tumor is exophytic and occurs as a fungating mass. Others are principally infiltrating. Extensive destruction of penile tissue, including the urethral meatus, is observed in some patients. Microscopically, the typical features of a well-differentiated, focally keratinizing squamous cell carcinoma are observed. Squamous cell carcinoma of the penis spreads to the inguinal lymph nodes, then to the iliac nodes, and ultimately, to distant organs.

☐ **Clinical Features:** Most squamous cell carcinomas are confined to the penis at the time of initial presentation, but occult metastases to the inguinal lymph nodes are not uncommon. The majority of patients with stage I cancer (superficial lesion of the glans or prepuce) can be cured, but the prognosis progressively worsens when the cancer grows more extensive. Treatment is partial or complete amputation of the penis.

CHAPTER *18*

The Female Reproductive System

Stanley J. Robboy
Maire A. Duggan
Robert J. Kurman

(continued)

Chronic Endometritis	Theca Lutein Cysts
Adenomyosis	**Polycystic Ovary Syndrome (Stein-Leventhal Syndrome)**
Endometriosis	**Tumors**
Dysfunctional Uterine Bleeding	Epithelial Tumors
Tumors	Germ Cell Tumors
Endometrial Polyps	Sex Cord/Stromal Tumors
Endometrial Hyperplasia and Adenocarcinoma	Tumors Metastatic to the Ovary
Leiomyoma	**PLACENTA**
Leiomyosarcoma	**Chorioamnionitis**
FALLOPIAN TUBE	**Toxemia of Pregnancy (Pre-eclampsia and Eclampsia)**
Salpingitis	**Gestational Trophoblastic Disease**
Ectopic Pregnancy	Complete Hydatidiform Mole
OVARY	Partial Hydatidiform Mole
Ovarian Cysts	Invasive Hydatitiform Mole
Follicular Cysts	Choriocarcinoma
Corpus Luteum Cysts	

Sexually Transmitted Genital Infections

Infectious diseases of the female genital tract are common and are caused by a wide variety of pathogenic organisms (Table 18-1). These diseases are also discussed in Chapter 9.

BACTERIAL INFECTIONS

Gonorrhea

Gonorrhea is caused by infection with *Neisseria gonorrhoeae*, which is a fastidious, gram-negative diplococcus. It is also a frequent cause of acute salpingitis and pelvic inflammatory disease (Fig. 18-1). The organisms ascend through the cervix and endometrial cavity to the fallopian tube, where they elicit a pronounced, acute, fibrinous, and inflammatory reaction (acute salpingitis). The infection spreads to involve the ovary, thereby creating a tubo-ovarian abscess.

Condyloma Acuminatum

■ *Condyloma acuminatum is a benign, exophytic, and squamous lesion that occurs on the skin or mucous mem-*

branes of the lower female genital tract and is caused by infection with human papillomavirus (HPV). The lesion may also involve the urethra, bladder, and rectum. Condylomata grow as papules, plaques, or nodules and, eventually, as spiked or cauliflower-like excrescences. On microscopic examination, a striking papillomatous proliferation of squamous epithelium is noted (Fig. 18-2). A characteristic finding is the **koilocyte,** which is an epithelial cell with a perinuclear halo and a wrinkled nucleus that contains HPV particles. Parakeratosis, dyskeratosis, and sometimes, hyperkeratosis may also occur.

Herpesvirus

Herpes simplex virus type 2, which is a double-stranded DNA virus, is a common cause of sexually transmitted genital infections. After an incubation period of 1 to 3 weeks, small vesicles develop on the vulva and erode into painful ulcers. Similar lesions occur in the vagina and cervix. In the biopsy specimen of a lesion, epithelial cells adjacent to intraepithelial vesicles show ballooning degeneration, and many contain large nuclei with eosinophilic inclusions.

Genital herpes tends to become latent, with the virus remaining in the sacral ganglia. Reactivation of the virus during pregnancy can result in its transmis-

TABLE   18-1.   Infectious Diseases of the Female Genital Tract

Organism	Disease	Diagnostic Feature
Sexually Transmitted Diseases		
Gram-Negative Rods and Cocci		
Calymmatobacterium granulomatis	Granuloma inguinale	Donovan body
Gardnerella vaginalis	*Gardnerella* infection	Clue cell
Haemophilus ducreyi	Chancroid (soft chancre)	
Neisseria gonorrhoeae	Gonorrhea	
Spirochetes		
Treponema pallidum	Syphilis	
Mycoplasmas		
Mycoplasma hominis	Nonspecific vaginitis	
Ureaplasma urealyticum	Nonspecific vaginitis	
Rickettsiae		
Chlamydia trachomatis type D-K	Various form of PID[a]	
Chlamydia trachomatis type L_{1-3}	Lymphogranuloma venereum	
Viruses		
Human papilloma virus	Condyloma acuminatum/planum	Koilocyte
	Neoplastic potential	
Type 6, 11, 42, 43, and 44	Low risk	
Types 31, 33, 35, 45, 51, 52, and 56	Intermediate risk	
Types 16 and 18	High risk	
Herpes simplex type 2	Herpes genitalis	Multinucleated giant cell
Cytomegalovirus	Cytomegalic inclusion disease	
Molluscum contagiosum	Molluscum infection	Molluscum body
Protozoa		
Trichomonas vaginalis	Trichomoniasis	
Selected Nonsexually Transmitted Diseases		
Actinomyces and Related Organisms		
Actinomyces israelii	PID (one of many organisms)	Sulfur granules
Mycobacterium tuberculosis	Tuberculosis	Necrotizing granulomas
Fungi		
Candida albicans	Candidiasis	

[a] *PID*, pelvic inflammatory disease.

sion to the newborn during passage through the birth canal, a complication that is often fatal.

PELVIC INFLAMMATORY DISEASE

■ *Pelvic inflammatory disease describes an infection of the pelvic organs that follows extension of a variety of microorganisms beyond the uterine corpus* (see Fig. 18-1). Ascent of the infection results in bilateral acute salpingitis, pyosalpinx, and tubo-ovarian abscesses. *N. gonorrhoeae* is the principal single organism causing pelvic inflammatory disease, but most infections are polymicrobial. The incidence is far greater in sexually promiscuous women than in those who are monogamous.

Patients with PID usually present with lower abdominal pain. Complications include (1) rupture of a tubo-ovarian abscess, which may result in life-threatening peritonitis; (2) infertility from scarring of the healed tubal plicae; and (3) intestinal obstruction owing to fibrous bands and adhesions.

Vulva

BARTHOLIN GLAND CYST

The paired Bartholin glands produce a clear, mucoid secretion that continuously lubricates the vestibular surface of the vulva. The ducts are prone to obstruction, however, and consequent cyst formation. In turn, infection of the cyst leads to abscess formation. Bartholin gland abscess is frequently caused by infection with staphylococci and anaerobes. Treatment consists of incision, drainage, marsupialization, and appropriate antibiotics.

DERMATOLOGIC DISEASES

Dermatologic conditions of the vulva usually present as white lesions and occur predominantly in middle-aged or older women.

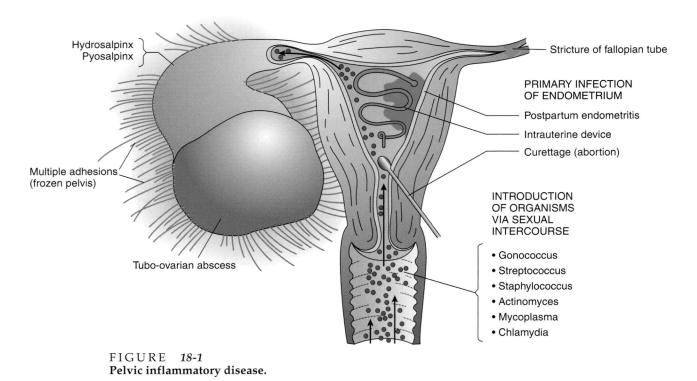

Hydrosalpinx
Pyosalpinx

Stricture of fallopian tube

PRIMARY INFECTION
OF ENDOMETRIUM

Postpartum endometritis

Intrauterine device

Curettage (abortion)

Multiple adhesions
(frozen pelvis)

INTRODUCTION
OF ORGANISMS
VIA SEXUAL
INTERCOURSE

Tubo-ovarian abscess

• Gonococcus
• Streptococcus
• Staphylococcus
• Actinomyces
• Mycoplasma
• Chlamydia

FIGURE 18-1
Pelvic inflammatory disease.

Lichen Sclerosus

■ *Lichen sclerosus, an abnormal growth of the vulvar skin, is characterized by white plaques, skin atrophy, and a parchment-like or crinkled appearance.* Occasionally, the disorder is marked by contracture of the vulvar tissues (kraurosis). Histologically, there is hyperkeratosis, blunting or loss of rete ridges, and a homogeneous, acellular zone in the upper dermis. A band of chronic inflammatory cells typically lies beneath this layer. Itching is the most common symptom, and dyspareunia (painful intercourse) is frequent. Although insidious and progressive, lichen sclerosus is not premalignant.

Squamous Hyperplasia

The squamous epithelium of the vulva may become hyperplastic (acanthosis), in which case enlargement and confluence of the epidermal rete ridges are noted. The thickened epithelium displays a marked increase in superficial keratin (hyperkeratosis), which imparts a white appearance to the vulva. Because squamous carcinomas may also appear as white plaques, the previously used term, **leukoplakia,** has caused considerable confusion and is no longer preferred.

MALIGNANT TUMORS AND PREMALIGNANT CONDITIONS

Vulvar Intraepithelial Neoplasia

■ *Vulvar intraepithelial neoplasia (VIN) reflects a spectrum of neoplastic changes that range from minimal cellular atypia to the most marked cellular changes short of invasive cancer.* The epidemiologic characteristics of women with VIN and cancer of the vulva are similar to those of women with cervical intraepithelial neoplasia (CIN) and cervical cancer. **VIN (like CIN) is considered to be the precursor lesion of squamous cell carcinoma.**

□ **Pathology:** VIN has a variable gross appearance. Lesions may be single or multiple, and may be macular, papular, or plaque-like. Microscopically, the grades are labeled as VIN I, II, and III, which correspond to mild, moderate, and severe dysplasia. Class III also includes carcinoma in situ. Despite local excision, VIN often recurs (25%), in which case it may progress to invasive squamous cell carcinoma (6%).

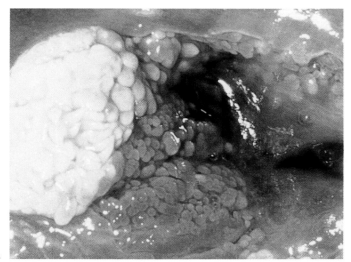

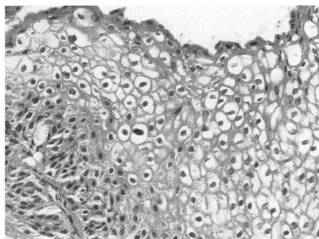

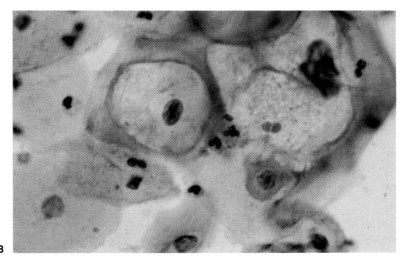

FIGURE 18-2
Human papillomavirus-induced condyloma-tous infections. (A) Condyloma acuminatum on the cervix, which is visible to the naked eye as cauliflower-like excrescences. (B) A cervical smear contains characteristic koilocytes, with a perinuclear halo and a wrinkled nucleus containing viral particles. (C) Biopsy specimen of the condyloma shows koilocytes, with perinuclear halos but lacking nuclear atypia.

Squamous Cell Carcinoma of the Vulva

Squamous cell carcinoma of the vulva (Fig. 18-3) is the end result of a multistep process that has its origin in VIN. This tumor accounts for 3% of all genital cancers in women, and it is the most common cancer of the vulva (85%). In the past, it mainly affected older women, but like VIN, it now occurs with an increasing frequency in younger women. Two-thirds of larger tumors are exophytic; the others are ulcerative and endophytic. Pruritus of long duration is commonly the first symptom, and ulceration, bleeding, and secondary infection may develop. The tumors (1) grow slowly; (2) extend to the contiguous skin, vagina, and rectum; and (3) metastasize to the superficial inguinal and then to the deep inguinal, femoral, and pelvic lymph nodes.

The survival rate for patients with vulvar carcinoma approaches 90% when the nodes are uninvolved. Two-thirds of women with inguinal node metastases survive for at least 5 years, whereas only one-fourth of those with pelvic node metastases live that long.

Verrucous Carcinoma

■ *Verrucous carcinoma of the vulva is a distinct variety of squamous cell carcinoma that presents as a large, fungating mass resembling a giant condyloma acuminatum.* HPV, usually type 6, is commonly identified. The tumor is very well differentiated, being composed of large nests of squamous cells with abundant cytoplasm and small, bland nuclei. Verrucous carcinoma invades locally but typically does not metastasize. Wide local surgical excision is the treatment of choice, and recurrence usually results from inadequate previous excision.

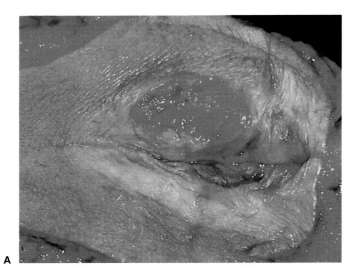

A

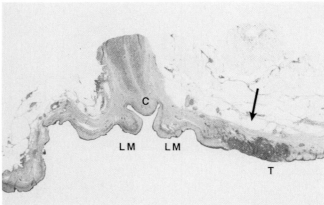

B

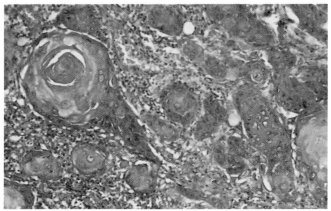

C

FIGURE   *18-3*
Squamous cell carcinoma of vulva. (A) The tumor is situated in an extensive area of lichen sclerosus (*white*). (B) A cross-section of the vulva with a small squamous cell carcinoma (*arrow*) shows both halves of the perineum, including labia minora (LM) and clitoris (C). A 1-cm tumor (T) is confined to the dermis. (C) Small nests of neoplastic squamous cells, some with keratin pearls, are evident in this well-differentiated tumor.

Extramammary Paget Disease

Paget disease of the vulva is a rare neoplasm of the labia majora in older women. The lesions are large, red, moist, and sharply demarcated. Microscopically, large, pale, and vacuolated cells, termed **Paget cells,** are scattered throughout the epidermis. In contrast to Paget disease of the breast, which almost always is linked to an underlying duct carcinoma, extramammary Paget disease only rarely is associated with an adenocarcinoma of the skin adnexa. Wide local excision is usually curative.

Vagina

VAGINAL ADENOSIS

■ *Vaginal adenosis refers to replacement of the normal squamous epithelium of the vagina by a glandular epithelium.* Exposure to diethylstilbestrol (DES) during early

prenatal life is associated with development of multiple changes in the genital tract, including vaginal adenosis. Rare cases of **clear cell adenocarcinoma** of the vagina have also occurred in the daughters of women treated with DES.

☐ **Pathology:** Adenosis presents as red, granular patches on the vaginal mucosa. Microscopically, it comprises two types of cells, namely mucinous columnar cells, which resemble those lining the endocervix, and ciliated cells with eosinophilic cytoplasm, which are similar to those lining the endometrium and fallopian tubes. The glandular cells ultimately undergo squamous metaplasia.

SQUAMOUS CELL CARCINOMA

Squamous cell carcinoma of the vagina accounts for more than 90% of all primary malignant tumors of the vagina. It is generally a disease of older women, with a peak incidence occurring between the ages of 60 and 70 years. Vaginal intraepithelial neoplasia, which is a term replacing both vaginal dysplasia and carcinoma in situ, frequently occurs in conjunction with squamous cell carcinoma and may precede the development of invasive carcinoma. The 5-year survival rate for tumors confined to the vagina (stage I) is 80%, whereas this rate is only 20% for those with extensive spread (stage III/IV).

Embryonal Rhabdomyosarcoma (Sarcoma Botryoides)

■ *Embryonal rhabdomyosarcoma is a rare vaginal tumor that appears as confluent, polypoid masses resembling a bunch of grapes, hence the name sarcoma botryoides (Gk. botrys, "grapes").* It occurs almost exclusively in children younger than the age of 4 years and is composed of primitive spindle rhabdomyoblasts, some of which display cross-striations. Larger tumors are likely to have invaded adjacent structures and to metastasize to regional lymph nodes and spread hematogenously to distant sites. Even in advanced cases, half of the patients survive after radical surgery and chemotherapy.

Cervix

CERVICITIS

Both acute and chronic cervicitis result from infection with many micro-organisms, particularly the endogenous vaginal aerobes and anaerobes, *Streptococcus, Staphylococcus,* and *Enterococcus.*

In **acute cervicitis,** the cervix is grossly red, swollen, and edematous, with copious pus dripping from the external os. Microscopically, tissues exhibit an extensive infiltrate of polymorphonuclear leukocytes and stromal edema.

In **chronic cervicitis,** which is more common, the cervical mucosa is hyperemic, and there may be true epithelial erosions. Microscopically, the stroma is infiltrated by mononuclear cells, principally lymphocytes and plasma cells. Metaplastic squamous epithelium may extend into the endocervical glands, where they form clusters of squamous epithelium that must be differentiated from carcinoma.

ENDOCERVICAL POLYP

■ *Endocervical polyp, which is the most common cervical growth, appears as a single, smooth, or lobulated mass,* *typically less than 3 cm in its greatest dimension.* It occurs in less than 5% of adult women and often presents as vaginal bleeding or discharge. The lining epithelium is mucinous, with varying degrees of squamous metaplasia. The stroma is edematous and contains thick-walled blood vessels. Simple excision or curettage is curative. Cancer rarely arises in an endocervical polyp.

SQUAMOUS CELL NEOPLASIA

Fifty years ago, cervical cancer was the leading cause of death from cancer in American women, and it remains an important disease today. Although the mortality rate from cervical cancer has decreased substantially, improved surveillance has led to an increase in the incidence of its precursor lesions.

Cervical Intraepithelial Neoplasia

■ *Cervical intraepithelial neoplasia is a spectrum of intraepithelial changes that begins with minimal atypia and progresses through stages of more marked intraepithelial abnormalities to invasive squamous cell carcinoma.* CIN, dysplasia, and carcinoma in situ are synonymous terms today. **Dysplasia** in the cervical epithelium implies an alteration that carries the potential for malignant transformation. **Carcinoma in situ** refers to a malignant lesion that involves the entire thickness of the squamous epithelium but that remains confined to the epithelium. Importantly, the term *in situ* signifies that the underlying stroma has not been invaded. The term *cervical intraepithelial neoplasia* emphasizes that dysplasia and carcinoma in situ are points on a disease spectrum rather than separate entities.

The grades of CIN are related to the previous terminology as follows:

- **CIN-1.** Mild dysplasia.
- **CIN-2.** Moderate dysplasia.
- **CIN-3.** Severe dysplasia and carcinoma in situ.

☐ **Epidemiology and Pathogenesis:** The epidemiologic features of CIN and invasive cancer are similar. **Multiple sexual partners and early age at first coitus are the most important factors.** As a consequence, CIN is, in many cases, likely to be a sexually transmitted disease. The incidence of cervical cancer is also considerably higher in women who smoke.

A substantial body of both clinical and laboratory evidence strongly supports the view that infection with HPV is involved in the pathogenesis of CIN and cervical cancer (Fig. 18-4). Cells in high-grade CIN con-

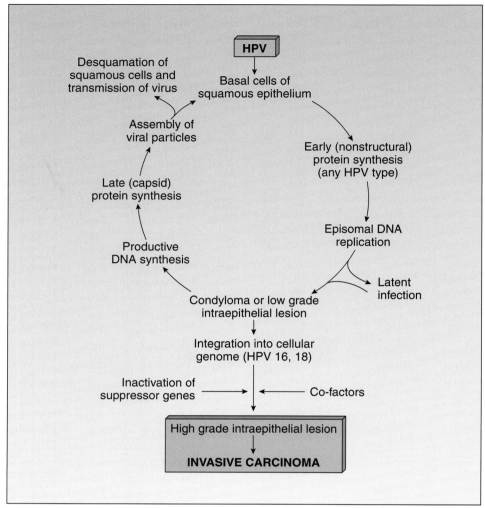

F I G U R E   *18-4*
Role of human papillomavirus (HPV) in the pathogenesis of cervical neoplasia.

tain HPV types 16, 18, 31, 33, or 35. **HPV types 16 and 18 are found in 70% of invasive cancers, and types 31, 33, and 35 are found in 20%. These types, therefore, are considered to be high-risk varieties.**

☐ **Pathology:**
  CIN-1: The most pronounced changes are seen in the basal one-third of the epithelium. Cells with abnormal nuclei migrate toward the surface and are sloughed. As a result, they are detected in Papanicolaou smears.
  CIN-2: Most of the cellular abnormalities are in the lower and middle one-third of the epithelium.
  CIN-3: Abnormal cells diffusely involve more than two-thirds of the epithelium (severe dysplasia) or appear as carcinoma in situ that involves all lay-

ers. Cytodifferentiation is minimal in patients with CIN-3.
  The sequence of histologic changes from CIN-1 to CIN-3 is illustrated in Figure 18-5. Half of the cases of CIN-1 regress, 10% progress to CIN-3, and less than 2% eventuate in invasive cancer. The frequency of progression is much greater in cases with initially higher grades of CIN. The average time for all grades of dysplasia to progress to carcinoma in situ is approximately 10 years. **At least 20% of the cases of CIN-3 progress to invasive carcinoma within 10 years.**
  Women with CIN-1 are often followed conservatively (repeated smears plus close follow-up). High-grade lesions are treated by cryosurgery, cervical conization (removal of a cone of tissue around the external os), laser vaporization, and rarely, hysterectomy.

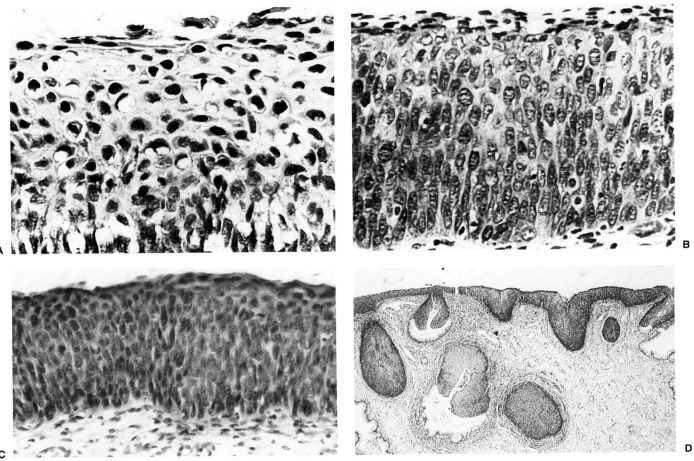

FIGURE *18-5*
Cervical intraepithelial neoplasia (CIN). (A) CIN-1. The cervical epithelium shows pronounced cellular atypia in the basal one-third. Some cells in the upper two-thirds of the epithelium have abnormal nuclei, but all show cytoplasmic differentiation. (B) CIN-2 to CIN-3. The lower two-thirds of the epithelium displays pronounced cell atypia. Although cytodifferentiation occurs in the upper one-third of the epithelium, it is less pronounced than in CIN-1. (C) CIN-3 (carcinoma in situ). Malignant cells are present throughout the entire epithelium. (D) CIN-3. Carcinoma in situ partially or completely replaces the columnar epithelium of the endocervical glands.

Microinvasive Squamous Cell Carcinoma

Microinvasive carcinoma is an early stage in the spectrum of cervical cancer (stage IA) and is characterized by minimal invasion of the stroma by neoplastic cells (Fig. 18-6). Approximately 7% of specimens removed for carcinoma in situ demonstrate foci of microinvasive cancer. Small clusters of cells or solid lesions in the stroma have the following characteristics:

- Invasion to a depth of less than 3 mm below the basement membrane
- Lack of vascular invasion
- No lymph node metastases
- A simple hysterectomy is sufficient to cure microinvasive squamous cell carcinoma of the cervix.

Invasive Squamous Cell Carcinoma

□ **Epidemiology:** Squamous cell carcinoma of the cervix has declined in frequency in the United States, but in Central and South America, parts of Asia, and Africa it remains a major cause of death from cancer. **The tumor generally evolves from precursor CIN.** The age at presentation peaks at 52 years, or approximately 25 years after the peak of CIN-1 and CIN-2 and approximately 10 to 15 years after CIN-3.

□ **Pathology:** Cervical cancer usually presents as a poorly defined, granular, and eroded lesion or as a nodular and exophytic mass (Fig. 18-7). On microscopic examination, the majority of tumors display solid nests of large, malignant squamous cells, with no more than individual cell keratinization. Most of the

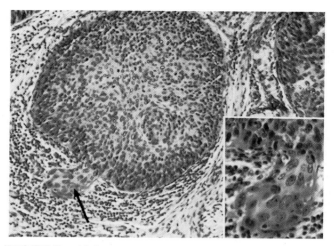

FIGURE 18-6
Microinvasive squamous cell carcinoma. A section of the cervix shows carcinoma in situ in an endocervical gland that has broken through the basement membrane (*arrow*) to invade the stroma. (Inset) A higher-power view of the microinvasive focus.

remaining cancers exhibit nests of keratinized cells that are organized in concentric whorls, or so-called keratin pearls.

Cervical cancer spreads by direct extension, through lymphatic vessels, and only rarely by the hematogenous route. Local extension into surrounding tissues results in ureteral compression; the corresponding clinical complications are hydroureter, hydronephrosis, and renal failure, with the last being the most common cause of death (50% of patients). Bladder and rectal involvement lead to fistula formation. Metastases to the regional lymph nodes involve the paracervical, hypogastric, and external iliac nodes.

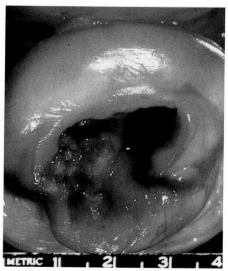

FIGURE 18-7
Squamous cell cancer. The cervix is distorted by the presence of an exophytic, ulcerated, squamous cell carcinoma.

□ **Clinical Features:** During the earliest stages of cervical cancer, patients complain most frequently of vaginal bleeding after intercourse or douching. With more advanced cancer, symptoms are referable to the route and degree of spread. Radical hysterectomy is favored for localized tumor, especially in younger women, whereas radiation therapy or combinations of radiation therapy and hysterectomy are used for more advanced tumors.

Adenocarcinoma

Adenocarcinoma of the endocervix accounts for 10% of malignant cervical tumors. The mean age at presentation is 56 years. Adenocarcinoma appears to share causative factors with squamous cell carcinoma of the cervix, and it spreads in a similar fashion. The tumors are often associated with adenocarcinoma in situ and are frequently infected with HPV types 16 and 18.

Uterus

MENSTRUAL CYCLE

Proliferative Phase

During the first 14 days of the menstrual cycle, the endometrium is under estrogenic stimulation. The superficial or functional zone exhibits tubular to coiled glands, which are evenly distributed and are supported by a cellular, monomorphic stroma (Fig. 18-8).

Secretory Phase

Ovulation occurs approximately 14 days after the last menstrual period, after which the graafian follicle that has discharged its ovum becomes a corpus luteum. Progesterone secreted by the corpus luteum transforms the endometrium after day 17 from a proliferative to a secretory state.

- **Days 17 Through 19.** The endometrial glands enlarge and become more coiled. The cells lining the glands develop abundant and prominent, glycogen-rich, subnuclear vacuoles.
- **Days 20 Through 22.** The glands dilate, have serrated borders, and are more tortuous.
- **Days 23 Through 27.** The stromal cells enlarge and exhibit large, round vesicular nuclei and abundant eosinophilic cytoplasm. These cells are precursors to the decidual cells of pregnancy.

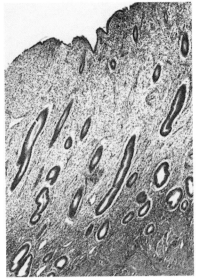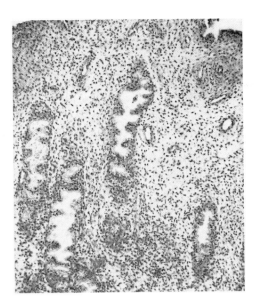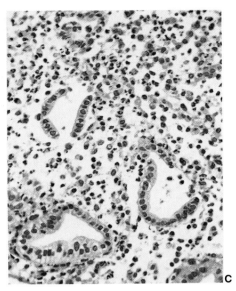

A,B   C

FIGURE   *18-8*
Endometrial phases of the normal menstrual cycle. (A) Proliferative phase. Straight tubular glands are embedded in a cellular, monomorphic stroma. (B) Secretory phase, day 24. Dilated, tortuous glands with serrated borders are situated in a predecidual stroma. (C) Menstrual endometrium. Fragmented glands, dissolution of the stroma, and numerous neutrophils are evident.

Menstrual Phase

As the corpus luteum degenerates, the levels of progesterone fall, the endometrium becomes desiccated, the spiral arteries collapse, and the stroma disintegrates. Menses commence on day 28, last from 3 to 7 days, and result in a flow of approximately 35 mL of blood. The denuded surface is re-epithelialized by extension of the residual glandular epithelium.

Endometrium of Pregnancy

During a normal pregnancy, the trophoblast begins to develop at approximately day 23. At that time, under the influence of human chorionic gonadotropin (hCG), which is secreted by the embryonic trophoblast, the corpus luteum increases its output of progesterone, thereby stimulating secretion by the endometrial glands. The hypersecretory endometrium of pregnancy is characterized by widely dilated glands that are lined by cells with abundant glycogen. These features can persist for as long as 8 weeks after delivery.

Atrophic Endometrium

After menopause, both the number of glands and the amount of stroma progressively decrease. Glands of the atrophic endometrium are often conspicuously dilated, an appearance that is termed *senile cystic atrophy of the endometrium.*

ENDOMETRITIS

Acute Endometritis

■ *Acute endometritis is the abnormal presence of polymorphonuclear leukocytes in the endometrium.* Most cases of acute endometritis are caused by an ascending infection from the cervix, such as occurs after the usually impervious cervical barrier is compromised by abortion, delivery, or medical instrumentation.

Chronic Endometritis

■ *Chronic endometritis is identified by plasma cells in the endometrium.* Chronic endometritis is associated with use of an intrauterine device, pelvic inflammatory disease, and retained products of conception after abortion or delivery. Patients usually complain of bleeding, pelvic pain, or both. The condition is generally self-limited.

ADENOMYOSIS

■ *Adenomyosis is the presence of endometrial glands and stroma deep within the myometrium.* As many as 20% of all uteri removed at surgery show some degree of adenomyosis.

□ **Pathology:** On gross examination, the my-ometrium contains small, soft, and red areas, some of which are cystic. Microscopic examination of these lesions reveals glands that are lined by mildly proliferative to inactive endometrium and surrounded by endometrial stroma.

□ **Clinical Features:** Although many patients with adenomyosis are asymptomatic, it is not uncommon for patients to present with varying degrees of pelvic pain, dysfunctional uterine bleeding, dysmenorrhea, and dyspareunia.

ENDOMETRIOSIS

■ *Endometriosis is the presence of benign endometrial glands and stroma outside the uterus.* It afflicts 3% of women of reproductive age and regresses following natural or artificial menopause. The sites most frequently involved are the ovaries (80%) and other uterine adnexae, including the uterine ligaments and rectovaginal septum. The pouch of Douglas and the pelvic peritoneum may also be affected (Fig. 18-9).

□ **Pathogenesis:** Several theories regarding the pathogenesis of endometriosis have been proposed, none of which are mutually exclusive. The most widely accepted theory holds that foci of the menstrual endometrium regurgitate through the fallopian tubes and implant on the various pelvic organs. Occurrence of endometriosis at distant sites such as the lungs and kidneys has been attributed to hematogenous spread from the endometrium. Endometriosis has also been proposed to arise by celomic metaplasia of the peritoneum.

□ **Pathology:** Early foci of endometriosis on the ovary or peritoneal surfaces are red or bluish ("mulberry") nodules, varying from 1 to 5 mm in diameter (Fig. 18-10). Because ectopic endometrial glands often participate in the menstrual cycle, repeated bleeding leads to deposition of hemosiderin and a grossly brown discoloration ("powder burns"). Fibrous adhesions often surround endometriotic foci and may cause adjacent structures, such as loops of the bowel, to adhere. In the ovaries, repeated hemorrhage may cause enlarged endometriotic foci to form cysts as large as 15 cm in diameter. These cysts often contain inspissated, chocolate-colored material (**chocolate cysts**).

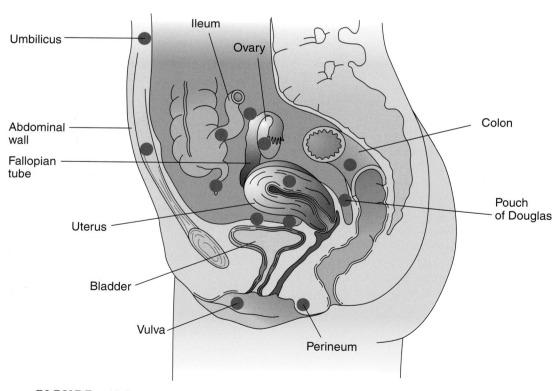

FIGURE **18-9**
Sites of endometriosis.

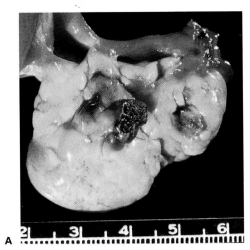
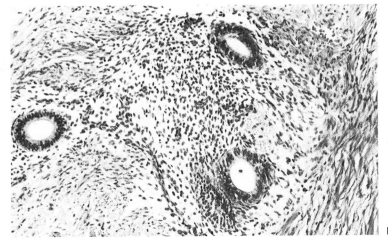

FIGURE   *18-10*
**Endometriosis. (A) Implants of endometriosis on the ovary appear as red-blue nodules.
(B) A microscopic section from the broad ligament shows endometrial glands and stroma
in the ovary.**

Microscopically, endometriosis is diagnosed by the presence of ectopic endometrial glands and stroma (see Fig. 18-10). On occasion, healed foci of endometriosis consist only of fibrous tissue and hemosiderin-laden macrophages.

☐ **Clinical Features:** The signs and symptoms of endometriosis depend on the location of the implants. The most common complaint is dysmenorrhea, which is related to implants on the uterosacral ligaments. **In fact, half of all women with dysmenorrhea have some degree of endometriosis.** Infertility is the primary complaint in one-third of women with endometriosis (Fig. 18-11).

DYSFUNCTIONAL UTERINE BLEEDING

■ *Dysfunctional uterine bleeding is defined as abnormal bleeding either during or between menstrual periods, in which the cause lies outside the uterus.* Most cases are related to an endocrine disturbance that involves the hypothalamic-pituitary-ovarian axis (Table 18-2). Ovarian dysfunction, especially anovulation, is usual.

TUMORS

Endometrial Polyps

■ *Endometrial polyps are benign, localized overgrowths that project from the endometrial surface into the endometrial cavity.* They occur most commonly during the perimenopausal period and are virtually unknown before menarche. Endometrial polyps are thought to arise from endometrial foci that are hypersensitive to estrogenic stimulation or unresponsive to progesterone. In either case, such foci would not slough during menstruation and, instead, would continue to grow.

☐ **Pathology:** Most endometrial polyps arise in the fundus, although they may originate in any location within the endometrial cavity. The majority are solitary, but 20% are multiple. They vary in size from several millimeters in length to a growth that fills the entire endometrial cavity.

Microscopically, the core of a polyp is composed of (1) endometrial glands, which often are cystically dilated and hyperplastic; (2) a fibromatous, endometrial stroma; and (3) thick-walled, coiled, and dilated blood vessels. A mantle of endometrial epithelium covers the polyp. The glandular epithelium is usually not at the same stage of the cycle as that of the adjacent normal endometrium.

☐ **Clinical Features:** Endometrial polyps typically present with intermenstrual bleeding owing to surface ulceration or hemorrhagic infarction. They are generally not preneoplastic, although as many as 0.5% harbor adenocarcinoma.

Endometrial Hyperplasia and Adenocarcinoma

■ *Endometrial hyperplasia and adenocarcinoma represent a broad spectrum of proliferative disease that consti-*

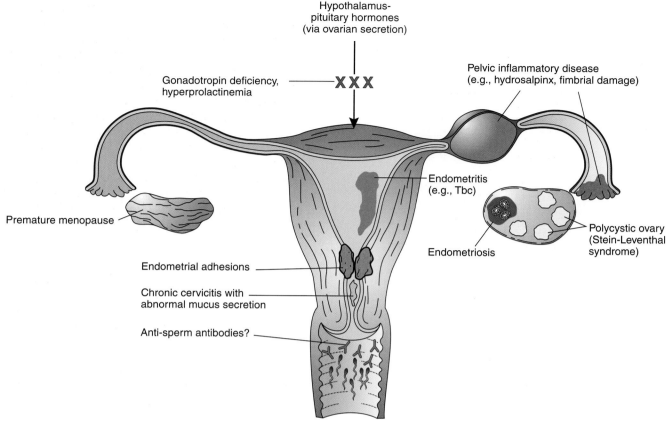

Hypothalamus-
pituitary hormones
(via ovarian secretion)

Gonadotropin deficiency,
hyperprolactinemia

Pelvic inflammatory disease
(e.g., hydrosalpinx, fimbrial damage)

Endometritis
(e.g., Tbc)

Premature menopause

Endometriosis

Polycystic ovary
(Stein-Leventhal
syndrome)

Endometrial adhesions

Chronic cervicitis with
abnormal mucus secretion

Anti-sperm antibodies?

FIGURE   *18-11*
Causes of acquired infertility.

tutes a morphologic and a biologic continuum, similar to multistep carcinogenesis in other tissues. The lesions often reflect either endogenous or exogenous hyperestrinism.

Endometrial Hyperplasia

■ *Endometrial hyperplasia refers to a morphologic continuum that ranges from simple glandular crowding to a conspicuous proliferation of atypical glands that are difficult to distinguish from early carcinoma.* The risk of developing carcinoma increases with progressively higher degrees of endometrial hyperplasia.

☐ **Pathology:** Endometrial hyperplasia is classified according to cytologic atypia and glandular architecture:

- **Simple Hyperplasia.** This is a proliferative lesion that shows minimal glandular complexity and crowding but no cytologic atypia. The epithelial lining is usually one cell layer in thickness, and the stroma between the glands is abundant. **One percent of the cases of simple endometrial hyperplasia progress to adenocarcinoma.**
- **Complex Hyperplasia.** This variant exhibits severe glandular complexity and crowding but no

cytologic atypia (Fig. 18-12). The stroma between the glands is scanty. **Three percent of such lesions progress to adenocarcinoma.**
- **Atypical Hyperplasia.** This lesion displays cytologic atypia and marked glandular crowding, frequently as back-to-back glands. The glands may have a complex architecture, with an intraluminal papillary arrangement or the appearance of budding glands in the stroma. **One-third of the cases of atypical endometrial hyperplasia progress to adenocarcinoma.**

Progression from hyperplasia free of atypia to invasive cancer requires approximately 10 years. The corresponding time for atypical hyperplasia is roughly 4 years.

☐ **Clinical Features:** Depending on the woman's age, endometrial hyperplasia may result from anovulatory cycles, polycystic ovary syndrome, an estrogen-producing tumor, obesity, or the intake of estrogenic drugs. Hysterectomy is usually considered to be the therapy of choice in women who have completed childbearing and in whom curettage reveals a significant degree of hyperplasia.

TABLE 18-2. Causes of Abnormal Uterine Bleeding (Including Uterine and Extrauterine Causes)

Newborn	Maternal Estrogen
Childhood	Iatrogenic (trauma, foreign body, infection of vagina)
	Vaginal neoplasms (sarcoma botryoides)
	Ovarian tumors (functional)
Adolescence	Hypothalamic immaturity
	Psychogenic and nutritional problems
	Inadequate luteal function
Reproductive age	Anovulatory
	Central: psychogenic, stress
	Systemic: nutritional and endocrine disease
	Gonadal: functional tumors
	End organ: endometrial hyperplasia
	Pregnancy: ectopic, retained secundines, abortion, mole
	Ovulatory
	Organic: neoplasia, infections (pelvic inflammatory disease), leiomyomas
	Polymeorrhea: short follicular or luteal phases
	Iatrogenic anticoagulants, (intrauterine device)
	Irregular shedding
Menopause	Organic: carcinoma, hyperplasias, polyps
Postmenopause	Organic: carcinoma, hyperplasias, polyps
	Endometrial atrophy

Endometrial Adenocarcinoma

Endometrial carcinoma is the most frequent cancer of the female genital tract in American women (7% of all cancers in women).

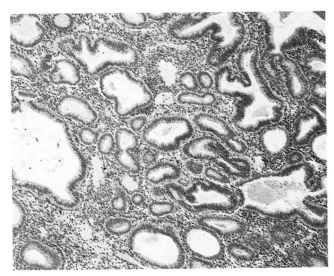

FIGURE 18-12
Complex endometrial hyperplasia. The endometrial glands, which are in the proliferative phase, are closely packed and display moderate architectural disarray (budding and branching). No cytologic atypia is present.

□ **Pathogenesis: Endometrial cancer is linked to prolonged estrogenic stimulation of the endometrium.** Exception for treatment of menopausal symptoms with exogenous estrogens, the most common risk factors for endometrial cancer are obesity, diabetes, hypertension, nulliparity, and late menopause. A high frequency of endometrial cancer is also found in women with estrogen-secreting granulosa cell tumors. Interestingly, cigarette smoking, which interferes with hepatic conversion of estrone to its active metabolite, estriol (see Chapter 8), is associated with a reduced risk of endometrial cancer. A high incidence of both endometrial carcinoma and breast cancer has been noted in closely related women, thereby suggesting a genetic predisposition to both diseases.

□ **Pathology:** Endometrial cancer may grow in a diffuse or a polypoid pattern (Fig. 18-13). Regardless of its site of origin, the tumor often involves multiple areas, because the anterior and posterior walls of the endometrium are in contact. Large tumors are often hemorrhagic and necrotic.

Pure, or Endometrioid, Adenocarcinoma of the Endometrium. This type of endometrial cancer is composed entirely of glandular cells and is the most common histologic variant (60%). The morphologic appearance varies from highly differentiated (grade 1) to poorly differentiated (grade 3; Fig. 18-14).

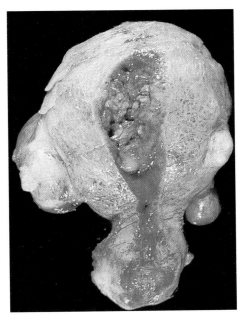

FIGURE 18-13
Adenocarcinoma of the endometrium. The uterus has been opened to reveal a partially necrotic, polypoid endometrial cancer.

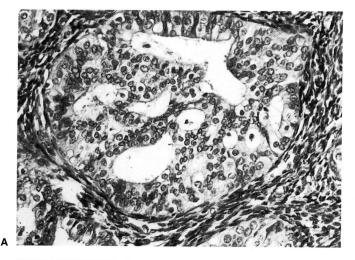

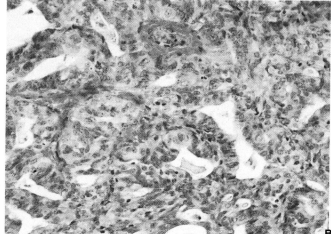

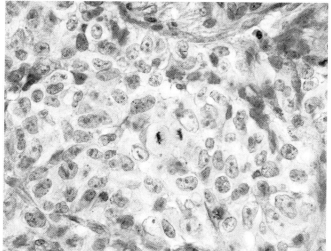

FIGURE *18-14*
Adenocarcinoma of the endometrium. (A) Grade 1. The tumor is well differentiated and composed entirely of glands. (B) Grade 2. The cancer is moderately differentiated and shows both glands and solid sheets of cells. (C) Grade 3. The tumor is poorly differentiated and composed entirely of sheets of cells. Numerous mitoses are present.

Endometrioid Adenocarcinoma with Squamous Differentiation. One-third of all endometrial carcinomas contain squamous cells in addition to the glandular element. If the squamous element is well differentiated and exhibits minimal atypia, the tumor is called **well-differentiated adenocarcinoma with squamous differentiation** (formerly adenoacanthoma). If the squamous element appears to be malignant, the tumor is labeled **poorly differentiated adenocarcinoma with squamous differentiation** (formerly adenosquamous carcinoma). These two variants represent 22% and 7% of all endometrial cancers, respectively.

Other types of endometrial carcinoma are less common and include **serous carcinoma, clear cell adenocarcinoma,** and **secretory carcinoma.**

☐ **Clinical Features:** Endometrial carcinoma typically occurs in perimenopausal or postmenopausal women. The chief complaint is usually abnormal uterine bleeding. Unlike cervical cancer, endometrial cancer may spread directly to the para-aortic lymph nodes, thereby skipping the pelvic nodes. Patients with advanced cancers may also develop hematogenous pulmonary metastases.

Patients with well-differentiated tumors confined to the endometrium are usually treated by hysterectomy. Postoperative radiation is administered if the tumor is poorly differentiated, the myometrium is more than superficially invaded, or the cervix is involved. The actuarial survival rate of all patients with endometrial cancer after treatment (regardless of any history of estrogen usage) is 80% after the second year and decreases to 65% after 10 years.

Leiomyoma

■ *Leiomyoma is a benign tumor of smooth muscle origin and the most common tumor of the female genital tract.* If minute tumors are included, leiomyomas occur in 75% of women older than 30 years of age. They are rare before the age of 20, however, and most regress after menopause.

☐ **Pathology:** Grossly, leiomyomas of the uterus are firm, pale-gray, whorled, and without encapsulation (Figs. 18-15 and 18-16). They range in size from 1 mm to more than 30 cm in diameter. Typically, the cut surface bulges, and the borders are smooth and distinct from the neighboring myometrium. Most leiomyomas are intramural, but some are submucosal, subserosal, or pedunculated. Leiomyomas with low mitotic activity and lacking nuclear atypia have little or no malignant potential. Microscopically, leiomyomas are composed of interlacing fascicles of uniform spindle cells, in which the nuclei are elongated and have blunt ends (see Fig. 18-16). The cytoplasm is abundant, eosinophilic, and fibrillar.

☐ **Clinical Features:** Submucosal leiomyomas may cause bleeding, an effect that results from ulceration of the thinned, overlying endometrium. Many intramural leiomyomas are symptomatic owing to sheer bulk, and large ones may interfere with bowel or bladder function. Leiomyomas usually grow slowly, but occasion-ally, they increase rapidly in size during pregnancy. Large symptomatic leiomyomas are removed by myomectomy or hysterectomy.

Leiomyosarcoma

■ *Leiomyosarcoma is a malignancy of smooth muscle origin and is generally identified by a high mitotic count* (discussed later). This cancer accounts for nearly 2% of uterine malignancies and is rare in comparison to its benign counterpart (1 : 1000 compared with leiomyoma). The pathogenesis of leiomyosarcomas is uncertain, but some appear to arise from within leiomyomas. Women with leiomyosarcomas are, on average, more than a decade older (age, >50 years) than women with leiomyomas, and the malignant tumors are larger as well (10–15 cm vs. 3–5 cm).

Leiomyosarcoma should be suspected if a "leiomyoma" is soft, shows areas of necrosis on gross examination, has irregular borders (invasion into neighboring myometrium), or does not bulge above the surface when cut. Microscopic evidence suggesting the diagnosis of leiomyosarcoma includes high mitotic activity and nuclear atypia. Because most leiomyosar-

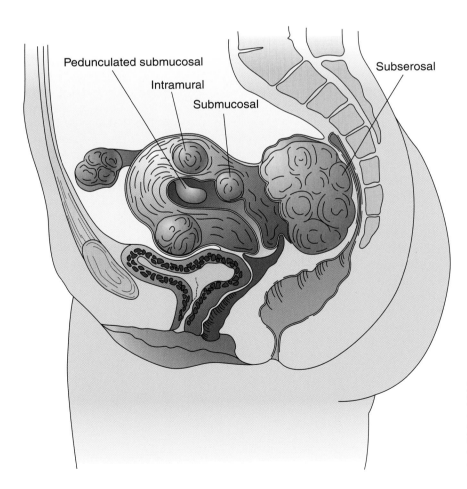

FIGURE *18-15*
Leiomyomas of the uterus. The leiomyomas are intramural; submucosal, with a pedunculated one appearing in the form of an endometrial polyp; and subserosal, with one compressing the bladder and the other compressing the rectum.

Labels on figure:
Pedunculated submucosal
Intramural
Submucosal
Subserosal

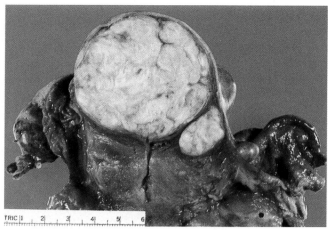
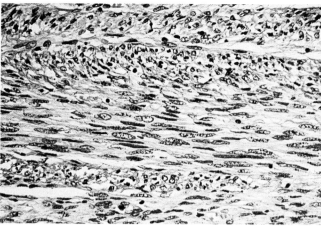

FIGURE   *18-16*
Leiomyoma of the uterus. (A) A bisected uterus displays a prominent, sharply circumscribed, and fleshy tumor. (B) Microscopically, smooth muscle cells intertwine in bundles, some of which are cut longitudinally (elongated nuclei) and others transversely.

comas are large and at an advanced stage when detected, they are usually fatal.

Fallopian Tube

SALPINGITIS

Both acute and chronic salpingitis typically result from ascending infections of the lower genital tract. The most common causative organisms are *N. gonorrhoeae, E. coli, Chlamydia,* and *Mycoplasma.* Chronic salpingitis usually develops only after repeated episodes of acute salpingitis. Inflammation of the fallopian tube is also the initial lesion in most cases of tuberculous genital infection.

☐ **Pathology and Clinical Features:** In patients with acute salpingitis, microscopic examination reveals a marked inflammatory infiltrate of polymorphonuclear leukocytes in association with marked edema and congestion of the mucosal folds (plicae). The inflammatory infiltrate in patients with chronic salpingitis is composed of lymphocytes and plasma cells. During the late stages, the fallopian tube may seal and become distended with pus (**pyosalpinx**) or an acellular transudate (**hydrosalpinx**). The adjacent ovary may also be involved in the process, sometimes giving rise to a **tubo-ovarian abscess.**

The damage wrought by chronic salpingitis often poses a mechanical obstruction to the passage of sperm, in which case infertility results. Chronic salpingitis is also a common cause of ectopic pregnancy,

because adherent mucosal plicae create pockets in which ova can become entrapped.

ECTOPIC PREGNANCY

■ *Ectopic pregnancy refers to any implantation that develops outside the endometrium.* More than 95% of ectopic pregnancies occur in the fallopian tube, mostly in the distal and middle one-thirds. An ectopic pregnancy results when passage of the conceptus along the fallopian tube is impeded, such as by mucosal adhesions or abnormal tubal motility secondary to inflammatory disease or endometriosis. Blood from the implantation site in the tube enters the peritoneal cavity, thereby causing abdominal pain. The thin tubal wall usually ruptures by the 12th week of gestation. Tubal rupture is life-threatening, because it can result in rapidly exsanguinating hemorrhage. Ectopic pregnancy, therefore, should be treated promptly with surgical intervention.

Ovary

OVARIAN CYSTS

Cysts are the most common cause of enlarged ovaries. Excluding cysts that arise from the invaginated surface epithelium of the ovary (serous cysts), almost all of these cysts arise from ovarian follicles.

Follicular Cysts

■ *Follicular cysts are thin-walled, fluid-filled structures that are lined internally by granulosa cells and externally by a layer of theca interna cells.* They are very common and occur at any age up to menopause. Follicular cysts are unilocular and may be single or multiple, unilateral or bilateral. They arise from ovarian follicles and probably relate to abnormalities in the release of pituitary gonadotropins. Follicular cysts rarely exceed 5 cm in diameter. The only significant complication is rupture of the follicular cyst, mild intraperitoneal bleeding, and abdominal pain.

Corpus Luteum Cysts

■ *Corpus luteum cysts result from delayed resolution of the central cavity of a corpus luteum.* Continued progesterone synthesis by the cyst leads to menstrual irregularities. A corpus luteum cyst is typically unilocular and 3 to 5 cm in diameter, with a yellow wall. Contents of the cyst vary from serosanguineous fluid to clotted blood. Microscopic examination shows numerous, large, luteinized granulosa cells. The condition is usually self-limited.

Theca Lutein Cysts

■ *Theca lutein cysts are multiple, bilateral, and luteinized follicular cysts.* They are commonly associated with conditions that are characterized by high levels of circulating gonadotropin (e.g., pregnancy, hydatidiform mole, choriocarcinoma, and exogenous gonadotropin therapy). Microscopically, the cysts show marked luteinization of the theca interna layer. Intraabdominal hemorrhage secondary to torsion or rupture of the cyst may require surgical intervention.

POLYCYSTIC OVARY SYNDROME (STEIN-LEVENTHAL SYNDROME)

■ *Polycystic ovary syndrome describes (1) persistent anovulation, (2) ovaries containing many small subcapsular cysts, and (3) clinical manifestations relating to secretion of excess androgenic hormones.* It was described initially as a syndrome complex of **secondary amenorrhea, hirsutism, and obesity.** However, it is now recognized that the clinical features associated with polycystic ovary syndrome are far more variable and even include amenorrheic women who otherwise appear to be normal. Three to 7% of women experience polycystic ovary syndrome, thereby making this condition one of the most common causes of infertility.

□ **Pathogenesis:** A simplified characterization of polycystic ovary syndrome holds that it is a state of chronic anovulation associated with luteinizing hormone (LH)–dependent ovarian overproduction of androgens (Fig. 18-17). Hormonal changes associated with polycystic ovary syndrome eventually result in abnormal maturation of the ovarian follicles, multiple follicular cysts, and a persistent anovulatory state.

□ **Pathology:** On gross examination, both ovaries are smooth and enlarged. Cut section reveals a thickened cortex and numerous subcortical cysts, which are typically less than 1 cm in diameter (Fig. 18-18). Microscopically, the following features are present: (1) numerous follicles in early stages of development, (2) follicular atresia, (3) stroma with luteinized cells (hyperthecosis), and (4) morphologic signs indicating an absence of ovulation (thick, smooth capsule and absence of corpora lutea and corpora albicantiae). Many of the subcapsular cysts are lined by thick zones of theca interna, some cells of which may be luteinized

□ **Clinical Features:** Patients with polycystic ovary syndrome are typically in their twenties and give a history of early obesity, menstrual problems, hirsutism, and infertility. Half of the women with polycystic ovary syndrome are amenorrheic, whereas most of the others have irregular menstrual periods. Unopposed, acyclic estrogen secretion results in an increased incidence of endometrial hyperplasia and adenocarcinoma. Treatment of polycystic ovary syndrome is mostly hormonal and directed toward interrupting the steady state of excess androgen production.

TUMORS

Cancer of the ovary is the second most frequent gynecologic malignancy after endometrial cancer, but in the United States, it carries a higher mortality rate than that from all other genital cancers combined. More than three-fourths of the patients already have extragonadal spread of tumor to the pelvis or abdomen at the time of diagnosis.

Epithelial Tumors

Tumors of common epithelial origin account for more than 90% of ovarian cancers and, if benign forms are included, nearly 60% of all ovarian tumors.

□ **Pathogenesis:** It is generally accepted that most common epithelial tumors arise from the surface ep-

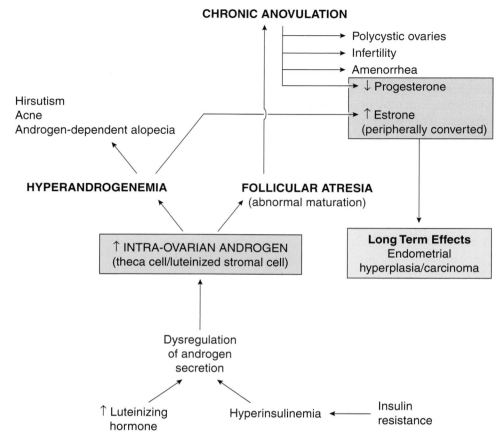

CHRONIC ANOVULATION

→ Polycystic ovaries
→ Infertility
→ Amenorrhea
→ ↓ Progesterone
→ ↑ Estrone
(peripherally converted)

Hirsutism
Acne
Androgen-dependent alopecia

HYPERANDROGENEMIA

FOLLICULAR ATRESIA
(abnormal maturation)

↑ INTRA-OVARIAN ANDROGEN
(theca cell/luteinized stromal cell)

Long Term Effects
Endometrial
hyperplasia/carcinoma

Dysregulation
of androgen
secretion

↑ Luteinizing
hormone

Hyperinsulinemia ← Insulin
resistance

FIGURE *18-17*
Pathogenesis of polycystic ovary syndrome.

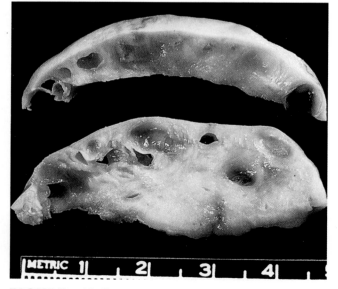

FIGURE *18-18*
Polycystic disease of the ovary. Cut sections of an ovary show numerous cysts embedded in a sclerotic stroma.

ithelium, or serosa, of the ovary. In order of decreasing frequency, the common epithelial tumors are:

- **Serous tumors,** which resemble the epithelium of the fallopian tube.
- **Mucinous tumors,** which mimic the mucosa of the endocervix.
- **Endometrioid tumors,** which are similar to the glands of the endometrium.
- **Clear cell tumors,** which consist of glycogen-rich cells that resemble endometrial glands in pregnancy.
- **Transitional cell tumors.**

Common epithelial neoplasms are associated with the repeated disruption of the epithelial surface that results from cyclic ovulation. Thus, these tumors most commonly afflict women who are nulliparous and, conversely, least often afflict women in whom ovulation has been suppressed (e.g., by pregnancy or oral contraceptives). A family history of ovarian carcinoma is occasionally elicited. Women with a history of ovarian carcinoma are also at greater risk for breast cancer, and vice versa. The same gene that is implicated in hereditary breast cancers, namely *BRCA-1* (17q12-q23), has been incriminated in the pathogenesis of familial ovarian cancers. Women with a mutated *BRCA-1* gene also tend to develop ovarian cancer considerably earlier than women with sporadic ovarian cancer.

Benign Epithelial Tumors

Benign common epithelial tumors are almost always serous or mucinous and generally arise in women between the ages of 20 and 60 years. They are frequently large, often growing to between 15 and 30 cm (or more) in diameter. Benign epithelial tumors are typically cystic, hence the term *cystadenoma*. **Serous cystadenomas** are more commonly bilateral (15%) than mucinous tumors, and they tend to be unilocular (Fig. 18-19). By contrast, **mucinous cystadenomas** are characteristically composed of hundreds of small cysts (locules; Fig. 18-20). As opposed to their malignant counterparts, benign epithelial tumors of the ovary tend to have thin walls and to lack solid areas. Microscopically, a single layer of tall columnar epithelium lines the cysts. Papillae, when present, consist of a fibrovascular core covered by a single layer of tall columnar epithelium identical to that of the cyst lining.

Pseudomyxoma Peritonei. As many as 5% of mucinous tumors of the ovary are complicated by the implantation of numerous mucus-producing cells on the peritoneal surfaces. These result in a massive accumulation of gelatinous material in the abdominal cavity similar to that seen in patients with pseudomyxoma peritonei associated with mucoceles of the appendix. Histologically, the peritoneal implants are composed of regular, mucus-containing columnar cells, without atypism or mitoses. Treatment of pseudomyxoma peritonei is primarily surgical and usually requires repetitive operations. Intraperitoneal alkylating agents have

also been used successfully. The 5-year survival rate is less than 50%.

Transitional Cell Tumor (Brenner Tumor)

■ *Transitional cell tumor (Brenner tumor) is a benign neoplasm composed of solid nests of transitional-like (urothelium-like) cells encased in a dense, fibrous stroma.* It occurs at all ages, with half of the cases presenting in women older than 50 years of age. The tumor size varies from a microscopic focus to masses as large as 8 cm or more in diameter.

Borderline Tumors (Tumors of Low Malignant Potential)

■ *Borderline tumors are a group of ovarian tumors that share an excellent prognosis, despite certain histologic features that suggest cancer.* A surgical cure is almost always possible if the tumor is confined to the ovaries. Even when it has spread to the pelvis or abdomen, 80% of these patients are alive after 5 years. Borderline tumors generally occur in women between the ages of 20 and 60 years.

Serous tumors of borderline malignancy are more commonly bilateral (34%) than are mucinous tumors (6%) or other types. Mucinous tumors sometimes achieve gigantic size (25 kg). In serous tumors of borderline malignancy, it is common to find papillary projections, which range from fine and exuberant growths to clusters of grape-like structures arising from one or several sites on the cyst wall. Microscopically, these foci resemble the papillary fronds in patients with benign cystadenomas but are distinguished from them by (1) epithelial stratification, (2) nuclear atypism, and (3) mitotic activity. The same criteria apply to borderline mucinous tumors, although papillary projections

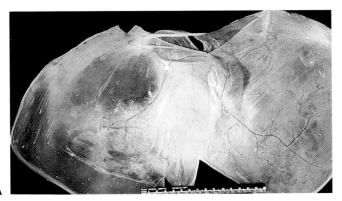

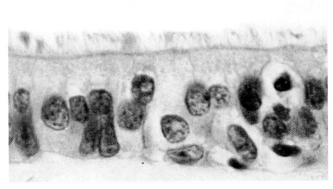

A   B

FIGURE **18-19**
Serous cystadenoma of the ovary. (A) The fluid has been removed from this huge, unilocular, serous cystadenoma. The wall is thin and translucent. (B) On microscopic examination, the cyst is lined by a single layer of ciliated, tubal-type epithelium.

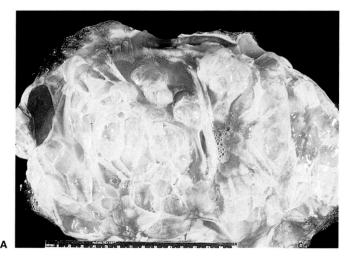

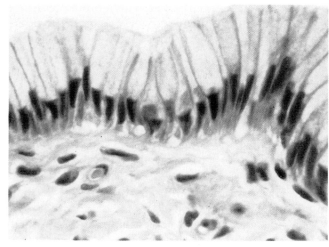

A   B

FIGURE *18-20*
Mucinous cystadenoma of the ovary. (A) The tumor is characterized by numerous cysts filled with thick, viscous fluid. (B) A single layer of mucinous epithelial cells lines the cyst.

are less conspicuous. **By definition, stromal invasion in the primary tumor removes it from the category of borderline malignancy and identifies it as being frankly malignant.**

Malignant Epithelial Tumors

Malignant epithelial tumors of the ovary are most common between the ages of 40 and 60 years and are rare before the age of 35. By the time a carcinoma reaches 10 to 15 cm, it often has already spread beyond the ovary and seeded the peritoneum.

Serous Cystadenocarcinoma. Serous cystadenocarcinoma is the most common malignant ovarian tumor, accounting for one-third of all cancers of the ovary. In half of the patients, the tumors are bilateral. On gross examination, serous cystadenocarcinomas usually present as multiloculated tumors, with soft, delicate papillae lining the entire surface. Solid areas, often with areas of necrosis and hemorrhage, are commonly present (Fig. 18-21).

Microscopically, serous cystadenocarcinomas vary from well-differentiated to poorly differentiated tumors. In the latter, the papillary pattern may be inconspicuous, with most areas being composed of solid sheets of malignant cells. Stromal and capsular invasion by the tumor cells is evident. Laminated calcified concretions, referred to as **psammoma bodies,** are present in one-third of the cases (see Fig. 18-21).

Mucinous Cystadenocarcinoma. Mucinous cystadenocarcinomas constitute as many as 10% of all ovarian cancers. They are among the largest tumors

recorded and, as previously noted for their benign counterpart, may attain a size of 50 cm in diameter. In one-fourth of the cases, bilateral tumors are present. Mucinous cancers are typically cystic and multilocular, with many solid areas and papillary projections. Microscopically, the appearance ranges from well differentiated to poorly differentiated, similar to that of serous cancers. Well-differentiated tumors are characterized by neoplastic glands that are lined by tall columnar, mucin-producing malignant cells (Fig. 18-22). Poorly differentiated mucinous adenocarcinomas show irregular nests and cords of tumor cells and numerous mitoses. Stromal invasion is the rule, and infiltration of the capsule is common.

Endometrioid Adenocarcinoma. Endometrioid adenocarcinoma is a tumor of the ovary that is identical histologically to carcinoma of the endometrium. Among epithelial tumors it is second only to serous cystadenocarcinoma in frequency, accounting for 20% of all ovarian cancers. The tumor occurs most commonly after menopause. **In contrast to serous and mucinous neoplasms, most endometrioid tumors are malignant.** One-third to one-half of endometrioid carcinomas are bilateral.

On gross examination, endometrioid carcinomas vary from 2 cm to more than 30 cm in diameter. They tend to be cystic, although some are completely solid and exhibit necrotic areas. A concomitant endometrial cancer has been encountered in 15% to 50% of cases. Overall, the survival rate of patients with endometrioid carcinoma is considerably better than that for patients with serous cystadenocarcinomas.

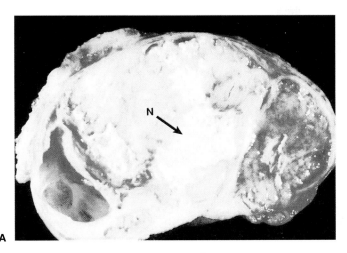

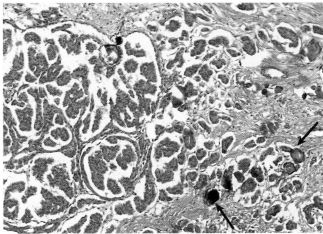

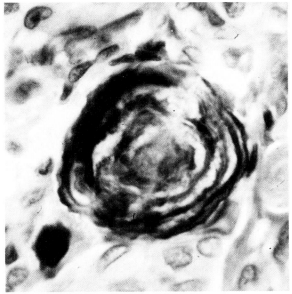

FIGURE *18-21*
Serous cystadenocarcinoma. (A) The ovary is enlarged by a solid tumor that exhibits extensive necrosis (N). (B) Microscopic examination shows a papillary cancer invading the ovarian stroma. Several psammoma bodies are present (*arrows*). (C) A higher-power view shows the laminated structure of a psammoma body.

Clear Cell Adenocarcinoma. Clear cell adenocarcinoma, which is thought to be closely related to endometrioid adenocarcinoma, is often found in association with endometriosis. It constitutes 5% to 10% of all ovarian cancers and usually occurs after menopause. Tumors range from 2 cm to 30 cm in diameter, and 40% are bilateral. The majority are partially cystic and exhibit necrosis and hemorrhage in the solid areas. Microscopically, clear cell adenocarcinoma is composed of sheets of malignant cells with clear cytoplasm, or tubules lined by cancer cells. The clinical course parallels that of endometrioid carcinoma.

☐ **Clinical Features:** The vast majority of ovarian tumors are nonfunctional—that is, they do not secrete hormones. However, an antibody to a cancer antigen (CA-125) in the serum detects a high proportion of nonmucinous epithelial tumors of the ovary. By the time these tumors are diagnosed, many have already metastasized.

Ovarian tumors have a tendency to implant in the peritoneal cavity on the diaphragm, lateral gutters, right paracolic gutter, and omentum. Lymphatic dissemination carries malignant cells to the para-aortic lymph nodes near the origin of the renal arteries and, to a lesser extent, to the external iliac (pelvic) or inguinal lymph nodes. Overall, the 5-year survival rate for malignant ovarian tumors is only 35%, because more than half of the tumors have spread to the abdominal cavity (stage 3) or elsewhere by the time they are discovered. The cornerstone to management of ovarian cancer is surgery. Adjuvant chemotherapy is used to treat distant occult sites of tumor spread.

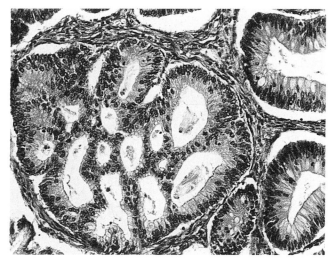

FIGURE *18-22*
Mucinous cystadenocarcinoma of the ovary. The malignant glands are arranged in a cribriform pattern and are composed of mucin-producing columnar cells.

Germ Cell Tumors

Tumors derived from germ cells of the ovary (Fig. 18-23) constitute one-fourth of all ovarian tumors. In adult women, germ cell tumors are virtually all benign (mature cystic teratoma, dermoid cyst), whereas in children and young adults, they are largely malignant. In children, germ cell tumors are the most common form of ovarian cancer (60%), but they are rare after menopause.

Dysgerminoma

■ *Dysgerminoma is the ovarian counterpart of testicular seminoma and is composed of primordial germ cells.* Although it accounts for less than 2% of all ovarian cancers, dysgerminoma is responsible for 10% of these cancers in women younger than 20 years of age. Most patients are between 10 and 30 years of age. The tumors are bilateral in 15% of cases.

On gross examination, dysgerminomas are often large and firm and have a bosselated external surface. The cut surface is soft and fleshy. Microscopic examination reveals large nests of monotonous tumor cells with a clear, glycogen-filled cytoplasm and irregularly flattened central nuclei. Fibrous septa containing lymphocytes traverse the tumor.

Dysgerminoma is treated surgically; when it is metastatic, radiation therapy and chemotherapy are also employed. The 5-year survival rate for patients with stage 1 tumors approaches 100%. Because the tumor is highly radiosensitive, 5-year survival rates for patients with higher-stage tumors still exceed 80%.

Teratoma

■ *Teratoma is a tumor of germ cell origin that shows differentiation toward somatic structures.* Most teratomas contain tissues representing at least two, and usually all three, of the embryonic layers.

Mature Teratoma (Mature Cystic Teratoma, Dermoid Cyst). The most common germ cell tumor, the mature cystic teratoma (dermoid cyst), is a benign neoplasm that accounts for one-fourth of all ovarian

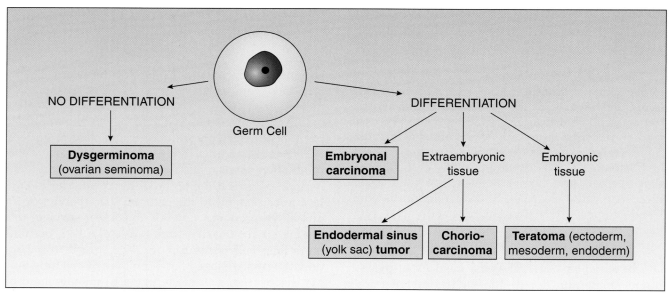

FIGURE *18-23*
Classification of germ cell tumors of the ovary.

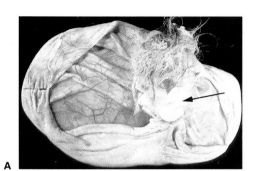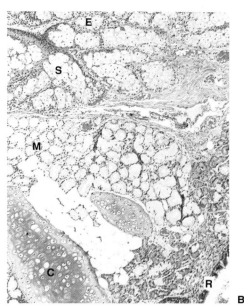

FIGURE *18-24*
Mature cystic teratoma of the ovary. (A) A mature cystic teratoma has been opened to reveal a solid knob (*arrow*), from which hair projects. (B) A photomicrograph of the solid knob shows epidermal and respiratory components. Tissue resembling the skin shows an epidermis (E) with underlying sebaceous glands (S). The respiratory tissue consists of mucous glands (M), cartilage (C), and respiratory epithelium (R).

tumors. The peak incidence occurs during the third decade of life.

The tumor is cystic, and more than 90% contain skin, sebaceous glands, and hair follicles (Fig. 18-24). Half of the tumors exhibit smooth muscle, sweat glands, cartilage, bone, teeth, and respiratory tract epithelium. Tissues such as gut, thyroid, and brain are encountered less frequently. **Struma ovarii** refers to a cystic lesion composed predominantly of thyroid tissue (5–20% of mature cystic teratomas).

A small minority (1%) of dermoid cysts undergo malignant transformation. Three-fourths of all cancers that arise in dermoid cysts are squamous cell carcinomas. The remainder include carcinoid tumor, basal cell carcinoma, thyroid cancer, adenocarcinoma, and others. The overall prognosis of patients with malignant transformation of a mature cystic teratoma is unfavorable, with less than one-third of these patients surviving for 5 years.

Immature Teratoma. Immature teratoma of the ovary is composed of elements derived from the three germ layers. However, unlike mature cystic teratoma, it contains embryonal tissues. Immature teratoma accounts for 20% of malignant tumors at all sites in women younger than 20 years of age, but it becomes progressively less common in older women.

Immature teratoma is predominantly solid and lobulated and contains numerous small cysts. Solid areas may contain grossly recognizable immature bone and cartilage. Microscopically, multiple tumor components are usually found, including those differentiating toward nerves (neuroepithelial rosettes and immature glia; Fig. 18-25), glands, and other structures found in mature cystic teratomas. Patients with well-differentiated immature teratomas generally have a fa-

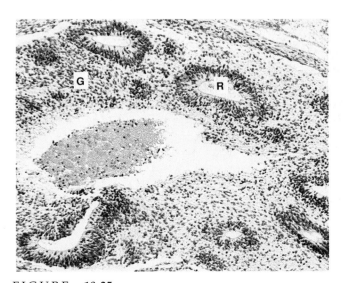

FIGURE *18-25*
Immature teratoma of the ovary. Immature neural tissue exhibits rosettes (R) with multilayered nuclei. Embryonal glia (G) display densely packed, atypical nuclei.

vorable outcome, whereas patients with high-grade tumors (predominantly embryonal tissue) have a poor prognosis.

Endodermal Sinus Tumor (Yolk Sac Carcinoma)

■ *Endodermal sinus tumor is a highly malignant tumor of women younger than 30 years of age that, histologically, resembles the mesenchyme of the primitive yolk sac.* Typically, endodermal sinus tumor is large and displays extensive necrosis and hemorrhage. The most common microscopic appearance is a reticular, honeycombed pattern of communicating spaces that are lined by primitive cells. **Schiller-Duval bodies,** which resemble the endodermal sinuses of the rodent placenta, are found in more than half of the tumors and are characteristic of the tumor. These structures consist of papillae that protrude into a space lined by tumor cells. Papillae are covered by a mantle of embryonal cells and contain a fibrovascular core and a central blood vessel.

Endodermal sinus tumor secretes α-fetoprotein, and detection of this protein in the blood is useful both for establishing the diagnosis and for monitoring the effectiveness of therapy. Before the era of chemotherapy, endodermal sinus tumor was nearly always fatal. Now, 5-year survival rates approach 80% for patients with stage 1 tumors.

Choriocarcinoma

■ *Choriocarcinoma of the ovary is a rare tumor that mimics the epithelial covering of placental villi, namely cytotrophoblast and syncytiotrophoblast.* Choriocarcinoma of germ cell origin generally presents in young girls as precocious sexual development, menstrual irregularities, or rapid breast enlargement.

The tumor is unilateral, solid, and extensively hemorrhagic. Microscopically, it is composed of an admixture of malignant cytotrophoblasts and syncytiotrophoblasts. The syncytial cells secrete hCG, which accounts for the frequent finding of a positive pregnancy test. The tumor is highly aggressive, but it is responsive to chemotherapy.

Sex Cord/Stromal Tumors

Sex cord/stromal tumors are derived from either the primitive sex cords or the mesenchymal stroma of the developing gonad. They account for 10% of all ovarian tumors, range from benign to low-grade malignant, and frequently, differentiate toward female (granulosa and theca cells) or male (Sertoli and Leydig cells) structures. **Sex cord/stromal tumors account for most of the clinically functional ovarian tumors.**

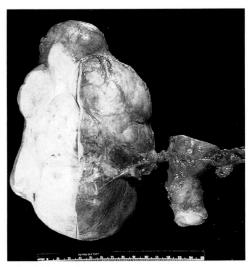

FIGURE   *18-26*
Fibroma of the ovary. The ovary is conspicuously enlarged by a firm, white, and bosselated tumor.

Ovarian Fibroma

Fibromas are the most common ovarian stromal tumors (76% of all stromal tumors and 7% of all ovarian tumors). They occur at all ages, with a peak during the perimenopausal period, and are virtually always benign. The tumors are solid, firm, and white (Fig. 18-26). Microscopically, the cells resemble stroma of the normal ovarian cortex, being composed of well-differentiated fibroblasts and variable amounts of collagen. Half of the larger tumors are associated with ascites and, rarely, with ascites and pleural effusions (Meigs syndrome).

Thecomas

■ *Thecomas are benign, functional ovarian tumors that arise in postmenopausal women.* In the majority of cases, they produce signs of estrogen production. Thecomas are solid tumors and are usually 5 to 10 cm in diameter. The cut section is yellow owing to the presence of many lipid-laden theca cells. Microscopically, the cells are large and oblong to round, with a vacuolated cytoplasm that contains lipid. Bands of hyalinized collagen separate nests of theca cells. Because of estrogen output by the tumor, thecomas commonly cause irregularity in menstrual cycles and breast enlargement. Endometrial hyperplasia or cancer may be complications.

Granulosa Cell Tumor

■ *Granulosa cell tumor is the prototypical functional neoplasm of the ovary associated with estrogen secretion.* This tumor should be considered as malignant because

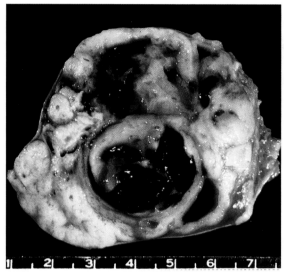 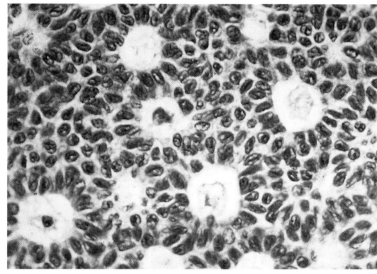

A · B

FIGURE 18-27
Granulosa cell tumor of the ovary. (A) Cross-section of the enlarged ovary shows a variegated, solid tumor with focal hemorrhages. The yellow areas represent collections of lipid-laden luteinized granulosa cells. (B) The orientation of tumor cells about central spaces results in the characteristic follicular pattern (Call-Exner bodies).

of its potential for local spread and the rare occurrence of distant metastases. Most granulosa cell tumors occur after menopause; they are unusual before puberty.

☐ **Pathology:** Granulosa cell tumors, like most ovarian tumors, are large and focally cystic to solid. Characteristically, the tumor has yellow areas representing lipid-laden luteinized granulosa cells, white zones of stroma, and focal hemorrhages (Fig. 18-27). Microscopically, granulosa cell tumors display an array of growth patterns: (1) diffuse (sarcomatoid), (2) insular (islands of cells), or (3) trabecular (anastomotic bands of granulosa cells). Orientation of the cells about a central space (**Call-Exner bodies**) results in a characteristic follicular pattern. The tumor cells are typically spindle-shaped and have a cleaved, elongated nucleus (coffee bean appearance).

☐ **Clinical Features: Three-fourths of granulosa cell tumors are functional—that is, they secrete estrogens.** Consequently, endometrial hyperplasia is a common presenting sign. Hyperplasia may progress to endometrial adenocarcinoma if the functioning granulosa cell tumor remains undetected. At initial diagnosis, 90% of granulosa cell tumors are confined to the ovary (stage I), and these patients have a 10-year survival rate of greater than 90%. Tumors that have extended into the pelvis and lower abdomen have a poorer prognosis, however, and recurrence after surgical removal is usually fatal.

Sertoli-Leydig Cell Tumors

■ *Sertoli-Leydig cell tumor (arrhenoblastoma or androblastoma) is a rare mesenchymal neoplasm of the ovary*

with low malignant potential. It resembles the embryonic testis and often secretes androgens. It occurs at all ages but is most common in young women of childbearing age.

☐ **Pathology:** Sertoli-Leydig cell tumors are unilateral and vary in size from microscopic foci to very large lesions, with most measuring between 5 and 15 cm in diameter. They tend to form lobulated, solid, and yellow or tan masses. Microscopically, the tumors vary from well to poorly differentiated, and some exhibit heterologous elements (e.g., papillae, glands, cartilage). The most characteristic features are large Leydig cells, which have abundant eosinophilic cytoplasm, and fine trabeculae of sex cords, which are immature solid tubules of embryonic Sertoli cells (Fig. 18-28).

☐ **Clinical Features:** Somewhat more than half of all patients with Sertoli-Leydig cell tumors exhibit no endocrine effects. Patients with functioning tumors present with signs of virilization, as evidenced by hirsutism, male escutcheon, enlarged clitoris, and deep voice. Virilization results from the secretion of testosterone and other androgenic hormones by the Sertoli-Leydig cell tumor. Well-differentiated tumors are virtually always cured by surgical resection, but poorly differentiated ones may recur and metastasize.

Tumors Metastatic to the Ovary

Some 3% of ovarian cancers (1% of all ovarian tumors) arise outside the ovary, with the most common primary sites being, in descending order, the breast, large intestine, stomach, and other genital tract organs. Of

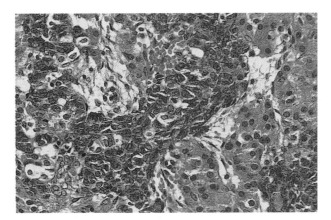

FIGURE   *18-28*
Leydig-cell tumor. Immature solid tubules of embryonic Sertoli cells are adjacent to clusters of Leydig cells, which exhibit abundant eosinophilic cytoplasm.

those metastatic tumors large enough to present clinically, the colon is the most frequent site of origin.

Krukenberg tumors are ovarian metastases in which the tumor appears as nests of mucin-filled, "signet-ring" cells within a cellular stroma derived from the ovary. The stomach is the primary site in 75% of the cases; most of the other Krukenberg tumors are from the colon.

Placenta

CHORIOAMNIONITIS

■ *Chorioamnionitis refers to inflammation of the placental amnion and chorion and of the extraplacental membranes.* It is usually the result of an ascending infection from the maternal birth canal, most commonly owing to premature rupture of the membranes. In this type of infection, the inflammatory process primarily affects the membranes (chorioamnionitis) rather than the chorionic villi.

☐ **Pathology:** The amniotic fluid is usually cloudy. The membrane walls are slightly opaque, edematous, and friable, and microscopically, they disclose a neutrophilic infiltrate, often with fibrin deposition. Microorganisms cultured from placentas with chorioamnionitis are group B streptococci, *E. coli, Gardnerella vaginalis,* and anaerobic organisms of the *Bacteroides* group.

☐ **Clinical Features:** Risks of chorioamnionitis to the fetus include (1) pneumonia after inhalation of infected amniotic fluid; (2) skin or eye infections from di-

rect contact with organisms in the fluid; and (3) neonatal gastritis, enteritis, or peritonitis from ingestion of infected fluid. Major risks to the mother are intrapartum fever, postpartum endometritis, and pelvic sepsis.

TOXEMIA OF PREGNANCY (PRE-ECLAMPSIA AND ECLAMPSIA)

■ *Toxemia of pregnancy defines a symptom complex of hypertension, proteinuria, pathologic edema, and in its most advanced stage, convulsions.* It occurs in 6% of pregnant women as **pre-eclampsia** during the last trimester, especially with the first child. If convulsive seizures appear, the disorder is termed **eclampsia.**

☐ **Pathogenesis:** A number of characteristic features of toxemia deserve emphasis:

- The first pregnancy carries a risk for the syndrome many times higher than that associated with subsequent pregnancies.
- Because toxemia also occurs with hydatidiform mole (discussed later), the responsible tissue is most likely the trophoblast.
- There is a marked reduction in maternal blood flow to the placenta.
- Renal involvement in toxemia leads to maternal hypertension and proteinuria.
- Platelet aggregation occurs early and plays a role in the development of disseminated intravascular coagulation.

Pathologic changes in the placenta reflect reduced maternal blood flow to the uteroplacental unit. The key factor resides in the spiral arteries of the uteroplacental bed, which never fully dilate in patients with toxemia of pregnancy. The arteries are smaller than normal and retain their musculoelastic wall, which ordinarily is replaced by a fibrinous material. Normally, extravillous trophoblast invades these arteries and destroys their vascular tone, thereby permitting vasodilatation. However, in patients with toxemia, as many as half of the spiral arteries escape invasion by endovascular trophoblastic tissue and, thus, are not dilated.

☐ **Pathology:** Extensive infarction of the placenta (>10% of placental parenchyma) is found in nearly one-third of patients with severe pre-eclampsia. Retroplacental hemorrhage occurs in as many as 15% of patients. Microscopically, the villi show signs of underperfusion: the cytotrophoblastic cells of the villi are hyperplastic, and the basement membrane is thickened. The kidney in patients with toxemia always demonstrates glomerular lesions (see Chapter 16). In fatal cases of toxemia, cerebral hemorrhages, ranging from petechiae to large hematomas, are common.

☐ **Clinical Features:** Toxemia usually begins insidiously after the 20th week of pregnancy, with excessive weight gain occasioned by fluid retention. Shortly thereafter, the maternal blood pressure tends to increase, with diastolic pressures of 110 to 120 mm Hg. At the same time, proteinuria appears and increases in severity as the disease progresses. In patients with severe toxemia (eclampsia), renal function declines, changes of disseminated intravascular coagulation appear, and convulsions and coma supervene. Preeclampsia is treated with antihypertensive agents and antiplatelet drugs, but the definitive therapy is removal of the placenta, ideally by normal delivery.

GESTATIONAL TROPHOBLASTIC DISEASE

■ *Gestational trophoblastic disease embraces the spectrum of trophoblastic disorders characterized by abnormal proliferation and maturation of trophoblast as well as neoplasms derived from trophoblast.*

Complete Hydatidiform Mole

■ *Complete hydatidiform mole is a placenta that has grossly swollen chorionic villi, resembling bunches of grapes, in which there are varying degrees of trophoblastic proliferation* (Table 18-3). The villi are enlarged and generally exceed 1 mm in diameter (Fig. 18-29). There is no embryo.

☐ **Pathogenesis:** Complete mole results from the fertilization of an empty ovum that lacks functional DNA. The haploid (23,X) set of paternal chromosomes duplicates to 46,XX. Hence, most complete moles are homozygous 46,XX, but all of the chromosomes are of paternal origin. Because the embryo dies at a very early stage, before placental circulation has developed, few chorionic villi develop blood vessels, and fetal parts are always absent.

☐ **Risk Factors:** The risk for development of hydatidiform mole is related to maternal age and has two peaks. Girls younger than 15 years of age have a 20-fold higher risk than women 20 to 35 years of age. The risk increases progressively for women older than 40 years of age. In fact, women older than 50 years have a risk 200-fold greater than that of women between 20

TABLE 18-3. Comparative Features of Complete and Partial Hydatidiform Mole

Features	Complete Mole	Partial Mole
Karyotype	46,XX	47,XXY or 47,XXX
Preoperative diagnosis	Mole	Missed abortion
Marked vaginal bleeding	3+	1+
Uterus	Large	Small
Serum hCG[a]	High	Less elevated
Hydropic villi	All	Some
Trophoblast proliferation	Diffuse	Focal
Atypia	Diffuse	Minimal
hCG in tissue	3+	1+
Embryo present	No	Some
Blood vessels	No	Common
Nucleated erythrocytes	No	Sometimes
Persists after initial therapy	20%	7%
Choriocarcinoma develops	2% after mole	No choriocarcinoma

[a] *hCG, human chorionic gonadotropin.*

and 40 years of age. The incidence of hydatidiform mole is many times higher among Asian women than among white women, reaching an incidence in Taiwan that is 25-fold greater than that in the United States. Women who have had a previous hydatidiform mole have a more than 20-fold greater risk than that of the general population to develop a subsequent molar pregnancy.

☐ **Pathology:** Molar tissue is voluminous and consists of macroscopically visible villi that are obviously swollen. Microscopically, many of the individual villi have cisternae, which are central, acellular, fluid-filled spaces devoid of mesenchymal cells. The trophoblast is hyperplastic and composed of syncytiotrophoblast, cytotrophoblast, and intermediate trophoblast. Considerable cellular atypia is present.

☐ **Clinical Features:** Patients with complete moles commonly present between the 11th and 25th weeks of pregnancy complaining of excessive uterine enlargement and, often, of abnormal uterine bleeding. These signs are sometimes accompanied by the passage of tissue fragments, which appear as small, grape-like masses. The serum hCG concentration is markedly elevated, and serial determinations disclose rapidly increasing levels.

Complications of complete hydatidiform mole include uterine hemorrhage, disseminated intravascular coagulation, uterine perforation, trophoblastic embolism, and infection. **The most important complication of hydatidiform mole is development of choriocarcinoma, which occurs in approximately 2% of**

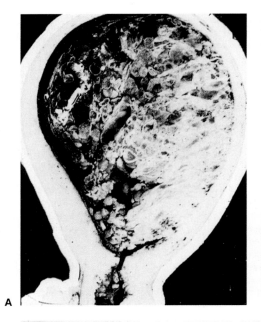

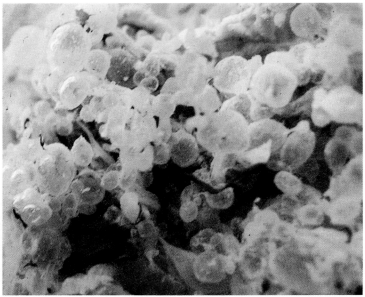

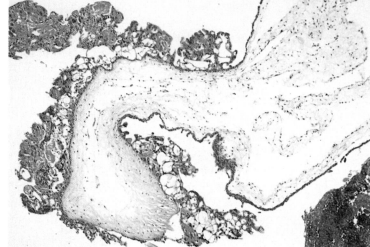

FIGURE   *18-29*
Complete hydatidiform mole. (A) Complete mole in which the entire uterine cavity is filled with swollen villi. (B) The villi are each 1 to 3 mm in diameter and grape-like in appearance. (C) Individual molar villi, many of which have cavitated central cisternal, exhibit considerable trophoblastic hyperplasia and atypia. The blood vessels of the villi have atrophied and disappeared.

patients after a complete mole has been evacuated. Treatment of hydatidiform mole consists of suction curettage of the uterus and subsequent monitoring of serum hCG levels.

Partial Hydatidiform Mole

Partial hydatidiform mole is now recognized to be a distinct form of mole. **It is important to distinguish this lesion from complete hydatidiform mole, because it does not evolve into choriocarcinoma** (see Table 18-2). The karyotype of a partial hydatidiform mole has 69 chromosomes (triploidy). This abnormal chromosomal complement results from the fertilization of a normal ovum (23,X) by two normal spermatozoa, each carrying 23 chromosomes, or by a single spermatozoon that has not undergone meiotic reduction and bears 46 chromosomes. The fetus associated with a partial mole usually dies at about 10 weeks of gestation, and the mole is aborted shortly thereafter. In contrast to a complete mole, fetal parts are present.

☐ Pathology: Partial moles have two populations of chorionic villi. Some villi are normal, whereas others are enlarged by hydropic swelling and may show central cavitation (Fig. 18-30). Unlike complete mole, the embryo is sometimes present.

Invasive Hydatidiform Mole

■ *Invasive hydatidiform mole is a mole in which the villous trophoblast has invaded the underlying myometrium.*

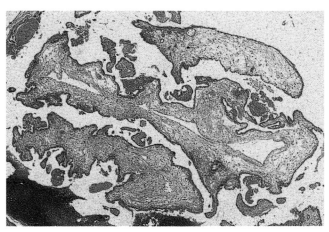

FIGURE *18-30*
Partial hydatidiform mole. Two populations of chorionic villi are evident. Some are normal, whereas others are conspicuously swollen. Trophoblastic proliferation is focal and less conspicuous than in a complete mole.

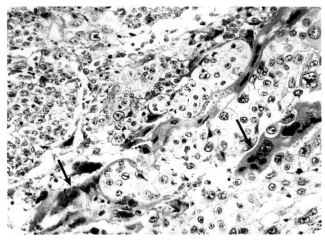

FIGURE *18-31*
Choriocarcinoma. Malignant cytotrophoblast and syncytiotrophoblast (*arrows*) are present.

□ **Pathology:** Invasive villi may extend only superficially into the myometrium or may penetrate the uterus. An invasive mole often enters dilated venous channels in the myometrium, and 25% to 40% of the cases involve spread to distant sites, most frequently the lungs. Unlike choriocarcinoma (discussed later), distant deposits of an invasive mole do not penetrate beyond the confines of the blood vessels in which they are lodged, and death from such spread is unusual.

Choriocarcinoma

■ *Gestational choriocarcinoma is a malignant tumor that derives from the trophoblast.* It is actually a tumor allograft in the host mother and, thus, is unique among human cancers.

□ **Epidemiology:** Choriocarcinoma occurs with a frequency of approximately 1 in 30,000 pregnancies in the United States, whereas in areas with a high incidence of hydatidiform mole (e.g., the Orient), the frequency is far greater. Although the risk that a hydatidiform mole will transform into a choriocarcinoma is only 2%, it is still several orders of magnitude greater than if the pregnancy were normal.

□ **Pathology:** The uterine lesions of choriocarcinoma range from microscopic foci to huge necrotic and hemorrhagic tumors. Histologically, the tumor consists of a dimorphic population of cytotrophoblast and syncytiotrophoblast, with varying degrees of intermediate trophoblast (Fig. 18-31). Rims of syncytiotrophoblast surround central cores of cytotrophoblast in addition to being arranged around maternal blood spaces. Choriocarcinoma invades primarily through venous sinuses in the myometrium. It metastasizes widely by the hematogenous route, especially to lung (>90%), brain, gastrointestinal tract, and liver.

□ **Clinical Features:** The most frequent initial indication of choriocarcinoma is abnormal uterine bleeding. Occasionally, the first sign is occasioned by metastases to the lungs or brain. In some cases, a choriocarcinoma only becomes evident 10 or more years after the last pregnancy.

Before the era of chemotherapy, the cure rate for choriocarcinoma limited to the uterus was only 30%, and metastatic choriocarcinoma was virtually always fatal. Today, survival rates of greater than 70% are now being achieved for tumors that have metastasized, and virtually 100% remission rates are to be expected if the tumor is localized. Serial serum hCG levels are used to monitor the effectiveness of treatment.

CHAPTER 19

The Breast

Sue A. Bartow

The breast has become biologically superfluous in advanced societies, and it is now a matter of choice whether to make use of its sole function—nursing the young. Nevertheless, cancer of the breast is common and remains one of the leading causes of death in women. It is, therefore, important to understand the biology of malignant tumors and of benign changes associated with an increased risk of cancer.

FIBROCYSTIC CHANGE

■ *Fibrocystic change of the breast refers to a constellation of morphologic features characterized by (1) cystic dilatation of terminal ducts, (2) a relative increase in fibrous stroma, and (3) variable proliferation of terminal duct epithelial elements.* The cause of fibrocystic change is unknown. It is most often diagnosed in women from their late twenties to the time of menopause, and some degree of fibrocystic change occurs in 60% to 80% of adult women in the United States. The frequency of diagnosis decreases progressively, however, after menopause.

Nonproliferative Fibrocystic Change

The morphologic hallmarks of nonproliferative fibrocystic change are an increase in dense, fibrous stroma and some degree of cystic dilatation of the terminal ducts (Fig. 19-1). Fibrocystic change always occurs in multiple areas of both breasts. Large cysts, as much as 5 cm in diameter, often contain dark, thin fluid, which imparts a blue color to the unopened cysts—the so-called **blue-domed cysts of Bloodgood.** Aspiration of a large cyst will usually cause it to collapse and then disappear.

On microscopic examination, the epithelium lining the cysts varies from columnar to flattened, or it may be entirely absent. A frequent concomitant of nonproliferative fibrocystic change is an alteration of the epithelial lining, termed **apocrine metaplasia.** The metaplastic cells are larger and more eosinophilic than the cells that usually line the ducts, and they resemble apocrine sweat gland epithelium. These cells are usually arranged in a single layer, but on occasion, they form papillary structures.

Proliferative Fibrocystic Change

The most common proliferative change in fibrocystic disease is an increased number of cells lining the dilated terminal ducts, which is referred to as ductal epithelial hyperplasia (see Fig. 19-1). The proliferation can, at times, become exuberant and form papillary structures within the lumen of the distended ductule (papillomatosis).

Hyperplasia of the duct epithelium involves the same cell type that gives rise to carcinoma of the breast. The morphologic spectrum ranges from cytologically benign hyperplasia to cytologic atypia to carcinoma in situ.

Sclerosing Adenosis

■ *Sclerosing adenosis is a variant of proliferative fibrocystic change and is characterized by the proliferation of small ducts and myoepithelial cells in the region of the terminal duct lobular unit (adenosis)* (Fig. 19-2). It is almost always associated with other forms of proliferative fibrocystic change. Because the lesion is commonly associated with fibrosis, the term **sclerosing** is added. Microscopically, the lobular units are deformed and enlarged by the proliferated epithelial cells, which appear as whorls and cords of tubules that are surrounded by fibrous stroma. Sclerosing adenosis is of significance primarily to the surgical pathologist, who must distinguish it histologically from invasive carcinoma.

Prognostic Significance

A number of conclusions can be drawn regarding the relationship of fibrocystic change to breast cancer:

- The presence of nonproliferative fibrocystic change in a biopsy specimen does not indicate an increased risk for the development of invasive breast cancer.
- The demonstration of proliferative fibrocystic change in a biopsy places a woman at a 1.5- to 2.0-fold increased risk for the development of invasive cancer.
- "Atypical" proliferative lesions increase the risk for the subsequent development of carcinoma of the breast to between four- to fivefold that of the general population. This risk is further increased if the woman has a first-degree relative (mother, sister, or daughter) with breast cancer.
- The proliferative lesions may be multifocal and bilateral, and the risk of subsequent carcinoma is equal in both breasts.

FIBROADENOMA

■ *Fibroadenoma, the most common benign neoplasm of the breast, is a tumor composed of epithelial and stromal ele-*

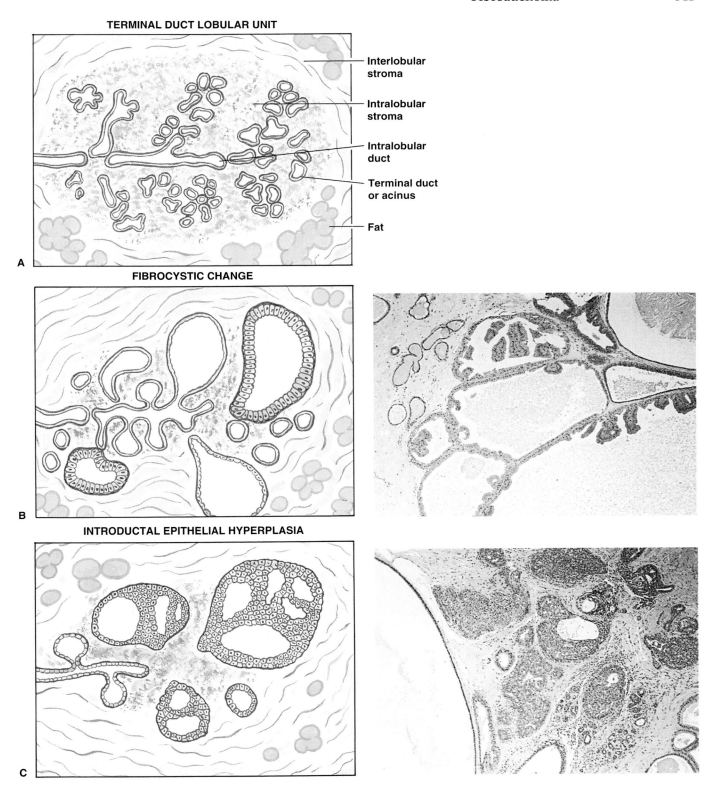

FIGURE *19-1*
Histology of fibrocystic change. (A) The normal terminal lobular unit. (B) Nonproliferative fibrocystic change: This lesion combines cystic dilatation of the terminal ducts with varying degrees of apocrine metaplasia of the epithelium and increased fibrous stroma. (C) Proliferative fibrocystic change: Terminal duct dilatation and intraductal epithelial hyperplasia are present.

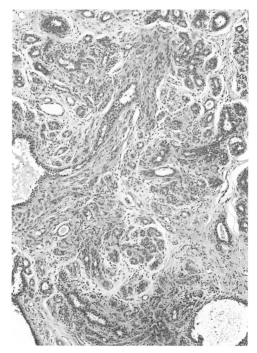

FIGURE *19-2*
Sclerosing adenosis. A proliferation of small, abortive, duct-like structures and myoepithelial cells both expands and distorts the lobule in which it arises.

ments that originates from the terminal duct lobular unit. Fibroadenomas are usually found in women between 20 and 35 years of age, although they also occur in adolescent girls. They commonly enlarge more rapidly during pregnancy and cease to grow after menopause. Women with fibroadenomas are reported to have a doubled risk of developing breast cancer.

☐ **Pathology:** Fibroadenoma is a round, rubbery tumor, usually 2 to 4 cm in diameter, that is sharply demarcated from the surrounding breast and, thus, is freely movable. The cut surface appears a glistening gray-white. On microscopic examination, the tumor displays a mixture of fibrous connective tissue and ducts (Fig. 19-3). The ducts may be simple and round or elongate and branching, and are dispersed within a characteristic fibrous stroma. This fibrous tissue, which forms most of the tumor, often compresses the proliferated ducts, thereby reducing them to curvilinear slits. Treatment is surgical excision.

CARCINOMA OF THE BREAST

Breast cancer is the most common malignancy of women in the United States, and the mortality rate from this disease is second only to that of lung cancer as a cause of death from cancer among women. Currently, 7% of American women may be expected to develop breast cancer by 70 years of age, and one-third of these women will die of the disease. Breast cancer is uncommon before 35 years of age.

☐ **Pathogenesis:** The pathogenesis of breast cancer is unknown, but a number of factors are associated with an increased risk.

Genetic Factors. The strongest association with an increased risk for breast cancer is a family history, specifically breast cancer in first-degree relatives (mother, sister, daughter):

- *BRCA1* **gene (breast cancer 1).** This gene, which is located on chromosome 17, has been implicated in the pathogenesis of hereditary breast and ovarian cancers. Germline mutations in the *BRCA1* gene place a woman at a remarkable 85% lifetime risk of breast cancer. It is suspected that mutations in this gene account for half of all cases of inherited breast cancer (as many as 10% of all breast cancers). Women with *BRCA1* mutations are also at a greater lifetime risk of ovarian cancer, which has been estimated to range from 20% to 60%.
- *BRCA2* **gene.** Mutations in this gene, which is situated on chromosome 13q, are incriminated in some 70% of the cases of inherited breast cancer that are not secondary to mutations in the *BRCA1* gene. Similar to the situation with *BRCA1*, women with *BRCA2* mutations also exhibit an increased risk of ovarian cancer.
- *p53* **tumor suppressor gene:** In the Li-Fraumeni familial cancer syndrome, mutations in the *p53* gene are responsible for breast cancer in young women. It is estimated that germline mutations in *p53* account for 1% of breast cancers among women in whom the tumor is detected before the age of 40 years.

Hormonal Status. Early menarche, late menopause, and older age at first-term pregnancy all increase the risk of breast cancer. Nulliparous women, or those who become pregnant for the first time after 35 years of age, have a two- to threefold increased risk of breast cancer compared with women whose first pregnancy occurred before 25 years of age. However, pregnancy transiently increases the risk of breast cancer for as long as 15 years, although this effect is overshadowed by a reduction in the long-term risk. The augmented susceptibility likely relates to the influence of female hormones on the proliferation or differentiation of the breast epithelium.

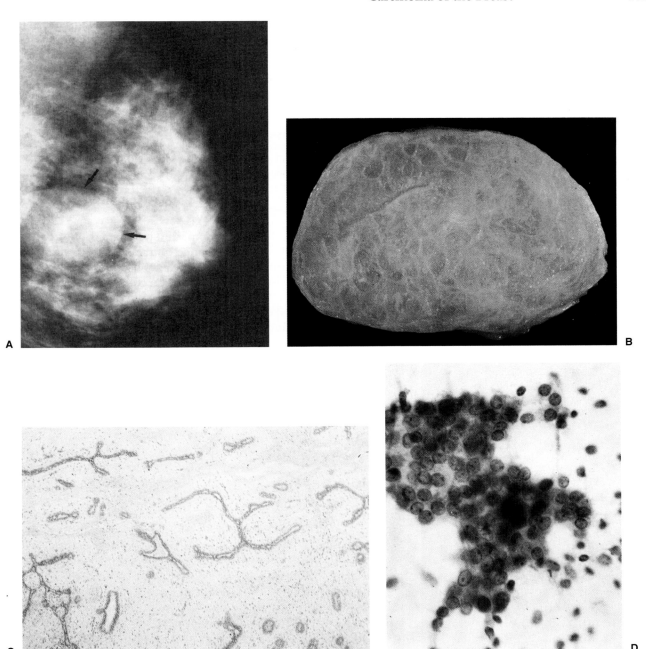

FIGURE 19-3

Fibroadenoma. (A) Mammogram. A dominant mass (*arrows*) with smooth borders is the same density as that of normal breast tissue in a young woman. (B) Surgical specimen. This well-circumscribed tumor was easily enucleated from the surrounding tissue. The cut surface is characteristically a glistening tannish-white and has a septate appearance. (C) Microscopic section. Elongated epithelial duct structures are situated within a loose, myxoid stroma. (D) Fine-needle aspiration. This cytologic preparation shows bland ductal cells arranged in cohesive clusters that have an irregular, "staghorn" shape.

Environmental Influences. There is a four- to five-fold greater incidence of breast cancer in Western industrialized countries than in less-developed countries or among Native Americans in the United States. Furthermore, women who migrate to the United States from countries where the incidence of breast cancer is low (e.g., Japan) manifest a cancer risk as high as that of the white American population within one or two generations. It has been suggested that dietary factors, particularly fat content, are responsible for these differences in the geographic distribution of breast cancer, but this concept remains controversial.

Fibrocystic Change. Women with fibrocystic change have an increased risk of breast cancer only in the presence of specific proliferative lesions.

Previous Cancer. Women who have previously had breast cancer are at a tenfold increased risk of developing a second primary breast carcinoma.

☐ **Pathology:** Cancers of the breast are almost always adenocarcinomas, which are derived from the glandular epithelium of the terminal duct lobular unit (Table 19-1).

Carcinoma in Situ (Noninvasive Carcinoma)

Carcinoma in situ, which is the preinvasive form of cancer, exhibits several histologic types: (1) intraductal, (2) lobular, and (3) papillary. Each of these types has an invasive counterpart.

Intraductal Carcinoma

Intraductal carcinoma is an in situ tumor that arises in the terminal duct lobular unit, greatly distending and distorting the ducts by its growth. Intraductal carcinoma in situ has two main histologic variants, namely comedocarcinoma and papillary-cribriform carcinoma.

Comedocarcinoma. This variant is composed of very large, pleomorphic cells that have abundant eosinophilic cytoplasm and irregular nuclei, commonly with prominent nucleoli. Comedocarcinoma typically grows in a solid pattern. It often becomes centrally necrotic, and the necrotic debris may undergo dystrophic calcification. On gross examination, the cut surface shows distended ducts containing pasty necrotic debris, resembling comedos (hence the term *comedocarcinoma*). Even though the malignant cells do not invade through the basement membrane of the

TABLE 19-1. Frequency of Histologic Subtypes of Invasive Breast Carcinoma

Subtype	Frequency (%)
Invasive ductal carcinoma	
Pure	50
Mixed with other types (including lobular)	30
Invasive lobular carcinoma (pure)	10
Medullary carcinoma (pure)	5
Mucinous carcinoma (pure)	2
Other pure types	2
Other mixed types	1

ducts, this form of carcinoma in situ commonly incites a chronic inflammatory and fibroblastic response in the surrounding stroma.

Papillary-Cribriform Carcinoma. This type of intraductal carcinoma, as its name indicates, tends to form papillary structures and small, regular fenestrations rather than a solid growth. Papillary-cribriform carcinoma is less likely than comedocarcinoma to incite a desmoplastic response in the surrounding tissue.

Intraductal carcinoma in situ, when treated only by biopsy, carries a 30% chance for development of invasive carcinoma in the same breast during the ensuing 20 years. The risk of cancer in the contralateral breast is also increased, but not to the same degree.

Lobular Carcinoma in Situ

Lobular carcinoma in situ also arises in the terminal duct lobular unit. In this type of in situ breast cancer, the cancer cells tend to be smaller and more monotonous than those of the ductal type, with round, regular nuclei and minute nucleoli. The malignant cells appear as solid clusters that pack and distend the terminal ducts, but not to the extent of in situ ductal carcinoma. Although lobular carcinoma in situ does not undergo the central necrosis seen in patients with intraductal carcinoma, it may also have microcalcifications in the ducts, which can be detected radiographically.

As with intraductal carcinoma in situ, 20% to 30% of women with lobular carcinoma in situ will develop invasive cancer within 20 years of diagnosis. In contrast to intraductal carcinoma in situ, however, approximately half of these invasive cancers will arise in the contralateral breast and may be either lobular or ductal cancers. Thus, lobular carcinoma in situ serves as a marker for an enhanced risk of invasive cancer in both breasts.

Invasive Carcinoma

Ductal Carcinoma

Invasive, or infiltrating, ductal carcinoma is the most common form of breast cancer (Fig. 19-4). In this tumor, stromal invasion by malignant cells usually incites a pronounced fibroblastic proliferation. In turn, this "desmoplasia" creates a palpable mass, which is the most common initial sign of ductal carcinoma. Invasive ductal carcinoma usually presents as a hard, fixed mass, which is often referred to as **scirrhous carcinoma**. On gross examination, the tumor is typically firm and shows irregular margins. The cut surface is pale gray, gritty, and flecked with yellow, chalky streaks.

Microscopically, invasive ductal carcinoma grows as irregular nests and cords of epithelial cells, usually within a dense fibrous stroma (Fig. 19-5). Well-differentiated cancers may form abortive glands, whereas the less-differentiated forms consist of solid sheets of neoplastic cells.

Paget Disease of the Nipple. Paget disease of the nipple is an uncommon variant of ductal carcinoma, either in situ or invasive, that extends to involve the epidermis of the nipple and areola (Fig. 19-6). This condition usually comes to medical attention because of an eczematous change in the skin of the nipple and areola. Microscopically, large cells with clear cytoplasm (Paget cells) are found, either singly or in groups, within the epidermis. The prognosis of Paget disease is related to that of the underlying ductal cancer.

Lobular Carcinoma

Invasive lobular carcinoma is the second most common form of invasive breast cancer (Fig. 19-7). The clinical presentation varies from a discrete, firm mass to a diffuse, indurated area. Microscopically, classic invasive lobular carcinoma consists of single strands of malignant cells infiltrating between stromal fibers, a feature that is termed **Indian filing**. Lobular carcinoma is as aggressive biologically as the ductal type.

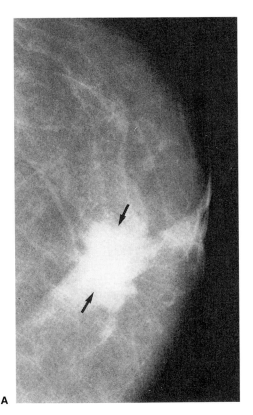

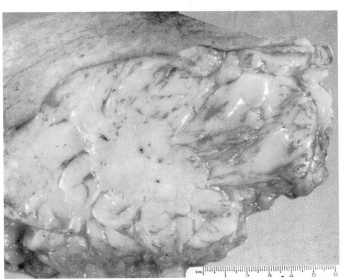

A   B

FIGURE **19-4**
Carcinoma of the breast. (A) Mammogram. An irregularly shaped, dense mass (*arrows***) is seen in this otherwise fatty breast. (B) Mastectomy specimen. The irregular white, firm mass in the center is surrounded by fatty tissue.**

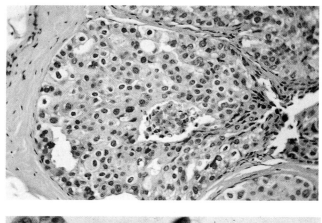

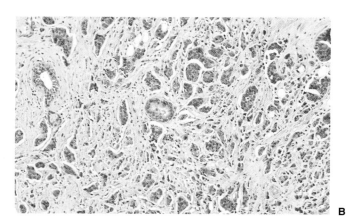

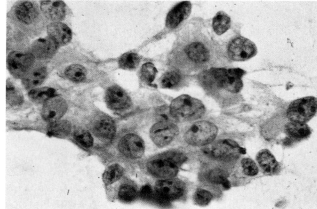

FIGURE 19-5

Ductal carcinoma. (A) Ductal carcinoma in situ. The terminal ducts are distended by carcinoma in situ (intraductal carcinoma). The tumor cells are large and have abundant cytoplasm. The center of the tumor mass is necrotic. (B) Invasive ductal carcinoma. Irregular cords and nests of tumor cells, derived from the same cells that compose the intraductal component in *panel A*, invade the stroma. Many of the cells form duct-like structures. (C) Fine-needle aspiration. This cytologic preparation shows tumor cells that exhibit nuclear pleomorphism and prominent nucleoli.

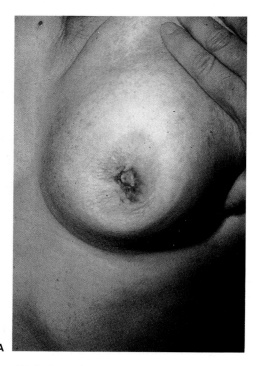

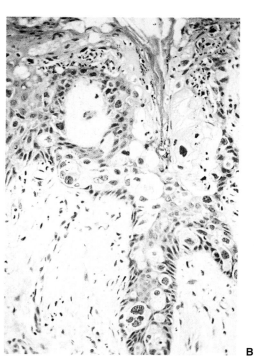

FIGURE 19-6

Paget disease of the nipple. (A) An erythematous, scaly, and weeping "eczema" involves the nipple. (B) The epidermis contains clusters of ductal-type carcinoma cells, which are larger and have more abundant pale cytoplasm than the surrounding keratinocytes.

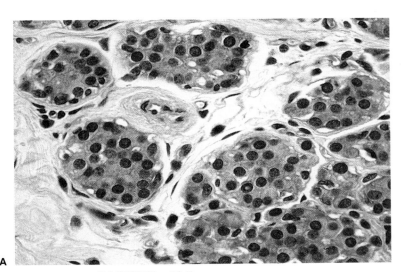
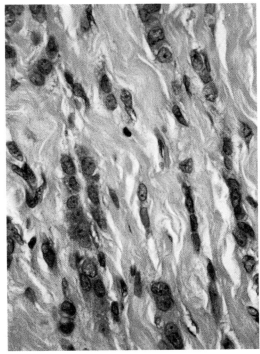

A   B

FIGURE   *19-7*
Lobular carcinoma. (A) Lobular carcinoma in situ. The lumina of the terminal duct lobular units are distended by tumor cells, which exhibit round nuclei and small nucleoli. The
cancer cells in the lobular type of carcinoma in situ are smaller and have less cytoplasm
than those in the ductal type. (B) Invasive lobular carcinoma. In contrast to invasive ductal carcinoma, the cells of lobular carcinoma tend to form single strands that invade between collagen fibers in an "Indian-file" pattern. The tumor cells are similar to those
seen with lobular carcinoma in situ.

Medullary Carcinoma

Medullary carcinoma is the third most common type of
breast cancer (after ductal and lobular carcinoma), accounting for 5% to 10% of invasive cancers. Clinically,
the tumor presents as a circumscribed mass, which on
mammography lacks calcifications. Medullary carcinoma has a distinctive gross appearance, being a well-
circumscribed, fleshy, and pale-gray mass. Microscopically, it is composed of sheets of cells that are
highly pleomorphic and have a high mitotic index (Fig.
19-8). The typical medullary carcinoma has a peripheral lymphoid infiltrate. In spite of the highly malignant histologic appearance of this neoplasm, it carries
a distinctly better prognosis than that of infiltrating
ductal or lobular carcinoma.

Metastatic Pattern of Breast Cancer

Invasive breast cancer spreads primarily through the
lymphatics to the regional lymph nodes, including the
axillary, internal mammary, and supraclavicular
nodes. In half of all patients with breast cancer, the tumor has already metastasized to the axillary nodes at
the time of diagnosis. The probability of spread to the
axillary nodes is directly related to the size of the primary tumor. Breast cancer also spreads to distant sites,
most commonly the lung and pleura, liver, bone,
adrenals, skin, and brain.

Prognostic Factors

Stage at Diagnosis

The most important prognostic factor in breast cancer
is the stage (the extent of tumor spread) at the time of
diagnosis. In general, small tumors localized to the
breast have an excellent prognosis, whereas those that
have spread to distant organs are incurable. Larger
primary tumors and those that have metastasized to
regional lymph nodes have an intermediate prog-
noses.

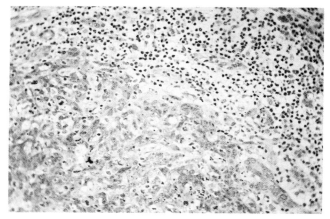

FIGURE   *19-8*
Medullary carcinoma. The malignant cells are pleomorphic and grow in solid sheets, forming a blunt margin. There is no gland formation. Numerous mitoses are present, and the tumor is surrounded by a dense, lymphocytic infiltrate.

Histologic Grade

In addition to the histologic subtype of the cancer, the cytologic grade of the primary tumor is also a useful prognostic indicator. Large, highly irregular nuclei with several prominent nucleoli suggest a poor prognosis.

Lymphatic and Vascular Invasion

The presence of lymphatic or vascular invasion also worsens the prognosis of breast cancer. Dermal lymphatic invasion is the pathologic criterion for making a diagnosis of **inflammatory carcinoma of the breast,** a condition that carries a particularly poor prognosis.

Estrogen and Progesterone Receptors

Approximately half of all breast cancers exhibit nuclear estrogen receptor protein. A smaller proportion of tumors also have progesterone receptors. Women whose cancers possess hormone receptors have longer disease-free and overall survival times than women with early stage cancers without these receptors.

Proliferative Capacity and Ploidy

In general, increased proliferative capacity is associated with a poorer prognosis. Several parameters are used to evaluate the proliferative capacity of breast cancers, including (1) mitotic index, as judged by histologic evaluation; (2) estimation of the proportion of cells in the S phase of the cell cycle, as judged by flow cytometry; and (3) immunohistochemical staining for nuclear proteins expressed in cells that are actively proliferating, namely the Ki67 or PCNA antigens. The presence of aneuploidy by flow cytometry, which is found in two-thirds of breast cancers, has also been associated with a worse prognosis.

Oncogene Expression

Recurrence of breast cancer and shortened survival time are correlated with amplification of (1) genes for growth factor receptors, (2) the related gene C-*erb* B2 (HER-2), and (3) the gene for epidermal growth factor receptor, as well as mutation and overexpression of the *p53* tumor suppressor gene.

Cathepsin D

The proteolytic enzyme cathepsin D is overexpressed by some breast cancers. Results of several studies show that high levels of cathepsin D have a negative prognostic impact.

PHYLLODES TUMORS (CYSTOSARCOMA PHYLLODES)

■ *Phyllodes tumor of the breast* is a proliferation of stromal elements accompanied by a benign growth of ductal structures. These tumors usually occur in women between 30 and 70 years of age, with a peak during the fifth decade of life. The original term for this tumor, **cystosarcoma phyllodes,** implies a malignant behavior, although only half of these tumors are capable of invasion and metastasis. Thus, current terminology refers to **phyllodes tumor,** with the additional designation of either benign or malignant.

☐ **Pathology:** Phyllodes tumor resembles fibroadenoma in its overall architecture and proportion of glandular and stromal elements. However, the stroma is hypercellular and has minor mitotic activity. The average tumor is about 5 cm in diameter.

The malignancy of a phyllodes tumor depends on the appearance of the stromal component. A malignant phyllodes tumor has an obviously sarcomatous stroma with abundant mitotic activity, and the stromal growth is out of proportion to the benign duct elements. It is usually poorly circumscribed, with invasion into the surrounding breast tissue. Malignant tumors may also have various sarcomatous tissue types, such as malignant fibrous histiocytoma, chondrosarcoma, and osteosarcoma.

Malignant phyllodes tumors tend to recur locally, and 15% eventually metastasize to both distant sites and axillary lymph nodes.

THE MALE BREAST

Gynecomastia

■ *Gynecomastia is an enlargement of the adult male breast* (Fig. 19-9). In men, gynecomastia is caused by an absolute increase in circulating estrogens or by a relative increase in the estrogen:androgen ratio. Excess estrogenic stimulation occurs with (1) intake of exogenous estrogens, (2) presence of hormone-secreting adrenal or testicular tumors, (3) paraneoplastic production of gonadotropins by various cancers, and (4) metabolic disorders, such as liver disease and hyperthyroidism, which are characterized by increased conversion of androstenedione into estrogens. Low levels of androgens may result from inadequate testicular secretion of testosterone (Klinefelter syndrome, castration, orchitis) or from androgen insensitivity (testicular feminization). Gynecomastia is often idiopathic, in which case it is commonly unilateral. **There is no evidence that gynecomastia is associated with an increased risk of cancer.**

Cancer of the Male Breast

Cancer of the male breast accounts for 1% of all cases of breast cancer. As in women, the most common subtype by far is infiltrating ductal carcinoma. For tumors of the same stage, the prognosis for breast cancer in men is similar to that of breast cancer in women. Predisposing factors for the development of breast cancer in men are largely unknown.

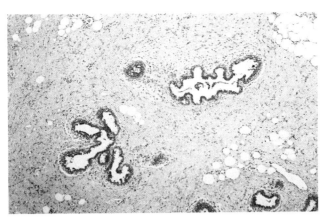

FIGURE **19-9**
Gynecomastia. There is a proliferation of branching, intermediate-size ducts. The ductal epithelium is hyperplastic, and mitoses are present. A concomitant increase in the surrounding fibrous tissue causes a palpable mass. Note the resemblance to the normal adolescent breast.

CHAPTER 20

The Blood and Lymphoid Organs

Hugh Bonner
Adam Bagg
Jeffrey Cossman

Cellular elements of the blood and lymphoid organs are responsible for a number of vital functions, including transport of oxygen, defense against micro-organisms and parasites, and preservation of vascular integrity. These cells all derive from a single pool of pluripotential stem cells in the bone marrow, which gives rise to two distinct types of multipotential stem cells, namely **hemopoietic stem cells,** which remain in the bone marrow, and **lymphopoietic stem cells,** which migrate to the lymphoid organs.

Hemopoietic stem cells differentiate into three committed progenitor cell lines: (1) erythroid, (2) granulocytic-monocytic, and (3) megakaryocytic. The lymphopoietic stem cells differentiate into two committed progenitor cell lines, thereby giving rise to the B- and T-cell lineages. Stimulated and regulated by various growth factors, the progenitor cells proliferate and undergo further differentiation to morphologically distinctive precursor cells and, in turn, to mature and circulating blood cells.

Functional Disorders of the Blood and Lymphoid Organs

ANEMIA

■ *Anemia is a reduction in the total circulating erythrocyte mass.* It is diagnosed on the basis of demonstrating below-normal values for the hemoglobin concentration, hematocrit, or erythrocyte count. A decreased erythrocyte mass leads to lesser transport of hemoglobin-bound oxygen from the lungs to the tissues and, in turn, to tissue hypoxia.

Classification of Anemias

Anemias can be classified either morphologically or pathophysiologically.

The **morphologic** classification divides anemias into three types: (1) macrocytic, (2) microcytic, and (3) normocytic (Fig. 20-1). For many anemias, however, the morphologic classification is less adequate.

The **pathophysiologic** classification divides anemias into two major groups, namely those caused by decreased production of erythrocytes and those caused by increased destruction of erythrocytes (Box 20-1).

Disorders of Stem Cells

Aplastic Anemia

■ *Aplastic anemia is a chronic disorder of hemopoietic stem cells that results in cellular depletion of the bone marrow and pancytopenia (decrease in all circulating formed elements).*

☐ **Pathogenesis:** Bone marrow aplasia can occur as an acute, self-limited event following exposure to radiation or chemotherapeutic drugs, but in aplastic anemia, marrow depletion continues indefinitely. In some patients, there is an initiating event, such as exposure to certain drugs, toxins, or viruses (Box 20-2). In most cases, however, no cause is found; the disorder arises in a previously healthy person with no known exposure to cytotoxic drugs or radiation. In such a situation, the disease is termed **idiopathic** and is assumed to have been triggered by an unknown event in a genetically susceptible person.

Because bone marrow transplantation for aplastic anemia may be curative, the defect must be intrinsic to the hemopoietic cells. The primary lesion is believed to involve an inability of stem cells to regenerate and repopulate the marrow. Successful therapeutic use of

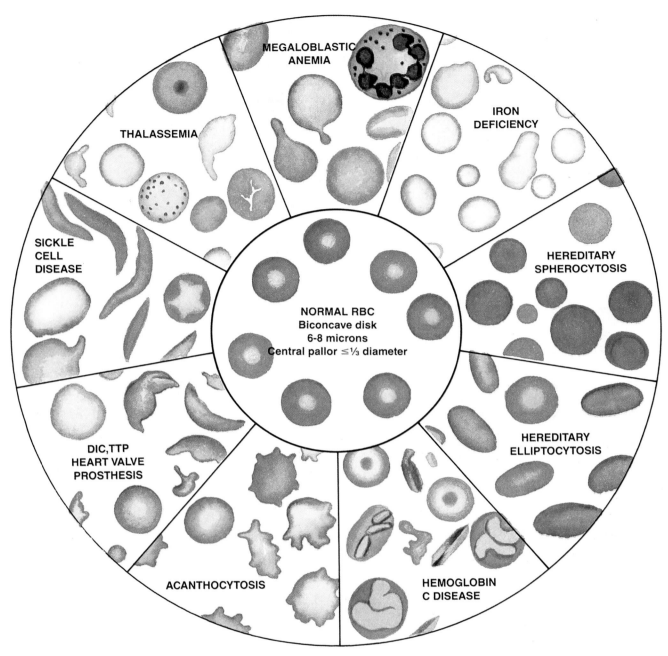

FIGURE *20-1*
The anemias. The pathophysiology of the characteristic morphologic features of the various anemias is shown, and the morphology of normal erythrocytes is contrasted in the central circle.

anti–T lymphocyte antibodies and other immunosuppressive agents for treatment of aplastic anemia suggests an immunologic component either in the pathogenesis of the disease or in its subsequent progression. However, monoclonal disorders may emerge, such as paroxysmal nocturnal hemoglobinuria, myelodysplastic syndromes, and acute leukemia.

☐ **Pathology:** The bone marrow in patients with aplastic anemia is, to a large extent, replaced by fat (Fig. 20-2). Thin strands of cells contain scant granulocytic and erythroid elements, lymphocytes, and plasma cells, as well as mast cells and macrophages. The peripheral blood invariably exhibits pancytopenia, which may be of varying severity. The anemia is usually macrocytic, with an increased erythrocyte content of fetal hemoglobin. Erythropoietin levels tend to be elevated, absolute granulocytopenia is always present, and the total lymphocyte count is often depressed. In addition, the platelet count is consistently reduced.

☐ **Clinical Features:** Untreated patients with severe aplastic anemia have a median survival time of 3 to 6 months, and only 20% survive for 1 year. Thera-

peutic use of blood components and immunosuppressive agents, and bone marrow transplantation have significantly improved the prognosis for patients with idiopathic aplastic anemia, although it still remains a life-threatening disease.

Paroxysmal Nocturnal Hemoglobinuria

■ *Paroxysmal nocturnal hemoglobinuria (PNH) is an acquired clonal stem cell disorder that affects all hemopoietic lineages and is characterized by the production of defective erythrocytes and abnormal platelets and granulocytes.* The defining characteristic of this condition is an unusual predisposition of the faulty erythrocytes to complement-mediated lysis.

☐ **Pathogenesis:** PNH is an acquired clonal stem cell disorder in which all blood cell lineages are defective. Not infrequently, the abnormal clone of PNH emerges in the marrow of patients with aplastic anemia. The erythrocyte defect in PNH relates to a deficiency of decay-accelerating factor on the erythrocyte membrane. These factors are membrane proteins that normally accelerate degradation of surface-bound complement, thereby preventing complement-induced hemolysis. In patients with PNH, the genes for these proteins are normal, but the protein anchorages are faulty. Defective synthesis of glycosyl phosphatidyl inositol, a lipid that anchors many proteins, is thought to be responsible.

☐ **Clinical Features:** PNH is characterized by intermittent or sustained periods of hemolysis and hemoglobinuria, often in a nocturnal pattern, during which patients excrete a red morning urine. In some patients, however, hemolysis occurs at random intervals. Patients with PNH are usually anemic, sometimes with hemoglobin levels of less than 5 g/dL. Because the membrane defect in PNH affects all hemopoietic

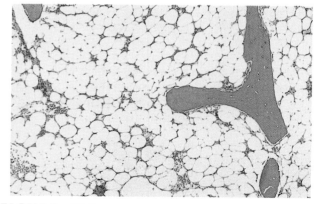

FIGURE *20-2*
Aplastic anemia. The bone marrow consists largely of fat cells and lacks normal hemopoietic activity.

cells, thrombocytopenia and granulocytopenia are ordinarily present.

Thrombotic complications are frequent, especially in the deep abdominal veins. In fact, PNH should always be considered in the differential diagnosis of Budd-Chiari syndrome (hepatic venous thrombosis). The reason for this thrombotic diathesis is poorly understood, but it may reflect complement-mediated activation of platelets.

The course of PNH is variable. Some patients succumb within months of the diagnosis, whereas others live for decades. Many patients eventually die from the complications of pancytopenia and thrombosis, and a few develop a myelodysplastic syndrome or acute leukemia. Bone marrow transplantation has produced long-term remissions in some patients.

Myelodysplastic Syndromes

■ *Myelodysplastic syndromes (MDS) encompass a heterogeneous group of disorders that are characterized by clonal proliferation of abnormal stem cells.* The progeny of these cells are usually defective, thereby resulting in pancytopenia of varying severity.

The cause of MDS is obscure, but some patients have evidence of occupational exposure to toxic chemicals. Benzene is the best defined of these agents, but gasoline and diesel fumes may also be causative agents. Use of chemotherapeutic agents, usually alkylating agents, is associated with a risk of subsequent MDS.

☐ **Pathology:** In patients with MDS, the cellularity of the bone marrow is either normal or increased. Erythroblasts tend to be megaloblastoid, with numerous immature forms (shift to the left) and nuclear fragmentation. Ringed sideroblasts, characterized by iron-laden mitochondria encircling the nucleus, may be present. Myeloid precursors may be morphologically normal, and the number of myeloblasts determines, in part, the classification. Megakaryocytes vary in number, and many have either hyposegmented or hypersegmented nuclei.

The circulating erythrocytes vary in both size and shape but display an increased mean volume. Basophilic stippling and nucleated erythrocytes are frequently observed. Hemoglobin abnormalities include an increased level of fetal hemoglobin and presence of $\beta 4$ complexes (acquired hemoglobin H disease). Granulocytes may show decreased nuclear lobation (**Pelger-Huet anomaly**), and there is often an increase in mature and immature monocytes. Large and atypically granulated platelets may also be encountered.

☐ **Clinical Features:** MDS may smolder for years and require only occasional transfusions or antibiotics.

Eventually, however, the disorder transforms into acute myelogenous leukemia in 20% to 40% of the patients. Attempts to modify this course with chemotherapeutic agents have not been successful. Bone marrow transplantation may offer the only hope for cure of this neoplastic disorder.

Disorders of Progenitor Cells

Pure Red Cell Aplasia

■ *Pure red cell aplasia (PRCA) is an autoimmune disease in which erythroid progenitor and precursor cells are suppressed.* As a result, secondary anemia occurs, but leukopenia and thrombocytopenia are absent. PRCA may present as an acute, self-limited disorder or as a chronic congenital or acquired disease.

Acute Red Cell Aplasia. The acute form of PRCA frequently follows a viral illness, especially infection with parvovirus B19, or exposure to one of several potentially toxic drugs. Parvovirus preferentially invades and destroys the erythroid progenitor cells. An immunologic attack on erythroid progenitors or precursor cells by antiviral antibodies may also play a role. In drug-induced cases of PRCA, the drug likely acts as an immunogenic hapten, inducing the formation of cytotoxic antibodies that are directed against erythroid precursor cells.

Acute PRCA usually becomes clinically apparent only in patients with underlying disorders characterized by a shortened life span of circulating erythrocytes, such as sickle cell anemia or hereditary spherocytosis. In such patients, a temporary decrease in the production of erythrocytes may cause a rapidly developing, yet brief, anemia, the so-called aplastic crisis.

Chronic Constitutional PRCA (Diamond-Blackfan Anemia). This condition is usually detected during the first year of life, and it is caused by the inheritance of defective erythroid progenitor cells. The progeny of these abnormal progenitor cells are macrocytic and have an increased content of fetal hemoglobin. The dramatic responsiveness to corticosteroids in the inherited type of PRCA suggests an immunologic component, but no firm evidence for this concept has been obtained.

Chronic Acquired PRCA. This disease usually presents in middle-age adults, and its intriguing relationship to thymomas (5% of cases) has attracted considerable attention. Most cases have strong evidence for an immunologic rejection of erythroid progenitor and precursor cells.

The marrow is usually depleted of erythroblasts, but some cases of acquired PRCA are marked by an arrest of maturation, with the presence of large, abnormal proerythroblasts. The myeloid and megakaryocyte cell lines are unaffected.

The anemia in patients with acquired PRCA is normochromic and normocytic or macrocytic. Reticulocytes are decreased or absent, and the serum iron level is elevated, with almost complete saturation of the iron-binding protein (transferrin). Thymic enlargement should be sought by computed tomography or magnetic resonance imaging, because removal of an abnormal thymus may result in clinical remission.

Use of corticosteroids and immunosuppressive agents has been of benefit therapeutically, with shorter or longer remissions having been induced in half of the cases. The median survival time for patients in acquired PRCA is now more than 10 years.

Anemia Associated with Chronic Renal Failure

A normocytic, normochromic anemia occurs in almost all patients with chronic renal disease. Its severity is roughly proportional to the degree of uremia, and most patients on a renal dialysis program are dependent on blood transfusions. The anemia results from both decreased production and increased destruction of erythrocytes, with the former playing the major role. Decreased production results primarily from inadequate synthesis of erythropoietin by the damaged kidneys.

The bone marrow usually appears normal in patients with chronic renal failure; it does not show the compensatory erythroid hyperplasia expected in patients with severe anemia. The circulating erythrocytes often show scalloped margins (burr cells) in patients with pronounced uremia and fragmentation in patients with severe renal hypertension. Widespread use of recombinant erythropoietin in the therapy for anemia of chronic renal disease has had a dramatic impact on this complication of uremia.

Anemia Associated with Chronic Disease

Anemia of chronic disease is one of the most common anemias worldwide, second only to iron deficiency anemia. Mild to moderate normochromic or hypochromic anemia, with a hemoglobin level of from 9 to 11 g/dL, is frequent in patients with (1) chronic inflammatory disorders (e.g., rheumatoid arthritis and systemic lupus erythematosus), (2) chronic infectious diseases (e.g., tuberculosis and acquired immunodeficiency syndrome [AIDS]), and (3) cancer. Fortunately, it is not severe enough to cause major symptoms, but it may render the underlying disorders more difficult to endure.

Although a decreased iron supply to the developing erythroblast plays an important pathogenic role, the anemia of chronic disease also results from a slightly shortened erythrocyte life span. Furthermore, there is impaired bone marrow response to erythropoietin and inadequate production of erythropoietin in response to anemia.

Disorders of Erythroid Precursor Cells
Megaloblastic Anemias

■ *Megaloblastic anemias are characterized by large, nucleated progenitors of red blood cells in the bone marrow and are mostly caused by impaired DNA synthesis owing to a deficiency of either vitamin B_{12} or folic acid.*

Vitamin B_{12} and Pernicious Anemia
Defective intestinal absorption of vitamin B_{12}, owing to a lack of production of intrinsic factor, causes pernicious anemia. This dramatic but treatable illness probably results from an autoimmune attack on the gastric mucosa, particularly the gastric parietal cells (see Chapter 13). Vitamin B_{12} deficiency can also be caused by (1) gastrectomy; (2) overgrowth of vitamin B_{12}–consuming micro-organisms in a surgically constructed, intestinal blind loop; (3) a variety of inflammatory and neoplastic disorders involving the ileum; (4) surgical removal of the site of absorption, the terminal ileum; and (5) intestinal infestation with a fish tapeworm (Diphyllobothrium latum) that consumes vitamin B_{12}.

Folic Acid Deficiency
The most common cause of folic acid deficiency is an inadequate dietary intake. Folic acid is a vital nutrient that is present in leafy vegetables, meat, and egg products. Folic acid deficiency occurs most commonly in persons with alcoholism and in recluses with poor nutrition. Impaired intestinal absorption of folic acid occurs in patients with celiac disease and tropical sprue and may be responsible, in part, for the deficiency observed in some patients taking anticonvulsive drugs (e.g., phenytoin).

Impaired DNA Synthesis
Regardless of the cause, a deficiency of either vitamin B12 or folic acid results in impaired DNA synthesis, which, in turn, leads to megaloblastic transformation of hemopoietic cells. The defect in DNA synthesis causes delayed nuclear maturation and abnormal mitotic activity. These consequences are mainly expressed in rapidly dividing cells, such as those in the bone marrow and the gastrointestinal epithelium.

☐ **Pathology:** In patients with macrocytic anemias, the defect in DNA synthesis produces large erythroid megaloblasts, with loose and immature nuclei, which often have satellite pieces (Fig. 20-3). The cytoplasm displays various degrees of maturation and hemoglobin synthesis. There is also a considerable degree of cellular destruction and ineffective erythropoiesis in the bone marrow. Circulating erythrocytes are large, often with an oval shape, and are associated with prominent poikilocytosis and a teardrop configuration.

Myeloid cells also show considerable changes. Large metamyelocytes with horseshoe-shaped nuclei are seen in the bone marrow, and neutrophils with five or more nuclear lobes circulate in the blood. The megakaryocytes display nuclear abnormalities, ranging from hyposegmentation to wide separation of the nuclear lobes.

☐ **Clinical Features:** Because all their cellular proliferation is defective, patients with vitamin B$_{12}$ or folic acid deficiency suffer from anemia, with a low reticulocyte count, neutropenia, and thrombocytopenia. Some patients with pernicious anemia experience degeneration of the posterior and lateral columns of the spinal cord, which is associated with irreversible ataxia and other neurologic defects (see Chapter 28).

Iron Deficiency Anemia

Paradoxically, although iron is the most abundant metal in the world, iron deficiency is the most common cause of anemia. Principal causes of iron deficiency are impaired intake owing to an iron-poor diet or excessive loss caused by hemorrhage, intravascular hemolysis, pregnancy, or lactation. In Western countries, dietary intake of iron is frequently inadequate among infants and young children who are on iron-deficient milk diets. In adults, the normal diet usually contains adequate iron, but there is little reserve to compensate for increased iron loss.

Loss of iron by blood loss is by far the most common cause of iron deficiency anemia in adults, because each 1 mL of packed erythrocytes contains 1 mg of iron. In women of reproductive age, iron loss usually results from menstruation or pregnancy, although the possibility of gastrointestinal or urinary blood loss should not be ignored. Iron deficiency anemia in an otherwise healthy man mandates a search for a gastrointestinal lesion that may be leaking blood.

☐ **Pathology:** On the peripheral blood smear, erythrocytes are hypochromic and microcytic. In patients with severe iron deficiency anemia, poikilocytosis (irregular shape) and anisocytosis (irregular size) can be observed (Fig. 20-4). The bone marrow smear reveals an increased number of small normoblasts, with poorly hemoglobinized or ragged cytoplasm.

Laboratory findings include a low serum iron level and an increased total iron-binding capacity. The most important finding is a decreased ferritin level (<20 ng/mL), which reflects a decrease in total tissue iron stores. A decrease in tissue iron can also be demonstrated by decreased or absent hemosiderin in macrophages, as demonstrated in Prussian blue-stained smears or biopsy samples of bone marrow.

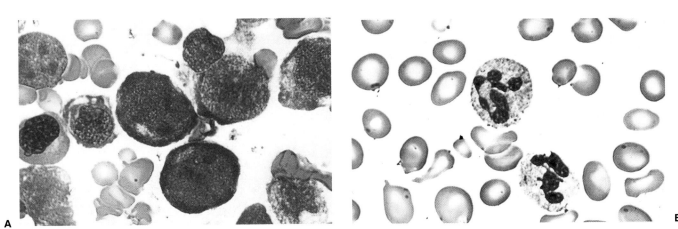

A   B

FIGURE *20-3*
Megaloblastic anemia. (A) A bone marrow aspirate from a patient with vitamin B$_{12}$ deficiency (pernicious anemia) shows prominent megaloblastic erythroid precursors. (B) In this peripheral blood smear from the same patient as *panel A*, the erythrocytes are large, often with an oval shape, and are associated with poikilocytosis and teardrop shapes. The neutrophils are hypersegmented.

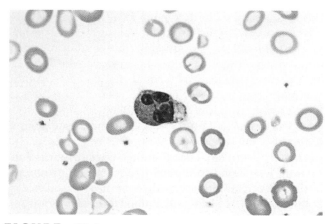

FIGURE   *20-4*
Iron deficiency anemia. A peripheral blood smear shows hypochromic and microcytic erythrocytes. Poikilocytosis (irregular shape) and anisocytosis (irregular size) are also observed.

Thalassemia

■ *Thalassemia syndromes are a heterogeneous group of heritable anemias that have in common defective synthesis of either the α or the β chains of the normal hemoglobin A tetramer ($\alpha_2\beta_2$; Fig. 20-5). In the β-thalassemias, synthesis of the β chain is impaired, whereas in the α-thalassemias, the defect involves the α chain.*

All forms of thalassemia are characterized by a hypochromic, microcytic anemia owing to reduced or absent synthesis of the complete hemoglobin molecule. In addition, accumulation of unmatched globin chains leads to their precipitation, with consequent damage to the membranes of both nucleated and mature erythrocytes.

□ **Epidemiology:** Thalassemia originally pertained to anemias observed among populations that inhabited the Italian and Greek coasts. However, in addition to the Mediterranean basin, thalassemias also occur in a belt that extends across the Middle East, through parts of Pakistan and India, to Southeast Asia. This belt also includes southern regions of the former Soviet Union, China, and the northern regions of the African continent. Importantly, sporadic mutations occasionally produce β-thalassemia among populations in whom the disease does not ordinarily occur.

β-Thalassemia

At the molecular level, the b-thalassemias are extremely heterogeneous, and more than 50 distinct mutations have been associated with this phenotype.

□ **Pathogenesis:** The β-thalassemias are caused by a point mutation on chromosome 11 or, less commonly, by a deletion of part of the gene. Defective β-globin synthesis causes anemia because of impaired production of erythrocytes (ineffective erythropoiesis) and hemolysis of circulating erythrocytes.

Heterozygous β-Thalassemia (β-Thalassemia Minor). The normal β-globin gene usually produces enough β or δ chains to bind most of the available α chains. The result is a moderate reduction in normal hemoglobin ($\alpha_2\beta_2$) and an increase in hemoglobin A_2 ($\alpha_2\delta_2$). There is usually a mild anemia, with some hypochromia, microcytosis, basophilic stippling, and target cells. The diagnosis is made on the basis of demonstrating an increased amount of hemoglobin A_2 (>5%).

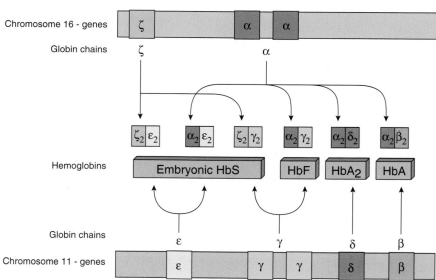

FIGURE   *20-5*
Assembly of subunit chains to form different hemoglobins.

The situation is somewhat different in patients with α,β-thalassemia. In such persons, α chain synthesis is released from its normal neonatal suppression, and γ chains bind excess α chains. The result is formation of an increased amount of fetal hemoglobin ($\alpha_2\gamma_2$).

Homozygous β-Thalassemia (Cooley Anemia). This severe disorder is caused by a pronounced reduction in or absence of β chain production. Hemoglobin electrophoresis reveals principally fetal hemoglobin. The hemoglobin A_2 concentration is either normal or moderately elevated. Because the excess unpaired α chains readily precipitate within the erythroid cells, they destroy both erythroid precursor cells (ineffective erythropoiesis) and circulating erythrocytes (hemolysis). Peripheral blood erythrocytes are hypochromic and microcytic and show marked anisocytosis, poikilocytosis, and target cell configuration (Fig. 20-6). Circulating nucleated erythrocytes are often observed, especially after splenectomy.

Facial and cranial bones tend to be enlarged or distorted because of severe bone marrow hyperplasia. Extramedullary foci of blood formation are present in the spleen, liver, and paraspinal regions. The spleen is increased in size because of both production and destruction of erythrocytes. The enlarged spleen may sequester and destroy both leukocytes and platelets.

Intensive transfusion therapy has diminished some of the effects of ineffective erythropoiesis and hemolysis in patients with Cooley anemia, and concomitant use of iron chelators (to prevent secondary iron overload) has resulted in a reasonably good prognosis for patients with this formerly lethal disease.

α-Thalassemia

α-Thalassemia comprises four distinct syndromes, each of which reflects the failure of one (or more) of the four α-gene loci on chromosome 16 to function. Both in utero and during the neonatal period, impaired synthesis of γ chains causes precipitation of unmatched γ chains as hemoglobin Barts (γ_4), whereas in children and adults, excess β chains are deposited as hemoglobin H (β_4).

The severity of the four α-thalassemias depends on the number of chains that are deleted:

- **The silent carrier** state is caused by deletion of only one gene.
- **α-Thalassemia trait** reflects deletion of two genes, which results in only a mild hemolytic anemia.
- **Hemoglobin H disease,** in which three genes are deleted, is characterized by a moderate hemolytic anemia, with hypochromia and microcytosis.
- **Deletion of all four α-chain genes** causes death either in utero or at the time of delivery. The pre-

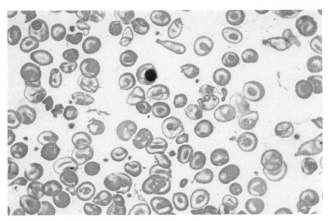

FIGURE   *20-6*
Thalassemia. The peripheral blood erythrocytes are hypochromic and microcytic and show anisocytosis, poikilocytosis, and target cells.

dominance of the high-affinity hemoglobin Barts produces severe impairment of oxygen delivery in utero.

Increased Destruction of Erythrocytes (Hemolytic Anemias) Associated with Hemoglobinopathies

Sickle Cell Disease

■ *Sickle cell disease refers to a group of hereditary hemoglobinopathies in which deoxygenated erythrocytes undergo transformation from the normal, biconcave disk to a sickle-shaped structure. This shape change, which results from the polymerization of sickle hemoglobin (HbS), leads to hemolytic anemia and occlusion of small blood vessels.*

Sickle Cell Anemia

☐ **Epidemiology:** Persons with sickle cell anemia are homozygous for the *HbS* gene. The disease is particularly common among blacks, and in some regions of Africa, as many as 40% of the population are heterozygotes. In the United States, 10% of blacks are carriers of the trait, and one in 650 persons among this population (50,000 persons) has sickle cell anemia. The gene is also encountered in parts of the Mediterranean basin, the Middle East, and India. It is noteworthy that the *HbS* gene is prevalent among areas in which falciparum malaria is endemic, thereby suggesting that heterozygosity for this gene confers a selective advantage in persons who become infected with malaria.

☐ **Pathogenesis:** HbS ($\alpha_2\beta S_2$) results from a point mutation in which valine is substituted for glutamic acid at the sixth position of the α-globin chain. HbS tends to aggregate and polymerize at low oxygen tension to form a rigid, filamentous gel (Fig. 20-7) that, in turn, renders the erythrocyte rigid and less deformable. The membrane contracts around aggregated polymers of HbS, and erythrocytes take on a characteristic appearance, resembling sickles or holly leaves (Fig. 20-8).

☐ **Pathology and Clinical Features:** In homozygous sickle cell anemia (hemoglobin SS), hemoglobin S constitutes 80% to 95% of the total hemoglobin, with hemoglobins F and A₂ constituting the remainder. **The predominance of hemoglobin S leads to both severe chronic hemolytic anemia and to vaso-occlusive disease.** Many afflicted persons are asymptomatic most of the time, only to suffer sudden episodes of sickle crises that, sometimes, can be fatal.

Infarctive Crisis. This is the most frequent form of sickle crisis, occuring either frequently or as uncommonly as once a year. Sickled erythrocytes obstruct small blood vessels in many organs, thereby producing severe pain, especially in the bones, abdomen, and chest. Repeated infarcts in the spleen cause progressive fibrosis, scarring, and eventually, splenic atrophy. By

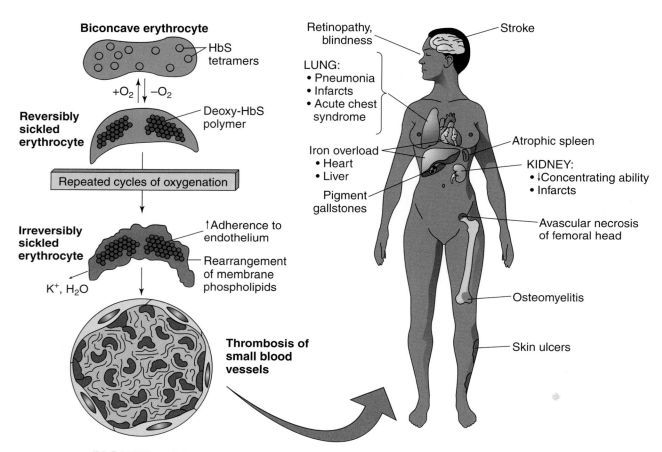

FIGURE 20-7
Pathogenesis of the vascular complications of sickle cell anemia. Because of the substitution of valine for glutamic acid, the charge on the surface of the hemoglobin molecule is altered. On deoxygenation, sickle hemoglobin tetramers aggregate to form poorly soluble polymers. A change in the shape of the erythrocyte, from a biconcave disk to a sickle form, accompanies polymerization of sickle hemoglobin (HgbS). This process is initially reversible on reoxygenation; however, with repeated cycles of deoxygenation and reoxygenation, the erythrocytes become irreversibly sickled. Such irreversibly sickled cells display a rearrangement of phospholipids between the outer and inner monolayers of the cell membrane, and particularly an increased number of aminophospholipids in the outer leaflet. Potassium and water are lost from the cells. The erythrocytes are no longer deformable and are more adherent to endothelial cells, which are properties that predispose to thrombosis of small blood vessels. The resulting vascular occlusions lead to widespread ischemic complications.

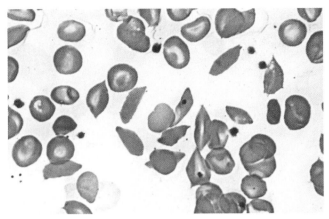

FIGURE *20-8*
Sickle cell anemia. A peripheral blood smear shows many sickled erythrocytes.

the time the affected person has reached adulthood, the spleen has been reduced to a small, functionless, and fibrous nodule that weighs as little as 10 g. Ulceration of the skin in the region of the ankles is common and results from obstruction of small dermal and subcutaneous vessels, with consequent infarctions of the skin. Infarcts of the femoral head are especially common because of its limited vascularization.

Aplastic Crisis. Lack of normal splenic function predisposes to bacterial infections, especially by pneumococci. Intercurrent infections, both viral and bacterial, tend to depress the normal rate of erythrocyte production. Because hemolysis continues unabated, the hemoglobin concentration falls rapidly, a condition termed *aplastic crisis.*

Sequestration Crisis. Intercurrent infections in young children with sickle cell anemia may cause reactive hyperplasia of the spleen, with a sudden pooling of erythrocytes and a rapid fall in hemoglobin levels to less than 6 g/dL. This complication accounts for most of the deaths from sickle cell anemia that occur during the early years of life.

Numerous organs demonstrate the ravages of sickle cell anemia.

- **Heart.** Chronic anemia leads to cardiac changes associated with the consequences of persistently increased cardiac output. This may be complicated by myocardial ischemia as a result of occlusive disease of the coronary microvasculature. Secondary iron overload, resulting from chronic hemolysis and multiple blood transfusions, may further compromise cardiac function. Thus, cardiomegaly and even congestive heart failure are not infrequent.
- **Lungs.** Pulmonary infarction and infections of the lungs are well-recognized complications of sickle

cell anemia. In addition, a rapidly progressive decrease in pulmonary function associated with radiologic infiltrates, termed **acute chest syndrome,** occurs in almost one-third of the patients and may be fatal.
- **Brain.** As many as 25% of the patients have some evidence of neurologic disturbances, including strokes (often preceded by transient ischemic attacks) and cerebral hemorrhage.
- **Kidney.** Because the microenvironment of the renal medulla is hypoxic, acidotic, and hypertonic, sickling in the vasa recta is common. Many patients lose the ability to concentrate urine. Hematuria is frequent, and renal infarcts and papillary necrosis are encountered.
- **Hepatobiliary System.** Chronic hemolysis predisposes to **pigment gallstones,** which are present in more than half of the adult patients and have been seen in children as young as 6 years of age. Massive hepatomegaly is occasionally observed, and secondary iron overload in the liver is common.
- **Bones.** A classic complication of sickle cell anemia is **osteomyelitis,** particularly with *Salmonella typhimurium.* The precise pathogenesis is not understood, but is thought to relate to poor splenic function and microinfarcts of the bone marrow.
- **Eye.** Occlusion of the retinal microvasculature is complicated by hemorrhage, proliferative retinopathy, retinal detachment, and eventually, blindness.

Sickle Cell Trait

The heterozygous form of sickle cell disease (hemoglobin SA) is termed *sickle cell trait*. It is a benign disorder found in 10% of American blacks. HbS constitutes one-third of the total hemoglobin of the erythrocyte, with the remainder consisting of normal hemoglobin A. The condition does not affect the life span of the patient, and no treatment is required.

Hemoglobin C Disease

Hemoglobin C (HbC) is the second most common abnormal hemoglobin, occurring in as many as one-fourth of West Africans. Among blacks in the United States, 2% to 3% are asymptomatic heterozygotes (hemoglobin AC). HbC results from the substitution of lysine for glutamic acid in the same sixth position of the hemoglobin β-globin chain that is involved in sickle cell anemia.

In homozygous hemoglobin C disease (hemoglobin CC), a chronic, mild hemolytic anemia is associated with dehydrated and rigid erythrocytes. The most prominent morphologic feature in homozygous hemoglobin C disease is the presence of numerous target cells.

Hemolytic Anemias Associated with Membrane Defects

The membrane of the erythrocyte consists of a lipid bilayer and a supporting protein cytoskeleton. A defect in any component of this skeleton renders the membrane unstable, thereby leading to a shortened erythrocyte life span.

Hereditary Spherocytosis

■ *Hereditary spherocytosis (HS) refers to a heterogeneous group of inherited, hemolytic anemias that are characterized by a genetic defect in the cytoskeleton of the erythrocyte.* The large majority of HS cases are autosomal dominant, but severe autosomal recessive forms are well documented.

☐ **Pathogenesis:** The heterogeneous molecular defects in HS involve one of four cytoskeletal proteins of the erythrocyte, including deficiencies of spectrin and ankyrin, protein 4.2 and band 3. As a result, the density of the cytoskeleton of the erythrocyte is decreased, and the membrane bilayer is destabilized. The cell surface area is progressively reduced owing to a loss of bilayer phospholipids. The decrease in surface:volume ratio is reflected in the formation of spherical erythrocytes (spherocytes), which are poorly deformable and trapped in the spleen. In that organ, the spherocytes are further damaged ("splenic conditioning") and, after several such splenic passages, are prematurely removed from the circulation.

☐ **Pathology:** The anemia of hereditary spherocytosis is normocytic and also hyperchromic, reflecting cellular dehydration. The mean corpuscular hemoglobin concentration is frequently greater than 36%. The peripheral blood smear shows a mixture of erythrocytes with decreased diameter, intense staining, and no central pallor (spherocytes); large, bluish erythrocytes (reticulocytes); and normal erythrocytes (Fig. 20-9). Hemolysis is reflected in decreased serum haptoglobin and increased lactic dehydrogenase levels. Bone marrow examination reveals marked erythroid hyperplasia. The spleen is enlarged owing to packing of the red pulp cords with macrophages and erythrocytes.

☐ **Clinical Features:** HS is characterized by jaundice, anemia, and splenomegaly. Because chronic hemolysis increases bilirubin production, pigment gallstones are present in half of the adult patients. **Because the spleen is primarily responsible for destruction of spherocytes, splenectomy is usually curative.**

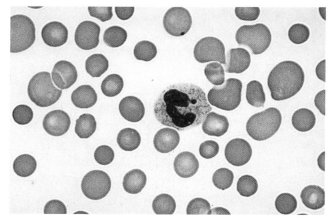

FIGURE *20-9*
Hereditary spherocytosis. A peripheral blood smear shows many erythrocytes with decreased diameter, intense staining, and no central pallor (spherocytes).

Hereditary Elliptocytosis

■ *Hereditary elliptocytosis is the common name for a group of autosomal dominant disorders that are characterized by the presence of elliptical or oval-shaped erythrocytes in the circulation.* Many different defects in the protein skeleton can cause elliptocytosis, and the clinical manifestations are equally varied.

In patients with hereditary elliptocytosis, more than 75% of the circulating erythrocytes appear to be elliptical (Fig. 20-10). Many patients, however, also have teardrop-shaped erythrocytes, fragmented cells, and stomatocytes, in which a wide slit or mouth-like area replaces the normal central pallor. Hemolysis is usually moderate, but if it is severe, splenectomy is curative.

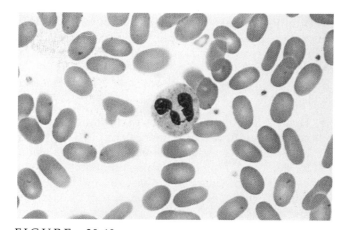

FIGURE *20-10*
Hereditary elliptocytosis. A peripheral blood smear reveals that virtually all of the erythrocytes have an elliptical shape.

Acanthocytosis

■ *Acanthocytosis refers to a group of anemias in which the membrane of the erythrocyte shows multiple, irregular projections caused by defects in the lipid bilayer.* A common cause of acanthocytosis is **liver disease,** in which free (nonesterified) cholesterol is deposited in the membrane. Acanthocytosis is also a feature of **abetalipoproteinemia,** an autosomal recessive lipid disorder. Acanthocytes, or spur cells, are morphologically impressive, but hemolysis is rarely pronounced (Fig. 20-11).

Glucose-6-Phosphate Dehydrogenase Deficiency

■ *Glucose-6-phosphate dehydrogenase (G6PD) deficiency refers to a large group of X-linked, hereditary, and hemolytic anemias in which inadequate activity of erythrocyte G6PD predisposes to episodes of hemolysis that are precipitated by drugs or infection.*

The distribution of G6PD deficiency shows both ethnic and geographic variations. For example, northern Europeans have a prevalence of less than 1 in 1000 persons, but as many as half of male Kurdish Jews are afflicted. This condition occurs in all populations but is particularly common among blacks of West African descent and among certain Mediterranean populations.

□ **Pathogenesis:** G6PD is an enzyme of the hexose monophosphate shunt pathway that maintains glutathione in its reduced (active) form. Erythrocytes that are deficient in G6PD are less resistant to oxidation caused by infections or exposure to oxidant drugs. Under such stress, hemoglobin is denatured and precipitates as Heinz bodies on the erythrocyte membrane.

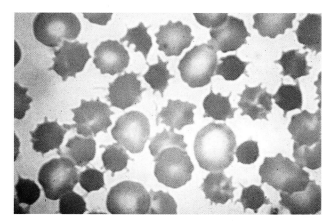

FIGURE **20-11**
Acanthocytosis. A peripheral blood smear from a patient with abetalipoproteinemia shows erythrocytes that display multiple, irregular projections from the surface.

These abnormal erythrocytes are then phagocytized in the spleen.

The gene for G6PD is located on the X chromosome, and the deficiency is expressed only in males. Among Mediterranean populations, a mutant gene encodes a severely deranged enzyme with barely detectable G6PD activity. Persons with this deficiency suffer sustained hemolytic anemia, which is aggravated by infections and drugs. Classically, these patients also develop a potentially lethal hemolysis after eating fava beans (**favism**).

Autoimmune Hemolytic Anemias

■ *Autoimmune hemolytic anemias are caused by autoantibodies with specificity for erythrocyte membrane proteins.* They are either warm-reacting, with maximal activity at 37°C, or, less commonly, cold-reacting, in which case the activity increases at temperatures below 37°C.

Warm-Reacting Autoantibodies

Hemolytic anemia caused by warm-reacting antibodies constitutes 80% of all autoimmune anemias. It occurs (1) as an idiopathic disorder, (2) in association with a variety of malignant or benign conditions, and (3) as a response to a number of drugs. Women are affected more than men, and the disease usually strikes in midlife.

□ **Pathogenesis:** Warm-reacting antibodies are usually of the immunoglobulin (Ig) G class and are often directed at the core antigen of the Rh locus. In hemolytic anemia mediated by warm-reacting antibodies, erythrocytes are mostly destroyed in the splenic sinusoids by macrophages with receptors for the Fc portion of immunoglobulins or for the C3b component of complement.

Half of the cases of warm autoimmune hemolytic anemia are idiopathic, and most of the remaining cases are associated with lymphocytic lymphoma and chronic lymphocytic leukemia. Autoimmune hemolytic anemia may also occur in association with collagen vascular diseases (particularly systemic lupus erythematosus), viral infections, some solid tumors (e.g., ovarian cancer), and certain inflammatory disorders (e.g., ulcerative colitis).

Drug-Induced Hemolytic Anemia. There are two pathogenetic variants of drug-induced autoimmune hemolytic anemia. In the first type, the drug changes the antigen permanently, thereby eliciting production of autoantibodies. These antibodies then react with the altered antigen in the absence of the drug and produce complement-mediated hemolysis. The principal offender is the antihypertensive drug α-methyldopa, which alters an antigen of the Rh family.

In the second type, the drug is only temporarily attached to an erythrocyte antigen, and antibodies are formed against the drug-antigen complex. These antibodies bind to this complex and destroy the cell, but only as long as the drug is present in the form of a drug-antigen complex. The principal offender is the antiarrhythmic agent quinidine.

☐ **Pathology and Clinical Features:** Anemia and jaundice are prominent clinical features of warm-reacting autoimmune hemolysis. The blood smear shows a characteristic mixture of normal erythrocytes, large and bluish reticulocytes, and small, intensely stained spherocytes. The haptoglobin level is decreased, the LDH level is increased, and most importantly, the Coombs test is positive. Immunosuppressive agents and splenectomy are effective in the treatment of warm-reacting autoimmune hemolytic anemia, but the prognosis in these patients generally reflects the underlying disorder.

Erythroblastosis Fetalis. This immune disorder is another example of hemolytic anemia induced by warm-reacting antibodies. Also termed **autoimmune hemolytic disease of the newborn,** erythroblastosis fetalis usually results from immunization of an Rh-negative mother by the erythrocytes of an Rh-positive fetus (see Chapter 6).

Cold-Reacting Autoantibodies

Cold-reacting autoantibodies account for 20% of the cases of autoimmune hemolytic anemia. These antibodies are usually of the IgM type, with specificity for the I antigen that is present on most adult erythrocytes. When blood is cooled in the extremities, IgM autoantibodies fix complement C3 to the erythrocyte membrane. However, at warmer body temperatures, the antibodies dissociate from the erythrocyte membrane and leave the erythrocyte coated only by complement. Because Kupffer cells have more receptors for complement than do splenic macrophages, the final erythrocyte destruction is hepatic rather than splenic.

Hemolytic anemia caused by cold-reacting autoantibodies occurs as an idiopathic, chronic disorder in elderly patients. Many of these patients eventually develop a malignant lymphoma. This disorder also occurs in younger persons with mycoplasmal pneumonia or infectious mononucleosis. The anemia tends to be mild, and the blood smear shows both reticulocytes and spherocytes, although not as pronounced as in the warm-reacting antibody type. The disease can be prolonged and difficult to treat, because immunosuppressive agents or splenectomy are rarely effective.

Hemolytic Anemia Secondary to Mechanical Erythrocyte Destruction

There are a number of circumstances in which otherwise normal erythrocytes are damaged, and their life span is shortened by mechanical impediments within the circulatory system. These situations are classified according to the mechanism by which the erythrocytes are traumatized.

Macroangiopathic Hemolysis. Circulating erythrocytes are vulnerable to shear forces exerted by intravascular prostheses in the heart and major arteries, particularly artificial heart valves. In such circumstances, erythrocyte fragmentation results in a macroangiopathic hemolytic anemia, which is characterized by the presence of many schistocytes (remnants of fragmented erythrocytes containing several spicules) on the blood smear.

Microangiopathic Hemolysis. Microangiopathic hemolytic anemia, which presents a morphologic picture similar to that of macroangiopathic hemolytic anemia (Fig. 20-12), is caused by the fragmentation of erythrocytes by fibrin strands in partially obstructed, small peripheral blood vessels. Disseminated intravascular coagulation (discussed later) is a frequent cause and is associated with a consumptive deficiency in platelets and coagulation factors.

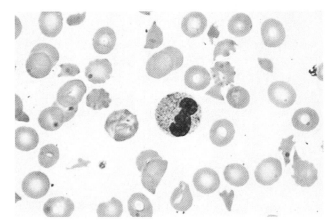

FIGURE   *20-12*
Microangiopathic hemolytic anemia. Irregular, fragmented erythrocytes (schistocytes) are seen in the blood smear of a patient with disseminated intravascular coagulation.

Hypersplenism. Hemolytic anemia associated with leukopenia and thrombocytopenia occurs in many patients with an enlarged spleen. This is especially true of patients with congestive splenomegaly, as occurs in cirrhosis and (less prominently) when the spleen is infiltrated by leukemic cells. An enlarged spleen causes pooling and sequestration of all cellular elements. The erythrocytes, which depend critically on active intermediary metabolism to maintain their shape and viability, are especially vulnerable to stasis and, therefore, are lysed in the congested splenic cords. The resulting anemia stimulates compensatory erythroid hyperplasia in the bone marrow.

ERYTHROCYTOSIS (POLYCYTHEMIA)

■ *Erythrocytosis, which is usually but not accurately termed* polycythemia, *encompasses a number of conditions that are characterized by an increased hematocrit.*

Relative Erythrocytosis. This condition is characterized by a normal erythrocyte mass with a decreased plasma volume. Dehydration is the most common cause of relative erythrocytosis.

Absolute Erythrocytosis. Absolute erythrocytosis is classified as being either primary or secondary. Primary absolute erythrocytosis (**polycythemia vera**) is a clonal stem cell disorder in which all progenitor cells continuously proliferate in the absence of growth-stimulating factors (discussed later).

Secondary erythrocytosis is induced by arterial hypoxia under the following conditions:

- High altitude with low ambient Po_2
- Pulmonary disease with impaired gas exchange
- Cardiac anomalies with a right-to-left shunt

In all three situations, the resulting renal tissue hypoxia causes the release of erythropoietin and, in turn, an increased rate of erythrocyte production.

QUANTITATIVE DISORDERS OF NEUTROPHILS

Neutropenia

■ *Neutropenia, or granulocytopenia, refers to an absolute neutrophil count of less than 1800 cells/μL.* However,

BOX *20-3* **Principal Causes of Neutropenia**

Decreased production
  Radiation
  Drug-induced (acute, chronic)
  Viral infections
  Congenital
  Cyclic
Ineffective production
  Megaloblastic anemia
  Myelodysplastic syndromes
Increased destruction
  Isoimmune neonatal
  Autoimmune
    Idiopathic
    Drug-induced
    Felty syndrome
    Systemic lupus erythematosus
    Complement activation–induced dialysis
Splenic sequestration
Increased margination

even at this level, there is an adequate number of granulocytes to defend against micro-organisms. A serious risk of infection is experienced with absolute counts of less than 500 cells/μL. The term **agranulocytosis** is reserved for severe granulocytopenias in which both the marginated pool and the bone marrow reserve have been depleted.

Neutropenia is caused either by decreased or ineffective production or by increased destruction of neutrophils (Box 20-3). Most cases of neutropenia are asymptomatic and unexplained, and the term **chronic benign neutropenia** is used.

Neutrophilia

■ *Neutrophilia is an increase in the absolute peripheral blood neutrophil count to more than 7000 cells/μL.* It has many causes (Box 20-4), and it reflects (1) increased mobilization of neutrophils from the bone marrow storage pool, (2) enhanced release of neutrophils from the peripheral blood marginal pool, or (3) stimulation of granulopoiesis in the bone marrow.

Leukemoid Reaction. In patients with acute infections, neutrophilia may be so pronounced that it can be mistaken for leukemia, in which case it is termed a *leukemoid reaction.*

BOX *20-4*   **Principal Causes of Neutrophilic Leukocytosis**

Infections (primarily bacterial)
Immunologic/inflammatory
    Rheumatoid arthritis
    Rheumatic fever
    Vasculitis
Tissue necrosis
    Infarction
    Trauma
    Burns
Neoplasia
Hemorrhage
Hemolysis
Metabolic disorders
    Acidosis
    Uremia
    Gout
Endocrinologic disorders
    Thyroid storm
    Glucocorticoids
Pregnancy
Toxins
Physical stimuli
    Cold
    Heat
    Stress
Emotional stress
Hereditary neutrophilia

QUALITATIVE DISORDERS OF NEUTROPHILS

If the functional competence of granulocytes is impaired, decreased resistance to infection may occur despite a normal granulocyte count.

Chronic Granulomatous Disease

■ *Chronic granulomatous disease (CGD) refers to a group of rare, inherited, X-linked or autosomal recessive disorders that are characterized by defects in the bactericidal function of phagocytic cells, including neutrophils and macrophages.* All forms of CGD reflect the inability of these cells to undergo a respiratory burst and to generate hydrogen peroxide upon phagocytosis of microorganisms. The basic defect in the X-linked variant is a deficiency of membrane-bound NADPH oxidase. In patients with autosomal recessive CGD, a cytosolic factor that activates this enzyme is lacking. CGD becomes symptomatic at any age, from infancy to adulthood, and recurrent infections lead to widespread microabscesses and granulomas.

Chédiak-Higashi Syndrome

■ *Chédiak-Higashi syndrome is a rare, autosomal recessive condition that is characterized by abnormal, giant lysosomes in leukocytes and numerous cells in other tissues.* In neutrophils, monocytes, and lymphocytes, the defect manifests by the presence of huge, cytoplasmic granules. Functionally, neutropenia is accompanied by decreased chemotaxis, impaired degranulation, and ineffective bactericidal activity. The underlying molecular defect is unknown but is presumably related to abnormal membrane fusion.

Clinically, patients with Chédiak-Higashi syndrome suffer recurrent bacterial and fungal infections, principally involving the skin, mucous membranes, and respiratory tract. Defective platelet aggregation is reflected in prolonged bleeding times. Oculocutaneous albinism (see Chapter 6) is related to the segregation of melanin in giant melanosomes.

LANGERHANS CELL HISTIOCYTOSIS

■ *Langerhans cell histiocytosis (LCH) refers to a spectrum of uncommon, proliferative disorders of Langerhans cells. The disease ranges from asymptomatic involvement of a single site, such as bone or lymph nodes, to an aggressive, systemic disorder that involves multiple organs.*

Langerhans cells are a component of the mononuclear phagocyte system that is derived from precursor cells in the bone marrow. They are found in the epidermis and other sites, such as the lymph nodes, spleen, thymus, and mucosal tissues. Langerhans cells ingest, process, and present antigens to T lymphocytes.

Certain eponyms were traditionally attached to the various presentations of LCH:

- **Eosinophilic granuloma** is the term used for the localized, usually self-limited disorder of older children (age, 5–10 years) and young adults (age, <30 years). It accounts for as much as 75% of all cases of LCH and afflicts males four times as frequently as females. The bones (Fig. 20-13) and lungs are the principal organs affected.
- **Hand-Schüller-Christian disease** is a multifocal and more indolent disorder, typically occurring in children between 2 and 5 years of age, which represents one-fourth of all cases of LCH. Boys and girls are affected equally. Bony lesions tend to predominate, and involvement of endocrine glands may be prominent.
- **Letterer-Siwe disease** refers to the rare (<10% of cases), acute disseminated variant of LCH in in-

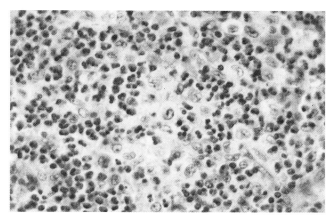

FIGURE   *20-13*
Eosinophilic granuloma. A section of an affected rib shows proliferated Langerhans cells and numerous eosinophils.

fants and children younger than 2 years of age. There is no sex predominance. Skin lesions and involvement of the visceral organs and hemopoietic system are characteristic (Fig. 20-14).

☐ **Pathology:** Langerhans cells that accumulate in these disorders are large (diameter, 15–25 μm), with round to indented nuclei, delicate vesicular chromatin, and small nucleoli. Marked nuclear folds and prominent grooves or creases are cytologic features lacking in other disorders of mononuclear phagocytes. The abundant cytoplasm is pink to red and, in patients with chronic disease, may contain lipid vacuoles.

By electron microscopy, a distinctive cytoplasmic inclusion, the **Birbeck granule,** is commonly observed in the Langerhans cells. This inclusion is rod-shaped or tubular, with a dense core and a double outer sheath. Frequently, one end is bulbous, in which case the granule resembles a tennis racquet.

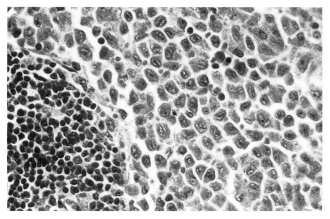

FIGURE   *20-14*
Letterer-Siwe disease. A section of the spleen illustrates sheets of proliferated Langerhans cells.

The infiltrating Langerhans cells are accompanied by variable numbers of inflammatory cells, principally eosinophils and less commonly plasma cells and neutrophils. There are characteristic histopathologic patterns of histiocytic infiltration in different organs:

- **The skin** initially shows involvement of the superficial papillary dermis. Invasion of the epidermis by Langerhans cells leads to secondary ulceration.
- **The lymph nodes** first exhibit involvement of the sinuses, although subsequent infiltration of the stroma is common.
- **The spleen** is infiltrated by Langerhans cells, predominantly in the red pulp.
- **The liver** displays Langerhans cells in the sinusoids.
- **The lungs** initially show infiltration in the alveolar septa and in the peribronchial and perivascular areas.
- **The bone marrow** is infiltrated in the hemopoietic stroma.

☐ **Clinical Features:** Clinical manifestations of LCH reflect the sites of tissue involvement. Skin involvement, principally in the Letterer-Siwe variant, takes the form of seborrheic or eczematoid dermatitis, most prominently on the scalp, face, and trunk. Painless localized or generalized lymphadenopathy and hepatosplenomegaly are frequent. Lytic lesions of bone cause pain or tenderness on palpation. Proptosis (protrusion of the eyeball) may be a complication of infiltration of the orbit. Diabetes insipidus occurs when the hypothalamic-pituitary axis is affected. The classic triad of diabetes insipidus, proptosis, and defects in membranous bones, however, occurs in only 15% of patients with Hand- Schüller-Christian disease.

The disorder is self-limited and benign in older persons (eosinophilic granuloma), whereas children younger than 2 years of age (Letterer-Siwe disease) tend to do poorly. Rarely, the clinical course is aggressive and indistinguishable from that of a malignant neoplasm.

REACTIVE HYPERPLASIA OF LYMPH NODES

Lymph nodes may exhibit hyperplasia of all cellular components or any combination of B lymphocytes, T lymphocytes, and mononuclear phagocytic cells in response to a variety of infectious, inflammatory, and neoplastic disorders.

- **Hyperplasia of the secondary follicles,** or germinal centers, and plasmacytosis of the medullary cords are indicators of B-lymphocyte immunoreactivity.
- **Hyperplasia of the deep cortex or paracortex** (interfollicular or diffuse hyperplasia) is characteristic of T-lymphocyte immunoreactivity.
- **Acute suppurative lymphadenitis** occurs in the lymph nodes that drain a site of acute bacterial infection. Suppurative lymph nodes enlarge rapidly because of edema and hyperemia. They also are tender owing to distention of the capsule. Microscopically, infiltration of the lymph node sinuses and stroma by polymorphonuclear leukocytes and prominent follicular hyperplasia are noted.

Follicular Hyperplasia

Nonspecific Reactive Follicular Hyperplasia. In this condition, prominent hyperplastic follicles occur principally in the cortex of the lymph node (Fig. 20-15). The follicles are round or irregular, and may be confluent. Activated B lymphocytes in the follicles range from small cells with irregular, cleaved nuclei to large immunoblasts. Numerous mitotic figures reflect the rapid proliferation of activated B lymphocytes. Scattered benign macrophages, with abundant pale cytoplasm containing pyknotic nuclear and cytoplasmic debris, impart the characteristic "starry sky" pattern of benign follicles. A well-defined mantle of normal, small B lymphocytes surrounds the follicles, thereby sharply demarcating them from the interfollicular regions.

The cause of nonspecific reactive follicular hyperplasia is frequently not known, although a viral or inflammatory cause is often suspected. The clinical course is typically benign, with rapid and complete resolution of the lymphadenopathy.

AIDS Lymphadenopathy. AIDS-associated lymphadenopathy is characterized by (1) marked follicular hyperplasia, with a distinctive loss of mantle zones; (2) infiltration of follicles by clusters of small lymphocytes; (3) foci of intrafollicular hemorrhage ("follicle lysis"); and (4) focal perisinusoidal or monocytoid B-cell hyperplasia. The lymph nodes in patients with AIDS show a high incidence of superimposed malignant neoplasms, including diffuse B-cell lymphomas, Hodgkin's disease, and Kaposi sarcoma.

Interfollicular Hyperplasia

Nonspecific Interfollicular Hyperplasia. In this condition, the lymph nodal paracortex is expanded by a heterogeneous, reactive cell population. On low-power microscopy, the infiltrate imparts a typical mottled ("salt-and-pepper") appearance, which reflects an admixture of small lymphocytes, variably activated lymphocytes, immunoblasts, and scattered macrophages (Fig. 20-16). Reactive nonspecific interfollicular hyperplasia most commonly results from viral infections or immunologic reactions. Although the precise cause is often not determined, the condition usually resolves promptly.

Infectious mononucleosis features immunoblastic cells in the lymph nodal sinuses.

Varicella-herpes zoster infection causes eosinophilic intranuclear inclusions, which are sur-

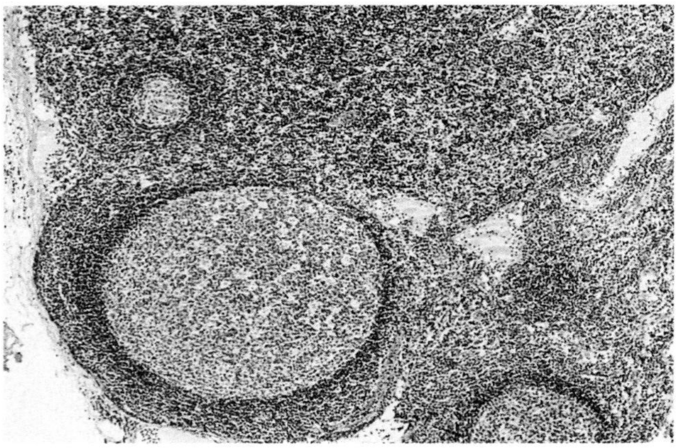

FIGURE *20-15*
Lymph node with reactive follicular hyperplasia. A section of a hyperplastic lymph node shows prominent follicles or germinal centers containing numerous macrophages with pale cytoplasm.

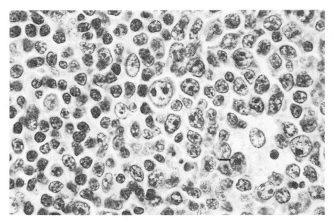

FIGURE *20-16*
Lymph node with reactive interfollicular hyperplasia. A high-power view of the T-dependent paracortex shows an admixture of small lymphocytes, variably activated lymphocytes, immunoblasts, and scattered macrophages.

rounded by a clear zone or halo (Cowdry type A inclusions), in endothelial cells.

Measles, in the prodromal phase, is characterized by scattered, multilobed or multinucleated lymphoid cells. These cells (**Warthin-Finkeldey cells**) display delicate chromatin, small punctate nucleoli, and scant, pale cytoplasm.

Cytomegalovirus lymphadenitis is distinguished by the presence in endothelial cells of large, round, eosinophilic, and intranuclear inclusions, which show a surrounding, clear halo.

Mixed Patterns of Reactive Hyperplasia of Lymph Nodes

Some infectious diseases are associated with mixed patterns of lymph node hyperplasia, in which several different features are prominent.

Toxoplasmosis. This form of lymphadenitis is characterized by (1) prominent follicular hyperplasia, (2) small collections of epithelioid macrophages in the interfollicular regions of the lymph node, which encroach on the follicles (Piringer-Kuchinka lesion), and (3) perisinusoidal monocytoid B-cell hyperplasia. Monocytoid B lymphocytes are medium-size lymphoid cells, with round to indented nuclei, bland chromatin, and moderate, pale cytoplasm.

Cat-Scratch Disease. This malady typically presents with lymphadenitis of the axillary and cervical lymph nodes, which is characterized by follicular hyperplasia and suppurative granulomatous foci. These areas consist of elongated or stellate abscesses, with an area of central necrosis containing polymorphonuclear leukocytes and cell debris and surrounded by palisaded macrophages and fibroblasts.

DISORDERS OF THE SPLEEN

Splenomegaly

The spleen is a prominent member of the lymphopoietic and mononuclear phagocyte systems, and splenomegaly is a common finding in a variety of unrelated pathologic situations (Box 20-5).

Reactive Splenomegaly

Reactive hyperplasia of the spleen occurs in a number of acute and chronic inflammatory conditions. It is probably caused by phagocytosis of blood-borne bacteria, with release of growth factors and other products of the inflammatory response. The spleen is moder-

BOX *20-5* **Principal Causes of Splenomegaly**

Infections
  Acute
  Subacute
  Chronic
Immunologic/inflammatory disorders
  Felty syndrome
  Lupus erythematosus
  Sarcoidosis
  Amyloidosis
  Thyrotoxicosis
Hemolytic anemias
Immune thrombocytopenia
Splenic vein hypertension
  Cirrhosis
  Splenic or portal vein thrombosis or stenosis
  Right-sided cardiac failure
Primary or metastatic neoplasm
  Leukemia
  Lymphoma
  Hodgkin disease
  Myeloproliferative syndromes
  Sarcoma
  Carcinoma
Storage diseases
  Gaucher
  Niemann-Pick
  Mucopolysaccharidoses

ately enlarged (≤400 g), and macrophages and neutrophils abound in the red pulp. Mild hyperplasia of the lymphoid white pulp is common.

In **acute and chronic parasitemias,** the red pulp may be engorged with parasites and their breakdown products. The spleen may be massively enlarged in chronic malarial infections (≤10 kg). It shows fibrous thickening of the capsule and trabeculae, with a slate-gray to black coloration of the pulp owing to the presence of phagocytosed malarial pigment (hematin).

In **chronic immunologic inflammatory disorders,** splenomegaly is caused by hyperplasia of the white pulp.

Systemic lupus erythematosus is characterized by fibrinoid necrosis of capsular and trabecular collagen and concentric ("onion skin") thickening of the penicilliary arteries and central arterioles of the white pulp.

In **infectious mononucleosis,** transformed lymphocytes (immunoblasts) prominently infiltrate the red pulp, whereas the white pulp may no longer be evident.

Congestive Splenomegaly

Chronic passive congestion of the spleen causes splenomegaly and hypersplenism. This is most common in patients with portal hypertension resulting from cirrhosis, thrombosis of the portal or splenic veins, or right-sided heart failure.

☐ **Pathology:** The spleen is modestly enlarged (300–700 g) and has a thickened, fibrotic capsule. The cut surface is firm, and the color varies from pink to deep red, depending on the extent of fibrosis. Microscopically, the parenchyma is fibrotic, and the red pulp is hypocellular. The white pulp tends to be atrophic.

Infiltrative Splenomegaly

The spleen may be enlarged by an increased number of cellular elements or the deposition of extracellular material, as in amyloidosis. Splenic macrophages accumulate in chronic infections, hemolytic anemias, and a variety of storage diseases, with Gaucher disease being the prototype (see Chapter 6). Splenomegaly is also caused by the infiltration of malignant cells in hematologic proliferative disorders (e.g., leukemias and lymphomas).

Disorders of Hemostasis

DISORDERS OF PLATELETS

Platelet abnormalities, whether qualitative or quantitative, result in a bleeding diathesis.

Thrombocytopenia is defined as a decrease in the platelet count to less than 150,000 cells/μL. A reduction in platelets to less than 50,000 cells/μL increases the hazard of bleeding from trauma or surgical procedures. Spontaneous bleeding can be expected with a platelet count of less than 20,000 cells/μL, and it is especially likely with a count of less than 10,000 cells/μL. Thrombocytopenia can result from decreased production of platelets, increased destruction of platelets, splenic sequestration, or dilution (Box 20-6).

Decreased Production of Platelets

A decreased number of megakaryocytes occurs in patients with aplastic anemia, infiltrative disorders of the marrow, or marrow hypoplasia produced by drugs, radiation, or viral infections. Chemotherapeutic agents are the most common drugs that cause a reduction in the number of megakaryocytes as a feature of general bone marrow hypoplasia.

Increased Destruction of Platelets

Two major mechanisms are responsible for an increased destruction of platelets. Many cases reflect immune-mediated damage and the removal of circulat-

ing platelets, as in idiopathic thrombocytopenic purpura and drug-induced thrombocytopenia. Alternatively, intravascular platelet aggregation may produce thrombocytopenia, such as in thrombotic thrombocytopenic purpura.

Idiopathic (Immune) Thrombocytopenic Purpura

■ *Idiopathic thrombocytopenic purpura (ITP) is a quantitative disorder of platelets that is caused by antibodies directed against platelet or megakaryocytic antigens.*

☐ **Pathogenesis:** ITP is related to antibody-mediated immune destruction of platelets or their precursors. In the large majority of patients, the autoantibodies are of the IgG class.

Acute ITP typically appears in children after a viral illness, and it is likely caused by viral-induced changes in platelet antigens that elicit autoantibodies.

Chronic ITP occurs predominantly in adults and is often associated with a collagen vascular disease (e.g., systemic lupus erythematosus) or malignant lymphoproliferative disease, especially chronic lymphocytic leukemia. As in patients with acute ITP, IgG antibodies bind to antigens on the platelet surface, after which complement is activated.

☐ **Pathology:** In patients with acute ITP, the platelet count is typically less than 20,000 cells/μL. In adult patients with chronic ITP, the platelet count varies from a few thousand to 100,000 cells/μL. The peripheral blood smear exhibits large platelets, which reflect an increased number of young platelets being released by the bone marrow. Accordingly, examination of the bone marrow reveals a compensatory increase in megakaryocytes, which tend to be young and mononuclear.

B O X *20-6* **Principal Causes of Thrombocytopenia**

Decreased production
   Aplastic anemia
   Bone marrow suppression by drugs or radiation
Ineffective production
   Megaloblastic anemia
   Myelodysplasias
   May-Hegglin disease
Increased destruction
   Immunologic (idiopathic)
   Drug-induced
   Consumptive (disseminated intravascular coagulation, thrombotic thrombocytopenic purpura)
Increased sequestration
   Splenomegaly
Dilutional
   Blood and plasma transfusions

☐ **Clinical Features:** Children with acute ITP experience the sudden onset of petechiae and purpura but are otherwise asymptomatic. Spontaneous recovery can be expected in more than 80% of patients within 6 months. If thrombocytopenia persists longer than 6 months, splenectomy cures the disease in a large majority of cases.

Chronic ITP in adults presents as bleeding episodes, such as epistaxis, menorrhagia, or ecchymoses. Although life-threatening hemorrhages may occur, they are uncommon. In those who fail to respond adequately to drug therapy within 2 to 3 months, splenectomy produces a complete or partial remission in 60% to 80% of patients.

Drug-Induced Thrombocytopenia

A number of drugs, especially quinidine, sulfonamides, penicillin, cimetidine, and digoxin, combine with surface proteins on platelets to produce neoantigens. The latter elicit antibodies and, in turn, platelet destruction. Heparin is a common cause of drug-induced thrombocytopenia, affecting as many as 5% of the patients treated with this anticoagulant. Thrombocytopenia tends to be severe and symptomatic, with platelet counts less than 20,000 cell/μL. The disorder usually resolves promptly after discontinuation of the drug.

Thrombotic Thrombocytopenic Purpura

■ *Thrombotic thrombocytopenic purpura (TTP) is a rare syndrome featuring the pentad of thrombocytopenia, microangiopathic hemolytic anemia, neurologic symptoms, fever, and azotemia.* Platelet aggregation leads to widespread deposition of platelets in the microvasculature as characteristic hyaline thrombi. Hemolytic-uremic syndrome is similar to TTP, and in its adult form, it is thought by many to be a variant of the latter (see Chapter 16).

☐ **Pathogenesis:** The pathogenesis of TTP is obscure, but the theory that has received the most attention involves the inappropriate release of von Willebrand factor multimers from injured endothelial cells. In patients with TTP, for unknown reasons, unusually large multimers of von Willebrand factor are present in the plasma, where they presumably mediate intravascular platelet aggregation. Although most cases of TTP arise in otherwise normal persons, the disease may also complicate autoimmune collagen vascular disorders, drug-induced hypersensitivity reactions, infections, cancer chemotherapy, and pregnancy.

☐ **Pathology:** The morphologic hallmark of TTP is deposition throughout the body of periodic acid-Schiff–positive, hyaline microthrombi in arterioles and capillaries, principally in the heart, brain, and kidneys. The microthrombi contain platelet aggregates, fibrin, and a few erythrocytes and leukocytes. On the peripheral blood smear, fragmented erythrocytes (schistocytes) are always evident.

☐ **Clinical Features:** TTP occurs at virtually any age. Clinical manifestations are described as a pentad: (1) fever, (2) thrombocytopenia, (3) microangiopathic hemolytic anemia, (4) azotemia, and (5) a constellation of mental and neurologic defects. The disease may be chronic and recurrent over a period of years or, more commonly, an acute and fulminant disease, which is often fatal. Most patients present with neurologic symptoms, including seizures, focal weakness, aphasia, and alterations in the state of consciousness. Widespread purpura are often present as well. Anemia is a constant feature and is often severe enough to reduce the hemoglobin to less than 6 g/dL.

Thrombocytopenia is invariable in patients with TTP, and more than half of the patients have a platelet count of less than 20,000 cells/μL. Before modern therapy, acute TTP was ordinarily fatal. However, with the use of plasma infusion and plasmapheresis, the cure rate has increased to 80%.

COAGULATION DISORDERS

Quantitative and qualitative disorders of all coagulation factors have been identified, which may be either hereditary or acquired. Of the hereditary deficiencies, only those of factor VIII (hemophilia A), factor IX (hemophilia B), and von Willebrand factor are common. Hemophilia A is discussed in Chapter 6.

Hemophilia B

■ *Hemophilia B (Christmas disease) is an X-linked, recessive bleeding disorder that results from a deficiency of factor IX activity.* Hemophilia B accounts for at least 10% of all cases of hemophilia. The hemorrhagic diathesis is clinically indistinguishable from that of hemophilia A.

Von Willebrand Disease

■ *Von Willebrand disease is the common name for a heterogeneous complex of hereditary coagulation disorders related to a deficiency or abnormality of von Willebrand factor (vWf).* This adhesive molecule is synthesized by endothelial cells and megakaryocytes as a 250-kd monomer that undergoes polymerization to multimers with molecular weights in the millions. vWf is stored in the cytoplasmic Weibel-Palade bodies of the endothelial cells and is released into the subendothelial tissues and plasma. After endothelial injury, subendothelial vWf binds to platelet glycoprotein receptors, thereby promoting adherence of platelets and sealing off the endothelial injury. In plasma, vWf binds to and protects factor VIII; its absence is always associated with deficient activity of factor VIII.

☐ **Clinical Features:** Most cases of von Willebrand disease are associated with only a mild bleeding diathesis. Easy bruising, epistaxis, gastrointestinal bleeding, and in women, menorrhagia are frequent. The presenting symptom is often excessive hemorrhage after trauma or surgery. The bleeding tendency in patients with all forms of von Willebrand disease is treated successfully with fresh-frozen plasma or with cryoprecipitate.

Vitamin K Deficiency

Vitamin K is a necessary cofactor for carboxylation and activation of prothrombin; factors VII, IX, and X; and the anticoagulant protein C. In most cases, vitamin K deficiencies are caused by elimination of vitamin K–producing bacteria in the gut after antibiotic treatment. In patients with liver disease, a deficiency of vitamin K–dependent factors does not result from vitamin K deficiency but, rather, from inadequate hepatic synthesis of the factors themselves.

Disseminated Intravascular Coagulation

■ *Disseminated intravascular coagulation (DIC) is an acquired disorder that is characterized by consumption of*

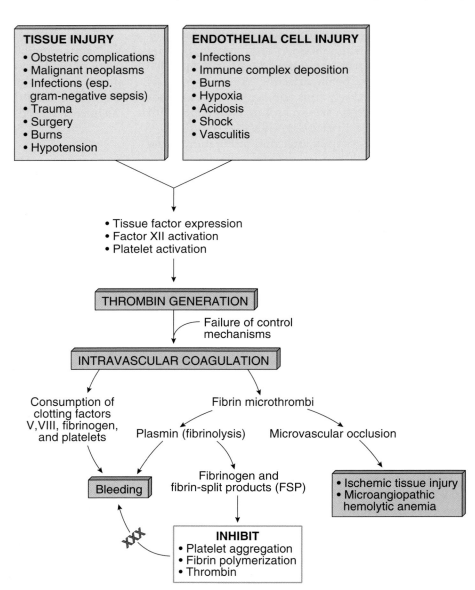

FIGURE 20-17
The pathophysiology of disseminated intravascular coagulation (DIC). The syndrome of DIC is precipitated by tissue injury, endothelial cell injury, or a combination of the two. These injuries trigger increased expression of tissue factor on cell surfaces and activation of clotting factors (including XII and V) and platelets. With the failure of normal control mechanisms, the generation of thrombin leads to intravascular coagulation.

platelets and coagulation factors, thereby resulting in a serious hemorrhagic diathesis. DIC is accompanied by widespread ischemic changes secondary to microvascular fibrin thrombi. It typically occurs as a complication of massive trauma, septicemia from numerous organisms, and obstetric emergencies. It is also associated with metastatic cancer, hemopoietic malignancies, cardiovascular and liver disease, and numerous other conditions.

☐ **Pathogenesis: The central event in the initiation of DIC is activation of the intrinsic or extrinsic clotting cascades within the vascular compartment by tissue injury, damage to the endothelium, or both.** The delicate balance between coagulation and fibrinolysis is disrupted, and the consumption of clotting factors, platelets, and fibrinogen ensues, with a consequent hemorrhagic diathesis (Fig. 20-17).

Procoagulant tissue factor is released into the circulation following trauma in a variety of circumstances. **Bacterial endotoxin** also stimulates macrophages to release tissue factor. **Certain neoplasms** are associated with DIC owing to the release of tissue factor by the cancer cells. As a consequence of the activation of the clotting cascade, intravascular fibrin is deposited as microthrombi in the smallest blood vessels. Stimulation of the fibrinolytic system by fibrin generates fibrin split products that possess anticoagulant properties and contribute to the bleeding diathesis.

Endothelial injury plays an important role in the pathogenesis of many cases of DIC. The normal endothelium has anticoagulant properties and shields platelets from activation by contact with the subendothelial connective tissue (see Chapters 2 and 10). The anticoagulant properties of the endothelium are impaired in the setting of widely varying injuries, including (1) tumor necrosis factor in gram-negative sepsis; (2) other inflammatory mediators, such as activated complement, interleukin-1, or neutrophil proteases; (3) viral or rickettsial infections; and (4) trauma (e.g., burns). As a result, platelet aggregates form in the microvasculature.

☐ **Pathology and Clinical Features:** Arterioles, capillaries, and venules in many parts of the body are occluded by **microthrombi,** which are composed of fibrin and platelets (Fig. 20-18). Microvascular obstruction is associated with widespread ischemic changes, particularly in the brain, kidneys, skin, lungs, and gastrointestinal tract. These organs are also the sites of bleeding, which, in the case of the brain and gastrointestinal tract, may be fatal.

Erythrocytes become fragmented (schistocytes) by passage through webs of intravascular fibrin strands,

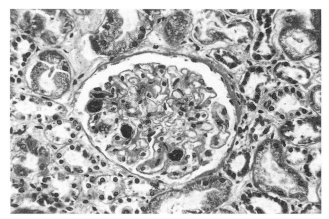

FIGURE *20-18*
Disseminated intravascular coagulation. A section of a glomerulus stained with phosphotungstic acid-hematoxylin, which colors fibrin deep purple, demonstrates several microthrombi.

thereby resulting in **microangiopathic hemolytic anemia**. Consumption of activated platelets leads to thrombocytopenia, whereas depletion of clotting factors is reflected in a prolonged prothrombin time and partial thromboplastin time and a decreased plasma fibrinogen level. Plasma fibrin split products prolong the thrombin time.

Ischemic changes in the brain lead to seizures and coma. Renal symptoms range from mild azotemia to fulminant acute renal failure. Acute respiratory distress syndrome may supervene, and acute ulcers of the gastrointestinal tract may cause substantial hemorrhage. The bleeding diathesis is evidenced by cerebral hemorrhage, ecchymoses, and hematuria. Patients with DIC are treated with heparin anticoagulation (to interrupt the cycle of intravascular coagulation) and replacement of platelets and clotting factors (to control the bleeding).

Neoplastic Disorders of the Blood and Lymphoid Organs

CHRONIC MYELOPROLIFERATIVE SYNDROMES

■ *Chronic myeloproliferative syndromes* comprise a group of interrelated, neoplastic disorders of multipotential hemopoietic stem cells. As a result, all cell lineages—erythroid, granulocytic, monocytic, and megakaryocytic—are involved. Four subtypes are recognized, each of which features a predominant cell lineage:

- **Polycythemia Vera**—Erythroid cells.
- **Chronic Myelogenous Leukemia**—Granulocytes.
- **Idiopathic Thrombocythemia**—Megakaryocytes.
- **Myelofibrosis with Myeloid Metaplasia**—All hemopoietic cell lines plus reactive marrow fibrosis (myelofibrosis).

Polycythemia Vera

■ *Polycythemia vera is a neoplastic disorder of multipotential hemopoietic stem cells in which the total body erythrocyte mass is markedly increased.* The disorder most commonly occurs in middle-age and elderly persons, although it may develop at any age.

☐ **Pathogenesis:** Polycythemia vera is thought to derive from malignant transformation of a single, multipotential hemopoietic stem cell with primary commitment to the erythroid lineage. Autonomous proliferation of the more mature cells confers a growth advantage to the neoplastic clone, because the increased erythrocyte mass suppresses the normal secretion of erythropoietin secretion and the function of the remaining normal progenitors.

☐ **Pathology:** The bone marrow is a homogeneous, red-purple color. The spleen is moderately enlarged, and its cut surface is also uniformly red-purple, with expansion of the red pulp and obliteration of the white pulp. The liver tends to be enlarged.

The principal histologic features in patients with polycythemia vera are outlined in Table 20-1. The bone marrow is hypercellular, with hyperplasia of all elements. Erythroid precursor cells predominate, however, and the myeloid:erythroid ratio is less than 2:1. Megakaryocytes typically are increased and tend to be enlarged.

The spleen exhibits a prominent accumulation of erythrocytes in the red pulp cords and sinuses. There may be myeloid metaplasia, with erythroid precursor cells, immature granulocytes, and megakaryocytes. The lymphoid white pulp is atrophic or obliterated. Myeloid metaplasia is also common in the sinusoids of the liver and in the sinuses and paracortex of the lymph nodes.

On the peripheral blood smear, the erythrocytes usually appear normal. The common initial laboratory findings are outlined in Table 20-2. The hemoglobin concentration may be greater than 20 g/dL, and the hematocrit may be greater than 60%. The erythrocyte count is 6 to 10 million cells/μL.

All formed elements of the blood are usually increased in patients with polycythemia vera. A mild to moderate leukocytosis of from 10,000 to 25,000 cells/μL occurs initially in two-thirds of the cases, but on occasion, neutrophil counts of more than 100,000 cells/μL may be observed. Thrombocytosis (400,000–800,000 platelets/μL) occurs initially in half of the cases. The platelets often exhibit abnormal morphologic features, including giant and hypogranulated forms.

☐ **Clinical Features:** The onset of polycythemia vera tends to be insidious. Plethora (from hypervolemia) and splenomegaly are early findings. Angina pectoris (secondary to disturbances of coronary artery blood flow) and intermittent claudication (caused by sluggish peripheral blood flow in the lower extremities) may be observed. Major thrombotic complications occur in one-third of the cases, including cerebrovascular accidents and myocardial infarction. Clinical features of polycythemia vera are outlined in Table 20-3.

The clinical course of polycythemia vera proceeds as a series of phases:

- **Proliferative Phase.** Most patients experience a prolonged proliferative phase, which is dominated

T A B L E   20-*1.*   Hematopathologic Features of Chronic Myeloproliferative Syndromes

	Polycythemia Vera	Chronic Myelogenous Leukemia	Myelofibrosis with Myeloid Metaplasia	Idiopathic Thrombocythemia
Bone Marrow				
Histopathology	Panhyperplasia (predominantly erythroid)	Panhyperplasia (predominantly granulocytic)	Panhyperplasia with fibrosis	Atypical megakaryocytes predominant
M:E ratio[a]	≤2:1	10:1 to 50:1	2:1 to 5:1	—
Marrow iron	↓ Or absent	Normal or ↑	Normal or ↑	Normal to absent
Marrow fibrosis	15–20%	<10%	90–100%	<5%
Liver and Spleen				
Extramedullary hemopoiesis (myeloid metaplasia)	Moderate (predominantly erythroid)	Moderate to marked (predominantly granulocytic)	Moderate to marked	Slight (predominantly megakaryocytic)

[a] Myeloid : erythroid ratio.

TABLE 20-2. Laboratory Features of Chronic Myeloproliferative Syndromes

	Polycythemia Vera	Chronic Myelogenous Leukemia	Myelofibrosis with Myeloid Metaplasia	Idiopathic Thrombocythemia
Hemoglobin	>20 g/dL	Mild anemia	Mild anemia	Mild anemia
Red-blood-cell morphology	Slight aniso- and poikilocytosis	Slight aniso- and poikilocytosis	Immature erythrocytes and marked aniso- and poikilocytosis	Hypochromic microcytes
Granulocytes	Normal to mildly increased, may show a few immature forms	Moderate to markedly increased, with spectrum of maturation basophilia	Normal to moderately increased, with some immature white blood cells	Normal to slightly increased
Platelets	Normal to moderately increased	Normal to moderately increased	Increased to decreased	Markedly increased with abnormal forms
Leukocyte alkaline phosphatase	Normal to increased	Decreased to absent	Variable	Variable
Cytogenetics	Aneuploid (25%)	Philadelphia chromosome (90%)	Aneuploid (50%)	Aneuploid (25%)

by erythroid proliferation and increased erythrocyte mass.

- **Spent Phase.** In 10% of the cases, excessive proliferation of erythroid cells ceases, thereby resulting in a stable or decreased erythrocyte mass.
- **Postpolycythemic Myelofibrosis with Myeloid Metaplasia.** An additional 10% of cases show progression to myelofibrosis, which is similar to that observed in patients with other chronic myeloproliferative syndromes (discussed later). At this stage, the prognosis is poor, with a mean survival time of only 2 years.
- **Acute Myelogenous Leukemia:** Acute myelogenous leukemia (AML) develops in 5% to 10% of patients with polycythemia vera.

The median survival time of patients with polycythemia vera is 13 years, and the most common causes of death are those associated with old age. Specific causes of death related to the disease itself include thrombosis, hemorrhage, acute myelogenous leukemia, and the spent phase. Therapeutic reduction of the erythrocyte mass, either by repeated phlebotomy or by drug therapy, constitutes effective management in most cases.

Chronic Myelogenous Leukemia

■ *Chronic myelogenous leukemia (CML) is a neoplastic disorder of multipotential hemopoietic stem cells that principally involves the granulocytic cell lineage.* Patients with CML display pronounced granulocytosis and immaturity of granulocytic elements, anemia, thrombocytosis, basophilia, and splenomegaly. CML constitutes 20% of all leukemias in Western countries. The disorder is most common in middle-age and elderly adults, with a median age at onset of 50 years, although it may occur at any age.

TABLE 20-3. Clinical Features of Chronic Myeloproliferative Syndromes

	Polycythemia Vera	Chronic Myelogenous Leukemia	Mylofibrosis with Myeloid Metaplasia	Idiopathic Thrombocythemia
Male:female ratio	1.2:1	3:2	1:1	1.2:1
Peak age range (years)	40–60	25–60	50–70	50–70
Clinical symptoms	Headache, dizziness, pruritus	Asymptomatic or LUQ[a] discomfort, fatigability	Asymptomatic or LUQ discomfort, fatigability	Asymptomatic or LUQ discomfort
Clinical signs	Bleeding, thrombosis	Easy bruising, bleeding	Weight loss, gouty arthritis	Bleeding, thrombosis
Splenomegaly	75%	90%	100%	30% (slight)
Hepatomegaly	40%	50%	80%	40% (slight)
Leukemic conversion	1–3%	70% (blast crisis)	15–20%	Uncommon
Median survival time (years)	13	3–4	3–4	Unknown

[a] *LUQ*, left upper quadrant.

☐ **Pathogenesis:** The cause of CML is not known. Survivors of the atomic bomb explosions in Japan and British patients treated with spinal radiation therapy for ankylosing spondylitis have suffered an increased incidence of CML. Myelotoxic agents (e.g., benzene) cause CML in a small minority of cases. In 90% of the cases of CML, the Ph[1] chromosome can be demonstrated in the karyotype (see Chapter 5).

Hyperplasia of granulocytic lineage elements in patients with CML is attributed principally to expansion of the multipotential stem cell pools. In addition, there may be abnormalities in the maturation and proliferation of the granulocytic precursor cells. Whatever the mechanism, the result is a 10- to 100-fold expansion of the total body pool of granulocyte cells.

☐ **Pathology:** The proliferation and expansion of neoplastic hemopoietic cells in patients with CML occur primarily in the bone marrow and secondarily in the spleen. Extramedullary proliferation (myeloid metaplasia) may also be identified in sites such as the liver and lymph nodes. The spleen is enlarged, often to massive proportions, and the cut surface is uniformly red-purple. The liver is moderately enlarged.

Microscopically, the bone marrow is conspicuously hypercellular owing to hyperplasia of all three lineages (Fig. 20-19). Granulocytic precursor cells predominate, and the myeloid:erythroid ratio is markedly increased. Megakaryocytes typically are numerous. The principal histopathologic features of CML are outlined in Table 20-1.

On peripheral blood smears, features are similar to those of bone marrow aspirates, and the entire spectrum of maturing granulocytic cells is observed. The spleen exhibits prominent myeloid metaplasia in the red pulp cords, and the lymphoid white pulp is generally obliterated. In the liver, foci of myeloid metaplasia in the sinusoids are common.

With progression to blast crisis, there is loss of the differentiation and maturation capacity of the granulocytic precursor cells. Medullary and extramedullary accumulation of primitive blast cells also occurs. The blast cells may have the morphologic features of any subtype of acute myelogenous leukemia. Destructive tumor masses consisting of myeloblasts and promyelocytes (**granulocytic sarcomas** or **chloromas**) may arise in sites such as the lymph nodes, bones, and meninges. The common laboratory findings in early CML are outlined in Table 20-2.

☐ **Clinical Features:** The onset of CML tends to be insidious. Hemorrhagic manifestations may be caused by thrombocytopenia or qualitative platelet defects, and thrombosis may occur secondary to thrombocytosis. The clinical course is characterized by an initially stable phase that lasts from 2 to 8 years (mean time, 3–4 years). During this period, the disorder is usually well tolerated. The salient clinical features of CML are outlined in Table 20-3.

In two-thirds of the cases of CML, the chronic stable phase is terminated by blast crisis, either abruptly or after an accelerated phase. The blast cells are of myeloid lineage in 70% of the blast crises and of lymphoid lineage in 30%. The mean survival time of patients in blast crisis is measured in months. Treatment of CML involves chemotherapy and administration of interferon-α to suppress the proliferation of hemopoietic progenitor cells. Good results have been obtained with bone marrow transplantation.

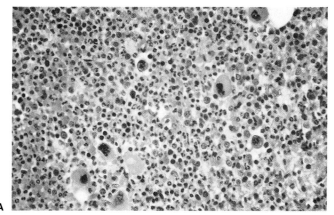
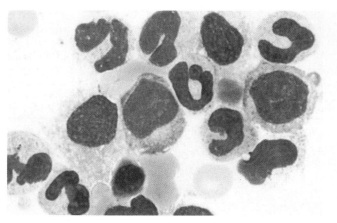

A   B

FIGURE   *20-19*
Chronic myelogenous leukemia. (A) The bone marrow is conspicuously hypercellular owing to increased numbers of granulocyte precursors, mature granulocytes, and megakaryocytes. (B) A smear of a bone marrow aspirate from the same patient as *panel A* reveals numerous granulocytes at various stages of development.

Myelofibrosis with Myeloid Metaplasia

■ *Myelofibrosis with myeloid metaplasia (MMM),* which was originally termed agnogenic myeloid metaplasia, is an uncommon neoplastic proliferation of multipotential hemopoietic stem cells in which the proliferation of all hemopoietic cell lineages stimulates a reactive fibrosis of the bone marrow. Myeloid metaplasia involves the sites of extramedullary hemopoiesis in the fetus, principally the spleen, liver, and lymph nodes. Abnormally shaped erythrocytes abound in the peripheral blood, and circulating immature erythroid and granulocytic cells (leukoerythroblastic reaction) are typical. The disease usually afflicts middle-age and elderly adults, with the median age at onset being 60 years.

□ **Pathogenesis:** As the name indicates, the cause of MMM is not known. One-third of the cases of polycythemia vera, and a lesser proportion of the cases of CML, progress to a condition that is indistinguishable from MMM.

A clonal disorder, MMM is thought to derive from the malignant transformation of a single, multipotential hemopoietic stem cell that has no selective commitment to any particular hemopoietic cell lineage. **Fibrosis of the bone marrow is thought to be reactive rather than neoplastic, because the marrow fibroblasts are polyclonal, and proliferation of clonal hemopoietic cells may occur before the onset of myelofibrosis.**

□ **Pathology:** At the time of presentation, the spleen is almost always conspicuously enlarged. Splenomegaly reflects myeloid metaplasia, erythrocyte pooling, and fibrosis. The liver is moderately enlarged as well. The marrow is often hypercellular, with decreased (or even absent) fat cells. The granulocytic and megakaryocytic cell lineages predominate, and the erythroid cell series is relatively, although not absolutely, decreased.

Cells of the granulocytic series show normal maturation. Megakaryocytes are increased and tend to be distributed in characteristic, cohesive clusters of more than five cells. Megaloblastoid change and hyperchromatic, irregular, or fragmented nuclei are dyspoietic features in erythroid precursor cells.

Myelofibrosis commonly involves the central flat bones and the proximal long bones. Biopsy specimens demonstrate a moderate to marked increase in reticulin fibers, which progresses to collagenous fibrosis (Fig. 20-20). The peripheral blood smear discloses a leukoerythroblastic reaction, with circulating, immature erythroid and granulocytic cells and giant platelets. The erythrocytes exhibit pronounced anisocytosis and poikilocytosis. Principal hematopathologic

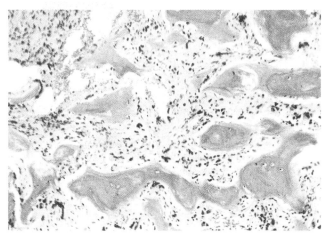

FIGURE *20-20*
Myelofibrosis with myeloid metaplasia. A section of bone marrow shows collagenous fibrosis, osteosclerosis, and numerous abnormal megakaryocytes.

findings in patients with MMM are outlined in Table 20-1. Common initial laboratory findings in patients with MMM are listed in Table 20-2.

□ **Clinical Features:** The clinical course of MMM is characterized by (1) progressively severe anemia, with gradually increasing transfusion requirements; (2) leukopenia with infections; and (3) thrombocytopenia with hemorrhages. The median survival time of patients with MMM is 5 years. Superimposed AML occurs in 5% to 10% of cases. Clinical features of MMM are outlined in Table 20-3.

Treatment of MMM is variable and includes chemotherapy, splenic radiation therapy, or splenectomy. Bone marrow transplantation is a promising therapy.

ACUTE MYELOGENOUS LEUKEMIA

■ *Acute myelogenous leukemia (AML),* also termed acute nonlymphocytic leukemia, *consists of a heterogeneous group of interrelated disorders in which the neoplastic transformation of a multipotential hemopoietic stem cell (or one of restricted lineage potential) results in the accumulation of granulocytes, monocytes, erythrocytes, or megakaryocytes.* In general, the neoplastic clone fails to mature beyond the blast-cell stage, thereby leading to a progressive accumulation of myeloblasts in the bone marrow.

In Western countries, AML constitutes 20% of all leukemias, with the large majority of these cases occurring in adults. In fact, whereas AML accounts for 20%

of the acute leukemias during childhood, it is responsible for 85% of the cases in adults.

☐ **Pathogenesis:** The cause of AML is not known. Risk factors include:

- **Myelotoxic Agents.** The most important myelotoxic agents are benzene and the antineoplastic alkylating agents.
- **Radiation.** In doses exceeding 100 rads (or cGy), there is a linear relationship between ionizing radiation and the development of AML.
- **Genetic Abnormalities.** Trisomy 21 (Down syndrome) is characterized by an increased incidence of AML, although most cases of leukemia in patients with this syndrome are acute lymphoblastic leukemia.
- **Hematologic Disorders.** Chronic myeloproliferative syndromes, myelodysplastic syndromes, aplastic anemia, and paroxysmal nocturnal hemoglobinuria all carry an increased risk for AML.

Cytogenetic abnormalities in the leukemic cells are demonstrated in most cases of AML. Common abnormalities include trisomies 8 and 21, monosomies 7 and 21, and loss of an X or Y chromosome. Nonrandom chromosomal translocations are also common.

The major problems associated with AML principally relate to the progressive accumulation in the marrow of immature myelogenous cells that lack the potential for further differentiation and maturation. Whereas leukemic myeloblasts replicate more slowly than normal hemopoietic precursor cells, their frequency of spontaneous cell death is less than normal. Thus, the expanded pool of leukemic blasts encroaches on the normal marrow and suppresses hemopoiesis. As a consequence, the major clinical problems in AML are granulocytopenia, thrombocytopenia, and anemia.

☐ **Pathology:** Nine morphologic variants of AML are recognized, reflecting the predominant lineage commitment of the neoplastic stem cells (Fig. 20-21). The most common subtypes are M2 and M4.

In patients with AML, the spleen and lymph nodes are moderately enlarged and firm. The cut surface of the spleen is uniformly red-purple, with a prominent red pulp and partial to complete obliteration of the white pulp. The liver tends to be enlarged, and its cut surface is gray-tan. The bone marrow in patients with AML is typically hypercellular (Fig. 20-22) but may be normocellular or, infrequently, hypocellular (hy-poplastic AML). Blast cells are increased (>30% of nucleated cells) and often efface the normal architecture.

Microscopically, the lymph nodes are initially infiltrated in the paracortex, which is a condition that may progress to complete obliteration of the nodal architecture. In the spleen, both the red pulp and the lymphoid white pulp are eventually obliterated by leukemic cells. The liver contains blasts in the sinusoids. Infiltration of any visceral organ, the skin (leukemia cutis), and other sites (e.g., central nervous system) may also occur.

☐ **Clinical Features:** The diagnosis of AML is established by demonstrating more than 30% myeloblasts in the bone marrow, with or without the presence of blasts in the peripheral blood. At the time of presentation, there is usually some degree of thrombocytopenia, neutropenia, and anemia.

If untreated, AML is a rapidly fatal disease, with the median survival time being less than 2 months. The most common causes of death are infection or hemorrhage. With current chemotherapeutic regimens, however, a complete clinical remission can be anticipated in 70% of the patients younger than 60 years of age. The disease relapses in most patients, but with maintenance chemotherapy, remissions of longer than 8 years—and possibly even complete cures—have been obtained in 15% of the cases. Bone marrow transplantation is the preferred therapy in many younger patients with AML.

CHRONIC LYMPHOCYTIC LEUKEMIA

■ *Chronic lymphocytic leukemia (CLL) is a neoplastic disorder that is characterized by the clonal proliferation of immunologically immature and functionally incompetent small lymphocytes.* B-cell lineage is demonstrated in more than 95% of the cases. The spectrum of B-cell malignant lymphoproliferative disease is outlined in Box 20-7, and the spectrum of T-cell disorders is given in Box 20-8.

In patients with CLL of B-cell lineage (B-CLL), the initial involvement is in the bone marrow, with the subsequent release of neoplastic lymphocytes to the peripheral blood. As the disease progresses, variable infiltration and enlargement of the lymph nodes, spleen, and less prominently, the liver occur. The

FIGURE **20-21**
Acute leukemia (French-American-British classification).

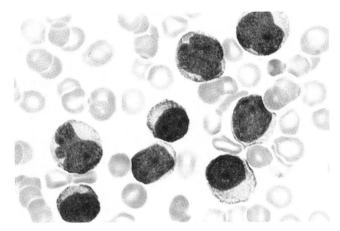

FIGURE 20-25
Acute lymphoblastic leukemia (L2 ALL). The lymphoblasts in the peripheral blood contain irregular and indented nuclei, with prominent nucleoli and a moderate amount of cytoplasm.

The pathogenesis of clinical disease in ALL relates principally to the progressive accumulation in the bone marrow of lymphoblasts that lack the potential for differentiation and maturation.

☐ **Pathology:** Both the spleen and liver are moderately enlarged. Microscopically, lymphoblasts vary from small to moderately large cells. They exhibit delicate and reticulated chromatin, one to several nucleoli, and scant, pale cytoplasm. Mitotic figures are numerous. The bone marrow is hypercellular, and the normal hemopoietic tissue is largely (or even completely) replaced by lymphoblasts.

The initial infiltration of the lymph nodes occurs in the paracortex following egress of lymphoblasts from the blood through the postcapillary venules. Eventually, the normal nodal architecture is completely effaced. Splenic involvement occurs predominantly in the red pulp, and the liver commonly shows infiltration of both the sinusoids and the portal areas.

Three cytologic subtypes of ALL are recognized (see Fig. 20-21). Immunologic markers define four major subtypes of ALL, three of B-cell origin and one of T-cell origin.

- **B-ALL.** Two subtypes of B-ALL are composed of B-cell precursors, namely pre-pre–B cell ALL (morphologically L1) and pre–B cell ALL (L2; Fig. 20-25). One subtype is composed of more mature B cells (L3).
- **T-ALL.** Twenty percent of the cases of ALL derive from T-cell precursors and are morphologically L2.
- **Null Cell ALL.** A small proportion of the cases of ALL lack distinguishing B- or T-lymphocyte lineage markers and are called null or unclassified ALL.

Terminal deoxynucleotidyl transferase (Tdt), a nuclear DNA polymerizing enzyme, is demonstrated in almost all (95%) of the cases of B-ALL and T-ALL. This enzyme is uniformly lacking only in the mature B cell, or L3, variant. Demonstration of Tdt activity suggests that a leukemic blast cell is of lymphoid rather than myeloid lineage, because the enzyme is demonstrated in only 5% to 10% of the patients of AML.

☐ **Clinical Features:** The diagnosis of ALL is established by demonstrating lymphoblasts in the bone marrow. If the leukocyte count is increased beyond normal, lymphoblasts are almost invariably present. Anemia, thrombocytopenia, and neutropenia are initially present in most cases.

Bleeding secondary to thrombocytopenia occurs in half of the cases. Less commonly, bacterial infections secondary to neutropenia bring the patient to medical attention. Generalized lymphadenopathy, which is particularly prominent in the cervical lymph nodes, is characteristic. Hepatosplenomegaly is also common. Involvement of the central nervous system, particularly the leptomeninges (leukemic meningitis), is frequent, even early in the course of the disease. Today, this complication is usually prevented by routine, prophylactic radiation therapy for the craniospinal axis following the diagnosis of ALL.

The two most important prognostic features of ALL are the age at onset and the initial blood leukocyte count (Table 20-4). Before the introduction of chemotherapeutic agents for the treatment of malignant diseases, the median survival time for patients after the diagnosis of ALL was only 2 months. The natural history of ALL has been dramatically altered, however, by modern, aggressive chemotherapy. **A complete clinical remission can now be achieved in more than 90% of the children with favorable prognostic features (age, 3–7 years; morphology, L1), and a permanent cure can be anticipated in the majority of such cases.** Although the prognosis in children with L2 and, especially, L3 ALL is less favorable, complete clinical remission can be achieved in most of these cases, and a cure is obtained in a substantial minority. In adults with ALL, complete clinical remission can be achieved in more than half of the patients, but a permanent cure occurs in only a few.

MALIGNANT LYMPHOMAS

■ *Malignant lymphomas are a heterogeneous group of solid tumors that are composed of neoplastic lymphoid cells.*

T A B L E   20-4.   Clinicopathologic Prognostic Features of Acute Lymphoblastic Leukemia

Clinicopathologic Features	Prognosis	
	Favorable	Unfavorable
FAB subtype	L1	L2, L3
Immunologic subtype B precursor ALL	Pre-B	Mature B
	Pre-pre–B	T
White blood cell count	<10,000 cells/μm	>50,000 cells/μm
Age (years)	3–7	<1
		>10
Sex	Female	Male
Race	White	Black
Organ involvement	Minimal or absent	Prominent

Their heterogeneity reflects the potential for malignant transformation at any stage of B- or T-lymphocyte differentiation. Malignant lymphomas constitute 3% of all malignancies in Western countries. These neoplasms have been termed non-Hodgkin's lymphomas to distinguish them from Hodgkin's disease, with which they share some clinicopathologic features. This designation is based on what lymphomas are not rather on what they are, however, and it will not be used in this discussion. Malignant lymphomas are characterized by:

- Homogeneous neoplastic cell population
- Characteristic patterns of tumor cell growth, either as cohesive cell aggregates called follicles or nodules or in a diffuse pattern
- Unpredictable or random spread of the disease
- Frequent presentation as a widespread or systemic disorder
- Pronounced clinicopathologic differences between children and adults

The histopathologic subtypes of the lymphomas can be broadly divided into three major subgroups: (1) low grade or clinically indolent, (2) intermediate grade, and (3) high grade or clinically aggressive.

☐ **Pathogenesis:** The cause of most malignant lymphomas is unknown. However, two uncommon subtypes are etiologically associated with specific viruses. First, there is evidence for infection with EBV in 95% of the cases of endemic Burkitt lymphoma in central equatorial Africa. By contrast, in cases of sporadic Burkitt lymphoma in the United States and other nonendemic areas, evidence for EBV infection is found in only 15%. Second, human T-cell leukemia/lymphoma virus type 1 (HTLV-1) is endemic in the southwestern islands of Japan and occurs sporadically in several other geographically restricted areas. Evidence for HTLV-1 infection is demonstrated in more than 90% of cases of T-cell leukemia/lymphoma in endemic areas of Japan.

Congenital and acquired immunodeficiency disorders are particularly associated with an increased risk for the development of aggressive B-cell immunoblastic lymphomas. This risk is further increased in situations involving both an immunodeficiency state and a long-term antigenic stimulation (Box 20-9).

Malignant lymphomas derive from the malignant transformation of a single lymphocyte that is arrested at a specific stage of B- or T-lymphoid cell differentiation. The neoplastic cells in the intermediate- and high-grade lymphomas have only a limited resemblance to normal lymphocytes, and their migratory and homing characteristics are generally lost.

☐ **Pathology:**

Lymph Nodes. The lymph nodes involved by malignant lymphoma are enlarged and soft. On cut section, they are a glistening gray-white, thereby imparting the so-called "fish-flesh" appearance (Fig. 20-26).

Microscopically, malignant lymphomas feature monotonous neoplastic lymphoid cells that infiltrate and, ultimately, obliterate the normal lymph nodal ar-

B O X *20-9* **Disorders with Increased Risk of Secondary Malignant Lymphoma**

Sjögren syndrome
Renal and cardiac transplant recipients
Acquired immunodeficiency syndrome
Congenital immune deficiency syndromes
    Chédiak-Higashi
    Wiskott-Aldrich
    Ataxia telangiectasia
    Immunoglobulin A deficiency
    Severe combined immune deficiency
α-Heavy-chain disease
Celiac disease
Hodgkin's disease (posttreatment)

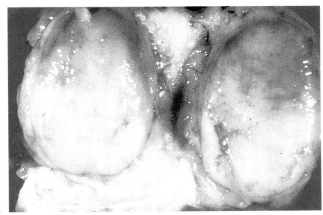
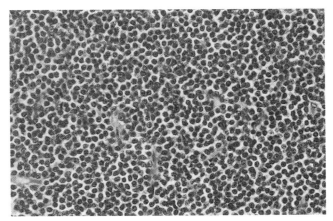

A   B

FIGURE   *20-26*
Small lymphocytic lymphoma. (A) The bisected, enlarged lymph node shows the characteristic uniform, glistening, gray color, which imparts a "fish-flesh" appearance. (B) On microscopic examination, the lymph nodal architecture is replaced by a diffuse infiltration of normal-appearing small lymphocytes.

chitecture and that of other tissues. The lymphoma cells exhibit abnormal cytologic features, except in the case of diffuse, small cell lymphocytic lymphoma, in which the cells resemble normal lymphocytes.

In adults, 40% initially show uniform, cohesive aggregates of neoplastic cells, which is termed the **follicular or nodular pattern** (Fig. 20-27). The neoplastic cells in follicular lymphoma progressively infiltrate the residual normal interfollicular areas, with subsequent progression to a mixed follicular and diffuse pattern and, in many cases, eventually to a uniformly diffuse pattern.

In 60% of adult lymphomas, the initial pattern of tumor cell growth is diffusely infiltrative, without formation of follicles or nodules. These diffuse lymphomas may be of B-cell (70%) or T-cell (30%) lineage. In children, virtually all malignant lymphomas are

high-grade, aggressive neoplasms with a diffuse pattern.

Spleen. The involved spleen is mildly to moderately enlarged, and the cut surface shows a generalized expansion of the white pulp, particularly in low-grade lymphomas. Discrete, variably sized tumors are characteristic of the more aggressive intermediate- and high-grade lymphomas. Microscopically, B-cell lymphomas initially involve the B cell–dependent germinal centers and mantle zones of the spleen. By contrast, T-cell lymphomas first infiltrate the periarteriolar lymphoid sheaths and, less frequently, the marginal zones.

Liver. The liver tends to be enlarged. There may be vague accentuation of the normal lobular pattern owing to widespread involvement of the portal tracts, particularly in patients with low-grade lymphomas. Alternatively, there may be discrete, gray-tan tumors in the liver, especially in patients with intermediate- and high-grade lymphomas. Both B- and T-cell lymphomas typically involve the portal tracts.

Bone Marrow. The pattern of lymphomatous involvement in the bone marrow may be focal, multifocal, or diffuse.

Classification of Lymphomas

The International Working Formulation (established in 1982) is based on correlating the microscopic features of lymphomas with their clinical features. It establishes three major subgroups in relation to overall survival:

- Low grade or clinically indolent
- Intermediate grade
- High grade or clinically aggressive.

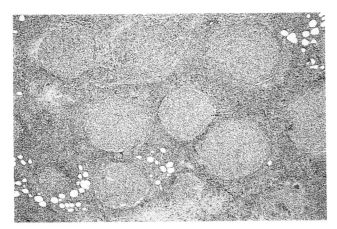

FIGURE   *20-27*
Follicular lymphoma. The lymph nodal architecture is replaced by homogeneous nodular aggregates of neoplastic B lymphocytes.

The International Working Formulation is particularly useful when assessing the clinical behavior of lymphomas, particularly their response to chemotherapy. In general, low-grade lymphomas follow an indolent course, but they are difficult to eradicate owing to a low proliferative index. By contrast, high-grade lymphomas are characterized by an aggressive clinical course but are often cured by appropriate chemotherapy. In this case, a high proliferative rate renders the tumor more susceptible to the effect of cytotoxic agents.

Low-Grade Malignant Lymphoma

Low-grade malignant lymphomas include (1) small lymphocytic, (2) small lymphocytic plasmacytoid, (3) follicular small cleaved, and (4) follicular mixed small cleaved and large cell lymphomas.

Small Lymphocytic Lymphoma

■ *Small lymphocytic lymphoma (SLL) is a diffuse lymphoma in which the neoplastic cells resemble normal small lymphocytes but are immunologically incompetent.* B-lymphocyte lineage is found in 95% of cases, whereas 5% exhibit a T-cell phenotype.

□ **Pathogenesis:** The cells of SLL are closely related to those of CLL, both morphologically and immunophenotypically. The only known difference in antigenic expression is the presence of the adhesion molecule LFA-1 (lymphocyte function-associated antigen) on the cells of SLL. Importantly, as many as one-third of the patients who present with SLL eventually develop peripheral lymphocytosis and a clinical syndrome indistinguishable from CLL.

□ **Pathology:** Microscopically, the normal architecture of the involved lymph nodes and other tissue sites is replaced by a monotonous population of small lymphocytes. Mitotic figures tend to be uncommon in patients with SLL, and more than 30 mitoses per 20 high-power fields predicts a more aggressive clinical course.

The clinical features of SLL resemble those of CLL.

Small Lymphocytic Lymphoma with Plasmacytoid Differentiation (Waldenström Macroglobulinemia)

■ *Waldenström macroglobulinemia is a diffuse lymphoma of small- to medium-size B lymphocytes that exhibit variable plasmacytoid differentiation, eccentric nuclei, and a moderate amount of purple cytoplasm and that secrete a monoclonal IgM.*

Waldenström macroglobulinemia occurs most commonly in middle-aged to elderly adults, and generalized lymphadenopathy and hepatosplenomegaly are common presenting signs. A leukemic distribution of circulating plasmacytoid lymphocytes occurs in 10% to 20% of the cases. Microscopic examination of the lymph nodes and bone marrow reveals diffuse infiltration by normal-appearing small lymphocytes and plasmacytoid lymphocytes.

Hyperviscosity syndrome in macroglobulinemia is secondary to a high-molecular-weight IgM paraprotein in the blood. Circulatory disturbances, principally in the central and peripheral nervous systems, are also observed, including peripheral neuropathy, headache, dizziness, deafness, paresis, and coma. A bleeding tendency, with severe nosebleeds and ecchymoses, is caused by a reduced level of factor VIII owing to the combination of that factor with IgM paraprotein. The clinical course of Waldenström macroglobulinemia is indolent, with a mean survival time of 3 to 4 years. The hyperviscosity syndrome is treated with plasmapheresis, and the lymphoma is treated with chemotherapy.

Heavy-Chain Diseases. These disorders are uncommon B-lymphocyte malignant lymphomas in which tumor cells secrete a portion of an immunoglobulin heavy chain. IgA, IgG, IgM, and IgD heavy-chain diseases have been described.

Low-Grade Follicular Lymphoma

Follicular Small Cleaved Cell Lymphoma. This disease is characterized by cohesive aggregates, or follicles, of neoplastic lymphocytes. It is the most common subtype (60%) of the follicular lymphomas. The tumor cells are atypical, small- to medium-sized (10–15 μm), lymphoid cells, with indented or cleaved nuclei, clumped chromatin, poorly defined nucleoli, and scant cytoplasm.

A translocation involving the long arms of chromosomes 14 and 18, t(14;18)(q32;q21), is identified in virtually every case of follicular lymphoma. This translocation involves the immunoglobulin heavy-chain locus on chromosome 14 and the proto-oncogene *bcl*-2 on chromosome 18. This oncogene seems to act in a unique manner, in that it prevents the programmed cell death (apoptosis) of B lymphocytes.

Follicular small cleaved cell lymphoma is typically an indolent disorder, with a median survival time of 10 years. Middle-aged and elderly adults of either sex are affected.

Intermediate-Grade Malignant Lymphoma

Follicular Large Cell Lymphoma. This is an uncommon disorder (10% of follicular lymphomas) in which the malignant follicles are composed of either large cleaved or noncleaved lymphocytes. As the disease evolves, the follicular pattern becomes progressively obliterated, and the neoplasm becomes a diffuse, large cell lymphoma. Thus, follicular large cell lymphoma is the only subtype of follicular lymphoma that is associated with an aggressive clinical course. The median survival time is 4 years.

Diffuse Small Cleaved Cell Lymphoma. This tumor features diffuse infiltrates of neoplastic cells, with cleaved or notched nuclei and scant cytoplasm (Fig. 20-28). The neoplastic cells are indistinguishable from those of follicular small cleaved cell lymphoma, and most cases, predictably, are of B-lymphocyte lineage.

Diffuse small cleaved cell lymphoma accounts for as much as 4% of malignant lymphomas in the United States and for twice that figure in Europe. The disease is more common in men than in women, and the median age at diagnosis is 60 years. The tumor is moderately aggressive; patients tend to present with advanced disease. The median survival time is 3 to 4 years, and cure is exceptional.

Diffuse, Mixed, Small and Large Cell Lymphoma. Diffuse lymphomas with mixed small and large cells are of B-lymphocyte lineage in two-thirds of the cases and of T-cell lineage in one-third.

B-cell diffuse mixed cell lymphoma is composed of neoplastic cells that are analogous to those of follicular mixed lymphomas. In most cases, the disease probably represents progression of a previously follicular tumor. The cells of diffuse, mixed, small and large cell lymphoma are predominantly small cleaved lymphocytes, with large, noncleaved, lymphoid cells comprising 20% to 50% of the neoplastic population (Fig. 20-29). Diffuse, mixed, small and large cell lymphoma

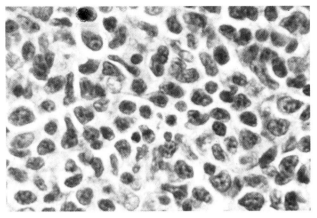

FIGURE   *20-29*
Diffuse mixed small and large cell lymphoma. The lymph nodal architecture is replaced by a diffuse infiltrate of small cleaved and large noncleaved neoplastic B lymphocytes.

is usually widespread at the time of presentation, but the potential for cure is greater in these patients than in those with the lower-grade, mixed follicular counterpart.

T-cell diffuse lymphoma of mixed cell type is composed of mature (peripheral), postthymic T cells. Unlike the B-cell diffuse mixed lymphomas, the neoplastic T cells do not resemble the cells of follicular lymphomas but, instead, are a mixture of atypical small and large lymphocytes. The characteristic features of T-cell diffuse mixed lymphomas include (1) diffuse infiltration by small to large lymphoid cells, with round to cerebriform nuclei and clear cytoplasm that produces a mosaic-like pattern owing to interlocking cytoplasmic margins; and (2) admixed inflammatory cells, including eosinophils and plasma cells. In general, the clinical course of T-cell diffuse mixed lymphoma is comparable to that of its B-cell counterpart, and the tumor is treated as an aggressive diffuse lymphoma.

Diffuse Large Cleaved and Noncleaved Cell Lymphoma. These tumors are composed of large, transformed lymphoid cells of either B-lymphocyte (70%) or T-lymphocyte (30%) lineage. The nuclear contours are either irregular or indented (cleaved) or round to oval (noncleaved). The nuclei show vesicular to coarsely reticulated chromatin and one to several nucleoli apposed to the nuclear membrane. Scant to moderate pink cytoplasm is also present, and numerous mitoses are typical.

Clinically, diffuse large cleaved and noncleaved cell lymphomas of both B- and T-cell types tend to behave aggressively. However, the large cleaved cell types often follow a more indolent course than the noncleaved variant. The disorder may occur at any age.

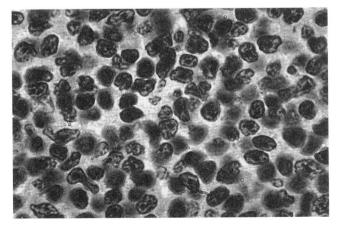

FIGURE   *20-28*
Diffuse small cleaved cell lymphoma. The lymph node demonstrates a diffuse infiltrate of neoplastic B lymphocytes with cleaved or notched nuclei and scant cytoplasm.

Lymph nodes and other lymphopoietic sites are most commonly first involved. However, extranodal sites of origin, such as the stomach, terminal ileum, thyroid gland, bone marrow, and skin, are the primary sites of involvement in as many as 30% of the cases of diffuse large cleaved and noncleaved cell lymphomas.

High-Grade Malignant Lymphoma

Large Cell Immunoblastic Lymphoma. Immunoblast is a morphologic term that refers to a transformed extrafollicular lymphoid cell that is three- to fourfold the size of a small lymphocyte and that displays a characteristically prominent nucleolus or nucleoli and abundant cytoplasm (Fig. 20-30). Immunoblastic lymphomas are high-grade tumors whose cells resemble normal immunoblasts, although there is no conclusive evidence that they arise from the latter.

Immunoblastic tumors are clinically aggressive, diffuse large cell lymphomas that arise in middle-aged or elderly persons of both sexes. They frequently occur in the setting of an immunodeficiency or disordered immune state, such as occurs in allograft recipients and patients with AIDS, chronic thyroiditis, and Sjögren syndrome. Most immunoblastic lymphomas are of B-cell lineage, and only a small minority derive from T cells. The International Working Formulation recognizes four morphologic variants of immunoblastic lymphomas: (1) plasmacytoid, (2) clear cell, (3) polymorphous (tumor giant cells), and (4) epithelioid cell.

Lymphoblastic Lymphoma. This variety of lymphoma is a clinically aggressive, diffuse, and high-grade neoplasm of primitive lymphoblasts. The neoplastic cells are morphologically indistinguishable from those of ALL and are medium in size, measuring from 10 to 15 μm in diameter. They have round or convoluted and cerebriform nuclei, with delicate chromatin, indistinct nucleoli, and scant cytoplasm. The mitotic rate is extremely high. The large majority ($\leq$90%) of cases are of T-lymphocyte lineage; the remaining 10% are derived from B cells. Tdt is demonstrated in almost all cases.

Lymphoblastic lymphomas initially present as soft-tissue masses and, subsequently, may progress to a leukemic distribution indistinguishable from ALL. T-lymphoblastic lymphomas occur most commonly in adolescent and young adult males, although the disease also occurs in young children and older adults. An anterior mediastinal mass occurs in at least half of the cases, apparently reflecting a thymic origin of the tumor. The clinical course is marked by rapid spread to the bone marrow, with secondary leukemic distribution and involvement of the central nervous system, particularly the leptomeninges. The prognosis is generally dismal.

Diffuse Small Noncleaved Cell Lymphoma (Burkitt Lymphoma). The diffuse small noncleaved cell lymphomas include Burkitt lymphoma and Burkitt-like lymphoma. Both of these tumors are high-grade, clinically aggressive neoplasms of B lymphocytes. They display extremely high mitotic rates and, in fact, are the most rapidly proliferative of all human tumors.

Diffuse small noncleaved cell lymphoma is composed of uniform, medium-size lymphoid cells from 10 to 25 μm in diameter and with round nuclei, coarsely reticulated chromatin, two to five small nucleoli, and a rim of dense, blue-purple cytoplasm. Scattered benign macrophages containing cellular debris impart a "starry sky" pattern (Fig. 20-31).

Morphologically, Burkitt lymphoma cells are indistinguishable from those of high-grade (L3) ALL (Burkitt leukemia). A characteristic chromosomal abnormality is translocation of the proto-oncogene c-*myc* on chromosome 8 to chromosome 14, which is noted in 80% of the tumors (see Chapter 5). In the remainder, the translocation involves chromosomes 8 and 2 or chromosomes 8 and 22. Whatever the translocation, the c-*myc* proto-oncogene is deregulated by its proximity to an immunoglobulin promoter sequence and by loss of its own regulatory elements. Such an event seems to be necessary, but not sufficient, for development of the malignant phenotype, and other genetic alterations are also probably involved.

Endemic Burkitt Lymphoma. This lymphoma is endemic in tropical equatorial Africa and in parts of New Guinea and occurs sporadically in other areas of the world as well. The EBV genome is identified in the neo-

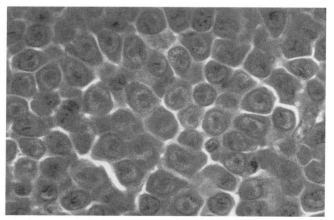

F I G U R E   *20-30*
Large cell immunoblastic lymphoma, plasmacytoid type. A lymph node displays uniform, large, and transformed lymphocytes with vesicular nuclei, prominent nucleoli, and abundant basophilic cytoplasm.

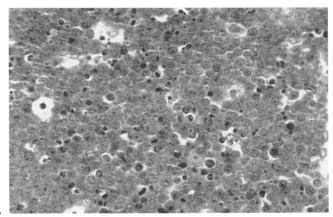
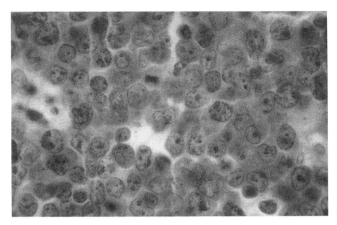

A   B

FIGURE *20-31*
Burkitt lymphoma. (A) A low-power view of a lymph node shows a uniform infiltrate of medium-size lymphoid cells, with scattered, benign macrophages that impart a "starry-sky" pattern. (B) A high-power view illustrates the neoplastic lymphocytes, which contain round nuclei with coarsely reticulated chromatin, small nucleoli, and abundant basophilic cytoplasm. Numerous mitoses are also evident, and large macrophages with abundant clear cytoplasm containing cell debris are prominent.

plastic cells in 95% of the cases. The median age at onset in endemic areas is 7 years, and the common sites of involvement include the jawbones (maxilla and mandible) and abdominal sites (e.g., ileocecal region of the small bowel, kidneys, and ovaries).

Sporadic Burkitt Lymphoma. In nonendemic areas, only 15% of the cases of Burkitt lymphoma harbor the EBV genome. The median age at onset is 11 years, and abdominal sites are commonly the first to be involved. Tumors of the jaw are rare.

Burkitt lymphoma (endemic or sporadic) is a highly curable cancer. Even in the case of advanced disease, 75% of the patients can be cured by chemotherapy, and the prognosis for those with involvement of the bone marrow or the central nervous system is not much worse.

Burkitt and Burkitt-like lymphomas are the most common (40%) lymphomas that occur in patients with AIDS. The remaining cases are divided equally between immunoblastic lymphoma and Hodgkin's disease.

Miscellaneous Lymphomas

Several distinctive subtypes of malignant lymphoma are included in a miscellaneous category by the International Working Formulation.

Cutaneous T-Cell Lymphoma (Mycosis Fungoides)

Cutaneous T-cell lymphoma (CTCL) is a primary lymphoma of the skin that is composed of mature, postthymic T-helper (CD4+) lymphocytes. CTCL is a chronic disorder, with a survival time of years to decades. It is characterized by three well-defined clinicopathologic stages:

- **The premycotic or eczematous stage** has a duration of several years and is not distinguishable from a variety of benign chronic dermatoses.
- **The plaque stage,** which follows the premycotic stage, is characterized by well-demarcated, raised cutaneous plaques. There is a dense, subepidermal, band-like infiltrate of lymphoid cells, with irregular nuclear contours and a spectrum of cell sizes. Distinctive, medium to large lymphoid cells with hyperchromatic nuclei and cerebriform nuclear contours, called **mycosis cells,** are typical.
- **The tumor stage** features raised cutaneous tumors, most commonly on the face and in the body folds, that frequently ulcerate and become secondarily infected. The name **mycosis fungoides** was initially derived from the raised, fungating, and mushroom-like appearance of these cutaneous tumors. Extracutaneous involvement, particularly of the lymph nodes, spleen, liver, bone marrow, and lungs, commonly occurs.
- **Sézary syndrome** is the leukemic variant of mycosis fungoides.

The predominant clinical manifestations in CTCL are extreme pruritus and recurrent cutaneous infections. Patients with early disease exhibit a 5-year survival rate of 90%, whereas those with advanced CTCL (visceral and lymph node involvement) have a median survival time of only 2 years. Infection and progressive lymphoma are the common causes of death. CTCL is treated with topical and systemic chemotherapy, photochemotherapy, and radiation therapy.

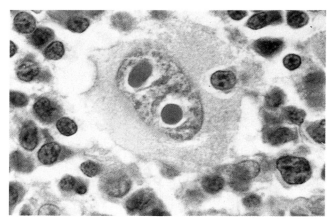

FIGURE *20-32*
Classic Reed-Sternberg cell. Mirror-image nuclei contain large eosinophilic nucleoli.

Adult T-Cell Leukemia/Lymphoma

Adult T-cell leukemia/lymphoma (ATL) is an aggressive malignancy that is endemic in the southwestern islands of Japan and that occurs with increased frequency in the Caribbean basin (including Florida) and West Africa. **ATL is the only human cancer thought to result from a retrovirus, namely HTLV-1** (see Chapter 5).

Cases of ATL are characterized by diffuse infiltration of many organs by (1) small lymphoid cells, (2) mixed small and large lymphoid cells, or (3) large lymphoid cells with irregular nuclear contours. The disease features involvement of the skin, lymph nodes, lungs, pleura, central nervous system, bone marrow, and blood. ATL carries a poor prognosis, although indolent variants have been described.

HODGKIN'S DISEASE

■ *Hodgkin's disease (HD) is a unique, malignant neoplasm originating in the lymphoid tissue that features characteristic Reed-Sternberg cells in association with an appropriate cellular background* (Fig. 20-32). Evidence is now accumulating that most cases of HD are neoplasms of B lymphocytes.

□ **Epidemiology and Pathogenesis:** HD is uncommon, with an annual incidence of only 3 per 100,000 persons in the United States. The disorder is somewhat more common in men than in women (4.0 : 2.5) and in whites than in blacks (3.5:2.0). There is a distinctive, bimodal age distribution, with a peak during the late twenties, a decrease during the fourth and fifth decades, and a gradually increasing incidence after the age of 50 years.

The cause of HD remains unknown. Although exposure to carcinogens or viruses has been proposed by

some and genetic or immune factors by others, none has been proved to be involved in the pathogenesis of HD. One subtype, namely nodular lymphocyte-predominant HD, appears to be a neoplasm of B-lymphoid origin, and the Reed-Sternberg cells of this variant express specific B-lymphocyte lineage markers. However, they lack the immunologic cell markers CD15 (Leu-M1) and CD30 (Ki-1), which are usually identified on the Reed-Sternberg cells in all other subtypes of HD.

□ **Pathology:**

Lymph Nodes. On gross examination, the consistency of lymph nodes involved by HD is variable. The cut surface is homogeneously gray-white, thereby producing a fish-flesh appearance. If tumor tissue extends beyond the confines of individual lymph nodes, groups of nodes may be matted together.

Spleen. The spleen is involved in one-third of the cases of HD at the time of diagnosis, although in most patients, the spleen is affected at autopsy. On cut section, the splenic white pulp is enlarged by HD, and the red pulp is affected only secondarily by direct extension from the white pulp. In the spleen, HD occurs first in the T cell–dependent, periarteriolar, lymphoid sheath of the white pulp or in the marginal zone between the white and the red pulp. As the disease progresses, single or multiple discrete tumor nodules or confluent multinodular tumor masses in the spleen are common (Fig. 20-33).

Liver. At autopsy, the liver is involved with HD in two-thirds of the patients, although such involvement is unusual at the time of presentation. The portal areas are first involved, but without significant macroscopic findings. With time, however, multiple gray-white tumor nodules, often resembling metastatic carcinoma, may appear in the liver.

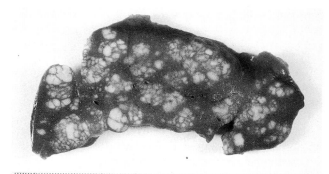

FIGURE *20-33*
Hodgkin's disease involving the spleen. Multinodular tumor masses replace the normal splenic parenchyma.

Bone Marrow. The initial changes in the bone marrow are characterized macroscopically by discrete foci of fibrotic tumor, without destruction of bony trabeculae. As the disease progresses, destruction of bone may produce an osteolytic appearance on radiologic examination.

Classification of Hodgkin's Disease

Four histopathologic subtypes of HD are recognized:

* **Lymphocyte-predominant HD**
* **Mixed cellularity HD**
* **Lymphocyte-depletion HD**
* **Nodular sclerosis HD**

In Western countries, nodular sclerosis HD accounts for 50% to 60% of the cases of HD, mixed cellularity HD for 30% to 40%, and lymphocyte-predominant and lymphocyte-depletion HD for 5% to 10% each. The ratio of normal small lymphocytes to neoplastic cells determines the sequence of HD, namely lymphocyte-predominant HD to mixed cellularity HD to lymphocyte-depletion HD. A decreasing number of normal lymphocytes is thought to correlate with a diminished host immune response to Reed-Sternberg cells and constitutes an adverse prognostic sign.

Lymphocyte-Predominant HD. Small lymphocytes are the predominant cell type in lymphocyte-predominant HD. Benign macrophages, either singly or in small clusters, may also be conspicuous. Reed-Sternberg cells have a single to multilobed nucleus. Reactive inflammatory cells, fibrosis, and necrosis are lacking or inconspicuous.

Mixed-Cellularity HD. This is the historic form of HD and exhibits (1) numerous, classic, binucleated

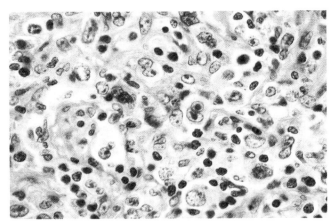

FIGURE   *20-34*
Hodgkin's disease, mixed cellularity. A photomicrograph of a lymph node shows classic and mononuclear Reed-Sternberg cells, lymphocytes, and mild diffuse fibrosis.

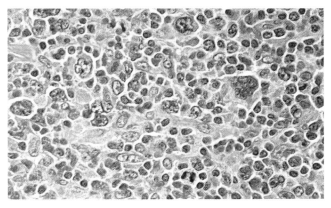

FIGURE   *20-35*
Hodgkin's disease, lymphocyte depletion. A photomicrograph of a lymph node shows numerous variants of Reed-Sternberg cells, whereas lymphocytes are sparse.

Reed-Sternberg cells and mononuclear variants; (2) an intermediate number of lymphocytes; and (3) a prominent component of inflammatory cells, particularly eosinophils and neutrophils (Fig. 20-34).

Lymphocyte-Depletion HD. This category features marked depletion of lymphocytes and inflammatory cells (Fig. 20-35). Advanced immunologic failure is common.

Nodular Sclerosis HD. This form of HD is a distinctive subtype that may be unrelated to the other varieties. It is characterized by (1) broad bands of dense collagen, which extend from a thickened capsule into the substance of the lymph node and circumscribe residual nodules of lymphoid tissue; and (2) a predominance of multinucleated Reed-Sternberg cells. Focal necrosis is a characteristic feature, typically with lacunar cell variants of Reed-Sternberg cells palisaded around the foci of necrosis.

☐ **Clinical Features:** HD usually presents as nontender, peripheral adenopathy involving either a single lymph node or groups of lymph nodes. The cervical and mediastinal nodes are involved in more than half of the cases. Less commonly, the axillary, inguinal, and retroperitoneal lymph nodes are initially enlarged.

So-called B signs and symptoms are found in 40% of the patients with HD. These include low-grade fever, which is occasionally cyclical (Pel-Ebstein fever), night sweats, and weight loss exceeding 10% of body weight in the 6 months before diagnosis. Pruritus (commonly generalized) occurs in 15% of the cases initially and in the large majority (85%) of the cases with disease progression. A deficiency of T-lymphocyte function is characteristic of HD. Anergy to skin test antigens is often noted early in the course of HD.

Lymphocyte-predominant HD is the most indolent type. Adult men younger than 35 years of age are most commonly affected (male:female ratio, 4 : 1). At the time of initial diagnosis, the disease is usually localized (stage I), with the high cervical or inguinal lymph nodes being most commonly involved. B signs and symptoms are typically lacking, presenting in only 20% of the cases. Visceral involvement is uncommon. **The prognosis of lymphocyte-predominant HD is excellent, with a cure rate exceeding 90%.**

Mixed-cellularity HD is most common during the fourth and fifth decades of life, although any age group may be affected. The majority of the patients are found to have stage II or III disease, and a minority have visceral involvement (stage IV). B signs and symptoms are present in half of the cases. **The prognosis is intermediate, with a cure rate of 75%.**

Lymphocyte-depleted HD is the most clinically aggressive type, and middle-aged to elderly men are most commonly affected. Advanced clinical stage (III/IV) and B signs and symptoms are characteristic, presenting in two-thirds of the cases. Patients commonly present with fever of undetermined origin, pancytopenia, and wasting. There is variable peripheral or mediastinal adenopathy. However, retroperitoneal adenopathy is frequently prominent, and involvement of the spleen, liver, and bone marrow is common. Profound immunodeficiency develops, and death commonly results from inanition or secondary infections. **The overall cure rate of lymphocyte-depleted HD is 40% to 50%.**

Nodular sclerosis HD is most common in young adult women from 15 to 34 years of age and usually presents as lower cervical, supraclavicular, and mediastinal adenopathy (stage II). B signs and symptoms occur in as many as 40% of cases. **The prognosis is good, with a cure rate of from 80% to 85%.**

If untreated, HD is a lethal disorder, with a 10-year survival rate of only 1%. With modern radiation therapy and chemotherapy, however, an overall cure rate of 70% can be achieved. Complications of HD include compromise of vital organs by progressive tumor growth and secondary infections owing to the primary defect in delayed-type hypersensitivity and to the immunosuppressive effects of therapy. Development of second malignancies as a consequence of therapy is of special concern, because more than 15% of the treated patients suffer this complication. AML develops in 5% to 10% of the cases, and aggressive malignant lymphomas occur in 1%.

PLASMA CELL NEOPLASIA

■ *Plasma cell neoplasia comprises a group of related, malignant disorders of terminally differentiated B lymphocytes (plasma cells).*

Multiple myeloma (90% of cases) is characterized by a multifocal infiltration of malignant plasma cells in the bone marrow. In patients with this condition, there are typically multiple destructive (lytic) lesions or diffuse demineralization of bone.

Solitary osseous myeloma (5% of cases) is a single destructive lesion of bone.

Extramedullary plasmacytoma (5% of cases) presents as an extramedullary, soft-tissue mass, most frequently in the upper respiratory tract.

In the large majority of cases, the neoplastic cells secrete a homogeneous, complete or partial immunoglobulin molecule termed an **M-component or paraprotein.** The most common M-component is IgG, followed by IgA. Other immunoglobulins are only rarely secreted by the tumor cells.

☐ **Epidemiology:** Plasma cell neoplasia constitutes 10% of all hematologic malignancies. The disorder is more than twice as common in blacks than in whites. The frequency increases with age, with the mean age at diagnosis of multiple myeloma being 65 years and that of solitary osseous myeloma and extramedullary plasmacytoma being a decade earlier. Male predominance is pronounced for solitary osseous myeloma and extramedullary plasmacytoma, with each having a male:female ratio of 3:1.

☐ **Pathogenesis:** A number of risk factors for plasma cell neoplasia have been identified:

- **Genetic predisposition** is suggested by the increased incidence of multiple myeloma in first-degree relatives of patients with plasma cell neoplasia and the higher frequency of multiple myeloma in blacks.
- **Ionizing radiation** has been incriminated as a cause of plasma cell neoplasia. Long-term survivors of the bombings of Hiroshima and Nagasaki suffered a fivefold increased incidence of multiple myeloma.
- **Chronic antigenic stimulation** may constitute a risk factor. For example, some cases of multiple myeloma have been associated with chronic infections (e.g., chronic osteomyelitis) and with chronic inflammatory disorders (e.g., rheumatoid arthritis).
- **Chromosomal abnormalities** have been reported in some cases of multiple myeloma, including translocations, trisomy, and monosomy.

☐ **Pathology:** On gross examination, the osseous and extraosseous tumors of plasma cell neoplasia are variably red, tan, or gray and have a consistency that ranges from fleshy to gelatinous. The bony lesions are well demarcated from the surrounding normal tissue (Fig. 20-36). The cortical bone may be destroyed, with direct tumor extension into the surrounding soft tissues.

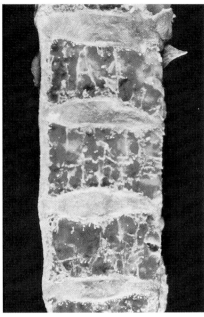

FIGURE   *20-36*
Multiple myeloma. Multiple lytic lesions of the vertebrae are present.

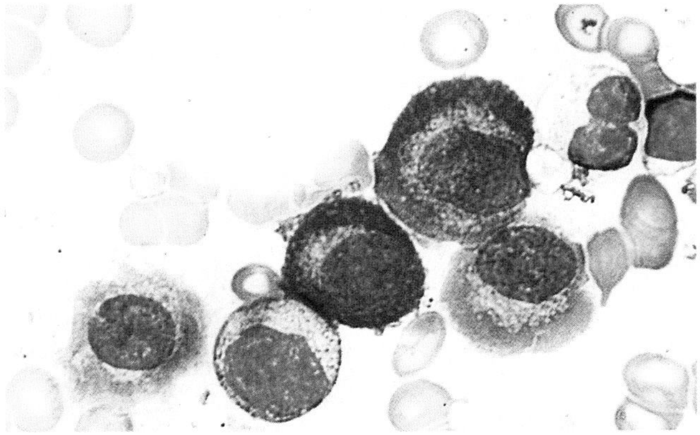

Microscopically, the morphologic hallmark of multiple myeloma in the bone marrow is the presence of diffuse sheets or nodular aggregates of plasma cells (Fig. 20-37). Ultimately, both normal hemopoietic tissues and fat cells are replaced by neoplastic plasma cells. In smears of marrow aspirates, neoplastic plasma cells usually exceed 25% of the nucleated cell elements.

FIGURE   *20-37*
Multiple myeloma. A smear of a bone marrow aspirate illustrates a cluster of three neoplastic plasma cells.

The malignant cells may be morphologically normal, but more commonly, they demonstrate cytologic atypia.

☐ **Clinical Features:** The diagnosis of multiple myeloma requires (1) the finding of uniform, diffuse sheets or nodular aggregates of plasma cells in the bone marrow; (2) in the large majority of cases, a significant monoclonal serum M-component (>3 g/dL) or a urine M-component (>150 mg/dL); and (3) radiologic demonstration of bone lesions. Lytic bone lesions of the skull and other flat bones, including the spine and ribs, are a characteristic (but not diagnostic) radiologic finding in patients with multiple myeloma (Fig. 20-38).

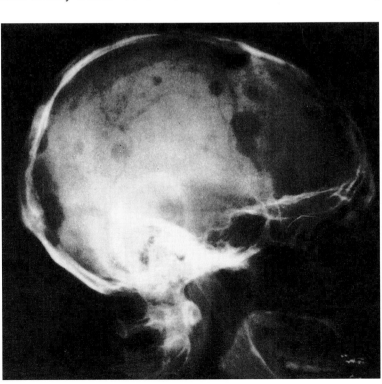

FIGURE   *20-38*
Multiple myeloma. A radiograph of the skull shows numerous "punched-out," radiolucent areas.

Multiple myeloma typically presents as bone pain, most commonly involving the vertebrae and ribs. Symptoms resulting from anemia, hypercalcemia, and renal insufficiency are frequent. Amyloidosis of light-chain origin (principally λ) occurs in 15% of cases and hyperviscosity syndrome in less than 5%. There is a "primary" distribution of amyloid, with deposition in such sites as the tongue, gastrointestinal tract, and heart.

Bence-Jones protein is present in the urine in as many as 75% of the cases of multiple myeloma and in a minority of the cases of solitary osseous myelomas and extramedullary plasmacytomas. The neoplastic clone of plasma cells may secrete excess light chains owing to an unbalanced synthesis of heavy and light chains. The light chains are rapidly filtered through the glomeruli and appear in the urine as Bence-Jones protein. A constellation of renal abnormalities is seen in many cases of multiple myeloma (see Chapter 16).

Humoral immune deficiency, with decreased levels of normal serum immunoglobulins, is characteristic of multiple myeloma. This defect results from the suppression of normal B lymphocytes by the neoplastic clone and from an increased catabolic rate of normal IgG. Because of the low levels of normal antibodies, patients with multiple myeloma are susceptible to a variety of infectious complications, particularly pneumonia and pyelonephritis.

Multiple myeloma is an incurable disease, with a mean survival time of 6 months in untreated patients and of 3 years in patients treated with chemotherapy. Death usually results from either infection or renal failure.

Solitary osseous myeloma presents as a single lytic skeletal lesion that most commonly involves the ribs, vertebrae, or pelvic bones. The natural history of solitary osseous myeloma is progression to multiple myeloma (70%), local extension or recurrence (15%), or extension to a distant skeletal site (15%). The overall 10-year survival rate ranges from 15% to 25%. Solitary osseous myeloma is treated with radiation therapy.

Extramedullary plasmacytomas occur in the upper respiratory tract, including the nasal sinuses, nasopharynx, and tonsils, in 80% of the cases. The remaining 20% occur in other soft-tissue sites, such as the lungs, breast, and lymph nodes. Extramedullary plasmacytoma is eradicated by surgery or local radiation therapy. In 20% of the cases, the condition progresses to multiple myeloma.

CHAPTER 21

The Endocrine System

Ernest A. Lack
John L. Farber
Emanuel Rubin

(continued)

Corticotropin-Independent Adrenal Hyperfunction	**Neuroblastoma**
Primary Aldosteronism (Conn Syndrome)	Ganglioneuroma
Metastatic Carcinoma	**THYMUS**
ADRENAL MEDULLA AND PARAGANGLIA	**Thymic Hyperplasia**
	Thymoma
Pheochromocytoma	Malignant Thymoma
Paraganglioma	Germ Cell Tumors

Pituitary Gland

The pituitary gland, also termed the **hypophysis,** resides within the sella turcica, which is located at the base of the skull within the sphenoid bone. The anterior lobe comprises 80% of the gland and is known as the **adenohypophysis.** The posterior lobe is termed the **neurohypophysis.**

Adenohypophysis. The glandular cells of the adenohypophysis are arranged in cords or nests within a highly vascular stroma. On the basis of staining with hematoxylin-and-eosin, these cells were classically divided into two groups of equal number, namely stainable cells and unstainable cells, with the latter being referred to as **chromophobe cells.** The cytoplasmic granules of the stainable cells were termed **acidophilic** (eosinophilic; 40%) or **basophilic** (10%). **However, the tinctorial properties of the granules have no relevance to their function, and the histologic classification has been replaced by one that defines these cells according to the hormone secreted.** The hormone-producing cells in the anterior pituitary are:

- **Corticotropes.** These basophilic cells secrete corticotropin (formerly termed adrenocorticotropic hormone or ACTH), which controls the adrenal secretion of corticosteroids.
- **Lactotropes.** Certain acidophilic cells secrete prolactin, which is essential for lactation and which has numerous other metabolic activities.
- **Somatotropes.** These acidophilic cells elaborate growth hormone and constitute half of all hormone-producing cells of the adenohypophysis.
- **Thyrotropes.** Thyroid-stimulating hormone (TSH) is produced by pale basophilic or amphophilic cells, which constitute only 5% of the cells of the anterior lobe.
- **Gonadotropes.** Follicle-stimulating hormone (FSH) and luteinizing hormone (LH) are secreted

by the same basophilic cell. FSH stimulates the formation of graafian follicles in the ovary, and LH induces ovulation and formation of corpora lutea in the ovary. LH also stimulates testosterone production in the testis.

Neurohypophysis. The posterior lobe of the pituitary gland is composed of pituicytes, a type of glial cell without secretory function, and unmyelinated nerve fibers containing antidiuretic hormone (ADH) and oxytocin. Both of these hormones are formed in the bodies of the nerve cells in the hypothalamus and are transported axonally to the neurohypophysis. ADH promotes water resorption from the distal renal tubules, whereas oxytocin stimulates the pregnant uterus to contract at term.

HYPOPITUITARISM

- *Hypopituitarism is the deficient secretion of one or more of the hormones produced by the pituitary.* In the most common situation, only one or a few of the pituitary hormones are deficient. Occasionally, however, a total failure of pituitary function occurs, in which case the term **panhypopituitarism** is applied. Symptoms of hypopituitarism relate to deficient function of the thyroid and adrenal glands and of the reproductive system. In children, growth retardation and delayed puberty are additional problems.

Pituitary Tumors. More than half of all the cases of hypopituitarism in adults are caused by pituitary tumors, usually adenomas. Even though the tumor itself may be functional, symptoms of hypopituitarism often result from the compression of adjacent tissue by the mass.

Sheehan Syndrome. Panhypopituitarism may be caused by ischemic necrosis of the gland. Commonly, but not exclusively, the condition follows hypotension induced by postpartum hemorrhage. Amenorrhea, hypothyroidism, and inadequate adrenal function are frequent consequences (Fig. 21-1). With modern obstetric care, however, Sheehan syndrome has become rare.

Pituitary Apoplexy. This term refers to hemorrhagic infarction of a pituitary adenoma. The condition usually has no endocrine effects, because sufficient functioning pituitary tissue remains. However, on occasion, pituitary apoplexy leads to hypopituitarism.

Iatrogenic Hypopituitarism. Radiation therapy administered to the pituitary itself or to lesions of the adjacent head and neck regions can result in hypopituitarism. Similarly, neurosurgical procedures may involve the pituitary.

Trauma. Basal skull fractures and other trauma to the sella turcica may injure the pituitary.

Isolated Growth Hormone Deficiency. Most dwarfs and midgets suffer from defects of nonpituitary origin, but a few are true pituitary dwarfs. Isolated growth hormone deficiency may be associated with a number of familial disorders that result from defective growth hormone genes. It may also occur secondary to hypothalamic dysfunction, either of unknown cause or caused by a variety of lesions. The availability of recombinant human growth hormone has permitted the safe and effective treatment of these children. African pygmies and, occasionally, other dwarfs (**Laron-type dwarfism**) have normal growth hormone secretion, but their target tissues are relatively unresponsive because of mutations in the growth hormone receptor. Because growth hormone acts by stimulating the production of insulin-like growth factor 1, administration of this hormone provides effective therapy for patients with Laron-type dwarfism.

Empty Sella Syndrome. This radiologic term describes an enlarged sella containing a thin, flattened pituitary at the base. Empty sella syndrome is secondary to a congenitally defective or absent diaphragma sellae, which allows transmission of cerebrospinal fluid pressure into the sella. Hormonal abnormalities are usually minor, although some women develop mild hypopituitarism.

PITUITARY ADENOMAS

■ *Pituitary adenomas* are benign neoplasms of the anterior lobe of the pituitary. They are often associated with excess secretion of pituitary hormones and evidence of corresponding endocrine hyperfunction. They occur in both sexes and at almost any age, but they are more common in men between the ages of 20 and 50 years. Small, apparently nonfunctioning pituitary adenomas are found incidentally in as many as 25% of adult autopsies. Pituitary adenomas range from small lesions that do not enlarge the gland to expansive tumors that erode the sella turcica and impinge on the adjacent cranial structure (Fig. 21-2). In general, adenomas smaller than 10 mm in diameter are referred to as **microadenomas,** whereas larger ones are termed **macroadenomas.** Microadenomas do not produce symptoms unless they secrete hormones; macroadenomas tend to cause both local symptoms, as a result of their size, and systemic manifestations, as a result of the overproduction of hormones. The mass effects of pituitary macroadenomas include (1) impingement on the optic chiasm, often with bitemporal hemianopsia and loss of central vision; (2) oculomotor palsies when the tumor invades the cavernous sinuses; and (3) severe headaches.

Lactotrope Adenomas (Prolactinomas)

■ *Lactotrope adenomas* are composed of cells that secrete prolactin. **Hyperprolactinemia is the most common endocrinopathy that is associated with pituitary adenomas.** Almost half of all pituitary microadenomas contain prolactin, but the number that secrete this hormone appears to be far lower. Symptomatic prolactin-

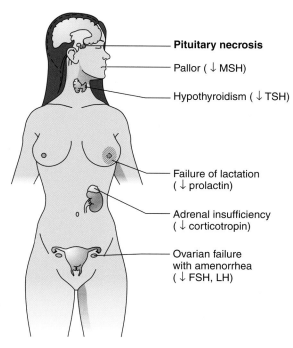

FIGURE **21-1**
Major clinical manifestations of Sheehan syndrome.

Pituitary necrosis

Pallor (↓ MSH)

Hypothyroidism (↓ TSH)

Failure of lactation
(↓ prolactin)

Adrenal insufficiency
(↓ corticotropin)

Ovarian failure
with amenorrhea
(↓ FSH, LH)

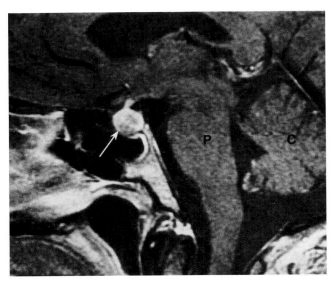

FIGURE   *21-2*
Pituitary adenoma. This magnetic resonance image, sagittal view, of the brain shows a distinct pituitary tumor (*arrow*). C, cerebellum; P, pons; V, lateral vetricle.

producing microadenomas are most often found in young women, whereas more than half of all macroadenomas elaborating prolactin occur in men.

☐ **Pathology:** Lactotrope adenomas tend to be chromophobic or slightly acidophilic. By immunohistochemistry, the Golgi region stains strongly for prolactin. Deposition of endocrine amyloid and the presence of psammoma bodies (calcospherites) are characteristic of lactotrope adenoma, but they are not pathognomonic.

☐ **Clinical Features:** In women, functional lactotrope adenomas lead to amenorrhea, galactorrhea, and infertility. The consistently elevated blood prolactin levels in these women inhibit the surge in the secretion of pituitary LH necessary for ovulation. Men tend to suffer from decreased libido and erectile dysfunction. Functional lactotrope microadenomas are successfully treated with dopamine agonists (bromocriptine) to inhibit prolactin secretion, whereas macroadenomas may require surgery or radiation therapy.

Somatotrope Adenomas

■ *Somatotrope adenomas secrete growth hormone and produce striking bodily changes.* **Gigantism** results when a somatotrope adenoma arises in a child or adolescent before the epiphyses close. **Acromegaly** results when a somatotrope adenoma becomes functional after the epiphyses of the long bones have fused and adult height has been achieved.

☐ **Pathology:** In patients with acromegaly, 75% have a somatotrope macroadenoma at the time of diagnosis, and most of the remaining patients have microadenomas. By light microscopy, somatotrope adenomas are either acidophilic or chromophobic. By electron microscopy, acidophilic tumors tend to contain abundant secretory granules, whereas chromophobic ones are sparsely granular. Acidophilic somatotrope adenomas usually grow slowly and remain within the sella.

Microscopically, sheets or trabeculae of regular eosinophilic cells are noted (Fig. 21-3). The chromophobic variant is typically faster-growing and invasive, and microscopically manifests both cellular and nuclear pleomorphism.

☐ **Clinical Features:** Acromegaly is distinctly uncommon. During the course of many years, patients with acromegaly gradually develop coarse facial features (Fig. 21-4). They exhibit overgrowth of the mandible (prognathism) and maxilla, with spaces between the upper incisor teeth, and a thickened nose. The hands and feet become enlarged, and the hat size becomes increased.

The incidence of cardiovascular, cerebrovascular, and respiratory deaths is increased among these patients. Most persons with acromegaly suffer from neurologic and musculoskeletal symptoms, including headaches, paresthesias, arthralgias, and muscle weakness. One-third have hypertension, and even half of nonhypertensive patients with acromegaly have increased left ventricular mass and may develop congestive heart failure in the absence of a defined cardiac condition. The viscera are also hypertrophied. Diabetes occurs in as many as 20%, and hypercalciuria and renal stones are present in another one-fifth of the patients. In half of the patients with acromegaly, hyper-

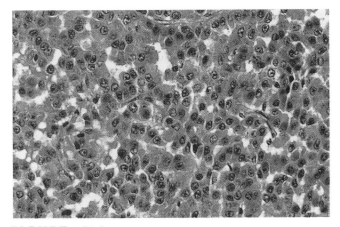

FIGURE   *21-3*
Pituitary somatotropic adenoma from a man with acromegaly. The tumor cells are arranged in thin cords and ribbons.

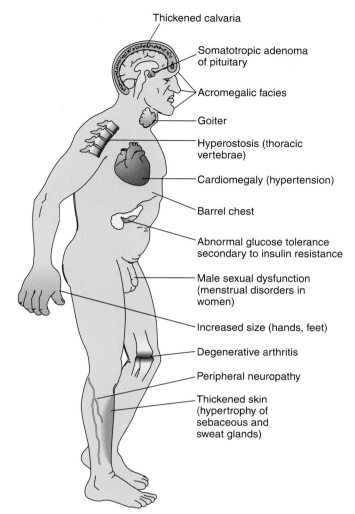

FIGURE **21-4**
Clinical manifestations of acromegaly.

Labels:
- Thickened calvaria
- Somatotropic adenoma of pituitary
- Acromegalic facies
- Goiter
- Hyperostosis (thoracic vertebrae)
- Cardiomegaly (hypertension)
- Barrel chest
- Abnormal glucose tolerance secondary to insulin resistance
- Male sexual dysfunction (menstrual disorders in women)
- Increased size (hands, feet)
- Degenerative arthritis
- Peripheral neuropathy
- Thickened skin (hypertrophy of sebaceous and sweat glands)

prolactinemia is severe enough to be symptomatic (discussed earlier).

The treatment of choice for somatotrope adenomas is transsphenoidal removal of the pituitary. Radiation therapy is an alternative when surgery is contraindicated. A long-acting antagonist of growth hormone is a useful adjunct to treatment.

Corticotrope Adenomas

■ *Corticotrope adenomas secrete corticotropin, which, in turn, induces adrenocortical hypersecretion to produce Cushing disease.*

☐ **Pathology:** In most cases, the tumor is a microadenoma that is intensely basophilic and stains positive with periodic acid-Schiff. Immunohistochemical analysis reveals not only the presence of corticotropin

but also that of related peptides (e.g., endorphins and lipotropin) in the cytoplasm. A few functional corticotrope adenomas are chromophobic and tend to be more aggressive than their basophilic counterparts.

Gonadotrope Adenomas

■ *Gonadotrope adenomas secrete LH and FSH.* Most of these tumors are macroadenomas and present in middle-aged men as (1) headache, (2) visual disturbance, and (3) acquired hypogonadism. Because LH normally stimulates testosterone production in the testis, hypogonadism in men with gonadotrope adenomas is seemingly paradoxical. This effect has seen attributed to inadequate bioactivity of the secreted LH or to abnormalities in the normal pulsatile pattern of LH release.

☐ **Pathology:** Gonadotrope adenomas are chromophobic or somewhat acidophilic. The tumor cells exhibit strong immunoreactivity for FSH, LH, or both. By electron microscopy, secretory granules are sparse, and no correlation is found between circulating levels of FSH or LH and immunoreactivity or ultrastructure. Surgical resection is the treatment of choice.

Nonfunctional Pituitary Adenomas

Approximately one-fourth of all pituitary tumors that are removed surgically do not secrete excess hormones and are not associated with endocrinopathies. The tumors are slowly growing macroadenomas that are diagnosed in older persons because of their mass effects.

POSTERIOR PITUITARY

Central diabetes insipidus (Fig. 21-5) is characterized by an inability to concentrate urine and consequent chronic water diuresis (polyuria), thirst, and polydipsia. The biochemical basis of the disease is a deficiency of vasopressin (antidiuretic hormone or ADH), which is secreted by the posterior pituitary under the influence of the hypothalamus. One-third of the cases of central diabetes insipidus are of unknown cause, and one-fourth are associated with brain tumors, particularly craniopharyngioma (Fig. 21-6). This tumor arises above the sella turcica from remnants of the Rathke pouch and then invades and compresses adjacent tissues. Trauma and hypophysectomy for anterior pituitary tumors account for most of the remaining cases. Polyuria may be controlled by powdered posterior pituitary or vasopressin administered as a nasal spray.

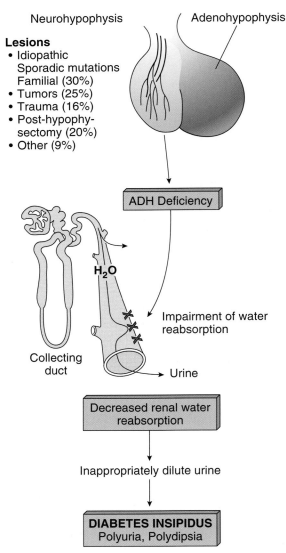

Lesions
- Idiopathic
  Sporadic mutations
  Familial (30%)
- Tumors (25%)
- Trauma (16%)
- Post-hypophy-
  sectomy (20%)
- Other (9%)

Neurohypophysis   Adenohypophysis

ADH Deficiency

H_2O

Collecting duct

Impairment of water reabsorption

Urine

Decreased renal water reabsorption

Inappropriately dilute urine

DIABETES INSIPIDUS
Polyuria, Polydipsia

FIGURE   *21-5*
Mechanism of diabetes insipidus.

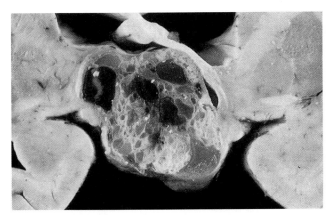

FIGURE   *21-6*
Craniopharyngioma. A coronal section of the brain shows a large, cystic tumor mass replacing the midline structures in the region of the hypothalamus.

Thyroid Gland

THYROGLOSSAL DUCT CYST

Failure of the thyroglossal duct to involute completely can result in a cystic, fluid-filled remnant anywhere along the route of that duct. These cysts, which are most common in children, are 1 to 3 cm in diameter and lined by squamous or respiratory-type epithelium. The presence of thyroid follicles in the wall or adjacent soft tissue distinguishes a thyroglossal duct cyst from a branchial cleft cyst. Surgical excision is curative.

NONTOXIC GOITER

■ *Nontoxic goiter (simple, colloid, or multinodular goiter) refers to an enlargement of the thyroid that is not associated with functional, inflammatory, or neoplastic alterations.* Thus, patients with nontoxic goiter are euthyroid. This disease is far more common in women than in men (8:1). The diffuse form frequently presents during adolescence and pregnancy, whereas the multinodular type usually presents in persons older than 50 years of age. Simple nodular enlargement of the thyroid tends to be familial, thereby suggesting a genetic contribution to the disorder.

□ **Pathogenesis:** These patients are thought to have a subtle impairment of iodine utilization and to respond in an exaggerated fashion to normal TSH levels. It is also possible, however, that the cause of the goiter has disappeared and that normal TSH levels simply maintain the enlargement of the thyroid.

□ **Pathology:** The size of nontoxic goiters ranges from a doubling in the size of the gland (40 g) to a massive enlargement, in which the thyroid weighs a few hundred grams (Fig. 21-7).

  Diffuse nontoxic goiter characterizes the early stages of the disease. The gland is diffusely enlarged, and microscopically exhibits hypertrophy and hyperplasia of the follicular epithelial cells.

  Multinodular nontoxic goiter evolves as the disease becomes more chronic. The enlarged thyroid assumes an increasingly nodular configuration, and the cut surface is typically studded with numerous irregular nodules. When nodules contain large amounts of colloid, they tend to be soft, glistening, and reddish. Nodules composed of smaller follicles containing little

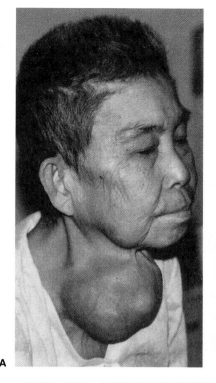

A

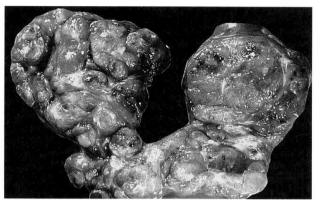

B

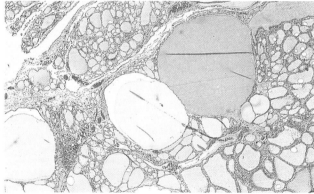

C

FIGURE *21-7*
Nontoxic goiter. (A) In a middle-aged woman with nontoxic goiter, the thyroid has enlarged to produce a conspicuous neck mass. (B) Coronal section of the enlarged thyroid gland shows numerous irregular nodules, some with cystic degeneration and old hemorrhage. (C) A microscopic view of one of the macroscopic nodules shows marked variation in the size of the follicles.

colloid are typically grayish-white and fleshy. Hemorrhagic, necrotic, and cystic areas are common, and fibrous bands often traverse the gland. Calcific foci, which impart a gritty surface, are also frequent.

Microscopically, the nodules vary considerably in both size and shape. Some are distended with colloid, whereas others are collapsed. The lining epithelial cells are flat to cuboidal and, occasionally, are arrayed as papillae that project into the follicular lumen. The individual follicles or groups of follicles are separated by dense fibrosis, and dystrophic calcification of necrotic foci is noted.

☐ **Clinical Features:** Patients with nontoxic goiter are typically asymptomatic and come to medical attention because of a mass in the neck. Large goiters may cause dysphagia or inspiratory stridor by compressing the esophagus or trachea. Pressure from the goiter on the neck veins leads to venous congestion of the head and face. Hoarseness may result from compression of the recurrent laryngeal nerve. Importantly, blood concentrations of T_4 and T_3, and usually of TSH as well, are normal.

Nontoxic goiter is most commonly treated with the administration of thyroid hormone to reduce TSH levels and, thus, stimulation to thyroid growth. In older patients with low TSH levels, further suppression by exogenous thyroid hormone may be ineffective, and radioactive iodine therapy is indicated. Although surgery is ordinarily contraindicated, it may become necessary if local obstructive symptoms become troublesome. Many patients with nontoxic goiter eventually develop hyperthyroidism, in which case the term **toxic multinodular goiter** is applied (discussed later).

HYPOTHYROIDISM

■ *Hypothyroidism refers to the clinical manifestations of thyroid hormone deficiency.* It can be the consequence of three general processes:

- Defective synthesis of thyroid hormone, with compensatory goitrogenesis (goitrous hypothyroidism)
- Inadequate function of thyroid parenchyma, usually because of thyroiditis or surgical resection of the gland or the therapeutic administration of radio-iodine
- Inadequate secretion of TSH by the pituitary or of TRH by the hypothalamus.

Hypothyroidism in Adults

Symptoms of hypothyroidism develop insidiously, and the first manifestations are often tiredness, lethargy, sensitivity to cold, and inability to concentrate. Many organ systems are affected, but all are hypofunctional (Fig. 21-8).

Skin. Alterations in the skin are almost universal among patients with clinically apparent hypothyroidism. Proteoglycans accumulate in the extracellular matrix, binding water and resulting in a peculiar form of edema termed **myxedema.** Patients with myxedema have boggy facies, puffy eyelids, edema of the hands and feet, and an enlarged tongue. A pale, cool skin reflects cutaneous vasoconstriction.

Nervous System. Hypothyroidism in pregnant women has grave neurologic consequences for the fetus, which are expressed after birth as cretinism (discussed later). Adults with hypothyroidism are lethargic and somnolent and suffer from memory loss and a general slowing of mental processes. Paranoid ideation or depression is frequent, and severe agitation, termed **myxedema madness,** may also develop.

Heart. In patients with early hypothyroidism, both the heart rate and stroke volume are reduced, thereby resulting in decreased cardiac output. Because vascular resistance is also increased, the peripheral circulation is impaired, thereby accounting for the cool, pale skin. In patients with untreated hypothyroidism, so-called **myxedema heart** develops, which is charac-

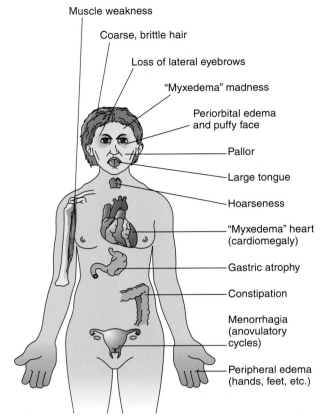

Muscle weakness
Coarse, brittle hair
Loss of lateral eyebrows
"Myxedema" madness
Periorbital edema and puffy face
Pallor
Large tongue
Hoarseness
"Myxedema" heart (cardiomegaly)
Gastric atrophy
Constipation
Menorrhagia (anovulatory cycles)
Peripheral edema (hands, feet, etc.)

FIGURE   *21-8*
Dominant clinical manifestations of hypothyroidism.

terized by a dilated heart and a pericardial effusion. Pathologically, the heart is flabby and microscopically shows interstitial edema and swelling of the myocytes. Coronary atherosclerosis is a common finding.

Gastrointestinal Tract. Constipation owing to decreased peristalsis is a common complaint. It may be severe enough to lead to fecal impaction (myxedema megacolon).

Congenital Hypothyroidism

Congenital hypothyroidism, also termed **cretinism,** may be endemic, sporadic, or familial. It is twice as frequent in girls as in boys. In nonendemic regions, 90% of the cases result from developmental defects of the thyroid (**thyroid dysgenesis**). The remaining cases have a variety of inherited metabolic defects.

Symptoms of congenital hypothyroidism appear during the early weeks of life. These infants are apathetic and sluggish. The abdomen is large and often exhibits an umbilical hernia. The body temperature is frequently less than 35°C (95°F), and the skin is pale and cold. Refractory anemia and a dilated heart are common. By 6 months of age, the clinical syndrome of congenital hypothyroidism is well developed. Mental retardation, stunted growth owing to defective osseous maturation, and characteristic facies are evident. Serum levels of T_4 and T_3 are low, and the serum level of TSH is elevated.

If thyroid hormone replacement therapy is not provided promptly, congenital hypothyroidism results in mentally retarded dwarfs. Children in whom hypothyroidism is detected early respond well to treatment with thyroid hormone and develop an apparently normal mental capacity. By contrast, children who are treated at a later age may be left with irreversible brain damage.

Primary Hypothyroidism

When the cause of thyroid failure is uncertain, the condition is termed **primary hypothyroidism.** Primary hypothyroidism is most common during the fifth and sixth decades of life, and like most thyroid disorders, it is more common in women than in men. Three-fourths of the patients have circulating antibodies to thyroid antigens, thereby suggesting that these cases represent the end stage of autoimmune thyroiditis (discussed later). Nongoitrous hypothyroidism may also result from antibodies that block either TSH itself or the TSH receptor without activating the thyroid. Some cases of primary hypothyroidism are part of multiglandular autoimmune syndrome, including insulin-dependent diabetes, pernicious anemia, hypoparathyroidism, adrenal atrophy, and hypogonadism.

Goitrous Hypothyroidism

There are a number of conditions in which thyroid enlargement (goiter) is associated with hypothyroidism. The causes are diverse, but in all of these cases, goiter is a compensatory response to the lack of adequate thyroid hormone secretion.

Endemic Goiter

■ *Endemic goiter refers to the goitrous hypothyroidism of dietary iodine deficiency that occurs in locales with a high prevalence of the disease.* In areas far from salt water and seafood, which are rich sources of iodides, goiters are (or were) common. The Great Lakes region of the United States, alpine Europe, central Africa, and the Himalayas are such places. Iodized salt is an effective preventive dietary measure, and its wide availability has essentially eliminated endemic goiter in many areas. Nevertheless, it has been estimated that more than 200 million persons worldwide are still afflicted with the disease.

The pathologic evolution of endemic goiter is comparable to that of nontoxic goiter (discussed earlier). However, in contrast to the latter, endemic goiter rarely eventuates in hyperthyroidism, presumably because iodine deficiency protects against this complication. Replacement therapy with thyroid hormone is indicated, and surgical resection may be necessary if local symptoms are severe.

Endemic Cretinism

■ *Endemic cretinism refers to congenital hypothyroidism that occurs in areas of endemic goiter.* Both parents are usually goitrous, and the disease encompasses two overlapping clinical presentations, namely a neurologic syndrome and a predominantly hypothyroid one.

Neurologic cretinism features (1) mental retardation, (2) ataxia, (3) spasticity, and (4) deaf-mutism. It is postulated that iodine deficiency during the first trimester of pregnancy may damage the developing nervous system independent of its effect on thyroid hormone production.

Hypothyroid cretinism is thought to arise from iodine deficiency during late fetal life and the neonatal period. The clinical course in these children is similar to that of other forms of congenital hypothyroidism (discussed earlier).

Goiter Induced by Antithyroid Agents

A number of drugs and naturally occurring chemicals in foods are goitrogenic owing to their suppression of thyroid hormone synthesis. The most commonly used goitrogenic drug is **lithium,** which is employed in the management of manic-depressive states. Other common goitrogenic drugs include phenylbutazone and *p*-aminosalicylic acid. Certain cruciferous vegetables (turnips, rutabaga, cassava) contain goitrogens, and their ingestion by persons with an iodine-deficient diet can produce goitrous hypothyroidism.

HYPERTHYROIDISM

■ *Hyperthyroidism refers to the clinical consequences of excessive circulating thyroid hormone.* In general, the signs and symptoms of hyperthyroidism reflect a hypermetabolic state of the target tissues. Prolonged hypersecretion of thyroid hormone usually results from the presence of an abnormal thyroid stimulator (Graves disease) or an intrinsic disease of the thyroid gland (toxic multinodular goiter or functional adenoma).

Graves Disease

■ *Graves disease is an autoimmune disorder that is characterized by diffuse goiter, hyperthyroidism, and exophthalmos* (Fig. 21-9). In the United States, Graves disease is the most frequent cause of hyperthyroidism in patients younger than 40 years of age.

☐ **Pathogenesis:** The cause of Graves disease is not fully understood, but it seems to involve the interplay between a number of factors.

Immune Mechanisms. Patients with Graves disease are hyperthyroid owing to the presence of immunoglobulin G (IgG) antibodies directed against components of the plasma membrane of the thyroid follicular epithelium, presumably the TSH receptor. These antibodies function as an agonist—that is, they stimulate the TSH receptor, thereby activating adenylyl cyclase and increasing thyroid hormone secretion. Under this continued stimulation, the thyroid becomes diffusely hyperplastic and excessively vascular.

Graves autoantibodies are actually heterogeneous, and those that stimulate the secretion of thyroid hormone represent only one component. Other antibodies seem to be cytotoxic and may account for the thyroid failure that often follows longstanding Graves disease. Sensitized T lymphocytes may also stimulate B cells to elaborate thyroid-activating immunoglobulins.

Genetic Factors. Graves disease exhibits a higher concordance rate in monozygotic twins than in dizygotic ones. Moreover, patients with Graves disease and their relatives both have a considerably higher incidence of other autoimmune diseases, including pernicious anemia and Hashimoto thyroiditis. White patients with Graves disease display an increased frequency of HLA-B8 and -DR3, whereas Chinese patients are more likely to manifest HLA-Bw46 and Japanese patients HLA-Bw35.

Sex. Like other autoimmune diseases, Graves disease is far more common (7–10-fold) in women than in men.

Emotional Influences. The onset of Graves disease often follows a period of emotional stress, such as separation anxiety, death of a loved one, or near-injury in an accident.

Ophthalmopathy. Exophthalmos is a common complication of Graves disease, but its occurrence and severity correlate poorly with the levels of thyroid hormone. A combination of humoral and cell-mediated immune mechanisms is likely to be involved. T lymphocytes that are sensitized to antigens shared by thyroid follicular cells and orbital fibroblasts accumulate around the eye, where they secrete cytokines that activate fibroblasts. There is also evidence for systemic or local production of antibodies that stimulate orbital fibroblasts to proliferate and produce both collagen and glycosaminoglycans.

☐ **Pathology:** The thyroid in patients with Graves disease is symmetrically enlarged and usually weighs from 35 to 40 g. The cut surface is firm and dark red. The tan translucence of the normal cut surface of the thyroid, which is attributable to stored colloid, is notably absent. Microscopically, the thyroid is diffusely hyperplastic and highly vascular. The epithelial cells are tall and columnar, and are often arranged as papillae that project into the lumen of the follicles. The colloid tends to be depleted and presents a scalloped or "moth-eaten" appearance where it abuts the epithelial cells (Fig. 21-10). Scattered lymphocytes and plasma cells infiltrate the interstitial tissue and may even aggregate to form germinal follicles.

Exophthalmos is caused by enlargement of the extraocular muscles within the orbit. The muscles themselves are normal, but they are swollen by mucinous edema, accumulation of fibroblasts, and infiltration by lymphocytes. The increased orbital contents cause forward displacement of the eye (proptosis).

☐ **Clinical Features:** Patients with Graves disease note a gradual onset of nonspecific symptoms, such as nervousness, emotional lability, tremor, weakness, and weight loss (Fig. 21-11). They are intolerant of heat,

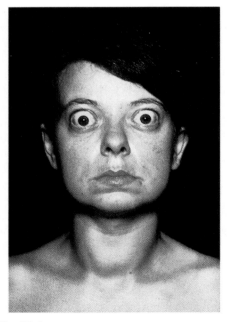

FIGURE *21-9*
Graves disease. This young woman with hyperthyroidism presented with a mass in the neck and exophthalmos.

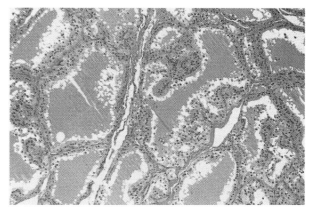

FIGURE   *21-10*
Graves disease. The follicles are lined by hyperplastic, tall columnar cells. Colloid is pink and scalloped at the periphery adjacent to the follicular cells.

seek cooler environments, and tend to sweat profusely. Almost all patients exhibit tachycardia, and many complain of palpitations. In patients with pre-existing heart disease, congestive heart failure may ensue. Women develop oligomenorrhea, which may progress to amenorrhea.

Physical examination reveals a symmetrically enlarged thyroid, often with an audible bruit and a palpable thrill. Protrusion of the eyeball and retraction of the eyelids expose the sclera above the superior margin of the limbus. The skin is warm and moist, and some

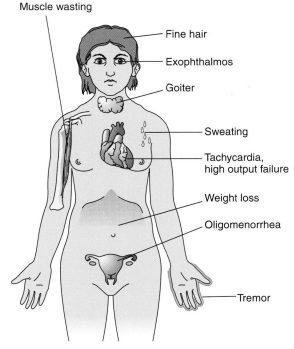

FIGURE   *21-11*
Major clinical manifestations of Graves disease.

patients exhibit Graves dermopathy, which is a peculiar, pretibial edema caused by the accumulation of fluid and glycosaminoglycans. The diagnosis of Graves disease is established by documenting an increased uptake of radioactive iodine by the thyroid and elevated serum levels of T_4 and T_3.

The course of Graves disease is characterized by exacerbations and remissions. Treatment of this disorder depends on many individual factors and includes use of antithyroid medication, destruction of thyroid tissue with radioactive iodine, and adjunctive therapy with corticosteroids and adrenergic antagonists. Unfortunately, despite successful relief of hyperthyroidism, exophthalmos often persists—and may even worsen.

Toxic Multinodular Goiter

Many patients with nontoxic multinodular goiter, who are usually older than 50 years of age, eventually develop functional autonomy of the nodules and a toxic form of the disease. Like its precursor disease, toxic goiter is 10-fold as frequent in women as in men.

□ **Pathogenesis and Pathology:** In some patients, uptake of iodine is diffuse and not affected by the administration of thyroid hormone. Microscopic examination of the thyroid shows groups of small, hyperplastic follicles mixed with other nodules of varying size that appear to be inactive.

Another pattern is characterized by the focal accumulation of radiolabeled iodine in one or more nodules. Hyperfunction of these nodules suppresses the function of the remainder of the thyroid. On microscopic examination, functional nodules are clearly demarcated from the inactive areas and consist of large, hyperplastic follicles, thereby resembling adenomas.

□ **Clinical Features:** Patients with toxic multinodular goiter usually have less severe symptoms of hyperthyroidism than those with Graves disease, and they never develop exophthalmos. Because patients with a toxic goiter tend to be older, cardiac complications, including atrial fibrillation and congestive heart failure, may dominate the clinical presentation. Serum T_4 and T_3 levels frequently are only minimally elevated, and the uptake of radiolabeled iodine may be within the normal range or only slightly increased. Radiolabeled iodine administration is the most common therapy for toxic multinodular goiter.

Toxic Adenoma

■ *Toxic adenoma is a solitary, hyperfunctioning, follicular neoplasm in an otherwise normal thyroid.* An infrequent cause of hyperthyroidism, such tumors display autonomous function. They are not dependent on TSH, and they are not suppressed by the administration of thyroid hormone. Hyperfunction of the toxic adenoma eventually suppresses the remainder of the thyroid, which then atrophies.

Toxic adenoma of the thyroid is most common during the fourth and fifth decades of life. Most patients do not suffer symptoms of hyperthyroidism until the adenoma has grown to a diameter of approximately 3 cm.

Because the normal thyroid tissue is suppressed, toxic adenoma is effectively treated with radiolabeled iodine. Alternatively, large nodules may be excised surgically.

THYROIDITIS

■ *Thyroiditis refers to a heterogeneous group of inflammatory disorders of the thyroid gland, including those that are caused by autoimmune mechanisms and infectious agents.*

Hashimoto Thyroiditis

■ *Hashimoto thyroiditis (lymphocytic thyroiditis) is an autoimmune disease that is characterized by circulating antibodies to thyroid antigens and features that are suggestive of cell-mediated immunity to thyroid tissue.* The disease arises most commonly during the fourth and fifth decades of life and afflicts women more often than men. **In regions where supplies of iodine are adequate, Hashimoto thyroiditis is the most common cause of goitrous hypothyroidism.**

□ **Pathogenesis:** Patients with Hashimoto thyroiditis exhibit high titers of circulating autoantibodies directed against thyroid peroxidase, thyroglobulin, and the TSH receptor. In addition, the intense infiltration of the thyroid parenchyma by lymphocytes and plasma cells suggests cell-mediated destruction of the gland.

A familial tendency for Hashimoto thyroiditis has been documented, and both patients and their relatives have a higher incidence of other autoimmune diseases, including insulin-dependent diabetes mellitus, pernicious anemia, Addison disease, and myasthenia gravis. Hashimoto thyroiditis is associated with an increased frequency of the HLA-B8 haplotype. In addition, HLA-DR3 is more common in those who progress to thyroid atrophy, and HLA-DR5 accompanies diffuse goiter. Interestingly, Hashimoto thyroiditis is particularly frequent in the context of Down syndrome.

□ **Pathology:** On gross examination, the gland in patients with Hashimoto thyroiditis is diffusely enlarged, firm, slightly lobular, and weighs from 60 to 200 g. The cut surface is pale tan and fleshy, and exhibits a vaguely nodular pattern. Microscopically, the thyroid displays (1) a conspicuous infiltrate of lymphocytes and plasma cells, (2) destruction and atrophy of the follicles, and (3) oxyphilic metaplasia of the follicular epithelial cells (Hurthle or Askanazy cells; Fig. 21-12). The inflammatory infiltrates are focally arranged in lymphoid follicles, often with germinal centers.

□ **Clinical Features:** In most cases of Hashimoto thyroiditis, the patient notes the gradual onset of a goiter. The majority of these patients are initially euthyroid, but a few are hypothyroid when they present for medical attention. Eventually, most cases progress to a

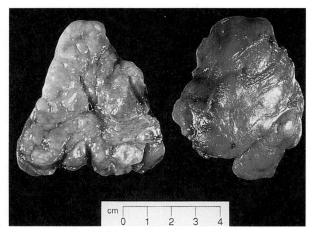
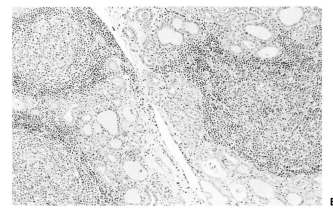

FIGURE *21-12*
Chronic autoimmune (Hashimoto) thyroiditis. The thyroid gland is symmetrically enlarged and coarsely nodular. **(A)** A coronal section of the right lobe shows irregular nodules and an intact capsule. **(B)** A microscopic section of the thyroid reveals a conspicuous chronic inflammatory infiltrate and many atrophic thyroid follicles. The inflammatory cells form prominent lymphoid follicles with germinal centers.

hypothyroid state, but on rare occasions, hyperthyroidism (hashitoxicosis) develops.

Many patients with Hashimoto thyroiditis require no treatment. Thyroid hormone is administered to alleviate hypothyroidism and to decrease the size of the gland. Surgery is reserved for patients who are unresponsive to suppressive hormone therapy or in whom pressure symptoms are troublesome.

Subacute Thyroiditis (DeQuervain, Granulomatous, or Giant Cell Thyroiditis)

■ *Subacute thyroiditis is an infrequent, self-limited viral infection of the thyroid that is characterized by granulomatous inflammation.* The disease typically occurs after upper respiratory tract infections, including those caused by influenza virus, adenovirus, echovirus, and coxsackievirus. Mumps virus has also been incriminated in some cases. DeQuervain thyroiditis principally affects women between 30 and 50 years of age.

☐ **Pathology:** The thyroid gland is enlarged to between 40 and 60 g, and the cut surface is firm and pale. Initially, microscopic examination reveals an acute inflammatory reaction, often with microabscesses. This is followed by the appearance of a patchy infiltrate of lymphocytes, plasma cells, and macrophages throughout the thyroid. Destruction of follicles allows the release of colloid, which elicits a conspicuous granulomatous reaction (Fig. 21-13). Numerous multinucleated giant cells of the foreign-body type, often containing colloid, are present. In most cases, the normal thyroid architecture is eventually restored.

☐ **Clinical Features:** Patients with subacute thyroiditis typically notice pain in the anterior neck, which is sometimes accompanied by fever. On physical examination, the thyroid is moderately enlarged and exquisitely tender. Subacute thyroiditis generally resolves within a few months and without clinical sequelae.

Riedel Thyroiditis

■ *Riedel thyroiditis is a rare disease that is characterized by dense fibrosis of the thyroid.* The term *thyroiditis* is something of a misnomer, because the disease also involves extrathyroidal soft tissues of the neck and is often associated with progressive fibrosis in other locations, including the retroperitoneum, mediastinum, and orbit. Riedel thyroiditis is primarily a disease of middle age, with a female:male ratio of 3:1. The cause

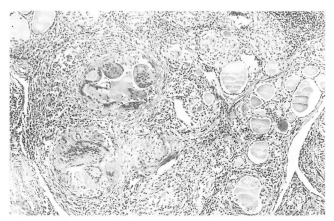

FIGURE *21-13*
Subacute thyroiditis. The release of colloid into the interstitial tissue has elicited a prominent granulomatous reaction, with numerous foreign-body giant cells.

is unknown but does not appear to be related to other forms of thyroiditis.

Patients with Riedel thyroiditis notice a gradual onset of a painless goiter. Subsequently, they may suffer from the consequences of compression of the trachea (stridor), esophagus (dysphagia), and recurrent laryngeal nerves (hoarseness). In the unusual cases that involve the entire thyroid, hypothyroidism ensues. Treatment is primarily surgical to relieve compression of the local organs.

FOLLICULAR ADENOMA OF THE THYROID

■ *Thyroid adenomas are benign neoplasms that exhibit follicular differentiation. They typically present as solitary, "cold" nodules—that is, tumors that do not take up radiolabeled iodine.* Follicular adenoma is an encapsulated tumor in which cells are arranged in follicles, resembling normal thyroid tissue, or mimic stages in the embryonic development of the gland. As many as 90% of palpable, solitary follicular lesions are actually the dominant nodule in a multinodular goiter, and follicular adenomas are correspondingly infrequent. Follicular adenoma is most common during the fourth and fifth decades of life, with a female:male ratio of 7:1.

☐ **Pathology:** On gross examination, follicular adenoma is a solitary, circumscribed nodule (diameter, 1–3 cm) that protrudes from the surface of the thyroid (Fig. 21-14). The cut surface of the tumor is soft and paler than the surrounding parenchyma. Hemorrhage, fibrosis, and cystic change are common. Histologically, a number of distinctive patterns are observed:

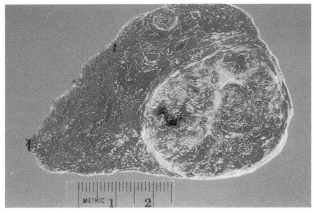

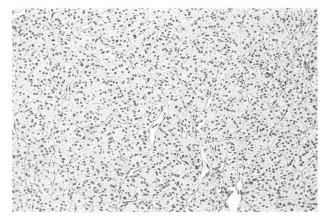

FIGURE *21-14*
Follicular adenoma of the thyroid. (A) Colloid adenoma. The cut surface of an encapsulated mass reveals hemorrhage, fibrosis, and cystic change. (B) Hürthle cell adenoma. The tumor is composed of cells with small, regular nuclei and abundant eosinophilic cytoplasm.

- **Embryonal adenoma** is distinguished by a trabecular pattern in which poorly formed follicles contain little or no colloid.
- **Fetal adenoma** features cells that are similar to those of embryonal adenoma but that tend to be arranged in microfollicles containing little colloid.
- **Simple adenoma** exhibits mature follicles with a normal amount of colloid.
- **Colloid adenoma** is similar to simple adenoma, except that the follicles are larger and contain more abundant colloid.
- **Hürthle cell adenoma** is a solid tumor characterized by oxyphilic cells, small follicles, and scanty colloid.
- **Atypical adenoma** is a follicular tumor that displays mitoses, excessive cellularity, nuclear atypism, or equivocal capsular invasion but in which a diagnosis of carcinoma cannot be established with certainty.

THYROID CANCER

Thyroid nodules are found in as many as 1% to 10% of the population, but malignant tumors of the thyroid account for only 1% of all cancers and 0.4% of cancer-related deaths.

The large majority of the cases of carcinoma of the thyroid occur between the third and seventh decades of life. The prognosis relates to the morphologic features of the tumor, ranging from a virtually benign clinical course to a rapidly fatal disease. The latter outcome, fortunately, is uncommon.

Papillary Thyroid Carcinoma

Papillary carcinoma is the most common thyroid cancer, accounting for more than three-fourths of all cases in the United States. The tumor is most frequent between the ages of 20 and 50 years, with a female:male ratio of 3:1. The reported incidence of this tumor has varied from 35% to 90% of all thyroid cancers, because some pathologists consider the most mature variant to be a papillary adenoma and others classify papillary tumors with follicular elements as being follicular carcinoma. **In this context, we consider all neoplasms with papillary elements to be papillary cancers.**

☐ **Pathogenesis:** Although the cause of papillary carcinoma of the thyroid remains to be established, a number of associations have been identified:

- **Iodine Excess.** Papillary thyroid cancer has been produced in animals by administering excess iodine.
- **Radiation.** External radiation to the neck of children and adults increases the incidence of later papillary carcinoma of the thyroid. Survivors of the atomic bomb explosions in Japan experienced more papillary cancers than would otherwise be expected.
- **Genetic Factors.** A concordance for papillary carcinoma of the thyroid has been described in monozygotic twins, and an association between this tumor and HLA-DR7 has been reported. Somatic rearrangements of the *RET* proto-oncogene on chromosome 10 are common in patients with papillary thyroid cancers. These rearrangements

cause fusion of the tyrosine kinase domain of *RET* with various other genes, creating the *RET/PTC* (papillary thyroid cancer) fusion oncogenes.

☐ **Pathology:** Papillary carcinomas of the thyroid vary from microscopic lesions to tumors larger than the normal gland itself. On gross examination, most papillary carcinomas are either pale and firm or hard and gritty lesions, with less than 10% being truly encapsulated (Fig. 21-15A).

Microscopic examination reveals branching papillae that are composed of a central, fibrovascular core and a single or stratified lining of cuboidal to columnar cells (see Fig. 21-15*B*). In most instances, irregularly shaped or tubular neoplastic follicles are present within the tumor, but the proportions of the papillary and follicular elements are highly variable. Nuclear atypism is an important diagnostic feature and includes clear ("ground-glass" or "Orphan Annie") nuclei, eosinophilic pseudoinclusions (representing invaginations of the cytoplasm into the nucleus), and nuclear grooves. Many papillary cancers show dense fibrosis, and calcospherites (psammoma bodies) are present in half of the cases. The latter feature, being rare in other conditions, is virtually diagnostic of papillary carcinoma. Vascular invasion is distinctly uncommon.

Papillary thyroid carcinoma typically invades the lymphatics and spreads to the regional cervical lymph nodes. Direct extension of papillary carcinoma into the soft tissues of the neck occurs in one-fourth of the cases. Although hematogenous metastases are less common than in other varieties of thyroid cancer, they occasionally do occur, most commonly to the lungs.

☐ **Clinical Features:** In general, the prognosis of patients with papillary carcinoma is excellent, and the life expectancy for these patients differs little from that of the general population. In fatal cases of papillary cancer, death is caused principally by metastases to the lungs or brain or by obstruction of the trachea or esophagus.

Follicular Thyroid Carcinoma

■ *Follicular carcinoma of the thyroid is a malignant neoplasm that is purely follicular and does not contain any papillary or other elements.* This tumor represents approximately 15% of all thyroid cancers. Most patients are older than 40 years of age, and the female:male ratio is 3:1.

☐ **Pathology:** Follicular carcinomas are subdivided into minimally invasive and widely invasive variants.

Minimally invasive follicular carcinoma is seen grossly as a well-defined, encapsulated tumor that, on cut section, is soft and pale tan to pink and bulges from the confines of its capsule. Microscopically, most of the

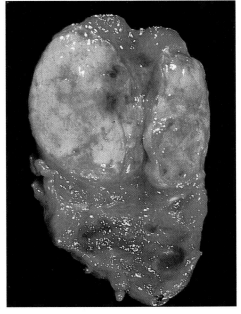
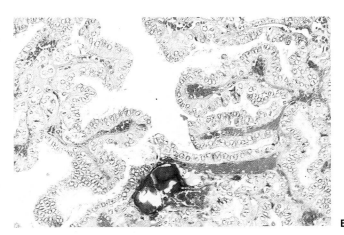

A **B**

FIGURE *21-15*
Papillary carcinoma of the thyroid. **(A)** The cut surface of a surgically resected thyroid displays a circumscribed, pale-tan mass with foci of cystic change. **(B)** Branching papillae are lined by neoplastic columnar epithelium containing clear nuclei. A calcospherite, or psammoma body, is evident.

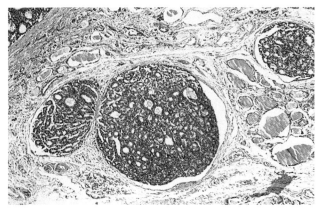

FIGURE   *21-16*
Follicular carcinoma of the thyroid. A microfollicular tumor has invaded veins in the thyroid parenchyma.

lesions resemble follicular adenoma, although they tend more toward a microfollicular or a trabecular pattern. Mitoses are commonly encountered, and this feature distinguishes follicular cancer from a benign adenoma. The principal distinction from adenoma, however, is in the interface of the capsule and the normal parenchyma. Carcinoma is diagnosed when the tumor extends into or through the capsule and invades small veins external to the capsule (Fig. 21-16).

Widely invasive follicular carcinoma presents few diagnostic difficulties, because it is not encapsulated, exhibits widespread infiltration of blood vessels, and often extends into the surrounding soft tissues.

Metastases are blood-borne rather than lymphatic, and they are directed principally to the bones of the shoulder and pelvic girdles, sternum, and skull. Whereas metastases in widely invasive follicular carcinoma are common, less than 5% of the minimally invasive variants metastasize.

☐ **Clinical Features:** Most follicular cancers of the thyroid are detected clinically as a palpable nodule or an enlarged thyroid, but in some patients, the presenting sign is a pathologic fracture through a bony metastasis or a pulmonary lesion. Both the primary tumor and the metastases have an affinity for radiolabeled iodine, which may be used therapeutically. Patients with minimally invasive follicular tumors have a 10-year survival rate of 85%, compared with a rate of only 45% for patients with the widely invasive form.

Medullary Thyroid Carcinoma

■ *Medullary carcinoma of the thyroid is a tumor derived from the parafollicular or C cells of the thyroid, which are distinguished by their secretion of the calcium-lowering hormone calcitonin.* This tumor represents no more than 5% of all thyroid cancers. The disease occurs in spo-

radic and familial forms, with the latter accounting for 20% of the cases. Patients having the familial form of medullary carcinoma are often afflicted with multiple endocrine neoplasia (MEN) type 2, which includes pheochromocytoma of the adrenal medulla and parathyroid hyperplasia or adenoma. Somatic mutations in the *RET* proto-oncogene have been detected in more than half of the cases of sporadic medullary thyroid carcinoma.

The mean age of patients with medullary carcinoma is 50 years, but familial cases appear earlier (mean age, 20 years). There is a slight female predominance (1.5:1). In familial cases, the inheritance is autosomal dominant, and the sex distribution is equal.

☐ **Pathology:** On gross examination, medullary carcinomas tend to arise in the superior portion of the thyroid (the regions that are richest in C cells). The cut surface is firm and grayish-white, and the histologic appearance is highly variable. Characteristically, the tumor is solid and composed of polygonal, granular cells that are separated by a distinctly vascular stroma (Fig. 21-17). **A conspicuous feature is the presence of stromal amyloid, which represents the deposition of procalcitonin.** The nests of tumor cells are embedded in a hyalinized, collagenous framework.

The histologic variability of medullary carcinoma is evidenced by different architectural patterns, including trabecular, tubular, follicular, carcinoid-like, or pseudopapillary arrangements. The neoplastic cells may exhibit peripheral nuclei (plasmacytoid pattern) or may be spindle-shaped, anaplastic, or oxyphilic.

By electron microscopy, the neoplastic C cells show dense-core secretory granules, which stain immunohistochemically for a variety of endocrine markers, including calcitonin, synaptophysin, chromogranin, and neuron-specific enolase. Almost all of these tumors are positive for carcinoembryonic antigen (CEA). Many cases are also positive for corticotropin, serotonin, substance P, glucagon, insulin, and human chorionic gonadotropin.

Medullary carcinoma extends by direct invasion into the soft tissues and metastasizes to the regional lymph nodes and to lung, liver, and bones. **The precursor lesion of the familial variety of medullary carcinoma is C-cell hyperplasia.** Thus, patients with MEN-2A and -2B (see the section on the adrenal medulla) who are at risk for development of medullary carcinoma of the thyroid are monitored by periodic measurements of serum calcitonin, CEA, and sometimes, chromogranin. When levels of these substances are elevated, the patient is subjected to total thyroidectomy.

☐ **Clinical Features:** Patients with medullary carcinoma often suffer a number of symptoms related to en-

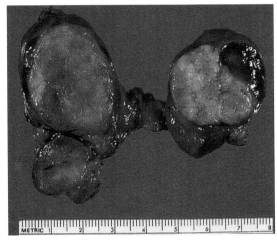

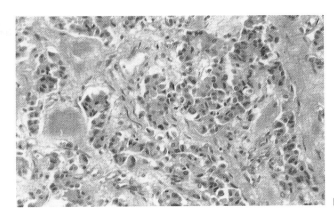

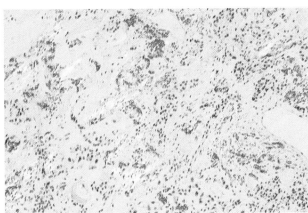

FIGURE *21-17*
Medullary thyroid carcinoma. (A) Coronal section of a total thyroid resection shows bilateral involvement by a firm, pale tumor. (B) The tumor features nests of polygonal cells embedded in a collagenous framework. The connective tissue septa contain eosinophilic amyloid. (C) A section stained with Congo red and viewed under polarized light demonstrates the pale green birefringence of amyloid.

docrine secretion, including carcinoid syndrome (serotonin) and Cushing syndrome (corticotropin). Watery diarrhea in one-third of the patients results from the secretion of vasoactive intestinal peptide, prostaglandins, and several kinins. In cases of familial medullary carcinoma, patients may exhibit hyperparathyroidism, episodic hypertension, and other symptoms attributable to the secretion of catecholamines by pheochromocytoma. Treatment is total thyroidectomy, but local recurrences follow in one-third of the patients. The 5-year survival rate is 75%.

Anaplastic (Undifferentiated) Thyroid Carcinoma

■ *Anaplastic (undifferentiated) carcinoma is a highly aggressive, undifferentiated thyroid cancer that is usually rapidly fatal.* This type of thyroid cancer principally afflicts women (female:male ratio, 4 : 1) older than 60 years of age. The tumor comprises 10% of thyroid cancers. At least half of the patients have a history of longstanding goiter. In addition, many cases of anaplastic carcinoma occur in patients with a history of lower-

grade thyroid cancer. Thus, it seems likely that anaplastic thyroid carcinoma often represents the transformation of a benign or low-grade thyroid neoplasm into a poorly differentiated, highly aggressive cancer. There is evidence that the risk of such an event is enhanced by external radiation.

☐ **Pathology:** Anaplastic carcinoma of the thyroid presents as large masses in the gland that are poorly circumscribed and, frequently, extend into the soft tissues of the neck. The cut surface is hard and grayish-white. The most common histologic pattern is a sarcoma-like proliferation of bizarre spindle and giant cells, with polyploid nuclei, many mitoses, necrosis, and stromal fibrosis (Fig. 21-18). Other specimens reveal distinct epithelial differentiation. The tumor tends to invade veins and arteries.

☐ **Clinical Features:** These highly malignant tumors compress and destroy local structures. Dysphagia and dyspnea are caused by tracheal compression or invasion. The prognosis is dismal, and widespread metastases are frequent. Less than 10% of the patients survive for 5 years.

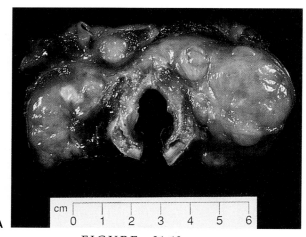
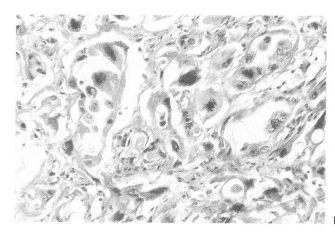

FIGURE   *21-18*
Anaplastic carcinoma of the thyroid. (A) The tumor in transverse section partially surrounds the trachea and extends into the adjacent soft tissue. (B) The tumor is composed of bizarre spindle and giant cells with polyploid nuclei and numerous mitoses.

Parathyroid Glands

HYPOPARATHYROIDISM

Hypoparathyroidism usually results from decreased secretion of parathyroid hormone (PTH) and, occasionally, from end-organ insensitivity to the hormone.

The most common cause of hypoparathyroidism is inadvertent surgical resection of the parathyroids as a complication of thyroidectomy. Symptoms of hypoparathyroidism relate to hypocalcemia, which causes increased neuromuscular excitability, and range from mild tingling in the hands and feet to severe muscle cramps, laryngeal stridor, and convulsions. Neuropsychiatric manifestations include depression, paranoia, and psychoses. Hypoparathyroidism is successfully treated with vitamin D and calcium supplementation.

Idiopathic hypoparathyroidism is a heterogeneous group of rare disorders, both sporadic and familial, that have in common deficient secretion of PTH.

Familial hypoparathyroidism is often part of a polyglandular syndrome that also includes adrenal insufficiency and mucocutaneous candidiasis. There is accumulating evidence that idiopathic hypoparathyroidism is an autoimmune disorder. The only pathologic changes are lymphocytic infiltration, parathyroid atrophy, and replacement of parenchymal cells by fat.

Pseudohypoparathyroidism designates a group of hereditary conditions in which hypocalcemia is caused by target-organ insensitivity to PTH. Most patients do not exhibit the normal increase in urinary excretion of cyclic adenosine monophosphate (AMP) on intravenous administration of PTH. The defect in these patients has been traced to mutations on the long arm of chromosome 20. These result in a decreased activity of the G protein that couples hormone receptors to stimulation of adenylyl cyclase in the renal tubular epithelium.

PRIMARY HYPERPARATHYROIDISM

■ *Primary hyperparathyroidism   is the syndrome caused by excessive secretion of PTH as a result of intrinsic parathyroid disease.*

Parathyroid Adenoma

Parathyroid adenomas accounts for 80% of all cases of primary hyperparathyroidism. They arise either sporadically or in the context of MEN-1 (discussed later). Rearrangements and overexpression of the cyclin D1 (*PRAD1*) proto-oncogene on chromosome 11 have been observed in some patients. The tumor is a circumscribed, reddish-brown, and solitary mass measuring from 1 to 3 cm in diameter. On microscopic examination, it is composed of sheets of neoplastic chief cells embedded in a rich capillary network. A rim of normal parathyroid tissue is usually evident outside the capsule and distinguishes an adenoma from parathyroid hyperplasia (Fig. 21-19). For the most part, the cells resemble normal chief cells, but some clear cells and occasional oxyphilic foci may also be present. With a functioning parathyroid adenoma, the other three glands tend to be atrophic. Surgical resection of the tumor relieves the symptoms of hyperparathyroidism.

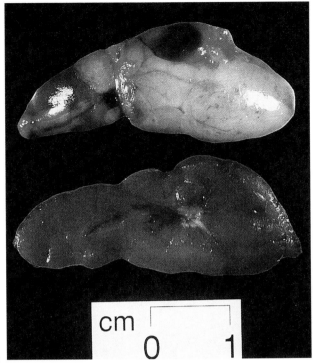

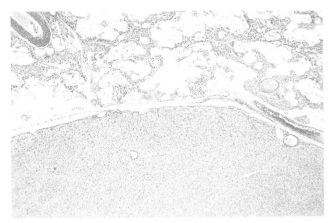

FIGURE   *21-19*

Parathyroid adenoma. (A) The external *(top)* and cross-section *(bottom)* show a tan, fleshy tumor. (B) The tumor consists of sheets of neoplastic chief cells and is separated from normal parenchyma by a thin capsule.

Primary Parathyroid Hyperplasia

Chief cell hyperplasia is responsible for some 15% of the cases of primary hyperparathyroidism. Of these, one-third are associated with familial hyperparathyroidism or MEN-1 and -2A. On gross examination, all four parathyroid glands are enlarged. In half of the patients, one gland is noticeably larger than the others, in which case the distinction from adenoma may be difficult. Microscopically, the normal adipose tissue of the gland is replaced by hyperplastic chief cells, which are arranged as sheets or in trabecular or follicular patterns (Fig. 21-20). An important feature that distinguishes hyperplasia from adenoma is the lack of cellular pleomorphism in the former.

Parathyroid Carcinoma

Parathyroid carcinoma accounts for 1% of all cases of primary hyperparathyroidism, occurring principally in those between 30 and 60 years of age. Similar to functioning parathyroid adenomas, overexpression of cyclin D1 has also been described in some parathyroid carcinomas. This cancer is usually a functioning tumor, and most patients present with symptoms of hyperparathyroidism. Carcinomas tend to be somewhat

larger than adenomas and appear as lobulated, firm, tannish, and unencapsulated masses that often are adherent to the surrounding soft tissues. Microscopically, most cases show a trabecular pattern, with significant mitotic activity and thick, fibrous bands. Capsular or vascular invasion is occasionally noted as well. Importantly, the cell atypism often encountered in parathyroid adenoma is unusual in parathyroid carcinoma.

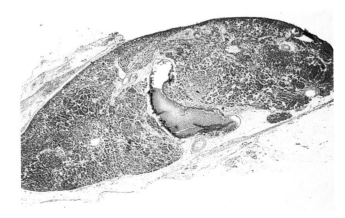

FIGURE   *21-20*

Primary parathyroid hyperplasia. The normal adipose tissue of the gland has been replaced by sheets and trabeculae of hyperplastic chief cells.

Despite surgical removal of the tumor, local recurrence is common, and one-third of the patients develop metastases to regional lymph nodes, lungs, liver, and bone. In fatal cases, the cause of death is most often hyperparathyroidism rather than carcinomatosis.

☐ **Clinical Features of Primary Hyperparathyroidism:** The clinical manifestations of primary hyperparathyroidism are highly variable, ranging from asymptomatic hypercalcemia detected on routine blood analysis to florid systemic, renal, and skeletal disease (Fig. 21-21). Hypercalcemia and hypophosphatemia are the characteristic biochemical abnormalities. Excessive PTH leads to increased loss of calcium from the bones and enhanced calcium resorption by the renal tubules. Production of the activated form of vitamin D (1,25[OH]$_2$D) by the renal tubules is also stimulated by PTH, thereby resulting in augmented intestinal absorption of calcium. The action of PTH on the kidney, together with hypercalcemia, leads to hypophosphatemia.

The classic bone lesions of hyperparathyroidism, termed **osteitis fibrosa cystica,** are encountered in a minority of patients with an accelerated and serious form of the disease. These patients present with bone pain, bone cysts, pathologic fractures, and localized bone swellings (brown tumors and epulis of the jaw).

Ten percent of the patients with primary hyperparathyroidism present with **renal colic** as a result of kidney stones. Hyperparathyroidism is often accompanied by **mental changes,** including depression, emotional lability, poor mentation, and memory defects. The incidence of **peptic ulcer disease** is increased in patients with hyperparathyroidism, possibly because hypercalcemia increases the level of serum gastrin, thereby stimulating secretion of gastric acid. **Chronic pancreatitis** is also a recognized complication of prolonged hypercalcemia, but the pathogenesis is not understood. **Hypertension** occurs in as many as half of the patients with hyperparathyroidism, although the underlying mechanism is not clear.

SECONDARY HYPERPARATHYROIDISM

■ *Secondary hyperparathyroidism refers to excess secretion of PTH as a response to chronic hypocalcemia.* Secondary parathyroid hyperplasia is encountered principally in patients with chronic renal failure, although it also occurs in association with vitamin D deficiency, intestinal malabsorption, Fanconi syndrome, and renal tubular acidosis (Fig. 21-22). Chronic hypocalcemia owing to renal retention of phosphate, inadequate production of 1,25(OH)$_2$D by diseased kidneys, and some degree of skeletal resistance to PTH, leads to compensatory hypersecretion of PTH. As a result, secondary hyperplasia of all four parathyroids occurs. In turn, the excess levels of PTH cause osseous manifestations of hyperparathyroidism, termed **renal osteodystrophy.** The morphologic appearance of the parathyroids in patients with secondary hyperplasia is similar to that of primary hyperplasia. Secondary parathyroid hyperplasia regresses after correction of the underlying condition producing the hypocalcemia.

Adrenal Cortex

CONGENITAL ADRENAL HYPERPLASIA

■ *Congenital adrenal hyperplasia (CAH) is a syndrome in which deficient synthesis of corticosteroids results in the unopposed action of corticotropin and, hence, adrenal hyperplasia.* CAH results from a number of autosomal recessive, enzymatic defects in the biosynthesis of cortisol from cholesterol. **More than 90% of the cases of CAH represent an inborn deficiency of 21-hydroxylase, or P450**$_{c21}$**,** a microsomal enzyme that converts 17-hydroxyprogesterone to 11-deoxycortisol. Deficient activity of this enzyme impairs the biosynthesis of cortisol, and the accumulated precursors are, instead, converted to androgens. The gene for P450$_{C21}$ is linked to the major histocompatibility complex locus on the short arm of chromosome 6 and is closely associated with HLA-B and some of the complement genes.

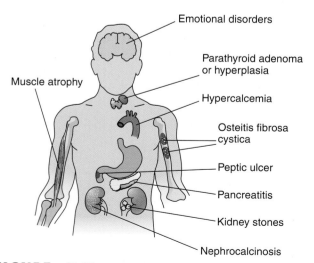

FIGURE 21-21
Major clinical features of hyperparathyroidism.

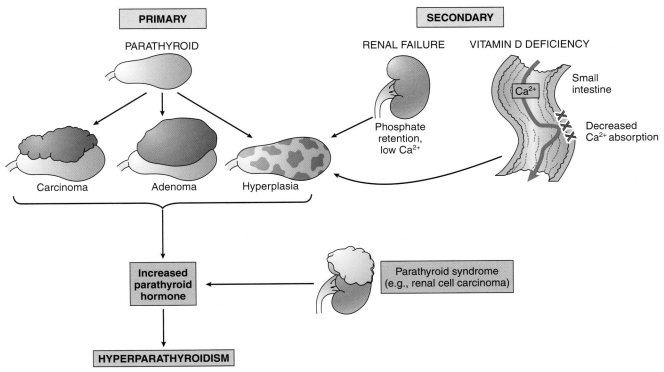

FIGURE 21-22
Major pathogenetic pathways leading to clinical primary and secondary hyperparathyroidism.

☐ **Pathology:** The adrenal glands are enlarged, weighing as much as 30 g (Fig. 21-23). The cut surface is either diffusely enlarged or nodular. Microscopically, the cortex is widened between the medulla and the zona glomerulosa. The hyperplastic zone is filled by compact, granular, and eosinophilic cells.

☐ **Clinical Features:** CAH caused by P450$_{c21}$ deficiency presents as two variants in newborns.

Simple Virilizing CAH. Female infants are afflicted with pseudohermaphroditism, whereas male infants exhibit no abnormalities of the sexual organs. Female newborns exposed to a large excess of adrenal androgens in utero are born with fused labia, an enlarged clitoris, and a urogenital sinus, which may be mistaken for a penile urethra. The sexual ambiguity may be so severe that the infant is mislabeled as being male. Infant boys exhibit sexual precocity. Eventually, the high levels of adrenal androgens lead to closure of the epiphyses and stunted growth. Adult women with CAH tend to be infertile, whereas adult men may, or may not, be fertile.

Salt-Wasting CAH. Owing to P450$_{c21}$ deficiency, synthesis of aldosterone may be impaired. As a result, hypoaldosteronism develops within the first few weeks of life in two-thirds of the newborns with CAH,

manifesting as hyponatremia, hyperkalemia, dehydration, hypotension, and increased renin secretion. These effects may be rapidly fatal if the disease remains untreated.

ADRENOCORTICAL INSUFFICIENCY

Deficient production of adrenocortical hormones can result from (1) destruction of the adrenal gland, (2) dysfunction of the pituitary or hypothalamus, or (3) intake of corticosteroids as treatment for chronic inflammatory diseases.

Primary Chronic Adrenal Insufficiency (Addison Disease)

■ *Primary chronic adrenal insufficiency (Addison disease) is a fatal, wasting disorder that is caused by failure of adrenocortical secretion.* This disease is characterized by deficiencies of glucocorticoids, mineralocorticoids, and androgens. If untreated, the disorder is characterized by weakness, weight loss, gastrointestinal symptoms, hypotension, electrolyte disturbances, and hyperpigmentation.

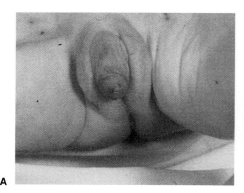

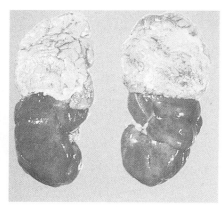

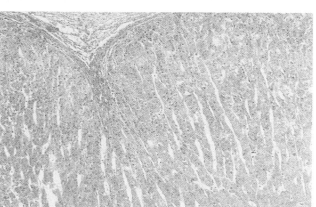

FIGURE 21-23
Congenital adrenal hyperplasia. (A) A female infant is markedly virilized with hypertrophy of the clitoris and partial fusion of labioscrotal folds. (B) A 7-week-old male died of severe salt-wasting congenital adrenal hyperplasia. At autopsy, both adrenal glands were markedly enlarged. (C) A microscopic view shows a widened cortex containing compact eosinophilic cells.

☐ **Pathogenesis:** Historically, the most common cause of Addison disease was tuberculosis of the adrenal glands. However, in advanced societies, autoimmune adrenalitis is today responsible for 75% of the cases. Autoimmune adrenalitis occurs as an isolated disorder or as a part of two different polyglandular autoimmune syndromes. Other causes of adrenal destruction include metastatic carcinoma, amyloidosis, adrenal hemorrhage, sarcoidosis, and fungal infections.

Antiadrenal antibodies that react with tissue from all three zones of the adrenal cortex have been reported in two-thirds of the patients with chronic adrenal insufficiency that could not be attributed to a specific cause.

Evidence for participation of cell-mediated immune mechanisms in the pathogenesis of primary adrenal insufficiency includes increased numbers of Ia-positive T lymphocytes in the blood and decreased function of suppressor T cells.

Half of the patients with autoimmune adrenal insufficiency also suffer from other autoimmune endocrine diseases, particularly those affecting multiple endocrine organs (polyglandular endocrine syndromes).

☐ **Pathology:** More than 90% of the adrenal gland must be destroyed before symptoms of chronic adrenal insufficiency appear. Autoimmune adrenalitis leads to a pale, irregular, and shrunken gland that weighs between 2 and 3 g or less. Microscopically, an intact medulla is surrounded by fibrous tissue containing small islands of atrophic cortical cells (Fig. 21-24). Depending on the stage of the disease, lymphoid infiltrates of varying density are encountered.

☐ **Clinical Features:** The first symptom of Addison disease is usually the insidious onset of weakness, which is followed by anorexia and weight loss. A diffuse, tan pigmentation of the skin usually develops. Melanocytes are stimulated by increased melanocyte-stimulating activity of pituitary pro-opiomelanocortin. Hypotension, with blood pressures in the range of 80/50 mm Hg, is the rule. Patients with Addison disease often exhibit marked personality changes and even organic brain syndromes.

The lack of mineralocorticoid secretion, together with other metabolic derangements, leads to low serum levels of sodium and elevated levels of potassium. Patients with Addison disease formerly survived for only 2 years, but today, such patients live a normal

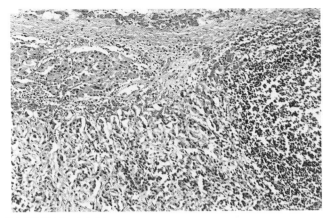

FIGURE 21-24
Autoimmune adrenalitis. This section of the adrenal gland from a patient with Addison disease demonstrates chronic inflammation and fibrosis in the cortex, an island of residual atrophic cortical cells, and an intact medulla.

life when treated with glucocorticoids and mineralocorticoids.

Acute Adrenal Insufficiency

■ *Acute adrenal insufficiency,* or adrenal crisis, is a *life-threatening medical emergency that reflects a sudden loss of adrenocortical function.* Symptoms relate more to mineralocorticoid deficiency than to inadequate glucocorticoids. Adrenal crisis occurs in three settings:

- **The abrupt withdrawal of corticosteroid therapy** in patients with adrenal atrophy secondary to chronic administration of these steroids is the most common cause of acute adrenal insufficiency.
- **The stress of infection or surgery** may precipitate a sudden and devastating worsening of chronic adrenal insufficiency.
- **Waterhouse-Friderichsen syndrome** refers to acute, bilateral, and hemorrhagic infarction of the adrenal cortex, most commonly occurring secondary to meningococcal or pseudomonal septicemia (see Fig. 7-24).

☐ **Clinical Features:** The initial manifestations of adrenal crisis are usually hypotension and shock. In the typical case of Waterhouse-Friderichsen syndrome, a young person suddenly develops hypotension and shock, together with abdominal or back pain, fever, and purpura. Adrenal crisis almost invariably is fatal unless the patient is promptly and aggressively treated with corticosteroids and supportive measures.

ADRENAL HYPERFUNCTION

Excess secretion of corticosteroids occurs in the context of adrenal hyperplasia or neoplasia (Fig. 21-25). Such hyperfunction may take one of two forms, namely hypercortisolism (Cushing syndrome) or hyperaldosteronism (Conn syndrome). Clinical features of hypercortisolism from any cause are referred to as **Cushing syndrome.** The term **Cushing disease** is restricted to corticotropin-dependent hyperadrenalism.

The most common cause of Cushing syndrome in the United States is long-term administration of corticosteroids in the treatment of immunologic and inflammatory disorders. The second most common cause is a paraneoplastic effect associated with nonpituitary cancers that inappropriately produce corticotropin. Cushing disease is fivefold more frequent than Cushing syndrome associated with adrenal tumors.

Corticotropin-Dependent Adrenal Hyperfunction (Cushing Disease)

Bilateral hyperplasia of the adrenal cortex is found in 85% of the patients with hyperadrenalism, with the exception of those resulting from administration of exogenous corticosteroids. **With few exceptions, adrenal hyperplasia is secondary to chronic stimulation by corticotropin.** Women, usually between 25 and 45 years of age, are five times more likely than men to develop Cushing disease.

☐ **Pathogenesis:** Corticotropin-dependent adrenal hyperfunction results from one of the following:

- **Primary hypersecretion of corticotropin by the pituitary** usually results from corticotrope microadenomas of the pituitary, although a few patients exhibit diffuse corticotrope hyperplasia.
- **Ectopic production of corticotropin by a nonpituitary tumor** accounts for most cases of corticotropin-dependent hyperadrenalism. Cancer of the lung, particularly small cell carcinoma, is responsible for more than half of the cases of ectopic corticotropin syndrome. The remaining cases are attributable principally to carcinoids and neural crest tumors (pheochromocytoma, neuroblastoma, medullary carcinoma of the thyroid), thymoma, and islet cell adenoma of the pancreas.
- **Inappropriate secretion of corticotropin-releasing hormone** (CRH) may occur in tumors arising outside the hypothalamus, with secondary pituitary hypersecretion of corticotropin. Ectopic production of CRH has been reported in patients with

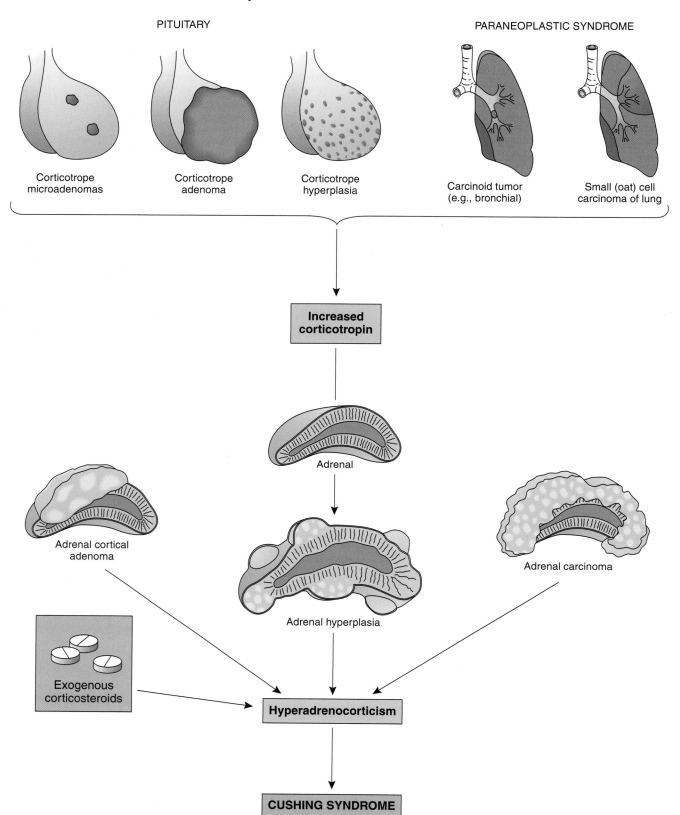

PITUITARY

Corticotrope microadenomas

Corticotrope adenoma

Corticotrope hyperplasia

PARANEOPLASTIC SYNDROME

Carcinoid tumor (e.g., bronchial)

Small (oat) cell carcinoma of lung

Increased corticotropin

Adrenal

Adrenal cortical adenoma

Adrenal hyperplasia

Adrenal carcinoma

Exogenous corticosteroids

Hyperadrenocorticism

CUSHING SYNDROME

FIGURE 21-25
Pathogenetic pathways of Cushing syndrome. The corticotropin-dependent pathway is referred to as Cushing disease.

medullary carcinoma of the thyroid, adenocarcinoma of the prostate, bronchial carcinoid, and intrasellar gangliocytoma.

□ **Pathology:** Cushing disease is characterized by bilateral, diffuse (75%) or nodular (25%) hyperplasia of the adrenal glands.

Diffuse adrenal hyperplasia features a grossly visible, broadened cortex that is composed of an inner brown layer and a yellow, lipid-rich cap. Microscopically, the inner one-third of the cortex features a compact cell layer, and the outer zone, which corresponds to the zona fasciculata, displays large, clear cells packed with lipid.

Nodular adrenal hyperplasia is a term reserved for grossly visible nodules as large as 2.5 cm in diameter. Bilateral, multiple nodules compress the overlying cortex, and the intervening parenchyma exhibits diffuse hyperplasia. Microscopically, the nodules are composed of large, lipid-laden, clear cells.

Corticotropin-Independent Adrenal Hyperfunction

A functional neoplasm of the adrenal cortex is a well-documented cause of Cushing syndrome. In adults, the incidence of adrenal carcinoma peaks at 40 years of age, and that of adenoma is greatest a decade later. In children, adrenal carcinoma accounts for fully half of the cases of Cushing syndrome, whereas adenoma comprises 15%. At all ages, the female:male ratio is 4 : 1.

Adrenal Adenoma

The typical adrenal adenoma is an encapsulated, firm, and yellow mass measuring some 4 cm in diameter (Fig. 21-26). These tumors usually weigh between 10 and 50 g, although weights as great as 100 g have been recorded. On cut section, the surface tends to be mottled yellow and brown. A thin rim of compressed, normal adrenal cortex surrounds the tumor. Necrosis and calcification may be present even in small tumors. Microscopically, adenomas exhibit clear, lipid-laden cells that are arranged in sheets or nests, often with interspersed clusters of compact, lipid-depleted, eosinophilic cells. The nontumorous cortex of the involved and contralateral gland is generally atrophic.

Adrenocortical Carcinoma

Most (80%) adrenocortical carcinomas are functional. They weigh more than 100 g, and weights as great as 5 kg have been recorded. Adrenal carcinomas are soft, encapsulated, lobulated, and bulky tumors (Fig. 21-27). The cut surface has a variegated pink, brown, or yellow color, often with necrosis, hemorrhage, and cystic changes. The tumor commonly invades locally, and remnants of normal adrenal tissue are difficult to identify. Microscopically, both clear and compact cells are present. Varying degrees of nuclear pleomorphism are seen, and mitotic figures and vascular invasion may, or may not, be apparent. In the case of functional carcinomas, the contralateral adrenal cortex is atrophic. Even with surgery, most patients only survive for 1 to 3 years.

Long-Term Administration of Corticosteroids

Today, corticosteroid treatment of a variety of immunologic and inflammatory diseases is by far the most common cause of Cushing syndrome. The synthetic hormones ordinarily employed (e.g., dexamethasone,

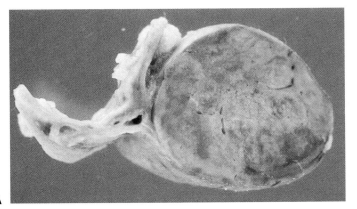
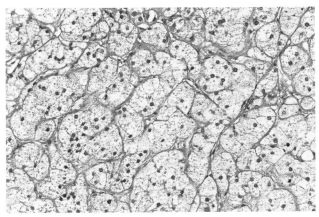

A   B

FIGURE **21-26**
Adrenal adenoma. (A) The cut surface of an adrenal tumor removed from a patient with Cushing syndrome is mottled yellow with a rim of compressed, normal adrenal tissue. (B) A microscopic view reveals nests of clear, lipid-laden cells.

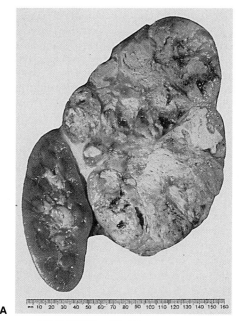
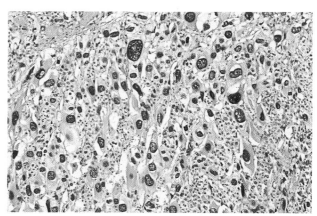

FIGURE *21-27*
Adrenal carcinoma. (A) A bulky, encapsulated tumor showing necrosis, hemorrhage, and cystic change is adherent to the upper pole of the kidney. (B) A microscopic section demonstrates marked anisocytosis and nuclear pleomorphism.

prednisone) have only glucocorticoid activity and little or no mineralocorticoid or androgenic effects. As a result, hypertension and hirsutism, which are commonly seen in patients with Cushing syndrome secondary to adrenal hyperplasia or neoplasia, are usually absent in patients with this iatrogenic disorder.

☐ **Clinical Features:** Clinical manifestations of Cushing syndrome are illustrated in Figure 21-28.

Obesity. Typically, the patient notes a gradual onset of obesity of the face (moon face), neck (buffalo hump), trunk, and abdomen (Fig. 21-29).

Skin. The skin is atrophic, and there is loss of subcutaneous fat. Enlargement of the abdomen and other areas of fat deposition stretches the thin skin and produces purplish striae, which represent venous channels that are visible through the attenuated dermis.

Musculoskeletal System. Increased bone resorption causes osteoporosis. Back pain is a common complaint, and as many as one-fifth of patients with Cushing syndrome have radiologic evidence of compression fractures of the vertebrae. Proximal muscle-wasting steroid myopathy causes weakness, which may be so severe that the patient cannot rise from a sitting position or climb a flight of stairs.

Cardiovascular System. Hypertension is a frequent feature of Cushing syndrome, often reflecting excessive mineralocorticoid activity.

Secondary Sex Characteristics. Females with Cushing syndrome tend to be virilized, showing increased facial hair, thinning of scalp hair, acne, and oligomenorrhea. Excess glucocorticoid levels in men cause impotence and, in both sexes, decreased libido.

Glucose Intolerance. Stimulation of gluconeogenesis by glucocorticoids leads to glucose intolerance and hyperinsulinemia. Diabetes mellitus supervenes in 15% of the patients, usually those with a family history of diabetes.

Psychologic Changes. Irritability, emotional lability, depression, and paranoia (even to the point of suicide) are common complications of Cushing syndrome.

Cushing syndrome is treated by (1) extirpation (surgery or radiation therapy) of pituitary, adrenal, or ectopic corticotropin-producing tumors; (2) discontinuation of corticosteroid therapy; or (3) administration of adrenal enzyme inhibitors (e.g., aminoglutethimide, ketoconazole, metapyrone). At one time, the 5-year mortality rate for patients with Cushing syndrome was 50%, but today, the prognosis is considerably better.

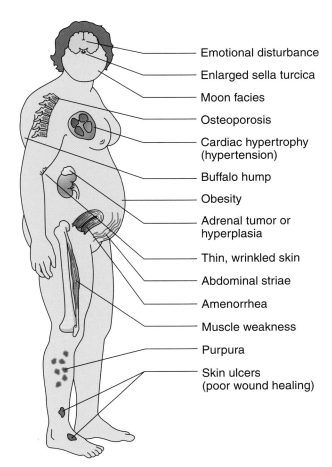

- Emotional disturbance
- Enlarged sella turcica
- Moon facies
- Osteoporosis
- Cardiac hypertrophy (hypertension)
- Buffalo hump
- Obesity
- Adrenal tumor or hyperplasia
- Thin, wrinkled skin
- Abdominal striae
- Amenorrhea
- Muscle weakness
- Purpura
- Skin ulcers (poor wound healing)

FIGURE 21-28
Major clinical manifestations of Cushing syndrome.

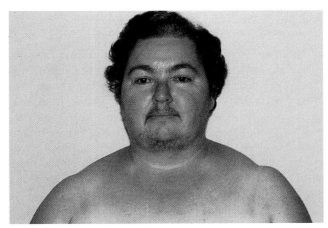

FIGURE 21-29
Cushing syndrome. This woman, who suffered from a pituitary adenoma that produced corticotropin, exhibits a moon face, buffalo hump, and increased facial hair.

With the exception of ectopic corticotropin syndrome and adrenal carcinoma, in which patients die from the cancer rather than from hypercortisolism, Cushing syndrome is highly curable.

Primary Aldosteronism (Conn Syndrome)

■ *Primary aldosteronism (Conn syndrome), which is characterized by hypertension and hypokalemia, is produced by inappropriate secretion of aldosterone by an adrenal adenoma or hyperplastic adrenal glands.* Aldosterone-secreting adenomas are more common in women than in men (3:1) and usually occur in those between 30 and 50 years of age.

☐ **Pathogenesis:** Solitary adrenal adenoma has been reported to account for as many as 90% of the cases of hyperaldosteronism. However, bilateral hyperplasia of the adrenal zona glomerulosa now accounts for as many as half of the cases in some university hospitals, perhaps reflecting a more careful evaluation of patients with hypertension.

Hypersecretion of aldosterone enhances sodium reabsorption by the renal tubules, thereby increasing the total body sodium level. Hypertension is caused not only by retention of sodium and consequent volume expansion but also by increased peripheral vascular resistance. Hypokalemia reflects aldosterone-induced loss of potassium in the distal renal tubule.

☐ **Pathology:** Most aldosterone-secreting adenomas measure less than 3 cm in diameter, weigh less than 6 g, and are yellow in color. However, the size is variable, and tumors as large as 50 g have been reported. On microscopic examination, the dominant cell is clear, lipid-rich, and arranged in cords or alveoli. In contrast to cortisol-producing adenomas, the nontumorous cortex in cases of hyperaldosteronism is not atrophic, because aldosterone does not inhibit corticotropin secretion by the pituitary.

☐ **Clinical Features:** Most patients with primary aldosteronism are diagnosed after the detection of asymptomatic diastolic hypertension. Muscle weakness and fatigue are produced by the effects of potassium depletion on the skeletal muscle. Polyuria and polydipsia result from a disturbance in the concentrating ability of the kidney, which probably occurs secondary to hypokalemia. Metabolic alkalosis and elevation of serum bicarbonate levels reflect the loss of hydrogen ions into the urine and their migration into potassium-depleted cells. Primary aldosteronism caused by an adenoma is cured by the surgical removal of the tumor.

METASTATIC CARCINOMA

Metastatic cancer to the adrenal glands commonly originates from carcinomas of the lung or breast or from malignant melanoma. The glands may be massively enlarged, even to between 20 and 45 g each, either unilaterally or bilaterally. They are largely replaced by carcinoma and often display necrosis and hemorrhage. Usually, enough adrenocortical parenchyma remains to ensure that Addison disease does not develop, particularly considering the limited survival of these patients.

Adrenal Medulla and Paraganglia

The adrenal medulla is entirely contained within the adrenal cortex and accounts for 10% of the weight of the gland. It consists of neuroendocrine cells, termed **chromaffin cells,** which derive from primitive pheochromoblasts of the developing sympathetic nervous system (Fig. 21-30). Chromaffin cells are so named because the catecholamines in their cytoplasmic granules have an affinity for chromium salts and darken on oxidation by potassium dichromate. These cells are also present at extra-adrenal sites of the sympathetic nervous system, such as the preaortic sympathetic plexuses and the paravertebral sympathetic chain.

PHEOCHROMOCYTOMA

■ *Pheochromocytoma is a rare tumor of chromaffin cells of the adrenal medulla that secretes catecholamines.* Such tumors also originate in extra-adrenal sites, in which case they are termed **paraganglioma.**

Pheochromocytomas are somewhat more frequent in women than in men. They are observed at any age, including infancy, although they are uncommon after 60 years. **Presenting symptoms relate to sustained or episodic hypertension.** Pheochromocytoma accounts for less than 0.1% of cases of hypertension, but it remains important to consider this tumor in the evaluation of any patient with hypertension. When detected early, pheochromocytoma is amenable to surgical resection, but when left untreated, the patient dies from the complications of prolonged hypertension.

□ **Pathogenesis:** The majority of pheochromocytomas are sporadic, and the cause is unknown. A minority of cases are familial and arise either alone or as part of the syndromes of MEN-2A and -2B. The gene for MEN-1 has been mapped to chromosome 11 but

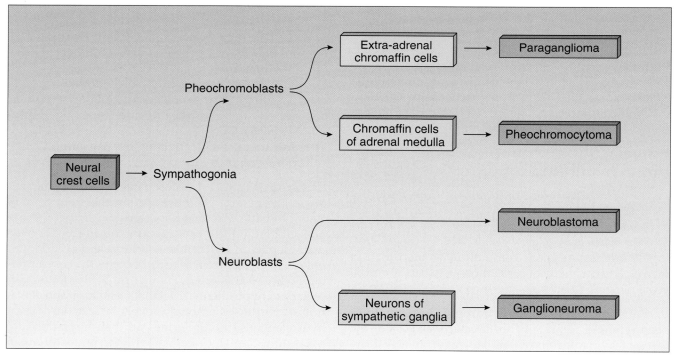

FIGURE   *21-30*
Histogenesis of tumors of the adrenal medulla and extra-adrenal sympathetic nervous system.

has not yet been identified. The *RET* proto-oncogene on chromosome 10, which codes for a receptor of the tyrosine kinase family, is responsible for MEN-2 syndromes. The most common mutation constitutively activates the receptor. The tumor is characterized by frequent deletions on chromosome 1, extrachromosomal double minutes, and homogeneously staining regions (HSRs) on chromosome 2. HSRs represent amplification of N-*myc*, an abnormality that plays a key role in determining the aggressiveness of neuroblastoma. The features of MEN syndromes are:

- **MEN-1 (Wermer syndrome)** includes adenoma of the pituitary, parathyroid hyperplasia or adenoma, and islet cell tumor of the pancreas. Two-thirds of the patients have adenomas of two or more endocrine systems, and one-fifth develop tumors of three or more systems.
- **MEN-2A (Sipple syndrome)** involves the combination of pheochromocytoma, medullary carcinoma of the thyroid, and parathyroid hyperplasia. A variety of neural crest tumors are occasionally seen in patients with MEN-2A, including gliomas, glioblastomas, and meningiomas.
- **MEN-2B** features pheochromocytoma, medullary carcinoma of the thyroid, and mucosal neuroma syndrome (neuromas of the conjunctiva, oral cav-

ity, larynx, and gastrointestinal tract). Mucosal neuromas are always encountered in patients with this syndrome, but only half of the patients express the full phenotype.

Adrenal medullary hyperplasia has been reported in some patients with both MEN-2 syndromes. Similar to C-cell hyperplasia as a precursor of medullary carcinoma of the thyroid, adrenal medullary hyperplasia is thought to antedate pheochromocytoma in these cases.

☐ **Pathology:** In sporadic cases of pheochromocytoma, 80% of the tumors are unilateral, 10% bilateral, and 10% in extra-adrenal locations. By contrast, two-thirds of those occurring in the context of MEN are bilateral. The tumors range in size from small lesions measuring 1 cm across to large masses of more than 2 kg. Most tumors are 5 to 6 cm in diameter and weigh from 80 to 100 g.

Pheochromocytomas tend to be encapsulated, spongy, and reddish masses with prominent central scars, hemorrhage, and foci of cystic degeneration (Fig. 21-31). The histologic appearance is highly variable. Typically, circumscribed nests (zellballen) of neoplastic cells are present. The tumor cells range from polyhedral to fusiform and show a granular, amphophilic or basophilic cytoplasm and vesicular nuclei. Eosinophilic globules are usually seen in the cytoplasm.

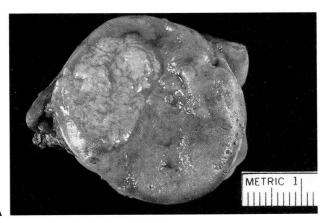

A

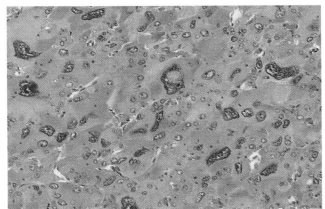

B

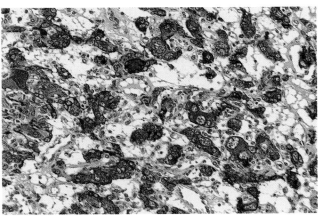

C

FIGURE **21-31**
Pheochromocytoma. (A) The cut surface of an adrenal tumor from a patient with episodic hypertension is reddish brown with a prominent area of fibrosis. Foci of hemorrhage and cystic degeneration are evident. (B) A photomicrograph of the tumor shows polyhedral tumor cells with ample finely granular cytoplasm. Note the enlarged hyperchromatic nuclei. (C) Many of the tumor cells show positive immunohistochemical staining for chromogranin A, a marker of neuroendocrine differentiation.

In 5% to 10% of the cases, pheochromocytoma proves to be malignant, although this figure may be higher for extra-adrenal tumors. There are no reliable histologic criteria with which to distinguish malignant from benign pheochromocytoma, and malignancy is determined only on the basis of the biologic behavior of the tumor, namely metastases. Metastases are most common in the regional lymph nodes, bone, lung, and liver.

☐ **Clinical Features:** Release of catecholamines by the tumor accounts for hypertension, which ranges from an asymptomatic condition to malignant hypertension (e.g., encephalopathy, papilledema, proteinuria). Episodic catecholamine release may lead to a paroxysm or crisis that is characterized by severe and throbbing headache, sweating, palpitations, tachycardia, abdominal pain, and vomiting. Elevated blood pressure, often to an extreme degree, is characteristic.

More than 90% of the patients with pheochromocytoma exhibit hypertension, which is sustained in two-thirds of the patients and is similar to essential hypertension. In one-third of the patients, the hypertension is only episodic but frequently becomes sustained.

Pheochromocytoma is diagnosed on the basis of finding increased urinary levels of catecholamine metabolites, particularly vanillylmandelic acid, metanephrine, and unconjugated catecholamines. The definitive treatment for pheochromocytoma is surgical extirpation of the tumor.

Paraganglioma

■ *Paragangliomas are pheochromocytomas that develop in paraganglia other than the adrenal medulla.* They arise in the retroperitoneum along the abdominal aorta, the posterior mediastinum, and the urinary bladder. They may also occur in the base of the skull, in the neck, in vagal or aortic bodies, or in any organ with paraganglionic tissue (e.g., larynx and small intestine). The tumors originate in paraganglia such as the glomus jugulare, carotid body, and other vasoreceptor bodies. **Carotid body tumor** is a prototypic paraganglioma that forms a palpable mass in the neck, which closely surrounds or envelops the carotid vessels. Compared with pheochromocytomas, paragangliomas are more often malignant.

NEUROBLASTOMA

■ *Neuroblastoma is a malignant tumor of neural crest origin that is composed of neoplastic neuroblasts.* It origi-

nates in the adrenal medulla or sympathetic ganglia. **Neuroblastoma is one of the most important malignant tumors of childhood, accounting for as much as 10% of all childhood cancers and 15% of deaths from cancer among children.** The peak incidence occurs during the first 3 years of life. The tumor is congenital in some cases and has even been found in premature stillborns. In fact, neuroblastoma accounts for half of all cancers diagnosed during the first month of life.

☐ **Pathogenesis:** The adrenal glands of fetuses during the third trimester of pregnancy contain microscopic nodules of primitive neuroblasts, which may even invade blood vessels. Persistence and transformation of these embryonal structures may relate to the pathogenesis of neuroblastoma.

☐ **Pathology:** Neuroblastoma can originate in any location at which cells derived from the neural crest are present—that is, from the posterior cranial fossa to the coccyx. One-third of the tumors occur in the adrenal gland, another one-third in other abdominal sites, and 20% in the posterior mediastinum.

Neuroblastomas range in size from minute, barely discernible nodules to tumors that are readily palpable through the abdominal wall. They are round, irregularly lobulated masses and weigh from 50 to 150 g or more (Fig. 21-32). The cut surface is soft and friable, with a variegated, maroon color. Areas of necrosis, hemorrhage, calcification, and cystic change are frequently present as well.

Microscopically, the tumor is composed of dense sheets of small, round to fusiform cells, with hyperchromatic nuclei and scanty cytoplasm, which are often compared with lymphocytes. Mitoses are frequent. Characteristic rosettes are defined by a rim of dark tumor cells in a circumferential arrangement around a central, pale, and fibrillar core. Pseudorosettes featuring tumor cells clustered radially around small vessels are also present. The electron microscopic appearance of neuroblastoma cells is distinctive. The malignant neuroblasts exhibit peripheral dendritic processes containing longitudinally oriented microtubules as well as neurosecretory granules and filaments in the cytoplasm.

Neuroblastomas readily infiltrate the surrounding structures and metastasize to the regional lymph nodes, liver, lungs, bones, and other sites.

☐ **Clinical Features:** The presenting sign of neuroblastoma is often an enlarging abdomen in a young child. Physical examination discloses a firm, irregular, and nontender abdominal mass. The tumor metastasizes to the liver and bones. Neuroblastomas arising in the thorax produce respiratory distress, and tumors

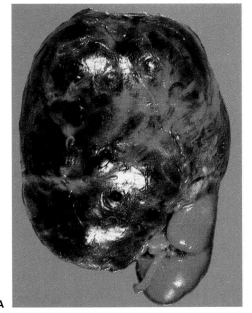 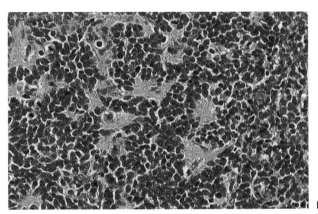

FIGURE   *21-32*
Neuroblastoma. (A) A large, lobulated, hemorrhagic, and cystic tumor adherent to the upper pole of the kidney was removed from a child who presented with an abdominal mass. (B) A photomicrograph illustrates the characteristic rosettes formed by small, regular, and dark tumor cells arranged around a central, pale fibrillar core.

arising in the pelvis obstruct the bowel and ureters. Spinal cord compression may lead to gait disturbance and sphincter dysfunction. Severe diarrhea may result from secretion of vasoactive intestinal peptide by the neuroblastoma.

Urinary excretion of catecholamines and their metabolites is almost invariably elevated in patients with neuroblastoma. The urine contains increased amounts of norepinephrine, vanillylmandelic acid, homovanillic acid, and dopamine.

The prognosis of neuroblastoma is influenced by its extraordinary propensity for spontaneous remission. Moreover, it may differentiate into a more mature, benign tumor—that is, ganglioneuroma. In general, the prognosis depends on the age of the patient and the stage of the tumor. The older the patient and more widespread the tumor, the poorer the prognosis. The catecholamine content of the tumor itself is not as great as that of pheochromocytoma, possibly because neuroblastoma cells metabolize these compounds.

Localized tumors are subjected to surgical resection alone. Patients with disseminated tumor are treated by chemotherapy and, sometimes, radiation therapy. Except for the most widely disseminated tumors, the prognosis for patients with neuroblastoma is good, with the large majority surviving more than 3 years without recurrence.

Ganglioneuroma

■ *Ganglioneuroma is a benign tumor of neural crest origin that occurs in older children and young adults.* It arises in sympathetic ganglia, typically in the posterior mediastinum. As many as 30% of these tumors occur in the adrenal medulla. Ganglioneuroma is the most mature variant of all the neuroblastic tumors.

Ganglioneuromas are well encapsulated and display a myxoid, glistening cut surface. Microscopically, they show well-differentiated, mature ganglion cells, which are associated with scanty spindle cells in a loose and abundant stroma.

Thymus

THYMIC HYPERPLASIA

■ *Thymic hyperplasia* refers to the presence of lymphoid follicles in the thymus, regardless of the size of the gland (Fig. 21-33). The total weight of the thymus is usually within the normal range, although it may also be increased. The follicles contain germinal centers; are composed largely of B lymphocytes, which contain IgM and IgD; and tend to both occupy and distort the medullary zones.

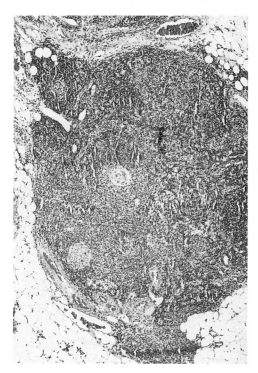

FIGURE *21-33*
Thymic hyperplasia. Lymphoid follicles with germinal centers are observed in this thymus from a patient with myasthenia gravis.

The best-known association of thymic hyperplasia is with **myasthenia gravis,** in which two-thirds of the patients exhibit this thymic abnormality. Thymic follicular hyperplasia may also be found in patients having other diseases in which autoimmunity is believed to play a role, including Graves disease, Addison disease, systemic lupus erythematosus, scleroderma, and rheumatoid arthritis.

THYMOMA

■ *Thymoma is a neoplasm of thymic epithelial cells, which occurs without regard to the presence or number of lymphocytes.* This tumor occurs during adult life, and the large majority (≤ 80%) are benign.

□ **Pathology:** Most thymomas are located in the anterosuperior mediastinum, although a few have been described in other locations with thymic tissue, including the neck, middle and posterior mediastinum, and pulmonary hilus. Benign thymomas are irregularly shaped masses that range from a few centimeters to 15 cm or more in greatest dimension. They are encapsulated, firm, and gray-to-yellow tumors that are divided into lobules by fibrous septa (Fig. 21-34).

On microscopic examination, thymomas consist of a mixture of neoplastic epithelial cells and nontumorous lymphocytes. The proportions of these elements vary among individual cases—and even among different lobules. The epithelial cells are plump or spindle-shaped and show vesicular nuclei. Among those cases in which epithelial cells predominate, they may exhibit an organoid differentiation, including perivascular spaces containing lymphocytes and macrophages, tumor cell rosettes, and whorls suggestive of abortive Hassal corpuscle formation. Many of the accompanying T lymphocytes are small, but others tend to be larger and have prominent vesicular nuclei, which are features suggestive of activation. Mitotic activity of the nonneoplastic lymphocytic component generally exceeds that of the neoplastic epithelial cells.

Myasthenia Gravis. The most conspicuous clinical association of thymoma is with myasthenia gravis: 10% of patients with myasthenia gravis also have thy-

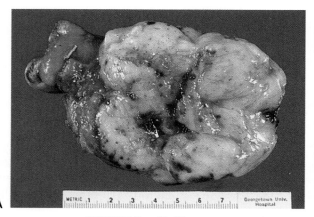
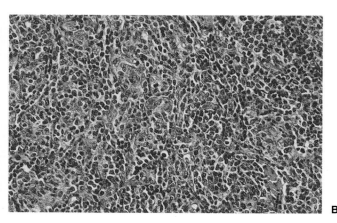

A   B

FIGURE *21-34*
Thymoma. (A) The tumor in cross-section is white-ish and has a bulging surface with areas of hemorrhage. Note the attached portion of normal thymus. (B) Microscopically, the thymoma consists of a mixture of neoplastic epithelial cells and nontumorous lymphocytes.

moma. Conversely, one-third to one-half of the patients with thymoma develop myasthenia gravis.

Other Associated Diseases. Thymoma is also associated with many other immune disorders. More than 10% of patients with thymoma are afflicted with hypogammaglobulinemia, and 5% suffer from erythroid hypoplasia. Other associated diseases include myocarditis, dermatomyositis, rheumatoid arthritis, lupus erythematosus, scleroderma, and Sjögren syndrome. Certain malignant tumors have also been associated with thymoma, including T-cell leukemia/lymphoma and multiple myeloma.

Malignant Thymoma

Roughly one-fourth of thymomas are not encapsulated and exhibit malignant features. Many of these invade locally within the thorax, and a few metastasize widely. Histologically, most malignant thymomas are virtually indistinguishable from encapsulated, benign thymomas. However, they penetrate the capsule, implant on pleural or pericardial surfaces, and may metastasize to the lymph nodes, lung, liver, and bone. An uncommon variant, termed **thymic carcinoma,** takes the form of squamous cell carcinoma, lymphoepithelioma-like carcinoma (identical to that found in the oropharynx), a sarcomatoid variant (carcinosarcoma), and a number of other, rare patterns.

Malignant thymoma is treated by surgical excision and radiation therapy. Chemotherapy is added in cases with distant metastases. The prognosis for patients with benign thymoma is excellent, and the presence or absence of myasthenic symptoms has little prognostic value. In patients with malignant thymomas, the prognosis correlates with the extent of the disease.

Germ Cell Tumors

Germ cell tumors in the thymus account for 20% of all mediastinal tumors. The migration of germ cells during embryogenesis is thought to leave misplaced germ cells in this location that, eventually, give rise to germ cell neoplasms. The spectrum of germ cell tumors in the mediastinum parallels that in the gonads (see Chapters 17 and 18). Mature cystic teratoma is the most common of these thymic tumors. Seminoma, embryonal carcinoma, endodermal sinus tumor, teratocarcinoma, and choriocarcinoma all occur as well. With the exception of mature cystic teratoma, which afflicts both sexes equally, all of the other tumors show a substantial male predilection, and thymic seminoma occurs only in men. In general, the prognosis for these patients is similar to that of patients with comparable gonadal tumors.

CHAPTER 22

Diabetes

John E. Craighead

Diabetes is a complex metabolic derangement that is characterized by either relative or absolute insulin deficiency. The two most common forms of diabetes are currently referred to as insulin-dependent (IDDM; type I) and noninsulin-dependent (NIDDM; type II) diabetes (Table 22-1).

Customarily, IDDM occurs in children and adolescents, but it also can develop in adults. By contrast, most cases of NIDDM appear during the later decades of life, although the disease is sometimes seen in young patients as well. IDDM is uncommon compared with NIDDM, which affects approximately 5% of adult Americans.

INSULIN-DEPENDENT DIABETES MELLITUS

■ *Insulin-dependent diabetes mellitus is characterized by few, if any, functional beta cells in the islets of Langerhans and substantially reduced or nonexistent insulin secretion.* As a result, body fat is metabolized as a source of energy. This oxidation produces ketone bodies (acetoacetic acid and β-hydroxybutyric acid), which are released into the blood and lead to metabolic acidosis. Hyperglycemia and glucosuria produce fluid and electrolyte imbalances, which can ultimately lead to coma and even death (Fig. 22-1). In fact, before insulin became commercially available, IDDM was usually fatal.

☐ **Pathogenesis:**

Genetic Factors. Many believe that susceptibility to IDDM is inherited as an autosomal recessive trait with variable penetrance, although this view is not universally accepted. Fewer than 20% of these patients with diabetes have a parent or sibling with the disease. In studies of identical (monozygotic) twins, in which

one or both were diabetic, both members of the pair were affected in only half of the cases. This lack of concordance suggests that environmental factors may contribute to development of the disease when superimposed on a heritable predisposition.

Of patients with IDDM, 95% express either HLA-DR3, HLA-DR4, or both, compared with only 20% of the general population. Recently, new evidence has pointed to the DQ locus and to point mutations at a specific site, codon 57, in the DQ β-chain domain. Fully 96% of patients with IDDM are homozygous for a mutation at this site that results in a lack of an aspartic acid residue, compared with only 19% of healthy, unrelated persons. Such a mutation could be the basis for an autoimmune response directed against the beta cell.

Autoimmunity. The concept of an autoimmune pathogenesis for IDDM is supported by the observation that patients who die shortly after the onset of disease often exhibit an infiltrate of mononuclear cells both in and around the islets of Langerhans (Fig. 22-2). Considerable evidence now suggests that sensitized cytotoxic T lymphocytes damage the beta cells in patients with IDDM.

Patients have now been successfully treated with drugs that depress cellular immunity, particularly when such agents are administered early in the course of the IDDM. Among patients with IDDM, 10% also manifest other organ-specific autoimmune diseases, including chronic thyroiditis and Graves disease, myasthenia gravis, Addison disease, and pernicious anemia.

Environmental Factors. Recently, viruses and chemicals have been implicated as being causative factors in at least some cases of IDDM. For example, the disease occasionally develops after measles. Group B coxsackieviruses can also infect the islets and result in the abrupt onset of diabetes. In addition, children and young adults who were infected in utero with rubella-

T A B L E   *22-1.*   Comparison of Type I and Type II Diabetes

	Type I	Type II
Age at onset	Usually before 20 years	Usually after 30 years
Type of onset	Abrupt, often severe	Gradual, usually subtle
Usual body weight	Normal	Overweight
Familial (parents or siblings with diabetes)	<20%	>60%
Monozygotic twins	50% discordant	90% concordant
HLA associations	+	0
Islet cell antibodies	+	0
Islet lesions	Early: inflammation Late: atrophy and fibrosis	Fibrosis, amyloid
Beta cells	Markedly reduced	Normal or slightly reduced
Blood insulin	Markedly reduced	Elevated or normal
Clinical management	Insulin and diet	Diet, occasionally drugs and/or insulin

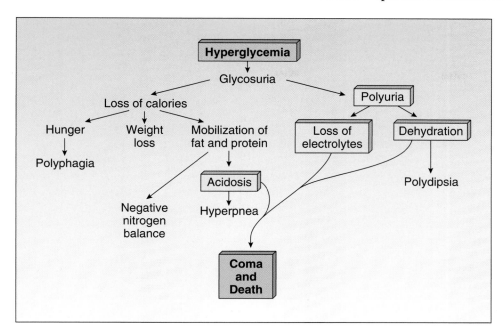

FIGURE 22-1
Symptoms and signs of uncontrolled hyperglycemia in patients with diabetes mellitus.

F I G U R E   *22-1*
Symptoms and signs of uncontrolled hyperglycemia in patients with diabetes mellitus.

virus occasionally develop diabetes, presumably owing to viral injury of the pancreas.

The role of chemicals in the initiation of human IDDM is more problematic, although agents such as alloxan and streptozotocin specifically destroy beta cells in experimental animals and produce acute diabetes. A rodenticide, Vacor, has caused diabetes in humans who have inadvertently consumed it.

Proteins contained in cow's milk may be an environmental trigger for IDDM. Epidemiologic data suggest that breast-fed children have a lower incidence of IDDM than children nurtured on cow's milk. It has been reported that a region of bovine serum albumin is homologous with subunits of major histocompatibility complex class II proteins. Thus, a hypothesis has been

presented that bovine milk proteins provide specific peptides that share antigenic epitopes with human cell surface proteins, thereby eliciting the production of autoreactive antibodies.

□ **Pathology:** In children who suffer the acute onset of IDDM, the most characteristic lesion in the pancreas is an infiltrate of lymphocytes in the islets, which is sometimes accompanied by a few macrophages and neutrophils (see Fig. 22-2). The term **insulitis** has been applied to these changes. As the disease becomes chronic, the beta cells of the islets become progressively depleted and, in many longstanding cases, eventually are no longer discernible. This loss of beta cells results in variably sized islets, many of which appear as ribbon-like cords that are difficult to distinguish from the surrounding acinar tissue. The amyloid deposition that is characteristic of NIDDM, which depends on beta cell secretion, is ordinarily absent.

□ **Clinical Features:** IDDM usually develops during childhood, with the peak incidence occurring at puberty. For this reason, IDDM was familiarly known as juvenile diabetes until a few years ago. However, we now know that some cases develop during the first years of life and a few during the later decades.

The lesions of IDDM develop slowly, and the clinical disease becomes apparent after an average of 3 years, when insulin deprivation becomes severe. It has been estimated that a metabolic abnormality appears only after at least 80% of the beta cells have been eliminated.

In many patients, diabetes is discovered at the time of hospitalization because of the signs and symptoms of metabolic acidosis, weight loss, dehydration, and

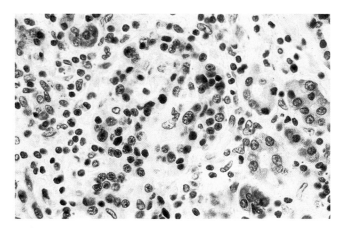

F I G U R E   *22-2*
Insulitis in patients with type I diabetes. A mononuclear inflammatory cell infiltrate is seen in and around the islet.

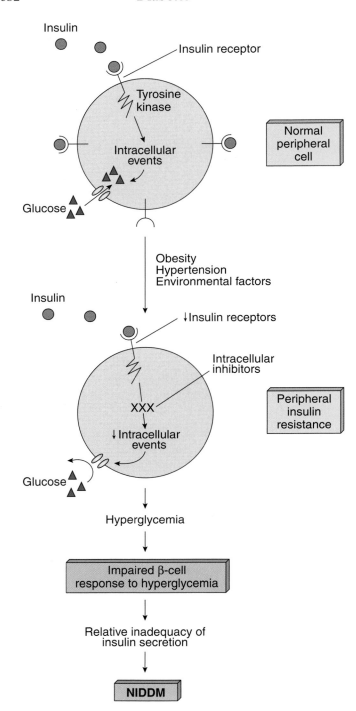

Insulin

Insulin receptor

Tyrosine
kinase

Normal
peripheral
cell

Intracellular
events

Glucose

Obesity
Hypertension
Environmental factors

Insulin

↓Insulin receptors

Intracellular
inhibitors

Peripheral
insulin
resistance

XXX

↓Intracellular
events

Glucose

Hyperglycemia

Impaired β-cell
response to hyperglycemia

Relative inadequacy of
insulin secretion

NIDDM

FIGURE 22-3
Pathogenesis of noninsulin-dependent diabetes mellitus (NIDDM). In the normal peripheral cell (e.g., adipocyte or skeletal muscle cell), the binding of insulin to its receptor activates the tyrosine kinase domain of the latter. In turn, protein phosphorylation leads to an intracellular response that allows glucose to enter the cell. Obesity, hypertension, and other environmental factors down-regulate the insulin receptors. In addition, intracellular inhibitors may interfere with intracellular signaling. As a result, the entry of glucose into the peripheral cell is reduced. The resulting hyperglycemia is normally countered by increased insulin secretion by pancreatic beta cells. In persons with a genetically determined impairment of the beta cell response to hyperglycemia, the secretion of insulin is inadequate to deal with the increased blood sugar, and NIDDM ensues.

electrolyte imbalance. Sometimes, these events occur unexpectedly and precipitously and prove to be life-threatening emergencies. Prominent symptoms include an increase in both urine output (polyuria) and thirst (polydipsia) owing to the diuresis resulting from glucosuria. In addition, many patients have an insatiable appetite (polyphagia) but, nonetheless, lose weight because of the inefficient energy utilization that results from defective carbohydrate metabolism.

NONINSULIN-DEPENDENT DIABETES MELLITUS

■ *Noninsulin-dependent diabetes mellitus is a heterogeneous disorder characterized by impaired insulin secretion and reduced tissue sensitivity to insulin.* Almost 10% of persons older than 65 years of age are affected, and 80% of patients with NIDDM are overweight.

☐ **Pathogenesis:** The current consensus holds that NIDDM is a genetically programmed failure of the beta cells to compensate for peripheral insulin resistance (Fig. 22-3). The pathogenesis of IDDM and NIDDM differs in most respects.

Genetic Factors: Multifactorial inheritance is a key factor in development of NIDDM. Sixty percent of patients have either a parent or a sibling with this disease. In some populations, notably the Pima Indians of Arizona and the natives of Nauru in the Gilbert Islands of the Pacific, one-third to one-half of all persons are afflicted with NIDDM. When one member of a monozygotic twinship has the disease, the second twin is almost invariably affected. However, an association with genes of the major histocompatibility complex, similar to that occurring in patients with IDDM, is not found. Despite the high familial prevalence of the disease, the precise mode of inheritance remains to be defined. Constitutional factors such as obesity and amount of exercise influence the expression of the condition and, thus, confuse genetic analyses.

Glucose Metabolism. Alterations in the metabolism of glucose appear to be critical factors in the development of NIDDM. In a normal person, the extracellular concentration of glucose is exquisitely controlled, even though the amount of exogenous glucose fluctuates and its utilization varies. This rigid control is mediated by the opposing actions of insulin and glucagon. Following a carbohydrate-rich meal, absorption of glucose from the gut leads to a hyperglycemia limited to 10 mM glucose; the fasting level of 5 mM glucose is restored within 2 hours. This response reflects stimulation of insulin secretion by the pancreatic beta cells and insulin-mediated increase in glucose uptake by the peripheral cells, principally adipose and muscle tissue. At the same time, insulin inhibits hepatic glucose production by antagonizing the release of glucagon from the islets and by blocking its effect on the liver. Persons with NIDDM manifest impaired insulin release by the β-cell in response to glucose stimulation. Despite this defect in insulin secretion, many patients with NIDDM exhibit an increased insulin concentration in the blood. This paradoxical situation is attributed to a reduction in the number of insulin receptors in the plasma membranes of the adipocytes and skeletal muscle cells. Thus, patients with NIDDM are hyperglycemic. Their cells are deficient in insulin, however, and they metabolize glucose inefficiently (see Fig. 22-3).

☐ **Pathology:** A variety of microscopic lesions are found in the islets of Langerhans of many, but not all, patients with NIDDM. Unlike IDDM, there is no consistent reduction in the number of beta cells, and no

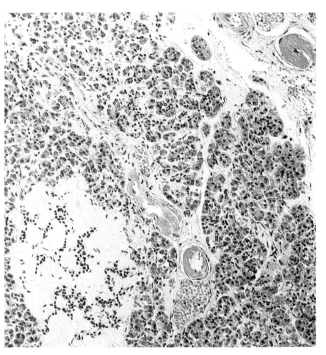

FIGURE 22-4

Amyloidosis (hyalinization) of an islet in the pancreas of a patient with type II diabetes. The blood vessel adjacent to the islet shows the advanced hyaline arteriosclerosis characteristic of diabetes.

morphologic lesions of these cells have been identified by light or electron microscopy.

In some islets, fibrous tissue accumulates, sometimes to such a degree that the islets are obliterated. In other patients, amyloid is present (Fig. 22-4), particularly in those older than 60 years of age. This type of amyloid is composed of a polypeptide molecule known as amylin, which is secreted with insulin by the beta cells (see Chapter 23).

COMPLICATIONS OF DIABETES

It is generally accepted that the development of secondary lesions in patients with diabetes (Fig. 22-5) relates largely to the severity and chronicity of hyperglycemia. From a practical perspective, control of blood glucose remains the major means by which development of diabetic complications can be minimized. Two distinct mechanisms have been proposed to account for the development of many of these changes.

Protein Glycosylation. Glucose binds to a wide variety of proteins, roughly in proportion to the degree of hyperglycemia. Protein adducts are found in hemoglobin, components of the crystalline lens, collagens,

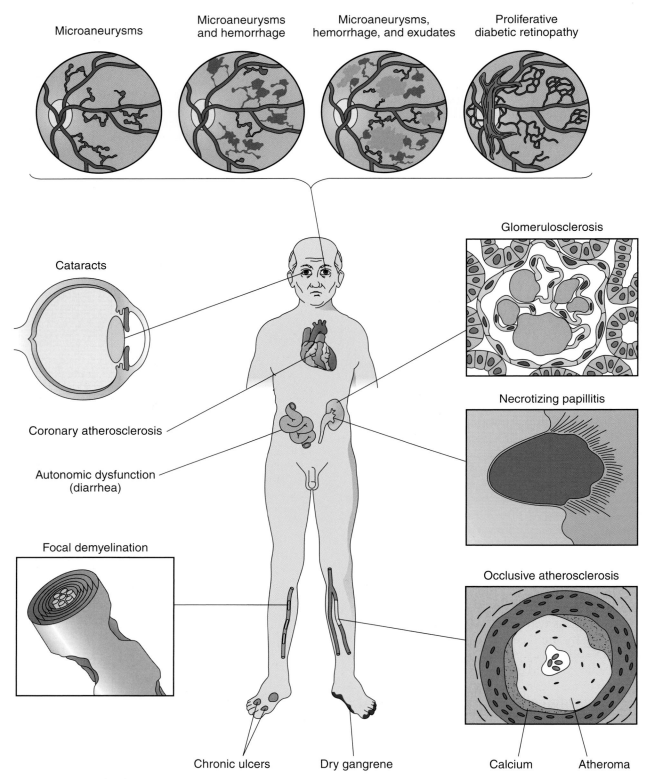

Microaneurysms

Microaneurysms and hemorrhage

Microaneurysms, hemorrhage, and exudates

Proliferative diabetic retinopathy

Glomerulosclerosis

Cataracts

Coronary atherosclerosis

Autonomic dysfunction (diarrhea)

Necrotizing papillitis

Focal demyelination

Occlusive atherosclerosis

Chronic ulcers

Dry gangrene

Calcium

Atheroma

FIGURE 22-5

Secondary complications of diabetes. The effects of diabetes on a number of vital organs result in complications that may be incapacitating (cerebral and peripheral vascular disease), painful (neuropathy), or even life-threatening (coronary artery disease, pyelonephritis with necrotizing papillitis).

myelin, fibrinogen, fibrin, cathepsin B, and antithrombin III. With time, these labile adducts undergo complex chemical rearrangements to form stable **advanced glycosylation products,** which not only inactivate the function of the proteins to which they are bound but also participate in the cross-linking of other proteins. This cross-linking of proteins is believed to contribute to the characteristic thickening of the vascular basement membranes in patients with diabetes.

The Polyol Pathway. Hyperglycemia also increases the uptake of glucose in tissues that are not dependent on insulin. The increased flux of glucose is handled by a number of metabolic pathways, of which the polyol pathway is the best characterized:

$$\text{glucose} + NADH + H^+ \xrightarrow{\text{aldose reductase}} \text{sorbitol} + NAD^+$$

Accumulation of sorbitol is suspected to be responsible for diabetic complications in a variety of tissues, including the peripheral nerves, retina, lens, aorta, and kidney. In the lens, accumulation of sorbitol may simply create an osmotic gradient, which, in turn, causes an influx of fluid and consequent swelling. Sorbitol may also be directly toxic. In experimental diabetic animals, drugs that inhibit aldose reductase also prevent the development of cataracts, retinal damage, peripheral neuropathy, and early functional derangements in the kidney. However, similar studies in humans have been inconclusive.

Atherosclerosis

Both the extent and severity of atherosclerotic lesions in large- and medium-size arteries are increased in patients with longstanding diabetes, and their development tends to be accelerated. As a result, atherosclerotic coronary heart disease is the major cause of death among adults with diabetes. Occlusions of the cerebral blood vessels, with resulting infarcts of the brain, are also common complications of diabetes. The vasculature of the lower extremities is compromised in many patients, and inadequate perfusion of the legs during exercise presents as the muscular pain of intermittent claudication. Vascular insufficiency also leads to ulcers and gangrene of the toes and feet, which are complications that ultimately necessitate amputation. Indeed, diabetes accounts for 40% of nontraumatic limb amputations in the United States today.

Diabetic Microvascular Disease

Hyaline arteriolosclerosis (see Fig. 22-4) and **capillary basement membrane thickening** are characteristic

vascular changes in patients with diabetes. Hypertension, when present, certainly contributes to development of the arteriolar lesions. In addition, increased deposition of basement membrane proteins occurs in patients with diabetes. Moreover, basement membrane proteins may also become glycosylated. Finally, aggregation of platelets in small vascular structures and impaired fibrinolytic mechanisms have also been suggested to play a role in the pathogenesis of diabetic microvascular disease.

Whatever the pathogenetic processes, the effects of disease in small vessels on both tissue perfusion and wound healing are profound. For example, microvascular disease is believed to reduce the flow of blood to the heart, which is already compromised by coronary atherosclerosis. Healing of the chronic ulcers that often develop from trauma and infection of the feet in patients with diabetes is commonly defective, in part because of microvascular disease. The major complications of diabetic microvascular disease, however, involve the kidney and the retina.

Diabetic Nephropathy

Of patients with IDDM, 30% to 40% ultimately develop renal failure. A somewhat smaller proportion of patients with NIDDM are similarly affected. The prevalence of diabetic nephropathy increases with the severity and duration of the hyperglycemia. Blacks with diabetes develop renal failure two- to threefold more often than whites with diabetes. Kidney disease caused by diabetes is now the most common reason for renal transplantation among adults.

The glomeruli in the kidney of patients with diabetes exhibit a unique form of sclerosis (Fig. 22-6), a lesion referred to as **Kimmelstiel-Wilson disease** or **diabetic glomerulosclerosis** (see Chapter 16). The mechanism whereby this unique lesion forms is not known, but ultimately, alterations of the glomerular tuft and its vasculature account for the progressive renal insufficiency.

The cause of diabetic nephropathy is unknown, but changes in the chemical composition of basement membrane components and renal hyperperfusion have been suggested as being causative factors. Regardless of the underlying mechanism, strict control of blood glucose levels will unquestionably retard development of diabetic nephropathy.

Diabetic Retinopathy

Diabetes is a leading cause of blindness. Ten percent of patients with IDDM of 30 years' duration are legally blind. Diabetic retinopathy is the most devastating

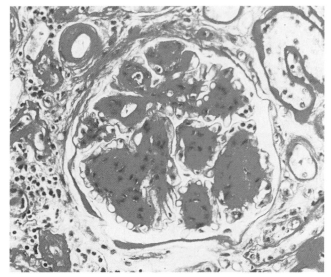

FIGURE 22-6
Diabetic glomerulosclerosis. A periodic acid-Schiff–stained section demonstrates nodular accumulations of basement membrane–like material in the glomerulus.

complication, although glaucoma, cataracts, and corneal disease occur with increased frequency in these patients (see Chapter 29). The prevalence of retinopathy relates to both the duration and control of diabetes.

Peripheral Neuropathy

Peripheral sensory and autonomic nerve dysfunction is one of the most common and distressing complications of diabetes. Because the symptoms are largely subjective and variable in their expression, it is difficult to quantitate the prevalence of this disorder. Changes in the nerves are complex, and abnormalities in the axons, myelin sheath, and Schwann cells have all been found. In addition, disease of the small blood vessels of the nerves contributes to the disorder.

Peripheral neuropathy is characterized by pain and abnormal sensations in the extremities. Fine touch, pain detection, and proprioception are ultimately lost. As a result, the patients with diabetes tends to ignore irritation and minor trauma to the feet, joints, and lower extremities. Thus, peripheral neuropathy can be a major factor in development of ulcers of the feet, which so commonly plague patients with severe diabetes. It also plays a role in the painless destructive joint disease that occasionally occurs.

Infections

Bacterial and mycotic infections complicate the lives of patients with diabetes in whom hyperglycemia is poorly controlled. Multiple abnormalities in the host response to microbial invasion have been described in such patients. Leukocyte function is compromised, and immune responses are blunted. During the preinsulin era, tuberculosis and purulent infections were life-threatening. Today, with good control, the patient with diabetes is much less susceptible to infections. However, urinary tract infections continue to pose a problem, in part because a dystonic bladder retains urine. Pyelonephritis is a constant threat for the patient with diabetes. Necrotizing papillitis may be a devastating complication of renal infection.

CHAPTER 23

Amyloidosis

Robert Kisilevsky

Amyloid **is a generic term that refers to a group of diverse, extracellular protein deposits that have (1) common morphologic properties, (2) affinities for specific dyes, and (3) a characteristic appearance under polarized light.** Although amyloid proteins vary in their amino acid sequence, all amyloid proteins are folded in such as way as to share common ultrastructural and physical properties.

Amyloid deposits are composed of at least three constituents:

- **A disease-specific fibrillary protein,** the nature of which varies with the underlying disease. The specific fibrillary protein in various types of amyloid is the determining factor in the classification of amyloid.
- **Amyloid P component (AP),** which consists of stacks of a pentagonal, doughnut-shaped protein. AP is derived from a normal circulating serum protein, which is termed *serum amyloid P component (SAP).*
- **Other molecular building blocks of basement membranes** are present in amyloid, including laminin, collagen type IV, and perlecan (a proteoglycan). The glycosaminoglycan side chain of perlecan is heparan sulfate, which provides the iodine-staining properties of amyloid.
- **Apolipoprotein E,** which is a normal constituent of high-density lipoproteins and plays a role in cholesterol transport, is present in amyloid.

It is important to emphasize that not all amyloids are the same, and that the protein responsible for the fibrillary characteristics varies significantly. For example, in amyloid associated with multiple myeloma, the fibrillary component is a product of immunoglobulin light chains produced by myeloma cells. In amyloid associated with inflammatory diseases, the fibrillary component is derived from the amino terminal two-thirds of an acute-phase protein, which is produced by the liver and is unrelated to immunoglobulins. In these two cases, amyloid is deposited systemically.

In other situations, amyloid is deposited only locally. Amyloid in medullary carcinoma of the thyroid is restricted to the tumor deposits, and its fibrillary component is derived from a polypeptide hormone that is related to calcitonin. In the pancreas, amyloid located either in an islet cell tumor or in the islets in type II diabetes is derived from a peptide hormone that is secreted with insulin (amylin).

Thus, amyloidosis is characterized by proteinaceous tissue deposits that have common morphologic, structural, and staining properties but variable protein composition.

DEFINITION OF AMYLOID

The staining and structural properties of amyloid allow for a general definition based primarily on its morphologic characteristics:

- All amyloid stains positively with Congo red and shows red-green birefringence when viewed under polarized light (Fig. 23-1).
- Ultrastructurally, all forms of amyloid consist of interlacing bundles of parallel arrays of fibrils, which have a diameter of 7 to 13 nm.
- Protein in the amyloid fibrils contains a large proportion of crossed, β-pleated sheet structure.

CLINICAL CLASSIFICATION OF AMYLOIDOSIS

The most common classification of amyloidosis is based on the clinical presentation of the patient.

■ *Primary amyloidosis refers to the appearance of amyloid de novo—that is, without any preceding disease.* In one-third of these cases, primary amyloidosis is the harbinger of frank **plasma cell neoplasia,** such as multiple myeloma or other B-cell lymphomas.

■ *Secondary amyloidosis is a complication of a previously existing,* **chronic inflammatory disorder,** *which may or may not have an immunologic basis.* Patients with rheumatoid arthritis, ankylosing spondylitis, and occasionally, systemic lupus erythematosus may develop secondary amyloidosis. Most other patients with secondary amyloidosis have conditions that are complicated by longstanding inflammation (e.g., lung abscess, tuberculosis, or osteomyelitis). Secondary amyloidosis is also seen in patients with specific cancers, such as Hodgkin's disease and renal cell carcinoma.

■ *Familial Mediterranean fever is an autosomal recessive disease characterized by polymorphonuclear leukocyte dysfunction and recurrent episodes of serositis, including peritonitis.* It is found predominantly in the Mediterranean basin among Jews, Turks, Armenians, and Arabs. Because there is recurrent inflammation, the type of amyloid protein deposited is the same as that in amyloidosis secondary to acquired inflammatory disorders. The gene for Mediterranean fever has been mapped to the short arm of chromosome 16; it encodes a protein that is expressed in neutrophils. The gene product is thought to be a transcription factor that regulates other genes in the suppression of inflammation.

The isolated forms of amyloidosis tend to involve single-organ systems.

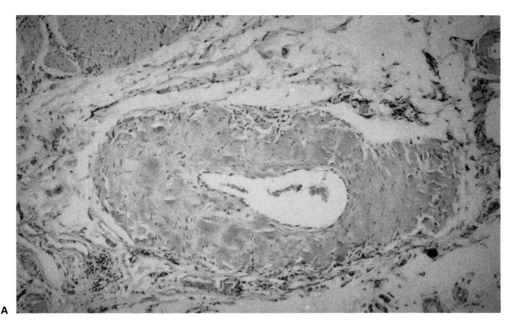

A

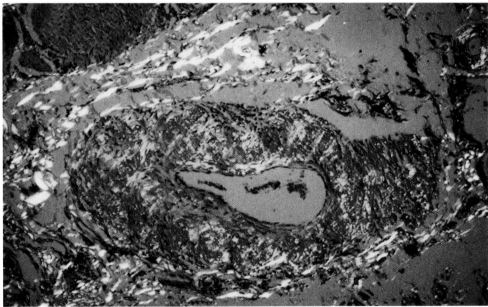

B

FIGURE *23-1*
AL amyloid involving the wall of an artery and stained with Congo red. The appearance under ordinary light (A) and polarized light (B) is shown. Note the red-green birefringence of the amyloid. Collagen has a silvery appearance.

Alzheimer Disease. In this widespread form of dementia, the amyloid (Aβ) is restricted to the brain and its vessels. The deposited β-protein is a fragment of a larger precursor (βPP), which is a normal constituent of the cell membrane. Mutations adjacent to the cleavage sites at the amino and carboxy terminal ends of β-protein are associated with several familial forms of Alzheimer disease, suggesting that amyloid is important in the pathogenesis of this malady.

Down Syndrome. The morphologic lesions that are characteristic of Alzheimer disease also occur in all patients with Down syndrome by 35 years of age. The senile plaques and cerebral blood vessels of Down syndrome contain the same β-amyloid protein found in patients with Alzheimer disease.

Diabetes. The amyloid deposited in the islets of Langerhans in type II diabetes is derived from a larger precursor, namely a peptide related to a variant of calcitonin, that is termed **islet amyloid polypeptide** or **amylin.** This novel hormone, like insulin, is produced by the beta cells of the islets of Langerhans.

Senile Cardiac Amyloidosis. Isolated amyloid deposition, which is derived from transthyretin, may oc-

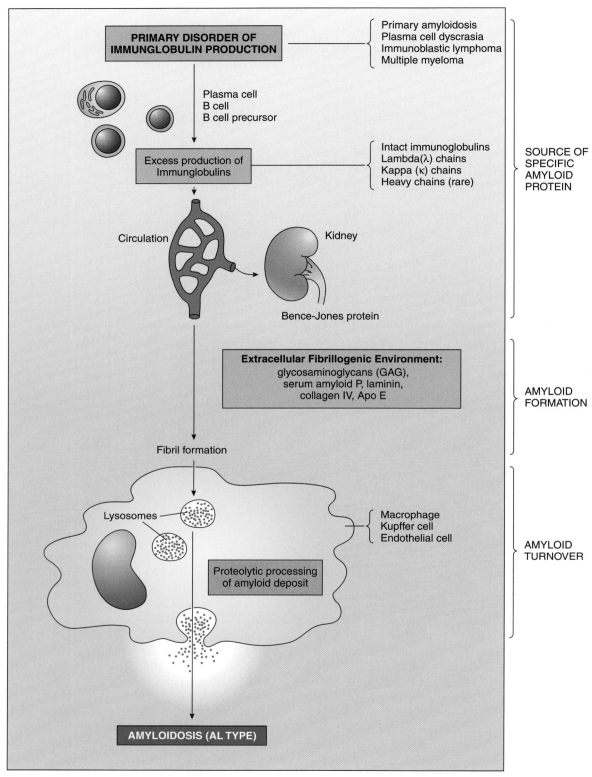

FIGURE   23-2
Mechanism of AL amyloid deposition.

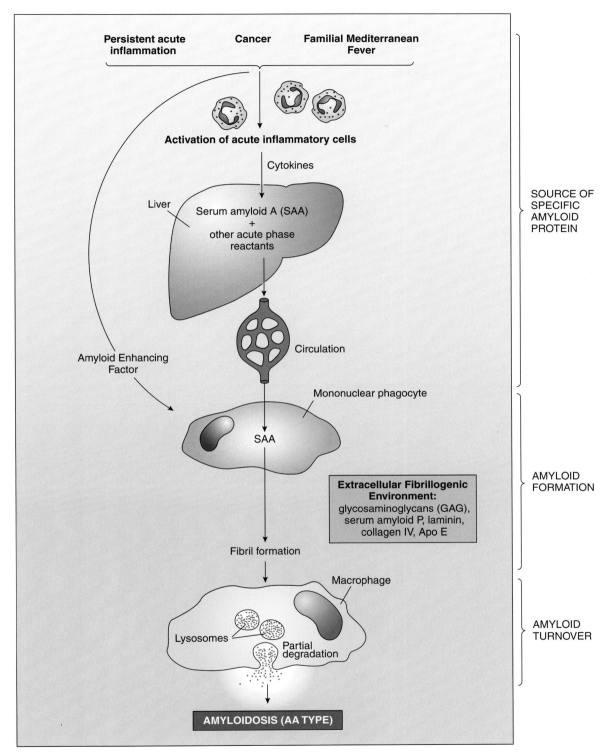

FIGURE   23-3

The mechanism of AA amyloid deposition. A variety of diseases is associated with the activation of polymorphonuclear leukocytes and macrophages, which, in turn, leads to the synthesis and release of acute phase reactants by the liver, including SAA. SAA in the presence of amyloid-enhancing factor (AEF) is likely released substantially intact by mononuclear phagocytes where, in a fibrillogenic environment, the released product complexes with glycosaminoglycans and SAP, as AA amyloid. This deposit is then processed by macrophages.

cur in the heart, particularly in men, after the age of 70 years. This disorder is usually asymptomatic.

Classification of Amyloidosis by Protein Type

The various amyloid proteins are designated as A (amyloid) followed by a letter or a word that refers to the specific origin of the protein.

AL Amyloid

AL amyloid usually consists of the variable region of immunoglobulin light chains (L = light) and can be derived from either the kappa or lambda moieties. Within an individual patient, the sequence of AL amyloid protein is constant, regardless of the organ from which the amyloid is isolated. Because AL amyloid represents the variable region of light chains (and, on rare occasions, portions of heavy chains), AL amyloid isolated from different patients differs in its amino acid sequence. AL protein is common to primary amyloidosis and amyloidosis associated with either multiple myeloma or B-cell lymphomas. However, only 10% to 15% of patients with multiple myeloma develop AL

amyloid. The mechanisms by which AL amyloid is deposited are summarized in Figure 23-2.

AA Amyloid

AA amyloid is derived from an acute-phase protein and is common to a host of seemingly unrelated, chronic inflammatory, neoplastic, and hereditary disorders that lead clinically to so-called secondary amyloidosis (Fig. 23-3). The 76 amino acids of the AA protein correspond to the amino terminal two-thirds of a naturally occurring serum protein called serum amyloid A (SAA). The serum concentration of SAA, an acute-phase protein, rapidly increases by as much as 1000-fold during any inflammatory process. In contrast to AL protein, the amino acid sequence of AA proteins is identical in all patients, regardless of the underlying disorder.

Persistent acute inflammation in animals induces not only the synthesis of the amyloid precursor SAA but also the appearance of a protein termed **amyloid-enhancing factor** (AEF). In such animals, amyloid deposition does not occur without the concomitant presence of AEF.

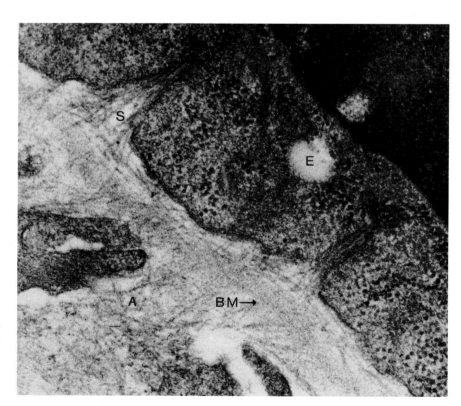

F I G U R E   *23-4*
Electron micrograph of glomerular amyloid (A) illustrating its location relative to the basement membrane (BM). Amyloid spicules (S) extend into the cytoplasm of the glomerular epithelial cells (E).

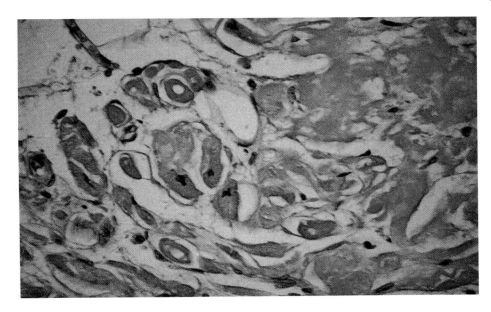

FIGURE 23-5
Myocardial amyloid (AL type). Note the encroachment on and strangulation of the individual myocardial fibers.

MORPHOLOGIC FEATURES OF AMYLOIDOSIS

Amyloid fibrils, when first deposited, are usually in close association with subendothelial basement membranes (Fig. 23-4). Regardless of whether amyloid is laid down in a systemic or a local fashion, the deposits tend to occur between parenchymal cells and their blood supply. Extension of these deposits eventually entraps the parenchymal cells, interferes with their nutrition, and leads to their strangulation and atrophy (Fig. 23-5).

CLINICAL FEATURES OF AMYLOIDOSIS

The symptomatology of amyloidosis is governed by both the underlying disease and the type of protein that is deposited.

Kidney. Patients with multiple myeloma, chronic and longstanding inflammatory disorders, or familial Mediterranean fever who develop nephrotic syndrome should be suspected of having amyloidosis.

Progressive glomerular obliteration may, ultimately, lead to renal failure and uremia.

Heart: Amyloid involvement of the myocardium should be suspected in patients with systemic forms of amyloidosis, in which congestive failure or cardiomegaly is associated with low voltage on the electrocardiogram. Entrapment of the conduction system may lead to arrhythmias, which, in turn, can result in sudden death.

Gastrointestinal Tract. The ganglia, smooth muscle vasculature, and submucosa of the gastrointestinal tract may all be involved by amyloid. Patients may complain of either constipation or diarrhea, occasionally in association with malabsorption.

In all systemic forms of amyloidosis, the course of the disease is usually unremitting and, ultimately, fatal. Patients with myeloma and AL amyloidosis generally die within 1 to 2 years, either from the malignancy itself or from the cardiac or renal complications of amyloidosis. Patients with AA amyloidosis secondary to longstanding inflammatory disease have a more protracted course, but death may be expected within 5 years of the diagnosis, usually from cardiac or renal failure.

CHAPTER 24

The Skin

Terence J. Harrist
Brian Schapiro
Timothy R. Quinn
Wallace H. Clark

Psoriasis

Pemphigus Vulgaris

Erythema Multiforme

Systemic Lupus Erythematosus

Urticaria and Angioedema

Melanocytic Neoplasia

Initial Lesion: Common Acquired Melanocytic Nevus

Melanocytic Nevus with Dysplasia

Intermediate Lesion: Radial Growth-Phase Melanoma

Vertical Growth-Phase Melanoma

Metastatic Melanoma

Verrucae

Benign Keratoses

Seborrheic Keratosis

Actinic Keratosis

Keratoacanthoma

Basal Cell Carcinoma

Squamous Cell Carcinoma

The skin serves as a protective barrier and is also vital in regulating temperature and protecting against ultraviolet (UV) radiation. A wide variety of sensory receptors communicates details related to the immediate environment. The skin also plays a role in immune regulation. Epidermal keratinocytes secrete prostaglandins, leukotrienes, and interleukin-1. The dendritic antigen-presenting cells of the skin, the Langerhans cells, express HLD-DR antigen, Fc, and complement receptors on their surface. Other cutaneous cells of immunologic importance include mast cells, lymphocytes, and macrophages.

PSORIASIS

■ *Psoriasis is a chronic, frequently familial disease characterized by large, erythematous, and scaly plaques, commonly on the extensor dorsal cutaneous surfaces.* The disorder is worldwide in distribution and affects 1% to 2% of the population. It may arise at any age and shows a peak incidence during late adolescence. Interestingly, the disease is absent among Native Americans and has a low incidence among Asians.

☐ **Pathogenesis:** The pathogenesis of psoriasis is poorly understood and may be multifactorial.

Genetic Factors. Psoriasis unquestionably has a genetic component, although only one-third of the patients with psoriasis have a positive family history for the disease. The genetic basis for psoriasis rests on a number of observations, including (1) an increased incidence of the disease among the relatives and offspring of patients with psoriasis, (2) a 65% concordance for psoriasis in monozygotic twins, and (3) an increased occurrence of certain HLA haplotypes in affected persons. HLA-B13, HLA-B17, HLA-Bw16, and particularly, HLA-Cw6 are all increased. In fact, persons with the HLA-Cw6 phenotype are 10- to 15-fold more likely to develop psoriasis than is the general population.

Environmental Factors. In patients with psoriasis, the entire skin, both in areas with lesions and in those without, is abnormal. A variety of stimuli, such as physical injury, infection, certain drugs, and photosensitivity, may produce psoriatic lesions in apparently normal skin.

Abnormal Cellular Proliferation. Although there is no universally accepted explanation for this unique response to injury, evidence suggests that a deregulation of epidermal proliferation and an abnormality in the microcirculation of the dermis are responsible (Fig. 24-1). Decreased activity of adenylyl cyclase in the lower proliferative compartment of the epidermis has been attributed to faulty β-adrenergic receptors. The consequent decrease in cyclic adenosine monophosphate (cAMP) alters cutaneous responses to trauma in complex ways that are not yet fully understood.

Microcirculatory Changes. The capillary loops of the dermal papillae become venular, showing multiple layers of basal lamina material, wide lumina, and "bridged" fenestrations between the endothelial cells. The vascular change, which occurs in concert with a striking increase in neutrophilic chemotactic factors, leads to diapedesis of many neutrophils at the tips of dermal papillae and subsequent migration into the epidermis. This unusual pattern of neutrophilic inflammation is responsible for the dense collections of neutrophils in the stratum corneum (**Munro microabscesses**) as well as for the scattering of neutrophils throughout the epidermis (spongiform pustules).

☐ **Pathology:** The epidermis in patients with psoriasis is thickened and displays both hyperkeratosis and parakeratosis. Parakeratosis may present as circumscribed, ellipsoidal foci, or it may be diffuse, in which case the granular layer is diminished or even absent. The nucleated layers of the epidermis are thickened severalfold in the rete pegs and, frequently, are thinner over the dermal papillae (Fig. 24-2). In turn, the papillae are elongated and appear as sections of cones, with their apices toward the dermis. In chronic lesions, the papillae tend to appear as bulbous clubs with short handles. The rete ridges of the epidermis have a profile reciprocal to that of the dermal papillae, thereby producing interlocked mesenchymal and epithelial clubs with alternatively reversed polarity. The capillaries of the papillae are dilated and tortuous.

Neutrophils may become localized in the epidermal spinous layer or in small Munro microabscesses in the stratum corneum, and they may be associated with circumscribed areas of parakeratosis. The dermis below the papillae exhibits a varying number of mononuclear inflammatory cells, mostly lymphocytes, about the superficial vascular plexus. There is little extension of the inflammatory process into the subjacent reticular dermis.

☐ **Clinical Features:** Psoriasis is a disease of intermittent activity and variable presentation. The severity of the disorder varies from annoying, scaly lesions over the elbows to a serious, debilitating disorder involving most of the skin and often associated with arthritis. A single lesion of psoriasis may be a small focus of scaly erythema or an enormous, confluent plaque covering much of the trunk. A typical plaque is 4 to 5 cm in diameter, is sharply demarcated at its mar-

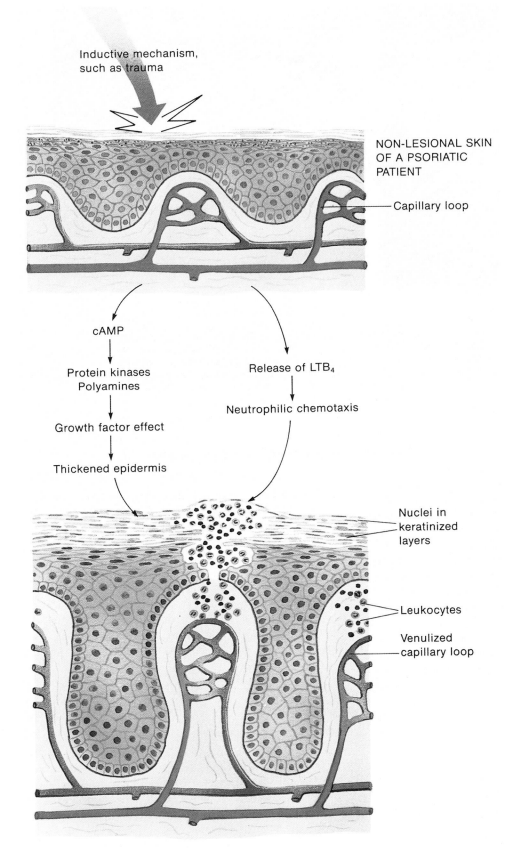

Inductive mechanism,
such as trauma

NON-LESIONAL SKIN
OF A PSORIATIC
PATIENT

Capillary loop

cAMP

Protein kinases
Polyamines

Release of LTB$_4$

Growth factor effect

Neutrophilic chemotaxis

Thickened epidermis

Nuclei in
keratinized
layers

Leukocytes

Venulized
capillary loop

FIGURE *24-1*
Pathogenetic mechanisms in psoriasis. This drawing depicts the deregulation of epidermal growth, the venulization of the capillary loop, and a unique form of neutrophilic inflammation. The altered epidermal growth is thought to result from defective epidermal cell surface receptors. In turn, this results in a decrease in cyclic adenosine monophosphate (cAMP), together with the effects indicated. The decrease in cAMP also likely relates to the increased production of arachidonic acid, which leads to activation of leukotriene B$_4$. This potent, neutrophilic chemotactic agent acts on a venulized capillary loop. Neutrophils then emerge from the tips of the capillary loop at the apex of the dermal papilla rather than from the postcapillary venule, as is the rule in most inflammatory skin diseases.

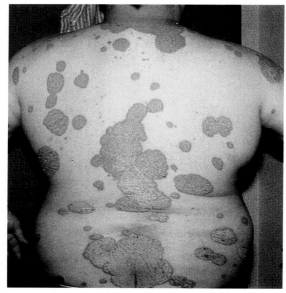 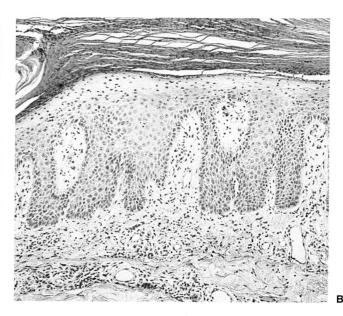

FIGURE 24-2
Psoriasis is the prototype of psoriasiform epidermal hyperplasia. (A) A patient with psoriasis shows large, confluent, sharply demarcated, and erythematous plaques on the trunk. (B) Microscopic examination of a lesion demonstrates that the rete ridges are uniformly elongated, as are the dermal papillae, thereby giving an interlocking pattern of alternately reversed "clubs." The dermal papillae are edematous and reside beneath a thinned epidermis (suprapapillary thinning), with striking parakeratosis. The parakeratosis is the scale that is observed clinically.

gin, and has a surface of silvery scales. When the scales are detached, pinpoint foci of bleeding dot the underlying glossy, erythematous surface.

Among patients with psoriasis, 7% develop **seronegative rheumatoid arthritis.** The tendency to arthropathy has a genetic component and is linked to several HLA haplotypes, particularly HLA-B27. Psoriatic arthritis closely resembles its rheumatoid counterpart, but it is usually milder and causes little disability.

Psoriasis has long been treated with coal- or wood-tar derivatives and anthralin (a strong reducing agent). More recently, it has been treated with derivatives of vitamins A and D. Topical and systemic corticosteroids have also been employed. Severe, generalized psoriasis justifies systemic treatment with methotrexate, although hepatic toxicity remains a threat. Phototherapy after the administration of psoralens (UV-absorbing compounds that bind to DNA) has proved to be effective in many severe cases.

PEMPHIGUS VULGARIS

■ *Pemphigus vulgaris is an autoimmune, blistering disease caused by the action of antibodies to surface antigens on stratified squamous cells.* It occurs most commonly in pa-

tients between 30 and 50 years of age, but it is reported in all age groups, including children.

☐ **Pathogenesis:** Circulating IgG antibodies in patients with pemphigus vulgaris react with an epidermal surface antigen, which is associated with desmosomes and is intimately bound to a protein known as plakoglobin. Antigen-antibody union results in dyshesion, which is augmented by the release of plasminogen activator and, hence, the activation of plasmin. This proteolytic enzyme acts on the intercellular substance and may be the dominant factor in dyshesion. Internalization of the pemphigus antigen-antibody complex, disappearance of attachment plaques, and perinuclear tonofilament retraction may all act in concert with proteinases to cause dyshesion and vesiculation. Pemphigus may be associated with other autoimmune diseases (e.g., myasthenia gravis and lupus erythematosus) and may be seen with benign thymomas.

☐ **Pathology:** The blister in pemphigus vulgaris results from separation of the stratum spinosum and outer epidermal layers from the basal layer. This suprabasal dyshesion produces a blister with an intact basal layer as a floor and the remaining epidermis as a roof (Fig. 24-3). The blister contains a moderate number of lymphocytes, macrophages, eosinophils, and

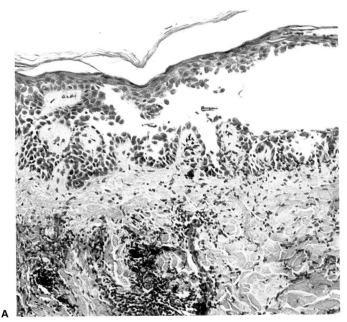
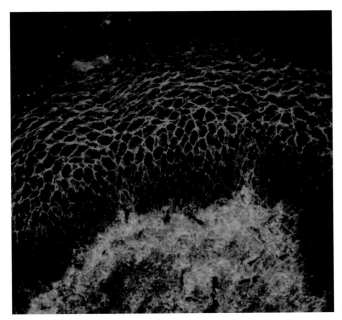

FIGURE 24-3
Pemphigus vulgaris. (A) Suprabasal dyshesion leads to an intraepidermal blister containing acantholytic keratinocytes. (B) Direct immunofluorescence examination of perilesional skin reveals antibodies, usually of the immunoglobulin G type, deposited in the intercellular substance of the epidermis, yielding a lace-like pattern that outlines the keratinocytes.

neutrophils. Distinctive, rounded keratinocytes, termed **acantholytic cells,** are shed into the vesicle during the process of dyshesion. The underlying dermis shows a moderate infiltrate of lymphocytes, macrophages, eosinophils, and neutrophils, predominantly about the capillary venular bed. Occasionally, eosinophils are particularly prominent.

☐ **Clinical Features:** The characteristic lesion of pemphigus vulgaris is a large, easily ruptured blister that leaves extensive denuded or crusted areas. The lesions are most common on the scalp and mucous membranes and in the periumbilical and intertriginous areas. Without corticosteroid treatment, the disease is progressive and usually fatal, and much of the cutaneous surface may become denuded. In addition to corticosteroids, immunosuppressive agents are useful for maintenance therapy.

ERYTHEMA MULTIFORME

■ *Erythema multiforme is an acute, self-limited disorder that varies from a few erythematous macules to a life-threatening, widespread ulceration of the skin and mucous membranes.* The disease is usually a reaction to a drug or infectious agent and is frequently associated with herpes simplex virus infection. Erythema multiforme is a common disorder, with a peak incidence during the second and third decades of life.

☐ **Pathogenesis:** The list of agents and disorders thought to invoke erythema multiforme is long and includes herpes simplex virus, *Mycoplasma,* and sulfonamides. However, a precipitating factor can be demonstrated in only half of the cases. In postherpetic erythema multiforme, deposition of viral antigens, IgM, and C3 can be identified in a perivascular distribution and at the epidermal basement membrane zone. The combined features of infiltrating lymphocytes and presence of apparent antigen-antibody complexes within the lesions suggests a combination of humoral and delayed-type hypersensitivity as pathogenetic mechanisms.

☐ **Pathology:** The dermis shows a sparse infiltrate of lymphocytes about the superficial vascular bed and at the dermal-epidermal interface. The most characteristic feature of the epidermis is the presence of shrunken keratinocytes, which have a pyknotic nucleus and an eosinophilic cytoplasm. Necrosis of keratinocytes may be extensive and associated with a subepidermal vesicle, the roof of which is an almost completely necrotic epidermis.

☐ **Clinical Features:** The characteristic target or iris lesions on the skin have a central, dark-red zone, occasionally with a blister, that is encompassed by a paler area. In turn, the latter is surrounded by a peripheral red rim. Urticarial plaques are common. The presence of vesicles and bullae, however, usually predicts a more severe course.

SYSTEMIC LUPUS ERYTHEMATOSUS

Systemic lupus erythematosus (SLE), the paradigm of immune complex disease, is characterized by a variety of autoantibodies and other immune abnormalities indicative of B-cell hyperactivity (see Chapters 4 and 16). Although cutaneous involvement may be severe and cosmetically devastating, it is not life-threatening.

Chronic Cutaneous Lupus Erythematosus. This form of lupus is usually a disease of the skin alone. The lesions of chronic cutaneous lupus erythematosus generally occur above the neck (on the face, scalp, and ears). They begin as slightly elevated, violaceous papules that have a rough scale of keratin. As they enlarge, they assume a discoid appearance, with a hyperkeratotic margin and a depigmented center. The cutaneous lesions may culminate in disfiguring scars. This form of the disease is not associated with the involvement of other organs.

Subacute Cutaneous Lupus Erythematosus. This is primarily a disease of young and middle-age white women. It may be accompanied by involvement of the musculoskeletal system, although severe disease of other organs is uncommon. The lesions are seen in the "V" area of the upper chest, upper back, and extensor surface of the arms, a distribution that suggests light may play a role in the pathogenesis of this form of the disease. Early lesions are scaly, erythematous papules, but they later enlarge into psoriasiform or annular lesions that, in turn, may fuse. Significant scarring does not occur.

Acute Cutaneous Lupus Erythematosus. This disorder is associated with the serious involvement of a variety of organ systems, especially progressive renal disease. Active SLE may be associated with inconspicuous and transient acute cutaneous lesions. Frequently, the only manifestation is the classic butterfly rash, which is a delicate erythema of the malar area of the face that may pass in a few hours or days.

☐ **Pathogenesis:** Although an impressive case can be made for the pathogenetic significance of immune complexes in renal diseases associated with SLE, they likely are not solely responsible for production of the cutaneous lesions. In this respect, immune complexes are present in both lesional and normal-appearing skin of patients with SLE. However, the deposition of immune reactants along the basement membrane zone of "normal" skin (positive lupus band test) is important in establishing the diagnosis of SLE.

Epidermal injury in cutaneous lupus erythematosus seems to be initiated by exogenous agents (e.g., UV light) and perpetuated by cell-mediated immune reactions, similar to those in graft-versus-host disease. The manifestations of epidermal injury include (1) vacuolization of basal cells, with some diminution in epidermal thickness and hyperkeratosis; (2) release of DNA and other nuclear and cytoplasmic antigen to the circulation; and (3) deposition of DNA and other antigenic determinants in the basement membrane zone (lamina densa and immediately subjacent dermis). Thus, epidermal injury, local formation of immune complexes, deposition of circulating immune complexes, and lymphocyte-induced cellular injury all seem to act in concert in the pathogenesis of cutaneous lupus erythematosus.

☐ **Pathology:** There is an inverse relationship between the prominence of skin pathology and the extent of systemic pathology in patients with lupus erythematosus. Chronic cutaneous (discoid) lupus erythematosus presents with distinctive histologic changes but is rarely associated with systemic pathology. The nucleated epidermal layers are either modestly thickened or somewhat thin, but hyperkeratosis and plugging of hair follicles are prominent. The rete-papillae pattern of the dermal-epidermal interface is partially effaced as well (Fig. 24-4).

Unique changes are seen in the basal cells and the basement membrane zone. The basal cells are vacuolated, and apoptotic bodies (death of individual keratinocytes) are noted. The lamina densa is greatly thickened and reduplicated, which reflects a response of the basal cells to damage. **The vacuolated basal cells, apoptotic bodies, and alterations of the lamina densa all suggest that injury to the basal keratinocytes is an essential pathogenetic characteristic of skin disease associated with lupus erythematosus.** The basal keratinocytic layer and basement membrane zone also show a diffuse, only moderately dense lymphocytic infiltrate, which focally penetrates the basal layer. Deeper in the dermis, a lymphocytic infiltrate may be the most prominent feature of discoid lupus erythematosus.

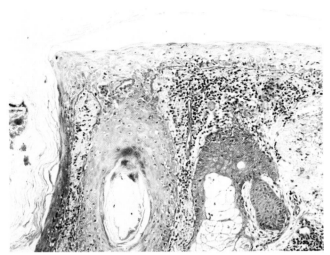

FIGURE *24-4*
Lupus erythematosus. A variably cell-rich to cell-poor, band-like lymphocytic infiltrate is present in the papillary and adventitial dermis. There is epidermal atrophy arising from damage to the epidermis mediated by infiltrating lymphocytes.

URTICARIA AND ANGIOEDEMA

■ *Uticaria and angioedema are immediate-type immunologic reactions (type I, anaphylactic, or IgE-dependent hypersensitivity) that result from the degranulation of mast cells sensitized to a specific antigen.*

Urticaria, or **hives,** are raised, pale, well-delimited, and pruritic papules and plaques, which appear and disappear within a few hours. They represent edema of the superficial portions of the dermis.

Angioedema is a condition in which edema involves the deeper dermis or subcutaneous adipose tissue, thereby resulting in an egg-like swelling. Both urticaria and angioedema are of rapid onset and may be simply annoying or reflect a life-threatening allergic reaction. The mainstays of treatment are avoidance of the offending agent and prompt administration of antihistamines.

□ **Pathogenesis:** Most cases of urticaria are IgE-dependent, and the final pathway is an exaggerated venular permeability owing to the degranulation of mast cells. Initially, cutaneous venules react to the degranulation of mast cells and the release of their stored vasoactive mediators with increased permeability, thereby resulting in rapidly forming edema. If the reaction persists, inflammatory cells are attracted to the area, and a persistent urticarial plaque (lasting for more than 24 hours) is the result.

□ **Pathology:** In urticaria, the collagen fibers and fibrils are pushed apart and separated by clear areas occupied by excess fluid. The lymphatic vessels are dilated, and the venules show margination of neutrophils and eosinophils, which is associated with a cuff of a few lymphocytes. Perivenular mast cell degranulation is an important feature.

MELANOCYTIC NEOPLASIA

The incidence of melanoma is increasing at a rate greater than that of any other form of human cancer. However, with proper awareness on the part of physicians and the general public, the mortality rate from melanoma should be less than 5%. UV light is one of the factors that have been causally related to malignant melanoma. Yet, exposure to light begins at birth, whereas malignant melanoma appears at a median age of 50 years. What of the intervening years?

Initial Lesion: Common Acquired Melanocytic Nevus

Most persons, regardless of their native skin color, who are exposed to a significant amount of light during the first 15 years of life develop some 10 to 50 moles on their skin. Melanocytic nevi begin to appear between the first and second years and continue to emerge for the first two decades. A mole is first recognized as a small, tan dot that does not exceed 0.2 cm in diameter. During a period of 3 to 4 years, the dot enlarges as a uniformly colored, tan to brown area. Later, the dark brown mole becomes sharply demarcated from the surrounding normal skin. During the next 10 years, the lesion begins to elevate, and its color diminishes slightly. Gradually, the mole becomes a tan skin tag.

□ **Pathology:** The histologic classification of melanocytic nevi distinguishes various stages of the lesion:

- **Lentigo.** The melanocytes of the lesion are limited to the basal layer of the epidermis.
- **Junctional Nevus.** Melanocytes form clusters at the tips of the rete ridges in the epidermis.
- **Compound Nevus.** Nests of melanocytes are seen in the epidermis, and the cells have migrated into the dermis (Fig. 24-5).
- **Dermal Nevus.** Intraepidermal melanocytic growth has ceased.

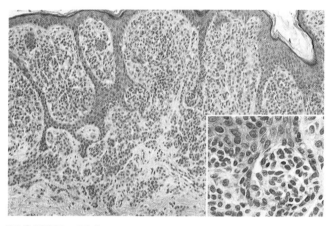

FIGURE *24-5*
Compound melanocytic nevus. Melanocytes are present as nests within the epidermis and dermis. (Inset) An intraepidermal nest of melanocytes is surrounded by keratinocytes.

- **Skin Tag.** The dermal component has differentiated into a delicate neuromesenchyme, and the lesion is indistinguishable from a small skin tag.

Melanocytic Nevus with Dysplasia

With time, melanocytes with large, atypical nuclei that have some similarities to cancer cells may appear. The combination of an abnormal pattern of growth and the cytologic abnormality of melanocytes (melanocytic nuclear atypia) defines a dysplastic nevus (Fig. 24-6). More than half of malignant melanomas that are 0.75 mm in thickness or larger display a precursor nevus with melanocytic dysplasia.

Intermediate Lesion: Radial Growth-Phase Melanoma

The appearance of intermediate lesions heralds the very beginnings of malignancy (malignant melanoma). Early lesions may have a slightly elevated and palpable border. The neoplasm is variably and haphazardly colored. For example, some parts are unusually black or dark brown, whereas lighter-brown shades are mingled with pink and light-blue tints. On the other hand, the entire lesion may be purely dark brown in color (Fig. 24-7).

On microscopic examination, large epithelioid melanocytes are dispersed in nests and as individual cells throughout the entire thickness of the epidermis (Fig. 24-8), with focal extension into the papillary dermis being the rule. The enlargement of such circular lesions is at the periphery, hence the term *radial growth phase*. **Importantly, melanomas in the radial growth phase have not been observed to metastasize.**

Vertical Growth-Phase Melanoma

After a variable time (usually 1–2 years), the character of growth of the radial growth phase changes focally. Melanocytes exhibit focal mitotic activity and grow as spheroidal nodules in a manner similar to the growth of metastatic nodules. The nodules expand more rapidly than the rest of the tumor in the surrounding papillary dermis (Fig. 24-9). The net direction of growth tends to be perpendicular to that of the radial growth phase, hence the term *vertical growth phase* (Fig. 24-10).

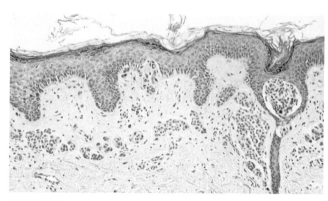

FIGURE *24-6*
Compound nevus with melanocytic dysplasia. A compound nevus (*right*) is apparent, with both intraepidermal and dermal components. Within the epidermis are single, atypical melanocytes (*left*) within the basal unit as well as incipient lamellar fibroplasia. Dermal melanocytes are present below.

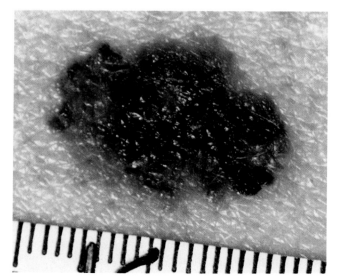

FIGURE *24-7*
Clinical appearance of the radial growth phase in malignant melanoma of the superficial spreading type. The larger diameter is 1.8 cm.

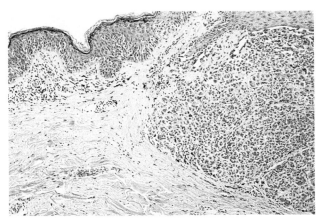

FIGURE *24-10*
Malignant melanoma of the superficial spreading type in the vertical growth phase. Vertical growth is manifested by the distinct, spherical tumor nodule (*right*). A focus of melanocytes clearly has a growth advantage (larger size) over other nests in the radial growth phase (*left*). The nodule distorts the papillary dermal–reticular dermal junction and, therefore, is level III.

Metastatic Melanoma

Metastatic melanoma, which is the final stage in tumor progression, arises from the melanocytes of the vertical growth phase. Initial metastases in malignant melanoma usually involve the regional lymph nodes, but spread through the bloodstream is also common. Hematogenous metastases are unusually widespread compared with other neoplasms, and virtually every organ may be involved.

Prognostic Features in Malignant Melanoma

The prognosis in patients whose tumor has entered the vertical growth phase is based on a number of different attributes.

Mitotic Rate. Patients whose tumors show no mitoses have a 12-fold greater chance of survival than that of patients in whom the mitotic rate is greater than six per square millimeter.

Lymphocytic Response. Patients whose tumors exhibit a brisk lymphocytic infiltrate have a probability of survival 11 times greater than that of patients whose melanoma lacks tumor-infiltrating lymphocytes.

Tumor Thickness. The thickness of a melanoma is measured from the outermost layer of the stratum granulosum to the deepest penetration of the tumor in the dermis. The 8-year survival rate varies from 93% in patients with tumors less than 0.76 mm deep to 33% in those with tumors thicker than 3.6 mm.

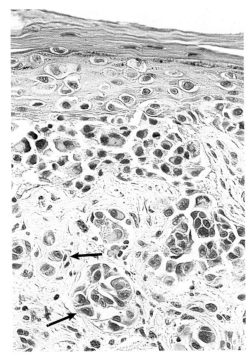

FIGURE *24-8*
Malignant melanoma of the superficial spreading type in the radial growth phase. Melanocytes grow singly within the epidermis at all levels and as large, irregularly sized nests at the dermal-epidermal junction. Tumor cells are present in the papillary dermis (*arrows*), but no nest shows preferential growth over the others.

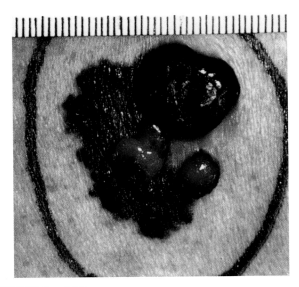

FIGURE *24-9*
Clinically, the radial growth phase in malignant melanoma of the superficial spreading type is represented by the relatively flat, dark, brown-black portion of the tumor. Three areas in this lesion are characteristic of the vertical growth phase. All are nodular in configuration. Two have a pink coloration, and the largest is a rich, ebony black.

Location. Melanomas on the extremities have a better prognosis than those on the head, neck, or trunk (axial). However, melanomas on the sole of the foot or the subungual region have a prognosis similar to or worse than that of axial lesions.

Sex. For every site and thickness, women have a better prognosis than men.

Levels of Invasion. Levels of invasion are not independent predictors of outcome, but level IV invasion may predict lymph node metastases and provide additional prognostic information for tumors thicker than 1.7 mm. Levels of invasion are categorized as follows:

- **Level I.** Tumor cells are situated entirely above the basement membrane zone (in situ).
- **Level II.** Invasive cells are present only in the papillary dermis. This level generally coincides with the radial growth phase.
- **Level III.** The tumor has entered the vertical growth phase and impinges on the reticular dermis, thereby forming small, expansile nodules that widen the papillary dermis.
- **Level IV.** Tumor cells clearly invade between the collagen bundles of the reticular dermis.
- **Level V.** The tumor extends into the subcutaneous fat.

When excising a melanoma in the radial growth phase, it is common practice to include a margin of 8 to 10 mm of normal skin around the lesion. Tumors in the vertical growth phase require excisions with a radius of at least 2.5 cm around the original lesion.

VERRUCAE

■ *Verrucae, or warts, are benign cutaneous tumors induced by infection with human papillomavirus (HPV).* The lesions are circumscribed, symmetric, epidermal neoplasms that are elevated above the skin and often appear to be papillary.

Verrucae Vulgaris. These lesions are elevated papules with a verrucous (papillomatous) surface. They may be single or multiple and are most frequent on the dorsum of the hands or on the face. Histologically, verruca vulgaris is characterized by hyperkeratosis and papillary epidermal hyperplasia (Fig. 24-11). Koilocytes (enlarged keratinocytes with a pyknotic nucleus surrounded by a halo) are observed within the upper epidermis, particularly on the sides of papillae. Several different HPV serotypes, including types 2 and 4, have been demonstrated in patients with verruca vulgaris.

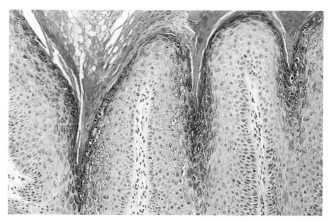

FIGURE *24-11*
Verruca vulgaris is the prototype of papillary epidermal hyperplasia. Squamous epithelial–lined fronds have fibrovascular cores. The blood vessels within the cores extend close to the surface of verrucae, which makes them susceptible to traumatic hemorrhage and the resultant black "seeds" that patients observe.

Plantar Warts. These painful lesions on the soles of the feet are hyperkeratotic nodules similar to a callus. On occasion, they may also appear on the palms (palmar wart). Histologically, plantar warts are endophytic or exophytic, papillary, squamous, epithelial proliferations. The cells contain strikingly abundant cytoplasmic inclusions that are similar to keratohyaline granules. The nuclei of keratinocytes near the base of these warts also show bright-pink nuclear inclusions. HPV type 1 is the causative agent.

BENIGN KERATOSES

■ *Keratosis refers to any horny growth or callosity that represents a benign, localized proliferation of keratinocytes.*

Seborrheic Keratosis

■ *Seborrheic keratoses are scaly, frequently pigmented, and elevated papules or plaques, the scales of which are easily rubbed off.* Although they are among the most common keratoses, the cause is unknown. The lesions generally present during the later years of life and tend to be familial. Microscopically, seborrheic keratoses appear tacked onto the skin and are composed of broad, anastomosing cords of mature, stratified squamous epithelium associated with small cysts of keratin, called horn cysts. Although these lesions are innocuous, they present a cosmetic nuisance.

Actinic Keratosis

■ *Actinic keratosis is an atypical, keratinocytic neoplasm that presents in sun-damaged skin as a circumscribed,*

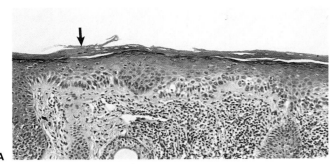
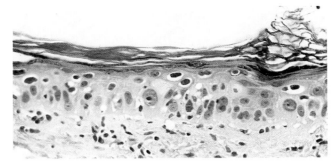

FIGURE *24-12*
Actinic keratosis. (A) Low-power examination reveals cytologic atypia within the stratum basalis and lower stratum spinosum, with loss of polarity. A lichenoid, band-like, lymphocytic infiltrate is frequently present. Parakeratosis is present here only in a small focus (*arrow*). (B) High-power examination of an actinic keratosis reveals striking cytologic atypia of the basal keratinocytes, which is the hallmark of actinic keratosis.

keratotic patch or plaque, commonly on the backs of the hands or on the face. Microscopically, the loose stratum corneum is replaced by dense parakeratotic debris as a result of the retention of nuclei in the stratum corneum. The underlying basal keratinocytes display significant atypia (Fig. 24-12). With time, actinic keratosis may evolve into squamous cell carcinoma in situ and, finally, into invasive squamous cell carcinoma. However, the early lesions are generally stable and may regress.

Keratoacanthoma

Keratoacanthomas are rapidly growing, keratotic papules on sun-exposed skin that develop over a period of 3 to 6 weeks into a volcano-like nodule with central umbilication. The lesion reaches a maximum diameter of 2 to 3 cm. Spontaneous regression usually ensues within 6 to 12 months, leaving an atrophic scar.

☐ **Pathology:** Histologically, keratoacanthoma is an endophytic, papillary proliferation of keratinocytes. The hyperplasia is cup-shaped, with a central, keratin-filled umbilication and overhanging edges. At the base of the keratin, the keratinocytes are large, with an abundance of homogeneous, eosinophilic ("glassy") cytoplasm. The lesions may be difficult to differentiate from squamous cell carcinoma because of cytologic atypia.

BASAL CELL CARCINOMA

■ *Basal cell carcinoma, the most common malignant tumor in persons with pale skin, derives its name from the histologic similarity of the constituent epithelial cells of the tumor to the normal basal keratinocytes.* Basal cell carcinoma is characterized by a singularly rare occurrence

of metastases. Although exposure to UV light is an important causative agent, there must be other pathogenetic factors. For example, basal cell carcinoma is unusual on the fingers and dorsum of the hands and is rare on hairless skin.

☐ **Pathology:** Basal cell carcinomas have prominent epithelial and mesenchymal components. Superficial basal cell carcinomas are composed of multiple nests of deeply basophilic epithelial cells, which are attached to the epidermis and protrude into the subjacent papillary dermis (Fig. 24-13). The central part of a nest is composed of closely packed cells with deeply basophilic nuclei surrounded by a small rim of cytoplasm. The periphery exhibits an organized layer of one or more palisaded columnar cells, although such palisading may be absent in deeply infiltrating basal cell carcinomas. In larger basal cell carcinomas, the epithelial nests are irregular and tend to fuse with each other.

☐ **Clinical Features:** Patients with basal cell carcinoma have a potentially serious disease. The tumor has the capacity for local tissue invasion, even though metastases are almost curiosities. Thus, the tumor should be promptly eradicated when the diagnosis is made.

SQUAMOUS CELL CARCINOMA

Squamous cell carcinoma (SCC) is second only to basal cell carcinoma in incidence. It is most common on the sun-exposed skin of fair persons with light hair and freckles, often in association with actinic keratoses. SCC is distinctly rare on normal black skin. The tumor is composed of stratified squamous epithelium, which tends to mimic the epidermis but, by definition, invades the underlying dermis. Invasion is usually su-

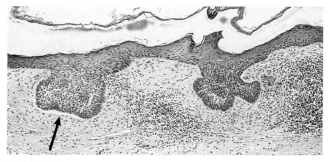

FIGURE *24-13*
Basal cell carcinoma of the superficial type. Buds of atypical, basaloid keratinocytes extend from the overlying epidermis into the papillary dermis. The peripheral keratinocytes mimic the stratum basalis by palisading. The separation artifact (*arrow*) is present because of poorly formed basement membrane components and the hyaluronic acid–rich stroma that contains collagenase.

perficial but, occasionally, may extend into the reticular dermis. SCC arising in sun-damaged skin has a very low propensity to metastasize (<2%).

☐ **Pathology:** The edge of most squamous cell carcinomas shows a precursor actinic keratosis in which the epidermis is variously thickened and parakeratotic, with significant atypia of the basal keratinocytes. In the tumor, atypical cells may involve all epidermal layers, and there are areas in which the atypical cells extend into the subjacent dermis (Fig. 24-14). SCC may also develop in chronic scarring processes, such as tracts of osteomyelitis and old burn scars. Tumors arising in the last setting as well as deeply invasive carcinomas have a greater propensity to metastasize than superficial, solar-related squamous cancers.

☐ **Clinical Features:** Lesions characteristically arise on the backs of the hands or the face, but they are also common on the lips and the ears. SCC tends to be more aggressive in the latter sites. Early lesions are small, often pruritic, erythematous nodules that may have a keratotic surface or may ulcerate. Small SCC lesions may be treated by electrosurgery, chemosurgery, or excision, whereas larger lesions require excision or radiation therapy.

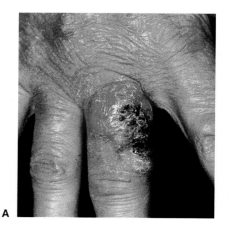

A

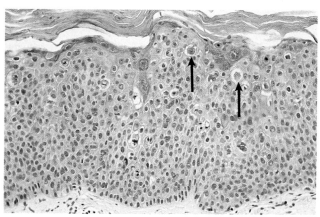

B

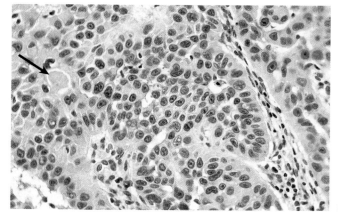

C

FIGURE *24-14*
Squamous cell carcinoma. (A) An ulcerated, encrusted, and infiltrating lesion is seen on the sun-exposed dorsum of a finger. (B) A microscopic view of the lesion periphery shows squamous cell carcinoma in situ. The entire epidermis is replaced by atypical keratinocytes. Mitoses and multinucleation of keratinocytes are apparent, as is apoptosis (*arrows*). (C) Squamous cell carcinoma with an invasive component. High-power examination reveals irregularly shaped lobules of strikingly atypical keratinocytes that have invaded to the level of the midreticular dermis. There is apoptosis (*arrow*). The pink, plate-like cytoplasm as well as intercellular bridges (desmosomes) are helpful diagnostic features for ex-
⸱ding other malignancies.

CHAPTER 25

The Head and Neck

Károly Balogh

Oral Cavity

INFECTIONS

The following terms describe localized inflammation of the oral cavity:

- **Cheilitis** (lips)
- **Gingivitis** (gums)
- **Glossitis** (tongue)
- **Stomatitis** (oral mucosa).

Aphthous Stomatitis (Canker Sores)

■ *Canker sores are a common disease characterized by painful, recurrent, solitary or multiple, small ulcers of the oral mucosa.* The causative agent is unknown. Microscopically, the lesion consists of a shallow ulcer covered by a fibrinopurulent exudate. The underlying inflammatory infiltrate is composed of mononuclear and polymorphonuclear leukocytes. The lesions heal without scar formation.

Pyogenic Granuloma

■ *Pyogenic granuloma is a highly vascular lesion of the oral cavity that results from minor trauma and subsequent invasion by nonspecific micro-organisms.* In the oral cavity, pyogenic granulomas, which range from a few millimeters to a centimeter, are most common on the gingiva. The lesion presents as an elevated, red or purple, soft mass with a smooth, lobulated, and ulcerated surface. Microscopically, the nodule consists of granulation tissue with varying degrees of acute and chronic inflammation (Fig. 25-1).

Acute Necrotizing Ulcerative Gingivitis (Vincent Angina)

■ *Acute necrotizing ulcerative gingivitis (Vincent angina) is an erosive lesion of the gums caused by infection with a fusiform bacillus and a spirochete* (Borrelia vincentii). The most important predisposing factors are inadequate nutrition, immunodeficiency, or poor oral hygiene. Vincent angina is characterized by punched-out erosions of the interdental papillae. The ulceration tends to spread and, eventually, to involve all of the gingival margins, which become covered by a necrotic pseudomembrane.

Candidiasis (Thrush or Moniliasis)

Candida albicans is a common surface inhabitant of the oral cavity, gastrointestinal tract, and vagina. To cause

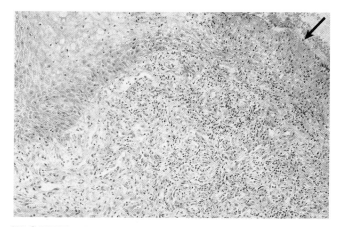

FIGURE   *25-1*
Pyogenic granuloma of the gingiva. The lesion displays vascular granulation tissue and inflammation. The epithelial surface is partly ulcerated (*arrow*).

disease, the fungus must penetrate the tissues, albeit only superficially. Oral candidiasis is most common among immunocompromised persons (e.g., those with acquired immunodeficiency syndrome) and diabetics. The lesions are white, slightly elevated, and soft patches that consist mainly of fungal hyphae.

Herpes Simplex Virus Type I

Herpes labialis (cold sores, fever blisters) and herpetic stomatitis are among the most common viral infections of the lips and oral mucosa. The disease starts with painful inflammation of the affected mucosa, which is followed shortly thereafter by formation of vesicles. These vesicles then rupture and form shallow, painful ulcers that range from a punctate size to a centimeter in diameter. Microscopically, the herpetic vesicle forms as a result of "ballooning degeneration" of the epithelial cells. Some epithelial cells show intranuclear inclusion bodies. The ulcers heal spontaneously without scarring. Herpes simplex virus type I survives in a dormant state in the trigeminal ganglion. It can be reactivated to cause recurrent herpetic lesions by trauma, allergy, menstruation, pregnancy, exposure to ultraviolet light, and other viral infections.

LEUKOPLAKIA

■ *Leukoplakia designates an asymptomatic, white patch on the surface of a mucous membrane.* A variety of diseases presents clinically as leukoplakia; these include various keratoses, hyperkeratosis, and squamous carcinoma in situ. Thus, leukoplakia is not a histologic diagnosis but, rather, a descriptive clinical term.

The causes of leukoplakia are diverse, with the most common factors being the use of tobacco products, alcoholism, and local irritation. The same factors also appear to be important in the pathogenesis of oral carcinoma. Leukoplakia occurs most often on the buccal mucosa, tongue, and floor of the mouth. The plaques may be solitary or multiple, and vary in size from small lesions to large patches.

It deserves emphasis that there is no correlation between the clinical appearance of leukoplakia and the microscopic diagnosis, although most cases show some abnormality of the squamous epithelium (Fig. 25-2). Biopsies have revealed dysplasia or carcinoma in situ in 10% of the cases and invasive carcinoma in 8%. In cases of leukoplakia without epithelial dysplasia, 20% eventually become malignant. **In view of these data, all cases of leukoplakia should be considered clinically to be precancerous.**

SQUAMOUS CELL CARCINOMA

Squamous carcinoma is the most common malignant tumor of the oral mucosa. It may occur at any site, but it most frequently involves the tongue and, in descending order, the floor of the mouth, alveolar mucosa, palate, and buccal mucosa. The male:female ratio is 2:1 for the gum but 10:1 for the lip. Predisposing factors in the pathogenesis of oral cancer include the use of tobacco products, alcoholism, iron deficiency (Plummer-Vinson syndrome), physical and chemical irritants, chewing of betel nuts, ultraviolet light on the lips, and poor oral hygiene (craggy teeth and ill-fitting dentures).

☐ **Pathology:** Invasive squamous carcinoma of the oral cavity is similar to the same tumor in other sites, and it is generally preceded by carcinoma in situ. Oral carcinoma metastasizes mainly to the submandibular, superficial, and deep cervical lymph nodes. More than half of the patients who die of squamous cell carcinoma of the head and neck have distant, blood-borne metastases, most commonly in the lungs, liver, and bones.

DENTAL CARIES (TOOTH DECAY)

■ *Dental caries is a chronic infectious disease of the calcified tissues of the teeth that leads to cavities and loss of teeth.*

☐ **Pathogenesis:** Dental caries results from the interaction of several factors.

Bacteria. Tooth surfaces are normally colonized by numerous micro-organisms, and unless the surface is cleaned thoroughly and frequently, colonies of bacteria coalesce into a soft mass known as **dental plaque.** Carious lesions result primarily from dissolution of mineral by acids that are produced during metabolism of food residues by bacteria on tooth surfaces. Indirect evidence points strongly to *Streptococcus mutans* as being the primary causative agent that initiates caries. In the deeper zones of the teeth, other organisms may be more capable of maintaining the destructive process.

Saliva. Saliva helps to neutralize acids in the mouth and contains potentially bacteriostatic factors, such as lysozyme, lactoferrin, and secretory immunoglobulins.

Dietary Factors. A high carbohydrate intake provides the substrate for the production of acid by bacteria. Raw and unrefined foods contain much roughage that cleanses the teeth.

Fluoride. The presence of fluoride in the drinking water protects against dental caries. It is incorporated into the enamel, where it forms fluoroapetite, a compound that is poorly soluble in acid.

☐ **Pathology:** Caries begins with the decalcification of enamel, which, in turn, leads to the accumulation of debris and bacteria. A small pit or fissure in the enamel then spreads to penetrate the dentin, after which a substantial cavity forms in the dentin (Fig. 25-3). Eventually, bacteria reach the dental pulp and cause pulpitis.

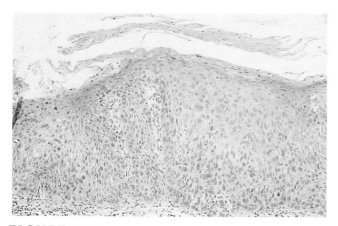

FIGURE   25-2
Leukoplakia. The lesion presented as a white patch on the buccal mucosa of a heavy smoker. Histologically, epithelial hyperplasia, marked atypia, and parakeratosis are evident.

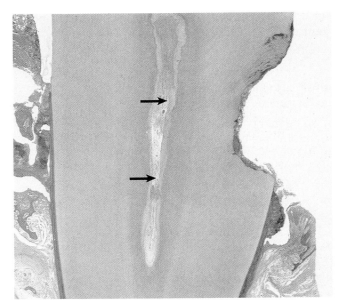

FIGURE 25-3
Dental caries. A large cavity close to the gingival margin is illustrated. *Arrows* point to the band of secondary dentin that lines the pulp chamber. This newly formed dentin is opposite the area of tooth destruction and was produced by the stimulated odontoblasts.

DISEASES OF THE DENTAL PULP AND PERIAPICAL TISSUES

The dental pulp consists of connective tissue enclosed within the calcified walls of dentin.

Pulpitis. Bacterial invasion of the pulp leads to the pain of acute pulpitis, which is caused by edema and exudate in the pulp chamber. The increased pressure in the chamber also facilitates the spread of inflammation. Acute or chronic pulpitis, if untreated, ultimately results in complete necrosis of the dental pulp.

Apical Granuloma. The most common sequel of pulpitis is the formation of chronically inflamed apical or periapical granulation tissue. This tissue is eventually surrounded by a fibrous capsule and squamous epithelium.

Periapical Abscess. As a result of pulpitis, an abscess may develop around the root of the tooth, either directly or after the formation of an apical granuloma.

Osteomyelitis. If a periapical abscess is not contained, the infection may extend to the adjacent bone, where it produces osteomyelitis. The bone infection may then spread to other areas of the head and neck and create fistulas to the skin or mucous membranes.

PERIODONTAL DISEASE

■ *Periodontal disease refers to bacterial infection and inflammation of the tissues surrounding the teeth. It results from extension of the gingival inflammation into the periodontium.* Chronic periodontal disease typically occurs in persons with poor oral hygiene or those with a strong family history of the disorder. **Chronic periodontitis causes loss of more teeth in adults than any other disease, including caries.**

☐ **Pathogenesis and Pathology:** Periodontal disease is caused by accumulation of bacteria under the gingiva in the periodontal pocket. As the mass of bacteria adhering to the surface of the tooth (dental plaque) ages and mineralizes, it forms **calculus** or **tartar.** The accumulated calculus stimulates chronic inflammation, which weakens and destroys the periodontium, causing loosening and eventual loss of teeth. Chronic periodontitis is associated strongly with *Bacteroides gingivalis,* although a few other bacterial species may participate in the process.

AMELOBLASTOMA

■ *Ameloblastoma is a tumor of the jaws that derives from odontogenic epithelium, most likely cell rests of the enamel organ.*

☐ **Pathology:** The large majority of ameloblastomas arise in the mandible, and most of these occur in the ramus or molar area. Ameloblastomas in the maxilla are most common in the molar area but can also involve the maxillary antrum or floor of the nasal cavity. The tumor tends to grow slowly, as a central lesion of bone. Radiographs show a multilocular cyst–like appearance, with a smooth periphery, expansion of the bone, and thinning of the cortex.

Microscopically, ameloblastoma resembles the enamel organ in its various stages of differentiation, and a single tumor may show various histologic patterns. Accordingly, the tumor cells resemble ameloblasts at the periphery of the epithelial nests or cords, where columnar cells are oriented perpendicularly to the basement membrane (Fig. 25-4). The centers of these cell nests consist of loosely arranged, larger, polyhedral cells that resemble the stellate reticulum of the developing tooth. Frequently, complete breakdown of these looser areas results in formation of microcysts.

The prognosis of ameloblastoma is favorable. Incompletely excised tumors recur but do not undergo malignant transformation.

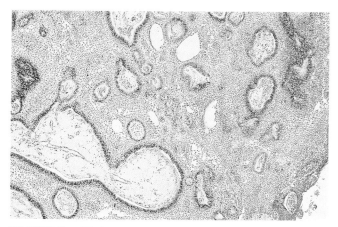

FIGURE   25-4
Ameloblastoma. A common histologic pattern is characterized by confluent islands of epithelium. The peripheral cells form bands that separate the tumor from the stroma.

Salivary Glands

The major and minor salivary glands are subject to a variety of inflammatory and neoplastic disorders.

XEROSTOMIA

■ *Xerostomia refers to chronic dryness of the mouth owing to lack of saliva.* It may result from mumps, Sjögren syndrome, drug toxicity, radiation, and any other inflammation that destroys the salivary tissue.

SIALOLITHIASIS

■ *Sialolithiasis refers to the presence of calcific stones in the salivary ducts, most commonly in the submandibular gland.* The cause of the disorder is unknown. Obstruction of the duct is followed by inflammation behind the occlusion.

PAROTITIS

Acute suppurative parotitis is caused by the ascent of bacteria, usually *Staphylococcus aureus,* from the oral cavity when the salivary flow is reduced. It is most common in debilitated or postoperative patients and in persons with sialolithiasis. Mumps is an acute viral parotitis, which spreads with infected saliva.

SJÖGREN SYNDROME

■ *Sjögren syndrome is a chronic inflammatory disease of the salivary and lacrimal glands, which may be restricted to these sites or may be associated with a systemic collagen vascular disease.* Involvement of the salivary glands leads to dry mouth (**xerostomia**), and disease of the lacrimal glands results in dry eyes (**keratoconjunctivitis sicca**). The pathogenesis and clinical features of Sjögren syndrome are discussed in Chapter 4; only the changes in the salivary glands are described here.

□ **Pathology:** The parotid glands and, sometimes, the submandibular glands in Sjögren syndrome are unilaterally or bilaterally enlarged, but their lobular appearance is preserved. Histologically, an initial, periductal, round cell infiltrate gradually extends to the acini, until the glands are completely replaced by a sea of polyclonal lymphocytes, immunoblasts, germinal centers, and plasma cells. Proliferating myoepithelial cells surround remnants of the damaged ducts and form so-called epimyoepithelial islands (Fig. 25-5). Late in the course of the disease, the affected glands become atrophic, with fibrosis and fatty infiltration of the parenchyma.

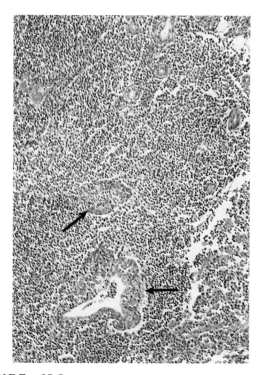

FIGURE   25-5
Sjögren syndrome. A massive lymphoid infiltrate and epimyoepithelial islands (*arrows*) in the parotid gland are shown. Marked acinar atrophy caused xerostomia.

PLEOMORPHIC ADENOMA

■ *Pleomorphic adenoma, a benign neoplasm with a tendency toward local recurrence after excision, represents the most common tumor of the salivary glands.* Two-thirds of all tumors of the major salivary glands, and half of those in the minor ones, are pleomorphic adenomas. This tumor is ninefold more frequent in the parotid than in the submandibular gland and usually arises in the superficial lobe of the parotid. It occurs most frequently in middle-aged persons and shows a female preponderance.

☐ **Pathology:** Pleomorphic adenoma presents as a slowly growing, painless, movable, and firm mass with a smooth surface. Microscopically, it shows a mixture of epithelial tissue intermingled with myxoid, mucoid, or chondroid areas (Fig. 25-6). The older term **mixed tumor** referred to this peculiar mixture of epithelial cells and mesenchymal ground substance. However, the neoplasm is now considered to be of epithelial origin, hence the label "adenoma."

The epithelial component of a pleomorphic adenoma consists of two cell types, namely ductal and myoepithelial cells. The cells lining the ducts form tubules or small cystic structures and contain clear fluid or eosinophilic, periodic acid-Schiff–positive material. Around the epithelial cells of the ducts are the smaller myoepithelial cells, which form well-defined sheaths, cords, or nests. Often, the myoepithelial cells are separated by a cellular ground substance, which resembles cartilaginous, myxoid, or mucoid material and appears to be the product of myoepithelial cells.

☐ **Clinical Features:** Pleomorphic adenomas tend to protrude focally into the adjacent tissues, thereby becoming nodular. At surgery, these projections can be missed if the tumor is not carefully dissected so as to leave an intact capsule and an adequate margin of surrounding glandular parenchyma. Tumor implanted during surgery or tumor nodules left behind continue to grow as recurrences in the scar tissue of the previous operation. When the recurrent tumor is removed, the facial nerve may have to be sacrificed. It is difficult to dissect the branches of this nerve, because they are embedded in dense scar tissue and surrounded by irregular, small nodules of nonencapsulated tumor. **Importantly, recurrence of pleomorphic adenoma represents local growth, not metastatic disease.**

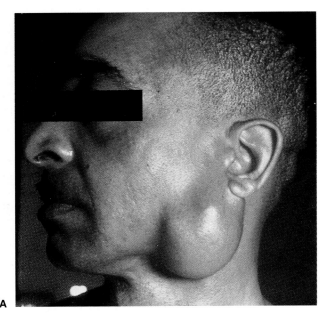

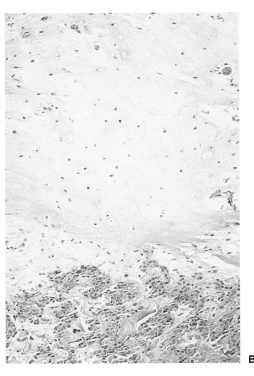

FIGURE   25-6
Pleomorphic adenoma of the parotid. (A) A conspicuous tumor mass is seen at the angle of the jaw. (B) A microscopic view shows myoepithelial cells embedded in a myxoid stroma adjacent to a chondroid area (*top*).

ADENOLYMPHOMA (WARTHIN TUMOR)

■ *Adenolymphoma (Warthin tumor) is the most common monomorphic adenoma of the parotid gland. It is composed of eosinophilic epithelial cells (oncocytes) embedded in dense lymphoid tissue with germinal centers.* Although it can be bilateral, or even multifocal within the same gland, the tumor is benign. Adenolymphoma is the only tumor of the salivary glands that is more common in men than in women. It generally occurs after the age of 30 years, with the majority arising after the age of 50. The tumor occurs almost exclusively in the parotid gland and is composed of glandular spaces, which tend to become cystic and to show papillary projections (Fig. 25-7). The cysts are separated by follicular lymphoid tissue and are lined by the characteristic eosinophilic oncocytes.

MUCOEPIDERMOID CARCINOMA

■ *Mucoepidermoid carcinoma is a malignant salivary gland tumor composed of a mixture of neoplastic squamous cells, mucus-secreting cells, and cells of an intermediate*

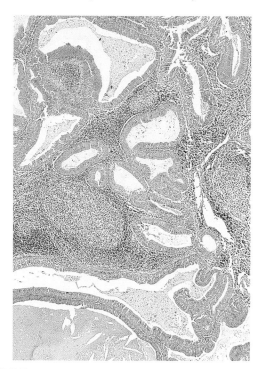

FIGURE   25-7
Adenolymphoma (Warthin tumor). Cystic spaces and duct-like structures are lined by oncocytes. Follicular lymphoid tissue is present.

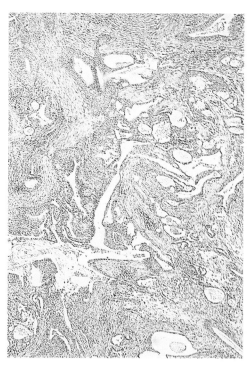

FIGURE   25-8
Mucoepidermoid carcinoma of a minor salivary gland. This tumor invades the fibrous stroma and forms irregular duct-like and cystic spaces. The cysts, lined by squamous and mucus-secreting cells, contain mucus.

type. Mucoepidermoid tumors probably originate from the ductal epithelium, which has a considerable potential for metaplasia. They account for 5% to 10% of major salivary gland tumors and for 10% of those in the minor salivary glands.

□ **Pathology:** Mucoepidermoid carcinoma grows slowly and presents as a firm, painless mass. Microscopically, well-differentiated tumors form irregular duct-like and cystic spaces that are lined by squamous or mucus-secreting cells (Fig. 25-8). Poorly differentiated carcinomas contain few mucus-secreting cells and resemble squamous cell carcinomas.

Even well-differentiated mucoepidermoid carcinomas can metastasize, but the 5-year survival rate is better than 90%, regardless of the primary site. Poorly differentiated mucoepidermoid carcinomas, however, have a much lower survival rate (20–40%).

ADENOID CYSTIC CARCINOMA (CYLINDROMA)

■ *Adenoid cystic carcinoma is a slow-growing, malignant neoplasm of the salivary gland that is notorious for its tendency to invade locally and to recur after surgical resec-*

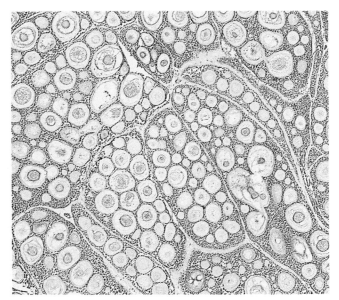

FIGURE   *25-9*
Adenoid cystic carcinoma of the palate. The tumor shows a cribriform arrangement, duct-like structures, and small groups of cells in a dense stroma.

tion. This cancer constitutes 5% of all major salivary gland tumors and 20% of all minor salivary gland tumors. Of all adenoid cystic carcinomas, one-third arise in the major salivary glands and two-thirds in the minor ones. These tumors not only occur in the oral cavity but also originate in the lacrimal glands, nasopharynx, nasal cavity, paranasal sinuses, and lower respiratory tract. They are most common in persons between 40 and 60 years of age.

☐ **Pathology:** Histologically, adenoid cystic carcinomas present with varying patterns. The tumor cells are small, have scant cytoplasm, and grow in solid sheets or as small groups, strands, or columns. Within these structures, tumor cells interconnect to enclose cystic spaces, thereby resulting in a cribriform (sieve-like) arrangement (Fig. 25-9). The tumor cells produce a homogeneous basement membrane material, which gives them the characteristic cylindromatous appearance. **Although adenoid cystic carcinomas do not metastasize for many years, they are difficult to eradicate completely, and their long-term prognosis is poor.**

Nose, Paranasal Sinuses, and Nasopharynx

NASAL POLYPS

■ *Nasal polyps are focal, inflammatory swellings of the mucosa of the nose or the paranasal sinuses.* Recurrent allergic reactions can cause chronic mucosal edema, thereby leading to formation of multiple smooth, pale, and rounded tumors (Fig. 25-10) that protrude into the airway and cause nasal obstruction. Microscopically, allergic polyps are lined externally by respiratory epithelium and contain mucous glands within a mucoid stroma, which is infiltrated by lymphoid cells and eosinophils. Nasal polyps can also arise in the setting of chronic rhinitis and chronic sinusitis, in which case they are not related to allergic diseases of the nose.

SINUSITIS

■ *Sinusitis refers to inflammation of the mucous membranes of the paranasal sinuses.* Any condition (e.g., inflammation, neoplasm, foreign body) that interferes with drainage or aeration of a sinus renders it liable to infection. Acute sinusitis is often associated with infection by *Haemophilus influenzae* and *Branhamella catarrhalis*. In chronic sinusitis, the purulent exudate almost always includes anaerobic bacteria. Complications of acute and chronic sinusitis include mucocele (accumulation of mucous secretions in the sinus), osteomyelitis, septic thrombophlebitis, and intracranial infections.

SCLEROMA

■ *Scleroma, a chronic inflammatory process caused by infection with* Klebsiella rhinoscleromatis, *usually begins in the nose and remains localized to that site.* However, it

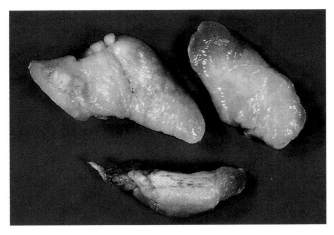

FIGURE   *25-10*
Nasal polyps. These smooth, pale, polypoid masses were removed from a patient with chronic rhinitis.

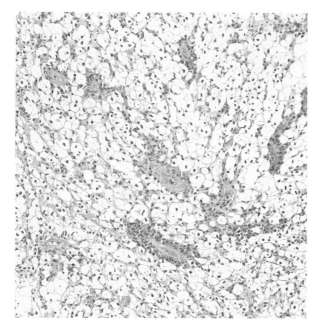

FIGURE 25-11
Scleroma. Granulation tissue contains numerous foamy macrophages (Mikulicz cells).

may extend slowly into the nasopharynx, larynx, and trachea. Scleroma is endemic in some Mediterranean countries and in parts of Asia, Africa, and Latin America. Indigenous cases have also been recognized in the United States. The disease occurs in both sexes and at any age. Poor domestic and personal hygiene are common to most patients, and epidemiologic evidence suggests that household relationships are the decisive factor in development of this disorder.

☐ **Pathology:** Infected tissues appear to be firm, greatly thickened, irregularly nodular, and often, ulcerated. Microscopically, the granulation tissue is strikingly rich in plasma cells, lymphocytes, and foamy macrophages (Fig. 25-11). The characteristic large macrophages, which are referred to as **Mikulicz cells,** contain phagocytosed bacilli. The disease is successfully treated with various antibiotics.

LETHAL MIDLINE GRANULOMA (POLYMORPHIC RETICULOSIS)

■ *Lethal midline granuloma is a type of peripheral T-cell lymphoma characterized by necrotizing, ulcerating mucosal lesions of the upper respiratory tract, which, if left untreated, is invariably fatal.*

☐ **Pathogenesis and Pathology:** The polymorphism of the atypical cells in lethal midline granuloma

is a characteristic feature that distinguishes it from a conventional lymphoma. Similar necrotizing infiltrates can also occur in the upper airways, lungs, and alimentary tract, but any organ may be involved, including the skin, lymph nodes, spleen, bone marrow, liver, kidneys, and central nervous system.

☐ **Clinical Features:** The nasal mucosa becomes focally swollen and indurated and, eventually, ulcerated. The ulcers are covered by a black crust, under which the lesions progress to erode and destroy both cartilage and bone. In turn, this destruction causes defects of the nasal septum, hard palate, and nasopharynx, with serious functional consequences. Frequently, the skin of the midface also becomes involved, hence the descriptive name. In half of the patients, the disease remains localized, but an equal proportion exhibit widespread dissemination of the lymphoma. Death results from secondary bacterial infection, aspiration pneumonia, or hemorrhage from an eroded, large blood vessel. The infiltrates of midline lethal granuloma are, at least initially, radiosensitive, and remission with use of cytotoxic agents has been reported.

NASOPHARYNGEAL CARCINOMA

■ *Nasopharyngeal carcinoma is an epithelial cancer often related to infection with Epstein-Barr virus (EBV), which is particularly common in southeast Asia and parts of Africa.* By far the most common cancer of the nasopharynx, nasopharyngeal carcinoma is the most frequent of all malignant tumors in the Chinese. In Hong Kong, this tumor represents 18% of all cancers, compared with a worldwide prevalence of 0.25%. Chinese born in the United States have a 20-fold greater mortality rate from carcinoma of the nasopharynx than persons of other races. There is also a high incidence in Tunisia and East Africa.

☐ **Pathogenesis:** Various environmental risk factors for carcinoma of the nasopharynx have been sought, but no association has been positively demonstrated. However, there is an association with the A2/sin HLA profile in the Chinese, thereby suggesting a genetic susceptibility.

Epstein-Barr virus is present in the tumor cells and B lymphocytes of patients with nasopharyngeal carcinoma. Moreover, 85% of the patients also have antibodies to EBV and have anti-EBV immunoglobulin A in the serum. Although a direct cause-and-effect relationship between EBV and nasopharyngeal carcinoma remains to be proved, the presence of the virus is a useful tumor marker.

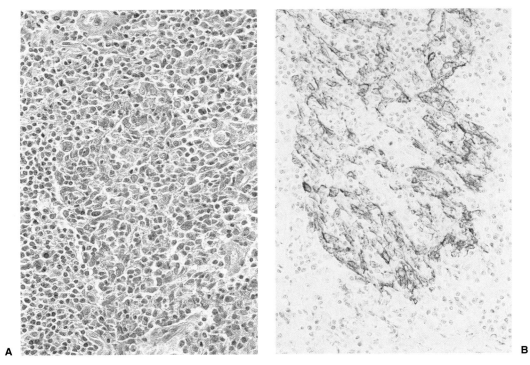

FIGURE *25-12*
Anaplastic nasopharyngeal carcinoma. (A) Poorly differentiated neoplastic cells are mingled with inflammatory mononuclear cells. (B) An immunohistochemical stain of the specimen in *panel A* reveals that the tumor cells contain abundant keratin.

□ **Pathology and Clinical Features:** Nasopharyngeal carcinoma is seen as either keratinizing (squamous cell) tumors or as nonkeratinizing tumors. Undifferentiated nonkeratinizing nasopharyngeal carcinoma is the type infected with HBV. It exhibits clusters of poorly delimited or syncytial cells bearing large, oval nuclei and scant eosinophilic cytoplasm (Fig. 25-12). The tumor is infiltrated by numerous lymphocytes. Anaplastic nasopharyngeal carcinoma infiltrates neighboring regions such as the parapharyngeal space, orbit, and cranial cavity. This locally aggressive growth results in various neurologic symptoms and disturbances of hearing. Invasion of the base of the skull leads to involvement of the cranial nerves. Neoplasms growing in the fossa of Rosenmüller and in the lateral wall of the nasopharynx produce symptoms referable to the middle ear, and obstruction of the eustachian tube is common. The rich lymphatic network draining the nasopharynx is the route of frequent and early metastases to the cervical lymph nodes.

Nasopharyngeal carcinomas are radiosensitive, and more than half of the patients with tumor restricted to the nasopharynx survive for 5 or more years. Metastasis to the cervical lymph nodes considerably lowers the survival rate, however, and cranial nerve involvement or distant metastases carry a dismal prognosis.

CHAPTER 26

Bones and Joints

Alan L. Schiller
Steven L. Teitelbaum

Juvenile Arthritis (Still Disease)	**Malignant Fibrous Histiocytoma**
Gout	**Tumors of Adipose Tissue**
Pathogenesis of Hyperuricemia	Lipoma
Pigmented Villonodular Synovitis	Liposarcoma
SOFT-TISSUE TUMORS	**Rhabdomyosarcoma**
Nodular Fasciitis	**Smooth Muscle Tumors**
Fibrosarcoma	**Synovial Sarcoma**

Bones

The functions of bone are classified as being mechanical, mineral storage, and hemopoietic. Mechanical functions include protection for the brain, spinal cord, and chest organs as well as rigid internal support for the limbs. Bone is the principal reservoir for calcium, but it also stores other ions, such as phosphate, sodium, and magnesium. Bone also serves as a host for the hemopoietic bone marrow.

Mechanical properties of bone relate to its specific type of construction and internal architecture. Although extremely light, bone has a high tensile strength. This combination of strength and light weight is a result of its hollow tubular shape, layering of bone tissue, and internal buttressing of the matrix.

ANATOMY

Cortical bone is dense, compact bone whose outer shell defines the shape of the bone.

Coarse cancellous bone (also referred to as spongy, trabecular, or marrow bone) is generally found at the ends of long bones within the medullary canal.

The **epiphysis** is the area of the bone that extends from the subarticular bone plate to the base of the epiphyseal cartilage plate (Fig. 26-1).

The **metaphysis** is the region from the side of the epiphyseal cartilage plate facing away from the joint to the area where the bone develops its fluted or funnel shape. The metaphysis contains coarse cancellous bone.

The **diaphysis** corresponds to the body or shaft of the bone, and it is the zone between the two metaphyses in a long tubular bone.

Endochondral ossification is the process by which bone tissue replaces cartilage.

Intramembranous ossification is the mechanism by which bone tissue supplants membranous or fibrous tissue laid down by the periosteum.

Gray or white marrow is deficient in hemopoietic elements and often is fibrotic. It is always a pathologic tissue in nongrowing bones in adults or in areas that are distant from the epiphyseal cartilaginous plate in children.

Cells of Bone Tissue

The cells of bone tissue (Fig. 26-2) have specific functions that relate to the formation, resorption, and remodeling of bone.

Osteoblast. Osteoblasts are the protein-synthesizing cells that make bone tissue. These large mononuclear and polygonal cells are arrayed in a line along the bone surface. Underlying the layer of osteoblasts is a thin, eosinophilic zone of organic bone matrix that has not yet been mineralized and is termed *osteoid*.

Osteocyte. Osteocytes are osteoblasts that are completely embedded in bone matrix and isolated in a lacuna.

Osteoclast. Osteoclasts are multinucleated cells that derive from hemopoietic mononuclear stem cells and that resorb bone. Osteoclasts are found on the surface of bones in a small depression termed a **Howship lacuna.**

Microscopic Organization of Bone Tissue

Microscopic examination reveals two types of bone tissue, namely lamellar bone and woven bone (Fig. 26-3). Both types may be mineralized or unmineralized, with the latter being termed **osteoid.**

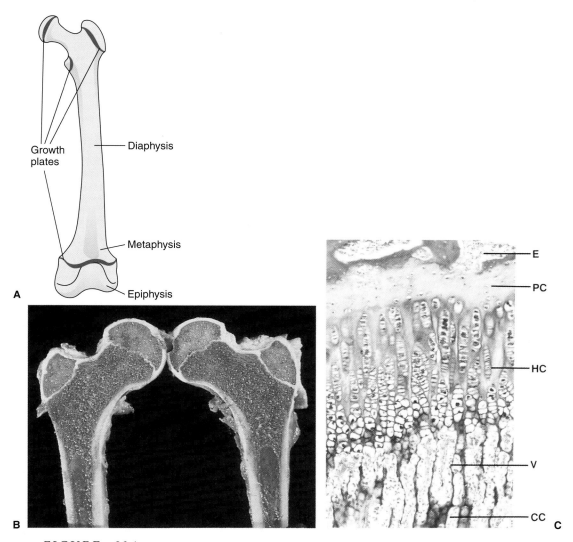

FIGURE   *26-1*

Anatomy of a long bone. (A) A diagram of the femur illustrates the various compartments. (B) A coronal section of the proximal femur illustrates the various anatomic parts
of a long bone. The epiphyses of the femoral head and the greater trochanter are separated from the metaphysis by their respective growth plates. The cortex and medullary
space are well visualized. The blood supply to the diaphysis and the femoral and
trochanteric epiphyses are separate. (C) A section of the growth plate of a long bone during active growth. At the top is a portion of the epiphysis with a zone of proliferating cartilage cells. Beneath this zone, the hypertrophic cartilage cells are arrayed in columns. At
the bottom, the calcifying matrix is invaded by blood vessels. *CC,* calcified cartilage; *E,*
epiphysis; *HC,* hypertrophic cartilage; *PC,* proliferative cartilage; *V,* vascular invasion.

Lamellar Bone. Lamellar bone is the stronger bone
tissue and forms the adult skeleton. **Anything other
than lamellar bone in an adult skeleton is abnormal.**
Lamellar bone is defined by three characteristics: (1) a
parallel arrangement of type I collagen fibers, (2) few
osteocytes in the matrix, and (3) uniform osteocytes in
the lacunae parallel to the long axis of the collagen
fibers.

Woven Bone. Woven bone is identified by (1) an
irregular arrangement of type I collagen fibers, hence
the term **woven;** (2) numerous osteocytes in the matrix;
and (3) variation in the size and shape of the osteocytes. **Woven bone in an adult skeleton always represents a pathologic condition and indicates that reactive tissue has been produced in response to some
stress in the bone.**

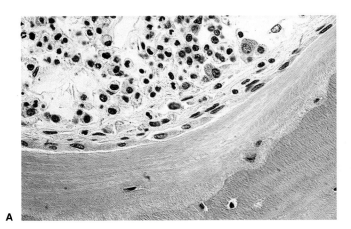

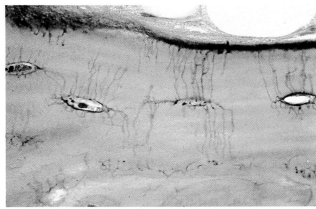

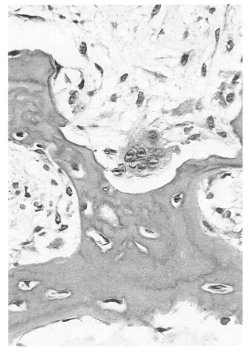

FIGURE   *26-2*
The cells of bones. (A) Osteoblast. A photomicrograph of bone reveals a layer of osteoblasts overlying an eosinophilic osteoid seam. Below the osteoid is mineralized bone. (B) Osteocyte. Osteocytes represent trapped osteoblasts embedded in a bony matrix. They are located in lacunae, and their cytoplasm extends into bony canals, termed *canaliculi*. (C) Osteoclast. Osteoclasts are multinucleated cells found on the surface of bones in a small depression, termed a *Howship lacuna*.

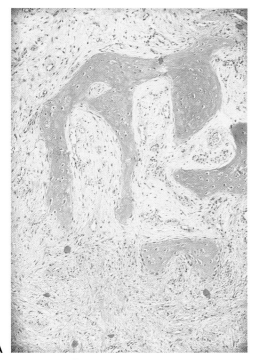

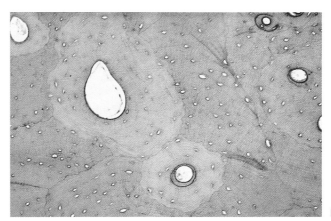

FIGURE 26-3
Woven and lamellar bone. (A) Woven bone is characterized by a random distribution of collagen fibers, numerous osteocytes, and variation in size of the osteocytes. (B) Lamellar bone shows a parallel and concentric arrangement of the collagen fibers and fewer osteocytes.

DISORDERS OF THE GROWTH PLATE

Achondroplasia

■ *Achondroplasia is an autosomal dominant trait that represents the most common inherited form of dwarfism, in which the zone of proliferative cartilage is either absent or attenuated.* The disorder reflects a mutation in the fibroblast growth factor-3 receptor (chromosome 4p16.3), which activates the receptor and suppresses growth at the epiphysis. The growth plate is greatly thinned, and the zone of provisional calcification, if present, undergoes endochondral ossification (but at a greatly reduced rate). A transverse bar of bone often seals off the growth plate, thereby preventing further bone formation and causing dwarfism. Because intramembranous ossification is undisturbed, the periosteum functions normally, and the bones become very short and thick. For the same reasons, the head of an affected patient appears to be unusually large compared with the bones formed from the cartilage of the face. The spine is of normal length, but the limbs are abnormally short. Patients with achondroplastic dwarfism have normal mentation and an average life span. However, some patients develop severe kyphoscoliosis and its complications.

SCOLIOSIS AND KYPHOSIS

■ *Scoliosis and kyphosis are curvatures of the spine.* **Scoliosis** *is an abnormal lateral curvature of the spine that usually affects adolescent girls.* **Kyphosis** *is an abnormal anteroposterior curvature. When both conditions are present, the term* **kyphoscoliosis** *is used.*

A vertebral body grows in length (height) from the end plates of the vertebrae, which correspond to the growth plates of the long tubular bones. As in tubular bones, the vertebral bodies increase in width because of appositional bone growth from the periosteum. In scoliosis, however, for unknown reasons, one portion of the end plate grows faster than the other, thereby producing a lateral curvature of the spine. Treatment is appropriate stress on the vertebral body through use of braces or internal fixation to straighten the spine. If kyphoscoliosis is severe, the patient may eventually develop chronic pulmonary disease, cor pulmonale, and joint problems, particularly involving the hip.

OSTEOCHONDROMA

■ *Osteochondroma is a developmental defect (hamartoma) of the skeleton that arises from an abnormality of the growth plate, in which epiphyseal cartilage grows laterally into the soft tissue.* Vessels originating in the marrow cavity of the bone extend into this mass of cartilage. If this process continues, a cartilage-capped, bony, and stalked osteochondroma results, which is in direct continuity with the marrow cavity of the parent bone (Fig. 26-4).

☐ **Pathology:** Osteochondromas tend to grow away from the joint. On radiographic examination, a cartilage mass is seen in direct continuity with the parent bone and is without an underlying cortex. On histologic examination, a cartilage-capped, bony mass is surrounded by a fibrous membrane, which actually represents the perichondrium. Active endochondral ossification deep to the cartilage cap allows the bony protuberance to lengthen.

Osteochondromas occur either as single lesions or as multiple lesions in an inherited syndrome. **Solitary osteochondroma** is the most common form of the lesion. It may need to be removed if it is cosmetically displeasing or presses on an artery or nerve.

Hereditary multiple osteochondromatosis is inherited as an autosomal dominant disorder and is characterized by multiple osteochondromas. It occurs predominantly in men and is primarily transmitted as a mendelian dominant trait. An unaffected woman from an afflicted family, however, may also transmit the disorder. In severe cases of hereditary osteochondromatosis, dwarfism may result because of lateral displacement of the longitudinal growth plate by the osteochondroma. Metacarpals may be shortened, and fixed pronation or supination may develop if lesions occur in the forearm and interfere with function of the wrist. Further orthopedic difficulties may be caused by unequal leg length and joint function because of the encroaching osteochondromas.

On gross and histologic examination, the lesions of multiple osteochondromatosis are identical to those of the solitary form. Especially in patients with multiple osteochondromatosis, there is a long-term increased risk of developing a chondrosarcoma in the cartilage cap, although this is a rare event.

OSTEOPETROSIS (MARBLE BONE DISEASE OF ALBERS-SCHÖNBERG)

■ *Osteopetrosis is a group of at least nine rare, inherited disorders, all of which are characterized by abnormally dense*

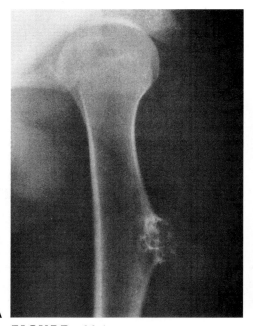
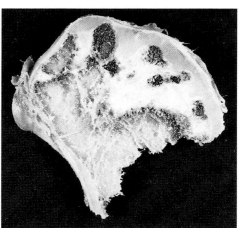

A   B

FIGURE **26-4**
Osteochondroma. (A) A radiograph of an osteochondroma of the humerus shows a lesion directly contiguous with the marrow space. (B) The cross-sectional appearance of an osteochondroma shows the cap of calcified cartilage overlying poorly organized cancellous bone.

bone. The autosomal recessive form is a severe and sometimes fatal disease affecting both infants and children. Death in infants with this severe variant is attributable to marked anemia, cranial nerve entrapment, hydrocephalus, and infections. A more benign form, which is transmitted as an autosomal dominant trait and presents during adulthood or adolescence, is associated with mild anemia or no symptoms at all.

☐ **Pathogenesis:** The cause of osteopetrosis is not known. The defect involves abnormal bone remodeling and, more specifically, **hypofunction of the osteoclasts.** The result is short, block-like, and radiodense bones, hence the term **marble bone disease** (Fig. 26-5). These bones are extremely radiopaque and weigh two- to threefold more than normal bone. However, they are basically weak, because the bone structure is intrinsically disorganized, not being remodeled along lines of stress. The mineralized cartilage is also weak and friable. As a result, the bones in patients with osteopetrosis fracture easily.

☐ **Pathology and Clinical Features:** On gross examination, the bones are widened in the metaphysis and diaphysis, thereby resulting in the characteristic "Erlenmeyer flask" deformity. Histologically, the bone tissue is extremely irregular, and almost all areas contain a core of cartilage.

The marrow cavity is severely attenuated, and the hemopoietic marrow is deficient, thereby resulting in severe and unremitting anemia. Cranial nerve involvement is secondary to lack of enlargement of the neural foramina. Subsequent strangulation of nerves leads to blindness and deafness.

To compensate for encroachment on the marrow space, extramedullary hemopoiesis occurs in the liver, spleen, and lymph nodes, with resultant enlargement of these structures. The only treatment currently employed for osteopetrosis is bone marrow transplantation, which may give rise to a new clone of functional osteoclasts.

DELAYED MATURATION

Osteogenesis Imperfecta

Osteogenesis imperfecta refers to a group of heritable disorders of connective tissue that tend to affect the skeleton, joints, ears, ligaments, teeth, sclerae, and skin. **The basic defect is synthesis of abnormal type I collagen.** The four types of osteogenesis imperfecta, each of which has a different mode of inheritance and clinical features, are described in Chapter 6.

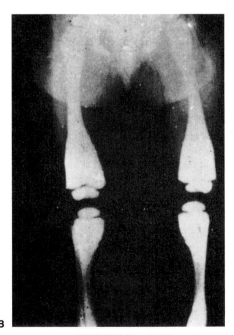
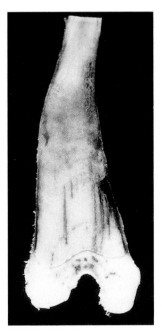
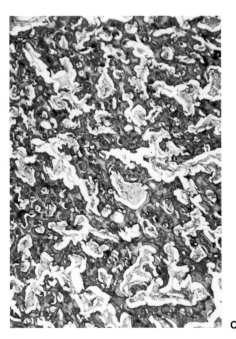

A,B   C

FIGURE 26-5
Osteopetrosis. (A) A radiograph of a child shows markedly misshapen and dense bones of the lower extremities, which are characteristic of "marble bone disease." (B) A gross specimen of the femur shows obliteration of the marrow space by dense bone. (C) A photomicrograph of the bone of a child with osteopetrosis reveals total disorganization of the bony trabeculae, most of which contain a core of calcified cartilage.

Enchondromatosis (Ollier Disease)

■ *Enchondromatosis is a condition in which the bones show multiple, tumor-like masses of abnormally arranged hyaline cartilage (enchondromas), with zones of proliferative and hypertrophied cartilage* (Fig. 26-6). Residual hyaline cartilage, anlage cartilage, or cartilage from the growth plate does not undergo endochondral ossification and remains in the bones. These cartilaginous masses tend to be located in the metaphyses, and as growth continues, the enchondromas settle in the diaphysis of adolescents and adults. **The cartilage nodules exhibit a strong tendency to undergo malignant change into chondrosarcomas during adult life.**

FRACTURE

■ *Fracture, which is defined as a discontinuity of the bone, is the most common bone lesion.* Healing of a fracture is divided into three phases: (1) the inflammatory phase, (2) the reparative phase, and (3) the remodeling phase (Fig. 26-7).

Inflammatory Phase. Rupture of blood vessels in the periosteum and adjacent soft tissue leads to extensive hemorrhage. There is also extensive necrosis of bone at the fracture site. The hallmark of dead bone is the absence of osteocytes and empty bone lacunae. Neovascularization begins to occur peripheral to the blood clot, which may extend deeply into the medullary cavity. Polymorphonuclear leukocytes, macrophages, and mononuclear cells accumulate, and by the end of the first week, most of the clot is organized by invasion of blood vessels and early fibrosis.

The earliest bone, which is invariably woven bone, is also formed after 7 days. In most fractures, cartilage is formed as well and is eventually resorbed. The granulation tissue containing bone cartilage is termed a **callus.**

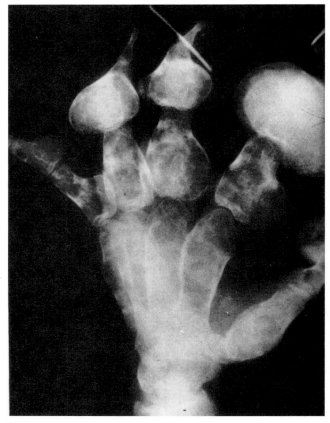

FIGURE   26-6
Multiple enchondromatosis (Ollier disease). A radiograph of the hand shows bulbous swellings that represent cartilage masses composed of hyaline cartilage, which is sometimes admixed with more primitive myxoid cartilage.

Reparative Phase. The reparative phase extends for months and involves both fibroblasts and osteoblasts. During this process, the blood clot is resorbed, and the callus bridges the fracture site.

Remodeling Phase. Several weeks after the fracture, the ingrowth of callus has sealed the bone ends. Remodeling then begins. The original cortex is restored, but remodeling may proceed for years.

FIGURE   26-7
Healing of a fracture. (A) Soon after a fracture is sustained, an extensive blood clot forms in the subperiosteal and soft tissue as well as in the marrow cavity. The bone at the fracture site is jagged. (B) The inflammatory phase of fracture healing is characterized by neovascularization and beginning organization of the blood clot. Because the osteocytes in the fracture site are dead, the lacunae are empty. The osteocytes of the cortex are necrotic well beyond the fracture site owing to the traumatic interruption of perforating arteries from the periosteum. (C) The reparative phase of fracture healing is characterized by formation of a callus of cartilage and woven bone near the fracture site. The jagged edges of the original cortex have been remodeled and eroded by osteoclasts. The marrow space has been revascularized and contains reactive woven bone, as does the periosteal area. (D) In the remodeling phase, during which the cortex is revitalized, the reactive bone may be lamellar or woven. The new bone is organized along stress lines and mechanical forces. Extensive osteoclastic and osteoblastic cellular activity is maintained.

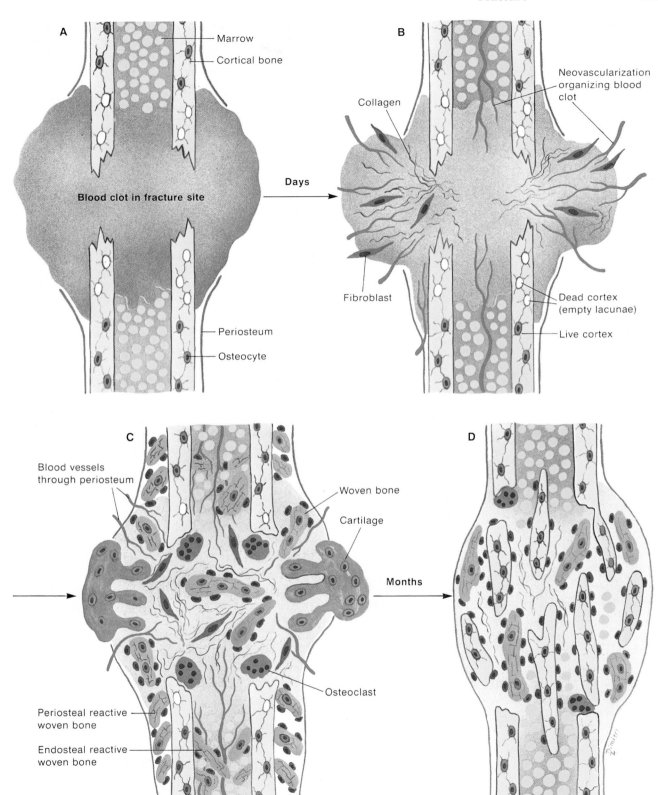

A

Marrow

Cortical bone

Blood clot in fracture site

Periosteum

Osteocyte

Days

B

Neovascularization organizing blood clot

Collagen

Fibroblast

Dead cortex (empty lacunae)

Live cortex

C

Blood vessels through periosteum

Woven bone

Cartilage

Osteoclast

Periosteal reactive woven bone

Endosteal reactive woven bone

Months

D

OSTEONECROSIS (AVASCULAR NECROSIS, ASEPTIC NECROSIS)

■ *Osteonecrosis refers to the ischemic death of bone and marrow in the absence of infection.* Causes of osteonecrosis include:

- **Trauma,** including fracture and surgery.
- **Emboli,** producing focal bone infarction.
- **Systemic diseases,** such as polycythemia, lupus erythematosus, Gaucher disease, sickle cell disease, and gout.
- **Radiation,** either internal or external.
- **Corticosteroid** administration.
- **Specific focal bone necrosis** at various sites, such as in the head of the femur (**Legg-Calvé-Perthes disease**) or in the navicular bone (**Köhler disease**).
- **Osteochondritis dissecans,** which is a condition of unknown cause in which a piece of articular cartilage and subchondral bone breaks off into a joint. It is thought that a focal area of bone necrosis occurs and, eventually, detaches.
- **Idiopathic factors,** such as in the high incidence of osteonecrosis of the head and the femur among chronic alcoholics.

MYOSITIS OSSIFICANS

■ *Myositis ossificans is a condition in which reactive bone forms in muscle as a result of injury.* It affects young persons and, although it is entirely benign, often mimics a malignant neoplasm. The lesion typically results from blunt trauma to the muscle and soft tissues, usually those of the lower limb. Peripheral neovascularization of the resulting hematoma leads, in a short time, to formation of bone spicules in the soft tissue, because the local environment is similar to that of an initial hematoma in a healing fracture. Since myositis ossificans often occurs near a bone, such as the femur or tibia, it may be misdiagnosed on the basis of radiographic results as being a malignant, bone-forming tumor.

OSTEOMYELITIS

■ *Osteomyelitis is an inflammation of bone caused by an infectious organism.* Despite the common use of antibiotics, osteomyelitis remains a major diagnostic and therapeutic problem. The most common pathogens are *Staphylococcus* sp., but other organisms, such as *Escherichia coli, Neisseria gonorrhoeae, Haemophilus influenzae,* and *Salmonella* sp., are also seen. These organisms are introduced either through the hematogenous route or by direct introduction of the organisms into the bone.

Direct Penetration. Infection by direct penetration or extension of bacteria is now the most common cause of osteomyelitis in the United States. Bacterial organisms are introduced directly into the bone by penetrating wounds, fractures, or surgery. Staphylococci and streptococci are commonly incriminated, but many other organisms can also produce such infections.

Hematogenous Osteomyelitis. Infectious organisms may reach the bone from a focus elsewhere in the body through the bloodstream. Often, the focus itself (e.g., a skin pustule or infected teeth and gums) poses little threat. The most common sites affected by hematogenous osteomyelitis are the ends of the long bones, such as the knee, ankle, and hip. The infection principally affects boys from 5 to 15 years of age, but it is occasionally seen in older age groups as well. Drug addicts may develop hematogenous osteomyelitis from infected needles.

☐ **Pathogenesis and Pathology:** Hematogenous osteomyelitis primarily affects the metaphyseal area (Fig. 26-8). If the organism is virulent and continues to proliferate, it creates increased pressure on the adjacent, thin-walled vessels, which further compromises the vascular supply in this region and produces bone necrosis. These necrotic areas then coalesce into an avascular zone, thereby allowing further bacterial proliferation.

If the infection is not contained, pus and bacteria extend into the endosteal vascular channels that supply the cortex and spread throughout the Volkmann and haversian canals of the cortex. Eventually, pus forms underneath the periosteum, shearing off the perforating arteries of the periosteum and further devitalizing the cortex. The pus then flows between the periosteum and the cortex, thereby isolating more bone from its blood supply, and may even invade the joint. Eventually, the pus penetrates the periosteum and skin to form a draining sinus, and a sinus tract that extends from the cloaca to the skin may become epithelialized by skin epidermis that grows into the sinus tract. When this occurs, the sinus tract invariably remains open, continually draining pus, necrotic bone, and bacteria.

Several lesions may develop:

- **Cloaca** is the hole formed in the bone during the formation of a draining sinus.

- **Sequestrum** is a fragment of necrotic bone that is embedded in the pus.
- **Brodie abscess** consists of reactive bone from the periosteum and endosteum that surrounds and contains the infection.
- **Involucrum** refers to a lesion in which periosteal formation of new bone forms a sheath around the necrotic sequestrum.

Vertebral Osteomyelitis

In adults, osteomyelitis frequently involves the vertebral bodies. Infections travel from one vertebra to the next by directly invading and traversing the intervertebral disk. The disk expands with pus and, eventually, is destroyed as the pus bores into the adjacent vertebral bodies. Half or more of the cases of vertebral os-

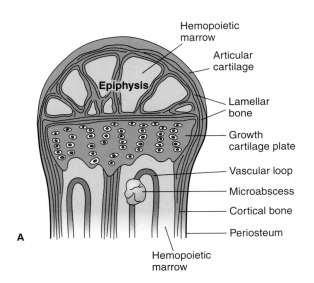

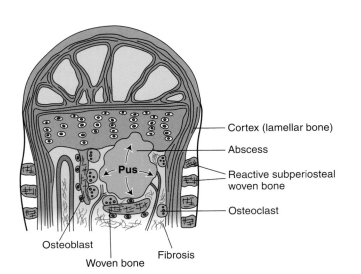

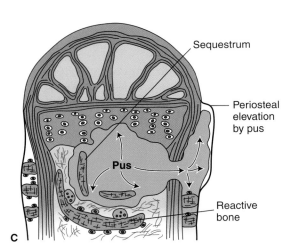

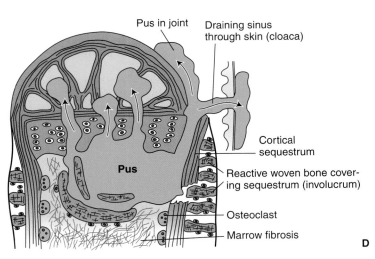

FIGURE 26-8
Pathogenesis of hematogenous osteomyelitis. (A) The epiphysis, metaphysis, and growth plate are normal. A small, septic microabscess is forming at the capillary loop. (B) Expansion of the septic focus stimulates resorption of adjacent bony trabeculae. Woven bone begins to surround this focus, and the abscess expands into the cartilage and stimulates reactive bone formation by the periosteum. (C) The abscess, which continues to expand through the cortex into the subperiosteal tissue, shears off the perforating arteries that supply the cortex with blood, thereby leading to necrosis of the cortex. (D) Extension of this process into the joint space, epiphysis, and skin produces a draining sinus. The necrotic bone is termed a *sequestrum*. The viable bone surrounding a sequestrum is termed the *involucrum*.

teomyelitis are caused by infection with *S. aureus*. Twenty percent represent infections with *E. coli* and other enteric organisms, many of which originate from the urinary tract.

Vertebral osteomyelitis may lead to (1) vertebral collapse with paravertebral abscesses; (2) spinal epidural abscesses, with cord compression from the abscess or displaced fragments of infected bone; and (3) compression fractures of the vertebral body, leading to neurologic deficits.

Complications

The complications of osteomyelitis include:

- **Septicemia.** Dissemination of organisms through the bloodstream may occur secondary to bone infection.
- **Acute Bacterial Arthritis.** Joint infection arises as a result of osteomyelitis in both children and adults and represents a medical emergency.
- **Pathologic Fractures.** Osteomyelitis may lead to fractures, which heal poorly and may require surgical drainage.
- **Squamous Cell Carcinoma.** This cancer develops in the bone or the sinus tract of patients with long-standing chronic osteomyelitis, often years after the initial infection. In such cases, squamous tissue arises from epithelialization of the sinus tract and, eventually, undergoes malignant transformation.
- **Amyloidosis.** This systemic disease was a common complication of chronic osteomyelitis during the preantibiotic era, and patients often would die of cardiac and renal disease.
- **Chronic Osteomyelitis.** Chronic infection of bone may follow acute osteomyelitis. Chronic osteomyelitis, especially that involving the entire bone, is incurable, because necrotic bone or sequestra function as foreign bodies in avascular areas and antibiotics do not reach these bacteria.

Therefore, chronic osteomyelitis is treated symptomatically, with surgery or lifelong use of antibiotics.

Tuberculous Spondylitis (Pott Disease)

Tuberculous spondylitis (infection of the spine) is a feared complication of childhood tuberculosis. The disease affects the bodies of the vertebrae, sparing the lamina and spines and the adjacent vertebrae. With antibiotic treatment, Pott disease is rare. The thoracic vertebrae are usually affected, especially the 11th thoracic vertebra, with the lumbar and cervical vertebrae being less commonly involved.

☐ **Pathology:** Tuberculous granulomas first produce caseous necrosis of the bone marrow, which, in turn, leads to resorption of the bony trabeculae. **Because there is little or no reactive bone formation, collapse of the affected vertebra is usual, after which kyphosis and scoliosis ensue.** The typical hunchback of bygone days was often the victim of Pott disease.

OSTEOPOROSIS

■ *Osteoporosis is a metabolic bone disease that is characterized by diffuse skeletal lesions in which normally mineralized bone is decreased in mass so that it no longer provides adequate mechanical support.* It is a type of metabolic bone disease (Fig. 26-9), which is a term that refers to generalized disorders involving all of the bones of the skeleton. Although reduced in mass, the bones in patients with osteoporosis display a normal ratio of mineral to matrix. Osteoporosis is the single most common bone disorder encountered by the practicing physician.

FIGURE   *26-9*
Metabolic bone diseases. (A) Normal trabecular bone and fatty marrow. The trabecular bone is lamellar and contains evenly distributed osteocytes. (B) Osteoporosis. The lamellar bone exhibits discontinuous, thin trabeculae. (C) Osteomalacia. The trabeculae of the lamellar bone have abnormal amounts of nonmineralized bone (osteoid). These osteoid seams are thickened and cover a larger-than-normal area of the trabecular bone surface. (D) Primary hyperparathyroidism. The lamellar bone trabeculae are actively resorbed by numerous osteoclasts that bore into each trabecula. The appearance of osteoclasts dissecting into the trabeculae, a process termed *dissecting osteitis*, is diagnostic of hyperparathyroidism. Osteoblastic activity is also pronounced. The marrow is replaced by fibrous tissue adjacent to the trabeculae. (E) Renal osteodystrophy. The morphologic appearance is similar to that of primary hyperparathyroidism, except that prominent osteoid covers the trabeculae. Osteoclasts do not resorb osteoid, and wherever an osteoid seam is lacking, osteoclasts bore into the trabeculae. Osteoblastic activity, in association with osteoclasts, is again prominent.

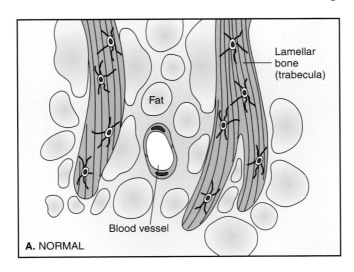

A. NORMAL

Lamellar bone (trabecula)

Fat

Blood vessel

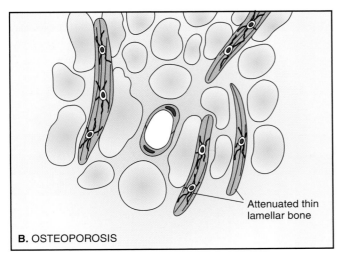

B. OSTEOPOROSIS

Attenuated thin lamellar bone

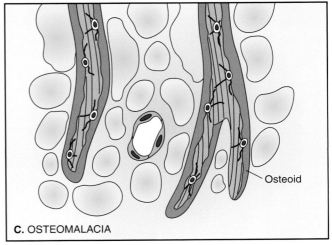

C. OSTEOMALACIA

Osteoid

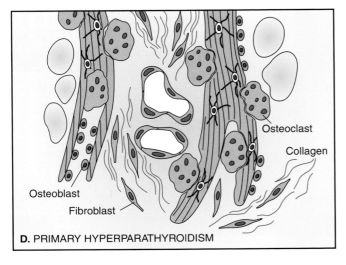

D. PRIMARY HYPERPARATHYROIDISM

Osteoclast

Collagen

Osteoblast

Fibroblast

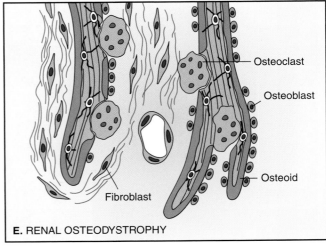

E. RENAL OSTEODYSTROPHY

Osteoclast

Osteoblast

Osteoid

Fibroblast

☐ **Epidemiology:** In normal persons, bone mass peaks between 25 and 35 years of age, after which time it inexorably declines. At a certain point, this loss of bone is sufficient to justify the label osteoporosis, and it renders weight-bearing bones susceptible to fractures. Among whites in the United States, 15% of persons have suffered a hip fracture by 80 years of age, and by 90 years of age, this figure rises to 25%. Women are at double the risk of hip fracture compared with men, although among blacks and some Asian populations, the incidence is equal among the sexes. The female sex predominance is particularly striking for vertebral fractures (Fig. 26-10), in which the female:male ratio is 8 : 1. A subset of women during the early postmenopausal years is at particular risk of vertebral fractures.

☐ **Pathogenesis:** Regardless of the cause, osteoporosis always reflects enhanced bone resorption relative to formation. Osteoporosis is classified as being either primary or secondary (Box 26-1). **Primary osteoporosis,** which is by far the more common variety, is of uncertain cause and occurs principally in postmenopausal women (postmenopausal osteoporosis) and elderly persons of both sexes (senile osteoporosis). **Secondary osteoporosis** is associated with a defined cause, including a number of endocrine and genetic abnormalities.

Primary osteoporosis has been linked to a number of factors that influence peak bone mass and rate of bone loss:

- **Genetic Factors.** Development of clinically significant osteoporosis relates, in part, to the maximum amount of bone in a given person, which is referred to as the **peak bone mass.** Determinants of peak bone mass are, to a large extent, genetic. In general, peak bone mass is greater in men than in women and in blacks than in whites.
- **Estrogens.** The decline in estrogen levels after menopause is associated with an accelerated rate of bone loss (postmenopausal osteoporosis).
- **Aging.** After the age of approximately 40 years, the rate of bone loss exceeds that of bone formation.
- **Calcium Intake.** The average calcium intake of postmenopausal women in the United States is less than the recommended value of 800 mg/day. Whether this possible dietary deficiency contributes to the development of osteoporosis, however, is controversial.
- **Exercise.** Physical activity is necessary for maintenance of bone mass, and athletes often have increased bone mass. By contrast, immobilization of a bone (e.g., prolonged bed rest, application of a cast) leads to accelerated bone loss.

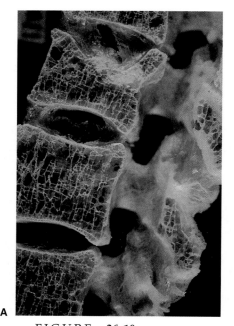

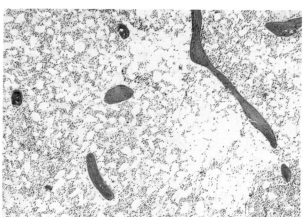

FIGURE   *26-10*
Osteoporosis. (A) A section of the vertebral column, in which the bone marrow has been washed out, demonstrates loss of bone tissue and compression fracture of a vertebral body (*top*). (B) A photomicrograph of a vertebral body shows very attenuated bony trabeculae.

BOX *26-1* **Classification of Osteoporosis**

Primary
Postmenopausal osteoporosis
Senile osteoporosis
Juvenile osteoporosis
Secondary
Primary biliary cirrhosis
Rheumatoid arthritis
Chronic pulmonary disease
Endocrine causes
    Hyperthyroidism
    Cushing syndrome (endogenous or exogenous)
    Diabetes
    Lactation and pregnancy
    Hypogonadism
    Hyperparathyroidism
Nutritional causes
    Intestinal malabsorption
    Protein malnutrition

Scurvy
Calcium deficiency (?)
Immobilization
Drugs
    Anticonvulsants
    Heparin
Heritable disorders of connective tissue
    Osteogenesis imperfecta
    Menkes syndrome
    Homocystinuria
    Adult hypophosphatasia
Neoplasms
    Multiple myeloma
    Myelomonocytic leukemia
    Systemic mastocytosis
    Waldenström macroglobulinemia

- **Environmental Factors.** Cigarette smoking in women correlates with an increased incidence of osteoporosis. The decreased level of active estrogens produced by smoking (see Chapter 8) may be responsible for this effect.

In summary, the two major determinants of primary osteoporosis are estrogen deficiency in postmenopausal women and the aging process in both sexes. Possible mechanisms for these effects are summarized in Figure 26-11.

☐ **Pathology:** The macroscopic features of osteoporotic bone are best appreciated radiologically, although abnormalities are detected only after 30% of the bone mass has been lost (at least in the vertebrae). Radiologically, osteoporotic bone is identified by loss of coarse cancellous bone and a thin, hollowed cortex, a condition labeled **osteopenia** ("little bone").

Histologically, osteoporosis is characterized by decreased thickness of the cortex and reduction in both the number and size of trabeculae of the coarse cancel-

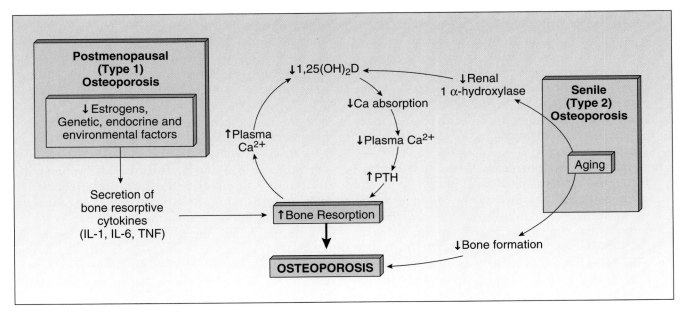

FIGURE *26-11*
Pathogenesis of primary osteoporosis.

lous bone. By contrast, the osteoid seams are of normal width. The trabecular bone loses its continuous arrangement so that isolated struts appear as minute, cigar-shaped fragments of bone.

□ **Clinical Features:** Postmenopausal osteoporosis usually becomes recognizable within 10 years after the onset of menopause, whereas senile osteoporosis generally becomes symptomatic after 70 years of age. Most patients are unaware of their disease until they suffer a fracture of a vertebra, hip, or other bone. Compression fractures of the vertebral bodies often occur after trivial trauma, and they may even follow the patient lifting a heavy object. With each compression fracture, the patient becomes shorter and may develop kyphosis (dowager hump). Serum calcium and phosphorus levels remain normal.

There is no complete cure for osteoporosis—despite virtually every mode of therapy having been tried. Estrogen treatment initiated at the time of menopause retards the development of postmenopausal osteoporosis, but it does not increase bone mass. A new class of inorganic compounds (bisphosphonates) seems to block bone resorption and appears to be promising. Dietary supplementation with calcium in elderly patients has reduced the risk of osteoporotic fractures by 30% to 70%.

Secondary Osteoporosis

Osteoporosis develops in association with many other conditions (see Box 26-1).

- **Corticosteroid Administration.** This is the most common form of secondary osteoporosis. Bone loss may also result from an excess of endogenous glucocorticoids, as in patients with Cushing disease. Corticosteroids inhibit osteoblastic activity, thereby reducing bone formation. They also impair vitamin D–dependent intestinal calcium absorption, thereby leading to secondary hyperparathyroidism and increased bone resorption.
- **Hematologic Malignancies.** A variety of hematologic cancers, particularly multiple myeloma, are accompanied by significant bone loss. The malignant plasma cells of multiple myeloma secrete osteoclast-activating factor, which presumably is responsible for secondary osteoporosis.
- **Malabsorption.** Gastrointestinal and hepatic diseases that cause malabsorption often lead to osteoporosis, probably because of impaired absorption of calcium, phosphate, and vitamin D.
- **Alcoholism.** Long-term alcohol abuse has been linked to development of osteoporosis. Alcohol is

a direct inhibitor of osteoblasts. It may also directly inhibit calcium absorption.

OSTEOMALACIA AND RICKETS

■ *Osteomalacia (soft bones) is a disorder of adults that is characterized by inadequate mineralization of newly formed bone matrix. Rickets is a similar disorder in children, in whom the epiphyses are open.* Thus, children with rickets manifest not only defective mineralization of bone but also of the cartilaginous matrix of the growth plate. Diverse conditions associated with osteomalacia and rickets include abnormalities in vitamin D metabolism, states of phosphate deficiency, and defects in the mineralization process itself.

Vitamin D Metabolism

An understanding of the pathogenesis of osteomalacia and rickets requires a brief discussion regarding the metabolism of vitamin D (Fig. 26-12). Vitamin D is ingested in food or is synthesized in the skin from 7-dehydrocholesterol under the influence of the ultraviolet component of sunlight. The vitamin is hydroxylated first in the liver and then in the proximal renal tubule, forming the active hormone $1,25(OH)_2D$. Ordinary exposure to sunlight provides sufficient vitamin D for bone growth and mineralization, even among persons with an inadequate dietary source.

Receptors for $1,25(OH)_2D$ are present in the intestine, bone, and kidney, and in numerous other cells in which no function of vitamin D is currently known. The effects of $1,25(OH)_2D$ on calcium metabolism relate to the intestine and the bones. In the intestine, $1,25(OH)_2D$ stimulates absorption of calcium and phosphate. Bone resorption is enhanced by $1,25(OH)_2D$, although the mechanism of this action is not clear. Some evidence suggests that this hormone promotes maturation of osteoclast precursors and interacts with osteoblasts to produce osteoclast-stimulating cytokines. **By its actions on the intestine and bone, $1,25(OH)_2D$ maintains the appropriate concentrations of calcium and phosphate in the blood that are required for proper bone mineralization.**

The principal determinant of the formation of $1,25(OH)_2D$ is the serum calcium concentration. A fall in the blood calcium level stimulates the release of parathyroid hormone, which augments the synthesis of $1,25(OH)_2D$ by the kidney.

Hypovitaminosis D can result from (1) inadequate exposure to sunlight, (2) deficient dietary intake, or (3) defective intestinal absorption. In addition, there are hereditary as well as acquired disorders of vitamin D metabolism.

Dietary Deficiency of Vitamin D and Inadequate Exposure to Sunlight

From the 17th through the 19th centuries, many urban children in the United States and Europe suffered from rickets because of insufficient exposure to sunlight and a poor diet. Although fortification of foods with vitamin D has virtually eliminated rickets in Western countries, it remains a problem in underdeveloped regions.

Intestinal Malabsorption

In the industrialized countries, osteomalacia most often results from diseases that are associated with intestinal malabsorption rather than from poor nutrition. Diseases of the small intestine, cholestatic disorders of the liver, biliary obstruction, and chronic pancreatic insufficiency are the most frequent causes of osteomalacia in the United States.

Malabsorption of vitamin D and calcium complicates a number of small intestinal diseases, including celiac disease, Crohn disease, scleroderma, and postsurgical blind loop syndrome. In patients with obstructive jaundice, the lack of bile salts in the intestine impairs the absorption of both lipids and lipid-soluble

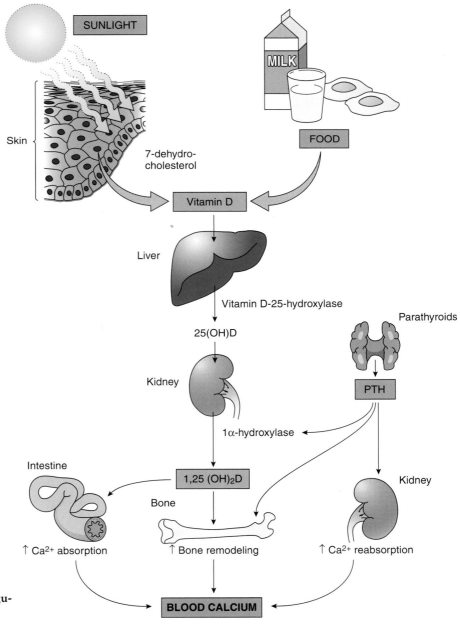

FIGURE *26-12*
Metabolism of vitamin D and the regulation of blood calcium.

substances, among which is the fat-soluble vitamin D. Furthermore, with sufficient liver damage, hydroxylation of vitamin D is reduced.

Disorders of Vitamin D Metabolism

There are both hereditary and acquired disorders of vitamin D metabolism that involve either defective 1-hydroxylation of vitamin D in the kidney or insensitivity of the target organ to $1,25(OH)_2D$. Two autosomal recessive diseases that are associated with rickets are, together, known as vitamin D-dependent rickets.

Type I vitamin D-dependent rickets results from an inherited deficiency of renal 1-hydroxylase activity. The clinical and biochemical changes of rickets appear during the first year of life, and these children exhibit hypocalcemia, hypophosphatemia, and high serum levels of parathyroid hormone and alkaline phosphatase. The disease is controlled by the administration of $1,25(OH)_2D$.

Type II vitamin D-dependent rickets represents inherited mutations of the vitamin D receptor that render end organs insensitive to $1,25(OH)_2D$. The manifestations of rickets usually become evident early in life, but they may appear at any time through adolescence.

Inherited Renal Disorders of Phosphate Metabolism

Both rickets and osteomalacia may result from impaired reabsorption of phosphate by the proximal renal tubules, with resulting hypophosphatemia.

X-Linked Hypophosphatemia. This condition is also termed **vitamin D-resistant rickets** or **phosphate diabetes.** It is inherited as a dominant trait, and it is the most common type of hereditary rickets. Hypophosphatemia is caused by impaired transport of phosphate across the luminal membrane of proximal renal tubular cells.

Fanconi Syndromes. These inborn errors of metabolism are characterized by renal wastage of phosphate, glucose, bicarbonate, and amino acids. They are also all characterized by **renal tubular acidosis** and result in rickets and osteomalacia. Fanconi syndromes include Wilson disease, tyrosinemia, galactosemia, glycogen storage disease, and cystinosis.

☐ **Pathology and Clinical Features:**

Osteomalacia. Osteomalacia, like osteoporosis, causes an osteopenic radiologic pattern. The only find-

ings may be compression fractures of the vertebrae and decreased bone thickness, as occur in patients with osteoporosis. Histologically, defective mineralization results in **exaggeration of the osteoid seams,** both in thickness and in the proportion of the trabecular surface that is covered (Fig. 26-13). In patients with mild forms of the disease, only slowly progressive changes in bone are seen, and many of these patients are totally asymptomatic for years. In advanced cases, however, poorly localized bone pain and tenderness are common, especially in the spine, pelvis, and proximal parts of the extremities. In such patients, the diagnosis of osteomalacia may be established only after an acute fracture, the most common sites of which include the femoral neck, pubic ramus, spine, or ribs.

Rickets. Rickets is a disease of children and, therefore, results in extensive changes at the growth plate (Fig. 26-14). This structure does not become adequately mineralized. In addition, the calcified cartilage and zones of hypertrophy and proliferative cartilage continue to grow, because osteoclastic activity does not resorb the cartilage growth plate. As a consequence, the growth plate is conspicuously thickened, irregular, and lobulated. Endochondral ossification proceeds very slowly and preferentially at the peripheral portions of the metaphysis. The net result is a flared, cup-shaped epiphysis. The largest part of the primary spongiosum is composed of lamellar or woven bone, which remains unmineralized.

On histologic examination, the growth plate exhibits striking changes. The resting zone is relatively normal, but the zones of proliferating cartilage are greatly distorted. Ordered progression of helix-form-

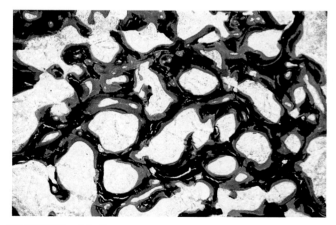

FIGURE   *26-13*
Osteomalacia. The surfaces of the bony trabeculae (*black*) are covered by a thicker-than-normal layer of osteoid (*red*) with the von Kossa stain, which colors calcified tissue black.

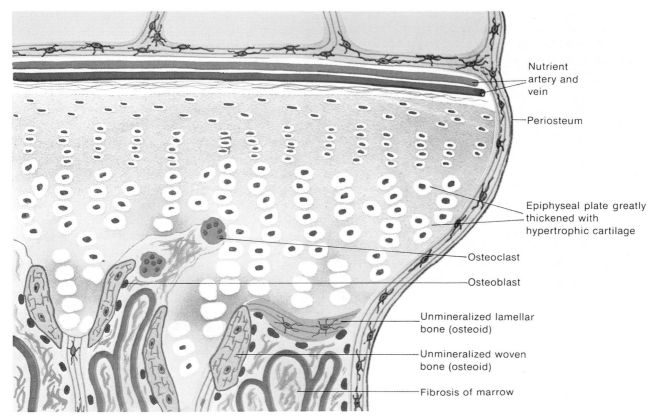

Nutrient artery and vein

Periosteum

Epiphyseal plate greatly thickened with hypertrophic cartilage

Osteoclast

Osteoblast

Unmineralized lamellar bone (osteoid)

Unmineralized woven bone (osteoid)

Fibrosis of marrow

FIGURE 26-14

The growth plate in rickets. The growth plate is thickened and disorganized, with a large zone of hypertrophic cartilage cells. There is irregular perforation of the cartilage plate by osteoclasts, because there is little calcified cartilage. The woven bone on the surface of some of the primary trabeculae is unmineralized and, therefore, easily fractured. Such microfractures often lead to hemorrhage at the interface between the plate and the metaphysis.

ing chondrocytes is lost and replaced by a disorderly profusion of cells, which are separated by small amounts of matrix. The resulting lobulated masses of proliferating and hypertrophied cartilage are associated with an increasing width of the growth plate, which may be five- to 15-fold the normal width. The zone of provisional calcification is poorly defined, and only a minimal amount of primary spongiosum is formed. Masses of proliferating cartilage extend into the metaphyseal region without any apparent vascular invasion and with little osteoclastic activity.

Children with rickets are apathetic and irritable, and they have a short attention span. They are content to be sedentary, assuming a Buddha-like posture. Rachitic children are short and exhibit characteristic changes of bones and teeth. Flattening of the skull, prominent frontal bones (frontal bossing), and conspicuous suture lines are typical. There is delayed dentition, with severe dental caries and enamel defects. In

addition, the chest has the classic **rachitic rosary,** which is a grossly beaded appearance of the costochondral junctions resulting from enlargement of the costal cartilages and indentations of the lower ribs at the insertion of the diaphragm. **Pectus carinatum** ("pigeon breast") reflects an outward curvature of the sternum.

PRIMARY HYPERPARATHYROIDISM (VON RECKLINGHAUSEN DISEASE)

■ *Primary hyperparathyroidism is a metabolic bone disease that is characterized by generalized bone resorption caused by the inappropriate secretion of parathyroid hormone (PTH).* Primary hyperparathyroidism is prominently associated with bone disease, termed **osteitis fi-**

brosa cystica. In 90% of the cases, the disorder results from one or more parathyroid adenomas, whereas hyperplasia of all four glands accounts for only 10%. Rarely, hyperparathyroidism complicates a parathyroid carcinoma. Because PTH promotes excretion of phosphate in the urine and stimulates osteoclastic bone resorption, low serum phosphate and high serum calcium levels are characteristic.

Actions of Parathyroid Hormone

The principal function of PTH is regulation of the calcium concentration in the extracellular fluid. This task is accomplished by the effect of the hormone on the bone, the kidney, and (indirectly) the intestine.

Bone. PTH mobilizes calcium from bone, which is the major reservoir of calcium in the body. PTH increases bone resorption by inhibiting the function of osteoblasts and augmenting the activity of osteoclasts.

Kidney. PTH stimulates the tubular reabsorption of calcium. It also enhances tubular excretion of phosphate by directly inhibiting sodium-dependent phosphate transport. Finally, the hormone augments the activity of 1-α-hydroxylase in the proximal tubules.

Intestine. PTH indirectly stimulates intestinal absorption of calcium by increasing renal synthesis of 1,25(OH)$_2$D.

☐ **Pathogenesis and Pathology:** The histogenesis of osteitis fibrosa cystica may be classified into three stages:

- **Early Stage.** Initially, osteoclasts are stimulated by the elevated PTH levels to resorb bone. At the same time, collagen fibers are laid down in the endosteal marrow.
- **Osteitis Fibrosa.** In the second stage, trabecular bone is resorbed, and marrow is replaced by loose fibrosis, areas of hemorrhage from microfractures, hemosiderin-laden macrophages, and reactive woven bone. This combination of features constitutes the osteitis fibrosa portion of the complex.
- **Osteitis Fibrosa Cystica.** As primary hyperparathyroidism progresses and hemorrhage continues, cystic degeneration ultimately occurs, thereby leading to the final stage of the disease. Areas of fibrosis often display many giant cells of the foreign body type as well as osteoclasts. Because of its macroscopic appearance, this lesion has been termed a **brown tumor** (Fig. 26-15). This is not a true tumor but, rather, a repair reaction as an end stage of hyperparathyroidism.

On radiologic examination of a patient with hyperparathyroidism, the entire skeleton shows generalized osteopenia. The weakened bones are associated with deformities such as biconcave vertebrae, bowing of the long bones, and fractures. A classic feature of von Recklinghausen disease is the presence of multiple, localized, and lytic lesions, which represent hemorrhagic cysts or masses of fibrous tissue. These eccentric and well-demarcated lesions are separated from the soft tissue by a periosteal shell of bone.

☐ **Clinical Features:** The symptomatology of primary hyperparathyroidism relates to the abnormality

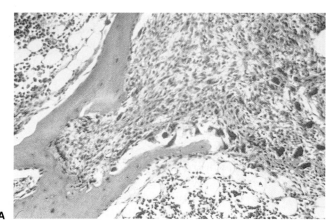
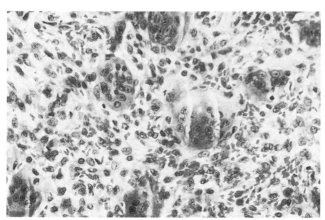

FIGURE 26-15
Primary hyperparathyroidism. (A) A section of bone shows a bony trabecula undergoing tunneling resorption. Numerous osteoclasts and marrow fibrosis are evident. (B) A section of tissue obtained from a "brown tumor" reveals numerous giant cells in a cellular, fibrous stroma. Scattered erythrocytes are present throughout the tissue.

of calcium homeostasis, and it is summarized as "stones, bones, moans, and groans." "Stones" refer to kidney stones and "bones" to the skeletal changes. "Moans" describe psychiatric depression and other abnormalities associated with hypercalcemia, whereas "groans" characterize the gastrointestinal irregularities associated with a high serum calcium level.

Primary hyperparathyroidism is treated by surgically removing the parathyroid adenomas. Among patients in whom parathyroid hyperplasia is the cause of the disease, three-and-a-half glands are usually removed. The remaining fragment is sufficient to ensure that the patient does not develop hypocalcemia.

RENAL OSTEODYSTROPHY

■ *Renal osteodystrophy is a complex, metabolic bone disease that occurs in the context of chronic renal failure.* Severe osteodystrophy is seen in patients who are maintained on long-term dialysis, because they live long enough to develop conspicuous bone disease.

☐ **Pathogenesis:** The pathogenesis of renal osteodystrophy is similar to that of osteomalacia, with secondary hyperparathyroidism exerting its influence by way of osteoclastic resorption of bone (see Fig. 26-9). The sequence of events leading to renal osteodystrophy may be summarized as follows:

1. In patients with chronic renal disease, a reduced glomerular filtration rate leads to retention of phosphate, thereby producing **hyperphosphatemia.**
2. Tubular injury causes a reduction in 1α-hydroxylase activity, with a resulting deficiency of $1,25(OH)_2D$.
3. Intestinal calcium absorption is, in turn, decreased, thereby producing **hypocalcemia.**
4. Hypocalcemia stimulates elaboration of PTH and, in severe cases, may lead to **secondary hyperparathyroidism.**

☐ **Pathology and Clinical Features:** As a result of these effects of chronic renal failure, renal osteodystrophy is characterized by varying degrees of osteomalacia, osteitis fibrosis cystica, and osteosclerosis. Microscopically, trabecular bone is increased and haphazardly arranged. Patients with terminal chronic renal disease and hyperphosphatemia may display metastatic calcification at various sites, including the eyes, skin, muscular coats of the arteries and arterioles, and periarticular soft tissues.

Management of cases of renal osteodystrophy involves not only treatment of renal failure but also the control of phosphate levels by appropriate drug therapy and infusions. Occasionally, parathyroidectomy is necessary to control hyperparathyroidism, and administration of vitamin D may also be necessary.

PAGET DISEASE OF BONE

■ *Paget disease is a chronic condition caused by disordered bone remodeling, in which excessive bone resorption initially results in lytic lesions that are followed by disorganized and excessive bone formation.*

☐ **Epidemiology:** Paget disease is common and generally affects men and women older than 60 years of age. In predisposed populations, 3% to 4% of elderly persons manifest the disease either at autopsy or on radiographic examination. The disorder has an unusual worldwide distribution, afflicting populations of the British Isles and following their migrations throughout the world. Persons of English descent living in the United States, Australia, New Zealand, and Canada have a high incidence of the disease. Northern Europeans also have a higher incidence of Paget disease than southern Europeans. The disorder is almost nonexistent in Asia, however, and in the indigenous populations of Africa and South America.

☐ **Pathogenesis:** Paget disease is of unknown cause. A hereditary predisposition is suggested by reports of almost 100 families in which Paget disease seems to be transmitted as an autosomal dominant trait. Recently, however, inclusions consistent with the structure of a virus have been demonstrated in the osteoclasts of Paget disease. Virtually all patients with Paget disease exhibit these inclusions, which are not found in any other skeletal disease except for giant cell tumors of bone (Fig. 26-16).

☐ **Pathology:** The lesions of Paget disease may be solitary or may occur at multiple sites. They tend to localize to the bones of the axial skeleton, including the spine, skull, and pelvis. The proximal femur and tibia may also be involved in the polyostotic form of the disease. **Paget disease is characterized by an uncoupling of osteoblastic and osteoclastic activities.** The disease is triphasic:

1. **"Hot" or Osteoclastic Resorptive Stage.** Radiologically, there is a characteristic, sharply defined, flame- or wedge-shaped lysis of the cortex, which often mimics a tumor.
2. **Mixed Stage of Osteoblastic and Osteoclastic Activity.** Radiologically, bones are generally larger than normal; in fact, Paget disease is one of two diseases that produces **larger-than-normal bones** (the other being fibrous dysplasia, which is discussed later). The cortex in the mixed phase is thickened,

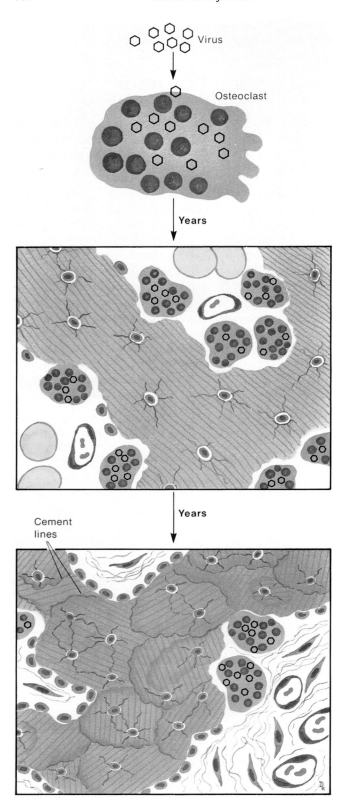

Cement
lines

and accentuation of the coarse cancellous bone makes the bone look heavy and enlarged (Fig. 26-17). Involvement of the vertebral bodies leads to a "picture frame" appearance, because the cortices and end plates become greatly exaggerated compared with the coarse cancellous bone of the vertebral body. Although the bone is abnormal, the distorted coarse cancellous bone and cortex still tend to align along stress lines. The pelvis is often thickened in the area of the acetabulum.

3. **"Cold" or Burnt-Out Stage.** This stage is characterized by little cellular activity and, radiologically, by thickened and disordered bones.

The diagnostic histologic feature of Paget disease is abnormal arrangement of lamellar bone, in which islands of irregular bone formation, resembling pieces of a jigsaw puzzle, are separated by prominent "cement lines" (Fig. 26-18). The result is a mosaic pattern in the bone. The osteoclasts are very large, with each possessing more than 12 hyperchromatic nuclei. Thus, they appear as large cells with dark, smeared nuclei. These are the cells that exhibit the virus-like particles by electron microscopy; however, the osteoclast precursor cells do not contain such particles.

☐ **Clinical Features:** The most common focal symptom of Paget disease is pain, although its cause is not clear. The pain may be related to microfractures, stimulation of free nerve endings by dilated blood vessels adjacent to the bones, or weight-bearing in weaker bones.

Skull Involvement. Involvement of the skull is particularly common in patients with Paget disease. The skull often exhibits localized lysis, generally in the frontal and parietal bones, which is termed **osteoporosis circumscripta.** Alternatively, there may be thickening of the outer and inner tables, which is most pronounced in the frontal and occipital bones.

Pagetic Steal. Occasionally, patients feel lightheaded, a symptom thought to result from the so-called pagetic steal, in which blood is shunted from the internal carotid system to the bones rather than being directed to the brain.

FIGURE **26-16**
Hypothetical viral pathogenesis of Paget disease of bone. A virus infects osteoclastic progenitors or osteoclasts and stimulates osteoclastic activity, thereby leading to excessive resorption of bone. During a period of years, the bone develops a characteristic mosaic pattern, which is produced by chaotically juxtaposed units of lamellar bone that form irregular cement lines. The adjacent marrow is often fibrotic, and there is a mixture of osteoclasts and osteoblasts on the surface of the bone.

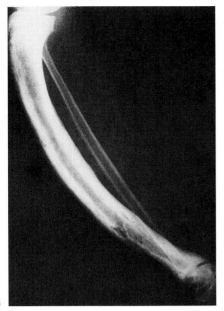
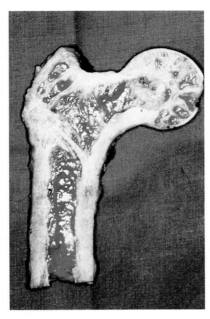
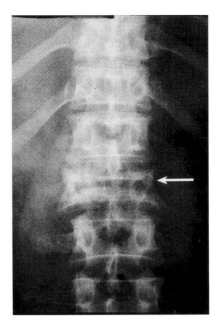

FIGURE 26-17

Paget disease. (A) A radiograph of the lower leg shows marked involvement of the tibia by Paget disease, with thickening and disorganization of the cortex. Note the normal appearance of the fibula. (B) The proximal end of a femur affected by Paget disease shows replacement of the normal cancellous architecture by coarse, thick bundles of trabecular bone. The cortical bone is irregularly thickened and exhibits a coarse, granular appearance instead of the normally smooth cortical bone. (C) A radiograph of the spine shows a vertebra (*arrow*) affected by Paget disease. The vertebra is shorter and wider than normal and displays the characteristic "picture frame" appearance.

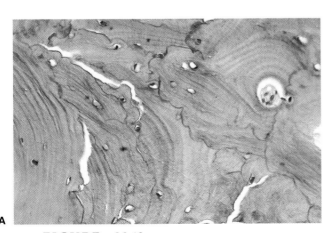
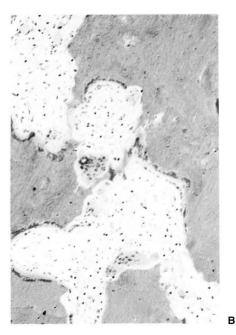

FIGURE 26-18

Paget disease. (A) A section of bone shows prominent basophilic cement lines with several microfractures. (B) In this Goldner-stained section, two osteoclasts are evident, each containing many more nuclei than normal. There are numerous osteoblasts together with new, unmineralized osteoid (*red*) and marrow fibrosis.

Fractures. Bone fractures are common in patients with Paget disease, the bones snapping transversely like a piece of chalk.

High-Output Cardiac Failure. In patients with extensive Paget disease, the flow of blood to bone and subcutaneous tissue is remarkably increased, which requires an increased cardiac output that may be severe enough to result in cardiac failure.

Sarcomatous Change. Neoplastic transformation may occur in a focus of Paget disease, usually in the femur, humerus, or pelvis. This complication occurs in less than 1% of all cases, however, and usually arises in patients with severe Paget disease. Interestingly, the skull and vertebrae, which are the bones most commonly involved in Paget disease, rarely undergo sarcomatous change. The sarcoma is usually osteogenic but may also be fibrogenic or cartilaginous.

Giant Cell Tumor. This lesion is not a neoplasm but, rather, a reactive phenomenon similar to the "brown tumor" of hyperparathyroidism. Giant cell tumor is thought to represent an overshoot of osteoclastic activity and an associated fibroblastic response. Radiation therapy for the giant cell tumor is curative in many cases.

Serum calcium and phosphorus levels are normal, even though the turnover rate of bone is increased more than 20-fold.

Fortunately, most patients with Paget disease are asymptomatic and, therefore, require no treatment. Fractures, osteoarthritis, and other orthopedic complications are treated symptomatically.

FIBROUS DYSPLASIA

■ *Fibrous dysplasia is a peculiar developmental abnormality of the skeleton that is characterized by a disorganized mixture of fibrous and osseous elements in the interior of affected bones.* It occurs in both children or adults and may involve a single bone (monostotic) or many bones (polyostotic). In 5% of the cases of fibrous dysplasia, skeletal lesions are associated with skin pigmentation and endocrine dysfunction, in which case the term **McCune-Albright syndrome** is applied.

Monostotic Fibrous Dysplasia. Monostotic fibrous dysplasia is the most common form of the disease and is most often seen during the second and third decades of life. Commonly involved bones are the proximal femur, tibia, ribs, and facial bones, although any bone

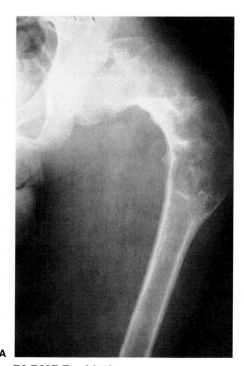

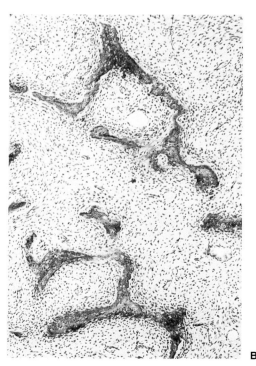

A   B

FIGURE   *26-19*
Fibrous dysplasia. **(A)** A radiograph of the proximal femur shows a "shepherd's crook" deformity, which is caused by fractures sustained over the years. There are irregular, marginated, ground-glass lucencies that are surrounded by reactive bone. The shaft has an appearance that has been likened to that of a soap bubble. **(B)** A photomicrograph reveals whorled fibrous tissue surrounding irregularly shaped spicules of woven bone.

may be involved. The disease may be asymptomatic, or it may lead to a pathologic fracture.

Polyostotic Fibrous Dysplasia. One-fourth of the patients with polyostotic fibrous dysplasia exhibit disease in more than half of the skeleton, including the facial bones. Symptoms usually present during childhood, and almost all patients suffer from pathologic fractures, limb deformities, or limb-length discrepancies. Polyostotic fibrous dysplasia is more common in females than in males. Sometimes, the disease becomes quiescent at puberty, whereas pregnancy may stimulate the growth of lesions.

McCune-Albright Syndrome. This condition is characterized by the association of fibrous dysplasia with endocrine dysfunction, including acromegaly, Cushing syndrome, hyperthyroidism, and vitamin D-resistant rickets. The most common endocrine abnormality is precocious puberty in females (males rarely have McCune-Albright syndrome). As a result, premature closure of the growth plates may lead to an abnormally short stature. The most frequent extraskeletal manifestations of McCune-Albright syndrome are the characteristic skin lesions. These are pigmented macules (café-au-lait spots) that are usually located over the buttocks, back, and sacrum.

☐ **Pathology:** The radiographic features of fibrous dysplasia are distinctive. The bone lesion has a lucent, ground-glass appearance, with well-marginated borders and a thin cortex. The bone may be ballooned, deformed, or enlarged, and involvement may be focal or encompass the entire bone (Fig. 26-19).

Histologically, benign fibroblastic tissue is arranged in a loose, whorled pattern (see Fig. 26-19). Irregularly arranged, purposeless spicules of woven bone, which lack osteoblastic rimming, are embedded in the fibrous tissue. In 10% of the cases, irregular islands of hyaline cartilage are also present. Occasionally, cystic degeneration occurs, with hemosiderin-laden macrophages, hemorrhage, and osteoclasts congregated about the cyst. Rarely (<1% of cases), malignant degeneration (osteosarcoma, chondrosarcoma, or fibrosarcoma) has been reported, but most of these cases involve previous exposure to radiation. Treatment of fibrous dysplasia consists of curettage, repair of fractures, and prevention of deformities.

NEOPLASMS OF BONE

A primary bone tumor may arise from any of the cellular elements of bone. Most neoplasms of bone occur near the metaphyseal area, however, and more than 80% of primary tumors occur in either the distal femur or the proximal tibia (Fig. 26-20).

Benign Tumors

Nonossifying Fibroma (Fibrous Cortical Defect)

■ *Nonossifying fibroma is a benign and usually solitary, fibromatous lesion of childhood that occurs in the metaphysis of a long bone, most commonly the tibia or femur.* The disorder is very common and may be present in as many as 25% of all children between 4 and 10 years of age, after which time it characteristically regresses. Most patients are asymptomatic, although pain or fracture through the thin cortex overlying the lesion occasionally may call attention to the condition.

☐ **Pathology:** Radiologically, nonossifying fibromas are identified by a cortical, eccentric position and by well-demarcated, central lucent zones that are surrounded by scalloped, sclerotic margins. On gross examination, the lesion is granular and dark red to brown. Microscopically, bland spindle cells are ar-

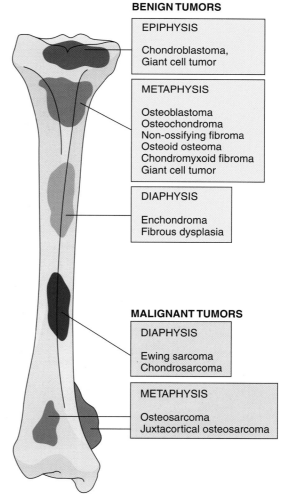

BENIGN TUMORS

EPIPHYSIS
Chondroblastoma, Giant cell tumor

METAPHYSIS
Osteoblastoma Osteochondroma Non-ossifying fibroma Osteoid osteoma Chondromyxoid fibroma Giant cell tumor

DIAPHYSIS
Enchondroma Fibrous dysplasia

MALIGNANT TUMORS

DIAPHYSIS
Ewing sarcoma Chondrosarcoma

METAPHYSIS
Osteosarcoma Juxtacortical osteosarcoma

FIGURE   *26-20*
Location of primary bone tumors in long tubular bones.

ranged in an interlacing, whorled pattern, in which multinuclear giant cells and foamy macrophages may be seen. The rare symptomatic lesions are treated by curettage and bone grafting.

Osteoid Osteoma

■ *Osteoid osteoma is a common, small, painful yet benign neoplasm of bone composed of osteoid tissue (the nidus) and surrounded by a halo of reactive bone formation.* The tumor occurs in persons ranging from 5 to 25 years of age, and males are more commonly affected than females (male:female ratio, 3 : 1). Osteoid osteoma frequently arises in the cortex of the diaphysis of the tubular bones of the lower extremity.

☐ **Pathology:** Osteoid osteoma is a spherical, hyperemic tumor of approximately 1 cm in diameter that is usually considerably softer than the surrounding bone (Fig. 26-21). It is easily enucleated at surgery. Microscopically, the tumor is composed of thin, irregular, osteoid trabeculae within a cellular granulation tissue containing osteoblasts and osteoclasts. The osteoid is more mature in the center, which is often partially calcified. Reactive, sclerotic bone (osteoma) surrounds the osteoid nidus.

☐ **Clinical Features:** Pain, typically nocturnal, is out of proportion to the size of the lesion. This pain is often exacerbated by the intake of alcoholic beverages and promptly relieved by the administration of aspirin, possibly because of the high prostaglandin content of the tumor. Surgical excision is curative—and leaves the patient very grateful to the surgeon.

Solitary Chondroma (Enchondroma)

■ *Solitary chondroma is a benign, intraosseous tumor that is composed of well-differentiated cartilage.* The diagnosis is made at any age, because many cases are entirely asymptomatic. Most cases of solitary chondroma occur in the metacarpals and phalanges of the hands, with the remainder occurring in almost any other tubular bone. The tumor is small and grows slowly. Radiologically, it appears as a well-delimited, osteolytic area.

On gross examination, a solitary chondroma has the semitranslucent appearance of hyaline cartilage, often with a few calcified areas. Microscopically, the cartilaginous tissue is well differentiated, with sparse chondrocytes being embedded in a myxoid stroma. Asymptomatic chondromas are best left untreated. When pain intervenes, however, curettage and bone grafting are the treatment of choice.

Malignant Tumors

Osteosarcoma (Osteogenic Sarcoma)

■ *Osteosarcoma is a highly malignant bone tumor that is characterized by the formation of neoplastic bone tissue.* It is also the most common primary malignant bone tumor, accounting for one-fifth of all bone cancers. Osteosarcoma is most frequent in adolescents between 10 and 20 years of age and affects males more often than females (male:female ratio, 2:1).

☐ **Pathogenesis:** More than two-thirds of the cases of osteosarcoma that have been studied exhibit muta-

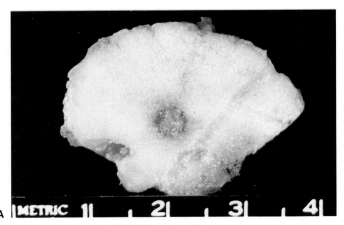

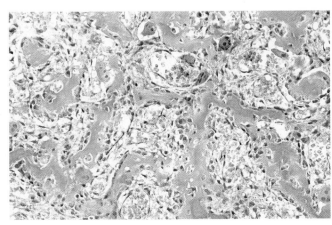

FIGURE   *26-21*
Osteoid osteoma. **(A) A gross specimen of an osteoid osteoma shows the central nidus, which is embedded in dense bone. (B) A photomicrograph of the nidus reveals irregular trabeculae of woven bone, which are surrounded by osteoblasts, osteoclasts, and fibrovascular marrow.**

tions in the retinoblastoma (*Rb*) gene (see Chapter 5). Mutations in the *p53* gene are also common. When the tumor arises in older persons, it is almost always as a complication of Paget disease or radiation exposure. For example, radium watch-dial painters who wetted their brushes with saliva developed osteosarcoma many years later because of the deposition of radium in their bones. Moreover, osteosarcoma has also developed in adults and children who have been subjected to external therapeutic radiation. Several pre-existing, benign bone lesions are associated with an increased risk of later osteosarcoma, including fibrous dysplasia, osteochondromatosis, and chondromatosis.

□ **Pathology:** Osteosarcoma often arises in the vicinity of the knee—that is, the lower femur (Fig. 26-22), upper tibia, or fibula—although any metaphyseal area of a long bone may be affected. The proximal humerus is second in incidence to the knee area as a site of osteosarcoma, and 75% of all these tumors arise adjacent to the knee or shoulder. The hands, feet, skull, and jaw are less common sites for this disease, being affected more frequently in persons older than 25 years of age.

Radiologic evidence of bone destruction as well as formation is characteristic, with the latter representing neoplastic bone. Often, the periosteum is elevated by reactive bone adjacent to the tumor. A "sunburst" pattern is often present as well. The cut surface of an osteogenic sarcoma may show any combination of hemorrhagic, cystic, soft, and bony hard areas. The neoplastic tissue may invade and break through the cortex, spread into the marrow cavity, elevate or perforate the periosteum, or grow into the epiphysis and even reach the joint space.

Histologic examination reveals malignant osteoblasts, producing osteoid and tumor bone (see Fig. 26-22). The neoplastic bone is usually woven and laid down haphazardly. Often, foci of malignant cartilage cells or malignant giant cells are intermixed.

Osteosarcoma spreads through the bloodstream to the lungs. In fact, almost all patients (98%) who die of this disease have lung metastases. Less commonly, the tumor metastasizes to other bones (35%), the pleura (33%), and the heart (20%).

□ **Clinical Features:** Osteosarcoma usually presents as mild or intermittent pain around the knee or other involved areas. As the pain becomes more intense, the involved area swells, and palpation is painful. Recent developments in chemotherapy and limb-sparing surgery have resulted in 5-year disease-free rates as high as 50%.

Chondrosarcoma

■ *Chondrosarcoma is a malignant tumor that originates from cartilage cells and maintains its cartilaginous nature throughout its evolution.* Most cases arise de novo; only a few patients have a history of a pre-existing benign cartilaginous lesion (e.g., osteochondromatosis). Chondrosarcoma is the second most common primary malignant bone tumor, occurring more commonly in men than in women (male:female ratio, 2:1). It is most frequently seen during the fourth to sixth decades of life (average patient age, 45 years).

□ **Pathology:** Chondrosarcoma occurs in three variants, which are classified according to location.

Central Chondrosarcoma. This type arises in the medullary cavity of the pelvic bones, ribs, and long bones, although any site may, on occasion, be affected.

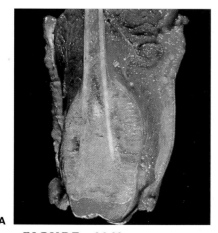
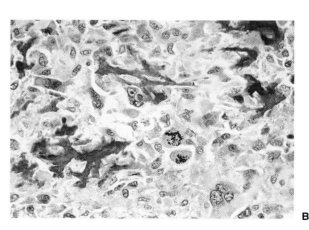

FIGURE *26-22*
Osteosarcoma. (A) The distal femur contains a dense, osteoblastic, malignant tumor, which extends through the cortex into the soft tissue and epiphysis. (B) A photomicrograph reveals pleomorphic malignant cells, tumor giant cells, and mitoses. The tumor produces bone matrix that is focally calcified.

The tumor may penetrate the cortex, but extension beyond the periosteum is uncommon. On gross examination, the neoplastic cartilaginous tissue is compressed inside the bone and exhibits areas of necrosis, cystic change, and hemorrhage. The cortex of the bone is infiltrated by the tumor.

Peripheral Chondrosarcoma. This form is less common than the central variety and arises outside the bone, either de novo or in the cartilaginous cap of an osteochondroma. It occurs in patients older than 20 years of age and never before puberty. The most frequent location of peripheral chondrosarcoma is the pelvis, followed by the femur, vertebrae (Fig. 26-23), sacrum, humerus, and other long bones. Macroscopically, peripheral chondrosarcoma tends to be a large, bosselated mass that surrounds the base of an osteochondroma and invades the bone.

Juxtacortical Chondrosarcoma. This is the least common variety of chondrosarcoma and is similar to central chondrosarcoma in its predilection for middle-aged men. It tends to be situated in the metaphysis of the long bones, lying on the outer surface of the cortex. Thus, it is probably of periosteal or parosteal origin.

Histologically, chondrosarcomas are composed of malignant cartilage cells in various stages of maturity (see Fig. 26-23). Occasionally, a well-differentiated chondrosarcoma is difficult to distinguish from a benign tumor on the basis of cytologic findings alone. Zones of calcification are often conspicuous and are seen on radiography as splotches or bulky masses.

Chondrosarcoma is one of the few tumors in which microscopic grading has significant prognostic value. In one study, the 5-year survival rate for patients with low-grade chondrosarcomas was 80%, for patients with moderate-grade tumors 50%, and for patients with high-grade tumors only 20%.

Chondrosarcoma expands by stimulating osteoclastic resorption of bone and often breaks through the cortex. Most chondrosarcomas grow slowly, but hematogenous metastases to the lungs are common in poorly differentiated variants. Wide excision is often necessary.

Giant Cell Tumor

■ *Giant cell tumor of bone is a locally aggressive, potentially malignant neoplasm that is characterized by the presence of multinucleated giant cells.* It usually occurs during the third and fourth decades of life, has a slight predilection for women, and seems to be more common in Asia than in Western countries. In older patients, giant cell tumors may also complicate Paget disease or exposure to radiation. Giant cell tumors are thought to arise from primitive stromal cells that have the capacity to modulate into osteoclasts.

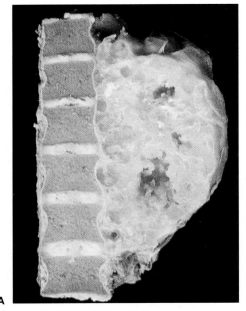
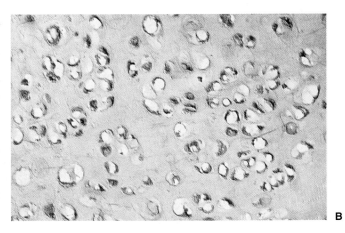

A   B

FIGURE   26-23

Chondrosarcoma. (A) A section through a chondrosarcoma of the vertebral column shows a glistening surface with focal calcification. (B) A photomicrograph of a chondrosarcoma demonstrates malignant chondrocytes with pronounced atypia.

□ **Pathology:** In the large majority of cases (90%), giant cell tumor of bone originates at the junction between the metaphysis and the epiphysis of a long bone, with more than half being situated in the knee area (distal femur and proximal tibia; Fig. 26-24). The lower end of the radius, humerus, fibula, and skull are also occasionally involved.

On gross examination, giant cell tumor is clearly circumscribed, and the cut surface is soft and light brown, without bone or calcification. Numerous hemorrhagic areas may result in the appearance of a sponge full of blood. In some cases, cystic cavities and necrotic areas are present. Giant cell tumor is often limited by the periosteum, although in patients with aggressive forms, it may penetrate the cortex and periosteum, even reaching the joint capsule and synovial membrane.

Microscopically, giant cell tumor exhibits two types of cells (see Fig. 26-24). The mononuclear ("stromal") cells are plump and oval, with large nuclei and scanty cytoplasm. Large osteoclastic giant cells, some with more than 100 nuclei, are scattered throughout the richly vascularized stroma. Diffuse interstitial hemorrhage is common.

Only the mononuclear cells are thought to be neoplastic. All giant cell tumors must be viewed as being potentially malignant, because as many as half recur locally after simple curettage and 5% to 10% metastasize to distant sites, particularly the lungs, after this procedure. Importantly, almost all cases of metastases have occurred after an initial surgical intervention. Thus, some believe that recurrence of the tumor reflects inadequate resection, and that distant metastases result from the dislodgment of tumor fragments during surgery.

□ **Clinical Features:** Giant cell tumors commonly present with pain, often in the joint adjacent to the tumor. Microfractures and pathologic fractures are common owing to thinning of the cortex. The tumor is usually treated with thorough curettage and bone grafting, although more aggressive management, including en bloc resection or even amputation, may be necessary.

Ewing Sarcoma

■ *Ewing sarcoma is an uncommon, malignant bone tumor that is composed of small, uniform, round cells, which*

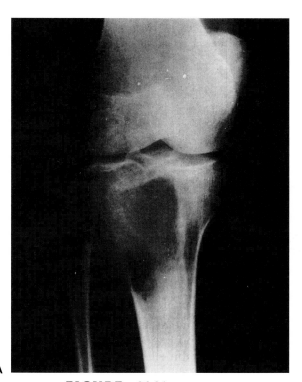
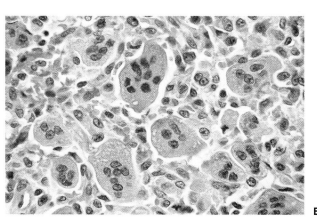

FIGURE   26-24
Giant cell tumor of bone. (A) A radiograph of the proximal tibia shows an eccentric lytic lesion, with virtually no new bone formation. The tumor extends to the subchondral bone plate and breaks through cortex into the soft tissue. (B) A photomicrograph shows osteoclast-type giant cells and plump, oval, mononuclear cells. The nuclei of both types of cells are identical.

belong to a family of primitive neuroectodermal tumors of childhood. It represents only 4% to 5% of all bone tumors and is found in both children and adolescents, with two-thirds of the cases occurring in patients younger than 20 years of age. Males are affected more often than females (male:female ratio, 2:1). Ewing sarcoma is believed to arise from primitive marrow elements or immature mesenchymal cells. Most Ewing sarcomas have a reciprocal translocation between chromosomes 11 and 22, which results in fusion of the Ewing sarcoma (*EWS*) gene to a transcription factor termed the *FLI-1* gene. The resulting chimeric gene product or fusion protein is an aberrant transcription factor and is also tumorigenic.

☐ **Pathology:** Ewing sarcoma is primarily a tumor of the long bones, especially the humerus, tibia, and femur, where it occurs as a midshaft or metaphyseal lesion. However, no bone is immune from involvement, and the tumor can also occur in the hands, feet, and other bones.

On gross examination, Ewing sarcoma is typically soft, grayish-white, and often studded by hemorrhagic foci and areas of necrosis. The tumor may infiltrate the medullary spaces without destroying the bony trabeculae. It may also diffusely infiltrate the cortical bone or form nodules in which the bone is completely resorbed. In many cases, the tumor mass penetrates the periosteum and extends into the soft tissues.

Microscopically, Ewing tumor cells typically appear as sheets of closely packed, small, round cells with little cytoplasm, which are as much as twice the size of a lymphocyte (Fig. 26-25). In some areas, the neoplastic cells tend to form rosettes, often with a central vessel. An important diagnostic feature is the presence of substantial amounts of glycogen in the cytoplasm of the tumor cells, which is well visualized with use of periodic acid-Schiff staining. Fibrous strands separate the sheets of cells into irregular nests. There is little or no interstitial stroma, and mitoses are infrequent.

Ewing sarcoma metastasizes to many organs, including the lungs and brain. Other bones, especially the skull, are also common sites for metastases (45–75% of cases).

☐ **Clinical Features:** Ewing sarcoma initially presents with pain, which becomes more intense and is

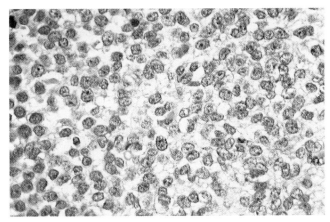

FIGURE   *26-25*
Ewing sarcoma. The tumor shows small, round cells with glycogen-filled, clear cytoplasm.

followed by swelling of the affected area. Use of chemotherapy combined with radiation therapy and surgery has led to a 5-year disease-free survival rate of 75%.

Metastatic Tumors

The most common malignant tumor of bone is metastatic cancer. Carcinomas, specifically tumors of the breast, prostate, lung, thyroid, and kidney, comprise the large majority of metastatic lesions to bone. Tumor cells usually arrive in the bone via the bloodstream; in the case of spinal metastases, they are often transported through the vertebral veins. It is estimated that skeletal metastases are found in at least 85% of the cases of cancer that have run their full clinical course. The vertebral column is by far the most commonly affected bony structure.

Some tumors (cancers of the thyroid, gastrointestinal tract, kidney, and neuroblastoma) produce mostly lytic lesions by stimulating osteoclasts. A few neoplasms (prostate, breast, lung, and stomach cancers) stimulate osteoblastic components to make bone; these appear radiographically as dense foci. However, most deposits of metastatic cancer in the bones have mixtures of both lytic and blastic elements.

FIGURE   *26-26*
Histogenesis of osteoarthritis. (A and B) The death of chondrocytes leads to a crack in the articular cartilage, which is followed by an influx of synovial fluid as well as further loss and degeneration of cartilage. (C) As a result of this process, cartilage is gradually worn away. Below the tide mark, new vessels grow in from the epiphysis. (D) At this point, fibrocartilage is also deposited. (E) The fibrocartilage plug is not mechanically sufficient and may be worn away, thereby exposing the subchondral bone plate, which then becomes thickened and eburnated. If there is a crack in this region, synovial fluid leaks into the marrow space and produces a subchondral bone cyst. Focal regrowth of the articular surface leads to formation of osteophytes.

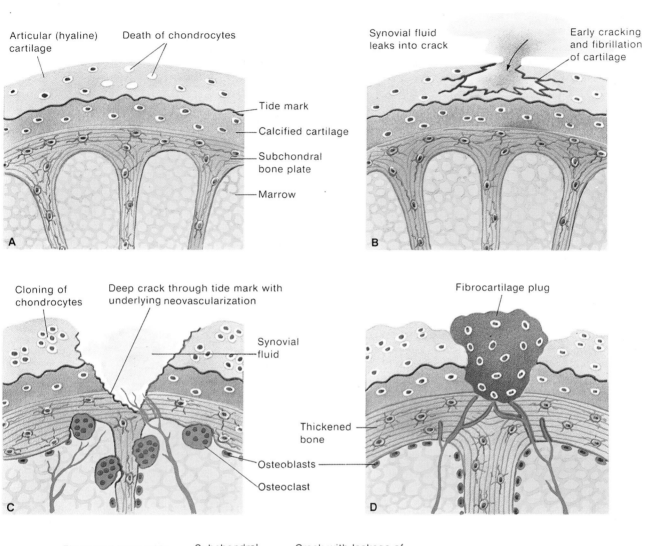

A — Articular (hyaline) cartilage; Death of chondrocytes; Tide mark; Calcified cartilage; Subchondral bone plate; Marrow

B — Synovial fluid leaks into crack; Early cracking and fibrillation of cartilage

C — Cloning of chondrocytes; Deep crack through tide mark with underlying neovascularization; Synovial fluid; Osteoblasts; Osteoclast

D — Fibrocartilage plug; Thickened bone

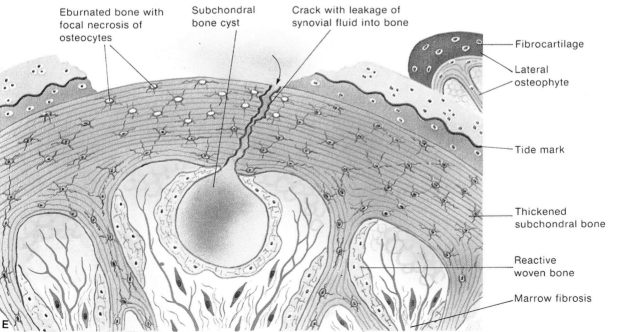

E — Eburnated bone with focal necrosis of osteocytes; Subchondral bone cyst; Crack with leakage of synovial fluid into bone; Fibrocartilage; Lateral osteophyte; Tide mark; Thickened subchondral bone; Reactive woven bone; Marrow fibrosis

Joints

OSTEOARTHRITIS

■ *Osteoarthritis is a slowly progressive degeneration of the articular cartilage that manifests in the weight-bearing joints and fingers of older persons or in the joints of younger persons subjected to trauma.* **Osteoarthritis is the single most common form of joint disease.** The disorder is not a single nosologic entity but, rather, a group of conditions that have in common the mechanical destruction of a joint.

Primary osteoarthritis is a disease of unknown cause in which destruction of the joints is believed to result from an intrinsic defect of the joint cartilage. Both the prevalence and severity of primary osteoarthritis increases with age, and persons who are 75 years of age have an incidence rate of 85%. Many cases of primary osteoarthritis seem to exhibit a familial clustering, thereby suggesting that hereditary factors may predispose to the disease. This form of osteoarthritis has variously been called "wear-and-tear" arthritis and "degenerative joint disease." Progressive degradation of articular cartilage leads to joint narrowing, subchondral bone thickening, and eventually, a nonfunctioning and painful joint. Although osteoarthritis is not primarily an inflammatory process, a mild inflammatory reaction may occur within the synovium.

Secondary osteoarthritis has a known underlying cause, including congenital or acquired incongruity of joints, trauma, crystal deposits, infection, metabolic diseases, endocrinopathies, inflammatory diseases, osteonecrosis, and hemarthrosis.

□ **Pathogenesis and Pathology:** Joints that are commonly affected by osteoarthritis are the proximal and distal interphalangeal joints of the upper extremity, knees, hips, and the cervical and lumbar segments of the spine. Radiologically, osteoarthritis is characterized by (1) narrowing of the joint space, which represents the loss of articular cartilage; (2) increased thickness of the subchondral bone; (3) subchondral bone cysts; and (4) large peripheral growths of bone and cartilage, called **osteophytes,** which represent the bone's attempt to grow a new articular surface. The progressive pathologic changes in patients with osteoarthritis can be arbitrarily divided into a number of stages:

1. The earliest changes of osteoarthritis are the loss of proteoglycans from the surface of the articular cartilage and the death of chondrocytes (Fig. 26-26).
2. Osteoarthritis may arrest at this stage for many years before proceeding to the next stage, which is characterized by fibrillation and development of surface cracks parallel to the long axis of the articular surface.
3. As fibrillations propagate, synovial fluid begins to flow into the defects and works its way deeper into the articular cartilage along the crack.
4. Later, the crack extends deeper, and neovascularization from the epiphysis and subchondral bone extends into the area of the crack, thereby inducing subchondral osteoclastic bone resorption. Adjacent osteoblastic activity also occurs, and the net result is thickening of the subchondral bone plate in the area of the crack. Fibrocartilage plugs form as a poor substitute for the articular hyaline cartilage (Fig. 26-27). The subchondral bone becomes exposed and burnished as it grinds against the opposite joint surface,

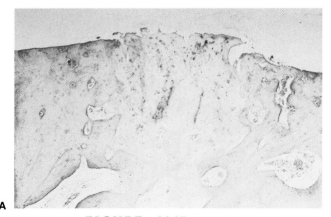

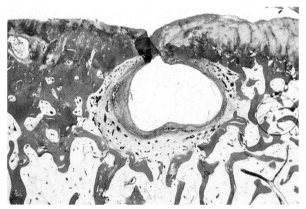

A   B

FIGURE *26-27*

Osteoarthritis. (A) A section of the femoral head from a patient with osteoarthritis shows a fibrocartilaginous plug extending from the marrow onto the joint surface. Eburnated bone is seen on both sides of the plug. (B) A section through the articular surface of an osteoarthritic joint demonstrates focal absence of the articular cartilage, thickening of subchondral bone (*right*), and a subchondral bone cyst.

which is undergoing the same process. These thick, shiny, and smooth areas of subchondral bone are referred to as **eburnated** ("ivory-like") bone (see Figs. 26-26 and 26-27).

5. The eburnated bone eventually cracks, thereby allowing synovial fluid to extend from the joint surface into the subchondral bone marrow, where it eventually leads to a **subchondral bone cyst** (see Figs. 26-26 and 26-27).

6. An **osteophyte** develops, usually in the lateral portions of the joint, when the mesenchymal tissue of the synovium modulates into osteoblasts and chondroblasts to form a mass of cartilage and bone. In the fingers, osteophytes at the distal interphalangeal joints are termed **Heberden nodes.**

☐ **Clinical Features:** The signs and symptoms of osteoarthritis relate to the location of the involved joints and both the severity and duration of the joint deterioration. The involved joints may be enlarged, tender, and boggy, and may also demonstrate crepitus. Deep, achy joint pain that follows activity and is relieved by rest is the clinical hallmark of osteoarthritis. Restriction of joint motion is a harbinger of severe disease and may result from joint or muscle contractures, intra-articular loose bodies, large osteophytes, and loss of congruity of the joint surfaces.

At present, there is no specific treatment to prevent or arrest osteoarthritis. Therapy is directed at specific orthopedic conditions and includes exercise, weight loss, and other supportive measures. In patients with disabling osteoarthritis, joint replacement may be necessary.

RHEUMATOID ARTHRITIS

■ *Rheumatoid arthritis is a systemic, chronic inflammatory disease in which chronic polyarthritis involves diarthrodial joints bilaterally.* The proximal interphalangeal and metacarpophalangeal joints, elbows, knees, ankles, and spine are commonly affected. The onset usually occurs during the third or fourth decade of life, but the prevalence increases with age until 70 years. However, rheumatoid arthritis may occur at any age. The disease afflicts 1% to 2% of the adult population, and its incidence is greater in women than in men (female:male ratio, 3 : 1). The course of the disease is variable and is often punctuated by remissions and exacerbations. The broad spectrum of clinical manifestations ranges from barely discernible signs and symptoms to destructive and mutilating disease.

It is now thought that classic rheumatoid arthritis probably comprises a heterogeneous group of disorders. Patients who are persistently seronegative for rheumatoid factor may have disease of a different cause than patients who are seropositive.

☐ **Pathogenesis:** The cause of rheumatoid arthritis is unknown, but a number of factors have been implicated.

Genetic Factors. A contribution of hereditary factors to patient susceptibility to rheumatoid arthritis is suggested by the increased frequency of the disease among first-degree relatives of affected persons and by concordance for the illness among monozygotic twins (30%). It is generally agreed that certain major histocompatibility (HLA) genes, especially a specific set of HLA-DR alleles, are expressed in a nonrandom manner among patients with rheumatoid arthritis.

Humoral Immunity. Lymphocytes and plasma cells accumulate in the synovium, where they produce immunoglobulins, mainly of the IgG class. In addition, immune complex deposits are present in the articular cartilage and synovium. Increased serum levels of IgM, IgA, and IgG may also be found in patients with rheumatoid arthritis.

As many as 80% of the patients with classic rheumatoid arthritis are positive for **rheumatoid factor.** The presence of rheumatoid factor in high titer is frequently associated with severe and unremitting disease, many systemic complications, and a serious prognosis. This factor actually represents multiple antibodies, principally IgM but sometimes IgG or IgA, that are directed against the Fc fragment of IgG. Such antibodies are known as anti-idiotype antibodies. Nevertheless, rheumatoid factor is not specifically diagnostic for rheumatoid arthritis, and significant titers are also found in patients with many other disorders.

Cellular Immunity. Abundant T lymphocytes in the rheumatoid synovium are frequently Ia-positive ("activated") and of the helper type. They are also often in close contact with HLA-DR-positive cells, which are either macrophages or so-called dendritic Ia-positive cells. In addition, patients with rheumatoid arthritis demonstrate a reactivity of T lymphocytes with collagen (types I and III).

Infectious Agents. There is a high incidence of circulating antibodies to a variety of Epstein-Barr virus (EBV) antigens in patients with rheumatoid arthritis. Most patients with rheumatoid arthritis develop antibodies against a nuclear antigen in EBV-infected B cells. This antigen is termed **rheumatoid arthritis–**

associated nuclear antigen, and it is closely related to the nuclear antigen that is encoded by EBV. The peripheral blood of many patients with rheumatoid arthritis contains an increased number of EBV-infected B cells.

A hypothetical scenario consistent with the evidence presented earlier might be constructed as follows:

1. In a genetically susceptible person, an unknown agent (possibly a virus, and possibly EBV) infects a joint or some other tissue and then stimulates the formation of antibodies.
2. These immunoglobulins act as new antigens—that is, they trigger the production of anti-idiotype antibodies (rheumatoid factor).
3. Immune complexes, which contain rheumatoid factor, are deposited in the synovium and activate the complement cascade. This results in increased vascular permeability and the uptake of immune complexes by leukocytes, which, in turn, release lysosomal enzymes, activated oxygen species, and other injurious products.
4. Activated macrophages in the synovium present unknown antigens to T cells, thereby stimulating the production of cytokines, which, in turn, amplify inflammation, tissue injury, and the proliferation of synovial cells.

☐ **Pathology:** The early synovial changes of rheumatoid arthritis are edema and the accumulation of plasma cells, lymphocytes, and macrophages (Fig. 26-28). There is a concomitant increase in vascularity and exudation of fibrin in the joint space, which may result in small fibrin nodules that float in the joint (**rice bodies**).

The synovial lining cells undergo hyperplasia, and multinucleated giant cells are often found among them. **The net result is a synovial lining thrown into numerous villi and frond-like folds that fill the peripheral recesses of the joint** (Fig. 26-29). The hyperplastic synovium creeps over the surface of the articular cartilage and adjacent structures to form a **pannus** (cloak). Lymphocytes aggregate into masses and, eventually, develop follicular centers (**Allison-Ghormley bodies**).

The pannus erodes the articular cartilage and adjacent bone, probably through the action of collagenase produced by the pannus. The characteristic bone loss of patients with rheumatoid arthritis is juxta-articular—that is, immediately adjacent to both sides of the joint. The pannus invades the joint and subchondral bones as if it were a neoplasm. Eventually, the joint is destroyed and undergoes fibrous fusion, termed **ankylosis.** Longstanding cases lead to a fused joint with bony bridging, called **bony ankylosis.**

Rheumatoid Nodules

Rheumatoid arthritis is a systemic disease that also involves tissues other than the joints and tendons. A characteristic lesion is termed the **rheumatoid nodule.** This structure has a centrally located core of fibrinoid necrosis, which is a mixture of fibrin and other proteins (e.g., degraded collagen). A surrounding rim of macrophages is arranged in a radial or palisading fashion. Peripheral to the macrophages is an outer circle of lymphocytes, plasma cells, and other mononuclear cells. The overall appearance resembles a peculiar granuloma surrounding a core of fibrinoid necrosis. Rheumatoid nodules, which are usually found in areas of pressure (e.g., the skin of the elbow and legs), are movable, firm, rubbery, and occasionally, tender. A large nodule may ulcerate, and recurrence following surgical removal is common. Rheumatoid nodules may also be found in visceral organs, such as the heart, lungs, intestinal tract, and even the dura.

☐ **Clinical Features:** The onset of rheumatoid arthritis may be acute, slowly progressing, or insidious. Diseased joints are frequently warm, swollen, and painful. The pain is heightened by motion and is most severe after periods of disuse. Unabated disease causes progressive destruction of the joint surfaces and periarticular structures. Eventually, patients manifest severe flexion and extension deformities, associated with joint subluxation, which may terminate in joint ankylosis.

The natural history of rheumatoid arthritis is variable, and in most patients, the activity of the disease will wax and wane. One-fourth of the patients seem to recover completely. Another one-fourth remain, for many years, with only slight functional impairment, whereas half experience serious progressive and disabling joint disease. Death from complications of rheumatoid arthritis is not uncommon. There is an increased mortality rate from a variety of infections, gastrointestinal hemorrhage and perforation, vasculitis, heart and lung involvement, amyloidosis, and subluxation of the cervical spine. In fact, the survival rate of patients with active rheumatoid arthritis is comparable to that observed in patients with Hodgkin's disease and diabetes.

Spondyloarthropathy

A number of clinical entities were formerly classified as being variants of rheumatoid arthritis but are now recognized as distinct disorders. These forms of arthritis are now termed **spondyloarthropathies** and include ankylosing spondylitis, Reiter syndrome, psoriatic arthritis, and arthritis associated with inflammatory bowel disease. These conditions have the following features in common:

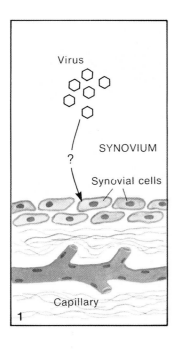

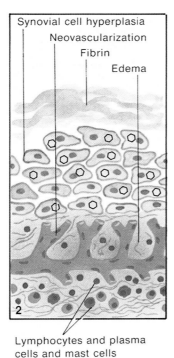

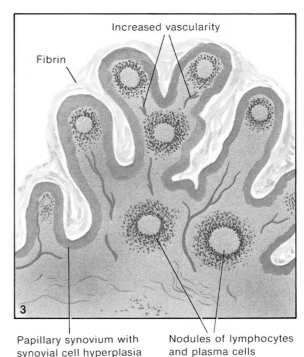

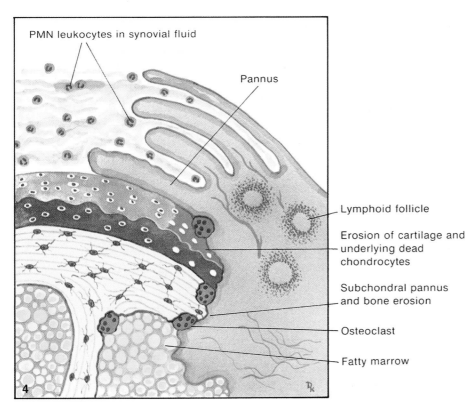

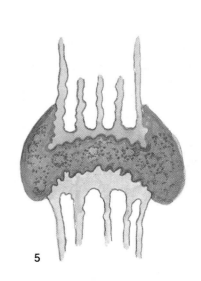

FIGURE *26-28*

Histogenesis of rheumatoid arthritis. (1) A virus or unknown stress stimulates synovial cells to proliferate. (2) The influx of lymphocytes, plasma cells, and mast cells, together with neovascularization and edema, lead to hypertrophy and hyperplasia of the synovium. (3) Lymphoid nodules are prominent. (4) The proliferating synovium extends into the joint space, burrows into the bone beneath the articular cartilage, and covers the cartilage as a pannus. The articular cartilage is eventually destroyed by direct resorption or deprivation of its nutrient synovial fluid. The synovial tissue continues to proliferate in the subchondral region and in the joint. (5) Eventually, the joint is destroyed and becomes fused, a condition termed *ankylosis*.

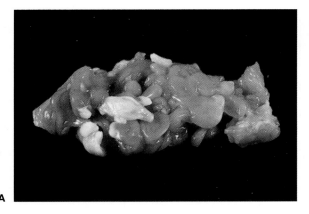

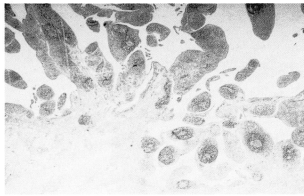

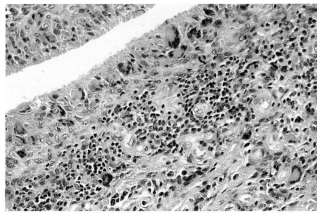

FIGURE *26-29*
Rheumatoid arthritis. (A) The hyperplastic synovium from a patient with rheumatoid arthritis shows numerous finger-like projections, with focal, pale areas of fibrin deposition. The brownish color of the synovium reflects hemosiderin accumulation derived from old hemorrhage. (B) A microscopic view reveals prominent lymphoid follicles (Allison-Ghormley bodies), synovial hyperplasia and hypertrophy, villous folds, and thickening of the synovial membrane by fibrosis and inflammation. (C) A higher-power view of the inflamed synovium demonstrates hyperplasia and hypertrophy of the lining cells. Numerous giant cells are noted both on and below the surface, and the stroma is chronically inflamed.

- Seronegativity for rheumatoid factor and other serologic markers of rheumatoid arthritis
- Association with class I histocompatibility antigens, particularly HLA-B27
- Preferential localization to the sacrum and vertebral column
- Asymmetric involvement of only a few peripheral joints
- Tendency to inflammation of periarticular tendons and fascia
- Systemic involvement of other organs, especially uveitis, carditis, and aortitis
- Preferential onset in young men

Ankylosing Spondylitis

■ *Ankylosing spondylitis is an inflammatory arthropathy of the vertebral column and sacroiliac joints.* It may be accompanied by asymmetric, peripheral arthritis (30% of patients) and by systemic manifestations. Ankylosing spondylitis is most common in young men, with the peak incidence occurring at approximately 20 years of age. **More than 90% of the patients are positive for HLA-B27 (normal, 4%–8%), although the disorder affects only 1% of persons with this haplotype.**

□ **Pathology:** Ankylosing spondylitis begins bilaterally at the sacroiliac joints and then ascends the spinal column by involving the small joints of the posterior elements of the spine. The net result is the ultimate destruction of these joints, after which the spine becomes fused posteriorly.

A few patients with ankylosing spondylitis usually have a rapid development of crippling spinal disease, but most can maintain their employment and live a normal life span. However, as many as 5% of the patients develop AA amyloidosis and uremia, and a few manifest severe cardiac involvement.

Reiter Syndrome

■ *Reiter syndrome refers to the triad of (1) seronegative polyarthritis, (2) conjunctivitis, and (3) nonspecific urethritis.* The disorder is almost exclusively encountered in men and usually follows venereal exposure or an episode of bacillary dysentery. As in ankylosing spondylitis, Reiter syndrome is associated with HLA-B27 antigen in as many as 90% of the patients. In most patients, Reiter syndrome remits within 1 year, but in 15% to 20%, progressive arthritis develops, including ankylosing spondylitis.

Psoriatic Arthritis

Approximately 7% of the patients with psoriasis, particularly those with severe disease, develop an inflammatory seronegative arthritis. HLA-B27 has been linked to psoriatic spondylitis and inflammation of the distal interphalangeal joints, and HLA-DR4 has been associated with a rheumatoid pattern of involvement.

Enteropathic Arthritis

Ulcerative colitis and Crohn disease are accompanied by seronegative peripheral arthritis in 20% of the cases and by spondylitis in 10%.

Juvenile Arthritis (Still Disease)

Juvenile arthritis refers to a number of different chronic arthritic conditions in children. In addition to rheumatoid arthritis, many children with juvenile arthritis eventually develop ankylosing spondylitis, psoriatic arthritis, and other connective tissue diseases. Juvenile arthritis can be classified as follows:

- **Seropositive.** Less than 10% of the children with arthritis are positive for rheumatoid factor and have a polyarticular presentation. These children are usually girls (80%), and 75% of these patients also exhibit antinuclear antibodies. There is an association with HLA-D4, and more than half eventually develop severe arthritis.
- **Polyarticular Disease Without Systemic Symptoms.** One-fourth of all patients with juvenile arthritis (90% girls) present with disease of several joints, are seronegative, and do not manifest systemic symptoms. Less than 15% of these patients eventually develop severe arthritis.
- **Polyarticular Disease with Systemic Symptoms.** Some 20% of children with polyarticular juvenile arthritis present with prominent systemic symptoms, which include high fever, rash, hepatosplenomegaly, lymphadenopathy, pleuritis, pericarditis, anemia, and leukocytosis. The majority (60%) of the patients are boys who are negative for rheumatoid factor, and one-fourth of these patients are left with severe arthritis.
- **Pauciarticular.** Children who present with involvement of only a few large joints (e.g., the knee, ankle, elbow, or hip girdle) account for half of all cases of juvenile arthritis. They fall into two general groups. The larger group includes mainly (80%) girls who are negative for rheumatoid factor but who exhibit antinuclear antibodies and are positive for HLA-DR5, -DRw6, or -DRw8. Of these patients, one-third have ocular disease that is characterized by chronic iridocyclitis (inflammation of the iris and ciliary body). Only a small minority of these children have residual polyarthritis or ocular damage.

The other children with a pauciarticular presentation are almost all boys, are negative for both rheumatoid factor and antinuclear bodies, and are positive for HLA-B27 (75%). A few have acute iridocyclitis, which resolves spontaneously. Some of these children subsequently develop ankylosing spondylitis.

GOUT

■ *Gout represents a heterogeneous group of diseases in which the common denominator is an increased serum level of uric acid and the deposition of urate crystals in the joints and kidneys.* Although all patients with gout display hyperuricemia, less than 15% of all persons with elevated serum uric acid suffer from gout.

Gout is characterized by both acute and chronic arthritis. **Primary gout** refers to hyperuricemia in the absence of any other disease, whereas **secondary gout** occurs in association with another illness that results in hyperuricemia. Of all cases of hyperuricemia, one-third are estimated to be primary and the remainder to be secondary.

Pathogenesis of Hyperuricemia

Uric acid is the end product of the catabolism of purines, which are derived either from the diet or synthesized de novo. In turn, uric acid is eliminated from the body in the urine. Gout can result from (1) overproduction of purines, (2) augmented catabolism of nucleic acids as a result of increased cell turnover, (3) decreased salvage of free purine bases, or (4) decreased urinary excretion of uric acid (Fig. 26-30).

Primary (Idiopathic) Gout

Most cases (75–90%) of so-called idiopathic gout result from an as-yet-unexplained impairment of uric acid excretion by the kidneys. In the remaining cases, there is a primary overproduction of uric acid, but only in a minority of cases has that underlying abnormality been identified. Primary gout is a disease of adult men, and only 5% of the cases occur in women. The peak incidence occurs during the fifth decade of life.

It is generally agreed that precocious gout exhibits a strong familial tendency, and hyperuricemia is common among the relatives of persons with gout. The overall consensus also holds that the level of serum uric acid is controlled by multiple genes.

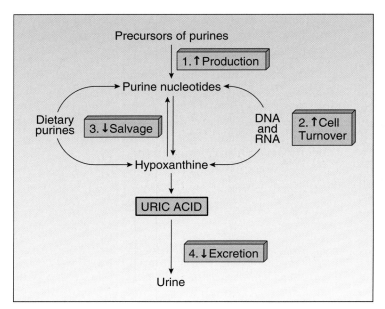

FIGURE   *26-30*
Pathogenesis of hyperuricemia and gout. Purine nucleotides are synthesized de novo from nonpurine precursors or are derived from preformed purines in the diet. Purine nucleotides are catabolized to hypoxanthine or incorporated into nucleic acids. Degradation of nucleic acids and dietary purines also produces hypoxanthine. Hypoxanthine is converted to uric acid, which, in turn, is excreted into the urine. Hyperuricemia and gout result from (1) increased de novo purine synthesis, (2) increased cell turnover, (3) decreased salvage of dietary purines and hypoxanthine, and (4) decreased uric acid excretion by the kidneys.

Secondary Gout

As in primary gout, secondary hyperuricemia may reflect urate overproduction or decreased urinary excretion of uric acid. Increased production of uric acid most commonly is associated with increased turnover of nucleic acids, as seen in patients with leukemias and lymphomas and after chemotherapy for cancer. Ethanol intake is a cause of secondary hyperuricemia, in part owing to accelerated adenosine triphosphate (ATP) catabolism and, to a lesser degree, decreased renal excretion of uric acid.

The most common causes of decreased urinary excretion of uric acid are chronic diseases that lead to a reduction in the functional renal mass. In patients with renal failure, the clearance of uric acid is decreased, and with a fall in the glomerular filtration rate, hyperuricemia ensues. Drugs that impair urate secretion by the renal tubules or that increase tubular reabsorption of uric acid are implicated in as many as 20% of patients with hyperuricemia.

☐ **Pathology:** The presence of long, needle-shaped crystals that are negatively birefringent under polarized light is diagnostic of gout. Urate crystals may be found intracellularly in leukocytes of the synovial fluid. Extracellular soft tissue deposits of these crystals (tophi) are surrounded by foreign-body giant cells and an associated inflammatory response of mononuclear cells (Fig. 26-31). These granuloma-like areas are found in cartilage, in any of the soft tissues around joints, and even in the subchondral bone marrow adjacent to joints.

Urate deposits in the kidney occur in the interstitium between renal tubules, especially at the medullary apices. These deposits are grossly visible as small, shiny, golden-yellow, and linear streaks in the medulla.

☐ **Clinical Features:** The clinical course of gout may be divided into four stages:

- **Asymptomatic hyperuricemia,** which often precedes clinically evident gout by many years.
- **Acute gouty arthritis,** which is a painful condition that usually involves one joint and is unaccompanied by constitutional symptoms. Later in the course of the disease, polyarticular involvement with fever is common. At least half of the patients first present with a painful and red first metatarsophalangeal joint (great toe), which is designated **podagra.** Eventually, 90% of all patients experience such an attack. Although the disease primarily affects the lower extremities, fingers, elbows, and wrists also become involved.

Commonly, a gouty attack begins at night and is exquisitely painful, thereby simulating an acute bacterial infection of the affected joint. An attack may be triggered by consuming a large meal or drinking alcoholic beverages, but other specific events (e.g., trauma, certain drugs, and surgery) may also be responsible. Even when untreated, an acute attack of gout is self-limited.

- **The intercritical period** is the asymptomatic interval between the initial acute attack and the subsequent attacks. These periods may last for as long as 10 years, but later attacks tend to be increasingly severe as well as prolonged, polyarticular, and febrile.

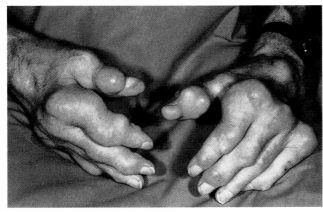

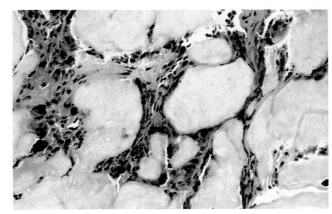

A   B

FIGURE   *26-31*
Gout. (A) Gouty tophi project from the fingers as rubbery nodules. (B) A section from a tophus shows extracellular masses of urate crystals with accompanying foreign-body giant cells.

- **Tophaceous gout** eventually appears among untreated patients in the form of tophi in the cartilage, synovial membranes, tendons, and soft tissues. A tophus is a chalky, cheesy, yellow-white, and pasty deposit of monosodium urate crystals. Classic locations of a tophus are the helix or antihelix of the ear. However, they can also occur on the hands, in the olecranon bursa, and in the Achilles tendon.

Renal failure is responsible for 10% of the deaths in patients with gout. One-third of patients with gout have mild albuminuria, a reduced glomerular filtration rate, and decreased renal concentrating ability. In patients with severe gout caused by inherited enzyme deficiencies and in those with a precocious presentation, urate nephropathy is a prominent feature of the clinical course.

Urate stones constitute 10% of all renal calculi in patients within the United States, and they affect as many as 25% of the patients with primary or secondary gout.

Treatment. The treatment of gout is designed to (1) decrease the severity of acute attacks, (2) lower the serum urate levels, (3) prevent future attacks, (4) promote the dissolution of urate deposits, and (5) decrease the urinary acidity to prevent stone formation. Colchicine has been used for hundreds of years and has been administered prophylactically during the intervals between gouty attacks to prevent recurrent episodes. Uricosuric drugs that interfere with urate resorption by the renal tubule include probenecid and sulfinpyrazone. Allopurinol is a competitive inhibitor of xanthine oxidase, the enzyme that converts xanthine and hypoxanthine to uric acid. This drug causes a prompt decrease in uricosemia and uricosuria.

PIGMENTED VILLONODULAR SYNOVITIS

■ *Pigmented villonodular synovitis, despite its obsolete name, is a benign neoplasm of the synovial lining that is characterized by exuberant proliferation of synovial lining cells with extension into the subsynovial tissue.* This tumor involves a single joint and usually occurs in young adults. It is equally distributed between males and females. The most common site (80%) is the knee, although pigmented villonodular synovitis also occurs in the hip, ankle, calcaneocuboid joint, elbow, and tendon sheaths of the fingers and toes.

☐ **Pathology:** Tumors arise on the synovium of tendon sheaths, bursae, and diarthrodial joints. The lesions of pigmented villonodular synovitis invade the joint and erode the bone. They may also insinuate through joint capsules into the soft tissue and encompass nerves and arteries, sometimes necessitating radical surgical excision. The synovium develops enlarged folds and nodular excrescences (Fig. 26-32). Microscopically, the tumor is composed of bland mononuclear cells, with scattered multinucleated giant cells, in which the nuclei are arrayed peripherally. Hemosiderin-laden macrophages reflect previous hemorrhage.

Treatment for pigmented villonodular synovitis is surgical. Radiation therapy produces fibrosis of the proliferating synovial tissue, but amputation is occasionally necessary.

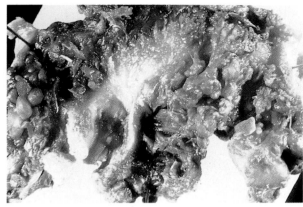
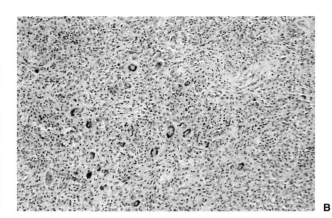

FIGURE   26-32
Pigmented villonodular synovitis. (A) A specimen of synovium exhibits the characteristic pigmented, thickened, opaque, and nodular appearance. (B) A microscopic section reveals bland mononuclear cells with interspersed giant cells.

Soft-Tissue Tumors

■ *Soft-tissue tumors refer to neoplastic conditions that arise in certain extraskeletal mesodermal tissues of the body, including the skeletal muscle, fat, fibrous tissue, blood, and lymphatic vessels.* Tumors of peripheral nerves are included in the category of soft-tissue tumors despite their derivation from the neuroectoderm. A few important general principles that relate to soft-tissue tumors are:

- Deep lesions tend to be malignant.
- The more superficial the location of the tumor, the more likely it is that the tumor is benign.
- Larger tumors tend to be malignant more often than small ones.
- A rapidly growing tumor is more likely to be malignant than one that develops slowly.
- Calcification may exist in both benign and malignant tumors.

NODULAR FASCIITIS

■ *Nodular fasciitis is a benign, reactive, soft-tissue lesion that probably occurs secondary to trauma and must be distinguished from a true neoplasm.* It commonly occurs on the forearm, trunk, and back. Histologically, nodular fasciitis may be mistaken for a sarcoma, because it is hypercellular and has abundant mitoses as well as numerous pleomorphic, spindle-shaped cells (Fig. 26-33). The true nature is defined when the entire "mass" is recognized as being the counterpart of granulation tissue in response to trauma. The lesion is self-limited and is cured by surgical excision.

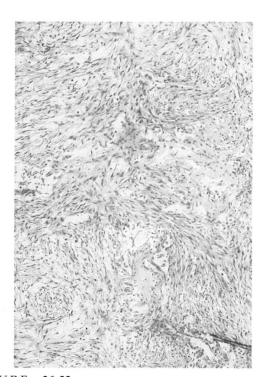

FIGURE   26-33
Nodular fasciitis. Swirls of tightly woven spindle cells and collagen are admixed with a few lymphoid cells and vascular channels.

FIBROSARCOMA

■ *Fibrosarcoma, a malignant tumor of fibroblasts, is most commonly found in the thigh, particularly around the*

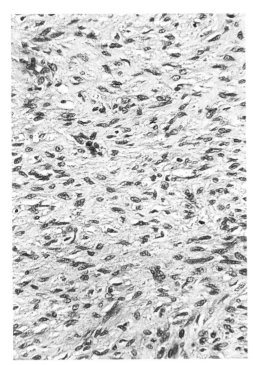

FIGURE   *26-34*
Fibrosarcoma. A photomicrograph demonstrates irregularly arranged neoplastic fibroblasts.

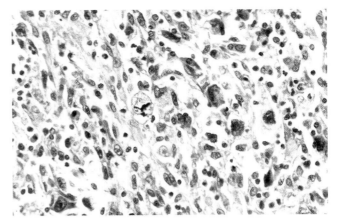

FIGURE   *26-35*
Malignant fibrous histiocytoma. An anaplastic tumor exhibits spindle cells, plump and lipid-laden histiocytes, tumor giant cells, an abnormal mitosis (*center*), and a mild chronic inflammatory infiltrate.

knee. This neoplasm typically occurs in adults, although it may be encountered in any age group and may even be congenital. Fibrosarcomas arise from connective tissue such as fascia, scar tissue, periosteum, and tendons. Macroscopically, the tumors usually are sharply demarcated and frequently exhibit necrosis and hemorrhage. They are characterized histologically by pleomorphic fibroblasts that form densely interlacing bundles and fascicles, thereby producing a "herring-bone" pattern (Fig. 26-34). The prognosis for patients with fibrosarcoma is guarded at best, with a 5-year survival rate of only 40% and a 10-year survival rate of 30%. Patients with poorly differentiated fibrosarcomas have a worse prognosis than patients with better-differentiated ones.

MALIGNANT FIBROUS HISTIOCYTOMA

■ *Malignant fibrous histiocytoma (MFH) is a malignant, soft-tissue tumor that contains foci of histiocytic (macrophage) differentiation.* It is the most common type of soft-tissue sarcoma and the most frequently encountered sarcoma after radiation therapy. MFH typically occurs in older adults, but cases have been recorded in patients at all ages. In half of the cases, MFH arises in the deep fascia or within a skeletal muscle. The tumor has also been reported in association with surgical scars and foreign bodies.

□ **Pathology:** Histologically, MFH displays a highly variable morphologic pattern, with areas of spindle-shaped tumor cells arrayed in an irregularly whorled (storiform) pattern adjacent to pleomorphic fields (Fig. 26-35). The spindle cells tend to be well differentiated and to resemble fibroblasts. There are occasional plump cells (histiocytes), abundant mitoses, a few xanthomatous (lipid-laden) cells, and a moderate chronic inflammatory reaction. Some tumors contain numerous tumor giant cells, which exhibit an intense eosinophilia. The extent of collagen deposition is variable and sometimes dominates the microscopic pattern. A few tumors reveal a conspicuous myxoid stroma.

The prognosis of patients with MFH depends on the degree of cytologic atypia. Almost half of the patients develop a local recurrence after surgery, and a comparable proportion later manifest metastatic disease, particularly in the lungs.

TUMORS OF ADIPOSE TISSUE

Lipoma

■ *Lipoma is a benign, circumscribed tumor that is composed of well-differentiated adipocytes.* It is the most common soft-tissue mass and can originate at any site that contains adipose tissue. Most lipomas appear in the subcutaneous tissues in the upper half of the body, especially on the trunk and neck. Lipomas are mainly encountered in adults, and patients with multiple tumors often have relatives with a similar history.

☐ **Pathology:** On gross examination, lipomas are encapsulated, soft, and yellow lesions, which vary in size and may become very large. Deeper tumors are often poorly circumscribed. Histologically, a lipoma is often indistinguishable from normal adipose tissue. Lipomas are adequately treated by simple local excision.

Liposarcoma

The second most common sarcoma in adults, liposarcoma accounts for 20% of all malignant soft-tissue tumors. The neoplasm arises in patients older than 50 years of age and is most frequent in the deep thigh and retroperitoneum. Liposarcomas tend to grow slowly but may become extremely large.

On gross examination, the typical liposarcoma measures from 5 to 10 cm in diameter, although examples measuring 40 cm in diameter and weighing in excess of 50 pounds have been encountered. On cut section, the appearance of the tumor is variable, depending on the proportions of adipose, mucinous, and fibrous tissue. Poorly differentiated liposarcomas appear similar to brain tissue and display necrosis, hemorrhage, and cysts. Microscopically, the most common pattern is one of variably differentiated, "signet ring" lipoblasts that are embedded in a vascularized myxoid stroma (Fig. 26-36). Poorly differentiated liposarcomas show uniform, round cells with vesicular nuclei, which may be difficult to distinguish from other small cell sarcomas. Well-differentiated liposarcomas can be confused with lipomas.

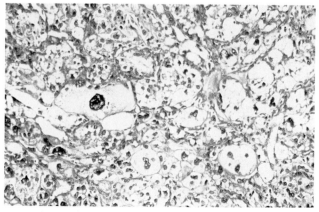

FIGURE   *26-36*
Liposarcoma. Large pleomorphic cells with bizarre nuclei and vacuolated cytoplasm are evident.

Local recurrence rates and metastases following surgery are high for round cell and pleomorphic liposarcomas, and the 5-year survival rate for patients with these tumors is less than 20%. By contrast, the 5-year survival for patients with well-differentiated and myxoid tumors exceeds 70%.

RHABDOMYOSARCOMA

■ *Rhabdomyosarcoma is a malignant tumor that displays features of striated muscle differentiation.* It is uncommon in mature adults but is the most frequent soft-tissue sarcoma in children and young adults.

☐ **Pathology:** Most cases of rhabdomyosarcoma can be classified according to four histologic categories.

Embryonal Rhabdomyosarcoma. This form is most common among children between 3 and 12 years of age and frequently involves the head and neck, genitourinary tract, and retroperitoneum. The morphologic appearance varies from that of a highly differentiated tumor containing rhabdomyoblasts, with a large eosinophilic cytoplasm and cross-striations (Fig. 26-37), to that of a poorly differentiated neoplasm.

Botryoid Embryonal Rhabdomyosarcoma. This tumor, which is also known as **sarcoma botryoides,** is distinguished by the formation of polypoid, grape-like tumor masses. Microscopically, the malignant cells are scattered in an abundant myxoid stroma. Botryoid foci may occur in any type of embryonal rhabdomyosarcoma but are most common in tumors of hollow visceral organs, including the vagina (see Chapter 18) and the bladder.

Alveolar Rhabdomyosarcoma. This neoplasm occurs less frequently than the embryonal type and principally affects young persons between 10 and 25 years of age. It is most common in the upper and lower extremities but can also be distributed in the same sites as the embryonal type. Typically, club-shaped tumor cells are arranged in clumps that are outlined by fibrous septa. The loose arrangement of cells in the center of these clusters leads to the "alveolar" pattern. The tumor cells exhibit an intense eosinophilia, and occasional multinucleated giant cells are identified. Malignant rhabdomyoblasts, which are recognizable by their cross-striations, occur less commonly in the alveolar variant than in embryonal rhabdomyosarcoma, being present in only 25% of the cases.

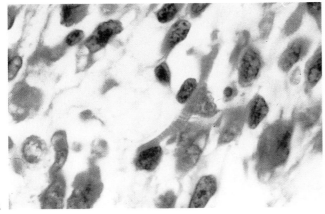

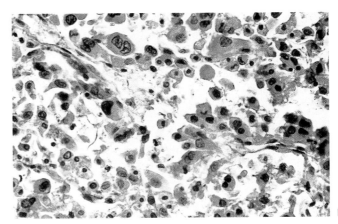

A   B

FIGURE   26-37.
Rhabdomyosarcoma. (A) Embryonal rhabdomyosarcoma. The center of the field shows a well-differentiated rhabdomyoblast with cross-striations. (B) Alveolar rhabdomyosarcoma. The neoplastic cells are arranged in clusters that display an alveolar pattern.

Pleomorphic Rhabdomyosarcoma. The least common form of rhabdomyosarcoma is found in the skeletal muscles of older persons, often in the thigh. This tumor differs from the other types of rhabdomyosarcoma in the pleomorphism of its irregularly arranged cells. Large, granular, and eosinophilic rhabdomyoblasts, together with multinucleated giant cells, are common. Cross-striations are virtually nonexistent.

The previously dismal prognosis associated with most rhabdomyosarcomas has improved during the past 20 years as a result of the introduction of combined therapeutic modalities, including surgery, radiation therapy, and chemotherapy. Today, more than 80% of patients with localized or regional disease are cured.

SMOOTH MUSCLE TUMORS

Leiomyoma. This benign soft-tissue tumor usually arises in the subcutaneous tissues or from the walls of blood vessels. Leiomyomas are painful lesions that appear as firm, yellow, and circumscribed nodules. Microscopically, intersecting fascicles of regular smooth cells are evident. Simple excision is curative.

Leiomyosarcoma. This malignant soft-tissue neoplasm is an uncommon tumor of adults and typically arises in the extremities from the wall of blood vessels. Macroscopically, leiomyosarcomas tend to be well circumscribed, but they are larger and softer than leiomy-

omas and often exhibit necrosis, hemorrhage, and cystic degeneration. Histologically, the tumor cells are arranged in fascicles, often with palisaded nuclei. Well-differentiated tumor cells have elongated nuclei and eosinophilic cytoplasm, whereas poorly differentiated ones may show severe nuclear atypism. Leiomyosarcoma is mainly differentiated from leiomyoma by a high mitotic activity, which is also an indicator of prognosis. The majority of leiomyosarcomas eventually metastasize, although dissemination may become evident as long as 15 or more years after resection of the primary tumor.

SYNOVIAL SARCOMA

■ *Synovial sarcoma is a highly malignant soft-tissue tumor that arises in the region of a joint, usually in association with tendon sheaths, bursae, and joint capsules.* Less than 10% of synovial sarcomas are intra-articular. Although the tumor bears a microscopic resemblance to the synovium, its origin from this tissue has not been established. Synovial sarcoma accounts for 6% to 10% of malignant soft-tissue tumors and occurs principally in adolescents and young adults. The tumor typically presents as a painful or tender mass, usually in the vicinity of a large joint, particularly the knee.

☐ **Pathology:** On gross examination, synovial sarcomas are usually circumscribed, round or multilobular masses that are attached to tendons, tendon sheaths, or the exterior wall of the joint capsule (Fig. 26-38). The tumors tend to be surrounded by a glistening pseudo-

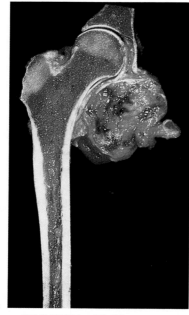

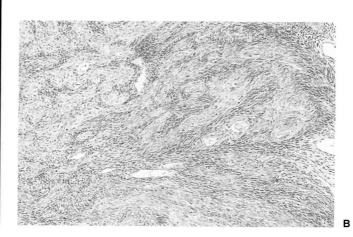

FIGURE   *26-38*
Synovial sarcoma. (A) A section of the upper femur and acetabulum reveals a tumor adjacent to the hip joint and neck of the femur. (B) A microscopic view demonstrates the biphasic appearance of a synovial sarcoma. Irregular spaces are lined by plump, synovial-like neoplastic cells. The intervening tissue contains cells with similar nuclei.

capsule and, in many instances, are cystic. They range from small nodules to masses of 15 cm or more in diameter (average diameter, 3–5 cm).

Microscopically, synovial sarcoma is classically described as having a **biphasic pattern** (see Fig. 26-38). Fluid-filled glandular spaces lined by epithelial-like tumor cells are embedded in a sarcomatous, spindle cell background. These elements vary in proportion,

distribution, and cellular differentiation, with the spindle cells usually being considerably more numerous than the glandular elements.

The recurrence rate of synovial sarcoma is high, and metastases occur in more than 60% of the cases. The 5-year survival rate for these patients is 50%, and those who die usually have extensive lung metastases.

CHAPTER 27

Skeletal Muscle

Arthur P. Hayes
Vernon W. Armbrustmacher

Duchenne Muscular Dystrophy

Myotonic Dystrophy

Inflammatory Myopathies

Myasthenia Gravis

Rhabdomyolysis

Denervation

DUCHENNE MUSCULAR DYSTROPHY

■ *Duchenne muscular dystrophy is a severe, progressive, X-linked, inherited degeneration of the skeletal muscle.* Boys with this disorder suffer progressive degeneration of muscles, particularly those of the pelvic and shoulder girdles. A milder form of the disease is known as **Becker muscular dystrophy** (see Chapter 6 for discussion of the molecular genetics in both diseases).

□ **Pathogenesis:** Duchenne muscular dystrophy is caused by mutations of a large gene on the short arm of the X chromosome. This gene codes for **dystrophin,** a protein that is localized to the inner surface of the sarcolemma. Dystrophin links the subsarcolemmal cytoskeleton through a transmembrane complex to an extracellular glycoprotein that binds laminin. Thus, dystrophin-deficient muscle fibers lack the normal interaction between the sarcolemma and the extracellular matrix.

□ **Pathology:** The disease sequence in Duchenne dystrophy proceeds as follows:

1. A relentless degeneration of muscle fibers.
2. A prolonged effort at repair and regeneration.
3. Progressive fibrosis.

The earliest pathologic changes in the muscle consist of irregularly distributed foci of degenerating and regenerating muscle fibers, together with scattered, large, and hyalinized dark fibers (Fig. 27-1). Myophagocytosis (infiltration of macrophages into degenerating muscle fibers) is almost invariable, but it does not reflect an inflammatory process. There is a brisk regenerative response to the muscle degeneration. These regenerating fibers have a basophilic sarcoplasm and large vesicular nuclei, with prominent nucleoli. Endomysial fibrosis develops early and, eventually, becomes prominent in patients with Duchenne dystrophy.

□ **Clinical Features:** Boys with Duchenne muscular dystrophy have markedly elevated serum creatine kinase levels from birth and morphologically abnormal muscle even in utero. Clinical weakness is not detectable during the first year of life but usually becomes evident during the third or fourth year. The weakness is noted mainly around the pelvic and shoulder girdles (proximal muscle weakness) and is relentlessly progressive.

The weak muscles eventually become atrophic and are replaced by fibrofatty tissue. Later, "pseudohypertrophy" of the calf muscles develops. Patients are usually wheelchair-bound by the age of 10 years and bedridden by 15 years. The most common causes of death are complications of respiratory insufficiency caused by muscular weakness or cardiac arrhythmia owing to myocardial involvement.

Myotonic Dystrophy

■ *Myotonic dystrophy, the most common form of adult muscular dystrophy, is an autosomal dominant disorder that is characterized by sustained muscle contractions and rigidity (myotonia) as well as progressive muscle weakness and wasting.* The age at onset and severity of symptoms show extreme variations.

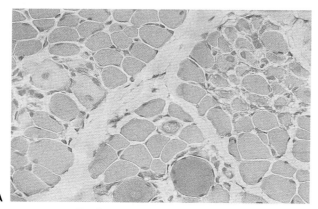
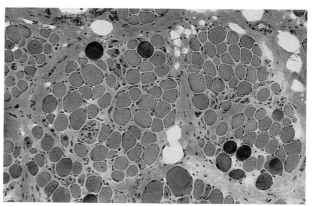

FIGURE *27-1*
Duchenne muscular dystrophy. **(A) Hematoxylin-and-eosin stain. A section of vastus lateralis muscle shows necrotic muscle fibers, some of them invaded by macrophages. The endomysial septa are thickened, indicating fibrosis. (B) Modified Gomori trichrome. A similar section demonstrates dark-staining enlarged fibers, which represent overly contracted fibers. Calcium influx across the defective surface membrane overwhelms mechanisms that maintain a low resting Ca^{2+} concentration and triggers excessive contraction. There is conspicuous perimysial and endomysial fibrosis.**

■ *Pathogenesis:* The gene for myotonic dystrophy has been localized to the long arm of chromosome 19, and most cases seem to be descended from one original mutation. An interesting genetic characteristic of this disease is the phenomenon of anticipation—that is, an earlier age at onset and increasing severity of symptoms in successive generations. Anticipation has been related to an unstable genomic segment (a CTG trinucleotide repeat) in the myotonic dystrophy gene. This segment enlarges through an increase in the number of repeats with successive generations, with the size of the gene (the number of repeats) correlating with the severity of the symptoms. Expansion of a trinucleotide repeat is a common mechanism in other human genetic disorders and has been observed in fragile X syndrome, Kennedy disease, and Huntington disease. The gene for myotonic dystrophy encodes a novel cyclic AMP–dependent protein kinase. Apparently, the excitability of the sarcolemma is altered as a result of abnormal phosphorylation of ion channels.

■ *Pathology:* The pathologic changes of myotonic dystrophy are highly variable, even in muscles from the same patient. Most cases display atrophy of type I fibers and hypertrophy of type II fibers. Internally situated nuclei are a constant feature, but necrosis and regeneration, although occasionally present, are not prominent (as they are in patients with Duchenne muscular dystrophy).

■ *Clinical Features:* Myotonic dystrophy can be separated into three clinical groups: (1) congenital, (2) classic adult onset, and (3) minimal symptoms with late onset.

Adult myotonic dystrophy presents with muscle weakness and stiffness, principally in the distal limbs. The facial and jaw muscles are virtually always affected, and ptosis can be severe. Extramuscular features of myotonic dystrophy are sometimes present and include cataracts as well as variable degrees of personality deterioration.

Congenital myotonic dystrophy is seen only in the offspring of women who themselves exhibit symptoms of myotonic dystrophy. These infants are born with muscle weakness. However, myotonia is inconspicuous or absent, although it does appear during later childhood. A significant number of these patients have some degree of mental retardation.

INFLAMMATORY MYOPATHIES

Inflammatory myopathies represent a heterogenous group of acquired disorders, all of which feature symmetric proximal muscle weakness, increased serum levels of muscle-derived enzymes, and nonsuppurative inflammation of skeletal muscle. Inflammatory myopathies are uncommon. Whereas dermatomyositis afflicts both adults and children, and women more commonly than men, polymyositis almost always occurs after the age of 20 years. The incidence of inclusion-body myositis is threefold greater in men than in women, and the disorder usually occurs after 50 years of age.

☐ **Pathogenesis:** Inflammatory myopathies are thought to have an autoimmune origin, but no specific target antigens on muscle or blood vessels have been confirmed.

Dermatomyositis. Muscle injury in patients with dermatomyositis is produced primarily by complement-mediated, cytotoxic antibodies directed against the microvasculature of skeletal muscle tissues. This microangiopathy leads to ischemia of individual muscle fibers, microinfarcts, and secondary inflammation. True infarcts may result from the involvement of larger intramuscular arteries.

Polymyositis and Inclusion-Body Myositis. These myopathies are related to direct muscle cell damage produced by cytotoxic T cells, and there is no evidence of a microangiopathy such as that found in dermatomyositis. In patients with these disorders, healthy muscle fibers are initially surrounded by CD8+ T lymphocytes and macrophages, after which the muscle fibers degenerate.

☐ **Pathology:** The most prominent histologic characteristics are (1) the presence of inflammatory cells (Fig. 27-2), (2) necrosis and phagocytosis of muscle fibers, (3) a mixture of regenerating and atrophic fibers, and (4) fibrosis.

Dermatomyositis. This disorder features perivascular or intrafascicular inflammatory infiltrates. The intramuscular blood vessels exhibit endothelial hyperplasia, fibrin thrombi, and obliteration of capillaries. Affected fibers are grouped in a portion of a muscle fasciculus, often as a result of microinfarcts within the muscle. Perifascicular atrophy, in which multiple layers of atrophic fibers are seen at the periphery of the fascicles, is diagnostic of dermatomyositis even in the absence of inflammation.

Polymyositis. In this inflammatory myopathy, infiltrates, mostly in the fascicles (endomysial inflammation), invade apparently healthy muscle fibers. Microvascular changes are absent. The degenerating fibers are scattered and not necessarily in areas of in-

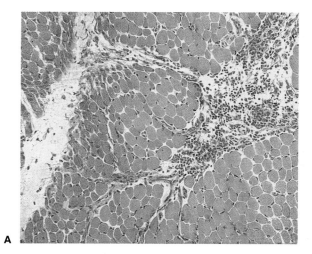

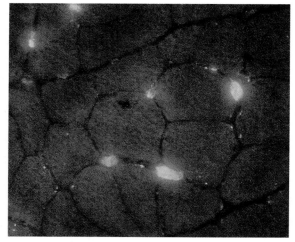

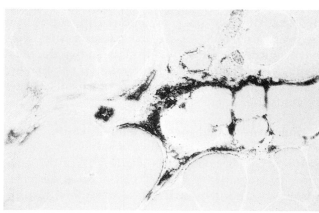

FIGURE 27-2
Dermatomyositis. (A) Hematoxylin-and-eosin stain. In dermatomyositis, the inflammatory cells infiltrate predominantly the perimysium rather than the endomysium. In addition, narrow, peripheral zones of muscle fascicles disclose atrophic fibers, a pattern referred to as perifascicular atrophy. (B) In this immunofluorescence photograph, the walls of many capillaries display C5b-9 (membrane attack complex). (C) Alkaline phosphatase stain. The abnormal staining of the tissue is located largely in the blood vessels of the endomysium, reflecting the altered microvasculature typical of dermatomyositis. A few small regenerating fibers are also stained by this method.

flammation. Perifascicular atrophy is characteristically not present in patients with polymyositis.

Inclusion-Body Myositis. Endomysial inflammation similar to that of polymyositis is noted in this variant. Basophilic granular inclusions are seen around the edge of slit-like vacuoles within the muscle fibers. Eosinophilic cytoplasmic inclusions and small groups of angulated fibers are present. Ultrastructurally, the pathognomonic feature of inclusion-body myositis is the presence of filamentous inclusions in the cytoplasm or nuclei of the muscle fibers.

☐ **Clinical Features:** All varieties of inflammatory myopathy discussed here present as the insidious development of both proximal and symmetric muscle weakness over a period of weeks to months. Dysphagia and difficulty in holding up the head reflect involvement of the pharyngeal and neck-flexor muscles.

As mentioned, the weakness progresses over weeks or months and leads to severe muscular wasting.

Dermatomyositis is distinguished from the other myopathies by a characteristic rash on the upper eyelids, face, trunk, and occasionally, other body surfaces. It may occur either alone or in association with scleroderma, mixed connective tissue disease, or other autoimmune conditions. **When dermatomyositis occurs in a middle-aged man, there is an increased risk for development of an epithelial cancer, most commonly carcinoma of the lung.** By contrast, polymyositis and inclusion-body myositis have only a chance association with malignant diseases.

Patients with inflammatory myopathies have moderate to markedly elevated serum creatine kinase levels and increases in other muscle enzyme levels. Treatment of dermatomyositis and polymyositis with corticosteroids is usually successful, but inclusion-body myositis is generally resistant to all therapy.

MYASTHENIA GRAVIS

■ *Myasthenia gravis is an acquired autoimmune disease that is characterized by abnormal muscular fatigability and is caused by circulating antibodies to the acetylcholine receptor at the myoneural junction.* It occurs in all races, and it is twice as common in women as in men. The disease typically begins during young adulthood.

☐ **Immunopathogenesis:** Myasthenia gravis is mediated by an immunologic attack on the acetylcholine receptor of the motor end plate. Polyclonal antibodies attach to various epitopes of the receptor protein, thereby blocking the binding of acetylcholine to its receptor and causing weakness similar to that produced by curare. The combination of partially blocked acetylcholine receptor sites in atrophic motor end plates, a decreased number of acetylcholine receptors, and widened synaptic space results in muscle weakness and abnormal fatigability.

The thymus clearly plays an important role in the pathogenesis of myasthenia gravis. As much as 40% of patients have an associated thymoma, and surgical removal is often curative. As many as 75% of the remaining patients have thymic hyperplasia, and in such cases, thymectomy is often effective treatment.

☐ **Pathology:** By light microscopy, pathologic changes in patients with myasthenia gravis are subtle, and at best, a muscle biopsy specimen may reveal atrophy of type II muscle fibers. Focal collections of lymphocytes may be present within the fascicles. By electron microscopy, most muscle end plates are abnormal, even in muscles that are not weakened.

☐ **Clinical Features:** Patients with myasthenia gravis show considerable variation in the severity of the condition, and similar to other autoimmune diseases, the symptoms tend to wax and wane. Weakness of the extraocular muscles is typically severe and causes ptosis and diplopia. In fact, myasthenia gravis may remain confined to these muscles. More frequently, however, the disease progresses to other muscles, such as those associated with swallowing, the trunk, and the extremities. Patients with myasthenia gravis also have a high incidence of other autoimmune diseases.

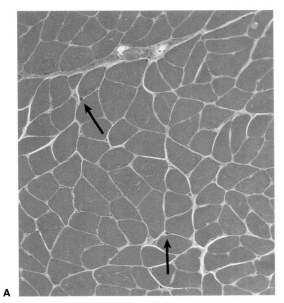
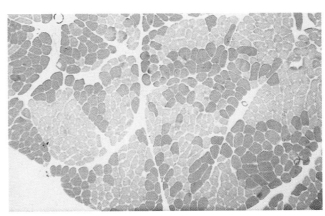

A

B

FIGURE 27-3
Type grouping. (A) This biopsy specimen of the biceps was obtained from a 27-year-old woman who had contracted poliomyelitis at the age of 7 years. A frozen section of the biceps stained with hematoxylin-and-eosin shows muscle fibers that vary slightly in size and shape. The scattered black "dots" (*arrows*) among some of the fibers are pyknotic nuclear clumps in extremely atrophic fibers that were not reinnervated. The fiber types cannot be distinguished with this stain. (B) A similar case stained for ATPase. Striking type grouping reflects reinnervation. Groups of type II fibers (*dark*) are adjacent to groups of type I fibers. As a result, there are fewer, but larger, motor units. The absence of angular atrophic fibers or target fibers suggests that there is no active denervation.

The overall mortality rate of myasthenia gravis is now less than 5%, often owing to respiratory insufficiency because of muscle weakness. In addition to thymectomy, corticosteroid therapy (with or without methotrexate) is helpful. Anticholinesterase drugs may be useful in controlling symptoms.

RHABDOMYOLYSIS

■ *Rhabdomyolysis refers to the dissolution of skeletal muscle fibers with release of myoglobin into the circulation, which may result in myoglobinuria and acute renal failure.* The disorder may be acute, subacute, or chronic. During acute rhabdomyolysis, the muscles are swollen, tender, and profoundly weak.

Occasionally, an episode of rhabdomyolysis may complicate or follow an influenza infection. Some patients develop rhabdomyolysis with apparently mild exercise; these persons probably have some form of metabolic myopathy. Rhabdomyolysis may also complicate heat stroke or malignant hyperthermia after administration of a triggering anesthetic agent (e.g., halothane). Alcoholism is occasionally associated with either acute or chronic rhabdomyolysis.

Pathologic changes in rhabdomyolysis are classified as being an active, noninflammatory myopathy, with scattered necrosis of muscle fibers and varying degrees of degeneration and regeneration. Clusters of macrophages are seen both in and around muscle fibers, but these are not accompanied by lymphocytes or other inflammatory cells.

DENERVATION

The pathology of denervation reflects lesions of the lower motor neuron. When a skeletal muscle fiber becomes separated from contact with its lower motor neuron, it invariably atrophies owing to progressive loss of myofibrils and myofilaments. On cross-section, the atrophic fiber has a characteristic angular configuration, being compressed by the surrounding normal muscle fibers. If the fiber is not reinnervated, the atrophy proceeds to complete loss of myofibrils and myofilaments, and the nuclei condense into aggregates. In longitudinal section, the end stage of atrophy consists of an aggregate of nuclei, connected by a thin strand of sarcoplasm to another group of nuclei. On cross-section, these nuclei are seen as pyknotic nuclear clumps. A section between clusters of nuclei may fail to demonstrate that a muscle fiber was even present. In a chronic denervating condition, reinnervation of the motor units is seen, but each surviving motor unit becomes larger. Thus, there is a tendency for a specific lower motor neuron to take over the innervation of a given field of fibers, and fiber groups of one type are seen adjacent to groups of another. This pattern is designated "type grouping," and it is pathognomonic of denervation followed by reinnervation (Fig. 27-3).

C H A P T E R **28**

The Nervous System

F. Stephen Vogel
Gregory N. Fuller
Thomas W. Bouldin

Central Nervous System

F. Stephen Vogel
Gregory N. Fuller

From an anatomic and a functional point of view, the nervous system is, perhaps, the most complex structure in the body. In some respects, the brain and spinal cord can be viewed as consisting of many distinct organs, which are nevertheless intimately interconnected and capable of exquisite and rapid communications. Thus, the sensory, motor, cognitive, memory, and autonomic functions of the nervous system have distinct anatomic correlates, although defects in one area may have significant effects on the functions of other regions. Despite this intricate organization, the nervous system is governed by the same principles that control the function of cells in the rest of the body. The field of neuropathology emphasizes the unique character of the nervous system and, at the same time, the responses that it shares with other tissues.

CELLS OF THE NERVOUS SYSTEM

Neurons

Mature neurons do not divide, and the nervous system loses neurons as a part of the aging process. Neurons of the central nervous system (CNS) cannot effectively regenerate axons. Thus, an infarct that transects the internal capsule creates a permanent motor deficit. Furthermore, neurons of the brain and spinal cord are not efficiently remyelinated after injury. Consequently, a plaque of multiple sclerosis establishes a lasting area of demyelination, which, in turn, creates a permanent functional deficit.

Anatomy. The centrally located nuclei are round and, particularly in large neurons, contain a prominent nucleolus. The cytoplasm is abundant, and the ribosome-studded endoplasmic reticulum forms prominent basophilic granules, which are known as **Nissl bodies** (Fig. 28-1). Some neurons (e.g., those in the substantia nigra or locus ceruleus) normally contain cytoplasmic pigment. The cytoplasm is also rich in neurofilaments, which are the counterparts of the intermediate filaments of other cells.

The surface of the neuronal cell body is disposed in numerous branching projections, termed **dendrites,** and this results in an enormous expansion of the surface area of the neuron. The cell body of a neuron leads into a single axon, which, depending on its location, may extend for more than a meter. Some axons are surrounded by a myelin sheath, whereas others are unmyelinated.

Chromatolysis. Swelling of a neuron in response to injury is termed **chromatolysis.** As the cytoplasm expands, the Nissl substance is displaced centrifugally and becomes marginated near the plasma membrane. In addition, the nucleus assumes an eccentric position (Fig. 28-2).

Atrophy. Loss of neurons in the brain may be appreciated on gross examination as a reduced weight or selective loss in specific regions (e.g., the caudate nucleus in Huntington disease). Atrophy may also refer to changes in a single neuron, in which case the cell shrivels and becomes hyperchromatic. Such damaged cells may ultimately disappear.

Neuronophagia. Aggregation of inflammatory cells about a dead neuron, coupled with phagocytosis, is termed **neuronophagia** (Fig. 28-3). Most phagocytic cells are polymorphonuclear leukocytes, although some are mononuclear macrophages.

Intraneuronal Inclusions. A variety of nuclear and cytoplasmic inclusions appear in neurons, particularly

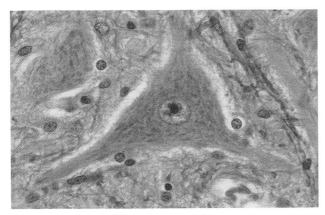

FIGURE *28-1*
Neuron. The neuron is a pyramidal cell with a rounded nucleus and prominent nucleolus. The granularity of the cytoplasm is imparted by rough endoplasmic reticulum (Nissl substance).

in patients with certain viral encephalitides and degenerative diseases. The characteristics of specific inclusions are described with the diseases they mark (Figs. 28-4 and 28-5).

Astrocytes

■ *Astrocytes are star-shaped cells of neuroectodermal origin that are distributed throughout the nervous system and play a prominent role in response to injury.*

Anatomy. **Fibrillary astrocytes** are located in the white matter, whereas **protoplasmic astrocytes** reside in the gray matter. Both types display a rounded nucleus with a diameter of 7 to 10 μm and a homogeneous chromatin pattern. The cytoplasm of "resting" astrocytes is not clearly evident. With silver impregnation, delicate and sinuous cytoplasmic processes ex-

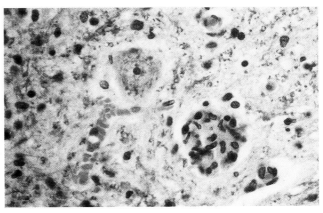

FIGURE *28-3*
Neuronophagia. Leukocytes may accumulate at sites of neuronal necrosis, as shown in this case of acute poliomyelitis.

tend in all directions from the cell body, often terminating in foot processes that rest on blood vessels (Fig. 28-6). Protoplasmic astrocytes tend to have flat, branching processes, whereas fibrillary astrocytes have longer, thinner, and less branched processes.

Reactions. Astrocytes multiply both in and about the localized sites of tissue injury (**astrogliosis** or simply **gliosis**), such as in contusions, penetrating wounds, abscesses, granulomas, metastatic tumors, infarcts, and cerebral hemorrhages (Fig. 28-7). Astrocytes form a "glial scar," which is composed predominantly of cell processes rather than collagen. Fibrillary astrocytes are prone to neoplastic transformation and are responsible for the dominant family of gliomas.

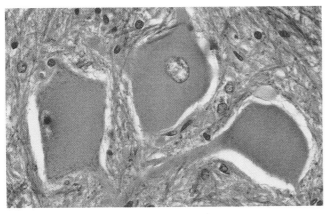

FIGURE *28-2*
Chromatolysis. An injured neuron has imbibed fluid and appears swollen, with a pale cytoplasm and Nissl substance marginated toward the plasma membrane.

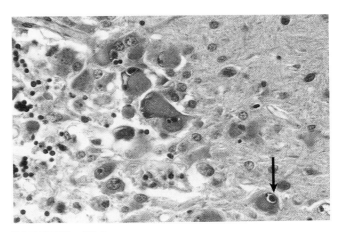

FIGURE *28-4*
Intranuclear inclusions. Cytomegalovirus induces intranuclear inclusions, which are made prominent by the presence of clear halos (*arrow*). These inclusions are demonstrated here in the Purkinje cells of a patient with acquired immunodeficiency syndrome.

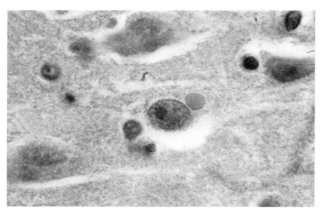

FIGURE 28-5
Negri body. Rabies encephalitis is characterized by round, eosinophilic cytoplasmic inclusions that resemble an erythrocyte.

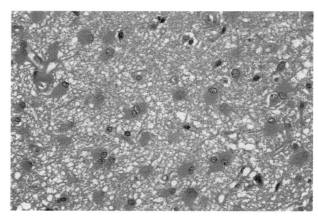

FIGURE 28-7
Astrocytes. In this section stained with hematoxylin-and-eosin, reactive astrocytes appear plump and display pink cytoplasm (gemistocytic astrocytes).

Oligodendroglia

■ *Oligodendroglia are the myelin-producing cells of the CNS that are related to astrocytes insofar as they are both of neuroectodermal origin.* They have dark, rounded nuclei, which resemble those of lymphocytes, and a thin rim of cytoplasm. In the gray matter, many oligodendroglia are satellites of neurons, residing in a small depression on the surface of the latter. In the white matter, oligodendroglia are arrayed longitudinally between myelinated fibers (Fig. 28-8).

Oligodendroglia synthesize myelin during the late gestational period and the first two postnatal years. Subsequently, they also maintain these lipid membranes throughout life. Damage to oligodendroglia results in demyelination, as in progressive multifocal leukoencephalopathy. These glial cells can undergo neoplastic transformation, but compared with astrocytes, they do so infrequently.

Ependyma

A single layer of ependymal cells lines the four ventricular chambers, aqueduct of Sylvius, central canal of the spinal cord, and filum terminale. These cells vary from cuboidal to flat and modulate the transfer of fluid between the cerebrospinal fluid (CSF) and the cells of the nervous system.

Microglia

■ *Microglia are phagocytic elements of the CNS and account for 5% of all glial cells.*

Anatomy. Resting microglia are identified by their hyperchromatic, elongated nuclei, which are surrounded by only a thin rim of cytoplasm (Fig. 28-9). In

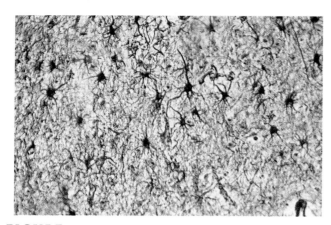

FIGURE 28-6
Astrocytes. Astrocytes have proliferated in the chronically injured brain of this patient with tertiary syphilis. The processes are well outlined with silver carbonate.

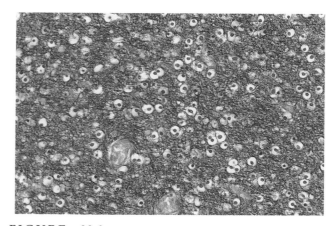

FIGURE 28-8
Normal white matter. In this section stained with luxol fast blue for myelin, the white matter is sparsely populated by oligodendroglia, which are aligned along the myelinated axons.

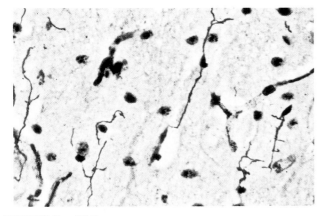

FIGURE *28-9*
Microglia. The native macrophages of the central nervous system, termed *microglia*, are elongated when resting and exhibit few "glial" processes as shown in this section stained with silver carbonate.

the gray matter, microglia may appear as isolated cells or as neuronal or vascular satellites. In the white matter, they are predominantly perivascular.

Reactions. Microglia proliferate and show reactive changes in areas of injury from almost any cause. **Microglial nodules** are formed of microglia and astrocytes and characterize viral, rickettsial, and protozoal infections (Fig. 28-10). Reactive microglia may exhibit a prominent elongated nucleus and are referred to as "rod cells." As befits their phagocytic nature, they become distended by lipid droplets and other cellular debris in response to tissue necrosis and are then designated "gitter cells."

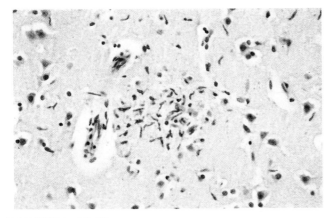

FIGURE *28-10*
Glial nodule. Microglia and astrocytes create cellular nodules in response to viral, protozoan, or rickettsial infections.

TRAUMA

Epidural Hematoma

■ *Epidural hematoma refers to the accumulation of blood between the calvarium and the dura.* This lesion usually results from a blow to the side of the head that fractures the temporal bone. Unless treated promptly, an epidural hematoma is generally fatal.

☐ **Pathogenesis:** The middle meningeal arteries occupy the theoretical space between the dura and the calvarium, and their branches splay across the temporoparietal area. The temporal bone is one of the thinnest bones of the skull and, therefore, is particularly vulnerable to fracture. Even trauma that seems to be inconsequential may be sufficient to fracture the temporoparietal bone and, thereby, transect branches of the middle meningeal artery. The result is life-threatening epidural hemorrhage (Figs. 28-11 and 28-12).

☐ **Pathology and Clinical Course:** Transection of the middle meningeal artery permits arterial blood to escape into the epidural space. This bleeding slowly separates the dura from the calvarium, and the hematoma relentlessly enlarges. During the initial 4 to 8 hours, the intracranial events are largely asymptomatic. Symptoms, which become evident when the hematoma attains a volume of 30 to 50 mL, reflect a space-occupying lesion. As the hematoma enlarges, the increased intracranial pressure exceeds the venous pressure, and the large venous sinuses are compressed. This collapse of the venous conduits creates circulatory stagnation, thereby causing cerebral ischemia and hypoxia.

Bleeding continues into the hematoma, which attains a size of approximately 60 mL within 6 to 10 hours. The brain is shifted laterally away from the side of the lesion, and the medial aspect of the temporal lobe on the side of the hematoma is compressed against the midbrain and displaced downward through the horseshoe-shaped opening of the tentorium, an event termed **transtentorial herniation.** Death is imminent, or if the supratentorial pressure is relieved, unconsciousness may be permanent. **Epidural hematomas are invariably progressive and, when not recognized and evacuated, are fatal in 24 to 48 hours.**

Subdural Hematoma

■ *Subdural hematoma is an accumulation of blood in the subdural space as a consequence of bleeding from torn bridging veins.* This lesion is a significant cause of death

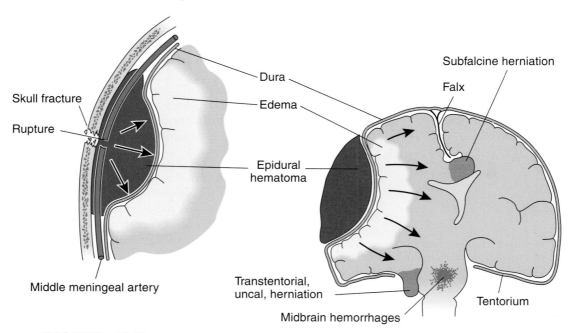

Skull fracture

Rupture

Middle meningeal artery

Dura

Edema

Epidural
hematoma

Subfalcine herniation

Falx

Transtentorial,
uncal, herniation

Midbrain hemorrhages

Tentorium

FIGURE   *28-11*
Development of an epidural hematoma. Transection of a branch of the middle meningeal artery by the sharp edge of a fracture initiates bleeding under arterial pressure. This bleeding slowly dissects the dura from the calvarium and produces an expanding hematoma. After an asymptomatic interval of several hours, transtentorial herniation becomes life-threatening.

following head injuries from falls, assaults, vehicular accidents, and sporting mishaps. Importantly, victims of child abuse also commonly suffer subdural hematomas.

☐ **Pathogenesis:** When the frontal or occipital portion of the moving head strikes a fixed object, or the stationary head is struck by a blunt object, the cerebral

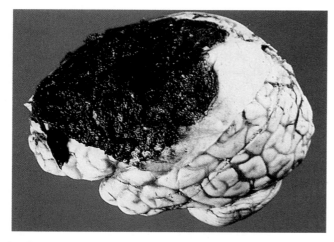

FIGURE   *28-12*
Epidural hematoma. A discoid mass of fresh hemorrhage overlies the frontoparietal cortex.

hemispheres impact forcefully against the inner aspect of the occipital or frontal bone. Because the dura is adherent to the skull and the arachnoid is attached to the cerebrum, the disparate movement of these membranes produces a shearing effect, which is localized to the subdural space. As a result, the cortical veins are torn where they pass across this theoretical subdural compartment (Fig. 28-13). This compartment is readily expansible, unlike the restricted epidural space. Fortunately, the bleeding, being venous in origin, usually stops spontaneously after an accumulation of 25 to 50 mL. Compression of the severed bridging veins by the hematoma (Fig. 28-14) initiates thrombosis. Because the brain is symmetric and a force applied in the sagittal plane similarly affects both hemispheres, it is not surprising that subdural hematomas are frequently bilateral.

☐ **Pathology:** A subdural hematoma, which is static in size and generally asymptomatic, has the potential for three routes of evolution:

- The hematoma may be reabsorbed, as occurs regularly when blood is introduced experimentally into the subdural space of a laboratory animal.
- The hematoma may remain static, with the potential for calcification.
- The hematoma may enlarge.

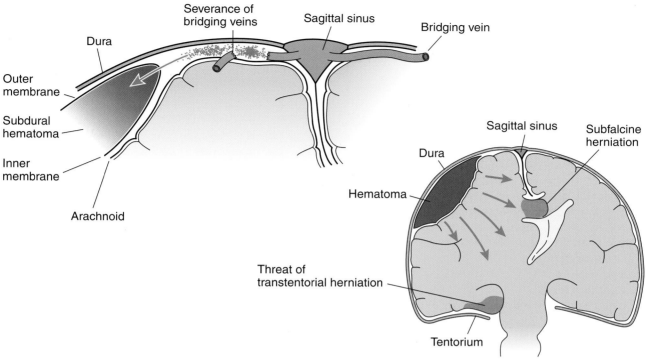

FIGURE   *28-13*
Development of a subdural hematoma. With head trauma, the dura moves with the skull and the arachnoid with the cerebrum. As a result, the bridging veins are sheared as they cross between the dura and arachnoid. Venous bleeding creates a hematoma in the expansile subdural space. Subsequent transtentorial herniation is life-threatening.

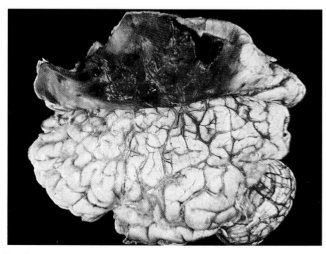

FIGURE   *28-14*
Subdural hematoma. The left leaf of the dura has been deflected upward to disclose a subdural hematoma, which is thinly encapsulated by an inner membrane.

Expansion of the hematoma and the onset of symptoms most often result from rebleeding, usually within 6 months.

☐ **Clinical Features:** The symptoms of a subdural hematoma are protean. Stretching of the meninges causes headaches. Pressure on the motor cortex produces contralateral weakness. Focal irritation of the cortex may initiate seizures. Diffuse and often bilateral subdural hematomas may impair cognitive function and lead to dementia, which invites the mistaken diagnosis of senility. One or several episodes of rebleeding may enlarge the mass and initiate a lethal transtentorial herniation.

Subarachnoid Hemorrhage

■ *Subarachnoid hemorrhage refers to bleeding into the subarachnoid space from any cause.* **Two-thirds of the cases of subarachnoid hemorrhages reflect the rupture of a pre-existing arterial aneurysm.** In 10% of the cases, an arteriovenous malformation is demonstrated. This type of hemorrhage may also be associated with traumatic head injuries (e.g., cerebral contusion or laceration). However, subarachnoid hemorrhage is rarely an isolated finding with trauma and usually complicates hemorrhage in other parts of the brain. The remaining cases are secondary to a variety of conditions, including blood dyscrasias, infections, vasculitis, and tumors.

Cerebral Contusion

> ■ *Cerebral contusion is a bruise of the cortical surface of the brain that virtually always is a result of head trauma.*

☐ **Pathogenesis:** Similar to subdural hematomas, cerebral contusions generally result from energetic anteroposterior displacement (when the moving head strikes a fixed object). Flotation of the cerebral hemispheres in the anteroposterior direction and the soft, gelatinous quality of the cerebral tissues create a vulnerability to bruising or laceration of the cortex by forces applied to the head, particularly those in the midsagittal plane.

When cerebral contusion occurs at the point of impact, the lesion is referred to as a **coup** contusion. When the occipital area strikes the ground in a backward fall, the resulting abrasions are prone to occur on the opposite side of the brain, opposite to the point of contact—that is, in the frontal or temporal cortex. Such lesions are designated as **contrecoup** contusions.

☐ **Pathology:** If the force is minimal, the contusion is limited to the gray cortex and restricted to the apex of the gyri. Greater forces destroy larger expanses of the cortex, thereby creating deeper, cavitary lesions that extend into the white matter or that lacerate the cortex and initiate cortical or subcortical hemorrhages (Fig. 28-15). The hemorrhage and edema associated with large contusions create a mass lesion, which threatens life by transtentorial herniation.

Contusions are permanent. The bruised, necrotic tissue is promptly phagocytized by macrophages and is ultimately transported, in large part, into the bloodstream. Mild astrocytic proliferation forms a local scar, and the lesion persists as a telltale crater.

CIRCULATORY DISORDERS

Vascular Malformations

Arteriovenous Malformation. This is the most common congenital vascular malformation and is of the greatest clinical significance (Fig. 28-16). Seizure disorders and intracranial hemorrhages, usually subarachnoid or intracerebral, supervene during the second or third decades of life.

Cavernous Angioma. This congenital anomaly is considerably less common than arteriovenous malformation. It is similar in structure to a cavernous angioma of the liver, being formed by large, vascular spaces that are compartmentalized by prominent fibrous walls. Most cavernous angiomas remain asymptomatic. However, a significant minority of patients suffer intracranial bleeding, epilepsy, or focal neurologic disturbances.

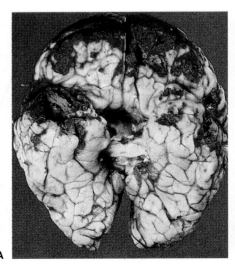
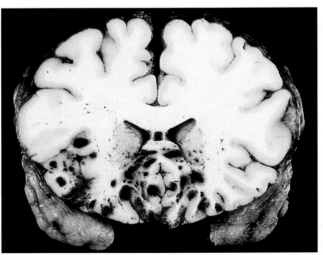

A   **B**

FIGURE   28-15
Recent cerebral contusions. (A) Multiple areas of hemorrhage mark the poles of the frontal and temporal lobes. (B) A coronal section of *panel A* shows underlying parenchymal hemorrhages.

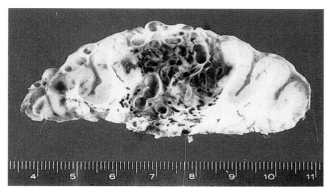

FIGURE *28-16*
Arteriovenous malformation. Abnormal blood vessels replace the cortical gray matter and extend deeply into the underlying white matter.

Aneurysms

Berry Aneurysm

■ *Berry aneurysms are saccular aneurysms that occur at branch points in the carotid system and result from developmental arterial defects.*

☐ **Pathology:** Berry aneurysms are approximately equally distributed at the unions of (1) the anterior cerebral and anterior communicating arteries, (2) the complex of the internal carotid/posterior communicating/anterior cerebral/anterior choroidal arteries, and (3) the trifurcation of the middle cerebral artery (Fig. 28-17). In 20% of the cases, multiple berry aneurysms are present. Careful autopsies have revealed that undetected berry aneurysms are found in as many as 25% of persons older than 55 years of age.

☐ **Clinical Features: Rupture of a berry aneurysm results in life-threatening subarachnoid hemorrhage, with a 35% mortality rate during the initial hemorrhage.** Rupture produces intracerebral or intraventricular hemorrhage in as many as one-third of the patients. A sudden, severe headache characteristically heralds the onset of subarachnoid hemorrhage and may be followed by coma.

Atherosclerotic Aneurysms

Aneurysms secondary to atherosclerosis are preferentially localized in the major cerebral vessels (vertebral, basilar, and internal carotid arteries), which are the favored sites of atherosclerosis (Fig. 28-18). Fibrous replacement of the media and destruction of the internal elastic membrane weaken the arterial wall and permit aneurysmal dilatation. Arteriosclerotic aneurysms are characteristically fusiform, and as they enlarge, the

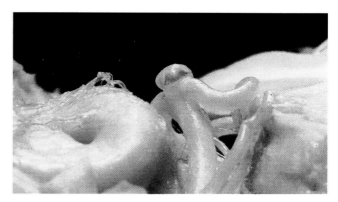

FIGURE *28-17*
Berry aneurysm. A thin-walled aneurysm protrudes from an arterial bifurcation in the circle of Willis.

vessel elongates. These aneurysms rarely rupture, and the major complication is thrombosis.

Cerebral Hemorrhage

Hypertensive intracerebral hemorrhage occurs at preferential sites, which are (1) the basal ganglia–thalamus (65%), (2) the pons (15%), and (3) the cerebellum (8%). The integrity of cerebral arterioles is compromised by hypertension through the deposition of lipid and hyaline material in their walls, an alteration referred to as **lipohyalinosis** (Fig. 28-19). The resulting weakening of the wall leads to formation of **Charcot-Bouchard aneurysms**. These small, fusiform aneurysms are located on the trunk of a vessel rather than at a bifurcation, and are disposed to rupture and hemorrhage.

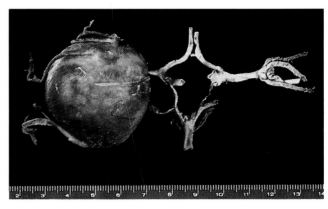

FIGURE *28-18*
Giant atherosclerotic aneurysm. In this patient, a large aneurysm of the middle cerebral artery created a mass lesion, which produced symptoms that were mistaken clinically for those of a tumor.

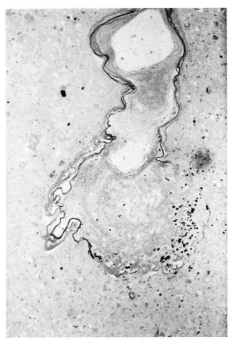

FIGURE   *28-19*
Charcot-Bouchard aneurysm. Chronic hypertension initiated the deposition of lipid in and the hyalinization of the arterial wall. A microaneurysm arises from the damaged wall of the arteriole, and the hemosiderin-laden macrophages attest to previous hemorrhage.

The onset of symptoms in patients with a hypertensive cerebral hemorrhage (hemorrhagic stroke) is abrupt, and weakness usually dominates. When hemorrhage is progressive—and it usually is—death occurs within a period of hours or several days. As the hematoma enlarges, it may cause death by transtentorial herniation, or it may rupture into a lateral ventricle and initiate massive intraventricular hemorrhage.

Intraventricular Hemorrhage. Rupture of a vessel into a ventricle rapidly distends the entire ventricular system with blood. The rush of blood through the ventricular system seemingly causes death by distention of the fourth ventricle and compression of the vital centers in the medulla.

Pontine Hemorrhage. In this catastrophic event, loss of consciousness reflects damage to the reticular formation, which is an injury that overshadows all other specific cranial nerve deficits. Patients rarely survive, and death usually occurs before arrival at the hospital.

Spontaneous cerebral hemorrhages have causes other than hypertension:

- Leakage from an arteriovenous malformation
- Erosion of vessels by a primary or secondary neoplasm

- A bleeding diathesis, as exemplified by thrombocytopenic purpura
- Endothelial injury by micro-organisms, notably rickettsiae
- Embolic infarction, with consequent hemorrhage into the area of necrosis.

Ischemia and Infarction

A generalized decrease in cerebral blood flow results in global ischemia, whereas vascular obstruction produces regional ischemia and a localized infarct. Lesions that follow global ischemia can also be produced by hypoxia (e.g., near-drowning, carbon monoxide poisoning, or entrapment in a burning building).

Global Ischemia

Watershed Infarcts. These ischemic lesions reflect the fact that the major cerebral vessels, notably the anterior, middle, and posterior cerebral arteries, provide overlapping circulations (Fig. 28-20). For example, whereas the anterior cerebral arteries principally supply the cortex on the medial aspects of both cerebral hemispheres, they also interface with the distribution of the middle cerebral arteries in the parasagittal cortex. However, the overlapping zone in the parasagittal cortex is not as richly vascularized as the regions that are supplied by the primary distributions of the anterior and middle cerebral arteries. A precipitous decline in cerebral blood flow (e.g., in shock) abruptly diminishes circulation in the overlapping branches of both the anterior and middle cerebral arteries. This inflicts a dual ischemic insult to the intervening circulatory zones, and watershed infarcts result (Fig. 28-21).

Laminar Necrosis. The cerebral gray matter receives its major blood supply through the "short penetrators," which take origin at right angles from larger vessels in the pia and then form a cascade as they penetrate the gray matter. In that location, they branch frequently and, finally, construct a rich plexus of capillaries deep in the gray matter, notably in the fourth to sixth neuronal cell layers. An abrupt loss of circulatory pressure selectively diminishes flow through this terminal capillary plexus. The necrotic zone is laminar, and the necrosis is, understandably, most severe in the deeper layers of the gray cortex (Fig. 28-22).

Regional Ischemia and Cerebral Infarction

Atherosclerosis predisposes to vascular thrombosis and embolic events, both of which result in localized ischemia and subsequent cerebral infarction (Fig. 28-23).

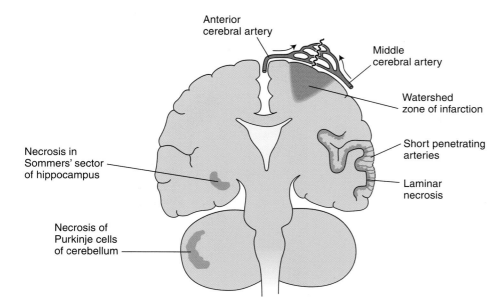

FIGURE *28-20*
Consequences of global ischemia. A global insult induces lesions that reflect the vascular architecture (watershed infarcts, laminar necrosis) and the sensitivity of individual neuronal systems (pyramidal cells of the Sommer section, Purkinje cells).

In general, infarcts resulting from embolization are the sites of hemorrhage, whereas those resulting from thrombotic occlusion in situ are largely ischemic. These differences are accounted for by the tempo of evolution. An embolus occludes the vascular flow abruptly, after which the ischemic region undergoes necrosis. The blood vessels that traverse the area of infarction also become necrotic and leak blood into that region. Because thrombosis in situ progresses more slowly, the collateral vessels also thrombose, thereby guarding against secondary hemorrhage.

A recent infarct of the brain transforms the cerebral tissue into necrotic, putty-like debris, which is ultimately phagocytized by macrophages. Unlike infarcts of the heart and kidneys, cerebral infarcts are not repaired by fibroblasts. As an early response, capillaries proliferate at the margin of the lesion and become numerous by the fifth day. Within months, the necrotic area is excavated by phagocytosis in proportion to the size of the lesion, and a permanent cyst is formed (Fig. 28-24).

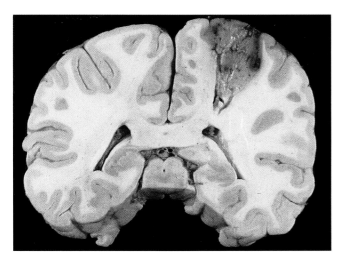

FIGURE *28-21*
Watershed infarct. A coronal section of the brain shows a recent infarct between the distributions of the anterior and middle cerebral arteries.

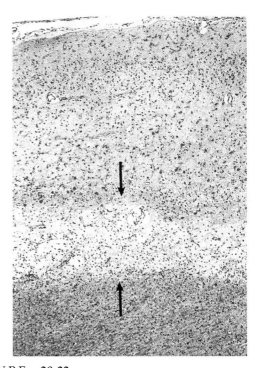

FIGURE *28-22*
Laminar necrosis. A microscopic view of Figure 28-21 shows that the zone of infarction (*arrows*) selectively involves the fourth to sixth cortical layers.

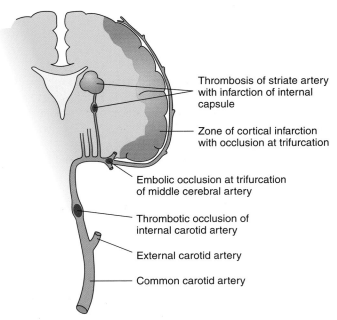

Thrombosis of striate artery with infarction of internal capsule

Zone of cortical infarction with occlusion at trifurcation

Embolic occlusion at trifurcation of middle cerebral artery

Thrombotic occlusion of internal carotid artery

External carotid artery

Common carotid artery

FIGURE 28-23
Distribution of cerebral infarcts. The normal geographic distribution of the cerebral vasculature defines the pattern and size of infarcts, and consequently, their symptoms. Occlusion at the trifurcation initiates cortical infarction, with motor and sensory loss, and often, aphasia. Occlusion of a striate branch transects the internal capsule and causes a motor deficit.

□ **Clinical Features:** Localized neurologic deficits are produced by occlusion of different cerebral vessels. For example, the lengthy and slender striate arteries, which take origin from the proximal middle cerebral artery, are commonly occluded by atherosclerosis and thrombosis. The resultant infarct often transects the internal capsule and produces hemiparesis or hemiplegia. Similarly, the trifurcation of the middle cerebral artery, which is a point of major stepdown in vascular caliber, is a favored site not only for the lodgement of emboli but also for atherosclerosis, which promotes thrombosis in situ. Occlusion of the middle cerebral artery at the trifurcation deprives the parietal cortex of circulation and produces motor and sensory deficits as well as aphasias when the dominant hemisphere is involved.

HYDROCEPHALUS

■ *Hydrocephalus, which may be either congenital or acquired, refers to an excessive amount of cerebrospinal fluid (CSF), with consequent dilatation of the ventricular system.* When the obstruction is within the ventricular chambers, the hydrocephalus is designated as being "noncommunicating" (Fig. 28-25). "Communicating" hy-

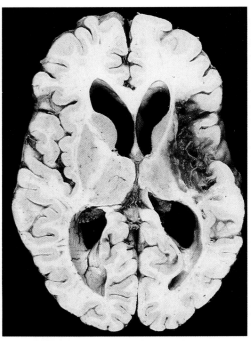

FIGURE 28-24
Remote cerebral infarct. A horizontal section of the brain demonstrates that the end stage of a cerebral infarct is a cyst traversed by atretic vessels.

drocephalus refers to the situation in which there is no obstruction in the ventricular system but in which the reabsorption of CSF by the arachnoid villi is impaired.

Noncommunicating Hydrocephalus. Flow through a ventricular chamber or foramen may be obstructed by (1) a congenital malformation, (2) a neoplasm, (3) inflammation, or (4) hemorrhage. The aqueduct of Sylvius is the most common location for an obstructive congenital malformation. Some tumors, notably papillomas or carcinomas of the choroid plexus and ependymomas, arise within a ventricular chamber. In that location, they can obstruct the flow of CSF and produce hydrocephalus. In addition to physical obstruction, neoplasms of the choroid plexus form excessive volumes of CSF. Parenchymal tumors, notably gliomas, compress the aqueduct or a ventricular chamber and cause hydrocephalus behind the point of stenosis. The ependyma is sensitive to viral infections, particularly during embryonic development; thus, ependymitis is believed to be a cause of congenital aqueductal stenosis.

Communicating Hydrocephalus. Impaired reabsorption of CSF, with resultant communicating hydrocephalus, can complicate subarachnoid hemorrhage, meningitis, and spread of tumor within the subarachnoid space. With only the rarest exception, communi-

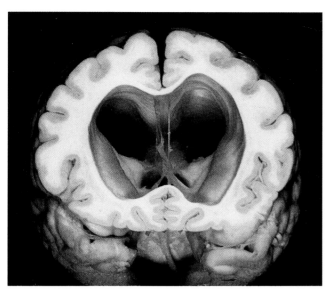

FIGURE 28-25
Hydrocephalus. A coronal section of the brain from a patient who died of a brain tumor obstructing the aqueduct of Sylvius shows marked dilatation of the lateral ventricles.

cating hydrocephalus is "acquired" and is predominantly a sequel to meningitis.

☐ **Pathology:** Similar pathologic changes occur in patients with hydrocephalus of all causes. The cerebral hemispheres are enlarged, and the ventricular system is dilated behind the point of obstruction. The external pattern of the gyri tends to be less prominent, because sulci are compressed. The white matter is reduced in volume, and the basal ganglia and thalamus are attenuated.

When hydrocephalus develops in utero or in early life, usually secondary to obstruction at the aqueduct of Sylvius, the ventricles expand behind the point of obstruction, and the cranial sutures separate. In addition, the head enlarges, and the cerebral cortex becomes attenuated. Without surgical drainage of the CSF from the ventricles, the hydrocephalus is slowly progressive, and the head may attain a huge size, with a circumference of 75 cm or more.

☐ **Clinical Features:** The infantile cranium expands easily, and the symptoms of increased intracranial pressure are generally absent. Convulsions are common, and in severe cases, optic atrophy leads to blindness. Weakness and incoordination are common. Insertion of shunts that link ventricles to the venous system has been successful at controlling hydrocephalus in some children.

In adults, the onset of hydrocephalus is usually marked by symptoms of increased intracranial pressure, including headache, vomiting, and shortly thereafter, papilledema (protrusion of the optic disc). If the obstruction is not relieved, mental deterioration eventually appears.

INFECTIOUS DISEASES

Meningitis

Leptomeningitis denotes an inflammatory process that is localized to the interfacing surfaces of the pia and arachnoid (Fig. 28-26). This compartment houses the CSF, which is an excellent culture medium for most micro-organisms.

Pachymeningitis refers to inflammation of the dura. It usually results from contiguous infection, such as chronic sinusitis or mastoiditis. The dura is a substantial barrier to infection, and inflammation is usually restricted to its outer surface.

Bacterial Meningitis

With few exceptions, all forms of meningitis are initiated by micro-organisms, with bacteria being the principal offenders. Among these, suppurative organisms predominate.

Suppurative Meningitis

- *Escherichia coli.* Among newborns, in whom resistance to gram-negative bacteria has not yet fully developed, *E. coli* is the prime cause of meningitis.
- *Haemophilus influenzae.* Environmental exposure to *H. influenzae,* also a gram-negative organism, is somewhat delayed, and the incidence of meningitis is maximal between 3 months and 3 years.
- *Streptococcus pneumoniae.* The pneumococcus predominates as a cause of meningitis later in life.
- *Neisseria meningitidis.* The meningococcus frequents the human nasopharynx, and airborne transmission in crowded environments causes "epidemic meningitis," which can be a serious event in military barracks. The initial phase of the infection is a bacteremia that manifests by fever, malaise, and a petechial rash. An intravascular coagulopathy may be associated with lethal adrenal hemorrhages (Waterhouse-Friderichsen syndrome). An untreated meningococcal bacteremia is prone to initiate an acute fulminant meningitis.

☐ **Pathology:** Gross examination of the brain discloses an exudate of leukocytes and fibrin that opacifies the arachnoid. A purulent exudate is most prominent over the convexity of the cerebral hemispheres (see Fig. 28-26), but it also extends along the base of the brain, where the interpeduncular fossa constitutes a reservoir of infection.

☐ **Clinical Features:** In patients with all forms of suppurative meningitis, headache, vomiting, and fever

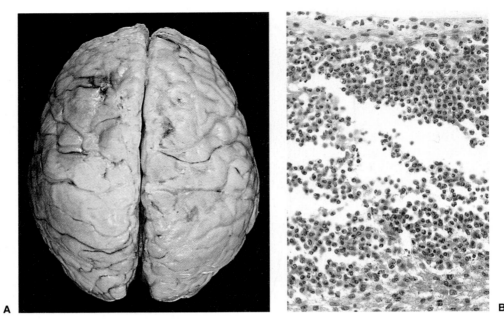

FIGURE 28-26
Purulent meningitis. (A) A creamy exudate opacifies the leptomeninges. (B) A microscopic section shows the accumulation of numerous neutrophils in the subarachnoid space.

are common. Convulsions frequently occur in children. The classic signs of meningeal infection include cervical rigidity, head retraction, pain in the knee when the hip is flexed (Kernig sign), and spontaneous flexion of the knees and hips when the neck is flexed (Brudzinski sign). In untreated patients, delirium often gives way to stupor, coma, and eventually, death.

Viral Meningitis

Infection of the meninges may be the most common viral disease of the CNS. The most common causative agents are the enteroviruses, including coxsackievirus B and species of echovirus. In addition, mumps virus, lymphocytic choriomeningitis virus, Epstein-Barr virus (infectious mononucleosis), and herpes simplex virus are probably responsible for sporadic cases.

Viral meningitis is predominantly a disease of children and young adults. A sudden febrile illness is characteristically marked by a headache that is out of proportion to the other symptoms. Unlike bacterial meningitis, viral meningitis is almost always a benign condition that leaves no sequelae.

Cerebral Abscess

The cerebral cortex and subjacent white matter contain the richest capillary bed in the brain. It is not surprising, therefore, that micro-organisms carried by the blood-stream lodge preferentially in this location. Here, they replicate and elicit an acute inflammatory reaction and regional edema termed **cerebritis.** Within several days, liquefaction necrosis converts the lesion to an expanding abscess (Fig. 28-27), which threatens life either by transtentorial herniation or by rupture into a ventricle.

Although astrocytes are ordinarily the predominant cell during cerebral repair, in this situation they yield the role of containment to fibroblasts, which knit a capsule around the abscess. Astrocytes multiply at the margin of the abscess outside the fibrous capsule, but their contribution to encapsulation is minimal.

If the abscess is not excised or drained, or if the infection is not restrained by antibiotic therapy, pressure builds within the abscess cavity. Edema is prone to develop in the underlying white matter, which is already vulnerable because of the normal paucity of blood vessels in this area. This region is further disposed to ischemia by the overlying position of the abscess, which compresses circulation through the deep penetrating vessels that course perpendicularly from the pia and into the depths of the white matter. Thus, the region below an abscess is susceptible to the growth of micro-organisms that escape from the "mother" abscess. Frequently, a "daughter" abscess forms beneath the primary lesion and, through one or several generations of contiguous abscesses, carries the inflammatory process inward with the threat of an intraventricular rupture. Purulent material liberated into the ventricle passes

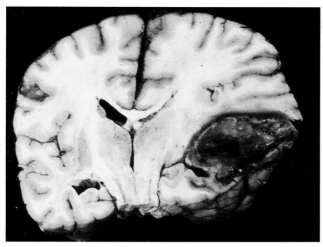

FIGURE 28-27
Cerebral abscess. A young man with chronic otitis media developed an abscess in the temporal lobe, which then ruptured into the temporal horn of the lateral ventricle.

through the chambers across the absorptive ependymal surfaces, through the foramina of Magendi and Luschka, and onto the meninges. Such an event is promptly fatal, presumably because of the absorption of toxic products.

Viral Encephalomyelitis

Manifestations of viral infections of the parenchyma of the CNS are heterogeneous. The attribute that permits recognition of viral infections, both clinically and pathologically, is their propensity for localization in specific areas of the nervous system (Fig. 28-28).

□ **Pathology:** The classic, though not universal, hallmark of viral infections in the CNS is the presence of **perivascular cuffs of lymphocytes** involving small arteries and arterioles (Fig. 28-29). A complementary and more diagnostic feature of viral infections of the brain is the formation of **inclusion bodies** (Figs. 28-30).

Poliomyelitis

■ *Poliomyelitis refers to any inflammation of the gray matter of the spinal cord but, in common usage, implies an infection with one of three strains of poliovirus (Brunhilde, Lancing, or Leon).* The organism is one of the enteroviruses, which are small, nonenveloped, and single-stranded RNA viruses. Persons infected with poliovirus shed large amounts of virus in their stools, and infection spreads by the fecal-oral route. Contaminated hands, food, and water transmit the virus to uninfected persons. The agent spreads most rapidly among children in close quarters, where there are the greatest opportunities for fecal-oral contact.

□ **Pathology:** Infected motor neurons undergo chromatolysis, after which they are phagocytized by macrophages (neuronophagia; see Fig. 28-3). The initial inflammatory response transiently features polymorphonuclear leukocytes, but these leukocytes soon yield to lymphocytes. The latter then surround blood

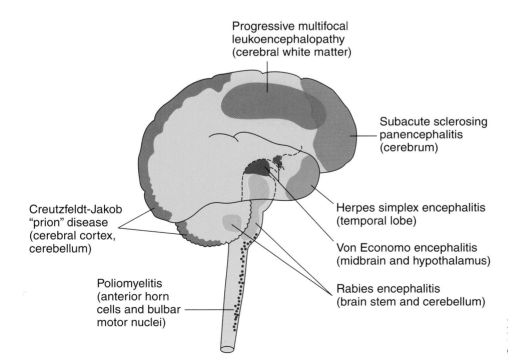

FIGURE 28-28
Distribution of the lesions of viral encephalitides.

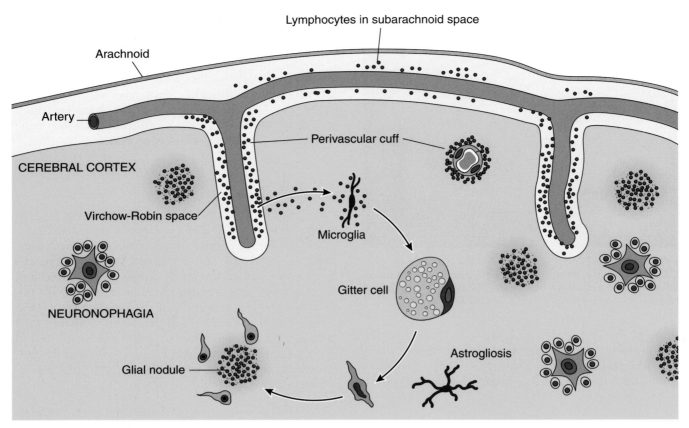

FIGURE   *28-29*
Lesions of viral encephalitis.

vessels in the anterior horns of the spinal cord and the medulla and may extend, in lesser degrees, into the meninges. Sections of spinal cord in cases of healed poliomyelitis show a paucity of neurons in the anterior horns of the affected regions, with secondary degeneration of the corresponding ventral roots and peripheral nerves.

☐ **Clinical Features:** After infection with poliovirus, nonspecific symptoms (e.g., fever, malaise, and headache) are followed in several days by signs of meningitis and, shortly thereafter, by paralysis. In severe cases, the muscles of the neck, trunk, and all four limbs may be powerless, and paralysis of the respiratory muscles may become life-threatening. Milder cases exhibit an asymmetric and patchy paralysis, which is most prominent in the lower limbs.

Improvement begins in approximately 1 week, and only some of the muscles that are affected at the outset remain permanently paralyzed. The mortality rate varies from 5% to 25%, with death usually resulting from respiratory failure. The development of effective vaccines against poliovirus during the 1950s has largely eliminated this disease; today, sporadic cases

occur only in nonimmunized children and young adults.

Rabies

■ *Rabies is an encephalitis caused by rabies virus, which is an enveloped, single-stranded RNA virus of the rhabdovirus group.* Carnivores (notably dogs, wolves, foxes, and skunks) are the principal reservoirs, but the infection also extends to bats and domestic animals, including cattle, goats, and swine. The infectious agent is transmitted to humans via contaminated saliva introduced through a bite.

☐ **Pathogenesis:** The virus enters a peripheral nerve and is transported by centripetal axoplasmic flow to the spinal cord and brain. The latent interval varies in proportion to the distance of transport, being as short as 10 days or as long as 3 months. Centrifugal, intra-axonal transmission of the virus contaminates visceral organs, especially the salivary glands, where the saliva becomes infectious.

☐ **Pathology:** Lymphocytes aggregate about small arteries and veins in the brainstem. Scattered neurons

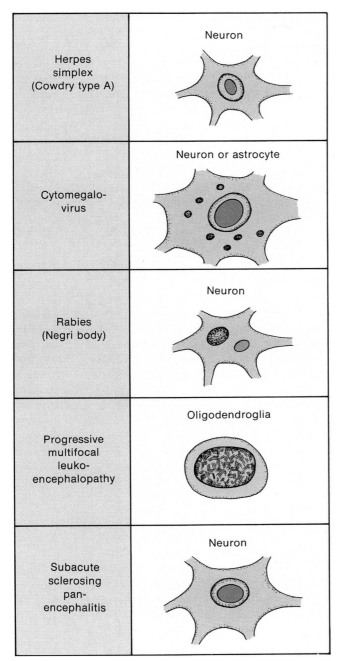

Herpes simplex (Cowdry type A)	Neuron
Cytomegalovirus	Neuron or astrocyte
Rabies (Negri body)	Neuron
Progressive multifocal leuko-encephalopathy	Oligodendroglia
Subacute sclerosing pan-encephalitis	Neuron

FIGURE **28-30**
Inclusion bodies in viral encephalitides.

show chromatolysis and neuronophagia, and glial nodules attest to the infectious nature of the process. The inflammation is centered in the brain stem and spills into the cerebellum and hypothalamus. The presence of Negri bodies (see Fig. 28-5) in the hippocampus, brainstem, and Purkinje cells of the cerebellum confirms the diagnosis of rabies.

☐ **Clinical Features:** Destruction of neurons in the brainstem by rabies virus initiates painful spasms of the throat, difficulty in swallowing, and a consequent tendency to aspirate fluids. Clinical symptoms also reflect a general encephalopathy, which is characterized by irritability, agitation, seizures, and delirium. The illness progresses to death during an interval of one to several weeks. Specific treatment of rabies is not available, but since the time of Pasteur, postexposure prophylaxis is accomplished by a series of vaccine injections and is usually effective.

Herpes Simplex Encephalitis and Related Infections

Herpesviruses include herpes simplex virus (HSV) types 1 and 2, varicella-zoster virus, cytomegalovirus, Epstein-Barr virus, and simian B virus.

HSV-1. Herpes encephalitis constitutes the most important viral infection of the human nervous system. In adults, this encephalitis is caused principally by HSV-1 and, curiously, is localized predominantly in one or both temporal lobes. HSV-1 is also largely responsible for the cold sore. The region of the vesicular lesion on the lip is innervated from the gasserian ganglion through its mandibular nerve trunk. HSV-1 may reside latently within the gasserian ganglion, where it proliferates during periods of stress and is transmitted centrifugally through the nerve trunk to the lip.

☐ **Pathology:** Herpes encephalitis is a fulminant infection. The temporal lobes become swollen, hemorrhagic, and necrotic, and the inflammatory exudate is predominantly lymphocytic and perivascular. The small arteries and arterioles characteristically become hemorrhagic and edematous (Fig. 28-31). Intranuclear inclusions occur in neurons but may also be found in astrocytes and oligodendrocytes. The inclusions are weakly eosinophilic, occupy less than half of the volume of a nucleus, and are usually surrounded by an inconspicuous halo.

HSV-2. In women, HSV-2 initiates a vesicular lesion on the vulva, which is coupled with a latent infection in the pelvic ganglia. Newborns acquire HSV-2 from the birth canal and, thereafter, suffer an encephalitis. At this age, the neural tissues are extremely vulnerable, and the infection promptly causes extensive liquefaction in the cerebrum and cerebellum.

Arbovirus Encephalitis

Arbovirus infections are zoonoses of both wild and domestic animals, and humans become accidentally in-

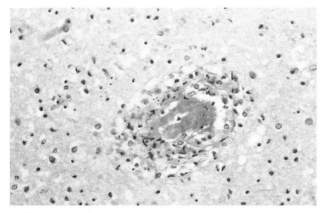

FIGURE   *28-31*
Herpes simplex encephalitis. A microscopic view shows necrotizing arteritis in a temporal lobe.

fected if bitten by an infected arthropod. The various encephalitides caused by arboviruses have been named principally for the geographic regions in which they were first noted (Table 28-1). These diseases include Eastern, Western, and Venezuelan equine encephalitis, St. Louis encephalitis, Japanese B encephalitis, and California encephalitis.

☐ **Pathology:** Lesions vary from a mild meningitis with scattered lymphocytes to a severe inflammation of the gray matter to a prominent necrosis. No inclusion bodies are present in the infected neurons. Perivascular lymphoid infiltrates are conspicuous, and in severe cases, thrombosis of small vessels occurs. In necrotic foci, neuronophagia is evident. Among patients in whom survival has been prolonged, areas of demyelination and gliosis may be apparent.

TABLE   28-*1*.   **Insect-Borne Viral Encephalitis**

Virus	Insect	Vector Distribution
St. Louis encephalitis	Mosquito	North and South America
Western equine encephalitis	Mosquito	North and South America
Venezuelan equine encephalitis	Mosquito	North and South America
Eastern equine encephalitis	Mosquito	North America
California encephalitis	Mosquito	North America
Murray Valley encephalitis	Mosquito	Australia and New Guinea
Japanese B encephalitis	Mosquito	Eastern and southeastern Asia
Tick-borne encephalitis	Tick	Eastern Europe and Scandinavia

☐ **Clinical Features:** The arthropod-borne encephalitides share many features, but each type has a different course. For example, Eastern equine encephalitis is commonly a fulminant disease that kills in a few days, whereas Venezuelan equine encephalitis tends to be benign. Mild cases of arbovirus encephalitis may manifest with no more than an influenza-like syndrome and are not even diagnosed as being encephalitis. In severe cases, however, the onset of disease is abrupt, with high fever, headache, vomiting, and meningeal signs. Shortly thereafter, lethargy and coma supervene, with most victims dying within 5 days. Young children often survive but may be left with mental retardation, epilepsy, and other neurologic sequelae.

Subacute Sclerosing Panencephalitis

■ *Subacute sclerosing panencephalitis (SSPE) is a viral infection of the brain caused by the measles virus.* Its features are (1) an encephalitis of insidious onset that predominates in childhood, (2) a protracted course, and (3) inflammation, principally in the cerebral gray matter. Occasional cases occur in adults, however, and may follow a more rapid course. Most patients with SSPE have a previous history of measles, usually before 7 years of age. The consistent association of SSPE with a measles-like virus argues strongly for a causative role of this agent.

☐ **Pathology and Clinical Features:** In tissue sections, the inflammation is highlighted by (1) prominent, haloed intranuclear inclusions within neurons and oligodendroglial cells; (2) marked astrogliosis in damaged areas of both the gray and white matter, thereby accounting for the term *sclerosing*; (3) patchy loss of myelin; and (4) ubiquitous perivascular cuffs of lymphocytes and macrophages. The classic protracted disease insidiously creates cognitive deficits, alters personality and behavior, inflicts motor and sensory deficits, and ultimately, causes stupor and death, all over a period of several years.

Progressive Multifocal Leukoencephalopathy

■ *Progressive multifocal leukoencephalopathy (PML) is a relentless, destructive focal disease caused by JC virus. It principally affects the white matter in all areas of the nervous system.* PML presents insidiously as dementia, weakness, visual loss, and ataxia, and most patients die within 6 months. The malady exemplifies many of the fundamental characteristics of neurotropic viruses: (1) opportunism; (2) selectivity for an individual cell species, notably oligodendroglia (Fig. 28-32); (3) capac-

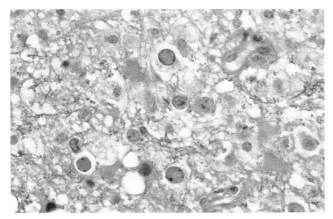

FIGURE 28-32
Progressive multifocal leukoencephalopathy. The oligodendroglia are enlarged and exhibit intranuclear inclusions.

ity to induce demyelination by damaging oligodendrocytes; and (4) oncogenicity.

JC virus, which is a papovavirus closely analogous to SV40 virus, is the causative agent of PML. With few exceptions, the encephalitis is a terminal complication in immunosuppressed patients, such as those being treated for cancer or lupus erythematosus, those receiving organ transplants, and those having acquired immunodeficiency syndrome (AIDS). In fact, PML is no longer a rare disease: it occurs in from 1% to 3% of patients with AIDS in the United States and among an even higher proportion of patients in studies from Europe.

□ **Pathology:** The typical lesions of PML appear as widely disseminated, discrete foci of demyelination near the gray-white junction in the cerebral hemispheres and brainstem. A pathognomonic feature of PML is a peripheral area of demyelination that contains enlarged oligodendrocytes, with homogeneously dense, hyperchromatic, and intranuclear inclusions that lack a halo and have a "ground-glass" appearance (see Fig. 28-32). Astrocytomas have developed in several patients with PML.

PRION DISEASES (SPONGIFORM ENCEPHALOPATHIES)

■ *Prion diseases are a group of neurodegenerative diseases that are characterized clinically by slowly progressive ataxia and dementia and pathologically by a peculiar vacuolization termed spongiform degeneration.*

Kuru. In 1956, a medical officer in New Guinea provided an account of kuru, which is a progressive

and fatal neurologic disorder, in members of an isolated, cannibalistic tribe. The transmission of kuru in New Guinea was linked to ritualistic cannibalism, wherein women and children consumed human brain. The incidence of kuru has sharply abated with the elimination of cannibalism.

Creutzfeldt-Jakob Disease. This rare subacute encephalopathy has a worldwide annual incidence of 1 per 1,000,000 persons. Symptoms begin insidiously, but within 6 months, the patient exhibits severe dementia and is usually dead within 1 year. There are reasons to assume that kuru and Creutzfeldt-Jakob disease (CJD) are variants of the same condition.

Sporadic CJD accounts for 75% of all cases of this disorder, whereas inherited CJD comprises 15%. New variant CJD, which is also known as bovine spongiform encephalopathy, has spread to humans who have eaten contaminated beef.

Other prion diseases include a familial form termed *Gerstmann-Straussler-Scheinker syndrome* and *fatal familial insomnia.*

□ **Pathogenesis:** Spongiform encephalopathies are transmissible diseases. Inadvertent human transmission of CJD has been observed as a consequence of the administration of contaminated human pituitary growth hormone, corneal transplantation from a diseased donor, insufficiently sterilized neurosurgical instruments, and surgical implantation of contaminated dura.

The putative "slow virus" of spongiform encephalopathies is not truly a virus at all but, rather, is an unprecedented protein that is not associated with nucleic acid. The term **prion** was introduced to differentiate these proteinaceous infectious particles from viruses.

The prion protein that causes scrapie is encoded by a host gene on chromosome 20. Its normal protein product has been labeled PrP^c. The infectious protein, PrP^{sc}, has the same amino sequence as PrP^c. The only differences that have been demonstrated between normal PrP^c and PrP^{sc} are infectivity, resistance to protease digestion of the latter, and differences in conformation and glycosylation. It is presumed that PrP^{sc} is derived from PrP^c by an as-yet-unidentified, posttranslational modification: the "replicative" process that produces the new infectious particles.

□ **Pathology:** The cardinal morphologic feature of CJD is spongiform degeneration—that is, the presence of small aggregates of microcysts (Fig. 28-33). These are most prevalent in the cortical gray matter, but they also involve the deeper nuclei of the basal ganglia, the hypothalamus, and importantly, the cerebellum. Involvement of the cerebellum adds ataxia to the predominant symptom of dementia and distinguishes CJD clinically

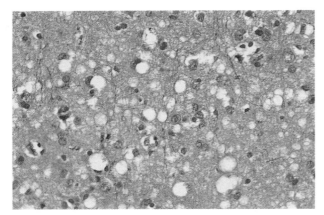

FIGURE　*28-33*
Creutzfeldt-Jakob disease. Spongiform degeneration of the gray matter is characterized by individual and clustered vacuoles, without evidence of inflammation.

from Alzheimer disease. Within the areas of spongiform degeneration, neurons disappear, and astrogliosis becomes prominent. The cortical spinal pathways also degenerate.

DEMYELINATING DISEASES

The category of demyelinating diseases is restricted to those disorders in which myelin is lost selectively, but other neural structures are preserved.

Leukodystrophies

Leukodystrophies are a heterogeneous group of inherited diseases that are characterized by profound disturbances in the formation and preservation of myelin.

Metachromatic Leukodystrophy

■ *Metachromatic leukodystrophy (MLD), the most common type of leukodystrophy, is an autosomal recessive disorder of myelin metabolism that is characterized by accumulation of a cerebroside (galactosyl sulfatide) in the white matter of the brain and peripheral nerves.* MLD predominates during infancy, but rare "juvenile" or "adult" cases have been described. The disorder is lethal within several years.

□ **Pathogenesis:** MLD results from a deficiency in the activity of arylsulfatase A, which is a lysosomal enzyme involved in the degradation of myelin. As a result of the inability of the mutant enzyme to hydrolyze sulfatides, there is a progressive accumulation of sulfatides within the lysosomes of Schwann cells and oligodendrocytes, which are the cells responsible for the maintenance of myelin.

□ **Pathology:** Metachromasia refers to a change in the color of a dye when it reacts with tissue. In patients with MLD, the accumulated sulfatides form cytoplasmic spherical granules with a diameter of from 15 to 20 μm that stain metachromatically with a variety of dyes, including acidified cresyl violet and toluidine blue.

At autopsy, the cerebral hemispheres and cerebellum feature a diffuse loss of myelin, with (1) accumulation of metachromatic material, principally in the white matter; (2) prominent astrogliosis; and (3) preservation of subcortical arcuate fibers.

Krabbe Disease

■ *Krabbe disease is a rapidly progressive, invariably fatal, and autosomal recessive neurologic disorder caused by a deficiency of galactocerebroside β-galactosidase.* The condition appears in young infants, and it is defined by the presence of perivascular aggregates of mononuclear and multinucleated **globoid cells** in the white matter. The globoid cells are macrophages that contain undigested galactocerebroside (galactosylceramide). Krabbe disease features an almost complete loss of oligodendroglia and myelin in the brain.

□ **Pathology:** At autopsy, the brain is small, and the loss of myelin is diffuse. However, the cerebral cortex is normal. Marbled areas of partial and total demyelination are present, and astrogliosis is typically severe. As demyelination proceeds, clusters of globoid cells are found around blood vessels. These cells measure as much as 50 μ in diameter and contain as many as 20 peripherally located nuclei. During the end stage of Krabbe disease, the number of globoid cells decreases, and in areas of severe myelin loss, only scattered globoid cells remain.

Krabbe disease appears during the early months of life and progresses to death within 1 to 2 years. Severe motor, sensory, and cognitive impairment reflects diffuse involvement of the nervous system.

Adrenoleukodystrophy

■ *Adrenoleukodystrophy (ALD) refers to an X-linked, inherited disorder in which dysfunction of the adrenal cortex and demyelination of the nervous system are associated with unusually high levels of saturated, very long-chain fatty acids (VLCFA) in tissues and body fluids.* ALD occurs in children between 3 and 10 years of age, and neurologic symptoms precede the signs of adrenal insufficiency. The disease progresses rapidly, and the body is quickly reduced to a vegetative state, which may persist for several years before death supervenes.

☐ **Pathogenesis:** A defect in the peroxisomal membrane prevents normal activation of free VLCFA by the addition of coenzyme A. As a result of the inability to degrade VLCFA, fatty acids of C24 or C30 (or more) accumulate as cholesterol esters in gangliosides and in myelin.

☐ **Pathology:** Tissue alterations of ALD are dominated by confluent and often bilaterally symmetric demyelination. The most severe lesions are in the subcortical white matter of the parieto-occipital region and, with time, extend in a rostral direction. The cerebral cortex is spared. Histologically, a severe loss of myelinated axons and oligodendrocytes is noted in the affected areas, together with astrogliosis. Peripheral nerves are also depleted of myelin, but to a lesser degree than occurs in the brain.

The adrenals are characteristically atrophic, and electron microscopy reveals pathognomonic cytoplasmic, membrane-bound, and curvilinear inclusions or clefts (lamellae) in the cortical cells. These lamellae contain VLCFA, probably in the form of cholesterol esters.

Multiple Sclerosis

■ *Multiple sclerosis (MS) is a chronic demyelinating disease of the CNS involving numerous patches of demyelination throughout the white matter.* MS is the single most common chronic disease of the CNS among young adults in the United States, with a prevalence approaching 1 in 1000 persons. The disorder affects both sensory and motor functions and, in most cases, is characterized by exacerbations and remissions over a period of many years.

☐ **Epidemiology:** MS is principally a disease of temperate climates, being rare in the tropics and increasing in frequency with distance from the equator. Persons who emigrate before the age of 15 years from areas with a low prevalence of MS to endemic areas acquire an increased risk of developing the disease, thereby suggesting involvement of an environmental factor that acts early in life. MS is acquired at a mean age of 30 years; an onset in children younger than 14 years and in adults older than 60 years is distinctly unusual. Women are afflicted almost twice as often as men.

☐ **Pathogenesis:** Experimental and clinical studies indicate a genetic predisposition to MS and a possible immunopathogenesis. Epidemiologic data suggest that an infection, presumably viral, may be acquired before 15 years of age and may play a pathogenetic role.

Genetic Factors. A genetic predisposition to MS is suggested by the results of studies showing a familial aggregation of the disease, with an increased risk in second- and third-degree relatives of patients with MS. Moreover, monozygotic twins show a 25% concordance for MS, whereas only 2% of dizygotic twins are both afflicted. Susceptibility is also associated with a number of MHC alleles, particularly HLA-DR2, which suggests that immune mechanisms are involved in the pathogenesis. Indeed, studies of siblings in which both suffered from MS have revealed a striking concordance for the same T cell-receptor haplotype.

Immune Factors. Chronic lesions of MS demonstrate perivascular lymphocytes and macrophages, and at the margins, numerous CD4-positive (helper-inducer subset) and CD8-positive T cells accumulate. CD4-positive T cells isolated from the CSF appear to be oligoclonal, thereby suggesting an immune response to a specific protein of the CNS.

Further support for the involvement of immune mechanisms in the pathogenesis of MS comes from the experimental production of an antigen-specific, T cell-mediated, autoimmune demyelinating disease, termed *experimental allergic encephalitis.* Injection of myelin basic protein into a variety of experimental animals, including nonhuman primates, results in relapsing or progressive paralysis and in demyelinating lesions of the CNS that exhibit perivascular lymphocytic infiltrates. As in MS, experimental allergic encephalitis is linked to class II immune response genes.

☐ **Pathology: The plaque is the hallmark of MS** (Fig. 28-34). Characteristically, plaques of variable size, though rarely more than 2 cm in diameter, accumulate in great numbers in the white matter of the brain and spinal cord. The lesion exhibits a preference for the optic nerves and chiasm and uniformly localizes to the paraventricular white matter of the corona radiata.

The evolving plaque is marked by the following morphologic hallmarks:

- Selective loss of myelin in a region of axonal preservation
- A few lymphocytes that cluster about small veins and arteries
- An influx of macrophages
- Considerable edema.

When neurons are encompassed by the boundaries of a plaque, the neuronal cell bodies are remarkably spared. The aging plaque acquires astrocytes, and with time, the tissue becomes dense with glial processes. This "scar" impairs the structural integrity of the axons.

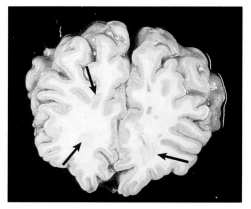

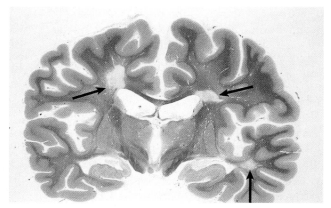

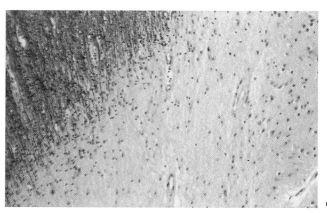

FIGURE *28-34*
Multiple sclerosis. (A) In this unfixed brain, the plaques of multiple sclerosis in the white matter (*arrows*) assume the darker color of the cerebral cortex. (B) A coronal section of the brain (stained for myelin) from a patient with longstanding multiple sclerosis shows discrete areas of demyelination (*arrows*), with characteristic involvement of the superior angles of the lateral ventricles. (C) A higher-magnification view of *panel B* shows the edge of a plaque and emphasizes the regional character of the lesion. Both motor and sensory fibers lose their myelin but retain axonal continuity as they traverse the lesion.

☐ **Clinical Features:** MS usually has its onset during the third or fourth decade of life. The disease is punctuated thereafter by abrupt and brief episodes of clinical progression interspersed with periods of relative stability. However, some patients with MS exhibit a relentless course, without any remissions. Each exacerbation expresses the formation of additional plaques of demyelination. The visual system and paraventricular areas are particularly vulnerable to the disease, whereas the peripheral nerves are uniformly spared.

Typically, MS begins with symptoms relating to lesions in the optic nerves, brainstem, or spinal cord. Blurred vision or loss of vision in one eye is often the presenting complaint. When the initial lesion is in the brainstem, the most troubling early symptoms are double vision and vertigo. Plaques within the spinal cord are reflected in weakness of one or both legs and in sensory symptoms in the form of numbness in the lower extremities.

In most patients with MS, the disease follows a chronic relapsing and remitting course. The degree of functional impairment is highly variable, ranging from minor disability to severe incapacity, with widespread paralysis, dysarthria, severe visual defects, incontinence, and dementia. Patients usually die of respiratory paralysis or urinary tract infections while in terminal coma. Most patients with MS survive 20 to 30 years after the onset of symptoms.

WERNICKE SYNDROME

■ *Wernicke syndrome is an encephalopathy resulting from a deficiency of thiamine (vitamin B$_1$) and arises most commonly in association with chronic alcoholism.* It may also appear in patients whose nutrition is sustained by infusions that lack thiamine. Typically, the onset of symptoms is precipitous and reflects lesions in (1) the hypothalamus and mamillary bodies (Fig. 28-35), (2) the periaqueductal regions of the midbrain, and (3) the tegmentum of the pons. These are evidenced clinically as a disturbance in thermal regulation, altered consciousness, ophthalmoplegia, and nystagmus.

Wernicke syndrome may progress rapidly to death, but in most cases, it is promptly reversible with administration of thiamine. In fatal cases, petechiae about small capillaries are conspicuous in the mamil-

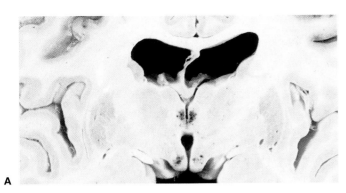

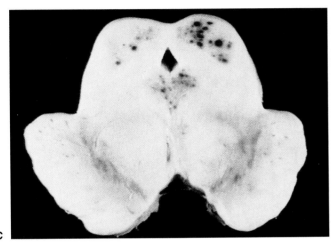

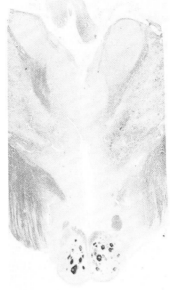

B

FIGURE 28-35
Wernicke encephalopathy. (A) The mamillary bodies and paraventricular regions exhibit petechiae. (B) A histologic section of *panel A* (stained with luxol fast blue) emphasizes selectivity for the mamillary bodies. (C) The quadrigeminal plate and periaqueductal regions display conspicuous petechiae.

lary bodies, hypothalamus, periaqueductal gray matter, and floor of the fourth ventricle. The previous occurrence of lesions is permanently marked by the presence of brown hemosiderin. Interestingly, neurons and myelin are spared in Wernicke encephalopathy; however, the mamillary bodies become atrophic.

The term **Wernicke-Korsakoff syndrome** is employed clinically to refer to a state of disordered memory for recent events, often compensated for by confabulation, in the setting of chronic alcoholism. When present, histologic changes are distinguished from those of Wernicke syndrome by chromatolysis and degeneration of neurons in the mediodorsal nucleus of the thalamus. Thus, Wernicke syndrome and Korsakoff psychosis occur concurrently in the setting of chronic alcoholism, but their causes may (or may not) be different.

DEGENERATIVE DISEASES

This heterogeneous group of disorders involves individual neuronal species (Parkinson disease) or select anatomic regions (Huntington disease). Alternatively, they affect the nervous system diffusely (Alzheimer disease; Fig. 28-36).

Parkinson Disease

■ *Parkinson disease (PD) is a neurologic disorder that is characterized pathologically by loss of neurons in the substantia nigra and clinically by tremors at rest and muscular rigidity.*

☐ **Epidemiology:** PD typically appears during the sixth to eighth decades of life. The disease is common, and more than 2% of the population in North America eventually develop PD. The prevalence has remained unchanged for at least the past 40 years, and no sex or racial differences are apparent. Genetic factors do not seem to be important, especially considering the low concordance rate in monozygotic twins.

☐ **Pathogenesis:** The vast majority of cases of PD are idiopathic, but the disease has been recorded after viral encephalitis (von Economo encephalitis) and after the intake of a toxic chemical (1-methyl-4-phenyl-1,2,3,6-tetrahydro-pyridine [MPTP]). Evidence is accumulating that the pathogenesis of PD may relate to both oxidative stress and a reduced ability to deal with

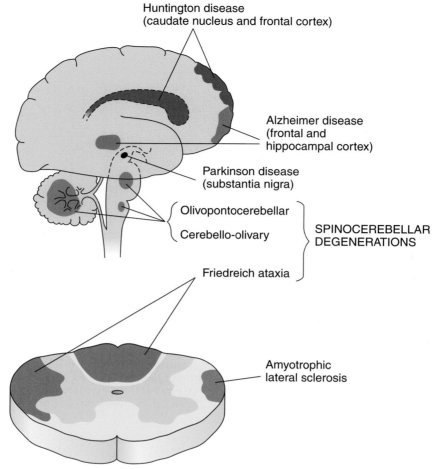

FIGURE   28-36
Distribution of degenerative diseases of the central nervous system.

it. Defects in mitochondrial electron transport have been described in patients with PD, and mitochondrial defects in the presence of oxidative stress could be lethal to dopaminergic neurons of the substantia nigra. In this respect, it is noteworthy that a byproduct of the illicit synthesis of meperidine analogues, MPTP, has induced a PD-like syndrome in intravenous drug users. MPTP is an inhibitor of mitochondrial electron transport and, thus, may produce parkinsonism by a mechanism similar to that of naturally occurring PD.

☐ **Pathology:** On gross examination, the brain has a loss of pigmentation in the substantia nigra and locus ceruleus (Fig. 28-37). On microscopic examination, pigmented neurons are scarce, and there are small extracellular deposits of melanin derived from necrotic neurons. Some residual nerve cells are atrophic, and a few contain spherical, eosinophilic, cytoplasmic inclusions, which are termed **Lewy bodies.**

☐ **Clinical Features:** PD is characterized by a slowness of all voluntary movements and a muscular rigidity throughout the entire range of movement. Most pa-

tients have a coarse tremor of the distal extremities that is present at rest and disappears with voluntary movement. The face is expressionless (mask-like), and a reduced rate of swallowing leads to drooling. There is an increased incidence of depression and dementia. In patients with early parkinsonism, substitution therapy with levodopa is beneficial. However, this therapy does not rectify the underlying disorder and, with the passage of several years, becomes ineffective.

Huntington Disease

■ *Huntington disease (HD) is an autosomal dominant, genetic disorder that is characterized by involuntary movements of all parts of the body, deterioration of cognitive functions, and often, severe emotional disturbance.* The disorder principally affects whites of northwestern European ancestry. Results of genealogic studies indicate that all cases of HD derive from the spread of an original focus in northern Europe, and the malady is notably rare in both Asia and Africa.

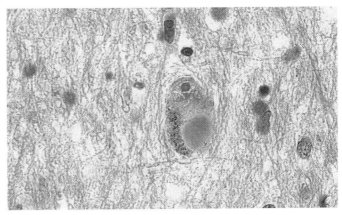

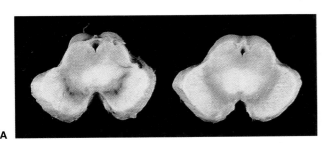

FIGURE 28-37
Parkinson disease. (A) The normal substantia nigra of the midbrain *(left)* is heavily pigmented, whereas the same region from a patient with long standing parkinsonism *(right)* has lost the pigment. (B) A microscopic section of the substantia nigra from a patient with parkinsonism shows a spherical eosinophilic inclusion within the cytoplasm of a pigmented dopaminergic neuron, termed a *Lewy body.*

The *HD* gene on chromosome 4 codes for a novel protein termed *Huntingtin,* and the mutation consists of an expanded and unstable trinucleotide (CAG) repeat. This places HD in a larger class of neurologic diseases termed *trinucleotide repeat expansion syndromes,* which include fragile X syndrome, Friedreich ataxia, myotonic dystrophy, and a number of other conditions. In most autosomal dominant diseases, heterozygotes tend to be less severely affected than homozygotes. **HD is a striking exception to this general rule and appears to be the only human disorder of complete dominance.**

The genetic injury remains latent for three to five decades, after which it manifests by progressive neuronal dysfunction. Interestingly, there is a strong influence of the parent's sex on the expression of HD. Inheritance of the HD allele from an affected father results in clinical disease 3 years earlier than inheritance of the HD allele from the mother. Moreover, children with juvenile-onset HD have almost always inherited the defective gene from the father. The mechanism for this departure from classic mendelian genetics is still debated, but genomic imprinting (an epigenetic process that differentially marks maternal and paternal chromosomes) is thought to play a role.

□ **Pathology:** On gross examination of the brain from patients who succumbed to HD, the frontal cortex is symmetrically and moderately atrophic, whereas the lateral ventricles appear to be disproportionately enlarged owing to a loss of the normal convex curvature of the caudate nuclei (Fig. 28-38). There is symmetric atrophy of the caudate nuclei, with lesser involvement of the putamen. Microscopically, the neuronal population of the caudate and putamen, particularly the small

neurons, is greatly depleted, and there is an accompanying moderate astrogliosis. The cortical neurons are also similarly, though less severely, depleted.

□ **Clinical Features:** Symptoms of HD usually present at approximately 40 years of age. Five percent

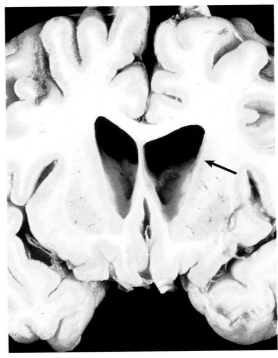

FIGURE 28-38
Huntington disease. The caudate nuclei *(arrow)* are markedly atrophic, thereby imparting a concave rather than the normal convex curvature to the lateral walls of the ventricles.

of those with the disorder develop neurologic signs before the age of 20, however, and a comparable proportion develop manifestations after the age of 60. Cognitive and emotional disturbances precede, sometimes by many years, development of abnormal movements in more than half of the patients. Because of the prominent involvement of the extrapyramidal system, the symptomatology inevitably features a choreoathetoid movement disorder, which progresses to total incapacitation. Subsequent involvement of the cortex leads to a severe loss of cognitive function and intellectual deterioration, often accompanied by paranoia and delusions. The interval from the onset of symptoms to death averages 15 years.

Amyotrophic Lateral Sclerosis

■ *Amyotrophic lateral sclerosis (ALS) is a degenerative disease of motor neurons that results in progressive weakness and wasting of the extremities and, eventually, impairment of the respiratory muscles.*

☐ **Pathogenesis:** ALS is a worldwide disease, with an incidence of 1 in 100,000 persons. The frequency of the disease peaks during the fifth decade of life and is rare in persons younger than 35 years of age. There is a 1.5- to 2.0-fold excess of ALS in men. Familial cases, with an autosomal dominant pattern, account for 5% of the total. The mutant gene in familial ALS is located on chromosome 21 and codes for superoxide dismutase 1. The disease is not, however, caused by a deficiency in superoxide dismutase activity. Rather, it results from a deleterious effect of the mutant protein. Restricted geographic areas with a particularly high incidence of ALS exist in Guam as well as in parts of Japan and New Guinea, but there is some question whether these cases represent the same disorder as found in the rest of the world.

☐ **Pathology:** ALS affects motor neurons in three locations: (1) the anterior horn cells of the spinal cord (Fig. 28-39); (2) the motor nuclei of the brainstem, particularly the hypoglossal nuclei; and (3) the upper motor neurons of the cerebral cortex. Injury to the motor neurons leads to degeneration of their axons, which is visualized as striking alterations in the lateral pyramidal pathways of the spinal cord (see Fig. 28-39).

The defining histologic change in patients with ALS is a loss of large motor neurons, which is accompanied by mild gliosis. This change is most evident in the anterior horns of the lumbar cord and cervical enlargements of the spinal cord and in the hypoglossal nuclei. There is also a loss of the giant, pyramidal Betz cells in the motor cortex of the cerebrum. The most striking secondary change in the spinal cord is a loss of

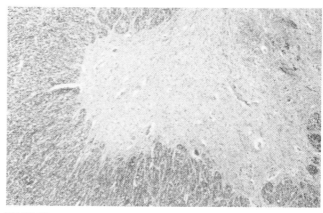

FIGURE *28-39*
Amyotrophic lateral sclerosis. A photomicrograph of the anterior horn of the spinal cord reveals severe loss of motor neurons, without evidence of inflammation.

myelinated fibers in the lateral corticospinal tracts, which imparts a pallor to these areas when viewed with myelin stains. The anterior nerve roots are atrophic, and the affected muscles are pale and shrunken.

☐ **Clinical Features:** ALS generally presents as weakness and wasting of the muscles of a hand, often accompanied by painful cramps of the muscles of the arm. Irregular rapid contractions of the muscles that do not move the limb (fasciculations) are characteristic. The disease is inexorably progressive, with increasing weakness of the limbs leading to total disability. Speech may become unintelligible, and respiratory weakness supervenes. Despite the dramatic wasting of the body, intellectual capacity is preserved to the end. The clinical course generally extends for more than a decade.

Alzheimer Disease

■ *Alzheimer disease (AD) is an insidious, progressive neurologic disorder that is characterized clinically by a loss of memory, cognitive impairment, and eventual dementia, and pathologically by amyloid-containing neuritic plaques and neurofibrillary tangles.*

☐ **Epidemiology: Alzheimer disease is the most common cause of dementia in elderly persons, accounting for more than half of all cases.** The prevalence of the condition is closely related to age. Before 65 years of age, the prevalence of AD is, at most, 1% to 2%, whereas after 85 years of age, it is 10% or greater. Women are affected twice as often as men. The large majority of cases of Alzheimer disease are sporadic, but a familial variant is recognized.

☐ **Pathogenesis:** Although the cause of AD has not been fully elucidated, significant advances have been made in our understanding of the origin of both AD-associated amyloid in the neuritic plaques and neurofibrillary tangles in the cytoplasm of neurons.

Amyloid β-Protein. Increasing evidence indicates the importance of deposition of amyloid β-protein (BAP) in the neuritic plaques of patients with AD. These plaques are located in areas of the cerebral cortex that are linked to intellectual function and are a constant feature of AD. The core of these plaques contains a distinct form of BAP that is 40 amino acids in length. BAP is derived by proteolysis from a much larger (695 amino acids), membrane-spanning amyloid precursor protein (APP). Full-length APP exhibits an extracellular region, a transmembrane sequence, and a cytoplasmic domain. The region comprising BAP anchors the amino-terminal portion of APP to the membrane. The physiologic function of APP is unknown, but the cytoplasmic portion of the molecule appears to be associated with the cytoskeleton and to be modulated by phosphorylation.

Normally, degradation of APP involves a proteolytic cleavage in the middle of the BAP domain, with the release of a fragment extending from the middle of the BAP domain to the amino terminal of APP. This fragment is lost to the extracellular fluid. By contrast, in patients with AD, and for reasons still to be determined, the APP molecule is cut at both ends of the BAP domain, thereby releasing an intact BAP molecule, which accumulates in the neuritic plaques as amyloid fibrils.

Neurofibrillary Tangles. Neurofibrillary tangles are composed of paired helical filaments that consist of an abnormal form of a normally occurring, microtubule-associated protein, which is termed *tau*. It is thought that tau stabilizes neuronal microtubules, a function that may be necessary for proper axonal transport. In patients with AD, phosphorylation of tau at aberrant sites results in a protein that does not associate with microtubules but, instead, aggregates in the form of paired helical filaments.

Apolipoprotein E. An increased risk of late-onset familial and sporadic AD is associated with inheritance of the apolipoprotein E4 allele, particularly the homozygous ε4/ε4 genotype. Apo E-ε4 specifically promotes amyloid fiber formation.

Presenilin. Mutations of the gene presenilin 1 (chromosome 14) and presenilin 2 (chromosome 1) occur in half of all cases of inherited AD. By altering the

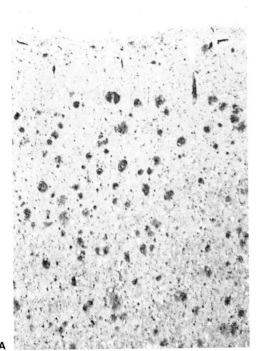

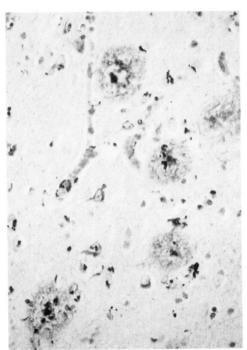

A   B

FIGURE   *28-40*
Alzheimer disease. (A) A section of the cerebral cortex impregnated with silver reveals neuritic plaques. (B) A higher-power view of *panel A* **shows the uniform size and spherical shape of the neuritic plaque, which contains a dense core of amyloid.**

processing of β-APP, these mutant proteins favor increased production and deposition of amyloid β-peptides.

☐ **Pathology:** The pathology of AD is dominated by the presence of (1) neuritic plaques, (2) neurofibrillary tangles, and (3) granulovacuolar degeneration. Identical morphologic alterations are also present, though in lesser intensity, in the cerebrum of a large proportion of elderly persons with symptoms as minor as forgetfulness. Indeed, the "disease process" is seemingly as inescapable in the aging human brain as systemic atherosclerosis.

During the course of AD, neurons and neuritic processes are lost. The gyri narrow, the sulci widen, and cortical atrophy becomes apparent. The brain loses approximately 200 g over a period of 3 to 8 years. The atrophy is bilateral and symmetric and targets both the frontal and the hippocampal cortex.

Neuritic Plaques. The most conspicuous histologic lesion, the neuritic plaque, is a discrete, spherical area of several hundred micrometers in diameter that, in severe cases, may occupy as much as half the volume of the gray matter of the cerebral cortex (Fig. 28-40). The neuritic plaque is argentophilic and contains abundant glial processes as well as deposits that stain positively for amyloid.

Neurofibrillary Tangles. The second member of the morphologic triad is the neurofibrillary tangle, which occupies the cytoplasm of pyramidal cells (Fig. 28-41). On light microscopy, neurofibrillary tangles are composed of argentophilic fibers, which are arranged in irregular bundles, knots, and curves. Electron microscopy reveals the tangles to be composed of paired helical filaments, with each filament being 10 nm in width.

Granulovacuolar Degeneration. The third constituent of the morphologic triad is largely restricted to the pyramidal cells of the hippocampus. Granulovacuolar degeneration refers to circular, clear zones in the cytoplasm of affected neurons, with each containing one or several basophilic and argentophilic granules (Fig. 28-42).

☐ **Clinical Features:** Patients with AD come to medical attention because of a gradual loss of memory and cognitive functions, difficulty with language, and changes in behavior. The disease is inexorably progressive, and during the late stages, previously intelligent and productive persons are reduced to pitifully demented, mute, incontinent, and bedridden patients. A terminal bronchopneumonia is the usual outcome.

NEOPLASIA

Intracranial tumors comprise only 2% of all "aggressive" neoplasms, but their frequency in childhood imparts a greater clinical significance. Gliomas account for 60% of primary intracranial neoplasms, meningiomas for 20%, and all others for 20% (Fig. 28-43).

Tumors Derived from Astrocytes

Neoplasms derived from astrocytes show a wide spectrum of differentiation, ranging from tumors with a histologic structure remarkably similar to that of normal brain tissue to highly aggressive growths that are hardly recognizable as being of glial origin. These tumors have been assigned three grades, in order of increasing anaplasia. The first two are astrocytoma (grade I) and anaplastic astrocytoma (grade II). The least-differentiated tumor derived from astrocytes (grade III) is referred to as glioblastoma multiforme.

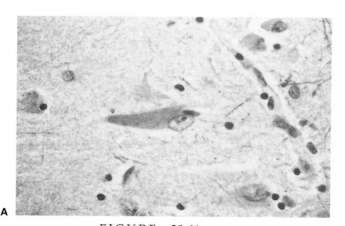
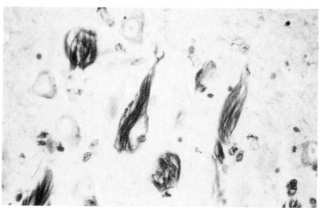

F I G U R E **28-41**
Alzheimer disease. (A) The cytoplasm of a neuron is distended by neurofibrillary tangles. (B) A silver stain of *panel A* **demonstrates the fibrillary character of the cytoplasmic inclusions.**

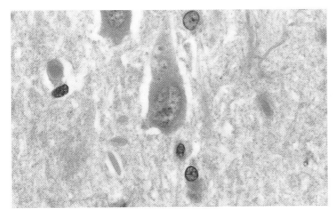

FIGURE 28-42
Alzheimer disease. A section of the hippocampus shows granulovacuolar degeneration of a pyramidal neuron as evidenced by clear cytoplasmic vacuoles containing granules.

Astrocytoma

Astrocytoma is a glioma composed of astrocytes and accounts for 20% of primary intracranial neoplasms. It frequents (1) the cerebral hemispheres in adults (Fig. 28-44); (2) the optic nerve, walls of the third ventricle, midbrain, pons, and cerebellum during the first two decades of life; and (3) the spinal cord, predominantly the thoracic and cervical segments, in young adults.

☐ **Pathology:** On gross examination, an astrocytoma is poorly defined and infiltrates the brain with an indistinct margin. Childhood astrocytomas of the cerebellar hemispheres are frequently cystic, and astrocytomas of the cerebrum often contain microcysts. An occasional astrocytoma contains sufficient calcospherites

to be visible radiographically. Microscopically, an astrocytoma is distinguished by a matrix of slender, glial, cytoplasmic processes in which the nuclei are dispersed randomly. There are several well-recognized morphologic variations of astrocytoma:

- **Fibrillary Astrocytoma.** Most astrocytomas, particularly those in the cerebral hemispheres of adults, have dense glial processes.
- **Gemistocytic Astrocytoma.** Abundant eosinophilic cytoplasm encases the tumor cell nuclei.
- **Juvenile Pilocytic Astrocytoma.** This tumor occurs in children and is characterized by abundant, hair-like glial processes.

The life expectancy of patients with astrocytoma, though widely variable, is approximately 5 years. Transformation to a higher degree of anaplasia, which often is glioblastoma multiforme, occurs in 10% of the cases and shortens life expectancy.

Anaplastic Astrocytoma

Anaplastic astrocytoma is distinguished from the other astrocytomas by (1) greater cellularity, (2) cellular pleomorphism, and (3) anaplasia. The topographic distribution parallels that of astrocytoma. Growth of the tumor is rapid, and life expectancy averages 3 years.

Glioblastoma Multiforme

Glioblastoma multiforme is the extreme expression of anaplasia among the glial neoplasms and accounts for 40% of all primary intracranial tumors. Most glioblas-

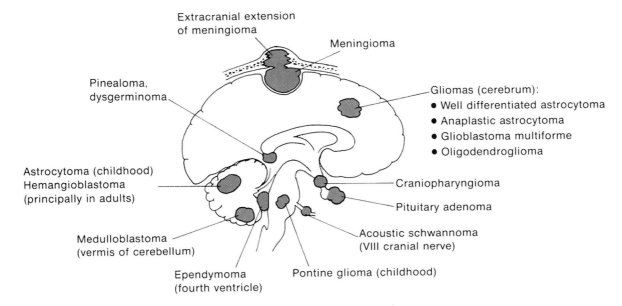

FIGURE 28-43
The distribution of common intracranial tumors.

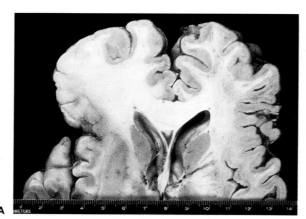
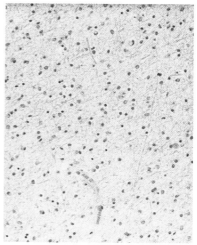

FIGURE   *28-44*
Astrocytoma. (A) A poorly demarcated, expansile mass occupies the left frontal lobe. (B) A microscopic section of a well-differentiated astrocytoma in the white matter shows an increased density of astrocytes, which exhibit only minimal deviation from their normal appearance.

tomas have constituent cells with recognizable astrocytic properties, but they also display (1) marked pleomorphism, (2) frequent mitoses, (3) regional zones of necrosis, and (4) endothelial proliferation.

Glioblastoma typically infiltrates extensively, and frequently crosses the corpus callosum to produce a bilateral lesion that has been likened to a butterfly in its gross configuration and mottled red-and-yellow coloration (Fig. 28-45). These colors are imparted by multiple areas of recent (red) and remote (yellow) hemor-

rhage. The cardinal histologic features of glioblastoma multiforme are:

- **Marked cellularity,** with variable degrees of cellular pleomorphism and multinucleated cells
- **Serpentine areas of necrosis** surrounded by zones of crowded tumor cells ("palisading"; Fig. 28-46)
- **Endothelial cell proliferation,** which creates clusters of small vessels that are referred to as "glomeruloid" formations.

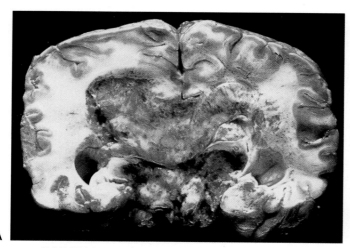
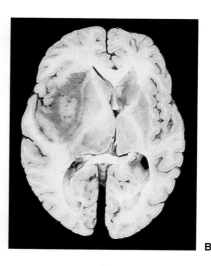

FIGURE   *28-45*
Glioblastoma multiforme. (A) The tumor occupies the splenium of the corpus callosum, with bilateral extension into the white matter, where it imparts variegated shades of red and yellow ("butterfly tumor"). (B) A horizontal section of the brain from another patient with a glioblastoma multiforme reveals a partially necrotic and edematous mass in the left insula.

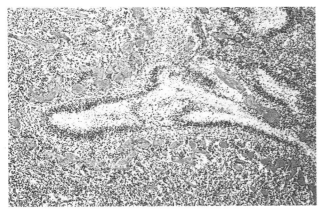

FIGURE *28-46*
Glioblastoma multiforme. A photomicrograph demonstrates a highly vascularized tumor with serpentine areas of necrosis, bordered by hypercellular zones (palisading).

The clinical course of glioblastoma multiforme rarely exceeds 18 months. The tumor predominates during the later decades of life and occurs twice as frequently as astrocytoma.

Oligodendroglioma

Oligodendroglioma, in accord with its cell of origin, arises in the white matter, predominantly in the cerebral hemispheres of adults. The histologic composition recreates the small, rounded nuclei of oligodendrocytes but introduces variable densities in cell population and cellular pleomorphism. Calcospherites, which occasionally are visualized radiographically, appear as grains of sand scattered randomly throughout the lesion. Slow growth is reflected by an absence of mitotic figures and necrosis.

Symptoms of oligodendroglioma are frequently ushered in by seizures. Although the lesion is infiltrative, its slow growth permits survival for 5 to 10 years.

Ependymoma

Ependymoma occurs most commonly in the fourth ventricle (Fig. 28-47), thereby producing obstruction and resulting in hydrocephalus. Ependymoma is also second only to astrocytoma as an intramedullary tumor of the spinal cord.

The cells of an ependymoma characteristically have an "epithelial" appearance, similar to that of normal ependymal cells. They possess ovoid nuclei, with coarse chromatin material and well-defined plasma membranes. The cells either form clefts or may arrange around blood vessels, thus creating an anuclear mantle of glial processes about the adventitia (see Fig. 28-47). The tumor generally grows slowly but can seed the subarachnoid space.

Medulloblastoma

Medulloblastoma, the most common intracranial neuroblastic lesion, is a cerebellar tumor that derives from the transient, external granular cell layer of neurons. It occurs with the highest frequency toward the end of the first decade of life. The tumor infiltrates aggressively and frequently disseminates through the CSF.

Medulloblastoma features hyperchromatic, round to oval nuclei and scant cytoplasm. The cells crowd together with no structural pattern. The neuroblastic character of the cells is occasionally expressed in rosette formation, which is a distinctive feature of embryonic and neoplastic neuroblasts.

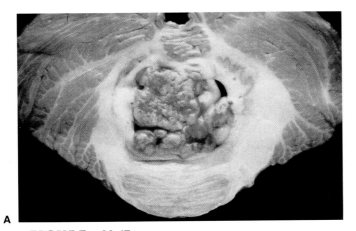
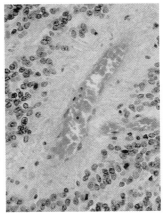

FIGURE *28-47*
Ependymoma. (A) A section through the fourth ventricle shows a fleshy lobulated mass. (B) A microscopic view reveals a highly cellular tumor, forming a perivascular pseudorosette, with an acellular mantle around the adventitia.

Children with medulloblastoma present with cerebellar dysfunction or hydrocephalus. Similar to embryonic neuroblasts, the tumor is highly sensitive to ionizing radiation, but unfortunately subarachnoid dissemination is frequent. The 10-year survival rate is only 50%.

Neoplasms of Mesenchymal Origin

Meningioma

Meningiomas account for almost 20% of all primary intracranial neoplasms. The peak frequency occurs during the fourth to fifth decades of life, but a significant incidence also occurs in youthful adults. These tumors take origin from the arachnoid villi and produce a globoid or discoid ("meningioma en plaque") mass (Fig. 28-48). Although meningiomas may occur at almost any intracranial site, they are most common in parasagittal areas, convexities of the cerebral hemispheres, the olfactory groove, and the lateral wing of the sphenoid. Meningiomas occur with a female:male ratio of 60 : 40, but in the spinal canal, this ratio approaches 10 : 1. The tumor has a propensity to erode contiguous bone.

Many sporadic meningiomas exhibit a loss, partial deletion, or mutation of chromosome 22, in the region of the *NF2* locus, thereby suggesting that inactivation of the *NF2* tumor suppressor gene is involved in the pathogenesis of this tumor. Meningiomas also occur in conjunction with several genetic syndromes, most importantly neurofibromatosis type II (NF2).

☐ **Pathology:** On gross examination, most meningiomas appear to be well-circumscribed, firm, and bosselated masses of variable size. The cut surface presents a gray, whorled pattern, which is similar to that of uterine leiomyomas. The histologic hallmark is a whorled pattern of "meningothelial" cells (Fig. 28-49) in association with psammoma bodies (laminated, spherical calcospherites). Although this morphologic appearance is distinctive, it is obscured in many meningiomas by a predominantly fibroblastic proliferation.

☐ **Clinical Features:** The indolent growth of meningiomas creates a symptomatic interval that often lasts for years. Well-differentiated lesions displace the brain, but they do not infiltrate it. Thus, seizures rather than neurologic deficits frequently characterize the clinical presentation. In some locations, meningiomas compress functional structures. Tumors of the olfactory groove produce anosmia, and those in the suprasellar region lead to visual deficits. Meningiomas in the cerebellopontine angle create cranial nerve palsies, and those in the spinal column produce dysfunction of the spinal nerve roots and spinal cord. The superficial position of meningiomas, coupled with neural displacement rather than infiltration, invites total surgical excision.

Metastatic Tumors

Metastatic tumors reach the intracranial compartment through the bloodstream, generally in patients with advanced cancer. Tumors of different organs vary in their incidence of intracranial metastases. For example, a patient with disseminated melanoma has a greater than 50% likelihood of acquiring intracranial metastases, whereas the incidence of such metastases for carcinoma of the breast and lung is approximately 35% and for cancer of the kidney or colon only 5%. Certain carcinomas, such as those of the prostate, liver, and adrenals, as well as sarcomas of all types, rarely estab-

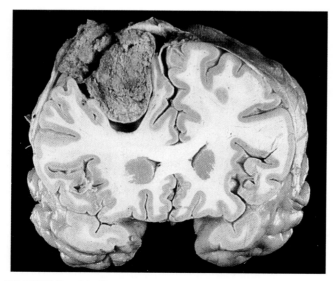

FIGURE   *28-48*
Meningioma. A tumor that arises from the arachnoid indents the underlying cortex.

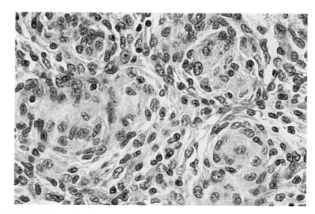

FIGURE   *28-49*
Meningioma. A microscopic section shows whorled meningothelial cells.

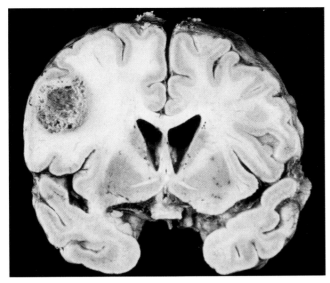

FIGURE 28-50
Metastatic carcinoma. A discrete, spherical lesion in the cerebral cortex is surrounded by edematous parenchyma.

lish intracranial metastases. Most metastatic lesions seed to the gray-white junction, reflecting the rich capillary bed in this area (Fig. 28-50).

Peripheral Nervous System

Thomas W. Bouldin

REACTIONS TO INJURY

Peripheral nerve fibers display only a limited number of reactions to injury (Fig. 28-51). The major types of nerve fiber damage are axonal degeneration and segmental demyelination. The peripheral nervous system differs from the CNS in that it has the capacity for functionally significant axonal regeneration and remyelination.

Axonal Degeneration

Degeneration (necrosis) of the axon occurs in many neuropathies and reflects significant injury of either the neuronal cell body or its axon. Axonal degeneration is quickly followed by breakdown of the myelin sheath and Schwann cell proliferation. Macrophages both infiltrate the nerve and clear the myelin debris. There are several types of axonal degeneration.

Distal Axonopathy. Peripheral neuropathies characterized by selective degeneration of distal axons are

A. INTACT MYELINATED FIBER

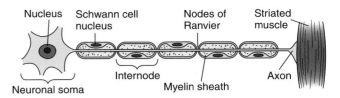

B. DISTAL AXONAL DEGENERATION

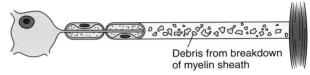

C. DEGENERATION OF CELL BODY AND AXON

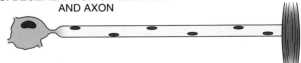

D. SEGMENTAL DEMYELINATION

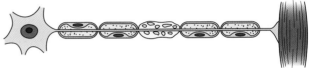

E. REMYELINATION

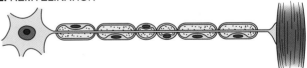

F. REGENERATING AXON

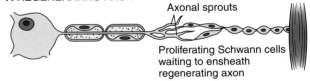

G. REGENERATED NERVE FIBER

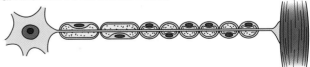

FIGURE 28-51
Basic responses of peripheral nerve fibers to injury.

known as **dying-back neuropathies** (distal axonopathies). They typically present as distal ("glove-and-stocking") neuropathies. In distal axonopathy, the neuronal cell body and proximal axon remain intact. Therefore, axonal regeneration and return of nerve function may be possible if the cause of the distal axonal degeneration can be identified and removed.

Neuronopathy. Axonal degeneration also may be secondary to degeneration of the neuronal cell body, as occurs in patients with poliomyelitis. Neuropathies showing selective degeneration of the neuronal cell body are referred to as **neuronopathies** and are much less common than distal axonopathies. There is little potential for recovery of function in patients with neuronopathy, because degeneration of the neuronal cell body precludes axonal regeneration.

Wallerian Degeneration. This term refers to the axonal degeneration that occurs in a nerve distal to a transection or crush of the nerve.

Segmental Demyelination

Loss of myelin from one or more internodes (segments) along a myelinated fiber is common in patients with many neuropathies and reflects Schwann cell dysfunction. Degeneration of the myelin sheath is unaccompanied by degeneration of the underlying axon. Macrophages infiltrate the nerve and clear the myelin debris.

PERIPHERAL NEUROPATHIES

■ *Peripheral neuropathy is a process that affects the function of one or more peripheral nerves.* The disease may (1) be restricted to the peripheral nervous system, (2) involve both the peripheral nervous system and CNS, or (3) affect multiple organ systems. Peripheral neuropathies are encountered in all age groups and may be either hereditary or acquired. The causes of peripheral neuropathy are diverse (Box 28-1). Pathologically, the involved nerves may show mainly axonal degeneration (**axonal neuropathy**), segmental demyelination (**demyelinating neuropathy**), or a mixture of both.

☐ **Clinical Features:** The major clinical manifestations of peripheral neuropathy are muscle weakness, muscle atrophy, alterations of sensation, and autonomic dysfunction. Motor, sensory, and autonomic functions may be equally or preferentially affected. The evolution of clinical manifestations may be acute

---

BOX **28-1** **Etiologic Classification of Peripheral Neuropathy**

Autoimmune
    Inflammatory demyelinating neuropathy
Metabolic
    Diabetic polyneuropathy
    Uremic neuropathy
    Hypothyroid neuropathy
    Hepatic neuropathy
    Porphyric neuropathy
    Neuropathy associated with multiorgan failure and
        sepsis
Nutritional
    Alcoholic neuropathy
    Beriberi neuropathy
    Neuropathy related to vitamin B_{12} deficiency
    Neuropathy related to vitamin E deficiency
    Neuropathy related to postgastrectomy state
    Neuropathy related to celiac disease
Ischemic
    Vasculitic neuropathy
    Neuropathy of peripheral vascular disease
    Diabetic mononeuropathy and polyneuropathy
Toxic neuropathy (see Table 28-2)
Paraneoplastic neuropathy
Amyloid neuropathy
Paraproteinemic neuropathy
Inherited neuropathy
Neuropathy associated with infections
    Herpes zoster
    Leprosy
    Diphtheria (toxin)
    Human immunodeficiency virus
    Lyme disease
Sarcoid neuropathy
Radiation neuropathy
Traumatic neuropathy
Cryptogenic neuropathy

(days), subacute (weeks), or chronic (months or years). The disease may be localized to one nerve (**mononeuropathy**) or to several nerves (**mononeuropathy multiplex**), or it may be diffuse and symmetric (**polyneuropathy**).

Inflammatory Demyelinating Neuropathy

Inflammatory demyelinating neuropathy is an acquired neuropathy that (1) may be sporadic; (2) may follow immunization, surgery, or viral and mycoplasmal infections; or (3) may complicate cancer. Current evidence suggests that the pathogenesis of demyelination may be immunologically mediated.

☐ **Pathology:** An inflammatory demyelinating neuropathy may involve all levels of the peripheral nervous system, including the spinal roots, ganglia, craniospinal nerves, and autonomic nerves. The involved regions show endoneurial infiltrates of lymphocytes and macrophages, segmental demyelination, and relative sparing of axons. The lymphoid infiltrates are often perivascular, but there is no true vasculitis. Macrophages are frequently found adjacent to degenerating myelin sheaths and have been observed to strip off and phagocytose the superficial myelin lamellae (macrophage-mediated demyelination).

☐ **Clinical Features:** Inflammatory demyelinating neuropathy usually presents as an acutely evolving, predominantly motor polyneuropathy, which is termed **Guillain-Barré syndrome.** In some cases, sensory or autonomic disturbances predominate. Resolution of Guillain-Barré syndrome begins 2 to 4 weeks after the onset, and most patients make a good recovery.

Diabetic Neuropathy

Peripheral neuropathy is a common complication of diabetes mellitus. The neuropathy may manifest as a distal sensory or sensorimotor polyneuropathy, autonomic neuropathy, mononeuropathy, or mononeuropathy multiplex. **Distal polyneuropathy is the most common form of diabetic neuropathy.**

Symmetric polyneuropathy of diabetes is characterized pathologically by a mixture of axonal degeneration and segmental demyelination, with the former being predominant. Axonal degeneration involves fibers of all sizes but, occasionally, preferentially involves the large myelinated fibers (large-fiber neuropathy) or the small myelinated and unmyelinated fibers (small-fiber neuropathy).

Toxic Neuropathy

A wide variety of drugs and toxic agents are recognized as being important causes of peripheral neuropathy (Table 28-2). Most toxic neuropathies are characterized by axonal degeneration, which is usually of the dying-back type.

Paraneoplastic Neuropathy

The remote effects of cancer on the nervous system include, among others, an encephalomyelitis, cerebellar degeneration, and peripheral neuropathy. It is not uncommon for a paraneoplastic disorder to precede clinical recognition of the underlying cancer. The most common type of paraneoplastic neuropathy is distal sensorimotor polyneuropathy. Pathologic examination

T A B L E 28-2. Agents Associated with Toxic Neuropathy

Drugs	Environmental Agents
Amiodarone	Acrylamide
Amytriptyline	Arsenic
Chloramphenicol	Buckthorn toxin
Dapsone	Carbon disulfide
Chlordecone	
Disulfiram	2,4-Dichlorophenoxyacetic acid
Glutethimide	
Gold	Dimethylaminopropionitrile
Hydralazine	Diphtheria toxin
Isoniazid	n-Hexane
Lithium	Methyl n-butyl ketone
Metronidazole	Lead
Misonidazole	Mercury
Nitrofurantoin	Methyl bromide
Perhexilene	Organophosphates
Phenytoin	
Platinum	Polybrominated biphenyls
Pyridoxine (vitamin B_6)	Tetrachlorobiphenyl
Thalidomide	Thallium
Vincristine	Trichloroethylene

of the nerves reveals evidence of axonal degeneration and, occasionally, demyelination.

TUMORS

Primary tumors of the peripheral nervous system are of neuronal or nerve sheath origin. Neuronal tumors (e.g., neuroblastoma and ganglioneuroma) usually arise from the adrenal medulla or the sympathetic ganglia. Common nerve sheath tumors are schwannoma and neurofibroma.

Schwannoma (Neurilemmoma)

■ *Schwannoma is a benign, slowly growing neoplasm of Schwann cells that may arise in any nerve, including the cranial nerves, spinal roots, or peripheral nerves.* These tumors usually present in adults.

Acoustic Schwannoma. With rare exceptions, intracranial schwannomas arise from the eighth cranial nerve (acoustic schwannoma), either within the internal auditory canal or at the meatus, and cause unilateral hearing loss and tinnitus. The slowly growing tumor enlarges the meatus, extends medially into the subarachnoid space of the cerebellopontine angle (**cerebellopontine angle tumor**), and compresses the fifth and seventh cranial nerves, brainstem, and cerebellum. The posterior fossa mass may also lead to increased intracranial pressure, hydrocephalus, and tonsillar herniation. Bilateral vestibular schwannomas are a defining feature of neurofibromatosis type II.

Intraspinal Schwannoma. These tumors arise most often from the dorsal (sensory) spinal roots. They typically present as intradural, extramedullary tumors and produce radicular (root) pain and spinal cord compression.

☐ **Pathology:** Schwannomas tend to be oval and well demarcated, and vary in diameter from a few millimeters to several centimeters. The cut surfaces are firm and tan to gray and often show foci of hemorrhage, necrosis, xanthomatous change, and cystic degeneration. Microscopically, proliferating Schwann cells form two distinctive histologic patterns (Fig. 28-52):

- **Antoni type A pattern** is characterized by interwoven fascicles of spindle cells with elongated nuclei, eosinophilic cytoplasm, and indistinct cytoplasmic borders.
- **Antoni type B pattern** features spindle or oval cells with indistinct cytoplasm in a loose, vacuolated background.

Neurofibroma

■ *Neurofibroma is a tumor that represents a combined proliferation of all elements of a peripheral nerve, namely axons, Schwann cells, fibroblasts, and probably, perineurial cells.* Nevertheless, the Schwann cell is the principal constituent of a neurofibroma, which may be more hamartomatous than neoplastic. A distinction between neurofibroma and schwannoma is warranted, however, because of the close association of neurofibroma with von Recklinghausen neurofibromatosis and its potential for sarcomatous degeneration.

Neurofibromas may be solitary or multiple, and may arise on any nerve. They are found in both children and adults. Most commonly, neurofibromas involve the skin, major nerve plexuses, large deep nerve trunks, retroperitoneum, and gastrointestinal tract. The large majority of **solitary cutaneous neurofibromas** occur outside the context of neurofibromatosis and do not have the potential of their deeper counterparts for sarcomatous degeneration.

The presence of multiple neurofibromas is diagnostic of neurofibromatosis (see Chapter 6). The occurrence of one large plexiform neurofibroma or of bilateral acoustic schwannomas is also considered to be evidence of neurofibromatosis.

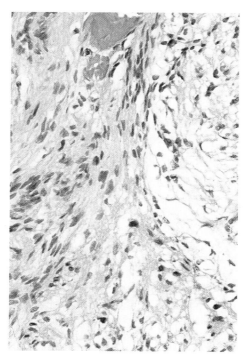

FIGURE   *28-52*
Schwannoma. A photomicrograph shows the characteristically abrupt transition between the compact Antoni type A histologic pattern (*left*) and the spongy Antoni type B histologic pattern (*right*).

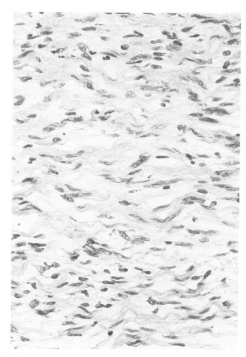

FIGURE   *28-53*
Neurofibroma. A photomicrograph shows that the proliferating, spindle-shaped Schwann cells form small strands that course haphazardly through a myxoid matrix.

☐ **Pathology:** On gross examination, a neurofibroma arising in a large nerve appears as a poorly circumscribed, fusiform enlargement of the nerve. Cutaneous neurofibromas arise from dermal nerves and present as soft, nodular or pedunculated skin tumors.

The cut surface of a neurofibroma is soft and light gray. Microscopically, a neurofibroma arising in large nerves is characterized by an endoneurial proliferation of spindle cells with elongated nuclei, eosinophilic cytoplasm, and indistinct cell borders. The spindle cells often aggregate to form tiny strands that course haphazardly through the tumor (Fig. 28-53). Interspersed among the spindle cells are wavy bands of collagen, an extracellular myxoid matrix, and residual nerve fibers.

A small, but clinically significant, proportion of neurofibromas exhibit sarcomatous transformation, with foci of neurofibrosarcoma (malignant schwannoma). The presence of increased cellularity and mitotic figures heralds malignant transformation.

Malignant Schwannoma (Neurofibrosarcoma)

The histogenesis of malignant schwannoma, which is a poorly differentiated, spindle cell sarcoma of the peripheral nerves, is uncertain. The tumor may arise either de novo or from malignant transformation of a neurofibroma. **Approximately half of these sarcomas occur in patients with neurofibromatosis.** There is an increased incidence of malignant schwannomas in areas of previous exposure to radiation.

Malignant schwannoma presents grossly as an unencapsulated, fusiform enlargement of a nerve. Microscopically, the neoplasm resembles fibrosarcoma. The tumor is prone to local recurrence and bloodborne metastases, and it carries a worse prognosis in the context of neurofibromatosis.

CHAPTER 29

The Eye

Gordon K. Klintworth

Disorders of the eye are common, and many afflictions of the eye result in blindness. The eye is exposed to a myriad of micro-organisms, antigens, and toxic chemicals as well as to solar radiation and adverse climatic conditions. The unprotected position of the eye also makes it vulnerable to a host of injuries. The eye is involved in numerous systemic diseases, and recognition of ocular abnormalities aids in establishing the diagnosis of many conditions.

EXOPHTHALMOS OF HYPERTHYROIDISM

Numerous conditions cause an abnormal forward protrusion of the eyeball, which is termed **exophthalmos** or **proptosis**. The most common cause is thyroid disease. Exophthalmos caused by Graves disease may precede or follow other manifestations of thyroid dysfunction. The disorder occurs during early adult life, especially in women (female:male ratio, 4:1). It may be severe and progressive, particularly in middle-aged persons, when exophthalmos no longer correlates well with the state of the thyroid function.

Exophthalmos results from an increased orbital tissue volume, which, in turn, is produced largely by an increase in orbital water, as a result of the osmotic pressure of glycosaminoglycans. Enlarged extraocular muscles, which are infiltrated with lymphocytes and other mononuclear cells, also contribute. Patients with hyperthyroidism and exophthalmos often manifest antibodies to the extraocular muscles, whereas those without eye disease do not. Exophthalmos may be an organ-specific autoimmune disease that is distinct from, but very closely linked to, Graves disease.

Sequelae of severe exophthalmos include several potentially blinding complications, namely corneal exposure with subsequent ulceration, secondary glaucoma, and optic nerve compression.

CORNEA

Herpes Simplex

Herpes simplex virus type 1 (HSV-1) has a predilection for the corneal epithelium, where it causes keratitis, but it can also invade the corneal stroma and, occasionally, other ocular tissues. Infection with HSV-1 causes multiple minute, discrete, intraepithelial corneal ulcers (superficial punctate keratopathy). Although some of these lesions heal, others enlarge and

eventually coalesce to form linear or branching fissures. The epithelium between the fissures then desquamates, thereby causing sharply demarcated and irregular geographic ulcers.

Corneal Dystrophies

■ *Corneal dystrophies encompass a heterogeneous group of hereditary, noninflammatory, and degenerative diseases of the cornea.* Traditionally, the corneal dystrophies have been classified according to the primary layer that is involved.

Epithelial Dystrophies. The different epithelial dystrophies are characterized by a variety of distinct abnormalities, including (1) microcysts or accumulations of anomalous material within the cytoplasm of the corneal epithelium, (2) defects in the epithelial basement membrane, and (3) deposition of a finely fibrillar substance in the Bowman layer. In some epithelial dystrophies, faulty desmosomes may permit the separation of adjacent epithelial cells, thereby leading to the accumulation of fluid-filled microcysts. There may be a slow decrease in visual acuity, but ordinarily, epithelial dystrophies do not cause blindness.

Stromal Dystrophies. The stromal dystrophies are clear-cut entities in which different substances, including amyloid, glycosaminoglycans, unidentified proteins, and a variety of lipids, accumulate within the corneal stroma because of an inherited metabolic disorder. Each stromal dystrophy causes a characteristic form of corneal opacification.

Endothelial Dystrophies. Several different endothelial dystrophies are recognized. They are usually accompanied by abnormalities in the Descemet membrane (the basement membrane of the corneal endothelium).

CATARACTS

■ *Cataract describes an opacification of the lens from many causes. It is a major cause of both visual impairment and blindness throughout the world* (Fig. 29-1). Cataracts can be caused by diabetes or vitamin deficiencies, genetic disorders, toxins, drugs, and physical agents (particularly ultraviolet light). However, the most common cataract in the United States is associated with aging (senile cataract). In patients with senile cataracts, clefts appear between the lens fibers, and degenerated lens material accumulates in these spaces

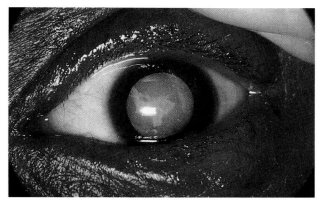

FIGURE 29-1
Cataract. The white appearance of the pupil in this eye results from complete opacification of the lens ("mature cataract").

(morgagnian corpuscles, incipient cataract). The degenerated lens material exerts an osmotic pressure, thereby causing the damaged lens to increase in volume by imbibing water. Such a swollen lens may then obstruct the pupil and cause glaucoma (phakomorphic glaucoma).

After the entire lens degenerates (mature cataract), its volume diminishes, because lenticular debris escapes into the aqueous humor through the damaged lens capsule (hypermature cataract). After becoming engulfed by macrophages, the extruded lenticular material may obstruct the aqueous outflow and, thus, produce glaucoma (phakolytic glaucoma). Fortunately, however, cataractous lenses can be surgically removed, and optical devices can be provided to focus light on the retina (spectacles, contact lenses, implanted prosthetic lenses).

UVEA

Inflammation of the iris and ciliary body typically causes a reddened eye, sensitivity to bright light (photophobia), moderate pain, blurred vision, pericorneal halo, dilated deep ciliary vessels (ciliary flush), and slight constriction of the pupil (miosis). Leukocytes aggregate on the posterior surface of the cornea as small clusters (keratinic precipitates), or if abundant, they settle to the bottom of the anterior chamber (hypopyon).

Posterior synechia, a sequel to iritis, refers to an adhesion that develops between the iris and the lens.

Peripheral anterior synechia describes an adhesion that develops between the peripheral iris and the anterior chamber angle. Both types of synechiae can cause glaucoma.

Sympathetic Ophthalmitis

■ *Sympathetic ophthalmitis is an autoimmune uveitis in which the entire uvea develops granulomatous inflammation after a latent period in response to an injury in the other eye.* Perforating ocular injury and prolapse of uveal tissue often lead to a progressive, bilateral, diffuse, and granulomatous inflammation of the uvea. This uveitis develops in the eye that was originally injured (the exciting eye) after a latent period of from 4 to 8 weeks. The uninjured eye (the sympathizing eye) becomes affected at the same time as the injured eye or shortly thereafter.

It is widely believed that sympathetic ophthalmitis is an autoimmune reaction to sensitization by uveal antigens. Results of experimental studies have suggested that the antigen responsible for sympathetic ophthalmitis resides in the photoreceptors of the retina (arrestin).

Sarcoidosis

Ocular involvement occurs in one-fourth to one-third of patients with sarcoidosis and is often the presenting clinical manifestation. Ocular involvement is usually bilateral and, most often, takes the form of a granulomatous uveitis.

RETINA

Hemorrhage

Retinal hemorrhages are a feature of many disorders, including hypertension, diabetes mellitus, and central retinal vein occlusion. Hemorrhage in the nerve fiber layer spreads between axons and causes a flame-shaped appearance on funduscopy, whereas deep retinal hemorrhages tend to be round. When located between the retinal pigment epithelium and the Bruch membrane, blood appears as a dark mass and, clinically, resembles a melanoma.

Retinal Occlusive Vascular Disease

Vascular occlusion results from thrombosis, embolism, stenosis (as in atherosclerosis), vascular compression, intravascular sludging or coagulation, or vasoconstriction (e.g., in hypertensive retinopathy or migraine). Certain disorders of the heart and major vessels (e.g., the carotid arteries) predispose to emboli that lodge in the retina and are evident on funduscopy at points of vascular bifurcation.

Retinal ischemia of any cause frequently results in the appearance of white, fluffy patches that resemble cotton (cotton-wool patches) on ophthalmoscopy. These spots consist of aggregates of swollen axons in the nerve fiber layer of the retina. Cotton-wool spots are reversible if the circulation is restored in time.

Central Retinal Artery Occlusion

Neurons of the retina, similar to those in the rest of the nervous system, are extremely susceptible to hypoxia. Central retinal artery occlusion (Fig. 29-2) may follow thrombosis of the retinal artery or embolization to that vessel. Intracellular edema, manifesting as retinal pallor, is prominent, especially in the macula, where the ganglion cells are most numerous. The foveola—that is, the vascularized choroid beneath the center of the macula—stands out, in sharp contrast, as a prominent, cherry-red spot. The lack of retinal circulation reduces the retinal arterioles to delicate threads. **Permanent blindness follows central retinal artery obstruction unless the ischemia is of short duration.** Unilateral blurred vision of a few minutes in duration (amaurosis fugax), occurs with small retinal emboli.

Central Retinal Vein Occlusion

Central retinal vein occlusion results in flame-shaped hemorrhages in the nerve fiber layer of the retina, especially around the optic disc. Edema of the optic disc and retina occurs because of impaired absorption of interstitial fluid. Vision is disturbed, but it may recover surprisingly well considering the severity of the funduscopic changes. An intractable closed-angle glaucoma, with severe pain and repeated hemorrhages, commonly ensues 2 to 3 months after central retinal vein occlusion. This distressing complication is caused by neovascularization of the iris and adhesions between the iris and the anterior chamber angle (peripheral anterior synechia).

Hypertensive Retinopathy

Elevated blood pressure commonly affects the retina, causing changes that can be seen readily on ophthalmoscopy and that relate to the severity of the hypertension (Fig. 29-3).

☐ **Pathology:** Features of hypertensive retinopathy include:

- Arteriolar narrowing
- Hemorrhages in the retinal nerve fiber layer (flame-shaped hemorrhages)
- Exudates, including some that radiate from the center of the macula (macular star)

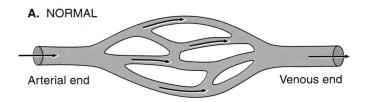

A. NORMAL

Arterial end   Venous end

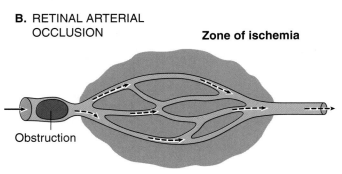

B. RETINAL ARTERIAL OCCLUSION   **Zone of ischemia**

Obstruction

Neuronal functional impairment → Visual loss
Edema → Pallor

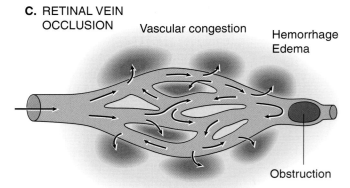

C. RETINAL VEIN OCCLUSION   Vascular congestion   Hemorrhage Edema

Obstruction

Mild ischemia: normal neuronal function

FIGURE   29-2
Occlusion of the retinal artery and vein. In the retina (A), as in other parts of the body, blood normally flows through a capillary network. When the retinal arteries become occluded, however, as with an embolus, a zone of retinal ischemia ensues. This is accompanied by impaired neuronal function and visual loss, and the ischemic retina becomes pale (B). Because the intravascular pressure within the ischemic tissue is low, hemorrhage is inconspicuous. On the other hand, with retinal vein occlusion (C), vascular congestion, hemorrhage, and edema are prominent, whereas ischemia is mild and neuronal function remains intact.

- Fluffy white bodies in the superficial retina (cotton-wool spots)
- Microaneurysms

In the eye, arteriolosclerosis accompanies long-standing hypertension and commonly affects the retinal arterioles and choroidal vessels. The lumen of the

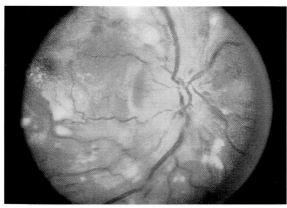

FIGURE   29-3
Hypertensive retinopathy. This photograph shows the ocular fundus in a patient with extensive retinopathy. The optic nerve head is edematous, and the retina contains numerous exudates and "cotton-wool" spots.

thickened retinal arterioles becomes narrowed, increasingly tortuous, and of irregular caliber. At sites where the arterioles cross veins, the latter appear to be kinked (arteriovenous nicking). This kinked appearance does not result from compression by a taut sclerotic artery. Rather, it reflects sclerosis within the venous walls, because the retinal arteries and veins share a common adventitia at sites of arteriovenous crossings. Small superficial or deep retinal hemorrhages often accompany retinal arteriolosclerosis. **Malignant hypertension** is characterized by a necrotizing arteriolitis, with fibrinoid necrosis and thrombosis of the precapillary retinal arterioles.

Diabetic Retinopathy

Diabetic retinopathy and glaucoma are the leading causes of irreversible blindness in the United States. Virtually all patients with type 1 (insulin-dependent) diabetes and many of those with type 2 (non–insulin dependent) diabetes develop some degree of background retinopathy (discussed later) within 5 to 15 years of the onset of diabetes (Figs. 29-4 and 29-5). The more dangerous proliferative retinopathy does not appear until at least 10 years after the onset of diabetes, after which the incidence increases rapidly. **The frequency of proliferative retinopathy correlates with the degree of glycemic control—that is, the better the control, the lower the rate of retinopathy.**

Retinal ischemia can account for most features of diabetic retinopathy. It results from narrowing or occlusion of the retinal arterioles (as from arteriolosclerosis or platelet and lipid thrombi) or from atherosclerosis of the central retinal or ophthalmic arteries.

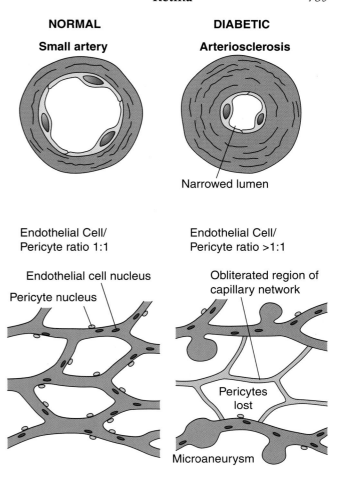

FIGURE   29-4
Diabetic retinopathy. In patients with diabetic retinopathy, the microvasculature is abnormal. Arteriosclerosis narrows the lumen of the small arteries. Pericytes are lost, and the endothelial cell:pericyte ratio is greater than 1. Capillary microaneurysms are prominent, and portions of the capillary network become acellular and show no blood flow. The basement membrane of the retinal capillaries is thickened and vacuolated.

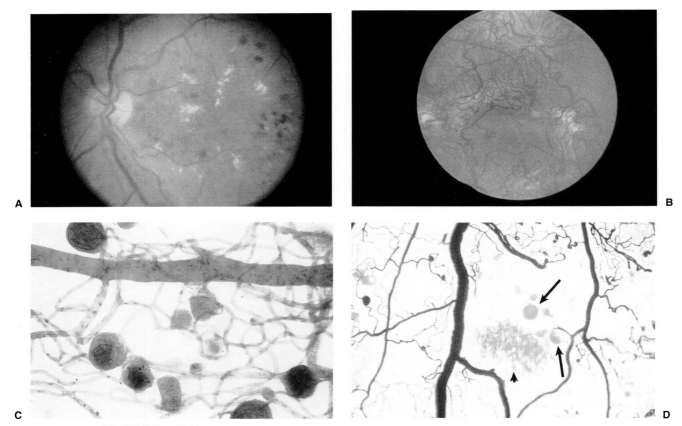

FIGURE *29-5*
Diabetic retinopathy. (A) View of the ocular fundus in a patient with background diabetic retinopathy. Several yellowish, "hard" exudates, which are rich in lipids, are evident, together with several relatively small retinal hemorrhages. (B) A vascular front has extended anterior to the retina in the eye with proliferative diabetic retinopathy. (C) Numerous microaneurysms are present in this flat preparation of a diabetic retina. (D) This flat preparation from a patients with diabetes was stained with periodic acid-Schiff after the retinal vessels had been perfused with India ink. Microaneurysms (*arrows*) and an exudate (*arrowhead*) are evident in a region of retinal nonperfusion.

☐ **Pathology:** The retinopathy of diabetes is characterized by background and proliferative stages.

Background (Nonproliferative) Diabetic Retinopathy. This stage exhibits venous engorgement, small hemorrhages (dot and blot hemorrhages), capillary microaneurysms, and exudates. On funduscopy, the first discernible clinical abnormality in patients with background diabetic retinopathy is engorged retinal veins, with localized, sausage-shaped distentions, coils, and loops. This is followed by small hemorrhages in the same areas. With time, exudates accumulate, chiefly in the vicinity of the microaneurysms. Because of the hyperlipoproteinemia of patients with diabetes, these exudates are rich in lipid and, hence, appear to be yellowish ("waxy" exudates).

Proliferative Retinopathy. After many years, diabetic retinopathy becomes proliferative. Delicate new blood vessels grow along with fibrous and glial tissue toward the vitreous humor. Neovascularization of the retina is a prominent feature of diabetic retinopathy. The newly formed friable vessels bleed early, and the resultant vitreal hemorrhages obscure vision. Proliferating fibrovascular and glial tissue contracts, often causing retinal detachment and blindness. However, **laser phototherapy early in the course of proliferative retinopathy has proved effective in controlling this complication.**

Retinal Detachment

The sensory retina readily separates from the retinal pigment epithelium when fluid (e.g., liquid vitreous humor, hemorrhage, or exudate) accumulates within the potential space between these structures. Such a separation is termed a *retinal detachment* and is a common cause of blindness. Factors predisposing to retinal detachment include retinal defects (from trauma or certain retinal degenerations), vitreous traction, diminished pressure on the retina (e.g., after vitreous loss), and weakened fixation of the retina.

Rhegmatogenous Retinal Detachment. This disorder is associated with a retinal tear and often with degenerative changes in the vitreous humor or peripheral retina. Retinal detachment follows intraocular hemorrhage (as after trauma) and is a potential complication of cataract extractions and several other ocular operations.

Tractional Retinal Detachment. In some instances, the retina is detached through being pulled toward the center of the eye by adherent vitreoretinal adhesions, as occurs in proliferative diabetic retinopathy, retinopathy of prematurity, and intraocular infection.

Retinitis Pigmentosa (Pigmentary Retinopathy)

■ *Retinitis pigmentosa is a generic term that refers to a variety of bilateral, progressive, and degenerative retinopathies that are characterized clinically by night blindness and peripheral visual field constriction, and pathologically by the loss of retinal photoreceptors (rods and cones) and pigment accumulation within the retina.*

☐ **Pathogenesis:** Multiple genetic abnormalities can result in retinitis pigmentosa. Although pigmentary retinopathies are often isolated ocular disorders, with autosomal dominant, autosomal recessive, or X-linked recessive inheritance, they are also associated with many neurologic and systemic disorders. Almost 12% of the autosomal dominant cases of retinitis pig-

mentosa have a mutation in the rhodopsin genes. Retinitis pigmentosa has also been mapped to two distinct loci on the X chromosome. Other cases have mutations in the genes for photoreceptor proteins and G proteins.

☐ **Pathology:** Retinal pigment epithelium migrates into the sensory retina (Fig. 29-6). Melanin appears within slender processes of spidery cells and accumulates mainly around small branching retinal blood vessels (especially in the equatorial portion of the retina), like spicules of bone. A gradual attenuation of the retinal blood vessels then ensues, and the optic nerve head acquires a characteristic waxy pallor. In a few cases, the macula becomes involved, and blindness ensues.

☐ **Clinical Features:** The clinical manifestations of retinitis pigmentosa, as well as the appearance and distribution of the retinal pigmentation, vary with the cause. As the condition progresses, contraction of the visual fields eventually leads to tunnel vision, but central vision is usually preserved.

Macular Degeneration

Perhaps the most common cause of reduced vision in the United States is age-related maculopathy. The center of the macula (the foveola) is the point of greatest visual acuity. With aging, in certain drug toxicities (e.g., chloroquine), and in several inherited disorders, the macula degenerates, and central vision is impaired. This condition is sometimes associated with bleeding into the subretinal space (hemorrhagic macular degeneration).

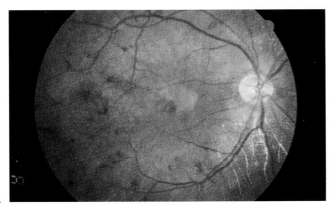
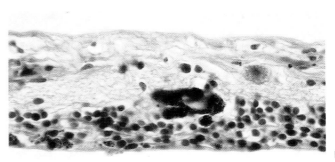

A   B

FIGURE 29-6. (A) **Fundus photograph shows the retina of a patient with pigmentary retinopathy (retinitis pigmentosa), with attenuated retinal vessels and foci of retinal pigmentation. (B) Microscopic appearance of a severely degenerated retina in pigmentary retinopathy. Note the focal accumulations of pigmented cells (derived from retinal pigment epithelium) within the retina.**

OPTIC NERVE

Papilledema

Papilledema, or optic disc edema, can result from various causes, the most important of which is **increased intracranial pressure.** Other causes include obstruction to the venous drainage of the eye (e.g., with compressive lesions of the orbit), infarct of the optic nerve (ischemic optic neuropathy), inflammation of the optic nerve close to the eyeball (optic neuritis, papillitis), and multiple sclerosis.

Edema of the optic nerve head is characterized by a swollen optic disc, which displays blurred margins and dilated vessels. Frequently, hemorrhages, exudates, and cotton-wool spots are seen, and concentric folds of the choroid and retina may surround the nerve head.

Acutely, papilledema results in few, if any, visual symptoms. As the condition becomes established, however, swelling of the disc enlarges the normal blind spot. After many months, atrophic changes lead to a loss of visual acuity.

Optic Atrophy

The axons within the optic nerve may be lost in many conditions. Longstanding papilledema, optic neuritis, optic nerve compression, glaucoma, and retinal degeneration are all possible causes. Optic atrophy can also be caused by some drugs (e.g., ethambutol and isoniazid). The optic disc is usually flat and pale in optic atrophy, but when this disorder follows glaucoma, the disc is excavated (glaucomatous cupping).

GLAUCOMA

☐ **Glaucoma** *refers to a group of disorders in which elevated intraocular pressure leads to atrophy of the optic nerve.* After being produced by the ciliary body, aqueous humor enters the posterior chamber (the space between the iris and the zonules) before passing through the pupil to the anterior chamber (between the iris and the cornea). From that site, it then drains into veins by way of the trabecular meshwork and the Schlemm canal (Fig. 29-7). A delicate balance between the production and drainage of aqueous humor maintains the intraocular pressure within its physiologic range (10–20 mm Hg). In certain pathologic states, however, aqueous humor accumulates within the eye, and intraocular pressure becomes elevated. Temporary or permanent impairment of vision results from pressure-induced degenerative changes in the retina and optic nerve head and from corneal edema and opacification.

Glaucoma almost always follows a congenital or acquired lesion of the anterior segment of the eye that mechanically obstructs the aqueous drainage. This obstruction may be located between the iris and the lens, in the angle of the anterior chamber, in the trabecular meshwork, in the Schlemm canal, or in the venous drainage of the eye. Glaucoma may develop in a person with no apparent underlying eye disease (primary glaucoma), or it may follow an antecedent or concomitant ocular disorder (secondary glaucoma).

Types of Glaucoma

Congenital Glaucoma (Infantile Glaucoma, Buphthalmos). This type of glaucoma results from an obstruction of the aqueous drainage by developmental anomalies, even though the intraocular pressure may not become elevated until early infancy or childhood.

Primary Open-Angle Glaucoma. Primary open-angle glaucoma, which is almost always bilateral, is the most frequent type of glaucoma and a major cause of blindness in the United States. The intraocular pressure becomes elevated insidiously and asymptomatically, and with time, damage to the retina and optic nerve causes an irreversible loss of peripheral vision. The angle of the anterior chamber is open and appears to be normal, but an increased resistance to the outflow of aqueous humor is present within the vicinity of the Schlemm canal.

Primary Closed-Angle Glaucoma. Primary closed-angle glaucoma occurs after the age of 40 years. It afflicts persons whose peripheral iris is displaced anteriorly toward the trabecular meshwork, thereby creating an abnormally narrow angle. When the pupil is con-

FIGURE   **29-7**
Pathogenesis of glaucoma. The anterior segment of the eye is affected differently in various forms of glaucoma. (A) Structure of the normal eye. (B) In primary open-angle glaucoma the obstruction to the aqueous outflow is distal to the anterior chamber angle, and the anterior segment resembles that of the normal eye. (C) In primary narrow-angle glaucoma, the anterior chamber angle is open but narrower than normal when the pupil is constricted (C1). When the pupil becomes dilated in such an eye, the thickened iris obstructs the anterior chamber angle (C2), thereby causing an increase in intraocular pressure. (D) The anterior chamber angle can become obstructed by a variety of pathological processes, including an adhesion between the iris and the posterior surface of the cornea (peripheral anterior synechia).

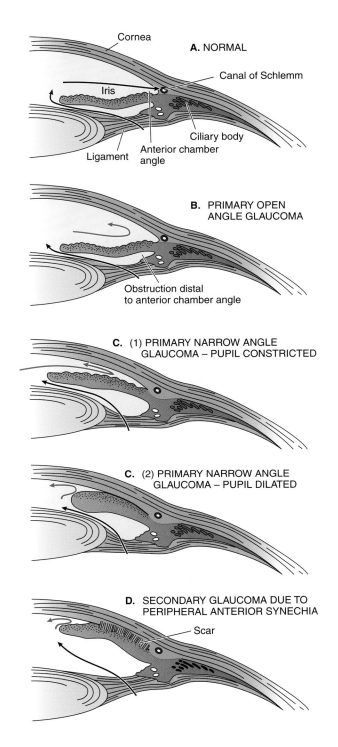

A. NORMAL

Cornea

Canal of Schlemm

Iris

Ciliary body

Ligament

Anterior chamber angle

B. PRIMARY OPEN ANGLE GLAUCOMA

Obstruction distal to anterior chamber angle

C. (1) PRIMARY NARROW ANGLE GLAUCOMA – PUPIL CONSTRICTED

C. (2) PRIMARY NARROW ANGLE GLAUCOMA – PUPIL DILATED

D. SECONDARY GLAUCOMA DUE TO PERIPHERAL ANTERIOR SYNECHIA

Scar

stricted (miotic), the iris remains stretched, so that the chamber angle is not occluded. When the pupil dilates (mydriasis), however, the iris obstructs the anterior chamber angle, thereby impairing aqueous drainage and resulting in sudden episodes of intraocular hypertension. **Acute closed-angle glaucoma is an ocular emergency, and it is essential to begin hypotensive**

treatment within the first 24 to 48 hours if vision is to be maintained.

Primary closed-angle glaucoma affects both eyes, but it may become apparent in one eye from 2 to 5 years before it is noted in the other. The intraocular pressure is normal between attacks, but after many episodes, adhesions form between the iris and the trabecular meshwork and cornea (peripheral anterior synechiae), and they accentuate the block to the outflow of aqueous humor.

Secondary Glaucoma. The causes of secondary glaucoma are many, and include inflammation, hemorrhage, neovascularization of the iris, and adhesions. In secondary glaucoma, the anterior chamber angles may be open or closed. Because the underlying disorder is generally limited to one eye, secondary glaucoma is usually unilateral.

Effects of Elevated Intraocular Pressure

Prolonged ocular hypertension has several effects on the eye:

- Elevated intraocular pressure leads to a characteristic, cupped excavation of the optic disc (glaucomatous cupping), which is accompanied by a nasal displacement of the retinal blood vessels.
- The cornea or sclera bulges at weak points, such as sites of scars in the outer coat of the eye.
- Optic atrophy follows the retinal degeneration and damage to the nerve fibers at the optic disc.
- The ganglion cell layer of the retina degenerates, thereby impairing vision.

PHTHISIS BULBI

■ *Phthisis bulbi refers to a nonspecific, end-stage eye that is characterized by atrophy of the eyeball* (Fig. 29-8). It most commonly occurs after trauma to or inflammation of the eye. The eye is small and soft, and the choroid and ciliary body are separated from the sclera. The sclera is thickened, wrinkled, and indented owing to the loss of intraocular pressure. The cornea is flattened, shrunken, and opaque. The intraocular contents are disorganized by diffuse scarring, and detachment of the sensory retina is invariably encountered. The lens is displaced and often calcified. A typical finding in patients with phthisis bulbi is intraocular bone formation, which seems to derive from the hyperplastic pigment epithelium. Eyes afflicted with phthisis bulbi should be enucleated.

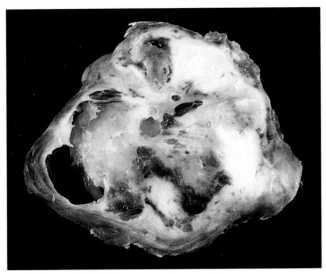

FIGURE　29-8

Section through an eye with phthisis bulbi exemplifying the markedly disorganized nature of the intraocular contents of such atrophic disordered globes.

MALIGNANT MELANOMA

Malignant melanoma is the most common primary intraocular malignancy. It may arise from melanocytes in any part of the eye, with the choroid being the most common site.

Choroidal melanomas are usually circumscribed and invade the Bruch membrane, thereby causing a stud-shaped or a mushroom-shaped mass (Fig. 29-9). In addition to hematogenous spread, uveal melanomas disseminate by traversing the sclera to enter the orbital tissues, usually at sites where blood vessels and nerves pass through the sclera.

The standard treatment of uveal melanoma is enucleation of the eye, and half of the patients survive for 15 years. More recently, early lesions have been successfully treated with radiation therapy or local excision. Anecdotally, the diagnosis of metastatic ocular melanoma has been made intuitively by astute clinicians who have discovered an enlarged liver in a patient with a glass eye.

RETINOBLASTOMA

Retinoblastoma is the most common intraocular malignant neoplasm of childhood (Fig. 29-10). The tumor arises from the retina and most frequently presents within the first 2 years of life, sometimes even at birth. Presenting signs include a white pupil (leukocoria), squint (strabismus), poor vision, spontaneous hyphema, or a red and painful eye. Secondary glaucoma is a frequent complication. Most retinoblastomas occur sporadically, but 6% to 8% are inherited. As many as 25% of the sporadic cases and most of the inherited retinoblastomas are bilateral.

Retinoblastomas are related to inherited or acquired deletions of, or mutations in, the retinoblastoma (*Rb*) tumor suppressor gene, which is located on the long arm of chromosome 13 (see Chapter 5).

☐ **Pathology:** Retinoblastoma is a cream-colored tumor that contains scattered, chalky-white, and calci-

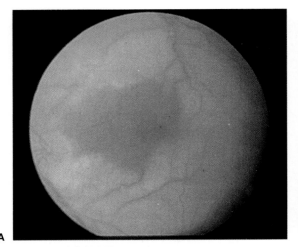
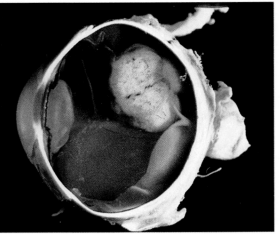

A   B

FIGURE　29-9

Malignant melanoma. (A) A malignant melanoma of the choroid is apparent as a dark mass visible beneath the retinal blood vessels. (B) A mushroom-shaped melanoma of the choroid is present in this eye. Choroidal melanomas commonly invade through the Bruch membrane and result in this appearance.

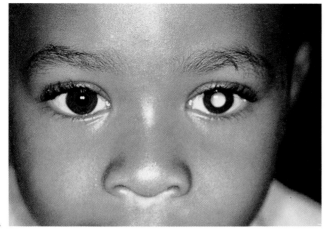
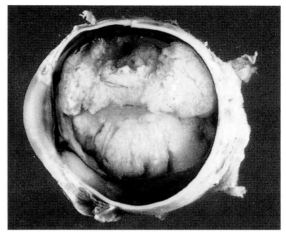

A   B

FIGURE   *29-10*
Retinoblastoma. (A) The white pupil (leucoria) in the left eye is the result of an intraocular retinoblastoma. (B) This surgically excised eye is almost filled by a cream-colored intraocular retinoblastoma with calcified flecks.

fied flecks within yellow necrotic zones that may be detected radiologically. They are intensely cellular and display several morphologic patterns. In some instances, densely packed, round neoplastic cells with hyperchromatic nuclei, scant cytoplasm, and abundant mitoses are randomly distributed. In other tumors, the cells are arranged radially around a central cavity (Flexner-Wintersteiner rosettes) as they differentiate toward photoreceptors.

Retinoblastomas commonly extend into the optic nerve, from where they spread intracranially. They also invade blood vessels, especially in the highly vascular choroid, before metastasizing hematogenously throughout the body.

Retinoblastomas are almost always fatal if left untreated. However, with early diagnosis and modern therapy, the survival rate is high (≈90%). As a consequence of the loss of *Rb* gene function, patients with inherited retinoblastomas have an increased susceptibility to other malignant tumors, including osteogenic sarcoma, Ewing sarcoma, and pinealoblastoma.

Index